# HAGAN'S INFECTIOUS DISEASES OF DOMESTIC ANIMALS

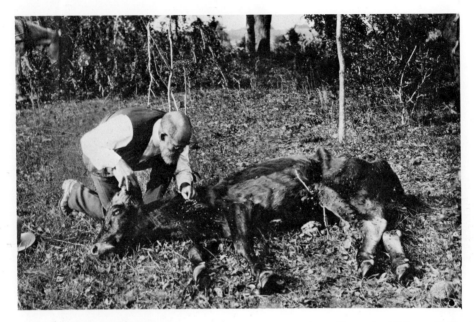

Dr. Cooper Curtice examining ticks on a cow dead of Texas fever. The work of Salmon, Smith, Kilborne, and Curtice on the causation and mode of transmission of Texas fever is one of the epochal accomplishments in the field of medical history, because it was the first to show that arthropods were capable of acting as carriers of diseases of mammals. Curtice championed the "tick theory" of the transmission of this disease and he was responsible in greater degree than any other person in proving that the southern cattle tick (*Boophilus annulatus*) was the sole carrier of this disease. (Courtesy *The Nation's Business*.)

# HAGAN'S INFECTIOUS DISEASES OF DOMESTIC ANIMALS

With Special Reference to Etiology, Diagnosis, and Biologic Therapy

**DORSEY WILLIAM BRUNER,** B.S., D.V.M., PH.D.

*Professor of Veterinary Microbiology Emeritus*
*New York State Veterinary College*
*Cornell University*

**JAMES HOWARD GILLESPIE,** V.M.D.

*Professor of Veterinary Microbiology*
*Chairman, Department of Veterinary Microbiology*
*New York State Veterinary College*
*Cornell University*

SIXTH EDITION

Comstock Publishing Associates, a division of
CORNELL UNIVERSITY PRESS | ITHACA AND LONDON

THE INFECTIOUS DISEASES OF DOMESTIC ANIMALS. First edition, 1943, by W. A. Hagan. Second edition, 1951, by W. A. Hagan and D. W. Bruner. Third edition, 1957. Fourth edition, 1961.

Fifth edition, 1966, entitled HAGAN'S INFECTIOUS DISEASES OF DOMESTIC ANIMALS by D. W. Bruner and J. H. Gillespie.

Sixth edition, 1973, published by Cornell University Press. Published in the United Kingdom by Cornell University Press, Ltd., 2–4 Brook Street, London W1Y 1AA.

*Second printing 1977.*


International Standard Book Number 0-8014-0752-4
Library of Congress Catalog Card Number 72-12909

Printed in the United States of America by Vail-Ballou Press, Inc.

*Librarians: Library of Congress cataloging information appears on the last page of the book.*

To
E. L. H., B. C. B.,
and V. A. G.

# Preface to the Sixth Edition

Following the death of William Arthur Hagan, in 1963, *The Infectious Diseases of Domestic Animals* became *Hagan's Infectious Diseases of Domestic Animals* and the fifth edition, which appeared in 1966, was authored by Bruner and Gillespie under the latter title.

It has been seven years since the fifth edition was completed. A massive amount of material relating to the infectious diseases of animals, especially in the areas of immunology and virology, has been published and this has had to be sifted and condensed in order that we might present the pertinent facts in a single volume. We have made every effort to make every facet of the book in accord with knowledge current at the time of writing in 1971. Inevitably a cutoff date had to be made in order to prepare the material for publication.

We have not changed the original plan of the book, but we have scrutinized each part and revised nearly every area. The main concern of the senior author has been with the first six parts of the text, and the junior author has revised completely the part dealing with rickettsial and viral diseases. Each of us has reviewed the work of the other and both share responsibility for the entire edition.

This is not a systematic discussion of disease-producing microorganisms, but rather a summation of the infectious diseases of animals with concern for etiological factors, diagnosis, prevention, and cure. Included with the bacterial diseases are those of fungal, protozoal, and viral origin. *Bergey's Manual* has been followed in general in the matter of bacterial nomenclature. For the other microorganisms current trends have been utilized. Where zoonoses are involved brief discussions of the nature of the disease in man are given.

Once again the authors wish to thank many colleagues and friends for their help in criticizing the manuscript, in calling attention to errors, in point-out omissions, and in allowing us to use some of their illustrative material. We hope that all who use this text will call our attention to its shortcomings so that, when another edition is prepared, we will be better able to improve its usefulness.

D. W. Bruner
J. H. Gillespie

*Ithaca, New York*
*September 1, 1971*

## PART 6.  THE PATHOGENIC PROTOZOA

# Contents

# Preface to the First Edition

This book is an outgrowth of a lecture course on pathogenic bacteriology and immunology which the author has given during the last twenty years to students of veterinary medicine. The work is less than a textbook of bacteriology in that a knowledge of the general principles of the subject is taken for granted and this part of the usual text is omitted. It is somewhat more, on the other hand, in that the fungi, protozoa, and viruses that are pathogenic for the domestic animals are included in addition to the bacteria. Also, somewhat greater consideration is given to the nature of the diseases produced by the various agents and to the biological products which are available for their diagnosis, prevention, and cure than is found in most texts of this type.

Since students of animal diseases are interested in microorganisms more because of what they do than for what they are, the work is not a systematic discussion of disease-producing organisms but rather a discussion of the infectious diseases of animals with special reference to their etiological factors.

With regard to the difficult matter of nomenclature of bacteria, *Bergey's Manual* has been followed in general except in the case of the Gram-negative enteric organisms for which the old name *Bacterium* is retained. This is done because it is felt that the numerous divisions which have been made in this group on the basis of cultural features are highly artificial. The newer methods of antigenic analysis do not support these divisions but rather suggest that we have a large group in which there are minor gradations from the colon bacillus at one end to the dysentery organisms at the other without sharp divisions anywhere. Until lines can be drawn more sharply it is felt that there is no justification for the creation of numerous genera within this group.

In instances in which the animal pathogens are transmissible to man, this fact is pointed out and brief discussions of the nature of the human diseases are given, together with what is known of the manner in which the transmission to man occurs. It is felt that veterinarians should be informed on these matters both for their own protection and for the assistance which they often can give to physicians in such cases.

The text will be used by the author in connection with his course in Infectious Diseases of Animals. It is hoped that it will prove suitable for such courses in other schools. In addition it is hoped also that the compilation of brief accounts of the biological characteristics of the etiological agents of all of the more important infectious diseases of animals in a single volume will make it useful to veterinary practitioners, laboratory workers who are called upon to make diagnoses of these conditions, and research workers who utilize animals in their daily work. Because of the wide scope of the field covered and the necessary limitations in a book designed for student use, the discussions are not exhaustive. Diseases which are known to occur in North America are treated more exhaustively than those which do not occur here. Since experience shows, however, that diseases which are thought to occur only in remote parts of the world often exist here in an unrecognized form, and that it is always possible that remote diseases may be imported, an effort has been made to include brief descriptions of all of the more important of such diseases and their causative agents. A few references are given at the end of each subject so those who wish to read more exhaustively may find the more important papers in the literature. Since most students and practitioners do not have a working knowledge of foreign languages, the greater part of the references are to papers published in English. By consulting the bibliographies given in most of these papers one can obtain leads which will open the entire literature to him.

The author is indebted to many friends for various kinds of assistance. The illustrations, in particular, have been borrowed from many sources, acknowledgment being made in each case. The author is especially grateful to Dr. William H. Feldman, of the Mayo Foundation, for reading and making numerous criticisms of the copy, criticisms which undoubtedly have contributed to greater clarity and greater accuracy in the volume. To all of those who have helped he wishes to extend his hearty thanks.

In a first edition of this kind many errors undoubtedly have been included. The author will appreciate having these called to his attention in order that they may be eliminated from future editions if the reception of the work warrants future revisions. In many instances it is realized that subjects are still in the stage of controversy. An attempt has been made not to be too didactic in the treating of such matters; however, in the interest of good pedagogical practice some sort of a stand usually is taken in such matters after it has been indicated that uncertainty exists.

W. A. HAGAN

*New York State Veterinary College*
*Cornell University, Ithaca, New York*
*June 1942*

# PART 1

# THE MECHANISMS OF INFECTION AND RESISTANCE

# I | The Causes of Disease

Disease may be defined as an alteration of the state of the body, or of some of its organs, which interrupts or disturbs the proper performance of the bodily functions. Functional disturbance soon is manifested by physical signs which the patient detects by his sensations and which usually can be detected by others. These signs are known as *symptoms*.

Disease may be of external or of internal origin. Little is known about the fundamental causes of the intrinsic diseases. These include metabolic and endocrine disturbances, degeneration of organs from age, neoplasms, and possibly autoimmunity. It is probable that many of these disorders are initiated by extrinsic causes as yet unrecognized. The external causes of disease may be living agents such as bacteria, protozoa, or viruses, or they may be nonliving agents such as traumatism, heat, cold, chemical poisons, or food deficiencies.

When living agents enter an animal body and set up a disturbance of function in any part, *infection* is said to have occurred. The word infection is derived from the Latin *inficere*, meaning "to put into." An *infectious disease* is one caused by the presence in or on an animal body of a foreign living organism, which creates a disturbance leading to the development of symptoms.

Most infections are caused by living organisms that have escaped from another individual of the same species, but sometimes they come from another species. This occurs when man develops rabies from a dog bite, or when a lap dog contracts tuberculosis from its consumptive master. Sometimes the infection is obtained indirectly, as when typhoid fever is contracted by a man from infected drinking water, or anthrax by a stable-fed horse in midwinter from hay that had been grown the previous summer on anthrax-infected soil. Some infections originate from organisms which normally live a free existence in nature, as, for example, the bacillus of tetanus. Presumably at some remote periods in evolutionary history, all the disease-producing organisms lived a free existence, becoming parasitic and pathogenic through gradual adaptation.

3

### The Fates of Infecting Organisms

Several possible fates await organisms that cause infections. This is a matter of considerable practical interest, because the transmission of the disease to other individuals depends upon the escape of the organisms from the infected one.

1. Some are destroyed by the host tissue. Infections are not accomplished without resistance on the part of the host, because the host-parasite relationship is not a natural one. The capacity of the host to destroy invading agents is so great that a large majority of the foreign living agents which manage to reach living tissues and fluids of the body are rapidly and completely destroyed. This process is going on at all times. Sometimes the resistance is not great enough entirely to prevent growth and multiplication in the tissues, but the infection does not become extensive and after a brief time is overcome, the invading organisms then being destroyed. Sometimes the agent persists and makes slow headway against the resistance of the host, in which case the infection is called *chronic*. In a few infections such as anthrax in the herbivorous animals, the resistance of the host is so quickly overwhelmed that the organism multiplies in all parts and early death of the host ensues. These cases are known as *acute*, or *peracute*.

2. Some usually are eliminated in the secretions or excretions of the host. Except in the peracute cases, when possibly no infecting organisms escape from the host, the diseased animal usually eliminates, in a manner that varies with the disease, the organism that causes it. The longer the disease lasts, i.e., the more chronic it is, the more likely is the host to eliminate large numbers of the infecting agent. Sometimes this agent is eliminated through pus, as when an abscess bursts or is lanced; sometimes through droplets which are coughed or sneezed out when the individual is suffering from one of the respiratory infections, as canine distemper, bovine tuberculosis, avian coryza, or human diphtheria; sometimes in the intestinal discharges (feces), as in the various forms of intestinal coccidiosis of animals and in the enteric infections of man; sometimes in the urine, as in cholera of swine and in typhoid fever of man. In some diseases that become extensive and even fatal, the causative organism may be eliminated in small numbers or not at all, as in some cases of tuberculosis. The more chronic the disease becomes, the less likelihood there is that the host will continue to retain all the infecting organisms. In some diseases the mechanism by which the infection escapes from one animal to another is peculiar, as, for example, in rabies, in which the seat of the infection is the central nervous system and the means of escape is through the salivary glands.

3. If the disease proves fatal to the host, many of the infecting organisms are destroyed with the carcass. Death of the host from infection always traps in the carcass a large number of the involved organisms. If the carcass is dis-

posed of properly by incineration or deep burial, these organisms perish. Improper disposal of the dead bodies of animals may result in serious outbreaks of disease.

4. In some instances the organism and host reach an impasse. The organism is unable to cause serious damage to the host, and yet the host is unable to eliminate the organism. This situation may continue to exist throughout the lifetime of the animal, or it may be terminated either by the final elimination of the infection or by a change in which the infection becomes more active and symptoms of disease are manifested by the host. In tuberculosis of both man and animals, the tubercle bacilli may become walled off by dense tissue in some of the organs and the case is said to be *arrested*. Such cases are not entirely cured because living tubercle organisms may continue to exist in the tissues and sometimes they break forth and cause a flare-up of the disease. In man, recovery from typhoid fever usually leaves the individual with many typhoid bacilli in his urine and stools, and these may persist for weeks, months, and years. Individuals who discharge virulent organisms with their excretions, although apparently normal otherwise, are said to be *carriers*. One who has had a recognized disease and who has not rid himself of the infecting agent is said to be a *convalescent carrier*. Sometimes individuals eliminate virulent infection although they have no history of ever having suffered from the disease themselves. These individuals are immune but are a source of great danger to others who lack the same amount of resistance. They are known as *immune carriers* or sometimes as *asymptomatic carriers*. At times individuals harbor and eliminate a dangerous organism that they have picked up from close contact with another individual. These are known as *contact carriers*.

The carrier is one of the great problems in the control of many infectious diseases. Animals that are obviously diseased may be recognized, but there is no simple way of recognizing the carrier.

### Sources of Infection

The courses by which infections reach new hosts often are indirect and complicated. Some of the more common ways by which infections are contracted by new hosts are as follows:

1. Direct or immediate contact with a diseased individual. This involves actual contact between a diseased and a normal surface, such as when a cow licks the external genitals of another animal and thus picks up the organism of Bang's disease or brucellosis, or when ringworm is contracted by an animal's rubbing against the affected skin of another, or when venereal infections are transferred through sexual contact, or when an infection is transmitted by an animal's bite.

2. Contact through fomites. *Fomites* (fomes) are inanimate objects that may serve to carry infections from one animal to another, such as a bran sack

which may convey dried discharge of an aborting cow to another cow, per-haps in a different herd; a railroad stock car; or a motor truck that has not been properly cleaned and disinfected after carrying diseased stock.

3. Contact with disease carriers. A disease carrier may infect others either directly or indirectly just as is done by a frankly diseased individual.

4. Infection from soil. Certain spore-bearing organisms which live in soil are able to produce disease in animals if chance carries them into the tissues, usually through wounds in the skin. Tetanus and gas gangrene infections are of this type.

5. Infections from food and water. Serious infections derived from food and water are more common in man than in animals, because animals do not suf-fer from the typhoid and dysentery organisms which are the principal men-aces to man. Water often is suspected of spreading animal diseases from one pasture to another when small streams flow between them, and occasionally the suspicion has been confirmed. Leptospirosis often is transmitted in this way. Anthrax is conveyed to animals through hay and straw raised on low-lands which are infected with anthrax spores. There have been a considerable number of reports of deaths of horses from eating ensilage which proved in-nocuous to cattle, and the organism of botulism has been incriminated in some of these cases.

6. Air-borne infections. Disease organisms do not spread very far through the air, though it was formerly believed they did. When individuals are close together and especially when indoors, droplets of moisture sneezed and coughed from the upper air passages often convey the organisms of respira-tory disease from diseased to well individuals. The common cold of man, in-fluenzal infections of man and animals, and glanders are good examples of diseases transmitted in this way. Tuberculosis of the lungs is usually passed on in this fashion. Dust particles less often convey viable disease-producing organisms, but there are some examples such as the anthrax spore (in woolsorter's disease), *Escherichia coli* (in hospital outbreaks of infant diarrhea), and spores of the higher fungi (in coccidioidomycosis and histo-plasmosis).

7. Infections from bloodsucking arthropods. Some diseases of man and ani-mals are normally transmitted through the bites of flies, fleas, mosquitoes, lice, or ticks. Malaria and yellow fever are good examples of such diseases of man, and Texas fever, anaplasmosis, anthrax, and the trypanosome diseases are examples in animals. In some instances, the infecting organism must pass a part of its life cycle in the invertebrate host, as, for example, the malaria and yellow fever parasites in the mosquito, in which case the arthropod is known as a *biological vector*. In other instances, such as anthrax, the black horsefly merely carries the bacillus mechanically, not being affected by it in any way. In these cases, the arthropod carrier is known as a *mechanical vec-tor*.

8. Infections from organisms normally carried. Pathogenic streptococci,

pneumococci, *Pasteurella,* and some other organisms can often be found on the mucous membranes of the head of apparently normal individuals. It is believed that infections sometimes occur from such organisms when the normal defensive forces of the body are weakened in any way. Many viral infections appear to pave the way for serious bacterial secondary infections.

9. Infections acquired in the laboratory. These usually appear in those who work with highly virulent and infectious microorganisms such as *Brucella melitensis, Pasteurella tularensis, Coxiella burneti,* and *Coccidioides immitis.*

### Infection and Contagion

A contagious disease is one that may be transmitted from one individual to another by direct or indirect contact. All contagious diseases are also infectious, but it does not follow that all infectious diseases are contagious. Tetanus and gas gangrene infections, caused by organisms which live in the soil, are infectious but not contagious, because they are not transmitted from one animal to another. The contagiousness of infectious diseases depends upon the way the parasites are eliminated from the body of the diseased animal and the opportunity they have of reaching others. Some infectious diseases are highly contagious, some are slightly contagious, and a few are not contagious at all.

### Properties of Pathogenic Organisms

**Virulence.** Virulence is an attribute of all pathogenic or disease-producing organisms. The word has reference to their disease-producing power or malignancy. A highly virulent organism has great malignancy, a slightly virulent has little, and a nonvirulent has none. The property of virulence varies greatly, both among different species of parasitic forms and among different strains of the same species. In some parts of the world smallpox is a highly malignant disease; in others it is very mild. In some years influenzal infections are mild; in others, severe. In the laboratory one may sometimes cause the death of a white mouse by inoculating it with as little as 0.001 ml of a strain of *Streptococcus,* whereas another strain of the same species of *Streptococcus* may not kill a mouse when 0.1 ml is inoculated. The one strain in this case may be said to be at least 100 times as virulent as the other.

**Alteration of Virulence.** The pathogenic power, or virulence, of many disease-producing organisms can readily be altered in the laboratory; others resist such alteration. It has been suggested that possibly the ability to change virulence is evidence that the organism has only recently acquired the property, and thus it is not a firmly fixed characteristic.

When the virulence of an organism is diminished, the process is known as *attenuation.* Attenuated organisms often are used as vaccines. Attenuation of virulence is readily accomplished in most instances; in fact the mere procedure of artificial cultivation is enough to attenuate most organisms in greater or less degree. When it is desired to reduce the disease-producing power of organisms, particularly of bacteria, many methods are available. Some of the more common are as follows:

1. Cultivating the organism at an unfavorable temperature. Pasteur found that anthrax bacilli quickly lost virulence when they were incubated at 42 to 43 C, a temperature about 5 degrees above their optimum.

2. Heating cultures or infective material for a short time to a point a little below the thermal death point of the organism.

3. Cultivating the organism on a medium rendered unfavorable by the presence of small amounts of acids, alkalies, metallic salts, dyes, or other substances. On such media many organisms may grow well if the concentration of the attenuating agent is gradually increased from day to day.

4. Plating the organism on a suitable medium and selecting a nonvirulent colony. Usually this is accomplished by picking the more granular-appearing type of colony. (See the next section, "Microbic Dissociation.")

5. Injecting the organism into a species of animal which is quite resistant naturally, or whose resistance has been increased by partial immunization, and recovering it after a sojourn there.

6. Injecting the organism into an animal and, after permitting its multiplication in this host for a time, passing it to a second individual of the same species. From the second animal it is carried in the same way to a third, and so on in a series of individuals. However, by such process some disease agents, particularly viruses, may be *adapted* to a certain animal species and become highly virulent for it. Frequently in the process of adaptation to the one species of animal, it loses much or all of its virulence for others. Tissue culture is another important means of producing attenuation through adaptation.

When an increase in the virulence of an organism is desired, all methods often fail, particularly if the organism has become highly attenuated. The procedure usually followed is to inoculate heavily an animal known to be highly susceptible, with the hope of overwhelming it with the infection. If this succeeds, another animal is immediately inoculated from the first, and so on. The virulence of some disease-producing agents may be enormously increased in this way. As a rule, the practice of growing avirulent bacteria in fresh animal serum, or in immune serum, fails to enhance virulence.

Burnet (4) in 1925 indicated that the cultivation of one species of microorganism in the presence of another enabled the first to acquire properties of the second. He called this phenomenon *entraînement*. In 1927 Frobisher and Brown (11) were able to cause a harmless *Streptococcus* from cheese to acquire the property of forming erythrogenic toxin (scarlet fever toxin) by growing it in contact with scarlet fever streptococci. In 1932 Alloway (1) found that extracts of dead, smooth Type 3 pneumococci would induce live, rough non-type-specific forms of Type 2 pneumococci to change into smooth Type 3 pneumococci. The new Type 3, like other Type 3 pneumococci, was highly virulent.

In 1951 Freeman (10) reported that it was possible to isolate virulent strains of *Corynebacterium diphtheriae* from avirulent cultures by exposing them to diphtheria bacteriophage. His studies indicated an association between lysogenicity and virulence (toxigenicity) in diphtheria bacilli.

Various methods have been devised for transmitting certain properties from one microorganism to another. In the *transformation* procedure genetic material (ribonucleic acid or deoxyribonucleic acid) is transmitted from one cell to another by contact between the cells, and in the *transduction* method the material is transferred in a virus particle (bacteriophage).

**Microbic Dissociation and Change of Virulence.** Certain growth phenomena which may be observed both macroscopically and microscopically are associated with change in virulence in many bacterial cultures. These were first described by Arkwright (2), in England, in 1920 and by De Kruif (7), in the United States, in 1921. Many of these phenomena had been seen earlier, but their significance had not been fully appreciated. The changes of the type of which we speak may easily be observed on ordinary culture media, especially of the solid type. When cells of a single bacterial culture are streaked on the surface of a solid medium, the colonies which develop are often not alike but may be differentiated into several types. The extremes of these are the so-called S-type (smooth type) and the R-type (rough type). Between these two there may be several intergrading forms. These types may be seen even when the culture is the progeny of a single bacterial cell; thus it is not a matter of a cultural mixture of types, except insofar as the progeny of single cells may vary from one another. In most cases certain other characters are associated with each of the colony types. The more important of these characters are described below.

*S-type colonies* are recognized by a smooth, glistening surface and rather regular margins. In consistency such colonies usually are soft and buttery. When grown in broth, these organisms usually produce uniform clouding of the medium, and, when suspended in physiological salt solution, uniform and stable suspensions are formed. Organisms of the smooth type usually are good antigens. They are excellent immunizing agents and, when agglutinated with specific antisera, produce large flocculi. If the organism is pathogenic, this form usually is highly virulent. Such organisms frequently produce capsules and are relatively resistant to phagocytosis.

*R-type colonies* differ from the preceding in that they have a rough or uneven contour, or at least show a granular structure under magnification and proper illumination that is not seen in the S-types. In consistency such colonies are friable or granular. When grown in a fluid medium, the growth usually is in the form of a pellicle and sediment, and when attempts are made to suspend such cells in salt solution, they usually fail because the cells form into flakes and clumps which settle out. While, in general, changed colony formation, stability in broth, and changed serological characteristics go hand in hand, many cultures produce colonies that are quite rough in appearance;

yet their broth cultures are stable and they retain most of their normal antigenic complex. In *Salmonella* studies the Pampana (15) trypaflavin test for the deduction of roughness follows the serological behavior of S and R antigens more closely than does any other test (9). If the parent culture was pathogenic, the R-type variant usually is not. Capsules are not produced and such cells usually are easily phagocytosed. Such strains usually are poor antigens, i.e., they immunize poorly.

*Intermediate types* usually have some of the characteristics of both R- and S-types. In some cultures several intermediate types may be recognized; in others they are not seen.

Dissociation of most bacterial cultures into S- and R-forms occurs naturally when the cultures are growing in culture media, and in many cases also when growing in tissues. Various ways have been found by which it is possible to force dissociation to occur in culture media when it does not occur readily otherwise. Many smooth strains, for example, can be made to develop the rough form by cultivating them in culture media to which immune serum has been added. In general, S-R dissociation takes place more rapidly in fluid than on solid culture media.

Spontaneous dissociation from the S- to the R-form occurs readily in most cultures, sometimes to the extent that the S-form disappears entirely. The R- to S-form of dissociation, however, is not often seen spontaneously and is not easily forced.

The significance of dissociation in relation to virulence is clear. It affords a possible clue to the reason why pathogenic bacteria in artificial culture tend to become less virulent, why such organisms in chronic infections often are attenuated in virulence, why vaccines sometimes are efficacious and sometimes not, and why some strains of organisms make satisfactory antigens for agglutination tests and others do not. If virulence is to be retained, if vaccines are to be effective, and if cultures are to make good agglutination antigens, means of keeping the strain in the S-form must be found. In many cases this is not difficult, it being necessary only to make frequent plate cultures and to select S-type colonies for propagating the strain. Inoculation of susceptible animals is another way to eliminate rough and intermediate variants from a culture. If the culture has not lost all virulence, the animal will act selectively, destroying the nonvirulent types and yielding finally only the smooth type.

**Evolution of Pathogenicity.** Many diseases apparently are not so destructive today as they once were. The reasons for this obviously are not simple, and probably they have to do with changes in both host and parasite. Mass immunization or "herd immunity," which gradually raises the resistance of populations, probably is a factor. It will be discussed later. Better nutrition and better hygienic conditions of many kinds probably have played a part. Genetic factors evidently are at work because destructive disease tends to eliminate the more susceptible and leave the resistant strains. Years ago Theobald Smith (17) suggested that it should be expected that infectious diseases would evolve into more chronic, less virulent forms in the course of time, even if the host resistance did not change in the meantime. The reasoning behind this conclusion was that in acute disease the parasite quickly destroys its host and thus quickly terminates its own chances of escaping to new hosts, whereas in chronic disease the opportunity for escape is much better because of the prolonged course of the disease. Under such conditions, Smith concluded that the chronic form had a much better chance of propagating itself and would, in time, become the predominating form.

### The Mechanism of Disease Production by Pathogenic Organisms

The possession of the property of virulence distinguishes pathogenic organisms from the nonpathogenic. In the final analysis virulence depends upon two properties of the organism:

(*a*) The ability to propagate in the tissues or on the surface of the body.

(*b*) The ability to form chemical substances that injure or destroy body cells, organs, or tissues.

**Ability to Propagate in Tissues.** The ability to grow in an animal body is something that an organism acquires in its evolution toward a parasitic existence. Obviously the organism has to "learn" how to protect itself against forces in the body which are antagonistic to it. Virulent organisms usually, but not invariably, are of the S-type, which means that they are more or less resistant to phagocytosis and often possess capsular or surface substances that serve to protect them from harmful influences in the tissue fluids.

The ability to invade and multiply in living tissues varies a great deal among disease-producing organisms. Some organisms that are malignant-disease producers have little invasive ability and do most of their damage while growing in restricted parts of the body, in which they generate powerful poisons, or toxins, that are absorbed and circulated throughout the body. The tetanus organism, for example, usually remains localized in a wound which may be very insignificant in size, but in this wound the tetanus toxin is generated, which is carried to the nervous system, where the damage is done. The organism of human diphtheria is rarely found in the internal organs but is usually restricted to the membranes of the throat, where the diphtheria toxin is generated. These bacteria produce systemic diseases only because of the absorption of their toxins.

The organisms that lack soluble toxins must have considerable powers of invasiveness if they are to produce systemic disease, or disease of any of the vital organs. Such organisms produce their principal damage at the points where they are multiplying. Sometimes they localize near the point where they enter the body and do not extend far from this site. These are known as *local infections*. Most wound infections are of this type. Others characteristically invade lymph and blood vessels, whence they are carried to many other parts of the body, a process known as *metastasis*, where secondary localizations occur. These are the *systemic* or *general infections*.

In speaking of invasiveness we should not develop the idea that organisms actively drive or bore their way into tissues. Many actively invading organisms are nonmotile. In most instances, bacteria probably enter the tissues in the same way that inanimate particles do. Organisms on mucous membranes are often picked up by wandering phagocytic cells which find their way back into the tissues carrying their bacterial load with them. These cells often destroy their bacterial meal, in which case nothing happens; but in other cases the bacterial load survives, destroys the cell which harbors it, and then proceeds to initiate an infection of the tissues where it finds itself. Other organisms colonize on surfaces and reach the subepithelial tissues by direct extension of growth through glands and hair follicles. Certain bacteria produce the enzyme hyaluronidase. This enzyme may aid in the spread of these bacteria throughout the tissues by hydrolyzing hyaluronic acid, a viscous mucopolysaccharide that binds water in the interstitial tissues, thereby holding cells together in a jellylike matrix and acting ordinarily as a physical barrier to invasion by foreign substances (14). This acid also is present in synovial fluid, and its destruction in joint cavities appears to be related to certain rheumatic diseases. If the organism possesses the property of virulence, it will go on from this point to produce an infection; if it does not, it will be picked up by the fixed or wandering phagocytic cells of the tissue and destroyed.

As a general rule, bacteria do not multiply in the circulating fluids of the body. When many bacteria are found in the blood, a condition which we call *bacteremia*, it means that there are foci in the tissues from which the organisms are being poured forth in such large numbers that the blood-clearing mechanism is temporarily overwhelmed.

At one time it was seriously believed that microorganisms might produce disease in a purely mechanical way, that is, by blocking capillaries or tissue spaces. This idea is untenable because it is known that the body has mechanisms for dealing with rather large amounts of foreign solids, more than the total bulk of bacteria present even in overwhelming infections. The damage caused by infecting organisms is clearly due to their metabolic activities.

**Ability to Form Poisons or Toxins.** *Endotoxins.* As to chemical poisons, it is clear that substances mildly poisonous to animal tissues are contained in most bacteria. Extracts of many purely saprophytic organisms often are distinctly poisonous when injected into animals. These substances apparently occur intracellularly as lipid-polysaccharide-polypeptide complexes and are structural components of the bacterial cell that represent O antigen and occur, for the most part, in the cell wall. Endotoxins may be extracted or they may be released by the mechanical disruption of bacterial cells. They are heat-stable and resistant to proteolytic enzymes, but are destroyed by mild acid hydrolysis. They produce a rise in body temperature on parenteral injection. For this reason they are sometimes known as *pyrogens.* They also increase capillary permeability, resulting in inflammation, hemorrhage, and shock. Actually the reaction to endotoxins is strikingly similar to the Shwartzman phenomenon (see p. 82). Endotoxins are excellent antigens in stimulating the formation of agglutinins and precipitins, but these antibodies fail to neutralize the toxic effects of the endotoxin, although they combine with it.

It is possible that the difference between a pathogenic and a nonpathogenic organism, if pathogenicity depends upon endotoxins, is that the former has the ability to penetrate into the body in the face of the resistance offered by the body's protective mechanism, to multiply and colonize in various tissues and organs, and there to release its poisons, while the latter lacks this ability. Pathogenic bacteria that do not form any recognizable poisons, other than endotoxins, must have the property of invasiveness.

*Exotoxins (True Toxins)*. Certain plants and animals and a few bacteria secrete or excrete substances that are highly poisonous to animals. These products have a number of properties in common, yet each toxin is highly distinctive or specific. The cardinal characteristic of all of these poisons is that they are *antigenic*, that is, that they will stimulate in animals *antibodies* which will neutralize them *in vivo* or *in vitro*. The endotoxic substances of bacteria do not have this property; they are not true toxins.

Toxins are divided into three groups according to the type of organism which produces them:

1. The phytotoxins, such as *ricin* of the castor bean plant, and the *amanita toxin* of the poisonous fungi of that name (toadstools).

2. The zootoxins, such as the venoms of certain snakes, spiders, and fish.

3. The bacterial toxins, such as those of the organisms causing diphtheria, tetanus, and botulism.

Toxins usually exhibit specific affinities for certain cells or tissues; thus we have *neurotoxins*, such as those of tetanus and botulism, *hemolytic toxins*, such as those of many streptococci and the organism of tetanus, and leukotoxins or *leukocidins*, such as those of the pyogenic staphylococci. The first type combines with and injures or destroys nerve cells, the second destroys erythrocytes, and the third destroys leukocytes. When toxins are injected into the blood of susceptible animals, they quickly disappear from it; furthermore, in diseases in which toxins play a predominating role, seldom can more than traces be found in the circulating blood. The reason for this is that toxins are quickly absorbed by the cells or tissues for which they have affinities. This can easily be demonstrated *in vitro;* suspensions of nerve cells will combine with and inactivate the neurotoxins, and erythrocytes will do likewise with the hemolytic toxins. Suspensions of other types of cells will not do this. It is interesting to note also that tetanus toxin will circulate for days in the blood of some cold-blooded animals, and diphtheria toxin disappears very slowly from the blood of rats. These animals are not susceptible to these toxins, and their tissues have little affinity for them.

**Physical Properties of Toxins.** 1. Most toxins are comparatively thermolabile. Heating to 58 to 60 C for 10 minutes will inactivate most toxins. A few are more resistant.

2. All toxins deteriorate with age. Some lose their potency very rapidly, while others deteriorate rather slowly. The speed of deterioration depends upon the conditions under which they are held. They usually keep best when stored in darkness and at a low temperature. If carefully dried and stored in a dry atmosphere, many toxins can be maintained with little change for long periods.

When toxins deteriorate, it is the poisonous portion that disappears first. Antigenicity is retained long after all traces of toxicity have been lost. Toxins that have lost their poisonous properties but have retained antigenicity are known as *toxoids*.

3. Toxins are composed of relatively large molecules. They will diffuse through parchment but not through the thicker collodion membranes. Their molecular size evidently is less than that of albumins and globulins but larger than that of the amino acids.

4. Most toxins require a "Period of incubation" before showing their poisonous effects. Many of the bacterial toxins, and some of the others, do not cause symptoms immediately after injection. Even when enormous doses are given to experimental animals, there usually is a delay of several hours before symptoms appear. This is quite different from the action of other highly active poisons such as prussic acid and strychnine, in which the symptoms of intoxication are immediate. Most poisons have small molecules and are readily diffusible; the toxins have large molecules and do not readily diffuse through membranes. Because poisoning does not occur until the poison has diffused into the susceptible cells, the lag shown by toxins can be explained on this basis. It is possible, too, that toxins have to be activated in some way before they become poisonous.

**Chemical Properties of Toxins.** 1. All toxins are antigenic poisons. It has already been stated that this is the prime, or cardinal, characteristic which separates these poisons from all others. The antibodies stimulated by the presence of toxin in the tissues of animals are always highly specific, i.e., they will neutralize only the type of toxin which caused their production.

2. Toxins can be precipitated from solution by concentrated alcohol, metallic salts, and ammonium sulfate. In these respects their reactions are like those of proteins.

3. Toxins can be concentrated and purified by adsorption on aluminum hydroxide gels and elution from them. In this respect they resemble enzymes.

4. Toxins can be crystallized. This is the highest degree of purification yet attained. Crystalline botulism toxin may be prepared by initial acid precipitation of the poison from solution, followed by shaking with chloroform, and salting out with ammonium sulfate (13). The crystals are in the form of needles and are pure protein, having the properties of globulin. Accordingly, certain toxins are protein in nature, but whether this applies to all toxins, or whether some of them are merely absorbed to proteins, remains to be answered.

5. Most toxins are readily destroyed by proteolytic enzymes. Peptic or tryptic digestion quickly destroys the majority of toxins. The toxin of *Clostridium botulinum*, which causes botulism because of its absorption through the digestive tract, is quite resistant.

6. Toxins can be changed to toxoids by chemical treatment. It has already been stated that toxins tend to deteriorate naturally into nonpoisonous substances called *toxoids*. The importance of toxoids lies in the fact that they retain the immunizing properties of toxins while losing their poisonous properties. Toxins can quickly be converted into toxoids by treatment with certain chemicals, notably formaldehyde. Formaldehyde-treated toxins are used for immunization against human diphtheria and against tetanus. Ramon (16), who developed the method, calls these products *anatoxins*, and they are so designated in the French literature. The term is used in English but the word *toxoid* is more common.

**Active Constituents or Products, Other Than Toxins, Produced by Pathogenic Bacteria.** Many years ago (1900), Bail (3) and his co-workers in Germany showed that sterile filtrates of the exudate which collect under the skin of animals after the injection of any of a number of pathogenic organisms had remarkable properties. The phenomena are highly specific for the organism used for injection. Several of the more important of these observations are as follows:

1. When the filtrate alone is injected into normal animals, no reactions are observed at the time, but later it can be shown that the animals have developed antibodies specific for the organism.

2. When the filtrate is injected with sublethal doses of the organism, the combination becomes lethal.

3. When the filtrate is injected with a dose of the bacterial culture which would have caused a chronic disease, the disease produced is acute.

4. When the filtrate is injected with a strain of the organism which has been attenuated so it no longer will produce infection when injected alone, the mixture will cause infection.

The agent in the exudate which apparently increases the virulence of the specific organism was called *aggressin*. Others called it *virulin*. It is now apparent that the word aggressin does not refer to a single substance secreted by bacteria, as Bail supposed, but to a property that is dependent upon the release from bacteria, in or out of the body, of substances such as capsular material, bacterial protein, secretions, excretions, enzymes, and toxins which have a deleterious effect upon the tissues of the host, thereby interfering with the host's defensive mechanism and permitting multiplication of the organism in the tissues.

Thus certain pathogenic *Staphylococcus aureus* strains were shown to produce a coagulase that accelerated the clotting of human and rabbit plasma (6), and Tillet and Garner (19) demonstrated an antigenic substance in hemolytic streptococci that dissolved human fibrin. This fibrinolysin behaves in many ways like an enzyme and is produced by most Group A, C, and G streptococci associated with suppurative and invasive types of human infection. For the most part these activities are broadly related to virulence.

Among the more important bacterial products can be listed the "spreading" or "diffusing" factors (Duran-Reynals, 8). These substances are elaborated by certain strains of staphylococci, streptococci, pneumococci, diphtheria bacilli, and clostridia. The identity of these bacteria-spreading factors with the enzyme hyaluronidase was suggested by Chain and Duthie (5). This enzyme hydrolyzes hyaluronic acid, an ingredient of the intercellular ground substance of mesodermal tissue, and by so doing permits the ready diffusion of fluid and bacteria through the intercellular spaces. In certain experimental infections it appears that the addition of hyaluronidase to the inoculum enhances the virulence of the organisms. However, the role of hyaluronidase in infections by organisms that produce this substance themselves is not entirely clear because there is no complete correlation between invasiveness and hyaluronidase production. In fact, this enzyme may even interfere with the virulence of certain encapsulated microorganisms by digesting their mucoid capsules.

Other enzymes besides those mentioned above also influence infection by alteration of the metabolism of the tissues.

## REFERENCES

1.    Alloway.   Jour. Exp. Med., 1932, 55, 91.
2.    Arkwright.   Jour. Path. and Bact., 1920, 23, 358.
3.    Bail.   Centrbl. f. Bakt., I Abt., 1900, 27, 10 and 517; 1902, 33, 343.
4.    Burnet.   Comp. rend. Soc. Biol. (Paris), 1925, 93, 1422.
5.    Chain and Duthie.   Brit. Jour. Exp. Path., 1940, 21, 324.
6.    Chapman, Berens, Peters, and Curcio.   Jour. Bact., 1934, 28, 343.
7.    De Kruif.   Jour. Exp. Med., 1921, 33, 773.
8.    Duran-Reynals.   Bact. Rev., 1942, 6, 197.
9.    Edwards and Bruner.   Ky. Agr. Exp. Sta. Cir. 54, 1942.
10.    Freeman.   Jour. Bact., 1952, 63, 407.
11.    Frobisher and Brown.   Johns Hopkins Hosp. Bul., 1927, 41, 167.
12.    Gay and Associates.   Agents of disease and host resistance. C. C Thomas, Springfield, Ill., 1935.
13.    Lamanna, McElroy, and Eklund.   Science, 1946, 103, 613.
14.    Meyer.   Physiol. Rev., 1947, 27, 335.
15.    Pampana.   Jour. Hyg. (London), 1933, 33, 402.
16.    Ramon.   Comp. rend. Soc. Biol. (Paris), 1922, 86, 661.
17.    Smith.   Jour. Am. Med. Assoc., 1913, 60, 1591.
18.    Smith, Conant, and Willett.   Zinsser microbiology. 14th ed. Appleton-Century-Crofts, New York, 1968.
19.    Tillet and Garner.   Jour. Exp. Med., 1933, 58, 485.
20.    Wilson and Miles.   Topley and Wilson's principles of bacteriology and immunity. 5th ed. Williams and Wilkins Co., Baltimore, 1964.

# II | The Protective Mechanisms of the Body

Animals are constantly in contact with many pathogenic organisms. Normal animals have rather effective mechanisms for protecting themselves against these organisms. The study of these mechanisms, in particular those of the tissues which we term the internal defenses, is known as *immunology*. The word *immunity* is used for the condition of enhanced resistance. Literally the word implies complete protection but actually it is used to indicate degrees of resistance varying from very slight to complete. The phrase *resistance to disease* is preferable to immunity from disease. On the other hand, the immunologist is interested in many phenomena which, so far as is known, have nothing to do with protection from disease. These will be discussed later.

The protective mechanisms of the body can conveniently be divided into two types:

1. Those that serve to hinder or prevent the passage of disease-producing agents into the tissues (*primary defenses*), and

2. Those that deal with such agents that have managed to enter the tissues in spite of the primary defense mechanism (secondary or parenteral defenses).

## The Primary Defenses

Before the tissues of the body can be reached, one of the epithelial coverings—the skin or a mucous membrane—must be penetrated. These integuments, the skin especially, serve as rather effective physical barriers, yet the matter evidently is more complicated than this. When cultures of many pathogenic organisms are swabbed on the skin, they die off very rapidly, much more rapidly than on the skin of cadavers and on other surfaces. The sweat contains chemical substances of unknown constitution which cause their destruction. Microbes of the normal-skin flora, resistant to these agents and having no pathogenic potential, may contribute to antimicrobial defense

17

against pathogens by the production of antagonistic metabolic substances.

The mucous membranes undoubtedly are protected by the mucus, which is constantly secreted. This material traps small particles of all sorts, including bacteria and subjects them to lysozyme and local antibodies, such as immunoglobulin A (IgA) in respiratory secretions and in feces. In the digestive tract mucus gathers into masses which are then carried through the canal with its contents. In the respiratory tract most of it is either coughed up or swept up into the pharynx by the action of the ciliated epithelium, whence it is swallowed.

Particles in the conjunctiva of the eye are washed away by tears or carried through ducts into the pharynx and swallowed. In the urinary tract foreign bodies usually are swept out with the urine. In the vagina there is no regular movement but the secretions appear to be unfavorable for the growth of most bacteria, and normally there are few bacteria there.

When organisms are swallowed, they immediately come in contact with the highly acid gastric juice. When much food is present, many of the ingested bacteria pass the stomach unharmed, but when it is relatively empty and thus there is little protection for them, most saprophytic and many pathogenic organisms are destroyed. The stomach thus stands guard at the beginning of the digestive canal to keep down the number of viable organisms entering it. In the beginning of the intestine, there likewise are few viable bacteria. It is only toward the end of the small intestine, and in the cecum and colon, that the intestinal flora becomes rich. It has long been known that gunshot and other penetrations of the anterior or upper portions of the bowel are not nearly so likely to lead to fatal peritonitis as when the wounds involve the lower portions.

### The Secondary or Parenteral Defenses

It has already been pointed out that some pathogenic organisms possess slight powers of invasiveness yet are capable of causing serious damage because of their potent toxins, whereas others must invade the interior of the body if they are to do damage. In the first case, the principal task of the defense mechanism is to inactivate or destroy the toxin, because its entrance cannot be prevented; in the second instance, the task is to hinder the multiplication and spread of the invading organisms and eventually to destroy them. The mechanism of defense is somewhat different in these areas.

**Biochemical Systems of Defense.** The enzyme lysozyme was discovered and named by Fleming (17). It is classified as a muramidase. Because all bacterial cell walls contain muramic acid, lysozyme is potentially able to attack any bacterium, but acting by itself it is less effective against Gram-negative than against Gram-positive bacteria. The former are protected from this enzyme by lipoprotein in their outer cell-wall layers. When these walls are acted upon by antibody and complement (C') the exposed inner walls become sensitive to the action of lysozyme.

Most animal tissues and fluids contain lysozyme. Exceptions usually are urine, cerebrospinal fluid, and sweat, but even these fluids may contain the enzyme when infections occur and lysozyme-rich leukocytes move in and undergo lysis.

A bactericidal system, not well characterized, but known as *beta-lysin* (*serum bactericidin*) is usually present in normal human serum. It appears that there are two essential components released during blood coagulation and that the system is only activated in sites where tissue damage occurs and fibrin is formed.

Many basic polypeptides are active primarily in inhibiting or killing Gram-positive bacteria. One of these, *leukin,* occurs in polymorphonuclear neutrophils (PMNs). Lysed PMNs also yield an antibacterial globulin (*phagocytin*) stable at 65 C for several hours and active particularly against Gram-negative enteric bacteria. Phagocytin kills, but does not lyse, and is most active in an acid environment.

*Spermine* has been isolated from renal tissue and from semen. It is a polyamine that possesses antibacterial activity against certain acid-fast bacilli, cocci, and *Bacillus anthracis.*

Organic acids and the iron porphyrins (*hematin* and *mesohematin*) possess antibacterial properties. *Peroxidase, thiocyanate,* and $H_2O_2$ form an antimicrobial system which inhibits the growth of a number of organisms. Those that accumulate $H_2O_2$ and lack catalase are inhibited by the addition of thiocyanate and peroxidase, whereas others that possess catalase are inhibited only if an $H_2O_2$-generating system is present in the reaction mixture. A so-called *Tillett factor* that is heat labile at 60 C for 1 hour and is bactericidal for beta-hemolytic streptococci has been observed in serum during the acute phase of various bacterial infections.

In viral diseases a mechanism that is responsible for the phenomenon of "interference" is called *interferon* and appears to be a low molecular weight protein secreted and released by many types of cells. Invasion by a virus stimulates the production of interferon which in turn interferes with virus replication. Some viruses require the presence of the mucolytic enzyme, *neuraminidase,* in order to penetrate the host's cells. Mucoproteins present in mucous secretions, serum, urine, and so on, may inhibit or block the action of the enzyme and prevent viral infectivity.

A high molecular weight serum protein called *properdin* is a constituent of normal mammalian sera (37). This factor, in conjunction with C' and $Mg^{++}$, participates in the destruction of certain bacteria, protozoa, and foreign red cells and in the inactivation of viruses. Properdin, complement, and $Mg^{++}$ constitute the so-called *properdin system* and the presence of these substances in normal serum suggests that this mechanism is one of the factors responsible for natural resistance. Pensky and colleagues (36) have demonstrated the existence of properdin as a unique serum protein, distinct from the known immunoglobulins or C' components that participate in certain immunologic reactions of human serum.

**Antitoxic Immunity.** Von Behring and Kitasato (51) were the first (1890) to show that the serum of animals that had received repeated sublethal doses of bacterial toxins developed the power of specifically neutralizing or inactivating the toxins, *in vitro* as well as *in vivo*. They worked with the toxins of the diphtheria and tetanus organisms. Ehrlich (12) later showed that antitoxic sera could be produced by injecting certain phytotoxins, ricin and abrin. Calmette (5) extended our knowledge by showing that antitoxins could be produced for zootoxins (antivenomous serum for cobra venom). In certain instances toxins are known to be enzymes, such as lecithinase a toxin of *Clostridium perfringens* and other bacteria.

Antitoxins can be produced only by stimulating animals with nonlethal doses of toxin, and the antitoxin produced is effective only for the toxin that stimulated its production. for the production of therapeutic sera, animals, usually horses, are given repeated doses of toxin. As antitoxin begins to develop in them, larger and larger doses of the toxin may be given. Finally, when the animal has tolerated enormous doses, it is bled, the serum is separated from the clot, and the globulin fraction of the serum is precipitated chemically. A solution of these globulins constitutes the antitoxin of commerce.

An animal that has suffered and recovered from a frank, or a mild unrecognized, infection by a toxin-producing organism has antitoxin in its blood for a long time thereafter. In practically all instances, however, the amount of antitoxin falls rapidly to a very low level after recovery. This amount usually is great enough to neutralize the toxin immediately if the individual should be infected with the same organism again. The toxin of the new infection is thus prevented from reaching and damaging the tissues that are susceptible to it. If a large dose of toxin is injected, experimentally, after the antitoxin level of the blood has become low, the animal can be fatally intoxicated because the blood is not capable of inactivating much toxin at one time. This situation cannot happen in the natural disease, however, because all infections have to have small beginnings, and it is in the beginnings that the blood antitoxin is effective.

When experimental animals are injected with toxin for the first time, antitoxin production is rather slow; it may be several weeks following a single injection before the maximum level is reached. On the other hand, when a dose is given to an animal that previously had been injected with the same material, even though it may have been many weeks, months, or years previously, the antitoxin content begins to rise much more quickly. This accelerated response, which is exhibited by animals treated with many other antigens in addition to toxins, is known as the *anamnestic* or remembering phenomenon. Nature evidently is not depending wholly on the small level of blood antitoxin for protection; the tissue cells are in readiness to produce more, when more is needed. Animals in this state are said to be *actively immune*. Other animals can be made *passively immune* by injecting blood or blood serum from actively immune animals into them. Such animals have heightened resistance only to the extent that it is conferred by the antitoxin which is introduced, and this is fleeting because the foreign antibodies are eliminated or destroyed within a period of several weeks. The tissues of such animals are not prepared to produce more antitoxin.

**Antibacterial Immunity.** The mechanisms that are involved in dealing with organisms that produce disease by actively invading the tissues are considerably more complicated and less is known about them than about those which have to do only with toxins. In general it appears that bacteria are treated by the body in much the same way as are inert particles of any kind.

Nonvirulent organisms are destroyed by these mechanisms. Large numbers of virulent organisms also are destroyed, but their ability to multiply in the body often enables virulent organisms to increase faster than they can be destroyed, in which case the defense mechanism sooner or later is broken down and the body is overwhelmed by the infection.

### Behavior of the Fluids and Tissues of Normal Animals Toward Foreign Particles

When suspensions of finely divided insoluble material, such as carmine or carbon (India ink), are injected into a vein of a normal animal, the material does not remain long in the circulation. After a few hours, at most, the greater part of it can be found deposited in certain organs, especially the liver, spleen, lymph glands, and bone marrow. It is fixed in these locations by being taken up from the circulating fluids by certain phagocytic cells that are known as *macrophages* or *histiocytes*. These cells are a part of what Aschoff (1) calls the *reticuloendothelial* system of the body. This system is a series of somewhat similar cells which are scattered through all parts of the body. Most of these cells are *fixed;* that is, they are permanently located in, and form a part of, the various organs. A smaller number are not so attached but are found wandering through the tissues and circulating in the blood and lymph. The sessile or fixed tissue macrophages include the endothelial cells lining the sinusoids of the liver (Kupffer cells) and those of the sinuses of the spleen, bone marrow, and lymph nodes, also the reticular cells, wherever they occur, which is largely in the spleen and lymph nodes. The circulating macrophages of the blood often are called large mononuclear leukocytes, or endothelial leukocytes. Besides those which are a part of the reticuloendothelial system, another kind of circulating blood cell, the polymorphonuclear or neutrophilic leukocyte, plays an important role in many infections.

Suspensions of inert material which are relatively stable before injection usually become unstable in the blood. This applies also to bacterial suspensions. The particles, or bacteria, are precipitated out of suspension and form masses which then lodge in some of the capillaries, particularly those of the lungs. This process is known as *agglutination*. Agglutinated masses are attacked by phagocytic cells, broken down gradually, and carried away piecemeal by the phagocytes.

When nonvirulent organisms are injected, they are taken up, like inert material, by the cells of the reticuloendothelial system, and especially by the endothelial cells of the liver and spleen. They are then destroyed by intracellular digestion.

Virulent organisms are taken up by the same cells but all of them are not destroyed. After a few hours the number of bacteria in the blood begins to rise because of their multiplication, and, from this point on, the outcome of the disease depends upon whether the phagocytic cells can remove the organisms as fast as they are produced. Table I, taken from Topley and Wilson (49), illustrates a typical experiment conducted by Wright, who studied the dissappearance from the peripheral blood of rabbits of nonvirulent, slightly virulent, and highly virulent pneumococci. In this experiment nearly 98 percent of the highly virulent culture had been removed from the blood by the end of 5 hours. It must not be supposed that the bacteria had been killed, however, because the subsequent behavior of the infection clearly showed that this had not been the case.

Table I.  NUMBERS OF PNEUMOCOCCI IN THE
PERIPHERAL BLOOD OF NORMAL RABBITS
AFTER SINGLE INTRAVENOUS DOSES *

| Time | Avirulent | Slightly virulent | Highly virulent |
|---|---|---|---|
| Immediately | 8,900,000 | 1,030,000 | 1,070,000 |
| 2 hours | 206 | 20,800 | 137,000 |
| 5 hours | 2 | 340 | 25,000 |
| 24 hours | 0 | 1,300 | 1,510,000 |
| 48 hours | — | 134 | Animal dead |
| 96 hours | — | 0 | — |

* From Topley and Wilson.

When inert particles, or bacteria, are injected into the body by other routes, they eventually are handled by the same types of cells that deal with them following intravenous injection. Often the load of foreign materials, after subcutaneous or intramuscular injection, is so slowly absorbed that the greater part of it is handled by the local macrophages, or by those of the neighboring lymph nodes. Animals frequently can be killed by smaller doses of pathogenic organisms when the organisms are injected into local areas than when they are introduced directly into the blood. When injected into the tissues they usually do not encounter the full strength of the protective mechanism as they do when they enter the blood, and thus they are enabled to multiply and establish a focus from which the blood later is flooded with organisms.

The peritoneum has a characteristic defensive mechanism. The peritoneal fluid usually has few cells in it. When bacteria or other particles are introduced into the cavity, there occurs an outpouring, for a few hours, of polymorphonuclear leukocytes, which phagocytose the particles. Within a few hours, these cells cease to take an active part in the situation; macrophages now appear in abundance and they not only take up any free particles which may be left, but also the polymorphonuclear cells which contain such particles. All of these cells then tend to collect on the surface of the omentum, which contracts into a mass in the anterior part of the cavity, usually coated with fibrin. In this mass, carbon particles or dead acid-fast bacilli can be recognized for months.

Bacteria or other particles pass very quickly from the peritoneal cavity into the lymph spaces, then into the lymph channels and the blood. Organisms introduced into the peritoneal cavity often can be found in the blood within a matter of minutes. It is believed that the pumping action of the diaphragm favors this passage.

Organisms that are introduced by mouth reach the tissues, in many instances, by invasion through the tonsillar crypts, whence they are carried to the neighboring lymph nodes. In other instances they pass into the intestine, through the intestinal mucosa into the lymphatics, and thence into the mesenteric lymph nodes, where they often lodge. After penetrating the mesenteric lymph nodes, they are washed into the thoracic duct and finally into the blood. It appears that the normal intestinal mucosa is remarkably resistant to penetration by bacteria, a fortunate circumstance, but there is no doubt that many organisms are constantly escaping through defects or injuries, if not through the normal epithelium.

## Behavior of Animals toward Injections of Organisms to Which They Have Been Immunized

Animals that have previously been treated with suspensions of living or dead organisms, or extracts of such organisms, behave toward virulent organisms in much the same way as untreated animals do toward the nonvirulent. Table II, from Topley and Wilson, showing the behavior of normal and immunized rabbits toward an intravenous injection of a virulent pneumococcus culture, illustrates this.

Table II.  NUMBERS OF VIRULENT PNEUMOCOCCI IN THE PERIPH-
ERAL BLOOD OF NORMAL AND ACTIVELY IMMUNIZED
RABBITS AFTER A SINGLE INTRAVENOUS DOSE *

| Time after injection | Normal | | Immunized | |
|---|---|---|---|---|
| | Rabbit 247 | Rabbit 248 | Rabbit 299 | Rabbit 300 |
| Immediately | 870,000 | 1,100,000 | 1,000,000 | 1,000,000 |
| 5 hours | 1,300 | 3,300 | 12 | 68 |
| 24 hours | 142,000 | 1,953,000 | 0 | 269 |
| 48 hours | 2,800 | Innumerable | 149 | 79 |
| 96 hours | Dead | Dead | 0 | 0 |

* From Topley and Wilson.

## Passive Transference of Antibacterial Immunity

It is possible to render an animal partially or wholly resistant to an infection by introducing into it the serum of another animal that has been actively immunized against it. The passive immunity is immediately effective after injection of the serum but is short-lived. The serum is cell-free, and because the passively immunized animal behaves toward the infection in essentially the same way as the actively immunized, or in the way that an unimmunized animal behaves toward a nonvirulent organism, it follows that there is something (antibodies) in the serum of the immunized animal which destroys the virulence of the organism. Protection in antibacterial immunity, therefore, is due to the co-operative effort of serum antibodies and the cellular mechanism which has been described. The effect of antibodies, passively transferred in serum, on the course of the infection by virulent pneumococci in the rabbit, is shown in table III. The immunized rabbits had been given antipneumococcus serum prior to the time of the test.

Table III.   NUMBERS OF VIRULENT PNEUMOCOCCI IN THE PERIPH-
ERAL BLOOD OF NORMAL AND PASSIVELY IMMUNIZED
RABITS AFTER A SINGLE INTRAVENOUS DOSE *

| Time after injection | Normal rabbit | Immunized rabbit | Immunized rabbit |
|---|---|---|---|
| Immediately | 2,300,000 | 2,300,000 | 2,000,000 |
| 5 hours | 43,000 | 2 | 52 |
| 24 hours | Dead | 8 | 14 |
| 48 hours | — | 0 | 1 |
| 96 hours | — | 0 | 0 |

* From Topley and Wilson.

## Effectiveness of Antibacterial Immunity

The effects of immunization so far described have been those which tended to keep the blood stream free of bacteria and thus to prevent fatal bacteremia. Although the blood may be kept free of organisms, it does not follow, necessarily, that the whole body has been freed from them. In many instances organisms continue to multiply locally, producing local damage which may be so extensive as to cause serious consequences, particularly when they are located in vital organs. Such animals must be regarded as only partially immunized. Antibacterial immunity is apt to be more partial, more variable, and less effective than antitoxic immunity.

## Types of Immunity

Immunity, or resistance to disease, may be divided into two categories, *innate* and *acquired*. Innate immunity is something that is inherent in an animal and is not due to the presence of antibodies. Acquired immunity is associated with the presence of antibodies. These are not inherent but are caused by contact with agents which have stimulated their formation.

**Innate Immunity.** One form of innate immunity is *species immunity*. This may be absolute or it may be relative. Man is absolutely insusceptible to hog cholera but only relatively insusceptible to foot-and-mouth disease. Horses are absolutely insusceptible to foot-and-mouth disease but only relatively resistant to tuberculosis. Species immunity appears to be due to a physiological incompatibility between host and parasite.

*Racial immunity* always is a relative matter. Races or breeds of plants and animals which have greater or less resistance to particular diseases than their parent stock may be developed by selection. Under natural conditions such races develop spontaneously.

*Individual immunity* of an innate nature always is relative and generally of slight degree. When epidemics of disease occur, all individuals of populations seldom contract them. This matter is complicated, of course, by the facts that acquired immunity generally is involved and that not all individuals are equally exposed.

**Acquired Immunity.** Acquired immunity may be *active* or *passive*. An active immunity is acquired by having suffered from an infection, either frank or unrecognized, or by having been artificially immunized by the injection of living or dead cultures, or by culture filtrates. These substances contain *antigens*, and because of stimulation by them the animal produces *antibodies*. Active immunity is relatively long-lived, and sometimes lifelong.

Passive immunity is attained by the transference of antibodies from another animal that has been actively immunized. The immunity in these cases lasts only so long as the antibodies remain in the body, which is a matter of several weeks only. Passive immunity usually is a state created artificially by the injection of antibody-containing serum. The only occasion when passive immunity occurs naturally is when antibodies pass to the fetus *in utero* or to the newborn through the first milk, or colostrum, of the mother.

**Immunity of Very Young Animals.** Before birth, animals of most species form little or no antibody. The reasons for this may be a lack of immunological maturity or because stimulation by foreign antigens is limited by the barrier of investing membranes. It has long been recognized that human infants usually are resistant to many of the common diseases during the first several weeks of their lives. The infant is resistant only to those diseases to which its mother is resistant, and the immunity is due to the passive transfer of antibodies, mainly immunoglobulin G (IgG), from the maternal blood to that of the fetus *in utero* through the placenta. In the case of children it is known that very young infants seldom contract diphtheria. Zingher (56) has shown that these infants usually are negative to the Schick test, which indicates that they carry antitoxin in their tissues. Ehrlich (11) was one of the first to show that antibodies could be transmitted through the placenta. Where maternal antibodies may fail to reach the infant in amounts sufficient to establish effective immunity, either active or passive immunization of mothers during the third trimester of pregnancy has been recommended.

Smith and Little (43) showed that calves are not passively immunized *in utero*. In this instance nature has made up for the defective mechanism by storing a rich supply of antibodies in the colostral milk of the mother, and the newborn must depend upon this material to provide the early immunity that it needs. The young animal usually suckles during the first hour after birth and thus takes in, quite promptly after birth, the antibodies (immunoglobulins IgA, IgG, and IgM) that are stored in the colostrum. These antibodies would not be absorbed unchanged from the intestine of the adult animal, but the intestine of the young calf permits them to pass freely. Within an hour after taking its first meal, antibodies can be detected in the blood of the calf. This absorptive capacity of the intestine may persist for only a day or two after birth, as in the equine and bovine species, or for 2 to 3 weeks, as in the rat.

Schneider and Szathmary (39) claimed that the transfer of antibodies *in utero* depends on the number of tissue layers between the maternal and fetal circulation. The presence of a few tissue layers allows antibody transmission through the placenta, but the occurrence of many layers necessitates the use of colostrum in the transfer of passive immunity to the newborn animal. Brambell (2) maintains that the tendency to call all fetal membranes "placenta" has led to confused statements with regard to *in utero* transmission of immunity. Actually this transfer takes place in the rabbit, guinea pig, and rat by way of the fetal yolk-sac, but follows the placental route in primates. There is also the opinion that the passage of maternal antibodies across the placenta is a highly selective process, more dependent on receptors provided by the antibody molecule than upon structural characteristics.

The findings of Ehrlich (11); Schneider and Szathmary (39); Famulener (14); Bruner, Edwards, and Doll (4); Bruner, Brown, Hull, and Kinkaid (3); Young, Erwin, Christian, and Davis (55); and Harding, Bruner, and Bryant (24) on the mechanism of transfer of antibodies from mother to offspring are given in table IV. It will be noted that the newborn of the common domestic animals obtain passive immunity through the colostrum.

Table IV. MECHANISM OF TRANSFER OF ANTIBODIES
FROM MOTHER TO OFFSPRING

| Wholly or largely *in utero* through the placenta or yolk-sac | Wholly or largely after birth through the colostrum |
|---|---|
| Man | Horses |
| Rats | Cattle |
| Guinea pigs | Sheep |
| Mice | Goats |
| Rabbits | Pigs |
| | Dogs |
| | Cats |

Table V presents the results of an experiment on the transfer of antibodies from a mare to its newborn foal. The mare was immunized against *Salmonella abortusequi* antigen, and although it carried an agglutinin titer of 1 to 5,000 for the homologous organism at the time of parturition, the foal showed no titer before it nursed. Within 2 hours after nursing, agglutinins for S. *abortusequi* appeared in the foal's serum and by the 12th hour its titer was 1 to 1,000.

The tissues of very young animals do not always react to antigenic stimuli in the same way as do those of older animals. Although suppression of antibody formation may be associated with the presence of maternally acquired passive antibodies in the neonatus, it may also be due to an imperfectly developed antibody-forming mechanism that has to mature after birth. It is known, for example, that some of the skin reactions to tuberculin are atypical, or they may fail to appear, in very young tuberculous animals, and that very young pigs do not react to injections of the virus of hog cholera in the same way that adult animals do. Smith and Ingram (42) have demonstrated immunological competence in 1-week-old calves following the injection of certain antigens even though the neonates had received colostrum; Levi *et al.* (30) showed that response to pertussis-diphtheria-tetanus vaccine was greater in babies with antibody in the umbilical-cord blood; and Jacoby *et al.* (25) decided that it was possible to elict humoral activity in fetal dogs at about the 40th day of gestation by injecting selected antigens. The intensity of the reaction increased with age. In general, it seems to be true that immunities induced in very young animals are not so enduring as those produced in mature individuals.

Table V.  TRANSFER OF PASSIVE IMMUNITY FROM A MARE IMMUNIZED AGAINST *SALMONELLA ABORTUSEQUI* TO ITS NEWBORN FOAL

|  | Titers *against* S. abortusequi *antigen* | | |
|---|---|---|---|
|  | Mare's serum | Mare's milk | Foal's serum |
| Before parturition | 5,000 | — | — |
| After parturition | | | |
|   Before nursing | 5,000 | 10,000 (Colostrum) | 0 |
| After nursing | | | |
|   12 hours | 5,000 | 200 | 1,000 |
|   1 week | 5,000 | 200 | 500 |
|   2 weeks | 5,000 | 100 | 500 |
|   1 month | 5,000 | 10 | 500 |
|   6 months | 200 | 0 | 10 |
|   1 year | 100 | 0 | 0 |

**Local Immunity.** The immunities so far discussed have been those of the animal as a whole. The question has often been raised as to whether or not it is possible for one part of the body to develop resistance to an infection while other parts remain susceptible. After an attack of erysipelas in man, it has often been observed that the skin of the affected area becomes relatively resistant to reinfection for a considerable time, while the skin of other parts of the body gives little or no evidence of heightened resistance. When certain toxins are injected into the skin, the injected area later becomes relatively insusceptible to a second injection, while other parts may be quite as susceptible as ever. These phenomena formerly were interpreted as evidence of specific resistance, but it is now known that the greater part, if not all, of this heightened resistance is due to the inflammatory reaction that has mobilized macrophages and left other changes which together make the area less sensitive. Injections of foreign serum, of egg albumen, and even of salt solution will render an area less sensitive to injections of irritating toxins or bacteria. It appears probable that an increase in specific resistance in such areas is a manifestation of general immunity, but the presence of antibodies, independent of serum antibodies, that occur in the intestine in enteric diseases and those found in the uterus of a cow following trichomonad infection may be classed as forms of local immunity.

## Influence of Stresses on Resistance to Disease

At times of food restriction during wars and famines, epidemic diseases of man and animals usually appear, and these frequently are more malignant than those seen at other times. In experimental animals inadequate diet may be correlated with increased susceptibility to a variety of bacterial diseases (53). It is possible that hypoproteinemia may contribute to the lowering of resistance to infection. In these cases there may not be protein in sufficient quantity to enable the animal to produce the phagocytes and antibodies that are necessary to prevent the development of disease (45).

A gross deficiency in *Vitamin A* is a factor that influences resistance to disease. Experimentally it has been shown by many workers that animals kept on diets that are deficient in this substance are much more susceptible to infectious diseases than animals that are fed adequately. This is especially true during the period of rapid bodily growth, when it appears that there is a marked increase in susceptibility to infection. Variations in the intake of *B vitamins* influence the course of infection by bacteria and viruses, but the direction of influence cannot be predicted. It may increase susceptibility or it may increase resistance. Undernourished rabbits are less susceptible than fully nourished rabbits to vaccinia virus, and pantothenic acid deficiency is reported to be associated with an increased resistance to experimental infection with Type I pneumococci (49). It is claimed that thiamine and riboflavin deficiency decreases resistance in rats to worm infection, and that biotin or folic acid (41) deficiency makes birds more susceptible to malaria. A diet deficient in either panothenic acid, pyridoxine, or thiamine produces a leukopenia with lymphopenia in rats (20). There also is evidence that lack of *Vitamin C* in animals such as guinea pigs, which have no power to synthesize it, will render them more susceptible to certain diseases, particularly pneumonia. The presence or absence of other vitamins appears to have little effect on bacterial infections.

It should be emphasized that these results are obtained with animals wholly deprived of these vitamins, and it is not clear whether slight deficiencies would have any serious effect. Animals or persons who are on a varied diet are seldom so deficient in any of the vitamins mentioned as to decrease appreciably their resistance to disease. There is little evidence, furthermore, that the feeding of vitamin concentrates will have any effect upon infections already started, or that the intake of quantities larger than meet the requirements of the body is of any service.

Mice were used by Schneider and Webster (40) in a study of host nutrition and natural resistance to *Salmonella enteritidis* infection. First it was determined that whole wheat, dried milk, and salt constituted a satisfactory diet when growth, fertility, fecundity, ability to rear young, and the growth of those young were used as criteria of nutritional performance. This Schneider and Webster called the "natural" diet. A "synthetic" diet consisting of casein, glucose, cystine, salts, and vitamins was devised. This contained all known dietary ingredients in adequate quantities, and it appeared to be satisfactory for prolonged use in rearing and maintaining mice. However, when numbers of mice from both groups were infected by stomach tube with S. *enteritidis*, 37.5 percent of those on the "natural" diet survived, whereas only 17.7 percent of those on the "synthetic" diet withstood the infection. Obviously, unknown protective factors were in the "natural" but absent from the artificial diet.

In general, it is only dietary deficiencies, whether of vitamins or foodstuffs, of a degree leading to manifest deterioration of the general bodily health which are definitely associated with depression of resistance to infection and inhibition of the cellular and antibody responses to the invading organisms.

*Fatigue* has long been recognized as a factor in increasing susceptibility to disease. This factor appears to be important in the so-called "shipping diseases" of animals.

*Heat* and *cold* evidently have an effect upon bodily resistance. In dogs held in rooms which were hot and humid, Arnold showed that the acidity of the gastric juice was diminished and that an increased passage of bacteria into the intestine from the stomach content occurred. Dogs under these conditions were much more easily poisoned by *Salmonella* toxins, given by mouth, than others under normal conditions. Chilling of the body surface sets up a train of physiological reactions that favor infection, particularly of the respiratory tract.

*Drugs* of the benzol groups are known to produce agranulocytosis and thereby favor infection. According to Hammond and Horn (23) there is a very high association between cigarette smoking and lung cancer in man.

*Irradiation* appears to modify bodily resistance in some instances. English workers (Colebrook *et al.*, 8) have observed that exposure of animals to ultraviolet light increases the native bactericidal activity of their blood against streptococci and staphylococci. Following the atomic bomb explosions in Japan it was reported (Leroy, 29) that injury to bone marrow caused by short wave irradiation and the consequent leukopenia that resulted favored the development of septic lesions of the gums, pharynx, and other tissues. On the other hand, the feeding of the flesh of lethally irradiated cows and sheep to dogs, albino rats, or chickens does not appear to be injurious or toxic to these animals (Wasserman and Trum, 52).

*Adrenal cortical hormones* seem to influence native as well as acquired resistance, but the direction of influence is at present subject to much question. The substances most studied have been cortisone (17-hydroxy-11-dehydrocorticosterone) and ACTH (anterior pituitary adrenocorticotrophic hormone). Treatment of tuberculosis with cortisone or ACTH appears to result in a wider distribution of lesions than ordinarily occurs (18, 32). On the other hand, Lurie *et al.* (31) claim that, although cortisone-treated rabbits develop more tubercles following inhalation of bacilli than do controls, and although the caseous contents of these tubercles swarm with bacilli, the tendency to dissemination is lessened.

In rabbits, suppression of antibody formation was reported as virtually complete with cortisone treatment (Germuth and Ottinger, 21) and partially so with ACTH (Fishell, 16). Human patients with pneumococcal pneumonia, while under treatment with cortisone and ACTH, proceeded to produce antibodies (Mirick, 33). Analogues of phenylalanine fed to rats before and after antigen injection will inhibit antibody response.

The use of *antibiotics* in feedingstuffs appears to influence the ability to resist disease in those animals consuming the feed. If disease is present, considerable benefit is derived from the supplementation of food with antibiotics. Animals kept under excellent conditions and free from disease apparently derive little benefit from antibiotic feeding, but young raised under *usual* farm conditions will respond to this feeding to a limited extent (10).

These are only a few of the more obvious conditions that have an effect upon bodily resistance to disease. It is clear that there are many others, such as finely divided solid material (calcium, silica) in the air which is breathed, noxious gases (mustard gases used in war), contact with and constant exposure to certain insecticides, and intercurrent diseases which may be quite trivial in themselves but pave the way for more serious infections by reducing the body's resistance. It is quite certain that an individual whose general health is weakened in any way is an easier prey for many infectious diseases than one who is enjoying good health.

### Antigens and Antibodies

The immunologist supposedly is concerned only with phenomena related to an increased resistance of the host against infection. Actually his work has led him to study a large number of phenomena having to do with interactions between body fluids and tissues, on the one hand, and various substances, principally foreign cells and organic bodies, on the other, many of which have nothing to do with protection against infection.

As defined by Topley (48), an *antigen* is "any substance that, when introduced parenterally into animal tissues, stimulates the production of antibodies and, when mixed with that antibody, reacts with it in some observable way."

The same author defines an *antibody* as "any substance that makes its appearance in the body fluids of an animal in response to a stimulus provided by the parenteral introduction of an antigen into the tissues and, when mixed with that antigen, reacts with it in some observable way."

The entire study of immunity is related to the interactions between antigens and antibodies. So far as resistance to disease is concerned, it is the antigens of the infecting organisms that stimulate the antibodies from which the protection is derived. These act directly in some cases, as when antitoxin neutralizes toxin, and indirectly in others, as when antibacterial antibodies so affect virulent bacteria as to render them susceptible to phagocytosis. But there are a great many substances having no relation to microorganisms or disease which are antigenic. When antibodies are produced by the injection of any of these, the serum is said to be immune. Instead of calling them by this name many prefer to use the word *antiserum*.

Bacterial and other cells contain a number of different antigenic materials. In the bacterial cell some of these antigens are associated with the flagella, others with the cell bodies, and still others with capsules and "envelopes." Upon injection each antigenic component induces the formation of antibody specific for it. Such antigens are referred to as *homologous antigens* and the antibodies that they induce are called *homologous antibodies*. Any other cell that possesses one or more of the same antigens will also react with this antiserum to the same or a lesser degree. In this case the adjective *heterologous* is applied to the antigen, the antibody, and the antiserum.

Most antigens are foreign to the animal in which they induce antibody formation. A few cells or substances are antigenic in the animal from which they are derived. Gonadal tissues and proteins from the crystalline lens of the eye may induce antibodies in other members of the same species or in the same individual. Formation of antibodies against substances from the same individual is known as *autoimmunization*. Antigens that produce *autoantibodies* are normally confined to certain cells or tissues and do not gain access to antibody-producing cells. In this sense the antigen is "foreign" to the antibody-forming lymphoid tissue of the animal and not to the animal as a whole. Erythrocytes of one individual may stimulate the formation of *isoantibodies* in another individual of the same species (see chapter 8). The tendency of an animal to produce antibodies against any foreign antigenic substance that is introduced parenterally has caused much concern in the surgical transplantation of tissues and organs. Unless the transplanted cells are homologous with those of the recipient, the antibody response elicited soon destroys the graft. Based on the donor's relationship to the recipient, grafts are designated as autografts (from same individual), syngrafts (from an identical twin or inbred individual), allografts (from a dissimilar member of same species), and xenografts (from another species). Three general procedures have been employed with limited success to suppress the recipients immune response. They are (a) exposure to immunosuppressive drugs such as cortisone; (b) x-irradiation; and (c) treatment with antilymphocyte serum. The third method shows promise for greater success in the future in the transplantation of tissues and organs.

Antibodies cannot be demonstrated except as they produce observable reactions when placed in contact with their specific antigens. There are at least five generally recognized kinds of antibodies:

1. *Antitoxins* are antibodies formed in response to the injection of toxins. When mixed with the homologous toxin they neutralize its poisonous qualities.

2. *Cytolysins* are antibodies that bring about a dissolution or lysis of bacterial and other cells.

3. *Opsonins* are antibodies that sensitize bacterial cells, thereby rendering them more susceptible to phagocytosis.

4. *Agglutinins* are antibodies that produce flocculation, or agglutination, when mixed with a suspension of suitable cells. This involves immobilization of motile cells, the formation of clumps, and the settling out of cells in suspension. Nonmotile cells merely form clumps and settle out of suspension.

5. *Precipitins* are antibodies that cause aggregates of the molecules of a soluble antigen to appear in the form of a precipitate.

Besides the five kinds of antibodies listed above, the provisional addition of ablastins, neutralizing antibodies, antienzymes, and mucoantibody can be made. Short discussions of these substances are given at this point because they are not treated in detail in subsequent chapters as are the antitoxins, cytolysins, opsonins, agglutinins, and precipitins.

*Ablastins* are antibodies that inhibit reproduction of invading microorganisms. Although the existence of an ablastin for bacteria has not been conclusively demonstrated, it appears that this factor develops in response to invasion with certain of the parasitic protozoa (46). The antibody can be differentiated from that of the coexisting cytolysin, but it need not be set apart as a specific inhibitor of reproduction because the union of antibody with antigen in the living organism might of itself inhibit the normal physiological function of cell division.

*Neutralizing antibodies* are those which render viruses innocuous. Neutralization is determined by mixing varying amounts of immune serum with one or more minimum infective doses of the specific virus and injecting the mixtures into susceptible animals. It is possible that this "virus neutralization" or "protective" capacity of immune serum can be accounted for on the basis of the combined activity of the known antibodies. Because it cannot be identified with any of the well-known antibodies, it is given a special name. The term *neutralizing antibody* is also used for antitoxin, because this antibody neutralizes the poisonous properties of the toxin.

*Antienzymes* are antibodies effective against homologous enzymes. All enzymes appear to be protein complexes and as such are antigenic and able to stimulate the production of specific antienzymes. Many enzymes are present in bacteria. Some are highly toxic and are referred to as toxins. That the bacterial enzyme hyaluronidase can provoke the formation of antihyaluronidase was shown by Thompson and Moses (47). They demonstrated that immune serum of patients with bacteremic pneumococcus infections inhibited penumococcic hyaluronidase.

It also appears that certain antienzymes differ from other antibodies in being less readily absorbable. Because some of the known enzymes are rather easily destroyed, or inactivated, bacterial antigens attenuated by heat or chemicals may be so altered in enzymic content that they are no longer able to adsorb antienzymes, but will adsorb other antibodies from an immune serum.

*Mucoantibody* occurs at various mucous surfaces where it is associated with local concentrations of antibody. In certain enteric diseases the type found in the intestine is referred to as *coproantibody* (19, 26). A variety of antibodies that apparently produce local immunities in the intestines are induced by dysentery bacilli, cholera vibrios, poliovirus, and the alpha-toxin of *Clostridium perfringens;* in the vagina by trichomonads; and in the urine by poliovirus.

As noted above, the various kinds of antibodies are named according to the way they are identified. This does not necessarily mean that each one is a separate and distinct type. There is abundant evidence, for example, that agglutinins and precipitins are the same antibody, and undoubtedly it is true that other antibodies also are identical. Some even believe that all antibodies are identical, but the present state of our knowledge does not warrant this assumption.

**The Nature of Antigens.** The chemical nature of antigenic substances has been greatly clarified by workers who have approached the problem by synthesizing relatively simple antigens. These are precipitated from their colloidal solutions by their specific antibodies, the antibody as well as the antigen being a part of the precipitate.

It was believed for many years that all antigens either were proteins or still more complicated chemical compounds having a protein component. This idea had to be abandoned when it was demonstrated that certain non-nitrogenous compounds derived from the polysaccharide of the pneumococcus could stimulate antibodies in horses and man, although not in the rabbit. Whatever their chemical nature, antigens are relatively large in size and, consequently, do not diffuse readily through organic membranes. Materials with a molecular weight of less than 10,000 are usually nonantigenic or only weakly effective.

Antibodies may be looked upon as nature's means of attacking, digesting, and removing the agents which otherwise could not be removed from tissues when accident carried them in.

The antibodies formed by the injection of highly purified, crystalline proteins are highly specific. Albumins can easily be distinguished from globulins, and egg albumen of the chicken can be distinguished from that of the duck, or of other birds, by immunological means. The fact that an antigen is widely distributed does not mean that it is nonspecific. Although an antigen known as the *Forssman antigen* (p. 35) is found in many animals and plants, it still possesses as great a specificity as other antigens that are confined to a very limited source.

It has been demonstrated that the immunological specificity of pure proteins can be changed by chemical means. If, for example, several proteins, such as the serum albumins of several species of animals, are halogenated or nitrated, the resulting compounds are still antigenic, but the species specificity of the albumins is lost and instead a new specificity is shared by the several nitrated, or by the several halogenated, albumins.

The synthetic antigens of Landsteiner and others are prepared in various ways, the most common being by utilizing the diazo reaction. Substances containing a benzene ring to which an amino group is attached are treated with nitrous acid to form a diazo compound. When this is mixed with certain proteins, the compound unites with the protein. If such a conjugated protein is used as an antigen, the resulting antiserum will react either with the original protein or with the conjugated compound. If the diazo compound is attached to two different proteins, the antiserum produced by the injection of either will react with both antigens. This proves, of course, that the reaction is dependent upon antibodies that have reacted with the diazo compound, because the proteins have nothing in common, immunologically. If the antibodies are mixed with the diazo compound alone, or with a diazo compound attached to a substance simpler than protein, such as tyrosine, no precipitate will occur. If later, however, the complete conjugated protein is added to such a mixture, precipitation will be inhibited. This proves that the diazo compound has united with the antibody and satisfied its combining powers even though precipitation did not occur.

In the definition of an antigen, it will be recalled that it has two properties: (a) the power of stimulating the formation of antibodies, and (b) the power of uniting with them, *in vitro*. To substances like the diazo compound, just discussed, which have the power of reacting with antibodies but cannot, alone, stimulate their formation, Landsteiner has given the name *haptens* or *partial antigens*. Haptens occur naturally. They may be of a carbohydrate nature, as the polysaccharides of the pneumococcus; they may be lipoidal; or they may be nitrogenous substances.

Landsteiner (27) recognizes three kinds of antigenic complexes:

1. *Simple haptens*, which, like the diazo compound alone, confer immunological specificity but are not precipitated by their antisera and do not have the power of stimulating antibody formation.

2. *Complex haptens*, which, like the pneumococcus polysaccharides, confer immunological specificity, are precipitated by their antisera, but do not have the power of stimulating antibody formation.

3. *Complex antigens,* like proteins or protein conjugates, which have immunological specificity, are precipitated by their antisera, and have the power of stimulating antibody formation.

Several workers have reported success in producing antibodies with nonprotein substances adsorbed on inert material such as collodion particles and finely divided carbon. Such studies, and even the work on synthetic antigens in which protein plays a part, suggest that antigenicity may not be so much a matter of structure as a matter of the manner in which the substance is presented to the tissues; that a carrier substance of high molecular weight is necessary.

*Heterophile antigens* are substances which stimulate the production of antibodies capable of reacting with tissues from a great variety of mammals, birds, reptiles, fish, bacteria, and plants.

In 1911 Forssman discovered an antigenic substance in the tissues of guinea pigs. Later it was designated *Forssman antigen.* This antigen acts like a hapten in its combining and immunizing power. It occurs in the guinea pig, sheep, horse, dog, cat, mouse, chicken, man, and many other animals. It is absent in cattle, rabbits, pigs, rats, geese, and deer. When present it is found in the organs or the erythrocytes, but usually not in both. It is also found in certain bacteria.

Forssman antigen and heterophile antigen are frequently used synonymously. The former should be limited to the antigen first discovered by Forssman in guinea pig tissues and the latter to a much broader group of antigens present in various plants and animals and possessing characteristics similar to those of the Forssman antigen (6).

In 1950 Coons and Kaplan (9) developed a technic for locating antigen in tissue cells. The method employs antibody-fluorescein conjugates as histochemical stains, the specific antigen-antibody precipitate being made visible under the fluorescence microscope. By means of this procedure antigens of viral and bacterial origin have been located in tissue cells and cultures of various microorganisms have been identified (35). The fluorescent-antibody technic is useful in the diagnosis of rabies (22), the serological grouping of streptococci (34), the identification of enteric bacteria in feces (7, 50), and in the study of many other viruses and bacterial forms.

**The Nature of Antibodies.** Antibodies may be defined as humoral globulins produced by the body in response to an antigen and capable of reacting with the antigen in some observable way. The serum of an immunized animal shows no characteristic chemical differences from that of a normal animal. The antibodies can, however, be precipitated from immune serum by reagents that precipitate the proteins and can be separated from the other proteins in the globulin fractions. Apparently, the antibodies of serum are present in the gamma globulin fraction. Most of these globulins have a molecular weight of about 160,000 and the five distinct globulins associated with antibody activity are designated as classes of *immunoglobulins,* abbreviated as IgG, IgM, IgA, IgD, and IgE and meaning *immunoglobulin G, immunoglobulin M,* etc. They may be assigned the letters γG, γM, γA, γD, and γE, abbreviations for *gamma globulin G, gamma globulin M,* and so on. Immunoglobulins contain variable amounts of covalently bound carbohydrates, associated with a polypeptide chain. The amount of carbohydrate is higher in IgA and IgM than in IgG.

Normal adult serum contains between 7 to 15 mg of IgG per ml and it appears that at least 80 percent of the serum antibodies directed against bacteria, viruses, and toxins belong to this class.

IgM comprises about 5 to 10 percent of the antibody protein in serum. In man heterophile antibodies, cold agglutinins, and certain antibodies effective against Gram-negative bacteria fall in this category.

In human serum the class IgA makes up about 10 percent of the gamma globulins. Globulins of this class are present in parotid saliva, colostrum, tears, and in nasal and bronchial secretions. Coproantibodies present in secretions of the intestine are most likely in this class.

IgD is present in small amounts in normal serum and its function is not known, while IgE is believed to be the source of the Prausnitz-Küstner (P-K) antibodies and is also present in a lesser amount.

**Function of Antibodies.** Immediately after an attack of a disease, or after active immunization by artificial procedures, antibodies usually are demonstrable in the circulating blood in appreciable amounts. If the animal succeeds in destroying the infecting organisms and clears the system of them completely, the antibody content of the serum diminishes rather rapidly. If this does not happen, it usually means that local foci of infection continue to exist.

The disappearance of antibodies in the circulating blood of an actively immunized animal does not mean that all immunity is lost; in a passively immunized animal it does have this significance. An actively immunized animal retains in its tissues a capacity for quickly producing more antibodies when the occasion demands. Sometimes it is said that *sessile* antibodies exist in the tissues. At any rate, the degree of resistance to a disease cannot be accurately measured by the amount of circulating antibody. Circulating antibodies indicate that resistance exists, but high degrees of active resistance, or immunity, may prevail when few or no antibodies can be demonstrated in the blood.

**The Origin of Antibodies.** In general, antibodies are most easily demonstrated in blood serum, but they also exist in milk and in various organs and tissues. Frequently the concentration of antibodies in the colostrum is higher than in the blood of the same individual. In milk they usually appear in lesser concentration, and normally they are not present in cerebrospinal fluid.

Although most animals are unable to form much antibody until some time after birth when they become immunologically more mature than in fetal life, it is possible to induce demonstrable antibody formation in certain fetuses before parturition.

Maturation of the thymus is believed to be the key to *immunologic maturation.* It appears that late in fetal life this organ secretes hormones or acts in some manner in the development of the lymphoid tissues in lymph nodes, spleen, bone marrow, and other sites.

In the chicken another lymphoid organ, the bursa of Fabricius, also contributes to immunologic maturation. In mammals the lymphoid tissue of the gastrointestinal tract may function in a similar manner. It is possible that, in mammals as well as birds, cells of the plasmacytic series (functional cells of the lymphocytic system) are concerned with humoral antibody production and depend in part on the bursa or bursa-equivalent lymphoid tissue, while thymus-dependent cells are related to cellular immunity and delayed sensitivities.

Except for the thymus, antibodies are synthesized in abundance by lymphoid cells located in the spleen, bone marrow, lymph nodes, and in other sites. This would include those cells found in granulomas and inflammations and would exclude areas lacking lymphoid elements. Although it is unlikely that macrophages synthesize antibody, they may aid by stimulating the proliferation of antibody-forming cells or by processing antigen to make it effective. There is evidence that both lymphocytes and macrophages are necessary for the primary antibody response, but it appears that the lymphoblasts, plasma cells, and various morphologic types of lymphocytes synthesize the antibodies.

The size and spacing of doses of antigen are of prime importance in the antibody response. A small dose usually will initiate the process while an excessive dose may cause *immunologic tolerance* (antigenic paralysis), a condition of complete suppression of antibody formation. The dangers of inducing immunologic tolerance in young infants by early vaccination are remote, but maternal antibody in the newborn mammal may have a dampening effect on the antibody response to newly administered antigen.

The injection of two or more antigens at or near the same time may reduce antibody formation against one or more of them, but to date competition among antigens has not interfered with antibody production in current practices of vaccination. In the universally employed *diphtheria-pertussis-tetanus* (DPT) vaccine the *pertussis* appears to enhance the production of antibodies against diphtheria and tetanus toxins. This stimulating action is sometimes called an *adjuvant* effect. *Adjuvants* such as kaolin, saponin, mineral oil, waxes, and dead bacteria have been added to antigens and vaccines to assist them in inducing antibody formation. Freund has prepared mixtures known as *Freund's incomplete* and *complete adjuvants* and *alum gels*. Part of the adjuvant's effectiveness depends on prolonging antigen absorption.

The injection of certain bacteria by the intracutaneous route produces a better and more lasting response than inoculation by any route other than an intravenous one. Clinical experience supports experimental findings that intradermal injections in lower animals have induced a higher degree of immunization against some diseases than have other methods, but in general it appears that a given dose of antigen is usually more effective when injected subcutaneously with an adjuvant or when injected as repeated small aliquants than when administered intravenously.

Having established the primary antibody response a secondary acknowledgment can be elicited readily at essentially any time during the lifetime of the animal. This has been called the *memory phenomenon, recall phenomenon,* or *anamnestic response.* Related to this is the so-called *Doctrine of original antigenic sin* (15). It is based on the observation that individuals who are given one type of vaccine may develop a much higher titer of antibodies against another related type, with which they have had previous experience, than against the type administered. This activity is believed to represent an anamnestic response to an antigen-determinant common to both types of the vaccine.

The acquisition of immunologic tolerance by exposure to antigen during fetal life is termed *fetal tolerance.* Its basis is either a destructive or a repressive action of antigen on inducible cells that would otherwise be capable of proliferating, differentiating, and producing antibodies specific for the antigen involved. Such tolerance is probably responsible for the high susceptibility of newborn animals to tumor production with oncogenic viruses. It may also permit microbes to establish *silent infections* and live in states of commensalism with their hosts. Artificially induced immunologic tolerance may develop in an immature animal through injection of antigens closely related to the animal's own antigens. A similar effect may be induced by the feeding of a hapten or an antigen. Such tolerance may be broken by x-irradiation or by treatment with a related antigen.

Immunoglobulin deficiencies also occur. Among these are hereditary agammaglobulinemia resulting from a lack of germinal centers and plasma cells, thymic aplasia where there is a faulty embryonic development of the thymus gland, and dysgammaglobulinemia where there may be an elevated level of IgM or IgD and a deficiency of IgA and IgG.

Certain agents are claimed to suppress antibody formation. Nitrogen mustard (2,2-dichloro-N-methyldiethylamine hydrochloride) is toxic for lymphocytes and thereby interferes with the production of antibodies (44). As mentioned previously, the adrenal cortical hormones seem to influence acquired resistance, some reports indicating that these substances suppress antibody formation while others present evidence to the contrary. $\beta$-3-thienylalanine also inhibits antibody formation (28). Antilymphocyte serum suppresses the production and release of antibody and exerts a dampening effect on the activity of antibody and immune cells. It is the best as well as the least toxic immunosuppressive agent available for clinical use in organ transplantation.

**Ehrlich's "Side-Chain" Theory for the Formation of Antibodies.** Paul Ehrlich was, by training, a chemist who became interested in bacteriological problems. Some of his earliest studies were with bacterial toxins and their antitoxins. These will be described later.

In 1885 Ehrlich (13) published a theory that he had developed to account for cellular nutrition. In this he postulated that before any cell could profit by a chemical nutrient with which it came in contact, the substance had to enter into chemical combination with it. In theorizing thus, he regarded the cells as having a central nucleus of matter, which differed with the different types of cells, and "receptors" or side chains, through which the chemical affinity for the nutrient was expressed. The matter generally is illustrated by comparing the situation to the chemical formula for the benzene ring:

$$
\begin{array}{c}
H \\
| \\
C \\
\diagup \quad \diagdown \\
H{-}C \qquad C{-}H \\
| \qquad\qquad | \\
H{-}C \qquad C{-}H \\
\diagdown \quad \diagup \\
C \\
| \\
H
\end{array}
$$

(Benzene)

The chemical nucleus of this compound is represented by the six carbon atoms, which are so firmly bound together that they cannot easily be broken down. The hydrogen atoms, representing the "receptors," are quite easily displaced by other chemical groupings such as $NO_2$, $OH$, $COOH$, $NH_2$, these completely altering the character of the compound, as, for example:

$$
\begin{array}{c}
H \\
C \\
\diagup \quad \diagdown \\
HC \qquad COH \\
| \qquad\qquad | \\
HC \qquad CH \\
\diagdown \quad \diagup \\
C \\
H
\end{array}
\qquad \text{or} \qquad
\begin{array}{c}
OH \\
C \\
\diagup \quad \diagdown \\
HC \qquad COOH \\
| \qquad\qquad | \\
HC \qquad CH \\
\diagdown \quad \diagup \\
C \\
H
\end{array}
$$

Phenol                                       Salicylic acid

The side chains thus represent affinities for other chemical groupings which combine with the chemical nucleus quite readily. Thus it is with the "side chains" or receptors of cells.

Ehrlich carried his nutritional theory into the field of immunity, where it became best known. His theory is no longer acceptable, but inasmuch as Ehrlich, in connection with it, coined a large number of the terms of immunology and since this terminology continues to be used in spite of the abandonment of the theory, it is well for every student of the subject to understand the concept.

Knowing that toxins were complicated chemical substances that affected some types of cells and had little or no effect on others, Ehrlich reasoned that the susceptible cells had affinities, or "receptors," for the toxin molecule and

*Table VI.* METHODS OF PRODUCING AN ARTIFICIAL IMMUNITY

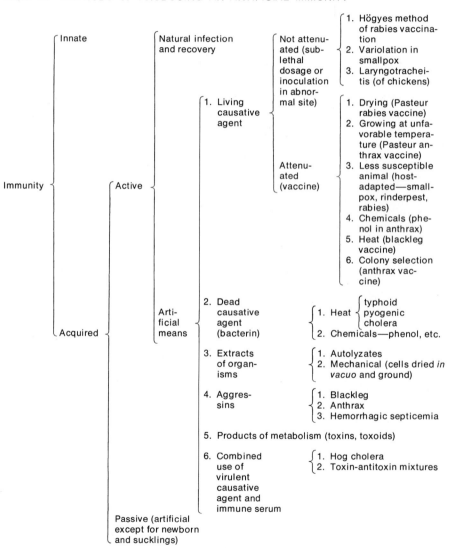

the nonsusceptible cells did not. But the toxins are substances that injure or even destroy the cells that have "receptors" for them. If the injured cells are not wholly devitalized by the experience, repair of the damage occurs, and in the course of this repair, nature tends to overcompensate for the damage done by producing more of the special "receptors" than previously existed or than the cells can use. These supernumerary receptors are then detached from the cells and pass into the fluids of the body. These free receptors retain their affinity for the toxin for which they are specific, unite with it when the opportunity is presented, and so neutralize or inactivate the toxin that it becomes harmless to the tissue cells. Animals with free receptors in their blood are immune to the toxin so long as there are enough receptors to unite with all the toxin present, and the blood serum of such animals, containing the receptors, can be used to protect other animals into which it is injected. The receptors of Ehrlich are what we call antibodies, in this case, antitoxin.

This is a bare outline of the concept of Ehrlich. He applied the theory to types of antibodies other than antitoxins, developing eventually an exceedingly complicated system made up of three orders, which will not be discussed. It may be seen, however, that Ehrlich's basic idea is that antibodies, the basis of artificial immunity, are produced by certain cells of the body as a result of a reaction to an injury. We might liken the process to the everyday experience of learning—for example, the baby burns his fingers on a stove and learns thereby not to repeat the process.

## REFERENCES

1. Aschoff. Ergebn. inn. Med. Kinderheilk., 1924, *26*, 1.
2. Brambell. Proc. Royal Soc. Med., 1961, *54*, 992.
3. Bruner, Brown, Hull, and Kinkaid. Jour. Am. Vet. Med. Assoc., 1949, *115*, 94.
4. Bruner, Edwards, and Doll. Cornell Vet., 1948, *38*, 363.
5. Calmette. Comp. rend. Soc. Biol. (Paris), 1894, *46*, 11, 120, and 204.
6. Carpenter. Immunity and serology. W. B. Saunders Co., Philadelphia, 1956.
7. Cherry and Ewing. Bact. Proc., 1959, *59*, 90.
8. Colebrook, Erdinow, and Hill. Brit. Jour. Exp. Path., 1924, *5*, 54.
9. Coons and Kaplan. Jour. Exp. Med., 1950, *91*, 1.
10. Editorial. Vet. Rec., 1953, *65*, 199.
11. Ehrlich. Zeitschr. f. Hyg., 1892, *12*, 183.
12. Ehrlich. Fortschr. Med., 1897, *15*, 41.
13. Ehrlich. Collected studies on immunity. Eng. trans., 2d ed. John Wiley and Sons, New York, 1910.
14. Famulener. Jour. Inf. Dis., 1912, *10*, 332.
15. Fazekas and Webster. Jour. Exp. Med., 1966, *124*, 347.
16. Fischell. N.Y. Acad. Med. Bul. 26, 1950, p. 225.
17. Fleming. Brit. Jour. Exp. Path., 1926, *7*, 174.
18. Freeman. Proc. 1st Clin. ACTH Conf. Blakiston Co., Philadelphia, 1950.
19. Freter. Jour. Inf. Dis., 1962, *111*, 37.

20. Furness and Axelrod. Jour. Immunol., 1959, *83*, 133.
21. Germuth and Ottinger. Proc. Soc. Exp. Biol. and Med., 1950, *74*, 815.
22. Goldwasser and Kissling. *Ibid.*, 1958, *98*, 219.
23. Hammond and Horn. Jour. Am. Med. Assoc., 1958, *166*, 1294.
24. Harding, Bruner, and Bryant. Cornell Vet., 1961, *51*, 535.
25. Jacoby, Dennis, and Griesemer. Am. Jour. Vet. Res., 1969, *30*, 1503.
26. Kono, Ikawa, Yaoi, Jr., Hamada, Ashihara, and Kawakami. Am. Jour. Epidemiol., 1966, *83*, 14.
27. Landsteiner. The specificity of serological reactions. C. C Thomas, Springfield, Ill., 1936.
28. LaVia, Uriu, Barber, and Warren. Proc. Soc. Exp. Biol. and Med., 1960, *104*, 562.
29. Leroy. Jour. Am. Med. Assoc., 1947, *134*, 1143.
30. Levi, Kravtzov, Levova, and Fomenko. Immunology, 1969, *16*, 145.
31. Lurie, Zoppasodi, Dannenberg, and Swartz. Science, 1951, *113*, 234.
32. Michael, Cummings, and Bloom. Proc. Soc. Exp. Biol. and Med., 1950, *75*, 613.
33. Mirick. Jour. Clin. Invest., 1950, *29*, 836.
34. Moody, Ellis, and Updyke. Jour. Bact., 1958, *75*, 553.
35. Moody, Goldman, and Thomason. *Ibid.*, 1956, *72*, 357.
36. Pensky, Hinz, Jr., Todd, Wedgwood, Boyer, and Lepow. Jour. Immunol., 1968, *100*, 142.
37. Pillemer *et al.* Ann. N.Y. Acad. Sci., New York, 1956, *66* [art. 2], 233–274.
38. Raffel. Immunity: Hypersensitivity-serology. Appleton-Century-Crofts, New York, 1953.
39. Schneider and Szathmary. Zeitschr. f. Immunitätsf., 1939, *95*, 465.
40. Schneider and Webster. Jour. Exp. Med., 1945, *81*, 359.
41. Seeler and Ott. Jour. Inf. Dis., 1945, 77, 82.
42. Smith and Ingram. Canad. Vet. Jour., 1965, *6*, 226.
43. Smith and Little. Jour. Exp. Med., 1922, *36*, 453.
44. Spurr. Proc. Soc. Exp. Biol. and Med., 1947, *64*, 259.
45. Steffee. Jour. Inf. Dis., 1950, *86*, 12.
46. Taliaferro. Am. Jour. Hyg., 1932, *16*, 32.
47. Thompson and Moses. Jour. Clin. Invest., 1948, 27, 805.
48. Topley. An outline of immunity. William Wood and Co., Baltimore, 1933.
49. Topley and Wilson. Principles of bacteriology and immunity. 4th ed. Williams and Wilkins Co., Baltimore, 1955.
50. Truant. Bact. Proc., 1959, *59*, 90.
51. Von Behring and Kitasato. Deut. med. Wchnschr., 1890, *16*, 1113.
52. Wasserman and Trum. Science, 1955, *121*, 894.
53. Watson. Jour. Hyg. (London), 1937, 37, 420.
54. Weiser, Myrvik, and Pearsall. Fundamentals of immunology for students of medicine and related sciences. Lea and Febiger, Philadelphia, 1969.
55. Young, Erwin, Christian, and Davis. Science, 1949, *109*, 630.
56. Zingher. Am. Jour. Dis. Children, 1923, *25*, 392.

# III | Toxins and Antitoxins

When toxin and its specific antitoxin are mixed *in vitro* in proper proportions, a union between the two agents occurs. This union is manifested in two ways: (a) the poisonous properties of the toxin are destroyed or inactivated, and (b) a precipitate is formed, consisting of the toxin-antitoxin combination. Presumably antibody prevents toxin from combining with its "biochemical target" on cells by blocking the "toxin site" on the toxin molecule through steric hindrance, and the process is much more complicated than a simple neutralization reaction.

Some of the first studies on toxin-antitoxin combinations were made by Ehrlich (5), who established the first units of measurement and gave names to them. The original studies were with diphtheria toxin and antitoxin, substances with which students of animal disease have little concern. The reason for describing them here is that the nomenclature, if not the unit sizes in every case, has been carried over from these studies to all toxin-antitoxin studies.

## Toxin Units (Diphtheria)

The simplest unit of toxin is the *minimum lethal dose* (MLD). This is the amount of toxin which will kill a 250-g guinea pig in about 96 hours after subcutaneous injection. Ehrlich formulated an antitoxin unit which is now of no importance except that it was with this unit that he discovered some of the peculiarities exhibited by neutralization experiments. The Ehrlich unit was based upon the antitoxin's ability to neutralize a test dose of toxin consisting of 100 MLD. Because this toxin deteriorated with age, and because deterioration was not accompanied by a change in its power to unite with antitoxin, it was found that a much larger quantity of antitoxin was required to neutralize 100 MLD of old toxin than of the freshly made. The reason for this is that the *toxoid*, formed by deterioration of the toxin, unites with antitoxin in the same

43

way as the toxin. A fresh toxin solution contains little toxoid, an old one a great deal. To obtain neutralization of a toxin solution, enough antitoxin must be added to combine with its toxoid content as well as with its toxin. The amount of antitoxin required to neutralize 100 MLD of a toxin in which there is also much toxoid to be satisfied will naturally be much greater than the amount required to neutralize 100 MLD of another toxin solution in which practically all of the combining power is in the form of toxin. This finding induced Ehrlich to formulate two additional units of toxin:

The $L_0$ dose of diphtheria toxin is the maximum amount of toxin that, when mixed with one unit of antitoxin, will be completely neutralized by it.

The $L_+$ dose of diphtheria toxin is the amount of toxin that, when mixed with one unit of antitoxin, will cause the death of a 250-g guinea pig in about 96 hours after subcutaneous injection.

The $L_0$ dose of toxin is determined by injecting guinea pigs, and because it is the largest quantity which, upon injection, produces no symptoms, the determination of this amount depends upon the acuity of the observer. The end point of the $L_+$ dose, because it is determined by the death of the animal, is not subject to this objection.

It should be noted that the $L_0$ dose of a toxin does not change materially as toxin deteriorates until practically all toxicity is lost, because there will be residual toxicity in a mixture of toxin and toxoid with antitoxin so long as both toxin and toxoid are not fully neutralized. In deteriorating, toxin changes to toxoid and the sum total of the two remains the same; consequently the amount of antitoxin required to neutralize the sum of the two will be constant. On the other hand, the $L_+$ dose is quickly affected by deterioration because even a small reduction in the amount of toxin will rob it of its ability to kill the guinea pig within the proper time interval.

In recent years the *median lethal dose*, $LD_{50}$, has come into use as a measure of virulence, not only of toxins, but also of other infective agents, especially viruses. This establishes an end point at the dose that kills approximately one-half of a group of animals rather than at one that kills all, thus equalizing individual differences in susceptibility. A simple procedure for the calculation of the $LD_{50}$ dose was published by Reed and Muench (9).

### Antitoxin Units

Antitoxin units vary in different countries. This causes much confusion; consequently attempts have been made to establish international units for the curative serums. In the United States the present unit of diphtheria antitoxin is the smallest amount that, when added to an $L_+$ dose of toxin, will neutralize the toxin sufficiently to cause a 250-g guinea pig to die in 96 hours after subcutaneous injection of the mixture. Inasmuch as this definition of a unit requires the use of a dose of toxin which can be arrived at only by having known units of antitoxin in the first place, the definition has no value unless a standard antitoxin of known unit value is kept, from which all new antitoxins can be standardized. Such a standard is kept by a governmental agency, as will be described later.

The unit of tetanus antitoxin is somewhat different. Tetanus toxin is relatively stable; hence it is possible to use it as a standard. The *official test dose* of tetanus toxin in the United States is 100 MLD (for a 350-g guinea pig) of a standard toxin produced by a governmental agency, designated by Congress for the purpose. The antitoxin unit is determined by titrating against this standard, and it may be defined as follows: The antitoxin unit (tetanus) is ten times the least quantity of antitoxin that will protect a 350-g guinea pig for 96 hours against the official test dose of toxin.

**Standardization of Diphtheria Antitoxin.** Standard *antitoxin* is maintained and distributed by the laboratories of the National Institutes of Health, Washington, D.C. An arbitrary unit was established by this laboratory when the antitoxin standardization work was begun many years ago, based upon a previous arbitrary unit established by Ehrlich. As new lots of antitoxin are made up for standardization purposes, each new lot is carefully compared with older lots so that the standard is kept unchanged. Commercial producing laboratories in the United States must obtain this standard antitoxin by which to standardize their own product. It is sent out, on request, in a dried state hermetically sealed in dark-glass containers. In this condition it is relatively stable.

The manufacturer first must produce his own toxin. He tests this toxin by mixing varying quantities with one unit of the standard antitoxin. In this way he learns the $L_+$ dose of his toxin. He now mixes varying quantities of the commercial antitoxin, which he has produced, with the amount of toxin that he has found to represent the $L_+$ dose and injects the mixtures into guinea pigs of 250 g in weight. Those that die in from 4 to 5 days indicate the dosage that contained the equivalent of one standard unit of antitoxin.

The manufacturer must state the unit value of his antitoxin on the trade packages. When used, allowance should be made for deterioration because of the date of manufacture; also the material should be kept cold. In the United States commercial diphtheria antitoxin must contain at least 350 units per ml.

*Ramon flocculation method of standardizing diphtheria antitoxin.* An entirely new method of standardizing diphtheria antitoxin was introduced by Ramon (7) of the Pasteur Institute in 1922. It depends upon the fact, previously observed by others, that, at the neutralization point of toxin with antitoxin, a flocculent precipitate is formed. The test is carried out in test tubes. Varying amounts of the unknown antitoxin solution are added to fixed amounts of a standard toxin solution. The tubes are incubated for a comparatively short time, and the characteristic coarse flocculation is looked for. The tube in which it appears indicates the quantity of antitoxin that has just neutralized the standard toxin solution.

The flocculation method gives data that correlate well with the combining powers of the toxin, but there is no such correlation with toxicity except in fresh toxins. In other words, deteriorated toxins flocculate the same as fresh ones.

The flocculation test has proved very useful as a preliminary test during standardization. Because it does not measure the ability of sera to neutralize toxin, the test is not likely to replace the animal tests.

*Intracutaneous method of standardizing diphtheria antitoxin.* This method is cheaper than the standard animal test and probably is more accurate.

When diphtheria toxin is injected intracutaneously (intradermally) in guinea pigs, an inflammatory reaction, manifested by swelling and redness, results. This reaction is the same as that obtained with the Schick test in a susceptible person.

In a white-skinned guinea pig, a reaction will be obtained with toxin solutions containing as little as about 0.002 MLD. The smallest amount of a toxin that will elicit a reaction is known as the MRD (minimum reacting dose). In intracutaneous testing, the $L_r$ dose corresponds to the $L_+$ dose, i.e., it is the smallest amount of toxin which, when mixed with one unit of antitoxin, will still give a reaction. The tests are made with fractions of units because the total amount injected at one site must not exceed 0.2 ml. Several dilutions may be tested simultaneously on the same animal.

*The use of the chick in titration of diphtheria antitoxin.* According to Branham and Wormald (2), diphtheria antitoxin can be successfully titrated in 8-day-old chicks. They claim that the chick test and the official guinea pig test produce approximately the same results.

**Standardization of Tetanus Antitoxin.** Like those for diphtheria antitoxin, the standards for tetanus antitoxin in the United States are maintained by the National Institutes of Health and furnished by that organization to commercial producers. The standard unit of antitoxin was determined for the United States by act of Congress in 1902. The official method of determining the unit was worked out by Rosenau and Anderson (10). The Institutes maintain both a standard toxin and a standard antitoxin. The two products are kept at uniform strength by measuring them against each other. The units of tetanus toxin and antitoxin are not the same as those of diphtheria.

Standard antitoxin is furnished the manufacturer on request. The smallest amount of his own toxin that, when mixed with 0.1 unit of the standard antitoxin, will kill a 350-g guinea pig in from 4 to 5 days after subcutaneous injection constitutes the $L_+$ dose. By mixing $L_+$ doses of his own toxin with varying amounts of his commercial antitoxin and injecting the mixtures into standard-weight guinea pigs, the manufacturer can determine the unit value of his product. The least quantity that protects the animals for 4 days constitutes 0.1 of a unit.

For prophylactic purposes, at least 1,500 units should be employed. For curative purposes, 50,000 or more units frequently are needed, and even these huge quantities often will not save the patients.

## Use of Toxoids for Immunization

Animals may be actively immunized to toxins by injecting quantities of toxins too small to kill, but this procedure is too heroic to be used practically. The severe local effects of toxins can be prevented, in part at least, by mixing them with antitoxin before injection. Toxins that have lost their poisonous properties through aging (toxoids) retain their immunizing properties and may be used for practical immunization. Better for the purpose are the toxoids produced by treating fresh toxins with formalin. This method was first described by Ramon (8) for diphtheria and by Descombey (4) for tetanus. The efficacy of these toxoids is enhanced by precipitating them with alum. Alum-precipitated toxoids are now frequently used for prophylactic immunization of man against both diphtheria and tetanus. The alum-precipitated toxoid also has proved very effective in immunizing horses against tetanus. It has been demonstrated that the antitoxin response of an animal injected with small daily doses of toxoid is greatly superior to that of one given the same total amount of toxoid in a single injection (3).

Toxoids are of no value in treating cases of disease because the immunity develops slowly. They should be used on children or young animals purely as prophylactic agents. For this purpose they have the advantage over antitoxin in that the immunity produced is more enduring. According to Fleming, Greenberg, and Beith (6), there is evidence that mixing toxoids derived from different species of bacteria does not increase the severity of reaction upon injection into infants, and that mixed antigens actually are more effective as immunizing agents. Combining diphtheria toxoid with tetanus toxoid enhances the efficiency of both. In fact, a stable quadruple antigen is now in use (11). Diphtheria and tetanus toxoids are combined with *Bordetella pertussis* and poliomyelitis vaccines (DPT polio vaccine).

By studying the antitoxin titers of individuals vaccinated with tetanus toxoid, Banton and Miller (1) determined that periodic booster doses of toxoid should be given at 3- to 4-year intervals in order to maintain an adequate residual antitoxin level. This has now been changed to 5 to 10 years. By keeping the proper level, a booster dose of tetanus toxoid given immediately after an injury will stimulate a high antitoxin titer within a few days. For further discussion of the use of tetanus toxoid on animals see page 366.

## REFERENCES

1. Banton and Miller.   New England Jour. Med., 1949, *240*, 13.
2. Branham and Wormald.   Jour. Immunol., 1954, *72*, 478.
3. Carlanfanti.   *Ibid.*, 1951, *66*, 311.
4. Descombey.   Comp. rend. Soc. Biol. (Paris), 1924, *91*, 239.
5. Ehrlich.   Collected studies on immunity. Eng. trans., 2d ed. John Wiley and Sons, New York, 1910.

6.   Fleming, Greenberg, and Beith.   Canad. Med. Assoc. Jour., 1948, *59*, 101.

7.   Ramon.   Comp. rend. Soc. Biol. (Paris), 1922, *86*, 661, 711, and 813.

8.   *Ibid.*, 1923, *89*, 2.

9.   Reed and Muench.   Am. Jour. Hyg., 1938, *27*, 493.

10.   Rosenau and Anderson.   The standardization of tetanus antitoxin. Hyg. Lab. Bul. 43, 2d ed., U.S. Treasury Dept., Government Printing Office, Washington, 1912.

11.   Wilson, Moss, Potter, and MacLeod.   Canad. Med. Assoc. Jour., 1959, *81*, 450.

# IV | The Lytic Antibodies: Bacteriolysins, Hemolysins, Complement Fixation

## The Lysins

In 1894 Pfeiffer (9) in Germany described the first of a series of studies in which it was shown that a bacterium, the *Vibrio* of cholera, was actually broken up, or lysed, by the cell-free fluids of guinea pigs which previously had been immunized with dead cultures of this organism. The observations were made by injecting the cultures into the peritoneal cavity and following the reactions by withdrawing the peritoneal fluid, from time to time, with a hypodermic needle. These observations are often known as the *Pfeiffer phenomenon*. The principal facts were as follows:

1. When a suspension of vibrios was injected into an *immunized* animal, the fluid withdrawn at intervals showed that the organisms were not multiplying, but instead were swelling and assuming abnormal shapes. Finally, all organisms underwent fragmentation and disappeared. The organisms had been lysed, and the animal remained well.

2. When the vibrios were injected into a *nonimmunized* animal, fragmentation and lysis did not occur. After a few hours the vibrios began to multiply, and eventually they overwhelmed the animal causing its death.

3. When the vibrios were mixed with serum from an *immunized* animal, and the mixture was injected into a normal animal, the vibrios behaved as in 1, and the animal lived.

4. When the vibrios were mixed with serum from a normal animal (*nonimmunized*) and the mixture was injected into a normal animal, the vibrios behaved as in 2, and the animal died.

Bordet (1) repeated the experiments of Pfeiffer, except that he conducted them *in vitro* instead of in living animals. Using the same organism, the following experiments were done:

1. When the vibrios were added to fresh *nonimmune* serum, there was only slight evidence of lysis of the organism. Eventually the organisms multiplied.

2. When the vibrios were added to fresh *immune* serum, lysis occurred.

3. When the vibrios were added to fresh *immune* serum, which had been heated at 60 C for a few minutes, lysis did not occur.

4. When the vibrios were added to a mixture of heated *immune* serum and fresh *normal* serum, lysis occurred.

### Mechanism of the Process of Serum Lysis

From the experiments just described, Bordet deducted that two factors were necessary for serum lysis:

1. A specific thermostable factor, which is not normally present in the body but which is produced by immunization (antibody).

2. A thermolabile factor, which is present in fresh, normal serum and is not increased by immunization.

These studies were further extended by Bordet, who showed that red blood cells (erythrocytes) could be lysed with serum produced by injecting the same kind of cells into a species of animal foreign to that from which they came, thus the erythrocytes of a rabbit could be lysed by serum from a goat that had received injections of rabbit erythrocytes. In these experiments it again was demonstrated that the antibodies produced by immunization required the assistance of the thermolabile substance of normal serum. When the blood cells were mixed with either of these constituents alone, lysis (hemolysis) did not occur. When the cells were placed in contact with the antibody (thermostable factor) alone for a time, were then carefully washed to remove the antibody, and afterward were placed in contact with the thermolabile factor, hemolysis occurred. When the thermolabile factor was used first and followed by the antibody, hemolysis did not occur. From these experiments it was evident that the blood cells were capable of absorbing the antibody, but not the thermolabile substance, and that the antibody injured or sensitized them so that the other agent caused their lysis.

In the case of blood cells and a few bacterial cells, the antibodies, working in co-operation with the other factor, do in fact cause lysis or dissolving of the cells for which they are specific. Such antibodies can be produced for any type of cell, but, in the vast majority of cases, the cells are not actually disrupted in the reaction. In these cases the mechanism might more properly be called *bactericidins* than *bacteriolysins;* however, the latter term is usually used whether or not the cells are dissolved.

**Amboceptor.** The antibodies that are demonstrated in the lytic phenomena were called *amboceptors* by Ehrlich because he visualized them as agents which united on the one hand with the antigenic cell and on the other with the thermolabile factor. Antibodies of this type were given the name *sub-*

*stance sensabilatrice* by Bordet. Ehrlich's name is generally used in this country.

**Complement.** The constituent of fresh normal serum which is required for the functioning of the lytic antibodies (the heat-labile substance of the foregoing discussion) was given the name *complement* by Ehrlich. Apparently it is identical with a substance previously studied by Buchner and which was named by him *alexin*. It is apparent that this substance is nonspecific; that is, it will function to injure, and often lyse, any kind of cell that has been acted upon or sensitized by antibodies.

Complement (C′) is a substance of mixed globulin composition which occurs in the serum of all normal animals. It quickly deteriorates in blood after it has been drawn, unless the blood is given special treatment. C′ is removed from whole blood in the serum portion. The serum can be lyophilized and stored as dried powder in sealed ampoules. The reconstituted powder acts like fresh serum. C′ also can be preserved in serum for years by freezing and maintaining it in a frozen state. It is easily destroyed or inactivated by chemical action and by heat, and it may be adsorbed from serum by many substances.

Methods of chemical separation together with inactivation have shown that C′ is composed of at least nine serum globulin components: C′1, C′2, . . . C′9. Certain components of C′ are highly labile to various physical and chemical agents. Those contained in C′1, 2, 5, 8, and 9 are destroyed by heating at 56 C for 30 minutes. It appears that C′1, 2, 3, and 4 constitute the activation mechanism, and that C′5, 6, 7, 8, and 9 the actual attack forces in complement-dependent cytolysis.

Many adult animals possess an abundant amount of C′, but its production during fetal life varies with the species. The tissue sources of the origin of the various C′ components are not known.

C′ of one species may differ from that of another. Some specimens react with certain antigen-antibody complexes but not with others. It appears that differences in activity of complements from various species are caused by altered proportions of the C′ factors in these animals. Reactions such as hemolysis and bacteriolysis require the co-operation of all components and cannot occur if one is too weak or missing. The horse, cat, and pig produce nonhemolytic complements and are therefore unsuited for the complement-fixation reaction. There is some evidence that this is due to low C′2 and C′4 content, but other components may be involved. Levy (7) has estimated that the hemolytic complement activities of the sera of the rat, hamster, and dog are the same as that of the serum of man; in guinea pigs it is seven times greater; in rabbit serum it is one-fourth and in mice one-sixtieth of that in man.

Appropriate antibodies that are capable of activating C′ can cause lysis of mammalian cells in the presence of C′. Many Gram-negative bacteria are killed by antibody and C′, and in some cases lysed. Lysozyme often augments the antibacterial action of C′.

**The Bordet-Gengou Phenomenon.** This name is given to an experiment conducted by Bordet and his pupil Gengou (3) to demonstrate that the same C′
could function equally well with a bacteriolytic and a hemolytic amboceptor.
The experiment is of great importance because it furnished the basis for the
complement-fixation test. The experiment seems rather complicated but this
really is not the case. It is easily understood if one understands the reagents
which are used. These are five in number, as follows:

1. An antiserum (bacteriolytic amboceptor) for some species of bacteria.
In the original study an antiserum for *Pasteurella pestis* was used. This serum
was inactivated (heated to 56 C for 30 minutes to destroy any complement
which may have been present).

2. A bacterial antigen homologous with this serum.
In this case a suspension of *Pasteurella pestis* in saline solution.

3. Complement (C′).
Fresh, unheated serum from a normal guinea pig.

4. Washed erythrocytes of a sheep.
Defibrinated blood from a normal sheep was centrifuged and the serum discarded. The sedimented cells were then shaken up in saline solution and centrifuged out, and this process was repeated several times until all trace of the
serum had been removed.

5. An antiserum (hemolytic amboceptor) for sheep erythrocytes.
A normal rabbit was injected several times with suspensions of washed
erythrocytes of a sheep. Finally the rabbit was bled and its serum obtained.
This serum was inactivated, to destroy its C′, before being used.

An outline of the experiment is as follows:

(a) Substances 1, 2, and 3 were mixed in a tube and placed in a water bath
for 1 hour. Substances 4 and 5 were now added; the tube was shaken and returned to the bath. Hemolysis did not occur.

(b) Substances 2 and 3 were mixed in a tube, and the tube was placed in a
water bath for 1 hour. Substances 4 and 5 were now added, and the tube was
returned to the bath after shaking. Hemolysis did occur.

Bacteriolysis had occurred in the first case, as would be expected, because
the three necessary constituents, antigen, 2, amboceptor, 1, and C′, 3, were
present. In the process the C′ had been used up or bound. When blood cells
with their hemolytic amboceptor were added, hemolysis did not occur because of lack of C′.

In the second instance, because of lack of amboceptor, 1, bacteriolysis did
not occur and the C′, 3, remained free after the first period of incubation.
When blood cells, 4, with their specific amboceptor, 5, were added, hemolysis
did occur because C′ was already present in a free condition.

In the one instance, a, the C′ was fixed by the bacteriolytic system and
hemolysis was prevented; in the other, there was no such fixation; hence the
C′ was free to enter into the hemolytic system. On the basis of this experiment Bordet and Gengou argued that C′ was a nonspecific substance because

it could function in the hemolytic or in the bacteriolytic system equally well.

The fact that some antigen-antibody systems do not fix C' suggests that certain stereochemical requirements are necessary. Antibodies of the classes IgA and IgE do not fix C'. While it appears that two molecules of IgG, properly spaced, are needed to activate the C'-reaction sequence, one molecule of IgM antibody can accomplish this and on a molar basis the latter is much more efficient than the former for hemolyzing erythrocytes and killing Gram-negative bacteria.

Components of C' are involved *in vivo* antigen-antibody reactions that include chemotaxis of neutrophils, opsonization, killing of mammalian cells and bacteria, generation of anaphylatoxin, certain sensitivity reactions, precipitation of antigen-antibody complexes, and the destruction of target cells by immune cells, but not all C'-components are required in each instance.

### The Complement-Fixation Test for the Diagnosis of Disease

The principle of this test is the same as that of the Bordet-Gengou experiment. Substances 3, 4, and 5 (which constitute the hemolytic system) are used irrespective of the disease being studied. The antigen (2) is a suspension or an extract of the causative agent of the disease for which the test is being made, e.g., a culture of *Actinobacillus mallei* when testing for glanders. Substance 1 is the sample of serum which is being tested. If this serum came from an infected individual, the amboceptors for that disease will be present; if the individual is not infected, the amboceptor will be absent. The test is run only after the various reagents have been carefully standardized (titrations). The

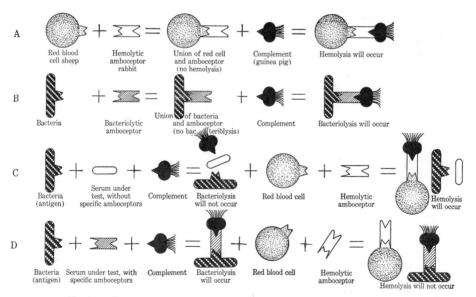

Fig. 1. A diagrammatic representation of the process of complement-fixation.

procedure in the final test is the same as that used by Bordet. If hemolysis results, the suspected serum must have been devoid of amboceptor, i.e., the test is negative. If hemolysis does not occur, the amboceptor for the suspected disease must have been present, i.e., the test is positive.

This method has been used more or less successfully for diagnosing nearly all infectious diseases. Some diseases in which the test has been effective in a practical way are syphilis, gonorrhea, tuberculosis, glanders, infectious abortion (of cattle), leptospirosis, coccidioidomycosis, histoplasmosis, leishmaniasis, trypanosomiasis, certain nematode infestations (12), and numerous viral infections.

The *Wassermann reaction* (11) is the complement-fixation test as applied to the diagnosis of syphilis. In the beginning the *Treponema* of syphilis had not been successfully cultivated and the antigen used was an extract of the liver of a syphilitic fetus. Later extracts of normal organs were found to function equally well. At present the acetone-insoluble fraction of an alcoholic extract of normal heart muscle, to which a small amount of cholesterol has been added, is considered the most satisfactory antigen.

The Wassermann reaction depends upon the fixation of complement by precipitates that are formed by the action of syphilitic antibodies on lecithin-containing lipoids. The test, then, is really a nonspecific one, and yet it has a remarkably high specificity for syphilis. For many years it was employed, almost alone, for the diagnosis of occult syphilis, but in recent years various precipitation tests have been developed which depend upon observing directly the precipitates that are detected by the Wassermann test. The precipitation tests are much simpler and appear to be fully as accurate as the more complicated test. The technics of Meinicke (8), Sachs and Georgi (10), and Kahn (6) have been used for the precipitation test. The Kahn test, in particular, has been very popular in recent years.

### Other Applications of the Complement-Fixation Test

When a known antigen is at hand, this test may be used to identify the homologous antibody. This is done when the method is used for testing serums for evidence of specific diseases. On the other hand, when a known serum is on hand, the homologous antigen may be identified. This procedure is followed occasionally in scientific work to identify unknown proteins, viruses, or organisms. The test may be used in medicolegal cases to identify blood stains or other protein-bearing substances, but the precipitin tests usually are preferred for this purpose because of their greater simplicity.

### Conglutination Complement-Absorption Test

As early as 1906 it was noted by Bordet and Gay (2) that sheep erythrocytes sensitized with heated normal bovine serum were aggregated (clumped) by the fresh serum of certain animals. This reaction was dependent upon the presence of C' in the fresh serum and was called *conglutination* to distinguish it from *agglutination*. The latter was accomplished without the aid of C'. Apparently two essential substances were furnished by the heated bovine serum: (1) a natural antierythrocyte antibody and (2) a clumping substance called *conglutinin*. Later it was shown that conglutination may be inhibited by the absorption of C' to an antigen-antibody complex in essentially the same manner as hemolysis is inhibited in the ordinary complement-fixation test, and the conglutination complement-absorption test was established.

Conglutination absorption was employed diagnostically by Hole and Coombs (5) to detect antibodies in horses convalescent from glanders. It is most useful in certain tests where for some unknown reason guinea pig complement fails to fix or is weakly absorbed. It can also be used to detect antibody too weak to cause agglutination. At present it is a valuable aid in investigations of some rickettsial and viral diseases.

Horse serum is the usual source of C' because it is well absorbed but is not hemolytic, and the actual test is conducted as follows: (a) incubate antigen, antibody, and horse C'; (b) add sheep erythrocytes sensitized with heated bovine serum; and (c) reincubate and read the test. No conglutination indicates positive fixation of the C' and a positive test. In the absence of antibody or antigen, C' remains free and conglutinates the erythrocytes.

## REFERENCES

1. Bordet. Studies on immunity. Eng. trans. John Wiley and Son, New York, 1909.
2. Bordet and Gay. Ann. l'Inst. Past., 1906, 20, 467.
3. Bordet and Gengou. *Ibid.*, 1901, 15, 289.
4. Carpenter. Immunity and serology. W. B. Saunders Co., Philadelphia, 1956.
5. Hole and Coombs. Jour. Hyg. (London), 1947, 45, 497.
6. Kahn. Arch. Dermatol. and Syphilol., 1922, 5, 570.
7. Levy. Proc. Soc. Exp. Biol. and Med., 1958, 99, 584.
8. Meinicke. Berl. klin. Wchnschr., 1917, 54, 613.
9. Pfeiffer. Zeitshcr. f. Hyg., 1894, 18, 1; 1895, 19, 75; 1895, 20, 198.
10. Sachs and Georgi. Med. Klin., 1918, 33, 805.
11. Wassermann and Bruck. *Ibid.*, 1905, 1, 1409.
12. Weber. Am. Jour. Vet. Res., 1958, 19, 338.
13. Weiser, Myrvik, and Pearsall. Fundamentals of immunology for students of medicine and related sciences. Lea and Febiger, Philadelphia, 1969.

# V | The Agglutinins and Precipitins

## The Agglutinins

Gruber and Durham (8; 1896) first observed the specificity of the phenomenon of agglutination of bacteria by antisera, using the typhoid bacillus and the serum of patients. Later it was discovered that cells other than bacteria, such as yeasts, fungi, protozoa, blood cells, and spermatozoa, will exhibit the phenomenon in the presence of specific antibodies.

The reaction may be observed *in vitro* as well as *in vivo*. It consists of a coming together of the cells in suspension to form aggregates, which finally may become so large as to be easily visible with the naked eye as granular masses or large flocculi, depending upon the conditions of the experiment and the substances present. The phenomenon is not a vital one; suspensions of dead cells, and of inanimate particles, may be flocculated. Agglutination depends upon antibodies. Complement need not be present. Red blood cells may be agglutinated by heated immune serum; the addition of guinea pig complement then induces lysis.

Agglutination is the result of the interaction of an antibody (or antibodies), known as an *agglutinin,* with an antigen (or antigens), known as an *agglutinogen,* contained in or on the cells. Agglutination of cells is believed to be the same phenomenon as precipitation of antigens in solution, the difference being that in one case the antigens are attached to, or are a part of, cells, whereas in the other they are free in solution. In agglutination the flocculation of the antigens by antibodies can occur only by clumping of the cells themselves. Emulsions of inert particles, such as collodion and carbon, can be agglutinated by antisera, after the particles have been treated with the homologous antigenic solution, followed by thorough washing to remove all antigen except that which is adsorbed by the particles. Because cells always contain more than one antigen, the agglutination reactions usually are quite complicated.

Agglutination is believed to be a physical reaction caused by changes occurring on the surfaces of the cells, probably produced by antibody molecules that bind to antigen molecules of the cells, How these combinations upset the normal stability of the suspensions is not known with certainty, but the cells, in the presence of specific antibodies, appear to act like hydrophobe instead of hydrophile colloids, and like the former become unstable and are precipitated in the presence of electrolytes.

Agglutination, as well as precipitation, does not occur in the absence of electrolytes. When both antigen and antiserum, in the case of precipitins, have been thoroughly dialyzed, the antigen-antibody reaction evidently occurs, but without evidence of flocculation. The addition of a small amount of salt to such mixtures will cause immediate flocculation. The presence of salts (electrolytes) has an effect upon the electric charge carried by the cells, or other particles in suspension. The electric charge, or potential, of the particles is the factor that keeps them apart (dispersing factor) and thus maintains the suspension. Anything that reduces the potential on the surface of the cells, or particles, reduces the dispersing factor and permits clumping or agglutination. The normal bacterial cell in suspension carries a negative potential. If this is reduced by adding acid in small increments, the stability of the suspension will be reduced gradually to zero, at which clumping occurs, and this is at the *isoelectric point* at which the potential of the cells has been wholly discharged. If additional acid is added, stability is restored because the cells resume a potential, but it now is a positive charge that is carried. Agglutination of bacteria, at their isoelectric point, is called *acid agglutination*. Serum agglutination is not dependent upon the isoelectric point, because the reaction occurs at a wide range of pH. Acid agglutination suggests, however, that serum agglutination may have to do with an alteration of the surface potential of the cells.

**Cellular Antigens.** It can easily be shown that most cells carry multiple antigens. Flagellated bacteria, for example, usually have one or more antigens located in the flagella (*flagellar antigens*), and these are different from those that are found in the body of the cell (*somatic antigens*). An antiserum prepared against flagellated organisms will agglutinate suspensions of the flagella, as well as of the cells from which the flagella have been removed, by virtue of the fact that it contains both flagellar and somatic agglutinins. An antiserum prepared against a suspension of the flagella will agglutinate the flagellated organism but not the cells from which the flagella are removed, and an antiserum against the deflagellated organism will agglutinate the flagellated organism but not the flagella alone.

Weil and Felix (19), while studying an organism of the *Proteus* group in 1916, observed two types of colonies, one a typical spreading type and the other a dissociant of the first which was nonspreading. The first was rapidly motile, the latter, nonmotile. Suspensions of these two types agglutinated differently because the first contained a flagellar antigen whereas the other possessed only the somatic. To the flagellar antigen, they attached the name H-antigen; to the somatic, O-antigen. These names are frequently used in the literature in this way.

The somatic antigens often are numerous. Some of these are thought to lie at or near the surface of the cell (surface and envelope antigens), while others are deeply embedded in the cytoplasm (deep antigens). Antisera prepared against the superficial antigens will readily agglutinate cells of the type from which they were extracted, but antisera for the deep antigens often will not agglutinate the cells, unless they have been treated by methods that remove the more superficial parts and expose the deeper to the action of the antibodies.

**Group Agglutinins.** Although antibodies are quite specific for the antigens that stimulated their formation, phenomena are sometimes observed which seem to indicate lack of specificity. Thus it frequently happens that agglutinins formed by stimulating with one organism will agglutinate other organisms as well as the homologous one. These are known as *group agglutinins.* The best-known examples of group agglutinins are those of organisms of the enteric group. If agglutinins are stimulated by injecting into rabbits certain species of this group, these antibodies will agglutinate other members of the enteric subgroups. That is, agglutinins prepared against a selected species of the genus *Escherichia* not only will agglutinate the homologous strain, but also will agglutinate members of the genus *Salmonella* as well as members of the genus *Proteus.* Usually, although not always, the heterologous organisms are not so susceptible to the antibodies as is the specific organism, and they are affected only when greater concentrations of serum are used.

Bacterial cells contain more than one antigenic substance, and group agglutinins may be explained by assuming that related organisms have some antigens in common. Suppose, for example, that three bacilli were in a related group and that *Bacillus* I contained antigens A, B, and C; *Bacillus* II, B, C, and D; and *Bacillus* III, D, E, and F. An antiserum for *Bacillus* I containing agglutinins a, b, and c would be expected to agglutinate *Bacillus* II but not *Bacillus* III. An antiserum prepared with *Bacillus* II on the other hand, would be expected to agglutinate all three organisms.

**Agglutinin Absorption.** It has been shown that there are two steps in the phenomenon of agglutination: (a) union of the agglutinogen with the agglutinin (antibody), and (b) flocculation of the organisms.

Some organisms cannot be flocculated with immune serum, and flocculation is impossible to determine in others because the organism does not normally form a uniform suspension in fluids. In either of these cases, it is impossible to demonstrate a satisfactory agglutination reaction. It can be shown, however, that binding of the agglutinin has occurred when such organisms are mixed with their specific antisera because, if the bacterial cells are removed by centrifugation, the fluid that remains will be freed of its agglutinin. This can be determined by testing the supernatant fluid with an organism that is known to agglutinate properly.

Agglutinin absorption has proved to be a more reliable test for distinguishing between closely related forms of bacteria than the straight agglutination reaction. In some instances, group agglutinins are present in such large amounts that by the ordinary agglutination reaction it is impossible to distinguish between the specific and the group agglutinins, for the specific organism may be agglutinated in no greater degree than the closely related one. In this case, absorption of the serum with the two organisms under consideration will generally tell which is the specific one. The specific organism should absorb all the agglutinins, while the closely related one is able to absorb only partially.

Suppose, to use as an example the organisms mentioned under "Group Agglutinins," *Bacillus* I, containing antigens A, B, and C, had been used for immunizing an animal and it had been found that *Bacillus* II was agglutinated by the antiserum to the same degree as the homologous strain. The serum would contain antibodies for each of the antigens in the bacillus injected. These will be indicated as a, b, and c to correspond to the antigens. If a large excess of *Bacillus* I is incubated for a time in a portion of this serum, and if these are then removed by centrifugation, the absorbed serum should then be free of antibodies, for each antigen would be expected to absorb its own antibody, and it would be removed with the organisms. No reaction should occur when this serum is again tested for agglutinins. On the other hand, if *Bacillus* II, containing antigens B, C, and D, is used for absorbing the serum, agglutinins b and c would be removed, but agglutinin a would remain. When this absorbed serum is tested for agglutinins, with the homologous organism, some agglutination should occur due to the presence of agglutinin a. This would indicate that *Bacillus* I is the homologous one, and *Bacillus* II, the heterologous.

**Normal Agglutinins.** The blood serum of normal animals frequently contains small quantities of agglutinins for a variety of bacteria. Young animals do not possess these antibodies so frequently as do older animals, a fact which suggests that they may have developed as a result of infections, perhaps so mild as to be undetected. In diagnostic work it is necessary to know the range of normal agglutinins for the organism and species concerned in order that reactions within this range may not be interpreted as of diagnostic significance. These so-called *normal* agglutinins may sometimes be a result of previous low-grade infections, possibly of group reactions in some cases, but in others they appear to be unrelated to agglutinins produced by antigenic stimuli (9).

**Zone Phenomena.** Some sera, particularly those that have been kept for some time and those that have been heated to 60 to 70 C, behave peculiarly in that agglutination fails in the lower dilutions (proagglutinoid zone) but occurs in the higher. This phenomenon has been extensively studied and various explanations have been postulated. It is generally believed now that some kind of protective colloid is the interfering factor and that agglutination occurs in the higher dilutions because this colloid has been diluted out. Occasionally a serum is encountered in which agglutination will occur in low and very high dilutions, but will fail in intermediate dilutions. No adequate explanation has been given for this parodoxical behavior.

**Practical Uses of the Agglutination Test.** The agglutination test is widely used for the diagnosis of disease. Theoretically it may be used for any disease caused by microscopic organisms; practically there are difficulties in the way of its use for some, as, for instance, when the organism grows characteristically in the rough form and, therefore, is spontaneously unstable in suspension. It has been used with a large measure of success in typhoid and the other enteric fevers of man, in undulant fever, and in tularemia. In animals it has its widest uses in brucellosis and pullorum disease. When the test is used for the diagnosis of disease, suitable identified cultures are suspended in a fluid. This suspension is commonly known as *antigen.* Definite amounts of the antigen are mixed with multiple dilutions of the serum of the patient, either in a test tube or in the form of drops on a glass surface. The reaction may develop immediately or it may require some hours for completion, depending upon the conditions under which the test is conducted.

**The Hemagglutinin and Hemagglutination-Inhibition Tests.** In 1941 Hirst (10) demonstrated that influenza virus was able to agglutinate the red blood cells of chick embryos and that the addition of influenza antiserum would inhibit this agglutination. Since that time hemagglutination-inhibition (HI) tests have been described for a number of viral and rickettsial diseases including mumps, vaccinia, scrub typhus, variola, fowl plague, encephalomyelitis, encephalomyocarditis, and pneumoencephalitis (Newcastle disease). A positive diagnosis in these tests depends on the ability of the homologous antiserum to prevent agglutination of erythrocytes in the presence of the specific virus.

The mechanism that makes the red blood cells of certain animal species susceptible to agglutination by some of the viruses is not understood at this time. It has been suggested that the combining elements of the erythrocytes belong to the mucoprotein class of compounds and that these substances are also present to some degree in normal serum (11).

That the hemagglutination-inhibition test must be used with great caution in the diagnosis of virus diseases is attested by the findings of various workers. The Commission on Acute Respiratory Diseases, Fort Bragg, North Carolina (3), noted the appearance of hemagglutinin in the amniotic fluid of normal chick embryos between the 11th and 13th days of incubation. The erythrocytes of 13 of 18 animal species were agglutinated. Mouse and rabbit cells were clumped to the highest titer and those of guinea pigs also were affected, but chicken cells were not. This hemagglutinin was associated with the globulin fraction of egg white and gained access to the amniotic fluid when the content of the albumen sac ruptured into the amniotic sac between the 11th to 13th days of embryonic development. Svec and Forster (18) found that filtrates and autolysates of Type 1 and Type 2 pneumococcus cultures inhibited the agglutination of chicken red cells by influenza virus. Human erythrocyte extracts and normal sera of man, guinea pigs, and rabbits were also shown to be capable of inhibiting agglutination of chicken red cells by influenza virus. The presence of a cholinesterase in each of these agents was shown, and it is possible that this enzyme was responsible for the inhibition.

Griffitts (7) and Lamanna (14) showed that certain toxins and bacterial suspensions caused hemagglutination and that these reactions were inhibited by specific antisera. Similar tests have been utilized in studying hydatid disease (6) and other worm infestations. The findings of all such tests have greatly extended the range of diagnostic applications of the HI test.

Modifications of the straight hemagglutination test are also used in the diagnosis of numerous diseases. By the exposure of erythrocytes to an extract from a strain of *Salmonella typhi* that possesses Vi antigen it is possible to sensitize the red cells for specific hemagglutination tests with sera containing Vi antibodies. Erythrocytes can also be treated with extracts of tubercle bacilli, *Escherichia coli,* or other bacteria and then be used as antigens in diagnosing infections caused by these organisms. Hemagglutination of the treated red cells is obtained with sera that contains antibodies specific for the adsorbed extracts. Hemagglutination is usually more sensitive than straight bacterial-cell agglutination. In tuberculosis hemagglutinins can be detected before agglutinins are found for the tubercle bacillus. The technic of the test can be modified by adding complement to the treated erythrocytes and specific antiserum. Then hemolysis rather than hemagglutination will appear.

Solomon and Hoff (17) have developed a test for the detection of pregnancy in the mare based on the immunologic properties of pregnant mare serum. Gonadotropin is present in the serum of the pregnant mare from approximately the 40th to the 150th day of gestation. In response to parenteral injections of purified pregnant mare serum gonadotropin (PMSG) rabbits produce antiPMSG antibodies. These will cause sheep erythrocytes, sensitized by serum from a mare pregnant for at least 44 days, to hemagglutinate.

Methods have been developed whereby formalin is used in binding proteins to erythrocytes. Such cells yield a stable, highly sensitive antigen and retain their original serologic activity after storage in the refrigerator for as long as 15 months (13). Other procedures recommended in preparing erythrocytes have been reported by Butler (2), Csizmas (5), and Hubert, Dalmanson, and Guze (12).

**The Precipitins**

When an antigen in solution is mixed in the proper amount with its antiserum, a flocculent precipitate is formed. This precipitate consists largely of the globulins that constitute the antibody, but the antigenic substance is also included in it. The antigen used in precipitin tests is known as *precipitino-*

*gen,* the antibody as *precipitin.* Precipitins undoubtedly are the same as agglutinins and probably the same as the amboceptor of the lytic antibodies.

Most proteins will serve as precipitinogens; so also will the other substances mentioned in the discussion on the nature of antigens. Gelatin, which lacks the aromatic amino acids, will not produce precipitins, and proteins that have been treated with alkali (racemized) lose their power to produce precipitins. Precipitins, like agglutinins, will not exhibit their characteristic properties in the absence of electrolytes, and in most other respects they exhibit the phenomena that have been discussed under "The Agglutinins."

**Practical Uses of the Precipitin Test.** The precipitin test is a very useful one for identifying antigenic substances of all kinds. It may be used for the diagnosis of disease, but, when it is feasible, the agglutination test will give the same information and is preferable because of its greater simplicity. The Kahn and other precipitin tests for human syphilis already have been discussed. In veterinary medicine, the Ascoli (1) test for anthrax is perhaps its most important use.

The *Ascoli test* has been used in Europe for detecting dried hides that have come from anthrax-infected animals. An antiserum for anthrax protein is kept on hand. Bits of the dried hides are snipped off, minced, and soaked in water or extracted in other ways. The extract is filtered to clarify it; then it is layered in small tubes on the precipitating serum. If the animal from which the hide came was infected with anthrax, there will be enough of the protein in the hide extract to form a cloudy ring at the line of junction of extract and antiserum.

The precipitin test often is used in medicolegal cases for identifying blood stains, determining deer meat or other game taken out of season, or for identifying proteins of any kind. Identification can be made of such antigens even though they may have been dried for many years. It has been claimed that muscle tissue taken from Egyptian mummies has given precipitin reactions for human protein.

For identifying the species of origin of any antigen, the laboratory must have on hand specific antisera for the protein of as many species as may be called into question. The stain, or the dried tissue, is merely soaked in water until it has been well extracted, the extract is clarified by filtration and then layered in narrow tubes with the series of antisera. A precipitate at the place where the layers come in contact will identify the homologous antigen.

**Gel-Diffusion Tests.** A very useful tool in demonstrating precipitation is the gel precipitin or the gel-diffusion test. Antigen and antiserum are allowed to diffuse toward each other through a layer of agar. When these substances meet in equivalent proportions, an obvious precipitate forms (15). The phenomenon involved is known as immunodiffusion. The double diffusion technic was developed by Ouchterlony. He placed antigen and antibody in wells in an agar gel and allowed them to diffuse toward one another to form a band of precipitate. A similar method utilizes strips of filter paper soaked in anti-

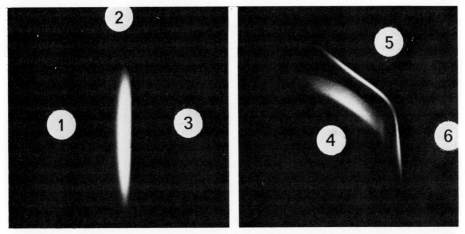

*Fig. 2.* Ouchterlony's double diffusion analysis of some strains of bovine *Mycoplasma*. (*Left*) Wells 2 and 3 contain the soluble antigens of different strains prepared by the ultrasonic disruption of whole cells. Well 1 contains rabbit antiserum for the strain in well 3. Notice that only the homologous system has formed a band of precipitate, indicating the absence of soluble antigens in well 2 that are identical with, or related to, those of well 3. (*Right*) Soluble antigens of different strains in wells 5 and 6. Well 4 contains antiserum for the strain in well 5. One common antigen is present as is indicated by the connected precipitin bands (reaction of identity). (Courtesy J. Michael Kehoe.)

gen solution and in antiserum. These are placed on the surface of an agar gel. Another procedure allows just one of the reactants to diffuse into a mixture composed of agar and the other reactant (20).

Immunodiffusion may be combined with electrophoresis. This is carried out by preparing a gel, commonly agar, in a thin strip on a glass microscope slide, applying the antigen in a well in the gel and separating the components of differing mobility, the gel serving as the supporting medium. The separated material is treated with antiserum placed in a trench extending the length of the separation. Bands of precipitate occur about the separated antigenic components (4).

Assay of antigen, or antibody, mixtures by precipitation in gels is based not only on the formation of successive bands of precipitate, but also on the rate at which they diffuse through the gel.

The immunoelectrophoresis test has the great advantage of identifying antigens which have different electrophoretic mobilities but similar diffusion properties. The test has proved to be sufficiently sensitive to detect over 35 proteins in human serum.

**Zoological Species Relationships as Determined by Precipitins.** An interesting use of the precipitation test was made by Nuttall (16), who tested the blood proteins of a large series of animals against an antiserum specific for human protein. He found that the blood serum of the chimpanzee gave practically as good reactions with it as human serum, and some of the other anthropoid apes gave good reactions but not so good as the chimpanzee. Other animals did not react. He regarded the results as another proof that man is not far removed from the apes on the phylogenetic tree.

## REFERENCES

1. Ascoli.   Centrbl. f. Bakt., I Abt. Orig., 1911, 58, 63.
2. Butler.   Jour. Immunol., 1963, 90, 663.
3. Commission on Acute Respiratory Diseases, Fort Bragg, N.C.   Proc. Soc. Exp. Biol. and Med., 1946, 62, 118.
4. Crowle.   Immunodiffusion. Academic Press, New York, 1961.
5. Csizmas.   Proc. Soc. Exp. Biol. and Med., 1960, 103, 157.
6. Garabedian, Matossian, and Djanian.   Jour. Immunol., 1957, 78, 269.
7. Griffitts.   Proc. Soc. Exp. Biol. and Med., 1948, 67, 358.
8. Gruber and Durham.   Münch. med. Wchnschr., 1896, 43, 285.
9. Hess and Roepke.   Proc. Soc. Exp. Biol. and Med., 1951, 77, 469.
10. Hirst.   Science, 1941, 94, 22.
11. Hirst.   Jour. Exp. Med., 1948, 87, 30.
12. Hubert, Dalmanson, and Guze.   Jour. Bact., 1963, 86, 569.
13. Ingraham.   Proc. Soc. Exp. Biol. and Med., 1958, 99, 452.
14. Lamanna.   Ibid., 1948, 69, 332.
15. Lazear, Killinger, Hays, and Engelbrecht.   Vet. Med., 1958, 53, 229.
16. Nuttall.   Blood immunity and blood relationship. Cambridge Univ. Press, Cambridge, Eng., 1904.
17. Solomon and Hoff.   Jour. Am. Vet. Med. Assoc., 1969, 155, 42.
18. Svec and Forster.   Proc. Soc. Exp. Biol. and Med., 1947, 66, 20.
19. Weil and Felix.   Wien. klin. Wchnschr., 1917, 30, 1509.
20. Wilson.   Jour. Immunol., 1958, 81, 317.

# VI | Phagocytosis

Of the phagocytes of the circulating blood, the granuloycte known as the neutrophilic leukocyte or as the polymorphonuclear leukocyte (PMN), is the most active against bacteria. It is a very mobile cell and may be found wandering through almost all tissues of the body. In acute inflammatory processes, it usually is conspicuous. The pyogenic bacteria have a powerful attraction for it, and pus always contains large numbers of these cells. For this reason, the neutrophilic leukocyte is often called the *pus cell*. It readily phagocytoses many bacteria and destroys them by intracellular digestion. This cell may be easily studied *in vitro*, and, as a result, more is known of its phagocytic activity than of any other type. Eosinophils are also able to ingest inert particles and bacteria, but do so less efficiently than neutrophils (1). According to Hirsch (5) the activity of the granulocytes is enhanced by the presence of *phagocytin,* a protein limited in distribution to these cells. This substance is able to destroy certain Gram-positive as well as Gram-negative bacteria. In many instances, the PMNs, with their bacterial loads, are engulfed and digested by the fixed cells of the reticuloendothelial system. Substances, other than phagocytin, that are derived from phagocytes and also from these fixed tissue cells and possess bactericidal effect are the arginine-rich fraction of calf thymus (histone B, 4) and the leukins (12).

The phenomenon of phagocytosis, the engulfing by ameboid activity of foreign particles of all sorts which happen to get into the tissues, was first described by Metchnikoff (8) in 1883. In a series of studies lasting throughout the greater part of his lifetime, this worker discovered most of the facts which we now have about this interesting group of cells. The magnitude of total leukocyte response to localized bacterial infection is conditioned by the neutrophil-lymphocyte (N:L) ratio in health. The N:L ratio for dogs was determined by Schalm (11) to be 3.5, for cats 1.8, for horses 1.1, and for cattle 0.5. Dogs develop total leukocyte counts of 50,000 to 100,000 or greater in severe local-

65

ized infection, while cattle develop initially a leukopenia and later may carry total counts of 30,000 or more. Cats and horses show leukocytosis intermediary in magnitude.

It was recognized quite early that the activity of phagocytic cells against foreign materials depended in large degree upon the fluid in which the cells were suspended. When suspended in animal serum, phagocytes were much more active than when in physiological saline solution. The substance in serum which was supposed to stimulate phagocytosis was given the name *stimulin*.

Denys and LeClef (1895) showed that phagocytosis of streptococci was carried out equally well by the phagocytic cells of normal and of immunized individuals. In other words, it was shown that immunization did not alter the phagocytes and make them more active, as had formerly been supposed, but altered the stimulating power of the body fluids in which they were suspended. Thus, in a particular immune serum, leukocytes that were derived from normal individuals behaved precisely the same as those which came from immune individuals. These experiments were carried out *in vitro*. Denys and LeClef also concluded that the effect of immune serum on phagocytosis was not in stimulating the phagocytes but rather in rendering the organisms more susceptible to phagocytosis.

Wright and Douglas (14; 1903) studied the mechanism of phagocytosis, and it was from their studies that the greater part of our knowledge of this process was obtained. Using a *Staphylococcus* that was only slightly affected by the normal lytic power of serum, these authors found that this organism appeared to have little attraction for normal leukocytes when both were suspended in serum-free fluid or in normal serum that had been heated to destroy the complement. In fresh complement-containing normal serum, phagocytosis of the organism was active; in fresh immune serum, the process was greatly accelerated. Assuming that the stimulating substance which was present in the normal serum was the same as that which had been increased by immunization, they concluded that it was an antibody and gave it the name *opsonin*.

Experiments were conducted to determine whether opsonins affected the organism or the phagocyte. When leukocytes were treated with immune serum, thoroughly washed, and then placed in contact with the specific organism, little or no phagocytosis occurred. When, however, the organism was treated with immune serum, thoroughly washed, and then placed in contact with phagocytes, active phagocytosis occurred. From this it was deduced that the immune body (opsonin) affects the bacterium and not the phagocyte. The manner by which immune opsonin affects cells, rendering them more susceptible to phagocytosis, is presumed to be by coating them with the antibody globulin, thereby lowering the surface tension.

The opsonin that is present in normal serum is heat-labile, quickly deteriorates with age, and is removed by substances which absorb complement. For these reasons it has been thought that normal opsonin was the same as com-

plement although it is possible that it is another substance which, like an amboceptor, requires the presence of a complement. The antibody that is produced by immunization is not heat-labile, although it also operates much
better in the presence of complement. Neufeld and Rimpau (9), who studied
this problem practically simultaneously with Wright and Douglas, gave the
name *bacteriotropin* to the heat-stable antibody. In common usage today the
term *opsonin* is usually used for both the normal and the immune agents.

If PMNs can ingest and destroy an invading microbe it loses its ability to
produce disease. Where the parasite is not suppressed or destroyed infection
proceeds and macrophages mobilize to provide a secondary phagocytic defense system. Whereas PMNs are short-lived and usually succumb in a few
hours after a phagocytic event, macrophages are long-lived and can carry on
a chronic long-term attack with pathogenic microbes. In this case a lesion may
develop characterized by the accumulation of epitheliod cells and is recognized as a *granuloma*.

The reticuloendothelial system (RES) includes the large circulating mononuclear cells of the blood (monocytes) and the fixed-tissue phagocytes
(macrophages or histiocytes) such as the Kupffer cells of the liver and
microglial cells of the brain.

Macrophages may arise from monocytes of the blood and progenitors in the
bone marrow. They may develop from mesenchymal tissue elements and undergo mitosis in local lesions. Macrophages mobilize at an accelerated rate
when the immune host encounters a given microbe for the second time. This
response is seen in granulomatous diseases like tuberculosis, actinomycosis,
and coccidioidomycosis. In these diseases, specific immunity does not reside
in the serum, but is macrophage-associated. Because immunity to these granulomatous diseases can be passively transferred with immune macrophages,
but not with any of the known serum immunoglobulins, it is referred to as *acquired cellular* immunity.

That phagocytosis may be influenced by factors not readily correlated with
acquired immunity has been claimed by numerous investigators. Glenn (3)
showed that moderate exposure of a portion of the skin of a rabbit to x-rays
caused an increase in opsonic activity against staphylococci, and Kina *et al.*
(6) demonstrated that leukocytes obtained from rats well fed for 4 weeks
prior to a 36-hour period of starvation engulfed three times the number of
bacteria that leukocytes from continuously well-fed rats did. By giving high
doses of either cortisone or ascorbic acid, Marcus *et al.* (7) reported that they
enhanced phagocytic activity in mice. On the other hand, Crepea *et al.* (2)
claimed that treatment with cortisone or ACTH decreased phagocytic activity
in 9 out of 10 human patients.

In 1955 Pollack and Victor (10) found a factor in dog leukocytes, but not in
guinea pig leukocytes, that had the ability to sensitize bacteria for phagocytosis. Sensitization resulted from direct contact of *Brucella suis* with the leukocytes. The sensitizer differed from opsonin in that it was liberated from blood

cells, was not fixed to sensitized bacteria, and required plasma, not opsonin, for its action. This finding might help to explain why dogs are more refractory to brucellosis than are guinea pigs.

## The Opsonic Index

As a means of estimating the resistance of the body to certain infections in which immunity depends mostly upon phagocytosis, Wright and Colebrook (13) devised a technic for determining the "opsonic index." Using special narrow, elongated pipettes, they mixed emulsions of the specific bacterium, suspensions of phagocytes from normal individuals, and serum of the individual under test, and incubated the entire pipette after sealing. As a control, the second pipette was filled with the same bacterial suspension, with the same leukocytic suspension, but with normal serum, preferably a pooled sample from several supposedly normal individuals. After incubation, both pipettes were removed from the incubator and broken open, and the contents were spread on slides in the form of films. After the films were stained, a careful examination was made of a large number (at least 100) of PMNs, the number of organisms engulfed by each cell being noted. In this way the average number of bacteria engulfed by the leukocytes was determined. The ratio which existed between the average number engulfed while under the influence of the serum of the patient to that engulfed by the same suspension when under the influence of normal serum was termed the *opsonic index.*

Wright used the opsonic index to determine the dosage of vaccines. The size of the injections was gauged so that the index remained above one. If the doses were too large or were repeated too frequently, the patient went into the "negative phase," i.e., the index became less than one, and this was considered harmful. At the present time the opsonic index is not considered to be of much value in clinical work. An exception to this statement may possibly have to be made in brucellosis or undulant fever of man, in which Huddleson claims that the opsonic index has diagnostic importance. This is discussed more fully on page 227.

## REFERENCES

1. Cline, Hanifin, and Lehrer. Blood, 1968, *32*, 922.
2. Crepea, Magnin, and Seastone. Proc. Soc. Exp. Biol. and Med., 1951, 77, 704.
3. Glenn. Jour. Immunol., 1946, *53*, 95.
4. Hirsch. Jour. Exp. Med., 1958, *108*, 925.
5. Hirsch. *Ibid.,* 1960, *111*, 323.
6. Kina, Blattberg, and Reiman. Proc. Soc. Exp. Biol. and Med., 1951, 77, 510.
7. Marcus, Esplin, and Hill. *Ibid.,* 1953, *84*, 565.
8. Metchnikoff. Immunity in the infectious diseases. Eng. trans. Cambridge Univ. Press, Cambridge, Eng., 1907.
9. Neufeld and Rimpau. Deut. med. Wchnschr., 1904, *30*, 1458.
10. Pollack and Victor. Proc. Soc. Exp. Biol. and Med., 1955, *89*, 561.

11. Schalm. Jour. Am. Vet. Med. Assoc., 1962, *140*, 557.
12. Sparnes and Watson. Bact. Rev., 1957, *21*, 273.
13. Wright and Colebrook. Technique of the teat and capillary glass tube. 2d ed. Constable and Co., London, 1921.
14. Wright and Douglas. Proc. Royal Soc. (Brit.), 1904, *73* (B), 1904.

# VII | Hypersensitization

The subject of hypersensitizations has been studied by a great many workers, but, in spite of this, much controversial material about it exists. In the immune reactions, so far discussed, previous contact with antigenic substances serves generally to lessen the sensitivity or susceptibility to them. Heightened resistance is the essence of immunity. In hypersensitiveness we appear to have the exact antithesis of immunity. In spite of this, it is quite certain that the mechanism involved is the same as that which functions in immunity.

The nomenclature in this field is confusing. The word *hypersensitization* is used in a broad sense to cover the entire subject without implications as to the mechanisms involved. Anaphylaxis, serum sickness, allergy, and hypersensitivity of infection, all are forms of hypersensitization. *Anaphylaxis* is a type of hypersensitization which can easily be produced experimentally in certain types of animals and which, therefore, is fairly well defined. *Allergy* includes types of hypersensitization which cannot readily be induced experimentally, and, for this reason, some have argued that allergy has nothing to do with anaphylaxis. Zinsser, admitting certain differences between them, nevertheless felt that their many similarities constituted sufficient evidence to regard all hypersensitivities as having a similar basic mechanism.

### Anaphylaxis

Reactions now known to have been anaphylactic in nature were described from time to time in the early literature. In 1839 Magendie described a typical anaphylactic shock in a dog that had received two injections of egg albumen. In 1894 Flexner (20) clearly described a similar situation.

Hericourt and Richet (24; 1898) observed that repeated injections of eel serum into dogs resulted in increased susceptibility instead of increased resistance as had been expected. These authors coined the word *anaphylaxis,* meaning decreased resistance, as opposed to *prophylaxis,* which means increased resistance.

70

Theobald Smith (1904) observed that guinea pigs that had previously been injected with diphtheria antitoxin could be killed by injecting them several weeks later with a dose of antitoxin that was harmless for normal animals. Ehrlich was told of these observations, and he had Otto, one of his students, study the matter thoroughly. Otto found that the reaction was caused by the horse serum and not by the diphtheria antibodies *per se*. Otto referred to the matter as the *Theobald Smith phenomenon*. Rosenau and Anderson (37) studied the reaction in guinea pigs that had been injected with horse serum and did much to clarify the nature of the reaction. Their first paper appeared in 1906.

These observations were repeatedly and consistently confirmed by later workers, and the active sensitization of animals by the injection of substances, usually protein in nature, became known as *anaphylaxis*. This type of hypersensitiveness may readily be produced experimentally in a number of species of animals and certainly is concerned with an antigen-antibody reaction. The condition can best be explained by describing the essential experimental facts about it.

When any foreign antigenic substance, which may be harmless in itself, is injected parenterally into an animal and a time interval is allowed to elapse thereafter (incubation period), an altered condition is established in the animal whereby a second injection of the same antigen may precipitate a train of symptoms which is known as *anaphylactic shock*. The symptoms vary according to the species of animal concerned, the size of the shocking dose, and the mode by which it is administered. The reaction is specific; that is, it occurs only when the substance to which the animal has been sensitized is reinjected. The symptoms of shock are the same irrespective of the nature of the antigen to which the animal is hypersensitive.

It should be pointed out that anaphylactic shock is a condition which usually requires the interfering agency of man. Animals may be perfectly protected by their immune mechanism against small doses of the specific antigen or against doses as large as could enter under natural conditions, but may be even more vulnerable than usual to large doses of the antigen introduced artificially and suddenly.

Exceptions might be the hypersensitivity that develops following a bee sting. Schenken *et al.* (38) have claimed that a protein antigen in the stinger mechanism of the bee sensitizes the person stung. Subsequent stings may produce severe or even fatal anaphylactic shock in the individual, depending on his state of hypersensitivity. Cross sensitization exists among protein antigens of the bee, wasp, and ant. In 1963 Antin (2) reported a case of fatal anaphylactic shock in a dog due to a bee sting and McCormick (30) reviewed the literature on severe and fatal reactions in man to *Hymenoptera* stings. He cited the death of a human patient following two stings by the common paper wasp, *Polistes fuscatus*. Thomlinson and Buxton (44) have indicated that edema disease of pigs results from anaphylactic shock which is caused by the rapid absorption of certain specific *Escherichia coli* polysaccharides from the organisms present in the animals' intestines. Certain cows apparently resorb their own milk and develop *milk allergy* (anaphylaxis) (11).

**Haptens in Anaphylaxis.** The production of anaphylaxis is not confined entirely to the more complex protein substances. Anaphylactic shock may be produced by injecting the polysaccharide of the pneumococcus. However, the animals cannot be sensitized by this substance alone. Thus, haptens assume the same role in anaphylaxis as they do in other immune reactions.

**Symptoms of Anaphylactic Shock.** Anaphylactic shock can be demonstrated readily in the guinea pig, rabbit, and dog but is not so easily induced in apes. In man, anaphylactic shock is most often an unnatural event. Current widespread practices of injecting drugs, vaccines, antisera, antibiotics, and so forth, are resulting in an increasing number of cases of severe anaphylaxis and death. Anaphylactic sensitivity to penicillin arises in patients exposed to this antibiotic, especially in those who have a history of Prausnitz-Küstner (P-K) reactivity with other allergens and it appears that P-K antibodies in man belong to the class IgE which in turn represent the one and only molecular class of antibodies anaphylactogenic for man. Cattle may be rendered anaphylactic readily by the injection of horse serum. In all animals, anaphylactic shock is manifested by a fall in blood pressure and by a subnormal temperature. The most striking signs are due to the effects upon the smooth muscles. These vary in different animals.

In the *guinea pig* there is evidence of extreme respiratory embarrassment due to the contraction of the abundant supply of smooth muscles in the bronchioles, and death is due to suffocation.

The *rabbit* does not show marked signs, as a rule, except those of collapse. Death is due to heart failure. The muscles of the pulmonary arteries cause constriction of these vessels, with blocking of the pulmonary circulation. The right side of the heart is dilated by the back pressure.

The *dog* shows epileptiform seizures, coma, and death after preliminary symptoms of restlessness, diarrhea, and vomiting. The liver and intestines are congested.

*Cattle* show uneasiness, labored breathing, edematous swellings around the eyes, udder, anus, and vulva, and diarrhea. Cattle seldom die as the result of the shock.

In *man* signs usually begin with itching of the scalp, flushing of the skin, headache, difficulty in breathing, edema of the glottis, rapid fall of blood pressure, and unconsciousness.

**Recognition of the Anaphylactic State.** The anaphylactic condition may be recognized in two ways, viz.:

1. By the production of shock. If the shocking dose is fairly large and is administered intravenously, death of a susceptible animal may result in a few minutes. Smaller doses, or doses given by routes in which absorption is slower, may result in less severe reactions.

2. By the Dale (18) method. Virgin female guinea pigs are used for this work. When ready for the test, the animal is destroyed and a piece of smooth muscle (a strip of the uterus) is removed and immersed in Ringer's solution held at body temperature. After the strip has been connected with a kymograph needle, some of the protein, toward which the animal is supposed to be hypersensitive, is added to the Ringer's solution. If the animal is anaphylactic toward the substance, the uterine muscle will exhibit its sensitiveness by contractions, which will be recorded on the kymograph drum.

**Passive Transmission of Anaphylaxis.** True anaphylactic sensitization may be transmitted to normal animals by transfusing them with small amounts of blood or serum from the hypersensitive individual. The new individual does not become hypersensitive immediately, a few hours being required for this to take place. Such individuals may be shocked and even killed by a small dose of the specific antigen. Anaphylactic hypersensitivity also is passively transferred from sensitized female guinea pigs to offspring.

**Desensitization: Antianaphylaxis.** After an anaphylactic shock, animals are desensitized and remain in this state for a considerable length of time. Likewise, it is possible to forestall the development of the anaphylactic state by injecting large doses of the antigen before the expiration of the "period of incubation," in which case desensitization occurs without the appearance of shock. Also, animals may be desensitized, without the production of acute shock, by the administration of the antigen over a period of considerable time in multiple small doses. In certain cases nonspecific desensitization, or at least partial desensitization, can be induced by the administration of anesthesia, adrenalin, salicylates, aminopyrine, gamma-globulins (23), or histaminic substances.

Although the anaphylactic condition, as we see it in some species of animals, may not occur in man, crises similar in clinical semblance certainly appear. It is possible that their mechanism may be somewhat different. Physicians usually inquire about evidences of hypersensitiveness in patients who are to receive doses of serum from other species of animals. If it appears likely that a shock may occur, it is customary to divide the dose, giving minute amounts at first, waiting, and noting possible unfavorable reactions before proceeding with the entire amount. Small quantities injected intradermally usually will indicate hypersensitiveness by causing the development of a wheal, which quickly appears and just as quickly fades away.

**Mechanism of the Anaphylactic Reaction.** The mechanism of the anaphylactic reaction is a matter that has been under investigation for many years and is still far from settled. Two general theories have been advanced: (a) the humoral theory and (b) the cellular theory. There is general agreement that this is an immune reaction and that antibodies are concerned in it. In light of recent knowledge it seems probable that more than one essential mechanism is involved in the shock reactions designated as anaphylaxis. It is doubtful whether all forms of systemic anaphylaxis can be equated with local "cutaneous anaphylaxis" with respect to causal antibodies. In the rabbit there is reason to believe that more than one class of antibody contributes to systemic shock.

*The humoral or anaphylatoxin theory and anaphylactoid shock.* At one time this theory was in favor, but it has now lost its adherents. It postulated that the initial or sensitizing dose stimulates the formation of an immune or protective mechanism. After this is fully working, a large dose of the specific antigen when injected into the animal is rapidly attacked by the immune bodies in the fluids of the body and split into a toxic split-protein product, *anaphylatoxin,* which, acting on susceptible cells, gives rise to the characteristic syndrome. This explanation found support in the work of Vaughn and Wheeler (48), who obtained toxic products from the splitting of various proteins by chemical means *in vitro.*

However, it soon became clear that sera could be rendered toxic by a variety of procedures in which antigen and antibody played no part. Animals not sensitized by an initial dose of serum gave a reaction similar to, but not identical with, anaphylactic shock on injection of normal serum made toxic by treatment with kaolin, barium sulfate, talc, starch, inulin, or agar. These poisonous sera were termed *serotoxins,* and the syndromes that they induced were called *anaphylactoid reactions.* Ordinary commercial peptone is capable of producing anaphylactoid reactions. The mechanism of these reactions has not been satisfactorily explained. It has been suggested that some serum component (such as antitrypsin) may be absorbed, thereby upsetting the normal balance of constituents and, as a result, releasing some toxic fractions. Those who may not accept the histamine hypothesis as the true cause of anaphylactic shock would include histamine shock under the heading of anaphylactoid reactions. The reaction to the injection of bacterial endotoxins appears to be another example of anaphylactoid activity (51).

*The cellular theory.* This theory now is regarded as a more plausible one. It would be expected, reasoning according to the humoral theory, that the greater the concentration of antibodies in the circulating fluids of the body, the greater the speed and violence of the reaction when the shocking dose of antigen is introduced. This, however, is not the case; in fact, when there is a large content of circulating antibody, anaphylaxis almost never exists. Furthermore, when serum from an anaphylactic animal is transferred to a normal animal, nearly half of it disappears from the circulating blood within an hour. If, after this time, the animal is completely exsanguinated, its blood being replaced by that of a normal animal, the first animal will be fully sensitized anaphylactically. These facts and others point to the probability that anaphylaxis is due to *sessile antibodies,* i.e., antibodies which, in some way, are attached to tissue cells and do not circulate. In the presence of large numbers of circulating antibodies, these cells are protected from artificially introduced antigens, but when few or no free antibodies exist, these antigens reach and injure the tissue cells. There is only speculation as to the type of antibody concerned. Many believe that there is some connection between precipitins and anaphylactic sensitivity. It does not appear that C' plays an important role in "true anaphylaxis" in any species, but the systemic Arthus reaction (p. 81) does require this ingredient.

**Histamine Shock.** The symptoms of anaphylactic shock can be reproduced very faithfully by injections of histamine. This substance, according to Thorpe (45), is a normal constituent of many different tissues and presumably bound to protein.

We may then, in general terms, describe the acute anaphylactic reaction as consisting of two different but related effects: (a) cell injury determined by an antigen-antibody reaction occurring in or on those cells by which antibody has been fixed and (b) a series of secondary effects due to the liberation of various substances among which histamine, or a histaminelike substance, appears to predominate. Although there is no reason to believe that histamine is fixed primarily in smooth muscle cells, there is a high correlation between histamine sensitivity and the cells concerned in anaphylactic shock. Furthermore, the tissues affected in anaphylactic shock are those that show the highest content of histamine. Another reason for considering histamine important in anaphylaxis is the fact that antihistaminic activity markedly alters the symptoms of shock. The manner of liberation of histamine as a consequence of the union of antigen with sessile antibody is unknown. Although histamine may not be the sole mediator of anaphylaxis and probably is not the principal one in the mouse there is no convincing evidence at present to indicate that other mediators play a significant role.

## Serum Sickness

This term is used for certain phenomena that appear in man following the administration of therapeutic sera. It is a hypersensitiveness to the antigens in the serum (usually horse serum). The disease, except in very unusual cases, is not serious, but it is very distressing to the patient. The signs usually appear in from 3 to 12 days after the dose of serum or drug is given, and they consist of urticaria, joint pains, edematous swellings, fever, and sometimes glandular swellings, especially of the part where the injection is made. The illness usually is of short duration. In very rare instances the picture is of an entirely different character. In these cases the patient collapses immediately after the injection and dies.

There is considerable difference of opinion as to whether serum sickness is a result of a prior sensitization. In a great many cases there is no history of any previous contact with the inciting agent. When there has been contact either in the form of prophylactic or therapeutic treatments, the incidence of serum sickness is considerably increased and the reactions usually appear earlier and may be more severe. They are termed *accelerated reactions*.

The designation *serum sickness* is sometimes used for certain hypersensitivities resulting from treating human patients with penicillin, para-aminosalicylic acid, sulfanomides, and other drugs (25, 26, 40). It is evident that some of these episodes are frank cases of anaphylaxis.

Shulman *et al.* (41) reported that the treatment of human patients with cortisone or ACTH resulted in prompt and usually complete relief from symptoms of serum sickness. In contrast, the administration of multiple courses of ACTH sometimes induced allergic reactions of the serum-sickness type. This hormone usually is obtained from the bovine, ovine, or porcine species, and it appears that sensitivity is caused by the presence of protein from these animals.

Serum sickness is specifically antagonized by antihistamines and like anaphylactic shock is presumably a consequence of the sudden liberation of histamine in toxic amounts. As in anaphylaxis, desensitization can be accomplished by injecting small doses of serum over a period of time. The condition is perhaps best regarded as a form of anaphylaxis in man.

### Allergy

Apparently closely related to anaphylaxis is a long series of hypersensitizations which occur among animals. By common usage, this type of hypersensitiveness is called *allergy*. The majority of substances toward which this type of hypersensitization is manifested are proteins or contain protein, but some of the drugs that are concerned in allergy are not in this category.

**Differences between Anaphylaxis and Allergy.** Distinguishing features between anaphylaxis and allergy are rather of degree than kind. Some of these characteristics may be listed as follows:

1. Anaphylaxis is artificially produced, whereas allergy is naturally acquired.

2. In anaphylaxis, inflammatory edema is a minor factor and smooth muscle contraction a prominent feature, whereas the opposite is true in allergy.

3. Nonprotein agents rarely produce anaphylaxis, but they often incite allergy.

4. Anaphylactic hypersensitivity is of limited duration, whereas that of allergy persists for long periods.

5. Desensitization is effective in anaphylaxis, but usually difficult and incomplete in allergy.

6. Inheritance of predisposition to certain forms of allergy is often a determining factor in the appearance of the disease. This is not true in anaphylaxis.

In spite of the differences suggested above, an allergic reaction, like anaphylactic shock, appears to be a consequence of the union of antigen with sessile antibody. The antigen is often designated *allergen* and the corresponding antibody *reagin*. Coca (16) originally called the inciting substances of these allergies *atopens*, and the substances that react with them, *atopic reagins*. He looked upon the atopens as haptens rather than antigens.

**Atopens (Allergens).** The substances provoking allergy are quite varied in nature. Such things as pollens (43), horse dander, cutaneous debris from other animals, foods (strawberries, milk, eggs, etc.), and drugs (iodoform, barbiturate derivatives, opiates, sulfonamides, antibiotics, arsenicals, quinine, etc.) are included. Frequently, the drug allergies are referred to as drug *idiosyncrasies*. In spite of the varied nature of the exciting materials concerned, the syndrome induced shows an essential uniformity, though there are minor differences which seem to depend in the main on the particular route by which the reacting substance gains access to the tissues. In the case of a drug the response bears no relation to its pharmacologic action.

Certain plant pollens and other substances in suspension in the air when inhaled will cause coryza (hay fever) or asthma in hypersensitive persons. Some foods will cause diarrhea and vomiting or, more commonly, skin diseases of an eczematous nature. In some persons, contact with substances that are innocuous to most people will cause severe dermatitis. The range of substances which elicit allergic reactions in people is very large, few, if any, commonly used food substances having failed to be incriminated. A more recent addition to the list of allergens is the one found in house-dust mites (genus, *Dermatophagoides*) (49).

Many of the substances that function as atopens, especially certain drugs, are nonprotein in nature and are not antigenic in the complete sense. However, it was shown by Klopstock and Selter (27) that animals can be sensitized by arsenical compounds alone, and it seems probable (Landsteiner and Levine, 29) that in such cases a preliminary union occurs between the simple arsenical compounds and some serum or tissue protein. This complex then functions as a complete antigen. In a similar manner any allergen could act as an incitant.

**Allergic Reactions.** In man, and possibly also in animals, the allergic state often is manifested by local signs, but a complete study of the clinical syndrome usually shows mild to severe general reactions in the circulatory system. These consist of varying degrees of angiitis accompanied by hypereosinophilia, edema, and other tissue alterations, especially in the collagen system. In severe cases proliferation of epithelioid and giant cells may produce the so-called *allergic granulomas* (14).

Very little is known about allergic reactions in domestic animals except those that occur as a result of bacterial infections. Eczematous conditions of the skin of dogs are very common, especially during the summer months, and it is suspected that some, if not many, of these cases are manifestations of food allergy. Pomeroy (33), in one such case, showed that the animal was hypersensitive to substances found in canned salmon. Burns (8) reported the case of a dog that was allergic to tomatoes. Rather typical symptoms of "hay fever" have been seen in dogs, the coryza and swelling of the mucous membranes occurring annually during the pollen season (31), and in 1963 a case of spontaneous canine hypersensitivity to ragweed was reported by Patterson,

Pruzansky, and Chang (32). Heaves in horses and so-called *farmer's lung* are considered to be allergic phenomena related to inhalation of some component of moldy hay (46). There is evidence that the dermatitis appearing in animals following flea bites is an allergic manifestation (1, 4). Schroeder (39) demonstrated that a form of dermatitis and a coryzalike condition in a walrus was due to hypersensitivity to bovine milk protein. An allergic dermatosis was reported in a cow by Bradford and Bradford (6). In fact allergic diseases occur frequently in cattle and may be caused by milk, various grains, hay, silage, wild plants, and certain insect bites (10). Colitis X in horses and some cases of scours in piglets are suspected forms of allergy.

Allergic dermatoses are not unusual in small animals and present a problem to the veterinarian because reliable diagnostic tests, desensitization methods, and permanent cures are still lacking (28).

There is no question about the fact that human allergy occurs naturally and apart from any previous contact with the particular antigen to which the sensitive subject reacts. In some families allergic individuals occur more commonly than in others, suggesting that hereditary factors are concerned. Zinsser believed that allergy was not of itself inheritable, but that a predisposition to develop such conditions was. In families in which such cases are frequent, one individual may be hypersensitive to butter, another to potatoes, another to rose pollen, another to lobster, another to poison ivy, and so on. It is not usual for hypersensitization to the same substance to appear in more than one individual in the same family.

There is also good evidence that this condition frequently arises naturally, sometimes rather late in the life of the individual, as a result of frequent contacts with the inciting agents, a condition which suggests an acquired sensitization.

**Atopic Reagins (Reagins).** Although these substances may be classed as antibodies, they appear to be specialized types. In the sera of ragweed-sensitive individuals it is possible to show their presence by hemagglutination (22). The test involves coupling of the allergen to rabbit erythrocytes via stable azo bonds. The antigen-coated cells are then suspended in serum from sensitized individuals. This test has been shown to be specific and highly sensitive.

That hypersensitive persons possess reagins is seen when extracts of the allergen are injected intradermally. Normal persons usually give essentially no reaction at the injection site; allergic individuals react with a reddened, inflamed area. This reaction is utilized clinically to determine what substances are concerned in the hypersensitive state. Some lessening in the degree of hypersensitization may be brought about by injections of extracts of the allergen in many instances, but complete desensitization as is seen in anaphylaxis ordinarily cannot be accomplished.

Passive sensitization of the skin of a nonsensitive individual can be established by the injection of a small amount of serum from a hypersensitive one.

If a small quantity of serum from an allergic individual is injected into the skin of a normal one and, 24 hours later, an extract of the allergen is injected into the same site, a typical inflammatory reaction will result. The reaction will not be seen if the same extract is injected into the skin of other parts. This reaction has been called the *Prausnitz-Küstner* (34), or *P-K phenomenon*, taking its name from the discoverers of the reaction. Wright and Hopkins (54) described a more sensitive reaction depending on "reversed" passive sensitization, in which the skin site is injected first with antigen and, 24 hours later, with the serum.

Certainly reagins have a marked affinity for cutaneous tissue. They differ from the precipitating antibodies which are believed to be responsible for anaphylactic and Arthus (p. 81) reactions in that the reagins are thermolabile and do not pass the placental barrier. Therefore cutaneous sensitivity of this type is not congenitally acquired.

An experiment by Walzer and Glazer (50) places reagins in a somewhat different light. They collected viable leukocytes from atopic human subjects who responded with immediate whealing reactions to skin tests with common allergens. Upon intracutaneous injection of these leukocytes into the skin of normal recipients specific and local sensitization was obtained. Erythrocytes collected from the same donors lacked this skin-sensitizing property. Whether serum alone could transfer this atopic sensitivity was not stated.

**Antihistaminic Therapy.** It appears that the union of allergen and reagin in the human body results in the liberation of histamine or histaminelike substances. Allergic shock is antagonized by antihistamines. According to Tuft (47), it is possible to counteract the effects of histamine in some allergic reactions by desensitizing with histamine. The enzyme histaminase was not helpful clinically. The antihistaminic drugs seem to be quite beneficial in the symptomatic treatment of a number of conditions in man including urticaria; angioneurotic edema and allied disorders; serum, drug, and physical allergies; certain types of allergic and migraine headaches; and seasonal hay fever and pollen asthma. They have proved disappointing in nonseasonal asthma, allergic rhinitis, and allergic dermatitis of the contact variety. At times their unpleasant side effects may require discontinuance. In action they are palliatives and not curatives. According to Quin and Cooper (35), great care must be exercised in treating large animals with histamine or histaminic substances. Side effects from these drugs may range from digestive upsets and urticaria to quickly fatal anaphylactoid shock.

Other drugs reported to be of value in the treatment of allergies are cortisone and the cortisonelike steroids such as prednisone and prednisolone (7). Tranquilizing drugs are credited with therapeutic value in allaying tension and anxiety states in patients suffering from various allergic conditions (19), but it has also been suggested that some of these compounds may play a role in presensitization (5).

## Bacterial Allergy, Hypersensitivity of Infection, The Delayed or Tuberculin Type of Reaction

Experimentally it is possible to create anaphylactic sensitization of animals with the proteins of microorganisms as well as with those of other origin. Shock may be produced by injecting large doses of extracted proteins, but even large doses of suspended organisms usually fail because the protein content is relatively low and it is presented to the tissues in the form of cells from which it is yielded slowly.

A type of hypersensitization commonly develops in the course of infectious diseases, especially in those of a chronic nature, as a result of the presence of the microorganisms in the tissues. This is regarded as an allergy rather than a state of anaphylaxis for several reasons:

1. The condition cannot be transferred passively with blood serum or other body fluids.

2. When specific proteins are injected to provoke reactions, the manifestations of the sensitivity are inflammatory rather than anaphylactic in nature.

3. This type of sensitivity cannot be produced by previous injections of proteins alone, and it is difficult to produce it with killed organisms.

4. In general, success in producing this condition is achieved only when living virulent organisms are used and active infections established. There are some exceptions to this rule.

5. Tuberculin shock is not antagonized by histamine or histaminelike substances (Weiser, Evans, and St. Vincent, 52).

The allergy of disease differs from other types already described. When the reaction-inciting agents (bacterial proteins or protein derivatives) are applied, the ensuing inflammatory reactions do not occur almost immediately but are delayed for hours or days. The causative mechanisms of the shock that ensues have not been elucidated.

The *tuberculin* reaction is the classic example of this type. Others are the *mallein* reaction in glanders, the *brucellin* reaction in undulant fever, and the *johnin* reaction in paratuberculosis. Hypersensitivity to fungi also occurs, and *coccidioidin* and *histoplasmin* are used in skin reaction tests to detect *Coccidioides immitis* and *Histoplasma capsulatum* infections, respectively. Hypersensitivity occurs in certain virus diseases, and skin tests with mouse brain antigen or yolk sac cultures are possible. Likewise, fluid taken from hydatid cysts has been used in diagnosing parasitic infestations by *Echinococcus granulosus*. The allergic states may be detected by injecting whole cultures, culture extracts, culture filtrates, or extracts from the infectious agents into the dermis of the skin, the subcutaneous tissue, the peritoneal cavity, or the blood stream, or even by placing some of the inciting agents in the conjunctival sac. Allergic individuals react to the skin tests by the development of inflammatory swellings at the points of injection, to the ophthalmic tests by inflammation of the conjunctival mucous membrane, and to the parenteral tests by the development of fever, chills, and symptoms of general illness, which usually disappear after a few hours. Because the allergic tests are specific, they have diagnostic value.

The concept that the delayed type of allergy exists only in the presence of active disease may have to be modified in the light of recent discoveries. For example, Raffel (36) has shown that the tuberculin type of hypersensitivity can be produced in guinea pigs by injecting a mixture of the protein and wax fractions of the tubercle bacillus. Humoral antibodies are produced by the protein alone, but allergy does not appear. The typical tuberculin hypersensitivity seems to be associated with a stimulus in which both protein and wax are necessary. It is noteworthy that a tuberculous guinea pig possesses delayed sensitivity to tuberculoprotein and anaphylactic sensitivity to polysaccharides of the tubercle bacillus.

A series of interesting findings beginning with that of Chase (13) indicate that it is possible to transfer tuberculin hypersensitivity passively. Such a transfer cannot be accomplished by blood serum or other fluids but succeeds when normal guinea pigs are injected with cells of peritoneal exudates, lymph nodes, and spleen of sensitized animals. This type of sensitivity lasts only a few days. It is suggested that lymphocytes may be the main carriers of the hypersensitivity with possible involvement of macrophages because antilymphocyte serum dampens the allergic response.

### Special Allergic Phenomena

There are two well-known phenomena that belong in the field of hypersensitization but are difficult to classify. These are the Arthus and the Shwartzman phenomena.

**Arthus Phenomenon.** Arthus (3) observed that repeated injections of horse serum into rabbits decreased the latter's tolerance for this substance. The first injections were innocuous, but later injections gave rise to a characteristic reaction, involving infiltrations, edema, sterile abscesses, gangrene, and death upon subsequent inoculation. It is not necessary that the later injections be made in the same place as the earlier ones. This reaction is less easily obtained in guinea pigs and some other animals. In man severe Arthus reactions may occur following injections of various serums, vaccines, antibiotics, etc. In some instances they may lead to extensive necrosis and sloughing of tissues involving large areas of skin and muscle. Some believe that "pigeon-breeder's disease" is a manifestation of a form of Arthus reaction in man.

The Arthus type of hypersensitivity is specific. In the rabbit the reaction results from antigen and antibody precipitates which fix C'. Both IgG and IgM antibodies produce the sensitivity.

According to Germuth and Ottinger (21), cortisone or ACTH therapy inhibited the production of the active Arthus reaction in the rabbit, but had no effect on the passive local Arthus reaction when antibody was supplied to the animal. They concluded that the hormones acted to suppress antibody formation in the rabbit.

Although histamine is believed to be closely concerned with the production of the characteristic anaphylactic reactions, Croxatto (17) reported that the injection of this substance into the rabbit would not produce the Arthus phenomenon.

**Shwartzman Phenomenon.** Shwartzman (42) described a curious phenomenon connected with a nonspecific increase in sensitivity. He injected a rabbit intracutaneously with a small amount of cell-free filtrate from a suitable bacterial culture. Twenty-four hours later he gave this rabbit a larger dose of the same material intravenously. Within an hour or two after the intravenous injection a hemorrhagic lesion appeared at the site of the original intracutaneous injection. Later necrosis of the area occurred and an ulcer formed.

The reaction cannot be elicited with filtrates of all organisms, nor is the local sensitizing effect the result of a simple inflammatory reaction. Apparently the sensitizing, or *preparatory*, substance is thermostable, antigenic, relatively large in particle size, and often closely associated if not identical with the "complete antigens" or endotoxins of certain bacilli. Substances of non-bacterial origin appear unable to act as preparatory substances. On the other hand, the range of materials able to provoke a reaction in a "prepared" animal is much wider than the range of preparatory materials and includes starch, agar, preparations of bacteria that are incapable of preparing tissues, and animal sera. Accordingly, the reaction is not wholly specific, because it may occur when the first injection has been made with a filtrate of one organism and the second with that of another organism or substance not antigenically related to the first. Cluff and Bennett (15) attempted to transfer this type of resistance passively with homologous serum but were unsuccessful. Apparently the phenomenon is not immunologic in nature.

A number of substances including nitrogen mustard and the anticoagulants heparin and dicumarol inhibit the local Shwartzman reaction. In contrast, cortisone does not appear to influence the dermal response.

### The Relationship of Allergy to Immunity

Although many aspects of the allergic state are not understood, it is quite clear that antibodies or substances similar to antibodies are involved. The allergic reactions are manifestations of the union of these bodies with specific antigenic substances.

A difference of opinion long has existed on the question of whether or not the allergic state in disease is a manifestation of increased resistance or immunity—whether in tuberculosis, for example, a state of allergy is desirable or undesirable from the viewpoint of the patient. It is clear that a severe allergic reaction is not desirable from the patient's viewpoint. An infected guinea pig may even be killed by a large dose of tuberculin. This is an artificial situation. Under natural conditions an infected animal would never have to deal suddenly with a large amount of freshly introduced tuberculoprotein. A mechanism that may be a valuable protective force to the patient in neutralizing or destroying soluble products released slowly by the bacilli in his tissues may operate disastrously when faced with large amounts of the same substances deposited in his tissues by artificial means.

Animals injected with tubercle bacilli develop allergic hypersensitivity very early in the course of the infection. In guinea pigs this often occurs within 6 or 7 days. At this time other kinds of antibodies, such as those concerned with the fixation of complement, are not demonstrable. Later in the course of the infection, complement-fixing antibodies are demonstrable in large concentration, and allergic sensitivity persists. Very late in the course of the disease, however, when the animal is overwhelmed with the infection, when large numbers of organisms are present in the tissues, when massive destruction of organs has occurred, and when death is near at hand, the complement-fixing antibodies are still present in high concentration but allergic sensitization diminishes and often cannot be demonstrated.

It is well known, also, that the tuberculin test in cattle is much more reliable in detecting animals that have early, localized lesions than in those which have generalized infections. In tuberculosis of cattle, therefore, as in the disease of guinea pigs, it appears that there is no fixed relationship between the condition of allergy and the presence of other types of antibodies, or, if there is a relationship, it is an inverse one. The condition of allergy and state of resistance to infection in bovine tuberculosis certainly show a better correlation than can be observed between the presence of humoral antibodies and the state of resistance. This does not prove that allergy and resistance or immunity are related, but there are strong indications that this is the case.

## REFERENCES

1. Andrews. Jour. Parasitol., 1962, *48*, 3.
2. Antin. Jour. Am. Vet. Med. Assoc., 1963, *142*, 775.
3. Arthus. Comp. rend. Soc. Biol. (Paris), 1903, 55, 817.
4. Benjamini, Feingold, and Kartman. Proc. Soc. Exp. Biol. and Med., 1961, *108*, 700.
5. Bernstein and Klotz. Jour. Am. Med. Assoc., 1957, *163*, 930.
6. Bradford and Bradford. North Am. Vet., 1951, 32, 396.
7. Brown and Seideman. Jour. Am. Med. Assoc., 1957, *163*, 713.
8. Burns. Jour. Am. Vet. Med. Assoc., 1933, 83, 627.
9. Burrows. Textbook of microbiology. 16th ed. W. B. Saunders Co., Philadelphia, 1954.
10. Campbell. Cornell Vet., 1970, *60*, 240.
11. Campbell. *Ibid.*, 1970, *60*, 684.
12. Carpenter. Immunology and serology. W. B. Saunders Co., Philadelphia, 1955.
13. Chase. Proc. Soc. Exp. Biol. and Med., 1945, 59, 134.
14. Churg and Strauss. Am. Jour. Path., 1951, 27, 277.

15. Cluff and Bennett.   Proc. Soc. Exp. Biol. and Med., 1951, 77, 461.
16. Coca.   Arch. Path., 1926, 1, 96.
17. Croxatto.   Johns Hopkins Hosp. Bul., 1952, 90, 439.
18. Dale.   Jour. Pharmacol. and Exp. Therap., 1912, 4, 517.
19. Eisenberg.   Jour. Am. Med. Assoc., 1957, 163, 934.
20. Flexner.   Med. News, 1894, 65, 116.
21. Germuth and Ottinger.   Proc. Soc. Exp. Biol. and Med., 1950, 74, 815.
22. Gordon, Rose, and Sehon.   Jour. Exp. Med., 1958, 108, 37.
23. Halpern and Frick.   Jour. Immunol., 1962, 88, 683.
24. Hericourt and Richet.   Comp. rend. Soc. Biol. (Paris), 1898, 50, 137.
25. Hesch.   Jour. Am. Med. Assoc., 1960, 172, 12.
26. Kern.   Ibid., 1962, 179, 19.
27. Klopstock and Selter.   Zeitschr. f. Immunitätsf., 1929, 63, 463.
28. Kral.   Vet. Med., 1958, 53, 660.
29. Landsteiner and Levine.   Jour. Exp. Med., 1930, 52, 347.
30. McCormick.   Am. Jour. Clin. Path., 1963, 39, 485.
31. Patterson.   Jour. Am. Vet. Med. Assoc., 1959, 135, 178.
32. Patterson, Pruzansky, and Chang.   Jour. Immunol., 1963, 90, 35.
33. Pomeroy.   Cornell Vet., 1934, 24, 335.
34. Prausnitz and Küstner.   Centrbl. f. Bakt., I Abt., Orig., 1921, 86, 160.
35. Quin and Cooper.   Proc. Am. Vet. Med. Assoc., 87th Ann. Mtg., 1950, p. 57.
36. Rafel.   Jour. Inf. Dis., 1948, 82, 267.
37. Rosenau and Anderson.   U.S. Pub. Health Service, Hyg. Lab. Bul. 29, 1906.
38. Schenken, Tamisiea, and Winter.   Am. Jour. Clin. Path., 1953, 23, 1216.
39. Schroeder.   Jour. Am. Vet. Med. Assoc., 1933, 83, 810.
40. Shelly.   Jour. Am. Med. Assoc., 1964, 189, 985.
41. Shulman, Schoenrich, and Harvey.   Johns Hopkins Hosp. Bul., 1953, 92, 196.
42. Shwartzman.   Proc. Soc. Exp. Biol. and Med., 1928–29, 26, 207; Jour. Exp. Med., 1930, 51, 571.
43. Spain.   Pub. Health Rpts. (U.S.), 1953, 68, 885.
44. Thomlinson and Buxton.   Immunology, 1963, 6, 126.
45. Thorpe.   Biochem. Jour., 1928, 22, 94.
46. Thurlbeck and Lowell.   Amer. Rev. Resp. Dis., 1964, 89, 82.
47. Tuft.   Am. Practitioner, 1947, 2, 1.
48. Vaughan and Wheeler.   Jour. Inf. Dis., 1907, 4, 476.
49. Voorhorst, Spieksma, Varekamp, Leupen, and Lyklema.   Jour. Allergy, 1967, 39, 325.
50. Walzer and Glazer.   Proc. Soc. Exp. Biol. and Med., 1950, 74, 872.
51. Weil and Spink.   Jour. Lab. and Clin. Med., 1957, 50, 501.
52. Weiser, Evans, and St. Vincent.   Proc. Soc. Exp. Biol. and Med., 1950, 73, 303.
53. Weiser, Myrvik, and Pearsall.   Fundamentals of immunology for students of medicine and related sciences. Philadelphia: Lea and Febiger, 1969.
54. Wright and Hopkins.   Jour. Path. and Bact., 1941, 53, 243.

# VIII | Auto- and Isoantibodies

Early in the study of immunological reactions, the question arose as to whether or not an animal might produce antibodies against antigens contained in its own body. It was suggested, for example, that when blood cells escaped into tissues in the course of hemorrhage, the tissues might produce hemolytic antibodies. If this should happen, it would be easy to see how a condition of chronic or pernicious anemia might develop as a result of blood destruction by the new antibody.

The first to investigate the matter were Ehrlich and Morgenroth (26), who injected blood cells of certain goats into other goats. In some cases the serum of the recipient developed hemolysins that were active against the blood cells of the donor. Such sera were actively hemolytic for the blood corpuscles of some other goats, but did not affect those of still others. In no instance, however, were the blood corpuscles of the recipient affected by its own hemolysins. In other words, these workers did not induce *autoantibodies* against erythrocyte antigens; but there is evidence that the animal body may, under some circumstances, respond to its own constituents, and that subsequent reactions may eventuate in disease.

The mechanism by which an animal recognizes and responds immunologically to foreign antigens and at the same time ignores its own "accessible" intrinsic antigens (*self-marked antigens*) is not clear.

Autoimmune diseases appear to belong in two categories. There are the afflictions caused by antibodies directed against occult antigens, which do not normally reach the circulation and hence are presumed not to be self-marked. Such antigens may be released from an organ or a tissue that is situated in relative isolation from lymphatic and vascular channels. The antigen may be freed to stimulate antibody formation by trauma, an infectious agent, or a drug. An example would be sympathetic ophthalmia.

The second category of natural autoimmune diseases apparently results

85

from production of antibodies which react with antigens that are accessible to antibody-forming tissue and hence are presumed to be normally self-marked. An antibody response to such antigens would perforce demand some unusual change in the response of antibody-forming tissues or in the antigens themselves. It is also possible that an adjuvant may cause a homologous or autologous substance, which under ordinary circumstances has no capacities as an antigen, to become an effective stimulus. An example of a natural disease that falls in this second category is autoimmune hemolytic disease.

Autoimmune diseases that have been produced experimentally are encephalomyelitis, glomerulonephritis, allergic thyroiditis, orchitis, and adrenalitis. Other natural diseases suspected of being of autoimmune origin include ulcerative colitis, lupus erythematosus, rheumatoid arthritis, Hashimoto's thyroiditis, Schilder's disease, Sjögren's disease, mumps orchitis, pernicious anemia, and pancytopenia. In the serums of aged persons it is possible to find antibodies for thyroglobulin, parietal cell, skeletal muscle, and heart muscle (58), thereby raising much concern over the role of these acquired substances in certain specific disease complexes. An autoimmune hemolytic anemia is believed to occur rarely in dogs (5).

Antibodies that are effective against antigens from other individuals of the same species are known as *isoantibodies*. From a practical viewpoint, the most important of the isoantibodies are the *isoagglutinins* and the *isohemolysins*. These antibodies are of interest, and of legal and clinical importance in man. It is known, also, that such antibodies exist normally in some species of animals and can be produced experimentally in others. The blood groups of man are dependent upon the distribution of isohemagglutinins among the population.

### The Human Blood Groups

The human blood groups were discovered by Landsteiner (37) in 1901. Originally it was found that a limited group of human beings could be placed into three groups according to the behavior of their blood cells in the presence of sera of other individuals. Later a fourth group was found.

The behavior of human erythrocytes when mixed with serum of other individuals can be explained by assuming that two antigens (factors), which have been designated A and B, are present in human blood corpuscles, some individuals having one, some the other, some both, and some neither. Also present in man are the corresponding agglutinating factors, which are designated a and b. Like the antigenic factors, these are distributed among people in all possible combinations, but never are the homologous antigens and antibodies found in the same blood. When sera containing one or the other, or both, agglutinins come in contact with the corpuscles containing the homologous factor or factors, the corpuscles are agglutinated and sometimes hemolyzed.

The blood groups of man are designated by the factor or antigen contained in the corpuscles. Thus the following groups are recognized:

Group O: Contains neither A nor B antigen. Agglutinins a and b are present in the serum.

Group A: Contains the A antigen in the corpuscles. Agglutinin b is present in the serum.

Group B: Contains the B antigen in the corpuscles. Agglutinin a is present in the serum.

Group AB: Contains A and B antigens in the corpuscles. No agglutinins are present in the serum.

Because agglutination will take place when two bloods are mixed if one contains the corpuscular antigen and the other the corresponding serum antibody, disastrous results may occur when blood transfusions are made with such incompatible bloods. The following table indicates how the several human blood groups interact:

Table VII.   HUMAN BLOOD GROUPS

| | Corpuscles | | | |
|---|---|---|---|---|
| Serum | Group O | Group A | Group B | Group AB |
| Group O Serum factors ab | − | + | + | + |
| Group A Serum factor b | − | − | + | + |
| Group B Serum factor a | − | + | − | + |
| Group AB No serum factors | − | − | − | − |

+ indicates that agglutination would be expected.
− indicates that agglutination would not be expected.

**Compatibility Tests.** Before a blood transfusion is done on man, a preliminary test should always be made in which the corpuscles of the donor are tested with the serum of the recipient. It is well also to test the serum of the donor against the corpuscles of the recipient, although this is not of as much importance as the preceding test for reasons that will be given later. It is obvious from what has already been said that unless the donor and recipient are members of the same blood group, there will be agglutination one way or the other. For this reason an effort always is made to find a donor of the same blood group as the recipient. If such a donor is not available, a transfusion generally can be made safely with a donor whose serum agglutinates the corpuscles of the recipient, for the reason that the amount of blood introduced is rather small compared with the blood volume of the recipient and the agglutinins are so diluted that ordinarily they do not cause trouble. It is highly undesirable and often dangerous to transfuse from a donor whose corpuscles are agglutinated by the serum of the recipient, because in this case the corpuscles are in the presence of undiluted agglutinins, which may cause the formation of intravascular clumps of such size as to cause serious circulatory trouble and even sudden death.

Individuals of Group O are frequently called *universal donors* for the reason that their corpuscles are not agglutinated by the sera of any of the groups. The fact that Group O individuals always have agglutinins in their sera may be ignored, in emergencies, for the reasons stated above. Accidents sometimes happen when universal donors are used for transfusions into individuals of other groups because agglutinins may be present in unusual concentration, in which case they may not be wholly inactivated by the dilution which occurs. It is best always to use homologous donors when they are available. When O blood is used, it is now common practice to add blood-group-specific substances A and B to reduce the anti-A and anti-B isoagglutinins of the serum. These purified group-specific substances are polysaccharide-amino-acid complexes derived from the mucosa of porcine and equine stomachs (65).

The possibilities of safe transfusions among groups are indicated in the following simple diagram:

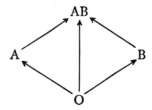

Interesting racial studies have been made on the basis of blood groups. The Hirschfelds (32), working in the Balkan countries where there is a very great mingling of racial types, showed that the several racial stocks differed considerably in the incidence of the A and B factors. The races can be divided roughly into three groups. The A : B ratio is highest among Nordic types, is intermediate among such races as the Japanese, Arabians, Russians, and Jews, and is lowest among African Negroes and some of the Asiatic races. The situation can be seen in the following table of the percentages of population of several typical groups which fall into each of the four blood groups.

Table VIII.   INCIDENCE OF A AND B FACTORS
IN CERTAIN RACIAL GROUPS

|  | Group O | Group A | Group B | Group AB |
|---|---|---|---|---|
| English | 45.4% | 43.4% | 7.2% | 3.0% |
| Turkish | 36.8% | 38.0% | 18.6% | 6.6% |
| African Negro | 43.2% | 22.6% | 29.2% | 5.0% |

**Inheritance of Blood Groups.** The factors A and B are not limited to the blood corpuscles but may be found in all cells of the body. They are somewhat variable very early in life, but after the human infant is a few months old his blood type becomes established and cannot be influenced by disease or medication. They are present in blood platelets, in the newly formed cells of tumors, and are transmitted through the germ plasm to the progeny.

Bernstein (3) has shown that blood factors A and B are inherited as triple allelomorphs, A and B being dominant to R, the allelomorph that determines O. From the mating of an A individual with a B, the offspring may be O, A, B, or AB. Two B individuals cannot produce offspring with the A factor; they are limited to B and O. When either parent is an AB, the offspring can be A, B, or AB, but never O. When either parent is an O, the offspring cannot be an AB.

Actually the ABO system is not quite as simple as it has been presented in introducing the principles of transfusion and inheritance. Among group A cells there are two antigenic types $A_1$ and $A_2$. Accordingly, the antigens in the red cells of the various groups are O, $A_1$, $A_1A_2$, $A_2$, B, $A_1B$, and $A_2B$. The gene $A_1$ is dominant over $A_2$. Furthermore, it appears that the antigens of the ABO system are derived from a single primitive gene called H, which determines the H antigen. It is regularly present in Group O and $A_2$ cells, variable in B cells, and weak or absent in $A_1$ cells. Consequently, some individuals of group $A_1$ or $A_1B$ possess high high titers against antigen H. Wiener and Ward (64) have modified the two agglutinogens and two corresponding isoagglutinins postulated for the classic interpretation of the ABO blood groups reactions by adding a third major isoagglutinin. Thus group O serum contains not merely a simple mixture of antiA and antiB isoagglutinins, but also carries, as a rule, a third isoagglutinin, antiC, specific for a blood factor (C) that is shared by agglutinogens A and B. AntiC appears to be the antibody most often responsible for ABO hemolytic disease of the newborn and it makes possible the recognition of certain rare individuals, who in ordinary test with antiA and antiB serums would be classified as group O, but whose erythrocytes nevertheless are agglutinated by most group O serums, apparently as a result of the antiC isoagglutinin present in group O serums.

Blood groups occasionally have medicolegal significance in questions of determining the legitimacy of children or in other questions of disputed parentage. Because of the great number of possibilities involved, it is not possible to identify positively the parents of a particular child through determination of their blood groups, or even to identify the second parent when one is known. It is possible in such cases, however, to exclude certain individuals. For example, if a child was found to belong to the A group and his mother to the O, the father could not have belonged to the O or B groups because he must have supplied the A factor. He could only be an A or an AB. Fresh blood is usually available for these determinations, and suspensions of the unknown erythrocytes are tested with known agglutinins. The latter may be isoagglutinins, hemagglutinins (usually sera from rabbits immunized with hemagglutinogens A and B), or special plant lectins (7) that contain agglutinins for factors A and B. In some instances the blood group of an individual must be determined from a blood stain. By the technic of Merkeley (43) isoagglutinins can be extracted from the stain and used with known erythrocytes in order to make the identification.

It is interesting that the natural antibodies of the ABO system are largely IgM antibodies while the "immune" ones are mostly IgG. Those of the molecular class IgA may occur in trace amounts as natural antibodies and to a greater degree as immune antibodies.

In 1954 Levine $et$ $al.$ (40) published a list of the known blood factors other than the major ones A and B. Their list includes $Rh_o$-$Hr_o$ (D-d), $rh'$-$hr'$ (C-c), $rh^w$ ($C^w$), $rh''$-$hr''$ (E-e), K-k, $Fy^a$-$Fy^b$, $Jk^a$-$Jk^b$, S-s, M-N, $Tj^a$, $Le^a$-$Le^b$, $Lu^a$, and P. The number of "minor blood group" systems has now reached more than forty. Some of these factors occur in only 1 percent of the population, whereas others appear in slightly less than 100 percent. Through their use subgroups have been identified among the four primary groups described above, thereby increasing the usefulness of blood type identification.

**The Rh Blood Factor.** It was shown in 1940 by Landsteiner and Wiener (38) that the serum of a rabbit immunized with the erythrocytes of the rhesus monkey contained hemagglutinins that would agglutinate the red cells of about 85 percent of the white population of New York City, regardless of blood groups. This hemagglutinogen was designated Rh or the rhesus factor.

Levine and Stetson (41) had suggested in 1939 that foreign protein from a fetus that had inherited its father's type of cells passed through the placenta and, acting as an isoantigen, immunized the mother. Then in 1940 Wiener and Peters (63) demonstrated that the new Rh factor when transferred into Rh-negative recipients could act as an isoantigen, and they indicated that certain transfusion reactions observed previously were caused by Rh incompatibility.

Levine, Burnham, Katzin, and Vogel (39; 1941) published on the role of isoimmunization in the pathogenesis of erythroblastosis fetalis. According to their findings, isoimmunization of an Rh-negative mother to the Rh antigen contained in her Rh-positive fetus, with subsequent passage of the immune anti-Rh agglutinin back across the placenta, caused certain cases of erythroblastosis. Because about 15 percent of the random population in the United States is Rh-negative, the combination of Rh-negative mother and Rh-positive fetus occurs in about 9.5 percent of all pregnancies in North America, and according to Mollison (45) only about once in 40 times does the potentially dangerous combination actually lead to morbidity.

It appears that the Rh-negative female becomes immunized to the Rh blood factor in several ways. A transfusion of Rh-positive blood can produce this condition as well as can a pregnancy in which the fetus is Rh-positive. Usually two or three pregnancies with Rh-positive fetuses are necessary in order to build up the Rh antibodies in the Rh-negative mother to the point where the effects of their action on the fetal red cells can be observed.

Whether the baby is born dead or alive depends on the amount of fetal red cell destruction before parturition.

Several different kinds of antibody may be found in the serum of a female isoimmunized against Rh antigens. The homologous Rh antibody is present, but it sometimes fails to bring about agglutination of Rh-positive red cells that are suspended in saline because so-called *blocking antibody* also is there and it prevents the clumping. If the serum dilutions are made in normal plasma instead of saline, or if the cells are tested while suspended in plasma, blocking antibodies do not interfere. The *blocking test* can be used to demonstrate the presence of these antibodies. A saline suspension of Rh-positive erythrocytes is mixed with suspect Rh antiserum. If no agglutination results, known Rh antiserum, diluted in saline, is added. No agglutination at this stage points to the presence of blocking antibodies in the suspect serum.

The Coombs (17) developing test produces similar results. Saline suspensions of Rh-positive erythrocytes are incubated with Rh antiserum and, if no agglutination results, they are washed with saline and mixed with antiglobulin serum. Rh antibody first combines specifically with its homologous agglutinogen, and, if unable to produce clumping in the presence of blocking antibody, it will then, as a globulin, react with the antiglobulin to cause hemagglutination.

Much of the Rh-typing sera in use today contains blocking antibodies, so saline must not be used as a diluent. Fresh whole blood or blood taken into a tube containing dry oxalate as anticoagulant is employed.

Although congenital hemolytic disease usually appears to be connected with the Rh factor, in very rare cases it can be caused by A-B isoimmunization (62), i.e., a mother belonging in group A may be sensitized by a fetus of group B. Wiener and Ward (64) have indicated that this may result because antiC isoantibodies are present. Isoimmunization induced by the arising of new blood factors through genetic mutations in tumor cells may also be a rare incitant, and the role of the Ch (chimpanzee) hemagglutinogen (13), which is present in most whites and Negroes, remains to be clarified.

Babies showing symptoms of erythroblastosis fetalis at birth have been treated successfully by simultaneous exsanguination and transfusion with suitable blood. Simpson *et al.* (55) recommend the use of ACTH in treating the newborn child, and Traina (60) has shown that ascorbic acid completely inhibits anti-Rh isoagglutination. Sussman *et al.* (57) have recommended that Rh-negative mothers should be given intramuscular injections consisting of small doses of high titer Rh immunoglobulin. This would prevent the female from developing a high titered Rh antiserum against Rh-positive fetal erythrocytes.

Further study of the Rh factor has shown it to be antigenically and genetically complex, and at least six genetic factors must be assumed to explain the inheritance of all the types observed. These factors are designated in the Fisher-Race system by the letters C-c, D-d, and E-e and in the Wiener system by the corresponding symbols rh'-hr', $Rh_o$-$Hr_o$, and rh"-hr". Each erythrocyte contains one or both antigens of each pair.

### Blood Groups in Domestic Animals

It has already been pointed out that the first work on isoantibodies was done by Ehrlich and Morgenroth on goats; hence it has been known from the beginning that group antigens existed in this species. Later workers have demonstrated the presence of group antigens in monkeys, chimpanzees, sheep, cattle, horses, swine, dogs, cats, mink, rabbits, ducks, chickens, turtles, and fish. It seems quite likely, in fact, that they occur in most, if not all, animal species. In apes the same group antigens and antibodies are found as in man. In other animals with few exceptions, the antibodies either are not normally present or they exist in very low concentration. This fact makes it possible to carry out single transfusions safely and indiscriminately within the species, without the formality of making compatibility tests.

Blood groups in animals usually become evident only when repeated transfusions are made. Between some individuals of the species numerous transfusions may be carried out without untoward results. In other cases severe and even fatal reactions may occur on second or subsequent transfusions from the same animal, apparently as the result of the formation of immune isohemolysins (50). This happens in dogs. Wright (67) and Melnick and Cowgill (42), who were studying plasma regeneration in dogs, found that a few animals reacted violently to second or later transfusions from a single dog when they had not reacted at all on the first transfusion. These animals showed muscular tremors, vomiting, bloody diarrhea, jaundice, hemoglobinuria, and signs of profound shock. Melnick and Cowgill report that the symptoms of shock are similar to those of anaphylaxis, even to the extent of being partially alleviated by intracardial injections of adrenalin. The symptoms, of course, are largely those associated with massive red cell destruction. Olson (48) studied compatibility tests on dogs that had not received blood transfusions and found that the plasma often agglutinated red cells, while serum from the same dogs did so only occasionally. Studies of blood groups in dogs by Young et al. (69) revealed six blood factors which were designated A, B, C, D, E, and F. A appears to be the most important factor. It is highly antigenic and is absent in about 37 percent of the dog population. When blood transfusions are given, differences between donor and recipient dogs with respect to antigenic factors other than A can usually be ignored, but to be entirely safe routine cross matching is recommended (66).

Ottenberg and Thalhimer (51) reported the development of immune isoagglutinins and isohemolysins in cats as a result of repeated transfusions. The cats showed no unfavorable reactions as a result of these antibodies except the development of hemoglobinuria. Kaempffer (34) divided swine into three groups according to the antigens and antibodies present. Only one antigen, designated A, and one antibody, homologous to this antigen and designated a, were identified. One group was characterized as Ao, another Oa, and the third Oo. Szymanowski and Frendzel (59) reported that anti-hog-cholera serum often contained a high concentration of a agglutinins, probably because of the hyperimmunization of Oa animals with blood from those of the Ao group. Later studies have indicated that blood groups in swine are much more complex and are formed by the distribution of A and 11 other red cell antigens (33).

Andersen (1) divided sheep blood into three groups which he called Ro, O anti-R, and Oo. The sheep agglutinogen R is related to, if not identical with, the agglutinogen A of human blood.

Ferguson (27) studied isoantibodies in cattle. He identified seven immune isolysins by repeated transfusions. In 1942 Ferguson, Stormont, and Irwin (28) described 23 additional antigens. Antibodies were produced by transfusions of whole blood among cattle and the antigens identified by agglutinin-absorption tests. Immune serum containing antibodies against some of these antigens also was obtained from rabbits. The behavior of the antigens suggests that each is controlled by a single gene and that immune isoantibodies can be used to prove breeding lineage in cattle. Each antigen appears to be dominant in character. In some of the cattle that were being injected a second or third time, anaphylaxislike symptoms appeared. These consisted of muscular trembling, dyspnea, salivation, lachrymation, depression, and hemoglobinuria. After 2 to 4 hours there often was a rise in temperature to 104 F or higher. All of Ferguson's animals recovered. A study by Kiddy and Hooven, Jr. (36) has shown that laboratory tests in cattle blood typing have become sufficiently standardized to render them highly accurate.

According to Schermer (54), erythrocytes of horses carry combinations of factors A, B, C, D, E, and F. These six antigens permit the formation of a large number of blood groups which frequently are hard to demonstrate owing to the presence of only small amounts of these substances. In 1949 Balakrishnan and Yeravdekar (2) claimed that horse blood could be classified into four blood groups analogous to those of human beings. This was confirmed in 1953 by Bruner and Doll (10), who concluded that the placing of horses in blood groups O, A, B, or AB had little practical significance because this system is based on two agglutinogens (A and B) and that the erythrocytes of horses contain additional red cell factors which must be considered when blood transfusions are needed. Further studies by Stormont et al. (56) have indicated that 16 reagents are needed to type horse blood and that subtyping relationships involve two trios of reagents, namely $A_1$-$A_2$-$A'$ and $P_1$-$P_2$-$P'$.

Isoantigens and immune antibodies have been studied by Saison (53) in mink; by Heard (31), Keeler and Castle (35), and Cohen and Tissot (15) in rabbits; by Wiener (51) and by Boyd and Alley (6) in fowls; and by Cushing (18) in fish, to mention only a few of the studies that have been made.

**Neonatal Isoerythrolysis (Hemolytic Icterus of the Newborn).** In 1947

Dimock, Edwards, and Bruner (20) suggested that certain cases of icterus in newborn foals indicated a condition similar to erythroblastosis fetalis in human infants. During the same year Bessis and Caroli (4) published a report on the involvement of blood factors in icterus of newborn mules. In 1948 Bruner, Hull, Edwards, and Doll (12) and Bruner, Hull, and Doll (11) demonstrated that cases of hemolytic disease in newborn foals occurred when mares isoimmunized to certain types of erythrocytes were bred to stallions which transmitted that type of blood cell to their offspring. The icteric condition developed in apparently normal foals after they obtained the specific erythrocyte-destroying antibodies from their dams' colostrum. These findings were confirmed by Coombs, Crowhurst, Day, Heard, Hinde, Hoogstraten, and Parry (16). The diagnosis of this disease in foals was discussed by Bruner (8).

Neonatal isoerythrolysis appears in normal foals within 12 to 96 hours after birth and usually terminates fatally within a short time after its appearance unless special treatment is administered. Anemia, icterus, and weakness are the usual symptoms, and postmortem examination reveals all the characteristics associated with abnormal destruction of erythrocytes.

The disease is caused by the specific erythrocytolysis that occurs because of the passive transfer of isoantibodies from the mare to the newborn foal. Present investigations indicate that it is not due to an Rh-like factor, but probably to an isoimmunization of pregnancy caused by intraspecies blood group factors. This was confirmed in part by Bruner and Doll (10), who showed that some sensitized mares belonged to group B of Balakrishnan and Yeravdekar and carried high isoantibody titers for antigen A. The identity of red cell factors that sensitized other mares was not determined. It is possible that the mare becomes isoimmunized through the breakdown and absorption of parts of the fetal placenta. Furthermore, the disease has not been encountered in first pregnancies, except in cases where vaccination with equine fetal tissues to prevent virus abortion has induced sensitization (24).

Neonatal isoerythrolysis can be prevented by breeding isoimmunized mares to stallions that carry erythrocytes compatible with the mares' cells. The appearance of the disease in a foal can be predicted if a rise in the isohemagglutinin titer of the mare is observed as parturition draws near or if the erythrocytes of the newborn foal, before it nurses, are exposed to the colostrum of the parturient mare. In these determinations the direct antiglobulin test of Coombs (22) is more reliable than straight cross-matching tests. Positive findings in either one or both of the tests indicate that the foal should not be allowed to nurse its dam. In the meantime the mare should be hand milked and the foal fed other milk. After 36 hours it can be allowed to nurse its dam without ill effects.

Treatment of a foal affected with hemolytic disease involves removal from its dam, withdrawal of about 1,500 ml of its isoantibody-laden blood, and replacement by approximately 2,000 ml of compatible blood. A method for exchange transfusion of the foal has been described by Roberts and Archer (52) and the mare's saline-washed erythrocytes have been used successfully in treating the foal (49).

In 1949 Young, Erwin, Christian, and Davis (68) reported on hemolytic disease in newborn dogs, and Bruner, Brown, Hull, and Kinkaid (9) demonstrated that hemolytic anemia could be induced in baby pigs by injecting gestating sows with the proper type of erythrocytes. In 1953 Buxton and Brookshank (14) recognized for the first time a naturally occurring case of neonatal isoerythrolysis in swine. One year later a report on the existence of this disease in Kentucky was made by Doll and Brown (23). Since then other cases have been reported (30, 44, 47), Goodwin (29) has published a paper on the clinical diagnosis of this disease in the newborn pig, and Edwards (25) has presented a plan for protecting piglets from developing it.

Morris (46), in 1959, experimentally induced hemolytic disease in young mice.

Neonatal isoerythrolysis has been described in cattle (19, 21), but it appears that all field cases have followed vaccination of cows to prevent the development of babesiosis or anaplasmosis. The vaccines employed contained bovine erythrocytes. Similar cases in sheep have not been reported.

## REFERENCES

1. Andersen. Zeitschr. f. Rassenphysiol., 1935, 7, 171.
2. Balakrishnan and Yeravdekar. Indian Vet. Jour., 1949, 26, 86.
3. Bernstein. Klin. Wchnschr., 1924, 3, 1495.
4. Bessis and Caroli. Comp. rend. Soc. Biol. (Paris), 1947, 141, 387.
5. Bone. Vet. Med., 1969, 64, 30.
6. Boyd and Alley. Jour. Heredity, 1940, 31, 135.
7. Boyd and Shapleigh. Jour. Immunol., 1954, 73, 226.
8. Bruner. Cornell Vet., 1950, 40, 11.
9. Bruner, Brown, Hull, and Kinkaid. Jour. Am. Vet. Med. Assoc., 1949, 115, 94.
10. Bruner and Doll. Cornell Vet., 1953, 43, 217.
11. Bruner, Hull, and Doll. Am. Jour. Vet. Res., 1948, 9, 237.
12. Bruner, Hull, Edwards, and Doll. Jour. Am. Vet. Med. Assoc., 1948, 112, 440.
13. Butts. Proc. Soc. Exp. Biol. and Med., 1953, 83, 701.
14. Buxton and Brookshank. Vet. Rec., 1953, 65, 287.
15. Cohen and Tissot. Jour. Immunol., 1965, 95, 148.
16. Coombs, Crowhurst, Day, Heard, Hinde, Hoogstraten, and Parry. Jour. Hyg. (London), 1948, 46, 403.
17. Coombs, Mourant, and Race. Brit. Jour. Exp. Path., 1945, 26, 255.
18. Cushing. Science, 1952, 115, 404.
19. Dennis, O'Hara, Young, and Dorris. Jour. Am. Vet. Med. Assoc., 1970, 156, 1861.
20. Dimock, Edwards, and Bruner. Cornell Vet., 1947, 37, 89.
21. Dimmock and Bell. Austral. Vet. Jour., 1970, 46, 44.

22. Doll.   Cornell Vet., 1953, *43*, 44.
23. Doll and Brown.   *Ibid.*, 1954, *44*, 86.
24. Doll, Richards, Wallace, and Bryans.   *Ibid.*, 1952, *42*, 495.
25. Edwards.   Vet. Rec., 1965, 77, 268.
26. Ehrlich and Morgenroth.   Berl. Klin. Wchnschr., 1900, *37*, 453.
27. Ferguson.   Jour. Immunol., 1941, *40*, 213; Jour. Am. Vet. Med. Assoc., 1940, 97, 544.
28. Ferguson, Stormont, and Irwin.   Jour. Immunol., 1942, *44*, 147.
29. Goodwin.   Vet. Rec., 1957, *69*, 505.
30. Goodwin, Heard, Hayward, and Roberts.   Jour. Hyg. (London), 1956, *54*, 153.
31. Heard.   *Ibid.*, 1955, *53*, 398.
32. Hirschfeld and Hirschfeld.   Lancet, 1919, *2*, 675.
33. Joysey, Goodwin, and Coombs.   Jour. Comp. Path. and Therap., 1959, *69*, 292.
34. Kaempffer.   Zeitschr. f. Immunitätsf., 1932, *61*, 261.
35. Keeler and Castle.   Jour. Heredity, 1934, *25*, 433.
36. Kiddy and Hooven, Jr.   Science, 1961, *134*, 615.
37. Landsteiner.   Wien. klin. Wchnschr., 1901, *14*, 1132.
38. Landsteiner and Wiener.   Proc. Soc. Exp. Biol. and Med., 1940, *43*, 223.
39. Levine, Burnham, Katzin, and Vogel.   Am. Jour. Obstet, Gynecol., 1941, *42*, 925.
40. Levine, Koch, McGee, and Hill.   Am. Jour. Clin. Path., 1954, *24*, 292.
41. Levine and Stetson.   Jour. Am. Med. Assoc., 1939, *113*, 126.
42. Melnick and Cowgill.   Proc. Soc. Exp. Biol. and Med., 1937, *36*, 697.
43. Merkeley.   Am. Jour. Clin. Path., 1953, *23*, 190.
44. Meyer, Rasmusen, and Simon.   Jour. Am. Vet. Med. Assoc., 1969, *154*, 531.
45. Mollison.   Post Grad. Med. Jour., 1944, *20*, 17.
46. Morris.   Jour. Path. and Bact., 1958, *75*, 201.
47. Newberne, Robinson, and Rising-Moore.   Jour. Am. Vet. Med. Assoc., 1956, *129*, 361.
48. Olson.   Am. Jour. Physiol., 1940, *129*, 433.
49. Osbaldiston, Coffman, and Stowe.   Canad. Jour. Comp. Med., 1969, *33*, 310.
50. Otte.   Brit. Vet. Jour., 1959, *115*, 71.
51. Ottenberg and Thalhimer.   Jour. Med. Res., 1915, *33*, 213.
52. Roberts and Archer.   Vet. Rec., 1966, *79*, 61.
53. Saison.   Jour. Immunol., 1962, *89*, 881.
54. Schermer.   12th Internat. Vet. Cong., 1934, *3*, 536.
55. Simpson, Akeroyd, Swift, and Geppert.   U.S. Armed Forces Med. Jour., 1951, *2*, 207.
56. Stormont, Suzuki, and Rhode.   Cornell Vet., 1964, *54*, 439.
57. Sussman, Uy, and Berk.   Am. Jour. Clin. Path., 1968, *50*, 287.
58. Svec and Veit.   Jour. Lab. and Clin. Med., 1969, *73*, 379.
59. Szymanowski and Frendzel.   Zeitschr. f. Immunitätsf., 1936, *88*, 397.
60. Traina.   Am. Jour. Clin. Path., 1951, *21*, 141.
61. Wiener.   Jour. Genetics, 1934, *29*, 1.
62. Wiener.   Lab. Digest, 1946, *10*, 1.
63. Wiener and Peters.   Ann. Internal Med., 1940, *13*, 2306.

64. Wiener and Ward.   Am. Jour. Clin. Path., 1966, *46*, 27.
65. Witebsky.   Ann. N.Y. Acad. Sci., 1946, *46,*, 887.
66. Wlodinger and Bruner.   Cornell Vet., 1963, *53*, 270.
67. Wright.   Proc. Soc. Exp. Biol. and Med., 1936, *34*, 440.
68. Young, Erwin, Christian, and Davis.   Science, 1949, *109*, 630.
69. Young, O'Brien, Swisher, Miller, and Yule.   Am. Jour. Vet. Res., 1952, *13*, 207.

PART **2**
## CHEMOTHERAPY

# IX | Chemotherapeutic Agents

At the beginning of the 20th century Ehrlich was busily engaged in seeking a "magic bullet," a compound strongly germicidal for *Trypanosoma equinum* yet sufficiently nontoxic to the host that it could be administered in effective concentrations. During this study he discovered *salvarsan 606*.

Throughout the early part of the century successful chemotherapy was confined to certain spirochetal and protozoan infections. The drugs generally used consisted of the arsenicals, the compounds of antimony and bismuth, dyes such as trypan red and the flavines, synthetic compounds such as plasmochin, and certain naturally occurring substances such as quinine. During this period no chemotherapeutic agents effective against bacteria were discovered.

In 1935 Domagk (11) demonstrated the value of a drug which he called *prontosil* for the treatment of *Streptococcus* infections. The active agent in prontosil is a para-aminobenzene sulfonamide, a name that has been shortened to *sulfanilamide*. In recent years many derivatives of para-aminobenzene sulfonamide have been prepared and used in chemotherapy, thereby establishing a group of "sulfa" drugs effective against certain bacteria and some protozoa.

Although the antibiotic substance pyocyanase had been known for years, the significance of the chemotherapeutic activity of the antimicrobial agents produced by certain microbes was overlooked until Fleming (18; 1929) discovered penicillin. It appears that Fleming realized the practical possibilities of his discovery but was not in a position to develop it more fully, and for some years its true value remained unrecognized. In 1939 Dubos (12) reported on the antibacterial substances secreted by *Bacillus brevis* and reawakened interest in Fleming's earlier findings on penicillin. This led to the work by Chain *et al.* (9) in which it was demonstrated that Gram-positive bacteria, including the streptococci, were susceptible to the action of penicillin. Many antimicrobial substances have been found in recent years and added to the ever-growing list. They are effective against many types of bacteria and closely related microorganisms but in general are less effective against protozoa and most viruses.

The dream of Ehrlich and his "magic bullet" continues to live, and the search for a new chemotherapeutic agent that will be a panacea for all illnesses continues. Many substances have been found, and some have proved to be quite effective in curing certain diseases. They include the synthesized drugs as well as the antibiotics derived from bacteria, molds, and actinomycetes. None has proved to be quite as effective as the earliest promoters predicted. In fact, the majority of the substances so far found are of little practical value. Many are too toxic for therapeutic use (13); others are too readily inactivated *in vivo*, are limited in potency or scope of activity, are not readily soluble, or have other undesirable properties. The usefulness of certain sulfonamides and some antimicrobial agents is limited because of the allergic reactions which they engender in individual animals. Furthermore, microorganisms originally sensitive to a sulfonamide or an antibiotic become resistant (drug-fast) on exposure to low and increasing concentrations of the drug and sometimes develop variants completely unaffected by it.

## CHEMOTHERAPEUTIC DRUGS

**Sulfonamides.** These compounds appear to be bacteriostatic rather than bactericidal and function *in vivo* by suppressing bacterial metabolism. It seems that para-aminobenzoic acid is required by certain bacteria in essential metabolic reactions, and it was suggested by Woods and by Fildes (Wooley, 60) that the sulfonamides react by combining with this acid, thereby suppressing bacterial multiplication and rendering the organisms readily susceptible to destruction by the body defenses, notably through phagocytosis. Furthermore, it has been shown that the bacteriostatic action of a wide variety of derivatives of sulfanilamide is nullified by the addition of para-aminobenzoic acid. This fact is utilized in isolating bacteria from fluids of individuals undergoing sulfonamide therapy. The addition of 5 mg of para-aminobenzoic acid per 100 ml of fluid neutralizes the effects of the drug. Although it is believed to aid the growth of some bacteria, it should be remembered that this acid is toxic for certain members of the rickettsiae, especially those of the spotted fever group (Hooten, Hooten, and Mitchell, 27).

It has also been postulated (59) that sulfonamides compete with para-aminobenzoic acid for the same enzyme and there is evidence that sulfonamide-inhibited organisms exhibit the metabolic signs of folic acid deficiency.

Names given to some of the sulfa drugs are sulfanilamide, sulfacetamide, sulfapyridine, sulfathiazole, sulfaguanidine, sulfadiazine, sulfamerazine, sulfadimidine (sulfamethazine), succinylsulfathiazole (sulfasuxidine), phthalylsulfathiazole, sulfasomidine, sulfafurozole, sulfamethoxazole, sulfamethizole, sulfamethoxypyridazine, sulfadimethoxine, sulfaphenazole, sulfamethoxydiazine, sulfasomizole, and sulfaquinoxaline. All are related but vary in toxicity, solubility, and efficacy. Sulfadiazine and sulfathiazole are valuable agents in treating infections caused by Gram-negative cocci. Sulfaguanidine and sulfasuxidine are not so soluble in the body as the others; they tend to remain in the intestine and to be excreted only in the feces. They are useful in treating intestinal diseases. As a group they inhibit the streptococci and related cocci. They are reported to be useful in treating some actinomycotic and fungus infections, as well as certain protozoan infections (24).

Although the sulfonamide drugs have a brilliant history as therapeutic agents, they are also dangerous. Certain animals are hypersensitive to these compounds and, following medication, may develop symptoms varying from mild allergic shock to acute prostration, which may even terminate in death. The most common adverse reactions are nausea, vomiting, headache, dizziness, drug fever, and sensitization from applications to the skin. The most serious are renal blockage from crystalluria, some systemic disorders which are probably of allergic origin and blood dyscrasias. Prolonged medication may result in kidney and liver damage, followed by icterus, anemia, and uremia (10, 20, 31, 37, 40, 42). Furthermore, an organism exposed to the action of one of these substances tends to become drug-fast.

**Sulfones.** Buttle *et al.* (7) described the therapeutic properties of 4,4'-diaminodiphenyl sulfone (DDS, DADPS, Dapsone) in 1937. This substance was obviously a very powerful chemotherapeutic agent, though unfortunately more toxic than the sulfonamides. Subsequently promin, promizole, promacetin, diasone, and sulphetrone were introduced. These are less toxic than diamino sulfone, and although in general they have not replaced the sulfonamides for the treatment of bacterial infections, since 1943 their use against leprosy has greatly increased and they have also been employed in the treatment of streptomycin-resistant cases of tuberculosis.

In recent years many of the chemotherapeutic drugs have been somewhat neglected as a consquence of the glamor of the antibiotics but in many instances they will do just as much as the antibiotics-and more cheaply. The sulfones, aminohydroxybenzoic acids, thiosemicarbazones, pyridine carboxylic acid compounds, and the sulfanomides continue to be useful in treating infectious diseases. Quinine and its derivatives such as atabrine (quinacrine), chloroquine, paludrine, pamaquine (plasmochin), pentaquine, and isopentaquine are used in malarial infections; sulfaguanidine, sufaquinoxaline, nitrofurazone (furacin), nitrophenide (megasul), and nicarbazin are recommended in coccidiosis; and drugs such as tartar emetic, tryparsamide, Bayer 205, pentamidine, and stilbamidine, *p*-arsenosophenylbutyric acid, antrycide methyl sulfate, and the phenanthridinium compounds are employed in leishmaniasis and trypanosomiasis. These compounds can produce toxic effects in domestic animals. Nitrofurazone has poisoned ducklings (22) and combinations of purine with pyrimidine analogs have been shown to suppress antibody formation (2).

**Combinations.** Various drugs and antibiotics are frequently used in treating bacterial infections. In general, antibiotics have replaced the drugs for this purpose although the use of Dapsone against leprosy has greatly increased since 1943. It has also been employed in the treatment of streptomycin-resistant cases of tuberculosis. By testing 21 individual metallic ions with 12 antibiotics (each ion with a single antibiotic) it was established that bacitracin and zinc formed a distinct compound with marked enhancement of antibacterial activity. The blending of lactose or dextrin to make a smooth and adhesive magma has resulted in an effective biologic antiseptic. Application of this thick paste prevents development of putrefactive and pathogenic bacteria by maintaining a vigorous growth of aciduric organisms.

## ANTIBIOTICS

Antibiotics have been defined by Waksman (54) as chemical substances produced by microorganisms that have the capacity to inhibit the growth of and even to destroy bacterial and other microorganisms. One of the distinguishing characteristics of the antibiotics is their selective action upon bacteria. Although some will act on fungi and upon rickettsiae, most antibiotics are less effective against viruses and protozoa. The antimicrobial action of these substances appears to depend on their ability (a) to suppress cell wall synthesis, (b) to interfere with protein synthesis, and (c) to disrupt lipoprotein membranes, thereby permitting the leakage of nucleic acid. Each antibiotic has its favored route of attack.

Antibiotics vary in their physical and chemical properties. The different penicillins are similar to one another but distinct from other antibiotic substances. Furthermore, certain microorganisms are capable of producing more than one antibiotic, i.e. *Penicillium notatum* produces not only different types of penicillin but also a different antibiotic designated *notatin*. Penicillin is also produced by more than one organism. It is formed by numerous strains of *Penicillium notatum, P. chrysogenum,* and *Aspergillus flavus* and by a variety of other fungi. The medium or the substrate may affect the anti-bacterial activity of an antibiotic. Some antibiotics are rapidly destroyed by varieties of bacteria, whereas others are not.

Antibiotics vary greatly in their toxicity for animals. Some, like actinomycin, are extremely toxic; others, like penicillin, have virtually no toxicity at all; most others fall between these two extremes. It is also true that sensitive bacteria develop resistance slowly against the antimicrobial action of penicillin but acquire resistance quickly against streptomycin (Waksman, 55). Because of these differences, antibiotics vary greatly in their chemotherapeutic potentialities. Although many antibiotics have now been described, very few of them have so far found practical application.

### Types of Antibiotics

Bacteria continue to receive attention as producers of antibiotic substances, but other fungi, actinomycetes, streptomycetes, algae, higher plants, protozoan forms, and other invertebrate animals are receiving much more consideration.

**Antibiotics of Bacteria.** Many antimicrobial substances have been isolated from bacteria. The *Bacillus subtilis* group is apparently capable of producing no end of antibiotics such as tyrothricin, subtilino, subtiline, subtilin, bacitracin, bacillin, subtilysin, eumycin, licheniformin, aerosporin, polymyxin, and nisin (55). Bacitracin and polymyxin have proved to be most useful. The low toxicity of most antibiotics of this group, their high antibacterial activity, and the effectiveness of some against Gram-negative bacteria and others against *Mycobacterium tuberculosis* enhance their importance.

Colicins are produced by certain enteric bacteria (Frederick and Levine, 19). Members of the genus *Shigella* are most sensitive to these products and *Aerobacter* and *Proteus* least. Their chemotherapeutic value is questionable. Numerous other bacteria produce antibiotic substances whose possibilities of usefulness are being investigated.

**Antibiotics of Eumycetes.** Much attention has been directed toward the fungi as producers of antibiotic agents.

*Phycomycetes.* A member of this group has yielded a product that is active against *Trypanosoma equiperdum* (Schantz, Magnuson, Waksman, and Eagle, 44).

*Basidiomycetes.* This group has produced the quadrifidins, polyporin, and clitocibin, substances believed to offer potentialities as chemotherapeutic agents, especially against *Myco. tuberculosis.*

*Ascomycetes.* This group has yielded the penicillins, griseofulvin, statolon (a nontoxic, prophylactic antiviral agent, 32), and a number of other antibiotics, many of which are quite toxic and offer little promise of becoming chemotherapeutic agents.

*Fungi Imperfecti.* Antibiotic substances have been isolated from some of the members of this group, especially the genus *Fusarium*, but their chemotherapeutic properties have not been established. Some of these substances are javanicin, enniatin, and lateritin. Others, credited with fungistatic and fungicidal activity, are lucensomycin (23) and mycobacillin (1).

**Antibiotics of Actinomycetes.** Actinomycin, nocardin, clavacin, and other antibiotics that inhibit Gram-positive bacteria and certain fungi are produced by these microorganisms. So far they have been of little value in chemotherapy.

**Antibiotics of Streptomycetes.** Members of the family *Streptomycetaceae* have yielded a number of useful antibiotics. The best known is streptomycin, produced by *Streptomyces griseus.* The streptomycin complex is made up of streptomycin (*n*-methyl-L-glucosaminido-streptosido-streptidine) and mannosido-streptomycin (D-mannosido-*n*-methyl-L-glucosaminido-streptosido-streptidine) (55).

Other antibiotics produced by this group are streptothricin, chloromycetin (chloramphenicol), aureomycin (chlortetracycline), neomycin, terramycin (oxytetracycline), viomycin, tetracycline, erythromycin (ilotycin), framycetin, novobiocin, vancomycin, kanamycin, paromomycin, lincomycin, magnamycin, candidin, fungicidin (nystatin), and gentamicin (obtained from *Micromonospora purpurea*). These are only a few of the antimicrobial agents secreted by members of this family.

It sometimes happens that scientists independently isolate, crystallize, and characterize the same antibiotic. This occurred with cycloserine and oxamycin—two substances which proved to bear the same formula (56). Welch and Wright (57) have established that cathomycin, streptonivicin, and cardelmycin, although isolated from different sources, are the same.

**Antibiotics from Other Natural Sources.** Mildews, the higher plants, and animals produce a variety of antibioticlike substances. Some of the plant products are allicin, raphanin, and tomatin, and among the animal products, lysozyme, erythrin, and lactenin. (55).

**Antibiotics from Synthetic Sources.** The chemical composition of a number of the important antibiotics has been determined, and in some cases it is possible to synthesize them. Shortly after the formula of penicillin was announced, the triethyl-ammonium salt of benzyl penicillin (G) was synthesized in the laboratory (Vigneaud *et al.*, 53). At present a synthetic oral penicillin is widely used. A synthetic chloromycetin was reported by Smadel, Jackson, Ley, and Lewthwaite (49) to be as effective in treating rickettsial and viral infections as that secreted by *Streptomyces*. Apparently some of the artificial antibiotics are as effective as those derived from natural sources, but most of the antimicrobial products presently used are produced by organisms. In many instances these organisms are fed precursors, substances that can readily be built into the desired agent.

### Production of Antibiotics.

The amounts of antibiotics secreted by various organisms are greatly modified by cultural conditions. Furthermore, the antimicrobial substances are found in the cultures mixed with other metabolic products and soluble ingredients of the substrate. In the production and purification of these agents suitable methods must be employed. For penicillin this involves cultivation of a mold (*Penicillium notatum*) under strictly aerobic conditions. This can be accomplished in special fluid medium in a vigorously aerated tank. The penicillin can be harvested after approximately 7 days of incubation (Johnson, 30). At this time the masses of mold growth are separated from the culture fluid by centrifugation and filtration. Pigment (chrysogenin) is removed from the clear liquid by adsorption on animal charcoal and filtration. The penicillin is extracted by ether and absorbed from the ether by $Al(OH)_3$ (For details see Stefaniak, 52.)

Chemical studies have showed that the penicillin obtained in this way is a mixture of related substances now designated as *penicillins X, G, F,* and *K,* and that the proportions of these substances present in lots of "natural" penicillin could be altered by changing the cultural conditions. Penicillin K is quite active *in vitro* but of less value *in vivo*. Penicillin X is best for treating streptococcal infections (Eagle, 14); G is used in treating syphilis. Natural impure penicillin greatly increases the activity of any of the pure F, G, X, or K penicillins when it is mixed with them. It is possible that some unknown substance in the untreated fluid is lost in the extracting processes.

**Assay and Standardization of Antibiotics.**

Penicillin was one of the first antibiotics for which a method of standardization was established. The original *Oxford unit* (Florey unit) is the least amount necessary to inhibit completely the growth of a certain strain of *Staphylococcus aureus* in 50 ml of a standardized meat extract broth. Later the cylinder-plate method was employed. A small, sterile, glass cylinder about 1 cm in diameter is sealed by touching it, while slightly heated, to the upper surface of the already inoculated solid agar. A measured quantity of penicillin is added to each cylinder. The Oxford unit is then expressed in terms of the width of the zone of inhibition of growth in the agar around the cylinder. One ml of the original unit, containing one unit as previously defined, produces a zone of inhibition exactly 24 mm in diameter. In 1944 a certain specimen of pure crystalline sodium penicillin G was adopted as a point of reference for international standardization. An international unit was then defined as 0.6 $\mu$g of the *international standard* sample, this quantity having been found to equal one Oxford unit. A calcium salt finally became the "working standard," and one unit of it contains 2.7 $\mu$g. Certain strains of *Staph. aureus* have been designated standard for assay work.

Methods of assay consist of the cylinder-plate method described above, the dilution method, and the agar streak method. In the dilution and the agar streak methods, standard bacterial types are exposed in broth or on the surface of agar plates to varying dilutions of penicillin, and the amounts needed to inhibit bacterial growth are determined. The general principles underlying the assay and standardization of the other antibiotics are closely analogous to those pertaining to penicillin, differing only in respect to cultural details and the technical procedures appropriate to the organism and substance involved.

**Hazards of Antibiotic Treatment.**

Although antibiotics have markedly reduced death rates attributable to infectious micoorganisms, the use of these substances is not without danger. Penicillin is a common cause of drug allergy, and severe and even fatal reactions to this antibiotic are occurring with increasing frequency (17). Penicillin should not be given for trivial conditions, and before it is administered the allergic state of the individual should be determined by skin test. Budd, Parker, and Norden (6) have reported the penicilloyl-polylysine (PPL) skin test to be highly accurate. According to Maslansky and Sanger (41), penicillin sensitivity can be decreased by injecting the antihistaminic agent chlorprophenpyridamine maleate (chlor-trimeton maleate).

Kligman (33) has stated that *Candida albicans* regularly emerges in abundance in the mouths and gastrointestinal tracts of those receiving certain wide-spectrum antibiotics. Others have reported similar results in the urogenital tract. Studies by Huppert and Cazin, Jr. (28), Seligman (45), and others have demonstrated that antibiotics such as aureomycin, neomycin, terramycin, and bacitracin as well as the hormone cortisone have the ability to stimulate the *in vitro* growth of *C. albicans*, while magnamycin, erythromycin, or a preparation of aureomycin which contains parabens (methyl- or propylparaben) does not. Furthermore, they indicated that the ability of the microorganism to establish itself and produce disease is enhanced by injecting it into animals in combination with the substances that show the stimulating activity.

The use of streptomycin is rarely followed by major complications, but its side effects include contact dermatitis, and the toxic effects on the eighth cranial nerve, though not life-endangering, are distressing. Dihydrostreptomycin appears to be less toxic. The tetracyclines can cause blood dyscrasia, severe liver and pancreatic dysfunction in pregnant women (58), and anaphylactic reactions, but the most serious major hazard is superimposed staphylococcic enterocolitis and wound infections. There is a definite association between chloramphenicol and aplastic anemia (25). Amphotericin B is an effective antifungal agent, but it may also cause anemia by suppressing erythrocyte production (5). When *Salmonella typhimurium* was used as a model, in order to compare the resistance of organisms isolated before 1948 and in the period of 1959–60 to tetracycline and chloramphenicol, it was found that no strains obtained prior to the former date were resistant. Among those isolated during the latter period over 13.9 percent were resistant to tetracycline, and for the first time cultures resistant to chloramphenicol were found (42). Another hazard of great concern has been the occurrence of antibiotic residues in milk after administration to cows.

Accordingly, antibiotics may be dangerous because they are toxic for the animal treated and because they may aid in the propagation of virulent strains of microorganisms that are resistant to their action. Their rational use in the future depends on practicing aseptic technic in treating patients, avoiding the use of drugs prophylactically for long periods of time, using drugs only periodically in a community, using combinations of drugs, and using the minimal effective dose of a drug for the minimal time (50).

### Antibiotics as Chemotherapeutic Agents

Antibiotics in general are much more active against Gram-positive organisms that against Gram-negative. In recent years the terms "broad spectrum" and "narrow spectrum" have come into use to indicate the range of effectiveness of antibiotics. It is frequently thought that broad-spectrum agents are useful against both Gram-positive and Gram-negative bacteria whereas those in the narrow-spectrum group are of value only against Gram-positive ones. This is only partially correct. Some antibiotics classed as narrow-spectrum types are effective against certain Gram-negative species, and none of the broad-spectrum types are useful against all Gram-negative types.

The mycotic, protozoan (40), and viral diseases have not, as a rule, responded as favorably as the bacterial diseases to antibiotic treatment. With the discovery of many additional antibiotics it now appears that effective therapeutic agents against at least some of these infections are at hand. One of these, statolon, has been reported to be an efficacious antiviral agent *in vivo* (32). Griseofulvin is important in the treatment of ringworm. This antibiotic is a metabolic product of a number of species of *Penicillium* and is sometimes called the *curling factor* because its fungistatic action is associated with malformation of the tips of growing hyphae (35). The use of this antibiotic as well as other effective ones will be discussed under the specific diseases.

The agents that cause psittacosis and lymphogranuloma are considered by some workers to be viruses, but they are sensitive to the action of both narrow- and broad-spectrum antibiotics. In this respect as in others (see p. 774) they differ from other viruses, and we have considered them with the rickettsiae.

## COMBINED CHEMOTHERAPEUTIC AGENTS

Combinations of antibiotic substances sometimes are used in treating infections. To obtain the best effect the combination must promote synergistic action. This cannot always be predicted accurately because the combined effect of two antibiotics may vary from synergism to antagonism depending upon the bacterium tested. In general, combinations which are predominantly synergistic are penicillin with streptomycin and aureomycin or terramycin with chloromycetin. In contrast, the mixing of chloromycetin with penicillin or streptomycin, aureomycin with penicillin or streptomycin, and terramycin with streptomycin usually produces antagonistic action (4, 29).

Streptococcic infection of the genital tract of the mare frequently is accompanied by *Escherichia coli* infection, and the use of penicillin alone will destroy the streptococci but not the *E. coli*. Combined penicillin-streptomycin treatment has sometimes been successful in eliminating both organisms.

Mixtures of antibiotics and sulfonamides frequently are used in treating bacterial infections. The synergistic action of streptomycin and sulfadiazine prevents rapid development of resistance of the bacteria to streptomycin. This treatment is used in brucellosis (Harris and Jett, 24). Combinations of penicillin and sulfonamides have greater antibacterial effectiveness than either used alone (46).

## USE OF CHEMOTHERAPEUTIC AGENTS

There are general rules which apply in the selection of chemotherapeutic agents for treating disease. These are useful when the diagnosis is obscure or the causative agent has not been determined. When the offending organism has been isolated, it should be subjected to a sensitivity test in order to determine which substance is most active against it. The isolate may be exposed to the action of picked chemotherapeutic substances by applying the blotting-paper-disc (26), the rapid dye-reduction test (3), or the tablet (39) method and then choosing the most effective agent.

Chemotherapeutic agents are not used solely for the treatment of infectious diseases. The addition of streptomycin, penicillin, and sulfanilamide to bull semen appears to increase its fertility, probably by reducing the bacterial content (15). Hormones, antibiotics, and antibiotic residues are incorporated in domestic stock diets and under certain conditions accelerate the growth rate of young animals (8, 16, 34, 48, 51, 61). Although the feeding of antibiotics is usually assumed to produce a beneficial effect, Slanetz (47) has stated that the prolonged use of these substances and their residues appears to interfere with antibody production. There also is evidence of an increase in drug-resistant microorganisms and in the occurrence of allergies ranging from urticaria to anaphylaxis when such feeding is practiced.

This chapter is designed to present briefly some general information about certain drugs and antibiotics used in veterinary medicine. Later in the book, sections on chemotherapy list the effective agents, insofar as they are known, for all the pathogenic organisms discussed.

## REFERENCES

1. Banerjee and Bose.   Jour. Bact., 1963, 86, 387.
2. Bieber, Elion, Hitchings, Hooper, and Nathan.   Proc. Soc. Exp. Biol. and Med., 1962, 111, 334.
3. Bieringer and Miale.   Am. Jour. Clin. Path., 1961, 36, 195.
4. Bliss, Warth, and Long.   Johns Hopkins Hosp. Bul., 1952, 90, 149.
5. Brandriss, Moores, and Stohlman, Jr.   Jour. Am. Med. Assoc., 1964, 189, 663.
6. Budd, Parker, and Norden.   Ibid., 1964, 190, 203.
7. Buttle, Stephenson, Smith, Dewing, and Foster.   Lancet, 1937, 1, 1331.
8. Cairy.   Vet. Med., 1955, 1, 339.
9. Chain et al.   Lancet, 1940, 2, 226.
10. Delaplane and Milliff.   Am. Jour. Vet. Res., 1948, 9, 92.
11. Domagk.   Deut. med. Wchnschr., 1935, 61, 250.
12. Dubos.   Proc. Soc. Exp. Biol. and Med., 1939, 40, 311.
13. Dubos.   Jour. Am. Med. Assoc., 1944, 124, 633.
14. Eagle.   Jour. Exp. Med., 1947, 85, 175.
15. Easterbrooks, Heller, Plastridge, and Jungherr.   North Am. Vet., 1951, 32, 394.
16. Editorial.   Vet. Rec., 1953, 65, 199.
17. Feinberg, Feinberg, and Moran.   Jour. Am. Med. Assoc., 1953, 152, 114.
18. Fleming.   Brit. Jour. Exp. Path., 1929, 10, 226.
19. Frederick and Levine.   Jour. Bact., 1947, 54, 785.
20. French.   Am. Jour. Path., 1946, 22, 679.
21. Garrod and O'Grady.   Antibiotics and Chemotherapy. 2d ed. The Williams and Wilkins Co., Baltimore, 1968.

22. Gibson. Vet. Rec., 1963, *75*, 90.
23. Graessle, Phares, and Robinson. Antibiotics and Chemother., 1962, *12*, 608.
24. Harris and Jett. Jour. Am. Med. Assoc., 1948, *137*, 363.
25. Herrell. *Ibid.*, 1958, *168*, 1875.
26. Hilson and Elek. Jour. Lab. and Clin. Med., 1954, *44*, 589.
27. Hooten, Hooten, and Mitchell. Va. Med. Monthly, 1949, *76*, 121.
28. Hubbert and Cazin, Jr. Jour. Bact., 1955, *70*, 435.
29. Jawetz, Gunnison, and Speck. Am. Jour. Med. Sci., 1951, *222*, 404.
30. Johnson. Ann. N.Y. Acad. Sci., 1946, *48*, 57.
31. Jones, Smith, and Roepke. Am. Jour. Vet. Res., 1949, *10*, 318.
32. Kleinschmidt and Probst. Antibiotics and Chemother., 1962, *12*, 298.
33. Kligman. Jour. Am. Med. Assoc., 1952, *149*, 979.
34. Klussendorf. North Am. Vet., 1953, *34*, 477.
35. Lauder and O'Sullivan. Vet. Rec., 1958, *70*, 949.
36. Lawrence and Francis. The sulfonamides and antibiotics in man and animals. H. K. Lewis and Co., London, 1953.
37. Lichtenstein and Fox. Am. Jour. Path., 1946, *22*, 665.
38. Long. The ABC's of sulfonamides and antibiotic therapy. W. B. Saunders Co., Philadelphia, 1948.
39. Lund, Funder-Schmidt, Christensen, and Dupont. Acta Path. et Microbiol. Scand., 1951, *29*, 221.
40. McVay, Laird, and Sprunt. Science, 1949, *109*, 590.
41. Maslansky and Sanger. Antibiotics and Chemother., 1952, *2*, 385.
42. More, McMillan, and Duff. Am. Jour. Path., 1946, *22*, 703.
43. Ramsey and Edwards. Appl. Microbiol., 1961, 9, 389.
44. Schatz, Magnuson, Waksman, and Eagle. Proc. Soc. Exp. Biol. and Med., 1946, *62*, 143.
45. Seligmann. *Ibid.*, 1953, *83*, 778.
46. Shlaes, Volini, Felsenfeld, and Burbridge. Antibiotics and Chemother., 1952, *2*, 25.
47. Slanetz. *Ibid.*, 1953, 3, 629.
48. Slanetz. Am. Jour. Pub. Health, 1954, *44*, 328.
49. Smadel, Jackson, Ley, and Lewthwaite. Proc. Soc. Exp. Biol. and Med., 1949, *70*, 191.
50. Smith. Vet. Rec., 1957, *69*, 749.
51. Smith. *Ibid.*, 1968, *83*, 143.
52. Stefaniak. Ind. Eng. Chem., 1946, *38*, 666.
53. Vigneaud, Carpenter, Holley, Livermore, and Rachele. Science, 1946, *104*, 431.
54. Waksman. Mycologia, 1947, *39*, 565.
55. Waksman. Biol. Rev., 1948, *23*, 452.
56. Welch. Antibiotics and Chemother., 1955, 5, 182.
57. Welch and Wright. *Ibid.*, 1955, 5, 670.
58. Whalley, Adams, and Combes. Jour. Am. Med. Assoc., 1964, 5, 357.
59. Woods. Brit. Jour. Exp. Path., 1940, *21*, 74.
60. Wooley. Physiol. Rev., 1947, *27*, 308.
61. Yeary. Medicated feed additives. A handbook on the safe use of feed additives and drugs for livestock and poultry. Ohio State Univ. Bul. 474, 1970.

# PART 3

# THE PATHOGENIC
# BACTERIA

# X | The *Pseudomonadaceae*

The important pathogenic members of this family belong in the genera *Pseudomonas* and *Aeromonas*. They are motile by means of polar flagella and are rod-shaped.

## THE GENUS *PSEUDOMONAS*

Certain members of this genus produce water-soluble pigments which diffuse through the medium. *Pseudomonas aeruginosa*, the so-called *bacillus of green pus*, is of especial importance in producing disease in man and animals. Other microorganisms within the genus that have been assigned pathogenic roles are *Pseudomonas pseudomallei* and *Pseudomonas maltophilia*.

### *Pseudomonas aeruginosa*

SYNONYMS:  *Pseudomonas pyocyaneus*, Bacillus of green pus

This is an organism of comparatively low virulence found frequently in suppurative processes in cattle and swine. It is also found occasionally in wound infections in man.

It can easily be isolated from many bodies of water, particularly when they are polluted with organic material. Apparently the organism is very common in nature, living generally as a saprophyte and only occasionally as a parasite. It is sensitive to chlorine and may be used to evaluate the effectiveness of this disinfectant in swimming pools (9).

**Morphology and Staining Reactions.** *Ps. aeruginosa* is a straight, slender rod of medium size. Young cultures are so rapidly motile that they can hardly be successfully watched under the microscope. Spores are not formed and there is no capsule. The organism is Gram-negative, and it stains readily with the ordinary dyes.

**Cultural Features.** This organism is readily recognized, as a rule, because of the bright-green pigment that it produces. There are really two pigments.

115

One of these is yellowish green when fresh and oxidizes to yellow. It is known as *fluorescein*. This pigment is produced by a number of organisms other than *Ps. aeruginosa* which have their habitat in water. The second pigment is a bluish green that oxidizes to brown. It is known as *pyocyanin*, and this pigment is produced by the green pus organism alone. One needs only to prove the existence of pyocyanin in a culture to know that *Ps. aeruginosa* is present. Both fluorescein and pyocyanin are water-soluble: hence in culture the green pigment diffuses throughout the medium. This is best seen when the organism is growing on a solid medium. Pyocyanin is soluble in chloroform to a greater degree than in water, whereas fluorescein is insoluble in chloroform. If a few drops of chloroform are added to a culture and thoroughly shaken through it, the chloroform, when it settles out, will be colored a deep blue. This is a rapid and reliable test for the presence of pyocyanin.

Both of the pigments of this organism are products of oxidation and do not appear unless the organism is growing under aerobic conditions. If the organism is cultivated under anaerobic conditions in a fluid medium and then exposed to oxygen by shaking the culture or blowing air through it, the colorless medium will assume the characteristic deep-green color within a few seconds.

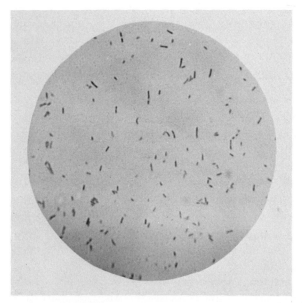

Fig. 3. Pseudomonas aerugi- nosa, from a culture on a slant agar incubated for 18 hours at 37 C. X 1,000.

*Ps. aeruginosa* may be cultivated upon the simplest of media. The growth is smooth, shiny, moist, and spreading. Colonies have thin, irregular margins, and the translucent centers are cream-colored although this often is disguised by the green pigment that stains the surroundings. An opalescent sheen characteristically appears on the surface of growths on solid media, and in old cultures crystals usually can be seen as needlelike structures radiating into the solid medium beneath the surface colonies. Of the common carbohydrate media, acid is produced only from glucose, and even this is sometimes disguised by simultaneous production of alkali from nitrogenous bodies. Milk is rapidly digested. If litmus is present, it becomes deep blue except near the surface, where the blue of the litmus is mixed with the green pigment of the organism. Gelatin and coagulated blood serum are rapidly liquefied. Cultures have a sweetish odor reminiscent of beeswax. Both cultures are heavily clouded and have a thin, iridescent, fragile pellicle.

*Ps. aeruginosa* produces a mild toxin against which it is possible to produce an antitoxin. Rather large doses are necessary to kill experimental animals. It also produces a lipoidal substance that has a strongly antagonistic and destructive influence on many other microorganisms. This substance has been called *pyocyanase*. It is heat-stable. Pyocyanase was probably the first known of our series of antibiotic agents.

By using precipitation tests in which trichloracetic acid extracts were used as antigen, Van den Ende (6) classified strains of *Ps. aeruginosa* into six serological groups. Verder and Evans (24) studied 326 cultures and by means of agglutination tests divided them into 10 O groups and 13 O types. Ten H factors were found to occur in eight distinct combinations. On the basis of these O and H antigens, 29 serotypes were established. In 1966 Muraschi *et al.* (16) employed the O antigens to correlate the two major serologic classifications (Habs'—European and Verder and Evans—North American).

**Pathogenicity for Experimental Animals.** Intraperitoneal injection of freshly isolated cultures into guinea pigs usually produces death within 24 hours. Rabbits are not so susceptible as guinea pigs; mice and pigeons are even less susceptible. According to Gorrill (13), the intravenous injection of *Ps. aeruginosa* in mice is followed either by (*a*) septicemic death within 24 to 48 hours, (*b*) renal-abscess formation and death in 3 to 14 days, or (*c*) survival. The results depend on the virulence and number of organisms injected. The extracellular slime layer of *Ps. aeruginosa* appears to be important in disease production in mice. It is suggested that the slime becomes toxic only after acid hydrolysis or enzymatic degradation (1). Liu (15) claims that lecithinase released by the bacterium produces edema, induration of the skin, and necrosis of the liver, while protease elicits hemorrhage, especially of the intestines and lungs, and also necrotic lesions.

**Pathogenicity for Domestic Animals.** This organism is often found in necrotic pneumonias of swine. Frequently it reaches these organs by aspiration of pus from necrotic rhinitis, a disease in which it is believed to be a secondary invader. The organism also appears in the intestinal lumen of swine in cases of necrotic enteritis. It often is found in foul-smelling abscesses of the spleen and liver of both swine and cattle. In traumatic pericarditis of cattle, this organism commonly accompanies the foreign body. In most abscesses other bacteria are present, and the responsibility of each of the organisms present is uncertain. Poels (19) has described a form of scours in calves in which *Ps. aeruginosa* was thought to be the causative agent. It was found in almost pure culture in the watery stools. Occasionally cases of septicemia are observed, the organism being found in pure culture in the blood and all organs shortly after death. It has been recognized in outbreaks of bovine mastitis and has been known to erupt from this gland into systemic infection (10). Tucker (22) has stated that some outbreaks of *Pseudomonas* mastitis have been caused by the introduction of the organism into the udder during administration of penicillin for infusion therapy. Heifers inseminated with semen containing this pathogen developed varying degrees of uteritis, cervicitis, and vaginitis (12). It has also been reported as the cause of sporadic abortions in cattle (18).

Chute (3) described an outbreak of *Ps. aeruginosa* infection in poults which resembled *Salmonella pullorum* disease. It has infected 1-day-old chicks inoculated subcutaneously with contaminated antibiotic solutions (25). Other outbreaks in turkeys, chickens, and ducks were described by Niilo (17). Keagy and Keagy (14) recorded an epizootic among chinchillas caused by *Ps. aeruginosa* and *Salmonella typhimurium*.

On two occasions *Ps. aeruginosa* was involved in equine abortions (Doll, Bruner, and Kinkaid, 5). This microorganism occurs infrequently in genital infection of mares. Once established in the uterus of the mare, it is difficult to eliminate, and mares infected with this bacterium usually fail to conceive.

In 1953 Farrag and Mahmoud (7) claimed that *Ps. aeruginosa* occurred in a high percentage of their cases of otorrhea in dogs, Cello and Lasmanis (2) described *Pseudomonas* infection of the eye of the dog following the use of contaminated fluorescein solution, and Ticer (21) reported on the role of this bacterium in chronic infertility in the dog.

Farrell *et al.* (8) studied an outbreak of hemorrhagic pneumonia in mink. It appears that enzootic infections resulting in heavy losses are produced in this animal by *Ps. aeruginosa*.

**Immunity.** The organism is not regarded as sufficiently important to call for specific immune treatment, and no commercial products for such treatment are available. Autogenous bacterins injected intradermally into infected mares are reported to be of some value in clearing up the infection. They have also been used successfully in treating certain outbreaks of mastitis in cattle (23).

**Chemotherapy.** Of the known chemotherapeutic agents, none has shown marked success in curing infections caused by *Ps. aeruginosa*, although aerosporin (polymyxin B) and neomycin show some promise when large doses are given. Farrag and Mahmoud (7) recommend the use of 1 percent acetic acid in treating otorrhea in dogs, and Scott and Denham (20) prescribe nitrofurazone ointment.

**The Disease in Man.** This bacterium is causally associated with a great variety of suppurative and other infections in man. It has been found in pure cul-

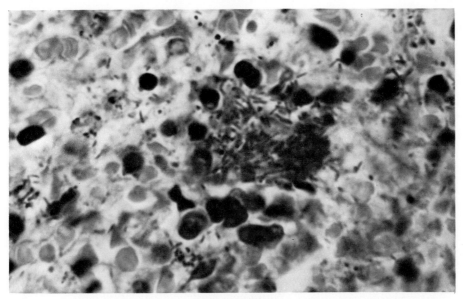

*Fig. 4.* A colony of *Pseudomonas aeruginosa* in a section of lung of mink with hemorrhagic pneumonia. X 650. (Courtesy Farrell, Leader, and Gorham, *Cornell Vet.*)

ture in abscesses of the middle ear and in cases of endocarditis and pneumonia, in which it appeared to be the sole responsible microorganism. It has also been reported in meningitis. Burns frequently become infected with this organism, and healing is prolonged partly because the pyocyanin produced by the bacteria is toxic for human skin (4). Without doubt it is pathogenic for man, although human infections appear not to be common. However, Yow (26) states that antibiotic therapy has increased the relative importance of *Ps. aeruginosa* and that cases of infection caused by this organism sometimes develop during or following such treatment. The relationship of the infection to the antibiotic therapy in most patients is believed to be a matter of change in the bacterial flora owing to the elimination of sensitive bacteria and the multiplication of resistant species.

## REFERENCES

1. Callahan, Beyerlein, and Mull.   Jour. Bact., 1964, *88*, 805.
2. Cello and Lasmanis.   Jour. Am. Vet. Med. Assoc., 1958, *132*, 297.
3. Chute.   Canad. Jour. Comp. Med., 1949, *13*, 113.
4. Cruickshank and Lowbury.   Brit. Jour. Exp. Path., 1953, *34*, 583.
5. Doll, Bruner, and Kinkaid.   Jour. Am. Vet. Med. Assoc., 1949, *114*, 292.
6. Ende, Van den.   Jour. Hyg. (London), 1952, *50*, 405.
7. Farrag and Mahmoud.   Jour. Am. Vet. Med. Assoc., 1953, *122*, 35.
8. Farrell, Leader, and Gorham.   Cornell Vet., 1958, *48*, 378.
9. Fitzgerald and DerVartanian.   Appl. Microbiol., 1969, *17*, 415.
10. Gardiner and Craig.   Vet. Rec., 1961, *73*, 372.

11.   Gay and Associates.   Agents of disease and host resistance. C. C Thomas, Springfield, Ill., 1935, p. 703.
12.   Getty and Ellis.   Jour. Am. Vet. Med. Assoc., 1967, *151*, 1688.
13.   Gorrill.   Jour. Path. and Bact., 1952, *64*, 857.
14.   Keagy and Keagy.   Jour. Am. Vet. Med. Assoc., 1951, *118*, 35.
15.   Liu.   Jour. Inf. Dis., 1966, *116*, 112.
16.   Muraschi, Bolles, Moczulski, and Lindsay.   *Ibid.*, 1966, *116*, 84.
17.   Nilo.   Canad. Jour. Comp. Med. and Vet. Sci., 1959, *23*, 329.
18.   Plastridge and Williams.   Cornell Vet., 1948, *38*, 165.
19.   Poels.   Berl. tierärztl. Wchnschr., 1901, *17*, 290.
20.   Scott and Denham.   Brit. Vet. Jour., 1963, *119*, 211.
21.   Ticer.   Jour. Am. Vet. Med. Assoc., 1965, *146*, 720.
22.   Tucker.   Cornell Vet., 1950, *40*, 95.
23.   Van Kruiningen.   *Ibid.*, 1963, *53*, 240.
24.   Verder and Evans.   Jour. Inf. Dis., 1961, *109*, 183.
25.   Williams and Newkirk.   Avian Dis., 1966, *10*, 353.
26.   Yow.   Jour. Am. Med. Assoc., 1952, *149*, 1184.

### *Pseudomonas (Malleomyces) pseudomallei*

SYNONYMS:   Bacillus of Whitmore, *Malleomyces whitmori*

*Ps. pseudomallei* produces melioidosis, a glanderslike disease originally described by Whitmore and Krishnaswami (26) in Rangoon. For many years it was thought to be primarily a disease of rodents, occasionally communicable to man, and limited in occurrence to southeast Asia. It is now known to occur in man in the Western Hemisphere and in orangutans (25), kangaroos (7), cattle (12), pigs, sheep, and goats in Australia (4, 15, 16) and in the Netherlands Antilles (24).

**Morphology and Staining Reactions.** It is a Gram-negative bacillus that closely resembles *Pseudomonas aeruginosa*.

**Cultural Features.** *Ps. pseudomallei* is related to *Ps. aeruginosa* in many of its culture features. A large number of strains produce a yellow pigment which has been described as water-soluble. The organism is more energetic than *Ps. aeruginosa* in attacking carbohydrates and produces acid from glucose, maltose, lactose, sucrose, and mannitol. According to reports by Colling *et al.* (3) and Heckly and Nigg (10), it produces an exotoxin.

**Pathogenicity.** The organism is pathogenic for rodents, cats, dogs, pigs, goats, sheep, horses, and man. The characteristic lesion produced is a small caseous nodule. These nodules may coalesce to form large areas of caseation or break down into abscesses. They may be found in lymph nodes, in the spleen, lungs, liver, joints, nasal cavity, and tonsils, and in fact in almost any tissue including the brain (18). Guinea pigs and rabbits are highly susceptible to infection, and inoculated male guinea pigs may produce the Strauss reaction (see p. 254). *Ps. pseudomallei* has been isolated from an aborted goat fetus (20). It has been reported as the cause of vertebral abscesses on the spinal cord of lambs, resulting in posterior flaccid paralysis (11). It has caused lumbar vertebral osteomyelitis in a macaque (*Macaca nemestrina*) (23).

Diagnosis of the disease depends on the isolation and identification of the organism rather than on clinical findings or serologic tests, although Olds and Lewis (15) reported some success with the melioidin test, and Nigg and Johnson (14) and Omar (17) have employed complement-fixation and agglutination tests with apparent success.

Dannenberg and Scott (6) have enhanced the resistance of mice and hamsters to melioidosis by vaccinating them with live avirulent strains of the organism.

**Mode of Transmission.** The disease occurs naturally in rodents, and transmission among these animals by biting insects such as mosquitoes and fleas has been reported (13). Studies by Strauss *et al.* (22) revealed no evidence to suggest that this microorganism requires the rat or any other animal as a maintenance host. They concluded that, in Malaysia, *Ps. pseudomallei* is a normal inhabitant of the soil and water. In man there is some evidence that melioidosis often follows trauma.

**The Disease in Man.** The first cases recognized in persons outside the endemic area in Asia were in Guam in 1946 (13). In the Western Hemisphere a number of cases have been diagnosed in military personnel who contracted the disease in the Far East following World War II, but the first case completely indigenous to continental United States appears to be the one described by Garry and Koch (9) in 1951. Other cases have been recorded (1), United States soldiers have picked up the infection in Vietnam (2, 19), and melioidosis pneumonitis has been recognized (21). The disease is not known to be transferred from man to man.

The infection often takes the form of an acute or subacute septicemia, with death resulting in 3 days to 4 weeks, but a chronic form also occurs in which death is delayed for months or years. Lesions consist of caseous nodules or abscesses which may be found in almost any part of the body except the brain. In the chronic form multiple sinuses usually are seen in the soft tissues together with extensive abscess formation. Mortality is said to be about 95 percent.

**Chemotherapy.** Cruickshank (5) recommends the use of sulfonamides in treating melioidosis. Eickhoff *et al.* (8) reported a favorable response from tetracycline, chloramphenicol, novobiocin, and sulfadiazine, with tetracycline the drug of choice. The organism is said to become streptomycin-resistant very quickly.

## REFERENCES

1. Beamer, Varney, Brown, and McDowell. Am. Jour. Clin. Path., 1954, *24*, 1231.

2. Brundage, Thuss, Jr., and Walden.  Am. Jour. Trop. Med. and Hyg., 1968, *17*, 183.
3. Colling, Nigg, and Heckly.  Jour. Bact., 1958, *76*, 422.
4. Cottew, Sutherland, and Meehan.  Austral. Vet. Jour., 1952, *28*, 113.
5. Cruickshank.  Brit. Med. Jour., 1949, *2*, 410.
6. Dannenberg and Scott.  Jour. Immunol., 1960, *84*, 233.
7. Egerton.  Austral. Vet. Jour., 1963, *39*, 243.
8. Eickhoff, Bennett, Hayes, and Feeley.  Jour. Inf. Dis., 1970, *121*, 95.
9. Garry and Koch.  Jour. Lab. and Clin. Med., 1951, *38*, 374.
10. Heckly and Nigg.  Jour. Bact., 1958, *76*, 427.
11. Ketterer and Bamford.  Austral. Vet. Jour., 1967, *43*, 79.
12. Laws and Mahoney.  *Ibid.*, 1964, *40*, 202.
13. Mirick, Zimmerman, Maner, and Humphrey.  Jour. Am. Med. Assoc., 1946, *130*, 1063.
14. Nigg and Johnston.  Jour. Bact., 1961, 82, 159.
15. Olds and Lewis.  Austral. Vet. Jour., 1954, *30*, 253.
16. *Ibid.*, 1955, *31*, 273.
17. Omar.  Brit. Vet. Jour., 1962, *118*, 421.
18. Omar.  Jour. Comp. Path. and Therap., 1963, *73*, 359.
19. Patterson, Darling, and Blumenthal.  Jour. Am. Med. Assoc., 1967, *200*, 447.
20. Retnasabapathy.  Vet. Rec., 1966, *79*, 166.
21. Spotnitz, Rudnitzky, and Rambaud.  Jour. Am. Med. Assoc., 1967, *202*, 950.
22. Strauss, Groves, Mariappan, and Ellison.  Am. Jour. Trop. Med. and Hyg., 1969, *18*, 698.
23. Strauss, Jason, Lee, and Gan.  Jour. Am. Vet. Med. Assoc., 1969, *155*, 1169.
24. Sutmöller, Kraneveld, and Van der Schaff.  *Ibid.*, 1957, *130*, 415.
25. Tammemagi and Johnston.  Austral. Vet. Jour., 1963, *39*, 241.
26. Whitmore and Krishnaswami.  Indian Med. Gaz., 1912, *47*, 262.

### *Pseudomonas maltophilia*

In 1960 Hugh and Ryschenkow (2) applied the name *Pseudomonas malto-philia* to a new species of pseudomonad isolated from human and animal sources, water, and milk. In 1966 Stainer *et al.* (3) described additional characteristics of cultures of this organism derived from human sources and in 1969 Gilardi (1) reported the results of a study of 22 strains.

The organism is a Gram-negative rod that is motile by means of flagella attached at one or both poles. It produces a brown diffusible pigment, green discoloration of blood, and no growth on SS agar. It liquefies gelatin but does not produce indol or utilize urea. It ferments glucose, fructose, mannose, and maltose, and most strains produce acid from lactose and sucrose.

In man pure cultures have been isolated from foot lesions, from the bladder, from periurethral and scrotal abscesses, and from wounds resulting from traumatic injuries. Gilardi (1) concluded that this pseudomonad must be considered a potential pathogen in the same manner as are *Ps. aeruginosa* and *Ps. pseudomallei.*

Antibiotics most effective against *Ps. maltophilia* proved to be methenamine mandelate, polymyxin, and colistin. Chloramphenicol, neomycin, and kanamycin were less active.

## REFERENCES

1. Gilardi. Am. Jour. Clin. Path., 1969, *51*, 58.
2. Hugh and Ryschenkow. Bact. Proc., 1960, *60*, 78.
3. Stanier, Palleroni, and Doudoroff. Jour. Gen. Microbiol., 1966, *43*, 159.

## THE GENUS *AEROMONAS*

The majority of species thus far described are from water or are known to be pathogenic for marine and freshwater animals such as fish and amphibians. The one apparently possessing the broadest zoological distribution is *Aeromonas hydrophila*. It is pathogenic for fish, salamanders, frogs, snakes, mice, guinea pigs, and rabbits.

### Aeromonas hydrophila

SYNONYMS: *Bacillus hydrophilus fuscus, Proteus hydrophilus*

The organism is a motile rod that possesses a single polar flagellum. It is Gram-negative. On solid medium it produces a yellowish to dirty brown-yellow coloration. In broth it develops a heavy pellicle. Gelatin is liquefied; indol, hydrogen sulfide, and catalase are produced; and nitrates are reduced. Urea is not utilized. Glucose, maltose, sucrose, and mannitol are fermented with acid and gas production. Lactose, arabinose, dulcitol, sorbitol, and inositol are not attacked. It is claimed that salicin is fermented at 22 C, but not at 37 C (1). Physiologically the *Aeromonas* organisms have identical characteristics with some of the enteric bacteria, but differ in flagellar arrangement and the former are less active in carbohydrate fermentation.

In fish, salamanders, frogs, mice, guinea pigs, and rabbits *A. hydrophila* produces hemorrhagic septicemia. The disease in frogs is sometimes called *red leg*. In snakes (2) the disease may result in ulcerative stomatitis (mouth rot) characterized by a chronic inflammation of the inner lips, gums, and palate and accompanied by copious quantities of yellow, caseous exudate within the mouth crevices. There may be a pneumonic form and a digestive involvement, but the acute type of the disease presents the pathological picture of a typical septicemic disease (3).

Control of *Aeromonas* infection in snakes would seem to depend on control and eradication of the snake mite, *Ophionyssus natricis*, which appears to be the transmitting agent (2).

Both sodium methazine (4) and tetracycline (3) have proved effective in treating mouth rot in snakes, but attention to hygiene and to control of the mite also are important in controlling the disease.

## REFERENCES

1. Breed, Murray, and Smith. Bergey's manual of determinative bacteriology. 7th ed. Williams and Wilkins Co., Baltimore, 1957.
2. Camin. Jour. Parsitol., 1948, *34*, 345.
3. Heywood. Cornell Vet., 1968, *58*, 236.
4. Page. *Ibid.*, 1961, *51*, 258.

# XI | The *Spirillaceae*

Within this family we find cells that are curved or spirally twisted rods. They are usually motile by means of a single flagellum or a tuft of polar flagella. The important pathogenic forms for man and the lower animals are found in the genus *Vibrio*.

## THE GENUS *VIBRIO*

This genus is composed of a group of short, curved, rigid rods, arranged singly or united into spiral forms. They are motile by a single or several polar flagella. They are nonsporing, usually Gram-negative, and aerobic to anaerobic; most species are saprophytic. Some forms are pathogenic for man and animals.

### Vibrio comma

The organism causing Asiatic cholera in man belongs in this group. It rarely occurs in the United States but is an ever-present danger in the Orient. A vaccine used in World War II seemed to be effective in controlling the disease in the Army of the United States. Immunity to this enteric disease appears to be concerned with *coproantibodies*, which are found in intestinal contents. Apparently these antibodies are independent of serum antibodies (Burrows *et al.*, 5). Gohar (18) recommends dihydrostreptomycin in combination with sulfaguanidine for treating cholera.

### Vibrio fetus

In 1909 McFadyean and Stockman (30), in an extensive report on cattle, referred to a form of abortion which had been discovered in English sheep, and which was shown to be caused by infection with a spirillum. Later several herds of cattle were found infected with the same organism. In 1918 Smith (53) found the disease in this country in cattle, and the following year Carpenter (6) found it in sheep. Since then it has been found to be widespread in the United States. It is known to be pathogenic for cattle, sheep, goats, pregnant guinea pigs, hamsters, and man.

**Morphology and Staining Reactions.** In infected tissues, the organisms are seen as comma-shaped or S-shaped bodies, occasionally as longer spirals. In young cultures the organisms are short, but in older cultures very long spirals are seen, many of them extending a considerable part of the way across the microscopic field. Granules may often be demonstrated by Giemsa or other polychrome strains. According to Rhoades (47), the comma forms have a single polar flagellum, but S forms may have bipolar flagella. The organism has no capsule and does not form spores. It stains readily with ordinary dyes and is Gram-negative. A detailed description of it is given by Smith and Taylor (54).

**Cultural Features.** V. *fetus* may be cultivated by any of the methods that succeed with *Br. abortus*, although it is a much more delicate organism than the latter and its growth in primary cultures is so meager that it may very easily be overlooked. McFadyean first cultivated it in tall tubes of serum agar that were inoculated while liquefied. Growth appeared in a zone beneath the surface in the manner of *Br. abortus*. Like the *Brucella* the organism is strictly aerobic but it will not grow in open tubes in primary culture unless they are incubated in an atmosphere of increased $CO_2$ content. Smith succeeded in obtaining cultures in tubes that were hermetically sealed with wax.

In making primary cultures Bacto-thiol * medium is very satisfactory (22). It is used in semisolid form and in 150-by-20-mm culture tubes filled to a depth of 4 to 5 cm. After being inoculated just through the surface, the tubes are incubated at 37 C in an atmosphere of 10 to 20 percent $CO_2$. *Vibrio* appear after 3 to 9 days of incubation as a layer of growth extending outward and downward from the point of inoculation. Another medium successfully employed in isolating V. *fetus* consists of cystine heart agar (Bacto) plates. After autoclaving 1,000 ml of this medium and cooling to 45 C, 10 percent of sterile whole citrated ox blood, 300,000 units of mycostatin, 2,000 micrograms of albamycin, and 2,000 units of bacitracin are added. Poured plates of this medium are streaked with suspect material.

Bacto-thiol medium is used in cultivating the organisms for antigen production. Two percent agar is used to make a solid medium. It is placed in flasks and allowed to solidify. Sterile beads and inoculum are added. Following incubation at 37 C under $CO_2$ tension, the beads are rotated over the surface of the agar to spread the organisms, and the flasks are reincubated to obtain maximum growth. Under the usual conditions the organism reproduces poorly in fluid medium, but Reich *et al.* (45) have shown that aerating a broth culture with 5 percent $CO_2$, 35 percent air, 10 percent $H_2$, and 50 percent helium results in rapid and heavy growth.

* Obtainable from Digestive Ferments Company, Detroit, Michigan.

It appears that pathogenic cultures of V. *fetus* can be divided into intestinal (V. *fetus* var. *intestinalis*) and venereal (V. *fetus* var. *venerealis*) types. The former are less fastidious than the latter, are weakly positive for $H_2S$, and grow in 1 percent glycine medium. The latter are both $H_2S$- and glycine-negative. Both types are catalase-positive, salt-sensitive, do not liquefy gelatin, produce indol, or ferment sugars. Colonies of V. *fetus* may be confused at times with those of V. *bubulus*, but the latter is strongly $H_2S$-positive, catalase-negative, and tolerant to 2.5 percent or more of sodium chloride. It is nonpathogenic.

According to Walsh and White (60) the *Vibrio* isolants may be classified into two groups based on biochemical and agglutination tests. Those in group I make up V. *fetus* type 1 and subtype 1, while those of group II comprise V. *fetus* type 2, V. *bubulus*, and some unclassified species.

**Resistance.** Stock cultures of this organism are hard to maintain unless they are given constant care or have been lyophilized. Evidently the resistance of this organism is not great.

**Pathogenicity for Experimental Animals.** Reports by Ristic and Morse (48) indicate that the pregnant guinea pig may be infected experimentally by intraperitoneal, subcutaneous, intravaginal, and oral routes. The animal may or may not abort. In the infected female the gross pathological changes consist of endometrial hemorrhage, edema, and necrosis. Nonpregnant guinea pigs do not become infected. Ristic *et al.* (49) also isolated V. *fetus* from the testes of male hamsters that were injected intraperitoneally and claimed that such males transmitted infection by coitus to noninfected female hamsters. V. *fetus* also appears to be pathogenic for the embryonating chicken egg. It produces congestion, hemorrhage, and sometimes necrosis in the chorioallantoic membrane, cutaneous tissues, liver, kidney, spleen, gizzard, and brain (61).

**The Natural Disease.** There is evidence that the intestinal type of V. *fetus* is the one that produces sporadic abortion in cattle and outbreaks of abortion in ewes. It is not generally transmitted by coitus. The venereal type is concerned in abortions and infertility in cattle and is carried and transmitted by the bull. In the nonpregnant cow or heifer the presence of V. *fetus* in the genital tract often results in infertility. Whether the organism damages the embryonic tissue or induces changes in the genital tract that interfere with conception, or both, is not known. As a herd problem vibriosis seems to be most important in increasing the number of services per conception and thereby lowers breeding efficiency. Probably early embryonic deaths occur frequently, but abortions are not uncommon and may occur at any time during the gestation period. In early abortions the embryo is usually expelled with membranes intact and the effects upon the dam are slight (41). In abortions that take place after the 5th month the membranes may be retained. Edema is the most common placental lesion, and pathologic changes in the fetus are superficial and variable. No lesions are found in bulls although these animals may carry V. *fetus* in their sheaths without showing signs of infection.

In outbreaks of ovine vibriosis the percentage of ewes having abortions or immature lambs may be high. The pathological changes observed in naturally infected sheep are chiefly confined to the uterus, placenta, and fetus. The uterine wall as well as the fetal membranes are edematous. The fetus shows edema of the subcutaneous tissues, and the peritoneal, pleural, and pericardial cavities may contain blood-tinged fluid. The presence of necrotic spots in the liver has also been reported. As a rule, ewes do not abort in the year following an outbreak and appear not to carry the infection, but Smibert (52) was able to isolate *V. fetus* var. *intestinalis* from the fecal and intestinal contents of clinically normal sheep.

Vibrionic abortion has been reported in goats (8), but the incidence of infection in these animals is in doubt at this time.

**Mode of Transmission.** Vibrionic abortion may be caused by the intestinal or by the venereal type of *V. fetus*. While the former is not considered to be a venereal disease the latter appears to be a true one because it is transmitted from bull to cow and from cow to bull during coitus. It may be transmitted by artificial insemination with untreated semen from infected bulls (27). Plastridge (41) believes that it can be transmitted from cow to cow and postulates that the activities of females in estrus may result in the transfer of organisms from the vulva of an infected animal to the vulva of other animals, but the experiments of McEntee *et al.* (29) do not confirm this.

Vibrionic abortion in sheep is produced by the intestinal type of *V. fetus*, sometimes called the *sheep type*, and the ram is not a factor in the transmission of ovine vibriosis (13). Outbreaks strike suddenly, often with no record of exposure of the flock to the disease, and disappear within the same year. It seems that ewes are susceptible in the late stages of gestation only and that infected ewes recover before the next breeding season. Ingestion is the most important route of infection in sheep (14, 35, 57). There is evidence that magpies (34, 59), ravens (7), and other carriers (12, 37) are concerned in spreading the disease and the possibility exists that sheep may be asymptomatic carriers (52).

**Diagnosis.** If the fetal membranes are available, a direct microscopic examination is made of the cotyledons. The finding of distinctly spiral-shaped organisms is regarded as positive evidence of the infection. Cultures are made, in serial dilution (22), on semisolid Bacto-thiol medium from stomach fluids, lungs, heart blood, amniotic fluid, and suspensions of ground cotyledons. The tubes are incubated under $CO_2$ tension at 37 C for 3 to 9 days and then examined for *V. fetus*. Careful culturing of cervicovaginal mucus, preputial samples by the millipore filter technic (43), or semen will sometimes reveal the organism in infected animals (21, 24, 42).

As a diagnostic aid, blood serum has been used in tube agglutination tests, but the results obtained have not been very satisfactory. The use of vaginal (cervical) mucus, instead of blood serum, seems to be helpful in the diagnosis of vibriosis in cattle (20). In this disease agglutinins appear in the vaginal mucus earlier than they do in the blood, and they persist for a longer period. A titer of 1:25 is usually considered to be positive, providing there is no blood in the mucus. Punga (44) recommends the use of erythrocytes sensitized with *V. fetus* antigen in detecting antibodies in bovine vaginal mucus and claims that the indirect hemagglutination test is more sensitive and accurate than bacterial agglutination. There is need for great care in selecting and maintaining the cultures used for antigen in the agglutination tests (27). Marked variation in sensitivity is shown among cultures of *V. fetus,* and serologic relations to *Br. abortus, S. pullorum,* and *Trichomonas fetus* have been reported in some strains.

In the diagnosis of vibriosis in sheep, isolation of the organism is necessary and the blood test is of limited value. Finkelstein and LaBrec (11) have described a procedure for the rapid identification of cholera vibrios by use of fluorescent antibody, and a similar technic is available for detecting *V. fetus.*

In bulls, the diagnosis of vibriosis is readily accomplished by immunofluorescence and cultural procedures (25, 26).

**Immunity.** Vibriosis tends to be self-limiting in female cattle and sheep. Although numerous strains of the organism have been studied by serologic methods, general agreement is lacking in the published results. On the basis of agar gel precipitin and passive hemagglutination reactions in which ultrasonic extracts were used as antigens, Winter and Dunne (62) concluded that an antigenic relationship exists among all strains of *V. fetus* and also between *V. fetus* and some noncatalase-producing vibrios (saprophytes). By means of whole-cell agglutination tests at least four serotypes have been demonstrated (1, 32).

It is evident that some degree of immunity is established in cattle and sheep naturally exposed to *V. fetus* and according to Hoerlein and Kramer (19) and Miller *et al.* (36) the use of adjuvant bacterins will enhance the resistance of cattle and sheep to *V. fetus* infection.

Frank *et al.* (16) have indicated that the vaccination of cows produces significant improvement in breeding efficiency, without attaining protection against infection.

Meinershagen *et al.* (33) obtained results confirming previous epizootiologic observations that indicated pregnant ewes involved or exposed in a vibriosis epizootic were immune during the following gestation, even though they had not aborted during the outbreak, and Storz *et al.* (56) presented data showing that yearly vaccination of replacement ewes, with a *V. fetus* bacterin, was an economical and highly effective method of maintaining an immune flock and prevented the occurrence of serious epizootics of vibriosis.

**Chemotherapy.** Infection tends to die out in females. This does not happen in the bull. McEntee *et al.* (28) have shown that the prevention of vibriosis in inseminated heifers is possible by treating the semen from infected bulls with penicillin, streptomycin, and sulfanilamide. Terramycin and streptomycin are believed to be effective in treating heifers, and the use of terramycin is suggested in areas where streptomycin is added to the semen in the hope that streptomycin-fast types will not develop. Frank *et al.* (15, 17) reported that the feeding of either chlortetracycline or furazolidone is effective in treating vibriosis in ewes.

**Control Measures.** Purchased cattle should be segregated and tested before being added to the herd. After vibriosis breaks out in a herd, suspend breeding, treat the animals with antibiotics, and then practice artificial breeding with streptomycin-treated semen. The findings by Storz *et al.* (56) suggest that outbreaks in sheep may be prevented by yearly vaccination.

**The Disease in Man.** The possibility of human infection was suggested by Vinzent (58), who isolated cultures regarded as *V. fetus* from the blood of three pregnant women. One of these aborted, one presented an immature birth, and one gave normal birth at term. The placenta was diseased in all three patients. Spink (55) reported the recovery of *V. fetus* from a case of febrile illness in a patient who worked in a meat-packing plant. The illness simulated brucellosis.

In 1969 Reyman and Silberberg (46) described two cases of septicemia in females caused by *V. fetus* and in 1970 Bokkenheuser (3) reported 10 new cases of vibriosis in man. He also stated that at least 74 confirmed cases had been recognized. The disease affected infants, pregnant women, and elderly individuals.

### Vibrio jejuni

*V. jejuni* has been described by Jones, Orcutt, and Little (23) as the causative agent of a disease in calves and older cattle which may occur in epidemic form during the autumn and winter months in stabled animals and is known as *winter dysentery* or *black scours*. The organisms are most abundant in the jejunum. The disease, which usually does not extend beyond the stage of simple, gastrointestinal catarrh, may in some instances be very severe. The exact role of *V. jejuni* in winter dysentery is not definitely known. MacPherson (31) believes the etiological agent to be a virus. According to Boyd (4), intestinal antiseptics have proved to be of greater value than sulfa drugs and antibiotics in treating this disease.

### Vibrionic Dysentery of Swine

In 1944 Doyle (9) described a vibrionic diarrhea in swine. The organism was obtained by streaking a small piece of the colonic mucosa on blood agar plates and incubating them in 10 to 15 percent carbon dioxide for 48 hours. The feeding of pure cultures of the *Vibrio* to eight pigs was followed by diarrhea in six. The diarrhea was less severe and contained less blood and mucus than in the naturally occurring disease. The findings of Roberts (50) in Australia in 1956 supported those of Doyle.

In 1949 Schmid and Klingler (51) isolated a *Vibrio* from an outbreak of severe dysentery in swine and in 1957 Birrell (2) described the finding of *Vibrio* in constant association with this type of disease. These workers were unable to find any proof that their isolates were the active pathogens. It appears that the etiology of this swine disease is also in doubt.

Miyat and Gossett (38) claim success in treating swine dysentery by using the antibiotic tylosin.

## Vibriosis of Fowl

*Avian vibrionic hepatitis* has been described by Peckham (39) and Winterfield (63). It is an infectious disease of chickens characterized by degenerative changes in the liver and, less frequently, in the heart and other organs. Bile is a good source of the infective agent and it can be isolated in artificial media or by means of chicken embryos. The finding of *Vibrio*-shaped organisms by direct phase microscopic examination serves as an aid in diagnosis (10). Furazolidone and erythromycin are effective therapeutic agents.

Peterson *et al.* (40) studied a condition of infertility and low hatchability of eggs of turkeys which they believed to be caused by *Vibrio* infection of the genital tract. They indicated that the feeding of oxytetracycline was beneficial.

## REFERENCES

1. Biberstein. Cornell Vet., 1956, *46*, 144.
2. Birrell. Vet. Rec., 1957, *69*, 947.
3. Bokkenheuser. Am. Jour. Epidemiol., 1970, *91*, 400.
4. Boyd. Jen-Sal Jour., 1950, *32*, 4.
5. Burrows *et al.* Jour. Inf. Dis., 1946, 79, 159; 1947, *81*, 151; 1948, 82, 232.
6. Carpenter. Rpt. N.Y. State Vet. Coll. for 1918–19, Legislative Doc., no. 8, 1920.
7. Dennis. Austral. Vet. Jour., 1967, *43*, 45.
8. Dobbs and McIntyre. Vet. Bul., 1951, *21*, 720.
9. Doyle. Am. Jour. Vet. Res., 1944, 5, 3.
10. Eleazer, Powell, Roebuck, and Bierer. Jour. Am. Vet. Med. Assoc., 1964, *144*, 380.
11. Finkelstein and LaBrec. Jour. Bact., 1959, 78, 886.
12. Firehammer, Lovelace, and Hawkins. Cornell Vet., 1962, 52, 21.
13. Firehammer, Marsh, and Tunnicliff. Am. Jour. Vet. Res., 1956, *17*, 573.
14. Frank, Bailey, and Heithecker. Jour. Am. Vet. Med. Assoc., 1957, *131*, 472.
15. Frank, Baron, Meinershagen, and Scrivner. Am. Jour. Vet. Res., 1962, 23, 985.
16. Frank, Bryner, and O'Berry. *Ibid.*, 1967, *28*, 1237.
17. Frank, Meinershagen, Scrivner, and Bailey. *Ibid.*, 1959, *20*, 973.
18. Gohar. Jour. Trop. Med. and Hyg. (London), 1953, 56, 289.
19. Hoerlein and Kramer. Am. Jour. Vet. Res., 1964, 25, 371.
20. Hughes. Cornell Vet., 1953, *43*, 431.
21. *Ibid.*, 1956, *46*, 249.
22. Hughes and Gilman. *Ibid.*, 1953, *43*, 463.
23. Jones, Orcutt, and Little. Jour. Exp. Med., 1931, 53, 853.

24.  Kuzdas and Morse.   Jour. Bact., 1956, 71, 251.
25.  Lein, Erickson, Winter, and McEntee.   Jour. Am. Vet. Med. Assoc., 1968, 152, 1306.
26.  Ibid., 153, 1574.
27.  McEntee, Hughes, and Gilman.   Cornell Vet., 1954, 44, 376.
28.  Ibid., 395.
29.  McEntee, Hughes, and Wagner.   Ibid., 1959, 49, 34.
30.  McFadyean and Stockman.   Rpt. Departmental Committee appointed by the Department of Agriculture and Fisheries to inquire into epizootic abortion. Part I, 1909, p. 15; Part III, 1913, p. 9.
31.  MacPherson.   Canad. Jour. Comp. Med. and Vet. Sci., 1957, 21, 184.
32.  Marsh and Firehammer.   Am. Jour. Vet. Res., 1953, 14, 396.
33.  Meinershagen, Frank, Hulet, and Price.   Ibid., 1969, 30, 203.
34.  Meinershagen, Waldhalm, Frank, and Scrivner.   Jour. Am. Vet. Med. Assoc., 1965, 147, 843.
35.  Miller, Jensen, and Gilroy.   Am. Jour. Vet. Res., 1959, 20, 677.
36.  Miller, Jensen, and Ogg.   Ibid., 1964, 25, 664.
37.  Miner and Thorne.   Ibid., 1964, 25, 474.
38.  Miyat and Gossett.   Vet. Med., 1964, 59, 295.
39.  Peckham.   Avian Dis., 1958, 2, 348.
40.  Peterson, Hendriz, and Worden.   Jour. Am. Vet. Med. Assoc., 1959, 135, 219.
41.  Plastridge.   In: Brandly and Jungherr. Advances in veterinary science. Academic Press Inc., New York, 1955, p. 326.
42.  Plastridge, Walker, Williams, Stula, and Kiggins.   Am. Jour. Vet. Res., 1957, 18, 575.
43.  Plumer, Duvall, and Shepler.   Cornell Vet., 1962, 52, 110.
44.  Punga.   New Zeal. Vet. Jour., 1959, 7, 72.
45.  Reich, Dunne, Bortree, and Hokanson.   Jour. Bact., 1957, 74, 246.
46.  Reyman and Silberberg.   Am. Jour. Clin. Path., 1969, 51, 578.
47.  Rhoades.   Am. Jour. Vet. Res., 1954, 15, 630.
48.  Ristic and Morse.   Ibid., 1953, 14, 399.
49.  Ristic, Morse, Wipf, and McNutt.   Ibid., 1954, 15, 309.
50.  Roberts.   Austral. Vet. Jour., 1956, 32, 27.
51.  Schmid and Klingler.   Schweiz. Arch. f. Tierheilk., 1949, 91, 232.
52.  Smibert.   Am. Jour. Vet. Res., 1965, 26, 320.
53.  Smith.   Jour. Exp. Med., 1918, 28, 701.
54.  Smith and Taylor.   Ibid., 1919, 30, 299.
55.  Spink.   Jour. Am. Med. Assoc., 1957, 163, 180.
56.  Storz, Miner, Olson, Marriott, and Elsner.   Am. Jour. Vet. Res., 1966, 27, 115.
57.  Tucker and Robertstad.   Jour. Am. Vet. Med. Assoc., 1956, 129, 511.
58.  Vinzent.   Presse Méd., 1949, 57, 1230.
59.  Waldhalm, Mason, Meinershagen, and Scrivner.   Jour. Am. Vet. Med. Assoc., 1964, 144, 497.
60.  Walsh and White.   Am. Jour. Vet. Res., 1968, 29, 1377.
61.  Webster and Thorp.   Ibid., 1953, 14, 118.
62.  Winter and Dunne.   Ibid., 1962, 23, 150.
63.  Winterfield.   Jour. Am. Vet. Med. Assoc., 1959, 134, 329.

# XII | The *Achromobacteraceae*

In the family *Achromobacteraceae* we find Gram-negative rods that may be salt-water, fresh-water, or soil forms and are less commonly found as parasites or pathogens. Some may be plant pathogens. Although there are five genera within this family (*Alkaligenes, Achromobacter, Flavobacterium, Agarbacterium,* and *Beneckea*), only *Alkaligenes* and *Flavobacterium* appear to be significant in veterinary medicine. The latter is sometimes pathogenic for fish and is not considered in detail, while the former is discussed briefly because of its broader area of activity.

## THE GENUS *ALKALIGENES*

Members of this genus are generally found in the intestinal tracts of vertebrates or in dairy products. *A. metalkaligenes, A. bookeri,* and *A. recti,* the inhabitants of the intestinal canal, are not ordinarily differentiated from *A. fecalis,* the type species of the genus. *A. viscosus* and *A. marshalli* are found in dairy products and produce a slimy alkalinity and ropiness in milk.

### *Alkaligenes fecalis*

The organism is a Gram-negative bacillus that is motile by means of peritrichous flagella. It alkalizes litmus milk, does not ferment carbohydrates, is aerobic, reduces nitrates, produces $H_2S$, does not liquefy gelatin, is oxidase- and catalase-positive, and indol-negative.

Actually *A. fecalis* is not highly pathogenic, but it has been reported as the cause of abortion of a 5-month-old bovine fetus (1) where it was found in pure culture in the stomach fluid and tissues. It has been found to be the cause of a disease closely resembling "red leg" in tree frogs (2). It has also appeared in man in cases of bacteremia, meningitis, infection of the gallbladder, renal tract, eye, lymph nodes, and appendix on occasion (3).

**REFERENCES**

1.  Bruner and Hughes.   Cornell Vet., 1955, *45*, 271.
2.  Miles.   Jour. Gen. Microbiol., 1950, *4*, 434.
3.  Weinstein and Wasserman.   New Eng. Jour. Med., 1951, *244*, 662.

# XIII | The *Enterobacteriaceae*

Members of the family *Enterobacteriaceae* are straight Gram-negative rods. They may be motile or nonmotile. The motile strains have peritrichous flagella. All species grow well on artificial media and attack glucose, with the formation of acid, or acid and gas. With some exceptions in the genus *Erwinia* they reduce nitrates to nitrites. Their antigenic composition constitutes a mosaic of interlocking serological relationships among the several genera. The family contains many animal parasites and some plant parasites. Frequently many of these bacteria occur as saprophytes in nature.

For the purpose of orientation the classification of the *Enterobacteriaceae* given by *Bergey's Manual of Determinative Bacteriology* is presented.

TRIBE 1. *Escherichieae*—Ferment lactose.
    Genus 1.   *Escherichia*—Inhabitant of the intestines of animals.
    Genus 2.   *Aerobacter*—Sometimes may be present in intestines of animals.
    Genus 3.   *Klebsiella*—Found in respiratory, intestinal, and urogenital tracts of animals.
    Genus 4.   *Paracolobactrum*—Opportunists, widely scattered in nature.
    Genus 5.   *Alginobacter*—Nonpathogenic organisms from soil.
TRIBE 2. *Erwinieae*—Ferment lactose.
    Genus 1.   *Erwinia*—Plant parasites.
TRIBE 3. *Serratieae*—Ferment lactose, rapidly liquefy gelatin.
    Genus 1.   *Serratia*—Chromogenic bacteria, nonpathogenic.
TRIBE 4. *Proteeae*—Do not ferment lactose. Decompose urea.
    Genus 1.   *Proteus*—Rarely pathogenic.
TRIBE 5. *Salmonelleae*—Rarely ferment lactose. Do not decompose urea.
    Genus 1.   *Salmonella*—Salmonellosis of man and animals.
    Genus 2.   *Shigella*—Shigellosis of man.

Table IX.  SOME DIFFERENTIAL CHARACTERISTICS OF ENTERIC GROUPS CONCERNED IN ANIMAL DISEASES

|  | Cultural features | | | | | | | | | | | | |
|---|---|---|---|---|---|---|---|---|---|---|---|---|---|
| Enteric groups | Semisolid motility medium | Gelatin | Hydrogen sulfide | Indol | Urea | Methyl red | Voges-Proskauer | Citrate medium | Glucose | Lactose | Sucrose | Salicin | KCN medium |
| *Escherichia coli* | v | – | – | + | – | + | – | – | ag | ag | v | v | – |
| *Klebsiella-Aerobacter* | (–) | (–) | – | – | s | v | v | + | ag | ag | ag | ag | + |
| "Paracolon bacilli" | | | | | | | | | | | | | |
| *Citrobacter* | +++ | – | + | > | s– | +++ | – | +++ | ag | > | > | > | ++ |
| *Providence* | +++ | – | – | + | – | +++ | – | +++ | ag | – | s | – | ++ |
| *Arizona* | +++ | s | +++ | + | (+) | – | – | – | av | s | – | – | + |
| *Proteus* | ++ | + | ++ | + | – | ++ | – | + | ag | – | av | – | – |
| *Salmonella* | | – | + | – | – | + | – | + | ag | – | – | – | – |
| *Shigella* | – | – | – | (–) | – | + | – | – | a– | (–) | (–) | – | + |

v = variable;  – = negative;  (–) = usually negative, but important exceptions occur;  + = positive;  s = slow utilization;  s – = slow utilization or negative;  ag = acid and gas;  av = acid with or without gas;  a – = acid without gas.

Biochemical and cultural reactions and antigenic structure have led to the more conventional groupings given below.

1. The *Escherichieae* tribe, consisting of the *Escherichia* (the classic colon bacillus, including alkalescens-dispar) and the *Shigella* (the dysentery bacilli).

2. The *Edwardsielleae*, containing the genus *Edwardsiella*.

3. The *Salmonelleae*, made up of the genera *Salmonella*, *Arizona*, and *Citrobacter* (including Bethesda-Ballerup).

4. The *Klebsielleae*, embracing the *Klebsiella*, *Enterobacter* (formerly *Aerobacter*, and including *Hafnia*), *Pectobacterium*, and *Serratia*.

5. The *Proteeae*, represented by the two genera, *Proteus* and *Providencia*.

In 1969, Niléhn (51) published an article on *Yersinia enterocolitica*, an organism that has been isolated from man, pigs, chinchillas, and hares. It is suggested that this organism belongs in the family *Enterobacteriaceae* and that it occurs in certain types of acute enteric infection in man.

For years the species and genera of the *Enterobacteriaceae* were characterized according to source of isolation and biochemical behavior. However, physiological characteristics proved to be variable even among members of the same species, and accurate identifications were impossible. Finally, recognition of the antigens possessed by the bacteria became the basis of identification, and serological methods have largely replaced the biochemical tests.

The isolation of enteric bateria is accomplished by means of various selective and enrichment mediums (19). Before attempting serological classification, a preliminary grouping based on certain physiological characteristics of the enteric isolate is often made. These groups are presented in table IX. It must be understood that the differences listed for each group are not fixed but tend to vary according to the species examined. At best, table IX presents only a very general biochemical classification of each group.

Polyvalent antiserums (7, 19) and bacteriophage (12) are useful tools in grouping members of the *Enterobacteriaceae*. The FA technic has not been especially helpful in selecting *Salmonella* types, but has proved to be useful in detecting enteropathogenic *Escherichia coli* types (14, 49). Wide-spectrum bacteriophages can be used to separate salmonellae from other enteric bacteria, but not to differentiate the serotypes (61).

In this chapter serological studies will be considered in the discussions of the various genera. Because the antigenic analysis of the *Salmonella* has received much study and is further advanced than that of the other genera in the family, it will be reviewed in greater detail when that genus is considered. For purposes of presentation the *Enterobacteriaceae* are diveded into the lactose-fermenting and non-lactose-fermenting groups.

## THE LACTOSE-FERMENTING GROUP

Among the organisms that ferment lactose are the members of the genera *Escherichia*, *Aerobacter* (*Enterobacter*), *Klebsiella*, *Paracolobactrum* (*Citro-*

*bacter* and *Arizona*), *Alginobacter* and *Erwinia* (*Pectobacterium*), and *Serratia*. Because the *Pectobacterium* are not animal paraisites, they are not discussed. Chromogenic *Serratia* have been reported in bovine mastitis (4) and in septicemias in man (29), but these bacteria usually are regarded as nonpathogens and of no concern in lower animal disease. In the genus *Escherichia* the type species is *E. coli*. It is quite strictly parasitic in its habits and is not found abundantly anywhere in nature except in intestinal tracts, in feces, and in materials that have been subjected to fecal pollution. Kauffmann (39) claims that the members of the genus listed in *Bergey's Manual* as *Klebsiella* are serologically identical with members of the *Aerobacter* genus. Accordingly, we will consider them as the *Klebsiella-Aerobacter* group. These species may be found in the alimentary tract of animals. Some members of the *Klebsiella-Aerobacter* group grow freely in nature on grains and plants, and others are found in the respiratory, intestinal, and genitourinary tracts of man and animals. Members of the genus *Paracolobactrum* ferment lactose slowly or in some instances not at all. They are often called *paracolon bacteria* and comprise a group that is widespread in nature and able to infect both warm- and cold-blooded animals. The members of the *Escherichieae* are frequently referred to as the *colon-aerogenes*, or the *coliform*, group of bacteria. Strains of this group are sought in bacteriological examination of water, and their presence is interpreted as evidence of fecal pollution.

In discussing *E. coli* (see below), especial emphasis will be given to the morphological and physiological characteristics of the species because, in general, its morphology and staining reactions as well as many of its cultural features are typical for all members of the enteric family. In subsequent discussions of the individual members of this family comments on morphological and physiological characters will be limited to the special cultural features of the type concerned.

## ESCHERICHIA COLI (BACTERIUM COLI)

This organism is a normal inhabitant of the lower bowel of all warm-blooded animals. It usually is absent from the intestines of fish and other cold-blooded animals. Few or none are found in the stomach and anterior portions of the bowel. Carnivora and omnivora usually harbor the organism in greater abundance than the herbivora. The feces of cows and horses frequently show very few.

According to Kauffmann (38), the ordinary *E. coli* strains are serologically divisible into a number of types. Certain of these types possess a particular pathogenicity and play an important role in various animal diseases. Within the group, cultural tests are of little value and type division rests on antigenic recognition. The three classes of antigens that are important in *E. coli* serology are: (*a*) the O antigens, or somatic antigens not inactivated by heat; (*b*) the K antigens, which are also somatic antigens but occur as sheaths, envelopes, or as capsules (they inhibit O agglutination and are inactivated by heat); (*c*) the H or flagellar antigens. (See page 149 for further details on H and O antigens.) Strains containing K antigen appear to be more toxic and resistant to phagocytosis and bactericidal action of antibody than those lacking this antigen.

**Morphology and Staining Reactions.** *E. coli* is a small rod-shaped organism that varies widely in morphology under varying conditions. Usually it is a short, plump rod; sometimes rather long filaments are seen. It may be motile or nonmotile. Spores are never formed, and capsular material is absent from most but not all strains. It stains readily and evenly with ordinary stains and is Gram-negative.

**Cultural Features.** *E. coli* grows readily on all ordinary media. Its optimum temperature is about that of the body, but it will grow through a wide range. It is aerobic and facultative anaerobic. Most strains show motility of a sluggish type.

In broth there is uniform clouding within 12 to 18 hours. On old cultures friable pellicles form, and very old cultures show considerable viscid sediment. Agar surface colonies are slightly raised, smooth, glistening, unpigmented, and circular in outline. Deep colonies usually are lenticular in shape and brownish. On slants the growth becomes confluent, and the water of syneresis, turbid. Gelatin colonies are thin, bluish-white, translucent, and glistening. The surface usually shows radial ridges, and the margins are somewhat irregular, giving the colonies the shape of a grape leaf. The gelatin is not liquefied. Growth on potato is less abundant than on agar, is brownish and rather dry. Some strains are strongly hemolytic, producing wide zones of Beta-type hemolysis around colonies on blood agar plates. Others have no hemolytic action. According to Smith (63) the hemolytic strains produce at least two hemolysins which he designates Alpha and Beta. The Alpha-hemolysin is filterable and the Beta-hemolysin is not. Litmus milk is acidified and coagulated within 24 hours at 37 C. The litmus is reduced except near the surface. Glucose and lactose are attacked by all strains, both acid and gas being formed. On other carbohydrate media, acid and gas are formed from some and not from others, depending upon the strain.

Indol is formed, usually in abundance; nitrates are vigorously reduced; and the Voges-Proskauer reaction is negative. This last reaction is considered valuable in distinguishing *E. coli* types from *A. aerogenes*, which give a positive reaction.

**Resistance.** *E. coli* is fairly resistant to drying and to the action of many chemical disinfectants. Usually it is destroyed by pasteurization, but certain heat-resistant strains may withstand this exposure (Stark and Patterson, 70).

**Pathogenicity.** Some strains of *E. coli* appear to be harmless parasites. That the organism may be pathogenic at times, or that certain serotypes may be pathogenic, has been known for a long time. Even the so-called *harmless types* that are normally found in the intestines appear to be opportunists— able to cause peritonitis following the abdominal operations, rupture of the intestines, and wounds perforating the digestive tract.

*E. coli* has been isolated from cases of mastitis. urogenital infections, abortions, diarrheal diseases of newborn animals (including man), and other pathologic processes. It is one of the most common organisms encountered in cultures made from animal tissues, especially when the tissues have been removed from the body some hours after death. This poses the question of whether the organism escaped from the digestive tract about the time of death and acted as a secondary invader of the tissues or whether it was primarily concerned in producing disease. Furthermore, the number of infections actually incited by types normally found in the intestinal tract in contrast to those caused by the so-called *pathogenic serotypes* is not known.

That certain serotypes are of major concern in infant diarrhea has been definitely established. The formulas of some of these types are O 111: B4, O 55: B5, and O 26: B6 (71). The somatic antigens are indicated by the letter O and figures and the K antigens are denoted by the letter B and figures. H antigens are also assigned figures. A formula that represents a motile type is O 26: B6: 11. It has also been demonstrated that adult human volunteers who were fed strain O 55: B5 obtained from infant diarrhea developed gastroenteritis, while those fed a strain of *E. coli* from a normal infant experienced no ill effects (36). Young *et al.* (77) studied an outbreak of gastroenteritis in infants and presented evidence to indicate that it was caused by serotype O 111: B4 uncomplicated by viruses or other microbial agents. Among the sources of infection for infants are unheated cow's milk (72) and household pets such as dogs and cats (46).

For years the question of the causal relation of *E. coli* to a disease in young calves commonly called *white scours* or *calf scours* has been debated. It now seems that certain serotypes are more important than others. In fact it was shown by Orskov (52) that type O 26: B6 occurs both in calf scours and in infant diarrhea. Wood (76) studied the epidemiology of white scours under experimental conditions and concluded that the disease was caused by enteropathogenic *E. coli*. In the most acute form of white scours the calf shows weakness, appears sleepy, and soon dies without other symptoms. In the usual form the calf shows a severe diarrhea, the fecal material often being full of gas bubbles and whitish because of lack of bile. The animal may die after a few days, or it may recover. In the more protracted cases, lameness may appear because of acute inflammation in one or more joints. In such joints the capsule is distended with a cloudy fluid in which there are myriads of colon bacilli. These animals nearly always die eventually. Calves that have passed through these infections frequently exhibit whitish fibrotic areas in the cortex of the kidneys.

Smith and Little (64) pointed out the interesting fact that calves that are deprived of the first milk (colostrum) of their dams nearly always develop *E. coli* septicemia. In a series of papers by Smith and his co-workers (44, 65–67), the mechanism of this septicemia is made clear. It appears that the function of colostrum is to carry to the digestive tract of the newborn calf protection against miscellaneous bacteria, principally colon bacilli, which are harmless to older animals but which rapidly invade the tissues of very young calves from intestinal canals that have not had the protection offered by colostrum.

It was shown by Smith and his co-workers that normal cow serum would function almost as well as colostrum in protecting the newborn calf. Normal cow serum contains antibodies for the colon bacillus; hence these antibodies rapidly appear in the blood of the calf when the serum is fed mixed with milk. The calf is protected best, however, when cow serum is both injected subcutaneously and fed.

Actually, white scours in calves appears to be the result of shifting the equilibrium between the young calf and *E. coli*. An upset favors the microorganism and enables it to invade the tissues. Whether or not it produces death depends on the virulence of the bacterium and other factors affecting the host (45). In controlling calf scours it should be remembered that colostrum as well as calf management is important. Changing the environment of the calf soon after birth or the environment of the cow shortly before parturition may be hazardous because the newborn calf may then meet bacteria against which it has no immunity.

Howarth (33) has reported a large outbreak of abortion in sheep in California in which an organism belonging to the colon group seemed to be the causative agent. Of a band of 820 ewes, abortions occurred in 219, and of the aborting ewes, 101 died shortly after the act. The organism was readily isolated from the body fluids and tissues of the fetuses and from the placentae, uterus, and uterine discharges of the ewes. With the cultures, abortions were readily produced by intravenous injection, but not by subcultaneous injection or by feeding. The flock had been forced to drink from stagnant pools containing a great deal of organic material, and it was thought that these pools had been the source of the infection. In cultural features the organism isolated from these ewes differed in no way from organisms found commonly in the intestinal canal. Serologic studies were not made. Roberts (55, 56) reported outbreaks of disease in lambs that resembled white scours in calves and Rees (54), in England, isolated pathogenic serotypes of *E. coli* from cases of septicemia and diarrhea in lambs. In South Africa, Botes (6) described colisepticemia in lambs, caused most frequently by serotype O 78: B80 and characterized by severe nervous symptoms, meningitis accompanied by excessive amounts of cerebrospinal fluid, ascites, hydropericardium, endo- and epicardial hemorrhages, and tumor hepatitis without any marked gastrointestinal disturbances.

In a 26-year study of infections in fetuses and foals, Dimock, Edwards, and Bruner (16) found that *E. coli* accounted for approximately 1 percent of the abortions observed in mares and for about 5 percent of the deaths of foals. Foals that succumbed to *E. coli* infection usually were ill at birth. They presented symptoms of increased temperature and pulse rate besides being dull and weak. Death frequently occurred within 24 hours after the onset of the disease. In foals examined before postmortem decomposition the microorganisms were isolated from the internal organs and frequently from the synovial fluid of the joints. It has been suggested that equine colitis X, an acute diarrheal disease accompanied by shock, may be caused by endotoxins of enteropathogenic *E. coli*.

*Coli-granuloma* or *Hjärre's disease* is a condition in chickens characterized by granulomatous lesions in the wall of the digestive tract and in the liver. It was described by Hjärre and Wramby (32) in 1945, who reported a coliform organism to be the causative agent. This condition is seen infrequently in this country and confirmation of the etiology has not appeared. That the inoculation of certain strains of *E. coli* into chickens produces aerosacculitis, fibrinous pericarditis, perihepatitis, salpingitis, and panophthalmitis was demonstrated by Gross (28). Harry (30) and Glantz *et al.* (25) have isolated pathogenic serotypes from outbreaks of septicemia and from cases of chronic respiratory disease and salpingitis in poultry. *E. coli* has been associated with coliform pericarditis in broiler chickens (31) and the organism usually is present in respiratory infections involving the *Mycoplasma*.

It appears that a disease known as *pig scours* is related to *E. coli* infection, but the etiology may be concerned with hypersensitivity rather than to a direct toxic effect or to a simple infective enteritis (37).

Nielsen *et al.* (50) claim that *piglet diarrhea, weanling diarrhea,* and *edema disease* comprise three distinct entities of enteric colibacillosis. In diarrheal diseases, *E. coli* produces a toxin which induces the movement of fluid into the intestinal lumen. In edema disease, the organism appears to elaborate a toxin which, when absorbed, causes neurologic disturbances and edema. On the other hand, Kashiwazaki *et al.* (37) list the three distinct entities in which *E. coli* plays a role in piglet diseases as *neonatal colibacillosis* (septicemic form), *pig scours* (hypersensitive state), and *edema disease* (anaphylactic shock).

*Edema disease of swine* (gut edema) occurs in young pigs, where it is acute and highly fatal. It is characterized by edema in one or more parts of the body of the affected animal, although this lesion may be absent.

The disease was first described by Shanks (60) in Ireland in 1938. Since then it has been recognized in a number of European countries, in the United States, and in Canada. According to Timoney (73) and Lamont *et al.* (41), four fairly constant conditions are associated with the occurrence of edema disease: (*a*) age—weanlings are most commonly involved, but occasionally pigs of any age may be affected; (*b*) change of feed—frequently a change either in feed or methods of feeding has been made; this is a natural occurrence at weaning time; (*c*) rapid growth—the disease is seen most frequently in thriving animals; (*d*) diarrhea—mild diarrhea often occurs a day or two before the attack.

There is still some doubt (24, 74) as to the etiology of the disease. Although Underdahl *et al.* (75) have indicated a viral cause there is also much evidence to indicate that specific hemolytic serotypes of *E. coli* (17, 42, 57, 69) are the cause. Ewing *et al.* (23) studied 38 *E. coli* cultures isolated in Ireland and the United States from cases of edema disease of swine. Two serotypes belonging to groups O 138: B81 and O 139: B82 occurred most frequently and were found in both countries. Kramer (40) has reported that the serotype found most frequently in Ontario and western Canada belongs in group O 141. Gregory (27) is of the opinion that stress triggers the appearance of edema disease and that it is a form of intestinal toxemia caused by the specific *E. coli* types.

The signs of the disease are variable. Pigs may be found dead without illness having been observed. More often they die after about 1 to 2 days of clinical sickness. Ill pigs rarely recover. The first symptoms are disturbance of locomotion in which the front, rear, or all four limbs may be involved. There is no increase in temperature. Paralysis and stupor are seen in the final stage. Edema of the eyelids and surrounding areas is common. The animals do not resist handling. The disease is most common in 8- to 20-week-old pigs.

Morbidity varies from about 4 to 37 percent and mortality from 50 to 70 percent. Edema is the characteristic lesion of the disease. It may occur in the eyelids and around the face. It is common in the stomach between the mucosa and the muscle layers. The gall bladder, perirenal areas, intestines, lungs, subcutaneous tissues, and the nervous system may show edema. It should be noted that in any animal only a part or an area may be edematous and this lesion may be absent in some cases.

An epizootic of food poisoning in mink was reported to be the result of feeding spoiled food contaminated with hemolytic *E. coli* and hemolytic *Paracolobactrum* spp. (47).

**Colon Bacillus Toxin.** Organisms of this group are regarded ordinarily as non-toxin-formers. Smith and Little (65), however, showed that filtrates of comparatively young broth cultures of certain strains of colon bacilli isolated from cases of calf septicemia were toxic to calves and older cattle when injected intravenously. Grave symptoms were often followed by death. The signs consisted of rapidly developing and severe dyspnea, and after death the lungs were found to be filled with a foamy, edematous fluid. Large doses of such filtrates did not produce symptoms when injected subcutaneously. The authors found that similar results could be obtained with filtrates of some paratyphoid bacilli. They did not determine the nature of the toxic material. Since the work of Smith and Little, Davis *et al.* (13) and Inukai *et al.* (34) have separated highly toxic fractions from strains of hemolytic *E. coli* that were associated with edema disease. Their substances were obtained by electrophoresis and by chromatography and appeared to be endotoxins.

Killed whole cultures of *E. coli* are especially toxic for horses, and intravenous injection of as much as 5 ml of a recently killed culture may be followed, within less than 24 hours, by the death of the animal.

**Immunity.** Calf scours serum made by immunizing horses or cattle with strains of colon bacilli isolated from calves suffering from white scours has been widely used as a means of treating animals suffering from this disease. The results reported have varied widely. It seems very doubtful that such sera have materially altered the course of the disease. Shortly after injection the calves frequently appear better for a time, but a similar effect can be obtained by injecting blood or blood serum from normal cattle.

Hemagglutination tests are of value in detecting *E. coli* infection, especially in infants. The antigen is prepared by subjecting sheep erythrocytes to protein extracts of *E. coli* strains.

There is evidence that inoculation of the dam with formalinized culture protects newborn pigs against the homologous strain, but not against heterologous serotypes. This makes vaccination impractical, because so many types are involved.

**Chemotherapy.** The antibiotic most effective against this organism seems to be dihydrostreptomycin. To treat edema disease Austvoll (2) recommends the use of vitamin $B_1$ and phthalylsulfathiazole (sulfathalidine) within the first day or so of sickness. Gouge and Elliott (26) report that acetozolamide sodium is effective. Furazolidone has proved to be efficacious and the use of erythromycin has been advocated, but Smith (62) cautions that antibiotics have a profound effect on the emergence of resistant strains of *E. coli*. With this in mind it now appears that polymyxin, nalidixic acid, sulfachloropyridazine, and kanamycin-ampicillin are among the more effective agents (9, 48, 68). The antihistamine (Allermin) has been reported to be highly efficacious in the treatment of naturally occurring edema disease of swine (53).

## THE *KLEBSIELLA-AEROBACTER* GROUP

Although certain members of this group are lacking in pathogenicity, some of the types are associated with mastitis (1), with respiratory and urogenital infections in man, with genital infections of animals, and possibly with endotoxemia in horses (11). The mucoid (encapsulated) types within the group, known as *klebsiellas*, are of most importance. In man, *Klebsiella pneumoniae* (Friedlander's bacillus) has been recognized in respiratory, urogenital, and intestinal (severe diarrheal) diseases.

Strains of *Klebsiella* have been classified serologically by Kauffmann (39). Among these encapsulated types is the organism *Klebsiella pneumoniae* var. *genitalium* described in 1927 by Dimock and Edwards (15) as the cause of a particular type of urogenital infection of mares.

### *Klebsiella pneumoniae* var. *genitalium*

**Morphology and Staining Reactions.** This microorganism is a Gram-negative, nonmotile, non-spore-bearing, encapsulated rod. The capsules are readily demonstrable and are responsible for an excessively mucoid form of growth on culture media.

**Cultural Features.** The organism grows readily on ordinary laboratory media. On agar slants there occurs an excessively dirty-white to slightly yellow growth that is moist, spreading, glistening, and very viscid. Agar colonies are large, raised, round, and entire. Broth becomes turbid, with a ropy sediment. A typical nailhead growth appears in gelatin; no liquefaction occurs. Acid and coagulation are produced in litmus milk. Nitrates are reduced to nitrites and ammonia. Indol is not formed. Most strains are methyl-red-negative and Voges-Proskauer-positive.

**Pathogenicity.** This bacterium is found infrequently in the genital tract of mares, where it causes a severe metritis. It has appeared in a high percentage of cases in individual groups and is exceedingly difficult to eliminate when once established in the uterus. It can readily be transmitted from infected to healthy mares by the stallion at time of service and by the hands and instruments of the individual who examines or treats the mares. It has also been found in ureteritis, mastitis, and septicemia in the moose and in mastitis in cattle (3, 18).

**Immunity.** None known at this time.

**Chemotherapy.** The organisms appear to be most sensitive to streptomycin (43).

## PARACOLON BACTERIA

These organisms belong in the family *Enterobacteriaceae* and possess features common to the well-established groups, but do not exactly fit into them. In general, they are motile or nonmotile enteric bacteria that produce hydrogen sulfide and seldom produce indol. Usually they are methyl-red-positive and Voges-Proskauer-negative. They produce acid and gas from glucose and vary in their ability to ferment sucrose or salicin. They often ferment lactose, either rapidly or after several days of incubation, and sometimes liquefy gelatin.

The *Citrobacter*—Bethesda-Ballerup group embraces a part of the species *Paracolobacterum intermedium* of Borman *et al.* (5), which in turn contains the organisms designated as the *Escherichia freundi* (8, 19, 22). This group as well as the others cited below were set up because of close serological relations among the members forming each lot. There is some slight sharing of antigens among the groups. The members have been associated with gastroenteritis in man and have been found in the feces of domestic animals. Their role in enteric infections is not clear. A paracolon type that proved to be closely related biochemically and serologically to certain members of the Ballerup subgroup has been isolated from cases of mastitis in a herd of dairy cattle. This bacterium was present in the udders of all the affected animals and appeared to be the causative agent (35).

The Providence group was proposed by Kauffmann (1951) for the paracolon bacteria type of 29911 of Stuart and co-workers (19). The members form an intermediate group of enteric bacteria that resemble certain species of the genus *Proteus*, but differ from them in failing to utilize urea rapidly. Bacteria of the group have been isolated from stools in sporadic cases and small outbreaks of diarrhea in man, but they occur also in the feces of normal individuals.

The Arizona group was established by Edwards *et al.* (21). Members of this group have been isolated from reptiles, fowls, rodents, swine, man, and egg powder. They are pathogenic and able to initiate infection in fowls. Their presence in the blood and internal organs of poults from flocks that have suffered heavy mortality, and the absence of any other known pathogenic organism or any recognized debilitating factor, indicate their primary role in the infection. It appears that these paracolon bacteria can be transmitted through the egg, a condition that is not uncommon in *Salmonella* infections of fowls. They have been isolated from cases of abortion in ewes (58) and from otitis media in a child (10). Details on studies of the Arizona group of paracolon bacteria were published by Edwards *et al.* in 1959 (20). Arizona bacterins have provided varying degrees of immunity in turkeys (59).

## REFERENCES

1.  Adler.   North Am. Vet., 1951, *32*, 96.
2.  Austvoll.   Vet. Rec., 1952, *64*, 135.
3.  Barnes.   Jour. Am. Vet Med. Assoc., 1954, *125*, 50.
4.  Barnum, Thackeray and Fish.   Canad. Jour. Comp. Med. and Vet. Sci., 1958, *22*, 392.
5.  Borman, Stuart, and Wheeler.   Jour. Bact., 1944, *48*, 351.
6.  Botes.   Jour. So. African Vet. Med. Assoc., 1966, *37*, 17.
7.  Bruner.   Cornell Vet., 1957, *47*, 491.
8.  Bruner, Edwards, and Hopson.   Ky. Agr. Exp. Sta. Bul. 543, 1949.
9.  Bulger and Roosen-Runge.   Am. Jour. Med. Sci., 1969, *258*, 7.
10. Butt and Morris.   Jour. Inf. Dis., 1952, *91*, 293.
11. Carroll, Schalm, and Wheat.   Jour. Am. Vet. Med. Assoc., 1965, *146*, 1300.
12. Cherry, Davis, Edwards, and Hogan.   Jour. Lab. and Clin. Med., 1954, *44*, 51.
13. Davis, Allen, and Smibert.   Am. Jour. Vet. Res., 1961, *22*, 736.
14. Davis and Ewing.   Am. Jour. Clin. Path., 1963, *39*, 198.
15. Dimock and Edwards.   Jour. Am. Vet. Med. Assoc., 1927, *70*, 469.
16. Dimock, Edwards, and Bruner.   Cornell Vet., 1947, *37*, 89.
17. Dunne.   Canad. Jour. Comp. Med. and Vet. Sci., 1959, *23*, 101.
18. Easterbrooks and Plastridge.   Jour. Am. Vet. Med. Assoc., 1956, *128*, 502.
19. Edwards and Ewing.   Identification of enterobacteriaceae. Burgess Publishing Co., Minneapolis, Minn., 1955.
20. Edwards, Fife, and Ramsey.   Bact. Rev., 1959, *23*, 155.
21. Edwards, West, and Bruner.   Ky. Agr. Exp. Sta. Bul. 499, 1947.
22. Edwards, West, and Bruner.   Jour. Bact., 1948, *55*, 711.
23. Ewing, Tatum, and Davis.   Cornell Vet., 1958, *48*, 201.
24. Gitter and Lloyd.   Brit. Vet. Jour., 1957, *113*, 212.
25. Glantz, Narotsky, and Bubash.   Avian Dis., 1962, *6*, 322.
26. Gouge and Elliott.   Vet. Med., 1959, *54*, 295.
27. Gregory.   Jour. Am. Vet. Med. Assoc., 1959, *135*, 321.

28. Gross. Am. Jour. Vet. Res., 1957, *18*, 724.
29. Haiby, McFarland, and Moore. Am. Jour. Clin. Path., 1961, *36*, 256.
30. Harry. Vet. Rec., 1964, *76*, 443.
31. Hemsley and Harry. *Ibid.*, 1965, 77, 103.
32. Hjärre and Wramby. Skand. Vet. Tidskr., 1945, *35*, 449.
33. Howarth. Cornell Vet., 1932, *22*, 253.
34. Inukai, Kodama, and Haga. Jap. Jour. Vet. Res., 1962, *10*, 57.
35. Johnson, Bruner, and Murphy. Cornell Vet., 1951, *41*, 283.
36. June, Ferguson, and Worfel. Am. Jour. Hyg., 1953, *57*, 222.
37. Fujiwara. Cornell Vet., 1969, *59*, 622.
38. Kauffmann. Jour. Immunol., 1946, *57*, 71.
39. Kauffmann. Acta Path. et Microbiol. Scand., 1949, *26*, 381.
40. Kramer. Canad. Jour. Comp. Med. and Vet. Sci., 1960, *24*, 289.
41. Lamont, Luke, and Gordon. Vet. Rec., 1950, *62*, 737.
42. Lemcke, Bellis, and Hirsch. *Ibid.*, 1957, *69*, 601.
43. Lemke and Gates. Jour. Lab. and Clin. Med., 1951, *38*, 889.
44. Little and Orcutt. Jour. Exp. Med., 1922, *35*, 161.
45. Lovell. Vet. Rev. and Annot., 1955, *1*, 1.
46. Mian. Jour. Am. Med. Assoc., 1959, *171*, 1957.
47. Mills and Radostits. Canad. Vet. Jour., 1970, *11*, 137.
48. Mongeau and Larivée. *Ibid.*, 1965, *6*, 220.
49. Nelson, Whitaker, Hempstead, and Harris. Jour. Am. Med. Assoc., 1961, *176*, 26.
50. Nielson, Moon, and Roe. Jour. Am. Vet. Med. Assoc., 1968, *152*, 1307.
51. Niléhn. Acta Path. et Microbiol. Scand., 1969, Sup. 206, pp. 5–45.
52. Orskov. *Ibid.*, 1951, *29*, 373.
53. Pan, Chen, and Morter. Canad. Jour. Comp. Med., 1970, *34*, 148.
54. Rees. Jour. Comp. Path. and Therap., 1958, *68*, 399.
55. Roberts. Austral. Vet. Jour., 1957, *33*, 43.
56. *Ibid.*, 1958, *34*, 152.
57. Roberts and Vallely. Vet. Rec., 1959, *71*, 846.
58. Ryff and Browne. Jour. Am. Vet. Med. Assoc., 1952, *121*, 266.
59. Sato and Adler. Avian Dis., 1966, *10*, 239.
60. Shanks. Vet. Rec., 1938, *50*, 356.
61. Silliker and Taylor. Jour. Lab. and Clin. Med., 1957, *49*, 460.
62. Smith. Vet. Rec., 1960, *74*, 1178.
63. Smith. Jour. Path. and Bact., 1963, *85*, 197.
64. Smith and Little. Jour. Exp. Med., 1922, *36*, 181.
65. *Ibid.*, 184.
66. *Ibid.*, 453.
67. *Ibid.*, 1927, *46*, 125.
68. Smith. Jour. Hyg. (London), 1966, *64*, 465.
69. Sojka, Erskine, and Lloyd. Vet. Rec., 1957, *69*, 293.
70. Stark and Patterson. Jour. Dairy Sci., 1936, *19*, 495.
71. Thomson. Jour. Hyg. (London), 1955, *53*, 357.
72. *Ibid.*, 1956, *54*, 311.
73. Timoney. Vet. Rec., 1950, *62*, 748.
74. Underdahl, Blore, and Young. Jour. Am. Vet. Med. Assoc., 1959, *135*, 615.

75.   Underdahl, Stair, and Young.   *Ibid.*, 1963, *142*, 27.
76.   Wood.   Jour. Path. and Bact., 1955, *70*, 179.
77.   Young, Warren, and Lindberg.   Proc. Soc. Exp. Biol. and Med., 1959, *100*, 579.

## THE NON-LACTOSE-FERMENTING ENTERIC ORGANISMS

In morphology and in many cultural features, these organisms are not unlike the bacteria discussed above; however, they ordinarily do not ferment lactose. The genera falling in this category are *Edwardsiella, Proteus, Salmonella,* and *Shigella,* although some rare lactose-fermenters occur in the group. Actually members of the genus *Providencia* (Providence group) belong in the non-lactose-fermenting category, but originally they were assigned to the paracolons and in this edition we have discussed them under *Paracolon Bacteria.*

A new genus of the *Enterobacteriaceae* was established in 1965 by Ewing *et al.* (22). The name *Edwardsiella* was selected for this serologic grouping that includes organisms sometimes referred to as *Asakusa* and *Bartholomew* types. The cultures studied were isolated from man and the lower animals, including cold-blooded species. They make up a group of serotypes whose IMViC reactions are similar to those of *Escherichia coli,* but they do not ferment lactose. Serologic studies have demonstrated over 21 serotypes.

Recent isolations of *Edwardsiella* from meningitis and diarrhea in man, as well as from snakes, sea lions, and alligators indicate that the organisms are widespread and that the main reservoir may be the cold-blooded vertebrates.

Organisms of the genus *Proteus* are readily differentiated from the *Salmonelleae* because of their ability to decompose urea. Another characteristic of *Proteus* strains is their tendency to *swarm* on solid media. This may be defined as progressive surface spreading by bacteria from the parent colony. Among motile *Proteus* cultures this spreading growth over the surface produces a uniform layer hardly distinguishable from the medium and makes the isolation of other enteric bacteria from a mixed culture very difficult. Organisms of the *Proteus* group are widely distributed in nature. Though often demonstrable in the feces of animals, especially in dogs and hogs, they rarely are found in large numbers except when the normal intestinal mechanism is deranged. Under certain conditions they apparently are able to grow in the animal body and even to give rise to pathological disturbances, but as a rule they are not important in animal diseases.

Some organisms of the *Salmonelleae* are associated with specific diseases, and many others are connected with septicemia, enteritis, and diarrhea of man and animals. Formerly it was customary to divide the organisms of this group into (*a*) those that form acid and gas from glucose (The Intermediate or Paratyphoid Group), and (*b*) those that form acid only (The Typhoid-Dysentery Group). This arrangement placed the typhoid organism in one group and the *Salmonella* (paratyphoid) organisms in another, a classification that cannot be justified by other criteria, and placed together the typhoid and dysentery organisms that are not closely related otherwise. On the basis of serologic classification (antigenic analysis) the typhoid organism of man is a *Salmonella.*

## THE GENUS *SALMONELLA*

Soon after the isolation of the "hog cholera bacillus" by Salmon and Smith (57) in 1885, paratyphoid bacteria were found by numerous workers in a variety of diseases of animals and in enteric fever and gastroenteritis of man. Smith and Stewart (66) in 1897 stated that these microorganisms "belong to one great group (or species) in virtue of the identity of their morphological and biological characters." However, the identity of the individual members was not clearly established until White (73) recognized the importance of considering bacterial variation in relation to the antigenic analysis of paratyphoid strains. The pioneer work of White, confirmed and greatly extended by Kauffmann (37), resulted in the Kauffmann-White schema for the rapid and exact identification of paratyphoid bacteria. Because Salmon and Smith (57) had isolated and described the first member of the group, the generic name of *Salmonella* was chosen and *Salmonella choleraesuis* became the type species.

## DEFINITION OF THE GENUS *SALMONELLA*

The *Salmonella* group consists of serologically related, Gram-negative, aerobic, nonsporing rods, corresponding to *Salmonella typhi* in staining properties and morphology and showing, with certain exceptions, a motile peritrichous phase in which they normally occur. They do not ferment adonitol, lactose, salicin, and sucrose, liquefy gelatin, produce indol, hydrolyze urea, or form acetylmethyl-carbinol. They regularly attack glucose with, but occasionally without, gas production. All members of the group have an antigenic structure by which they can be recognized, and all the known types are pathogenic for man, animals, or both.

## SEROLOGY OF THE GENUS *SALMONELLA*

Identification of *Salmonella* cultures is based on antigenic analysis, and in order to determine the antigenic constituents it is necessary to consider the variational phenomena to which the bacteria are subject. First among these is the H and O variation of Weil and Felix (71), who investigated the heat-stable and heat-labile antigens and their relation to the soma and the flagella of the bacilli. The H (flagellar) antigens are heat-labile and the O (somatic) antigens are heat-stable. Organisms like S. *pullorum* and S. *gallinarum,* which are nonmotile, possess only the O antigens. In the antigenic formulas assigned to *Salmonella* serotypes the O antigens are designated by Arabic figures. The first step in the identification of a culture is to determine its somatic antigens. Some of these antigens are specific and identify the O group, whereas others occur in several groups. Most animal types fall into one of four large somatic groups. They are called *B, C, D,* and *E.*

Once the somatic group of the *Salmonella* strain is established, its exact identity is determined by recognizing its H antigens. Here the phase variation of Andrewes (3) assumes importance. He found that the flagellar antigens may occur in a single unit (*monophasic type*), or in two separate units (*diphasic type*). In the diphasic type the H antigen units are designated *phase* 1 and *phase* 2. They have the property of transforming one into the other. Colonies of the two phases are identical in appearance and physical characters and differ only in their serological behavior. Antigens of phase 1 are assigned small letters, and antigens of phase 2 may be designated by Arabic numbers or by small letters. Thus the antigenic formula of S. *typhimurium* is 1,4,5,12: i-1,2 (diphasic type); that of S. *chester* is 4,5,12: e,h-e,n,x (diphasic type); that of S. *abortusequi* is 4,12: -e,n,x (monophasic type); that of S. *choleraesuis* is 6,7: c-1,5 (diphasic type); and that of S. *pullorum* is 9,12: – (nonmotile type).

Besides the variational phenomena mentioned above, other *variants* such as appear in "Rough" and "Smooth" (S-R) variation as well as those concerned with the "Vi" (virulence) envelope antigen and with changes in somatic antigens (form variation) occur and tend to complicate the typing procedure. Because complete antigenic analysis in this group requires a certain amount of technical training besides a rather elaborate set of typing sera, it probably will continue to be limited to a few laboratories especially equipped for this work.

The International *Salmonella* Typing Center is located in the State Serum Institute of Copenhagen, Denmark. In this laboratory are kept standard type cultures and sera. In the United States active typing of *Salmonella* cultures is being done at the Communicable Disease Center, Enteric Bacteriology Laboratory, Atlanta, Georgia, and at the National Animal Disease Laboratory, Ames, Iowa. Many laboratory workers concerned with animal diseases can identify and classify a high percentage of the *Salmonella* strains they encounter by the use of biochemical tests and a few of the standard typing sera (Kauffmann and Edwards, 39, and Kauffmann, 38). Phage typing of cultures of *Salmonella typhi* has been of marked value in epidemiological studies of typhoid fever and trials with a few serotypes within somatic group B have established stable phage varieties for the selected salmonellas (33).

### *SALMONELLA* INFECTIONS OF ANIMALS

Edwards, Bruner, and Moran (20) reported on the occurrence and distribution of *Salmonella* types in the United States. They studied 12,000 *Salmonella* cultures derived from outbreaks of salmonellosis in animals, including man. Cultures isolated from asymptomatic carriers and from water, food, and food products also were examined. For convenience these cultures may be grouped as in table X. In 47 animal species, 106 distinct serological types were recognized. Table XI lists the outbreaks that occurred in various animal species and the number of cultures isolated. Most of the cultures were obtained from

*Table X.   SALMONELLA* CULTURES

| Source | Outbreaks | Cultures |
|---|---|---|
| Man | 1,920 | 3,488 |
| Fowls | 4,245 | 6,387 |
| Other animals | 1,510 | 2,742 |
| Water and food |  | 327 |
| Totals | 7,675 | 12,944 |

fowls. Turkeys presented the highest number. Man was the next most frequent source of *Salmonella* cultures, and then came swine, chickens, pigeons,
and dogs. A 5-year (1963–1967) review on *Salmonella* surveillance in man in
the United States established the reported annual incidence at a level of 10.4
isolations per 100,000 population, but the actual incidence was estimated to
be as great as 100 times that amount (4). Studies on mortality and morbidity
in calves have indicated that the former may reach 18 percent and the latter
20 percent of the animals in certain cattle-raising areas.

*Salmonella* infections in animals, exclusive of man, may be grouped roughly
into two categories:

1. The diseases whose clinical manifestations are sufficiently characteristic
to permit recognition with a reasonable degree of certainty. Some of these are
equine abortion, fowl typhoid, and pullorum disease, and they are caused by
specific *Salmonella* types.

*Table XI.*   THE NUMBER OF *SALMONELLA*
CULTURES ISOLATED FROM
DIFFERENT ANIMALS AND THE
NUMBER OF OUTBREAKS FROM
WHICH THEY CAME

| Source | Outbreaks | Cultures |
|---|---|---|
| Man | 1,920 | 3,488 |
| Turkeys | 2,390 | 4,007 |
| Chickens | 1,603 | 1,956 |
| Pigeons | 109 | 210 |
| Ducks | 56 | 90 |
| Geese | 4 | 4 |
| Other domestic fowls | 2 | 2 |
| Pheasants | 23 | 29 |
| Other game birds | 17 | 30 |
| Canaries | 30 | 46 |
| Other birds | 11 | 13 |
| Horses | 51 | 77 |
| Cattle | 69 | 78 |
| Sheep | 43 | 44 |
| Other ruminants | 3 | 4 |
| Swine | 1,056 | 2,119 |
| Dogs | 73 | 103 |
| Cats | 16 | 34 |
| Other carnivora | 87 | 103 |
| Rats and mice | 52 | 88 |
| Guinea pigs | 46 | 76 |
| Other rodents | 14 | 16 |
| Totals | 7,675 | 12,617 |

2. The diseases whose clinical symptoms merely indicate a *Salmonella* infection. This type of outbreak occurs most frequently and can be caused by almost any one of the *Salmonella* types. The infections are septicemic in nature and are characterized by weakness, recumbency, and increased temperature. Pregnant animals may abort. Brain symptoms and convulsions may be observed in some cases in calves and in adult cattle. Blindness may appear in chicks (21). Diarrhea is usually one of the accompanying symptoms. In fact, experience has shown that most any tissue or joint-cavity may be involved.

Records of isolations show that outbreaks of salmonellosis are more common in young animals, and the mortality in these exceeds that of adults. While primarily a disease of immature animals, salmonellosis frequently appears in debilitating conditions of both young and adult animals. It usually assumes a septicemic condition in lower animals. Although it can do the same in the enteric (typhoid and paratyphoid) fevers of man, it frequently causes only a gastroenteritis. Asymptomatic carriers appear in both man and animals, and it is quite possible that some animals become carriers without

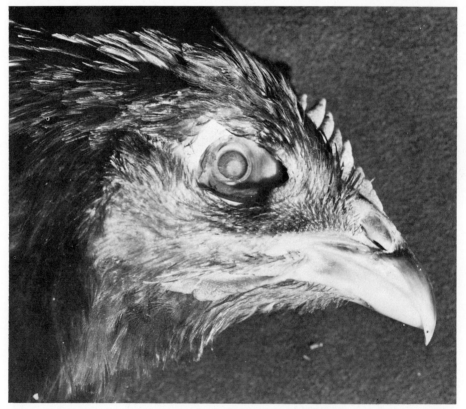

*Fig. 5.* A blind eye in a chick infected with salmonellosis. (Courtesy W. M. Evans, *Cornell Vet.*)

showing evidence of *Salmonella* infection. The main carriers of salmonellosis appear to be fowl, man, swine, and dogs (12). Dogs have been added to this group because numerous reports have shown that *Salmonella* infection in these animals is not as uncommon as once believed and that apparently healthy dogs are frequent carriers of these organisms (1, 5, 24). One source of the bacteria for dogs has been dehydrated dog meals (23).

It should be emphasized that practically all of the cultures from fowls were isolated from acute, fatal infections of young birds. A small number were derived from adult birds affected with acute infections and a somewhat larger number from the intestines of adult birds that were apparently normal carriers. However, a large majority of the strains were from birds a few days to 2 weeks of age. Most of the cultures were isolated from the blood or internal organs although a number were found in the intestinal content of birds affected with enteritis. Some strains were derived from unabsorbed yolks, cysts, and oviducts, but the number of these cultures was not large. Subsequent surveys have shown that wild birds may be common carriers of *Salmonella*.

The high incidence of *Salmonella* in egg powder reported by Solowey, McFarlane, Spaulding, and Chemerda (68) and by the Medical Research Council of Great Britain as well as the numerous accounts of the isolation of salmonellae from eggs leaves little doubt that outbreaks of infection in young birds often are egg-borne. There has been a great deal of discussion as to whether salmonellae other than S. *pullorum* were present in eggs as the result of ovarian transmission or whether organisms present in the intestinal tract contaminated the eggs. It is well known that salmonellae are able to penetrate the egg shell under favorable conditions (8). Because eggs may harbor *Salmonella* it sometimes happens that hatcheries become contaminated and chick fluff (50) from such commercial establishments frequently contributes to the spread of salmonellosis. It is also known that salmonellae other than S. *pullorum* are present in the ovaries of birds. It is evident that these methods of transmission are concerned in the appearance of salmonellosis in young birds. Other sources of infection for poultry are animal products used in feeds (9, 69). This is especially true of bone meal.

In 1951 McCullough and Eisele (48) found that *Salmonella* strains isolated from market samples of spray-dried whole egg powder readily induced clinical salmonellosis in human volunteers. It should be noted that egg powder can be used with safety providing it is subjected to thorough cooking immediately before it is eaten. The same rule applies to the flesh of the meat-producing animals that are carriers of *Salmonella*. From the public health aspect it appears that meat, eggs, and milk, products made from these materials, and domestic pets, including turtles, baby chicks, and various rodents, are the most important sources of *Salmonella* infections (14). Among the many products involved are imported meats (including canned meat), packaged foods, food supplements, raw coconut, powdered milk, animal-feeds that contain reduced offal, and plant foods. Reported sources of contamination are poultry-processing plants, abattoirs, butcher shops, rendering plants, home-produced meats, and caterer-delicatessen-restaurants.

Publications appearing since 1960 have indicated that salmonellosis is on the increase. This may be caused in part to changing food habits involving preparation, transportation, and dispensing. *Salmonella* types have been demonstrated in many processed foods prepared for human or for animal consumption. The finding that a cow with symptomless *Salmonella* mastitis caused a milk-borne outbreak of food poisoning (43) is significant because it has generally been believed that these organisms get into milk only after it is drawn and not before.

*Salmonella* do not produce spores and are killed by recommended pasteurization temperatures. They are ubiquitous, not fastidious in their growth requirements, and are able to survive for long periods under diversified conditions.

Edwards, Bruner, and Moran (20) in their studies encountered 106 distinct serological types in animals. Twelve of these types that appeared more frequently than the others are listed. The figures in parentheses indicate the number of cultures examined. They are as follows: S. *typhimurium* (3,238), S. *pullorum* (1,170), S. *choleraesuis* (1,121), S. *oranienburg* (645), S. *newport* (592), S. *derby* (513), S. *anatum* (506), S. *bareilly* (375), S. *muenchen* (353), S. *bredeney* (336), S. *montevideo* (325), and S. *paratyphi B* (262). Besides these 12 types, S. *gallinarum*, S. *enteritidis*, S. *typhi*, S. *paratyphi A*, S. *paratyphi C*, S. *sendai*, S. *abortusequi*, S. *abortusovis*, S. *dublin*, and S. *typhisuis* are included in the discussion because of host adaptation. They did not occur as frequently as some of the types that were omitted (see Edwards, Bruner, and Moran, 20). Cultures of the types not listed varied in occurrence from 1 to 250. It must be remembered that the figures given above do not represent the true incidence of the types. The figure for S. *pullorum* is certainly low, workers in animal disease laboratories readily recognized these types and did not forward them for identification. Figures compiled from the Cornell University Service Laboratories for New York State, whose isolates come for the most part from fowl, show that S. *typhimurium* ranks first in incidence and S. *pullorum* second.

In the description of serological *Salmonella* types, a division into host-adapted and non-host-adapted types is made and the infections of domestic animals are considered. Brief mention is made of *Salmonella* infection of man.

## HOST-ADAPTED *SALMONELLA* TYPES

S. *typhi* (typhoid bacillus, 9,12,Vi: d-), S. *paratyphi A* (1,2,12: a-), S. *paratyphi B* (1,4,5,12: b-1,2), S. *paratyphi C* (6,7: c-1,5), and S. *sendai* (1,9,12: a-1,5) are strictly human types that produce typhoid and paratyphoid febrile diseases, result in a relatively high carrier rate, and tend to become endemic in the population. S. *paratyphi C* rarely is found in the United States and is not very common along the shores of the Mediterranean Sea, where it is supposed to be endemic. S. *paratyphi* A and S. *sendai* have been found in the United States on very few occasions in recent years. S. *typhi* and S. *paratyphi* B appear frequently. The latter occurs as a diphasic, D-tartrate-negative type that produces enteric fever and as a monophasic, D-tartrate-positive type that usually is involved in gastroenteritis. Of the types listed above, S. *paratyphi B* alone shows some secondary host adaptation. In the studies of Edwards, Bruner, and Moran (20), it was found in man, turkeys, chickens, cattle, sheep, swine, a dog, a mouse, monkeys, a cockroach, and egg powder. Ninety percent of the cultures came from man. However, domestic animals may act as reservoirs of S. *paratyphi B*, and it is also possible that they may contract this type from man. S. *paratyphi B* rarely causes septicemia in lower animals, and its inclusion in bacterins for veterinary use is not warranted.

### Salmonella abortusequi (4,12: -e,n,x)

SYNONYMS: *Bacillus abortus-equi, Salmonella abortivo-equina, Salmonella abortivo-equinus, contagious equine abortion.*

Kilborne (41), in 1893, made cultures from the vagina of an aborting mare in Pennsylvania. These were turned over to Smith (64), who studied the pure culture that developed on the media. The organism was so like the hog cholera bacillus, with which he was then working, that he could not differentiate it with certainty. The same organism was isolated by Good (26) in Kentucky in 1911 and by Meyer and Boerner (49) in Pennsylvania in 1913. It has been isolated from aborting mares in several European countries, from Pennsylvania, Kentucky, Iowa, Illinois, Washington, and Minnesota in the United States, from the Province of Ontario in Canada, from South Africa, from South America, and from Japan.

**Special Cultural Features.** This strain grows less luxuriantly on ordinary laboratory media than do most *Salmonella* strains. It is a monophasic type.

**Incidence.** The organism is practically host-specific, the horse being the susceptible animal.

**Pathogenicity.** S. *abortusequi* apparently is spread mainly in the pasture. Infective discharges from aborting animals contaminate the grass, which then is eaten by susceptible animals. Abortion can readily be produced in mares by mixing pure cultures with their feed and by injecting cultures intravenously. Just before the act of abortion occurs, the affected mare usually shows fever and other signs of a general reaction. Some believe that the mare suffers a brief period of septicemia. If so, it disappears and the only lesions found after the abortion are in the fetal membranes, which are edematous and frequently show hemorrhages and areas of necrosis.

Within recent years there have been a few sporadic isolations of S. *abortusequi* in the United States, but outbreaks have occurred in South Africa and South America (20).

Rabbits and guinea pigs may be killed by parenteral injection. For small experimental animals this organism has about the same degree of virulence as the other members of the paratyphoid group.

In rare instances the organism has been incriminated in food poisoning in man (Bruner, 11).

**Diagnosis.** The specific organism may easily be cultivated by ordinary cultural methods from the placenta, fetus, or uterine exudate. Agglutinins are produced in the course of the infection, and the diagnosis may be obtained through them. According to Good and Corbett (27), normal animals may agglutinate the specific organism in dilutions of 1:200 and occasionally as high as 1:300. Infected animals usually agglutinate in dilutions from 1:500 to 1:5,000.

**Immunity.** Various workers have induced abortion in pregnant mares by injecting pure cultures of the organism intravenously. Against such a method of infection artificial immunization is not effective. Against natural modes of infection (ingestion) bacterin treatment has proved highly satisfactory as a prophylactic procedure (Good and Dimock, 28). This method of controlling abortion has been practiced successfully by the United States Army (Koon and Kelser, 44). Some European authorities, however, are skeptical of the immunizing value of dead cultures of this organism.

### Salmonella abortusovis (4,12: c-1,6)

SYNONYMS:  *Bacillus paratyphi abortus ovis, Bacillus enteritidis C* typ. *ovis*

This organism causes a highly contagious form of abortion in sheep. It was first isolated by Schermer and Ehrlich (59) and studied by Lovell (47). Fortunately this infection has not been found in the United States. It is not known to infect other animals.

### Salmonella choleraesuis (6,7: c-1,5)

SYNONYMS:  *Bacillus cholerae-suis,* "hog cholera bacillus," *Bacterium suipestifer, Salmonella suipestifer*

This organism was isolated and described by Salmon and Smith (57) in 1885 and was the first of the paratyphoid organisms to be recognized. It is because of this fact that these organisms are now known as the *Salmonella.* The authors believed the organism to be the cause of the destructive and prevalent disease known as hog cholera, but later work demonstrated that this is not the case, that hog cholera is caused by a filterable virus. Nevertheless this organism plays an important role in porcine pathology, principally as a secondary invader in the virus disease.

**Special Cultural Features.** On the basis of biochemical and serological properties S. *choleraesuis* is divided into two types. One type is diphasic, has the formula 6,7: c-1,5 and fails to produce hydrogen sulfide. The second type is monophasic, has the formula 6,7: -1,5 and produces abundant hydrogen sulfide. In the early years of this century the cultures isolated in the United

States were diphasic and failed to produce hydrogen sulfide. The type became known as the American type. Between the years 1920 to 1935 a distinct change occurred in the type of S. *choleraesuis* endemic throughout the United States, and now the monophasic, hydrogen-sulfide-positive Kunzendorf (western European) variety is found in over 95 percent of the isolations. These types do not ferment arabinose or trehalose and vary in their ability to attack dulcitol (Bruner and Edwards, 13).

**Incidence.** S. *choleraesuis* usually is considered a bacterium particularly adapted to swine, but its zoological distribution is broader than might be expected. It has been found in man, swine, a turkey, chickens, canaries, cattle, horses, sheep, dogs, foxes, a cat, mink, and guinea pigs. It has also appeared in mayonnaise and egg powder (20).

**Pathogenicity.** A majority of these cultures were isolated from the internal organs of hogs affected with cholera. The organism also occurs many times in septicemia of hogs following treatment with serum and virus. Its isolation from the intestine in cases of colitis is rare. In fact, in several instances S. *choleraesuis* has been isolated from the blood and parenchymal organs of hogs while other *Salmonella* types were isolated from the intestines of these animals. From these results it would seem that S. *choleraesuis* has no more relation to enteritis of swine than do a number of other *Salmonella* types. It appears that *Salmonella* are much more likely to be isolated from cases of acute enteritis in swine than from chronic, necrotic enteritis. The occurrence of S.

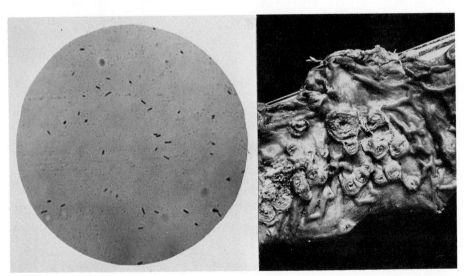

*Fig. 6 (left)*. *Salmonella choleraesuis,* from a culture on slant agar incubated for 18 hours at 37 C. X 950.

*Fig. 7 (right)*. The so-called *button ulcers* of hog cholera. These craterlike ulcers, their centers filled with caseous material, are sometimes caused by the activities of S. *choleraesuis. Spherophorus necrophorus* usually has an active part in their formation but is not primary.

*choleraesuis,* as well as other *Salmonella* types, in virus infections is well known.

In addition to those cases in which it is associated with hog cholera, S. *choleraesuis* is encountered occasionally in outbreaks of infection in suckling pigs and young hogs. In these cases no other infectious agent is found. In some of these outbreaks poor sanitation and diet inadequate in quantity or quality are evidently contributing factors because upon removal of the animals to clean quarters and institution of adequate feeding the losses quickly stop. S. *choleraesuis* is also found in sporadic cases of septicemia in older hogs, particularly in old brood sows. Upon necropsy the most frequently observed lesions are purple-red discoloration of the ears, limbs, and abdomen; splenomegaly; hepatomegaly; pulmonary hemorrhage; and colitis. The most common histologic lesion is the so-called *typhoid* nodules in the liver accompanied by vascular lesions (fibrinoid thrombi) in the lungs, kidneys, and brain.

S. *choleraesuis* occurs frequently in cattle and sheep. In these animals it is found in septicemias, abortions, and 'enteritis. This organism appears frequently in carnivorous animals and has been found in dogs, foxes, a cat, and mink. It possesses marked invasiveness for man, where it frequently produces fatal septicemias. However, human carriers of this microorganism rarely are found, and cases that appear among young children who have not eaten raw or insufficiently cooked pork suggest that household pets may be responsible. Furthermore, the occurrence of 30 *Salmonella* types in dogs and cats indicates that these animals should be considered in epidemiological studies of salmonellosis.

### Salmonella typhisuis (6,7: c-1,5)

SYNONYMS:   *Bacillus typhi-suis, Salmonella typhi-suis, ferkeltyphus* (German) bacillus

This organism is very similar to S. *choleraesuis* and probably should be regarded as a variety of that organism. Whereas S. *choleraesuis* fails to ferment arabinose and trehalose and ferments mannitol, S. *typhisuis* does just the opposite. Furthermore, it grows less luxuriantly on ordinary laboratory media than does S. *choleraesuis.* Its antigenic structure is the same. This organism has been reported in swine in Canada, Minnesota (6), and Massachusetts (55). In Europe it causes an intestinal disease of young pigs known as *ferkeltyphus.*

### Salmonella enteritidis (9,12: g,m-)

SYNONYMS: *Bacillus enteritidis, Klebsiella enteritidis, Bacterium enteritidis, Bacillus gaertner*

S. *enteritidis* was first isolated by Gärtner (25) from human feces in an epidemic of meat poisoning at Frankenhausen, Germany.

**Incidence.** Compared to certain other *Salmonella* types, S. *enteritidis* has a low incidence rate in the United States (20). It is included in the discussion because it is an old, established type rather than because it occurs frequently. Isolations have been made from turkeys, chickens, cattle, swine, rats, mice, guinea pigs, a beaver, a spider monkey, and man. It is primarily a rodent type because 70 percent of the total cultures of S. *enteritidis* were isolated from these animals, and 40 percent of the rodent cultures were S. *enteriditis*. However, it is not the most common type found in rodents. S. *typhimurium* made up 51 percent of the cultures derived from these animals.

**Pathogenicity.** As indicated above, S. *enteritidis* is quite pathogenic for rodents. In these animals this bacterium may cause outbreaks of epizootic proportions. It sometimes produces *Salmonella* infections in other animals and acute intestinal infection in man.

### Salmonella dublin (9,12: g,p–)

SYNONYMS: *Salmonella enteritidis*, Gärtner, type Kiel

This organism is recognized in many parts of the world as a type particularly adapted to cattle which often causes severe losses in young calves and which frequently is transmitted to man through milk. S. *dublin* holds an important position in salmonellosis of cattle in most parts of the world in contrast to its low incidence in the United States (20). A still more peculiar situation exists in the geographical distribution of the organism within the United States. All the cultures of S. *dublin* recognized in this country have been isolated in the Far West; not one has been found east of the Rocky Mountains. The organism has been derived from a turkey, a canary, cattle, foxes, and a man. Although this type is primarily adapted to cattle, it is the predominant type among western foxes. This predilection for foxes may be a secondary adaptation. In 1960 Rokey and Erling (56) reported on the natural occurrence of S. *dublin* in Arizona. They stated that it produces an extremely destructive disease of calves and that it has been isolated from horses, dogs, mice, chickens, and rabbits as well as from calves in this area. It caused an epizootic of diarrhea and abortion in a flock of pregnant ewes in Idaho. It has been recorded (61, 70) as the etiologic agent of outbreaks of abortion in Scotland. In South Africa, where S. *dublin* is a common cause of infection in calves, Henning (30) recommends the use of a formalinized bacterin precipitated by Al (OH)$_3$ to control the infection. It may be administered to the cow in order to protect the newborn calf, and later the calf itself is vaccinated. The antibiotic ampicillin was recommended by Kerr and Brander (40) for use in treating calves.

### Salmonella pullorum (9,12: –)

SYNONYMS: *Bacillus pullorum, Bacterium pullorum*

S. *pullorum* is the cause of *pullorum disease,* sometimes called *bacillary white diarrhea,* of young chicks. It frequently creates heavy losses to the industry. This organism was first isolated and described by Rettger (53) in 1909.

**Special Cultural Features.** The organism grows upon ordinary culture media, but the growth is never luxuriant. In semisolid medium the growth is confined to the line of stab, indicating a lack of motility. Acid and gas are produced from glucose, although anaerogenic strains occur. The organism does not ferment dulcitol and rarely ferments maltose.

**Incidence.** S. *pullorum* was isolated from turkeys, chickens, a pheasant, canaries, a parrot, a calf, swine, a dog, a fox, a mink, a cat, a chinchilla, and man (20). It occurs most frequently in chickens, less often in turkeys, and rather infrequently in man, although one rather large outbreak of gastroenteritis involved over 400 men. This organism is considered to be nearly host-specific and able to produce a well-defined disease in young chicks, but it also tends to produce symptoms of salmonellosis in other animals, as do most of the recognized *Salmonella* types.

**Pathogenicity.** S. *pullorum* is highly fatal if cultures are fed to young chicks during the first few days of life, and particularly if the chicks are allowed to become chilled by a lowering of the temperature of the brooder house. Older chicks become progressively harder to infect in this way, but occasionally even adult birds may be killed. Old birds can be infected by subcutaneous or intravenous injection. In these cases the infection may remain localized, or septicemia may result. Large doses, given intraperitoneally, will kill guinea pigs.

In its natural host, pullorum disease proceeds in cycles. The infection is carried in the ovaries of some hens, but there are no symptoms to indicate this fact. Some of the eggs laid by such hens will contain the organism in their yolks. If these eggs are incubated, many will fail to hatch but the ones that do will give rise to chicks that harbor the infection in their yolk sacs. Some of these chicks appear not to be seriously harmed by the presence of the organism and become in turn ovarian carriers of the disease when adult age is reached. Others, especially those that are shipped very young and that are chilled or otherwise devitalized, may become ill from an acute diarrhea accompanied by septicemia. The diarrheal discharges are highly contagious for the other chicks, and soon a large part of the birds associating with a few sick ones are infected with the disease. In incubator-raised chicks the disease is especially malignant, for the infected down from a few diseased chicks will be blown around the entire machine by the fan circulating the air, and all or many of the chicks will contract the disease by inhaling the organism.

The affected chicks huddle near a source of heat, they do not eat, they appear sleepy, they may show diarrhea, and they usually die within a few hours. The lesions vary according to the method of infection. The chicks that are hatched containing the infection usually show unabsorbed yolk sacs with dry cheesy material in them, the liver frequently appears pale and half-cooked, and the intestines are inflamed. Chicks infected by inhaling the organism usually show caseous areas in the lungs. Similar caseous areas often are seen in the wall of the gizzard and in the heart muscle. The losses vary

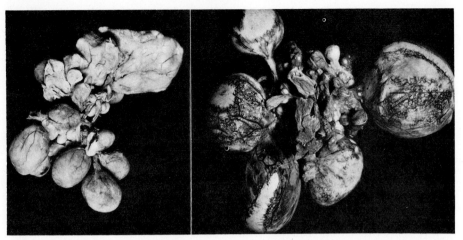

*Fig. 8.* Pullorum disease in the chicken ovary. The diseased ovary is depicted on the left. On the right is a normal ovary for comparison. The ova of the diseased bird are small, misshapen, discolored, and sometimes hemorrhagic.

greatly depending upon how the chicks are handled. It not infrequently occurs that a hatcheryman will have no trouble in chicks that he raises himself but there will be great losses in other chicks of the same lot that are shipped to distant points.

**Control Measures.** Treatment of the diseased chicks is impracticable because birds of a few days of age have very little resistance and quickly succumb. Efforts at control must be aimed at preventing the infection. Sanitation, including fumigation, of the incubators of commercial hatcheries helps, but the main effort must be directed toward the detection and elimination of the hens that are carrying the infection and laying infected eggs. Finding these hens necessitates the use of serological tests.

The poultry industry in the United States is highly specialized. Large numbers of chicks are hatched in commercial hatcheries and sold as day-old chicks. These chicks are raised, frequently in large groups, for replacements in laying flocks or for sale to meat markets. The traffic in day-old chicks is very great, and it is in this traffic that the greatest losses from pullorum disease occur. To aid in controlling poultry diseases the United States Department of Agriculture, in co-operation with poultry leaders, poultry breeders, and members of the breeder and commercial hatchery industry, has developed a program that is described in *USDA National Poultry Improvement Plan*, December 1954. This designates the regulatory procedure for establishing and maintaining pullorum-typhoid-clean flocks. It defines two classes as follows: (*a*) *U.S. pullorum-typhoid-passed* flocks which have been officially blood-tested within the past 12 months and are found to contain no reactors; (*b*) *U.S. pullorum-typhoid-clean* flocks which are found to contain no reactors on two consecutive official blood tests. This publication also lists the official tests and gives instructions for their uses and interpretations. Because it is constantly being revised and the classes of flocks redefined and changed, for up-to-date descriptions one must consult the revisions.

**Serologic Tests.** Agglutination tests are used in pullorum disease control. The birds are bled from the wing vein into small vials. The antigen is a suspension of S. *pullorum*. Three methods of performing the test are in use, viz.:

1. *The tube method.* This is the older and standard test. The serum is separated from the clot. The test may be set up in a number of tubes, using decreasing concentrations of serum as is done in the test for Bang's disease of cattle (see p. 203), but usually, to save expense, only a single tube is used. Into the clean, dry tube 0.05 ml of undiluted serum (some merely add one drop without bothering to measure the quantity more accurately) is placed. The suspension of bacilli (antigen) is then pipetted into the tube and caused to mix with the serum. If 1 ml of antigen is used, a dilution of 1:20 is obtained; if 1.5 ml, 1:30; if 2 ml, 1:40. Birds that react in dilutions of 1:25 or higher are regarded as infected.

Some chicken sera yield a flocculent, fatty material that floats on the surface of the fluid. This interferes with the reading of the test. These cloudy reactions can be avoided by making the antigen alkaline (pH 8.0) by the addition of NaOH just before the tests are set up.

2. *The serum-plate method.* This is done in the same way as the plate method for Bang's disease (see p. 205). When done by experienced operators, it is as accurate as the tube method.

3. *The whole-blood-plate method.* This method can be used while the birds are being held to await the outcome of the test. A drop of blood is collected on a clean glass slide and immediately mixed with a drop of the concentrated antigen that has been especially prepared for this test. The accuracy of the test may not be as great as that of the other methods, but it is frequently used because of the cheapness of the method.

Marked advances have been made in eradicating pullorum disease. With effective state and federal regulatory programs in operation it should be possible to eliminate this disease from the poultry industry.

**Form Variation in S. *pullorum*.** Younie (75) called attention to the occurrence of S. *pullorum* infection in the progeny of flocks that contained no reactors to the standard agglutination test. Cultures of S. *pullorum* recovered from the chicks of such flocks differed serologically from standard antigen strains of S. *pullorum*. Serums of chicks infected with these variant cultures failed to agglutinate the standard antigen strains but did agglutinate the infecting cultures in high dilution.

Edwards and Bruner (19) studied the "standard" and "variant" strains of S. *pullorum* and noted that the antigenic formula of S. *pullorum* is $9,12_1, (12_2),$ $12_3$. In normal cultures the $12_2$ factor is variable, and forms containing a large amount or a negligible amount of $12_2$ can be isolated from the same strain. It is possible for cultures to become fairly well stabilized in either form, thus giving rise to the so-called *standard* strains and *variant* or X strains. The standard strains contain only a small amount of $12_2$, but the X strains contain a large amount of the antigen. Although the $12_2$-lacking strains and the $12_2$-containing strains cross-agglutinate to a certain titer, each strain agglutinates to a much higher titer when exposed to its homologous serum. Therefore, the presence of the variant type of infection in a flock of birds necessitates the use of the variant antigen if the disease is to be eradicated by removing the agglutination reactors.

Although serological methods usually are employed in typing standard and variant strains of S. *pullorum*, William (74) proposed a simple method based on the ability of a solution of ammonium sulfate (330 g per L) to clear a suspension of the standard type and on its lack of effect on the turbidity of variant-type suspensions.

**Immunity.** No attempts have been made to immunize birds against S. *pullorum* infection.

**Chemotherapy.** Furazolidone has been tested widely in treating S. *pullorum* infection, and although it appears to have some beneficial effect it does not eliminate the disease (29, 67). Furaltadone has also been recommended as a water medication against S. *pullorum* infection in broilers (7).

### Salmonella gallinarum (9,12: –)

SYNONYMS: *Bacillus sanguinarium, Bacterium gallinarum, Eberthella gallinarum, Shigella gallinarum,* fowl typhoid bacillus

This organism was isolated and described by Klein (42) in 1889 as the cause of a disease known as *fowl typhoid*. In 1895 Moore (51) isolated an organism which later proved to be the same as Klein's from an outbreak of an acute disease in chickens which he named *infectious anemia*. Moore applied the name *Bacillus sanguinarium* to his organism because he was not aware that it was the same as the one with which Klein had worked. The name gallinarum has priority over Moore's name and therefore is the one now used.

**Special Cultural Features.** The organism grows much more luxuriantly than does S. *pullorum*. It is nonmotile. It ferments glucose with acid but with no gas production and for that reason formerly was included in the typhoid-dysentery group. The bacterium is serologically identical with S. *pullorum* but differs in being anaerogenic, growing more luxuriantly, and fermenting maltose and dulcitol. Differentiation between S. *pullorum* and S. *gallinarum* can also be made by means of bacteriophage (45).

**Incidence.** S. *gallinarum* has been isolated from turkeys, chickens, and man (20). Its distribution is limited almost entirely to the two species of fowls listed, and its occurrence in those species is considerably less than that of S. *pullorum*, S. *typhimurium*, S. *oranienburg*, and S. *bareilly*. It can be grouped in the host-specific types, and it produces a well-defined disease of adult fowls.

**Pathogenicity.** Fowl typhoid affects adult birds. The symptoms are those of an acute septicemic disease, that is, wasting, weakness, drowsiness, and diarrhea. There is rapidly developing anemia and a leukocytosis. In many cases the birds are found dead under the roosts in the morning before any symptoms have been noticed. The lesions consist of thin anemic blood, multiple small necrotic areas in the liver and heart, and an enlarged spleen. The best means of making a diagnosis is the isolation of the causative organism, which is easily accomplished.

Carcasses of birds that died of fowl typhoid have yielded viable bacteria from the liver up to 11 days and from the bone marrow up to 25 days after death. The organisms have also been obtained from maggots feeding on the carcasses (34).

Some workers have isolated this organism from diseased ovaries of hens, from eggs, and from outbreaks of typical bacillary white diarrhea in chicks. On the other hand, outbreaks of disease in adult birds which resemble fowl typhoid in every way have been attributed to S. *pullorum.*

Like other members of this group, pure cultures will usually cause fatal septicemia when injected into mice, guinea pigs, and rabbits.

**Immunity.** Killed cultures have been used in attempts to control this disease, but the evidence indicates slight success. Smith (65) has demonstrated that good immunity against oral infection with S. *gallinarum* can be obtained by vaccinating with attenuated cultures, but this procedure is not practical at present.

## THE MORE COMMON NON-HOST-ADAPTED *SALMONELLA* TYPES

### *Salmonella typhimurium* (1,4,5,12: i-1,2)

SYNONYMS:   *Bacterium aertrycke, Bacterium pestis-caviae, Bacterium psittacosis, Salmonella aertrycke,* etc.

This organism, frequently called the *mouse typhoid bacillus,* was first isolated by Loeffler (46). Later it was found in a variety of animals diseases and assigned a number of names before its identity was established.

**Special Cultural Features.** Anaerogenic strains of this serotype occur, and cultures from pigeons usually lack the somatic antigen 5. Actually there are many subserotypes of S. *typhimurium.* These can be demonstrated by antigenic analysis or by phage typing. The phage-typing scheme of Callow (15) initially defined 34 types of the organism.

**Incidence.** S. *typhimurium* occurs more often and is more widely distributed than any other type. Of 47 animal species that harbored *Salmonella* types, 36 presented S. *typhimurium* (20). This organism probably appears in all warm-blooded animals and is important in diseases of young and adult cattle, horses, swine, and sheep. It has been found in reptiles. It has been isolated from water and various foods. It is a common infection of birds and, like S. *pullorum,* can be transmitted through the egg.

**Pathogenicity.** Severe outbreaks of salmonellosis have been caused by this organism in all kinds of animals. Many of the laboratory animals are especially susceptible to infection with S. *typhimurium.* It can cause severe losses in young birds of the domestic varieties. In most species the infection is manifested by enteritis and diarrhea, with septicemia in fatal cases.

In pigeon lofts, losses from this organism often are very great. The losses are in the squabs. The squabs either die soon after hatching or develop swollen wing joints that render them unable to fly. The joint swelling is caused by the collection of a gelatinous exudate in the joint capsule. In this exudate the organism is readily found by making cultures. The adult stock shows no evidence of the disease ordinarily, but when it is destroyed for examination the ovaries of some of the females are found to be diseased. The organism can be found in many of the developing yolks and presumably passes in this way into the egg and then into the developing embryo. The pigeon fancier often calls this disease *megrims.*

The organism is frequently encountered both in sporadic cases and in outbreaks of gastroenteritis in man. In a recent outbreak involving 29 persons the probable source of the organism was Easter chicks (2).

**Immunity.** Cultures of the organism, killed with heat or chemicals, have been used in attempting to stop epizootics among mice and guinea pigs but without great success. Resistance can be enhanced in this way, but the protection usually is not great enough to stop outbreaks.

Attempts have been made to control the squab disease by using the agglutination test to detect infected adult female pigeons. The antibody content of the birds is so low, however, that the method has failed.

Hinshaw and McNeil (31) reported on the use of the agglutination test in an attempt to eradicate S. *typhimurium* infection from turkey flocks. They found that the use of an H (flagellar) antigen and an O (somatic) antigen in separate tests at a 1:25 finding dilution enabled them to reduce markedly the S. *typhimurium* infection in a community, but they doubted that they could eliminate it entirely by testing alone. For more details see DeLay *et al.* (17). According to Sieburth (62), the indirect hemagglutination test which employs chicken erythrocytes that have been exposed to S. *typhimurium* antigens is useful in detecting infected birds.

### *Salmonella derby* (1,4,12: f,g–)

SYNONYM: *Salmonella derbyensis*

This organism was isolated by Peckham (52) from a pork pie.

**Incidence.** S. *derby* appears frequently in man and animals. It has been recognized in turkeys, chickens, a duck, pheasants, cattle, a camel, a fawn, swine, a dog, cats, a mink, and man (20). Although the zoological distribution of this type is quite broad, almost one-half of the cultures came from swine.

**Pathogenicity.** The organism is associated with septicemias in animals and gastroenteritis in man. It is frequently connected with fatalities in poults.

In 1963 (58) this organism received much attention as the cause of outbreaks of hospital-associated infections. Its source was believed to be undercooked or raw eggs or person to person transmission. There is no reason to suspect that S. *derby* is any more likely to be transmitted through eggs than any other *Salmonella* serotype or that it shows predilection for hospitals or hospital patients.

### Salmonella bredeney (1,4,12,27: l,v-1,7)

This organism was isolated from cases of human gastroenteritis by Hohn and Herrmann and typed by Kauffmann (36).

**Incidence.** S. *bredeney* has been isolated from turkeys, chickens, ducks, a guinea fowl, quail, a partridge, a wood duck, a calf, a lamb, swine, dogs, cats, man, and egg powder (20). Although the zoological distribution of this type is rather wide, most of the isolates came from swine and fowls.

**Pathogenicity.** The organism is associated with septicemias in animals and gastroenteritis in man.

### Salmonella montevideo (6,7: g,m,s–)

The organism was isolated and typed by Hormaeche and Peluffo (32). The original culture came from a case of human gastroenteritis.

**Incidence.** S. *montevideo* has been isolated from turkeys, chickens, a duck, a pheasant, a pig, a dog, cats, foxes, a rat, man, egg powder, and chocolate-covered ice-cream bars (20). It occurs more frequently in man and fowls than in other animals.

**Pathogenicity.** This organism is usually involved in septicemic conditions of fowls and gastroenteritis of man. It has also been isolated from a number of asymptomatic carriers both in man and animals.

### Salmonella oranienburg (6,7: m,t–)

SYNONYM: *Salmonella oranienburgensis*

This organism was first isolated from a case of infant diarrhea. It was typed by Kauffmann (35).

**Incidence.** S. *oranienburg* has been derived from turkeys, chickens, pigeons, quail, pheasants, swine, dogs, cats, man, veal salad, and ice-cream bars (20). The major portion of the isolations came from man and fowls.

**Pathogenicity.** It causes fatalities in fowls, gastroenteritis in man, and appears in asymptomatic carriers in man and the lower animals.

### Salmonella bareilly (6,7: y-1,5)

The bacterium was isolated from cases of mild enteric fever in Bareilly, India (Bridges and Scott, 10).

**Incidence.** S. *bareilly* has been found in turkeys, chickens, a duck, a quail, swine, foxes, a dog, a cat, a mink, man, and egg powder (20). It occurs most frequently in man and fowls.

**Pathogenicity.** It follows the same pattern as S. *montevideo* and S. *oranienburg* above.

### Salmonella muenchen (6,8: d-1,2)

It was isolated first from a fatal case of enteric fever (Schütze, 60).

**Incidence.** S. *muenchen* has been isolated from turkeys, chickens, swine, dogs, reptiles, man, and egg powder (20). Over 66 percent of the cultures of this type came from swine. They were isolated from the intestinal contents and feces of hogs maintained under experimental conditions by the United States Department of Agriculture. It was found that in one group of animals this type frequently appeared. This condition partly accounted for the large number of S. *muenchen* cultures from swine.

**Pathogenicity.** It produces the same general salmonellosis pattern as described above.

### Salmonella newport (6,8: e,h-1,2,3)

SYNONYMS: Paratyphus B$_2$, *Bacillus paratyphosus B*,
*Salmonella newportensis*

The organism was isolated by Weil and Saxl (72) in 1917 from food poisoning in man.

**Incidence.** S. *newport* has been found in turkeys, chickens, ducks, cattle, swine, dogs, a mink, a raccoon, a mouse, a guinea pig, a tortoise, gopher snakes, man, water, egg powder, turkey dressing, and chocolate éclairs (20). It occurs most frequently in man and fowls.

**Pathogenicity.** This organism is important in *Salmonella* infections of poults. It has been incriminated in outbreaks of gastroenteritis in man. In a few instances it has caused fatalities in man. In general, salmonelloses caused by this organism follow the usual pattern.

### Salmonella anatum (3,10: e,h-1,6)

SYNONYMS: *Bacterium anatis, Escherichia anata*, etc.

In 1920 Rettger and Scoville (54) described S. *anatum* as the cause of a destructive disease of ducklings on Long Island and in Connecticut and Massachusetts. The disease was called *keel* by the duck raisers because many of the affected birds collapsed suddenly with few premonitory symptoms.

**Special Cultural Features.** Freshly isolated cultures of S. *anatum* frequently fail to ferment xylose but can be trained to do so.

**Incidence.** Next to S. *typhimurium*, this organism is the most widely distributed *Salmonella* type. It has been derived from turkeys, chickens, a pigeon, ducks, a goose, a canary, a horse, cattle, sheep, a goat, swine, dogs, foxes, cats, rats, a Gila monster, man, sewage, and egg powder (20). Although the original isolation came from a duckling and it is connected with *Salmonella* infection in this species, its zoological distribution is very wide. Furthermore, it produced only 11 percent of the *Salmonella* infections observed in ducks, whereas S. *typhimurium* accounted for 70 percent.

**Pathogenicity.** The disease produced in animals follows the pattern of other *Salmonella* infections. The organism produces gastroenteritis in man, but many of the cultures derived from man have come from asymptomatic carriers.

## OTHER *SALMONELLA* TYPES

Ninety-eight percent of the *Salmonella* types isolated in the United States from animals, exclusive of man, belonged to somatic groups B, C, D, and E of the Kauffmann-White schema. A few types outside these four groups appeared frequently enough to warrant notice. They are S. *worthington* (1,13,23: z-l,w) and S. *minnesota* (21: b-e,n,x). Neither one is host-specific (20).

In salmonellosis it is not uncommon to find that multiple serotypes are involved. This is especially true in fowl when types of somatic group E are concerned (18).

## BIOCHEMICAL TESTS THAT DISTINGUISH VARIETIES OF CERTAIN SEROLOGICAL TYPES

In a few instances biochemical characteristics are used to aid in distinguishing the varieties of a serological type. S. *pullorum* and S. *gallinarum* are serologically identical but differ markedly in certain cultural features. Physiological behavior also helps to differentiate varieties of S. *paratyphi* B and S. *choleraesuis*. Some of these differential characteristics are set forth in table XII.

*Table XII.* DIFFERENTIAL CHARACTERISTICS OF THE VARIETIES OF SOME SEROLOGICAL TYPES OF *SALMONELLA*

| Organisms | Cultural Features | | | | | | Antigenic Formula | | |
| | | | | | | | | H antigens | |
| | Hydrogen sulfide | D-Tartrate | Arab-inose | Tre-halose | Dul-citol | Mal-tose | O antigens | 1st phase | 2nd phase |
|---|---|---|---|---|---|---|---|---|---|
| S. paratyphi B | | | | | | | | | |
| Enteric variety | + | — | ag | ag | ag | ag | 1,4,5,12 | b | 1,2 |
| Gastroenteritis variety | + | + | ag | ag | ag | ag | 4,5,12 | b | — |
| S. choleraesuis | | | | | | | | | |
| American variety | — | + | — | — | v | ag | 6,7 | c | 1,5 |
| Kunzendorf variety | + | + | — | — | v | ag | 6,7 | — | 1,5 |
| S. pullorum | + | + | ag | ag | — | v | 9,12 | — | — |
| S. gallinarum | + | + | a | a | a | a | 9,12 | — | — |

ag = acid and gas;   a = acid without gas;   v = variable.

## IMMUNITY IN *SALMONELLA* INFECTIONS

S. *abortusequi* and S. *dublin* bacterins and the triple-typhoid-paratyphoid (S. *typhi*, S. *paratyphi* A, and S. *paratyphi* B) vaccine have been used with reasonable success as immunologic agents. Bacterins made from non-host-adapted serotypes, including S. *typhimurium* have been credited with some value in protecting lambs, calves, and foals against salmonellosis. None are highly effective.

**Control.** In most cases salmonellosis in animals runs its course or is eliminated by slaughter of the diseased and exposed animals and the application of extensive sanitary measures. In poultry it sometimes is possible, by good management, to raise a flock to market age and sell the birds at a profit even though infection has occurred in the young birds. However, the poultryman's big problem is the breeding flock, because carriers readily transmit *Salmonella* through the egg and are a constant source of danger to the highly susceptible baby bird. Pullorum testing is an effective aid in maintaining flocks free from this disease, but similar tests for other types of salmonellosis are not so successful. One of the most useful is the agglutination test for the detection of S. *typhimurium* in turkeys, and it is most effective only when circumstances permit complete replacement of all flocks shown to harbor carriers of the organism (16). Another test that may prove to be helpful is the indirect hemagglutination test in which chicken erythrocytes sensitized with polyvalent *Salmonella* antigens are employed. It is claimed that this test is useful for detecting salmonellosis in infected flocks (63).

The following principles have been advocated in setting up a control program for paratyphoid infection in turkey poults: (1) Stock the breeding ranch from a known clean source; (2) take bacteriologic samples of all poult mortality up to 21 days of age; (3) tube-agglutination test all potential breeding stock with S. *pullorum*, S. *typhimurium*, and Arizona paracolon antigens; and (4) make a routine bacteriologic examination of samples of 10-day-old dead embryos from the hatchery. Because it is quite clear that domestic animals constitute a major reservoir of infection, important also to the health of man, reduction of this source should be the concern of all veterinarians.

**Chemotherapy.** No specific drug or biological product has proved effective in completely arresting *Salmonella* infection. Some substances that ameliorate the course of the disease in domestic animals but do not eliminate the carriers are sulfa drugs, nitrofurazone, furazolidone, and furaltadone. Some antibiotics appear to enhance susceptibility to *Salmonella* infection while others are reasonably effective in controlling it. Among the latter are chloramphenicol, ampicillin, and tylosin.

## REFERENCES

1. Adler, Willers, and Levine.   Jour. Am. Vet. Med. Assoc., 1951, *118*, 300.
2. Anderson, Bauer, and Nelson.   Jour. Am. Med. Assoc., 1955, *158*, 1153.

3.  Andrewes.   Jour. Path. and Bact., 1922, *25*, 505.
4.  Aserkoff, Schroeder, and Brachman.   Am. Jour. Epidemiol., 1970, *92*, 13.
5.  Ball.   Jour. Am. Vet. Med. Assoc., 1951, *68*, 164.
6.  Barnes and Bergeland.   *Ibid.*, 1968, *152*, 1766.
7.  Bierer.   Avian Dis., 1961, *5*, 333.
8.  Bigland and Papas.   Canad. Jour. Comp. Med. and Vet. Sci., 1953, *17*, 105.
9.  Boyer, Bruner, and Brown.   Avian Dis., 1958, *2*, 396.
10.  Bridges and Scott.   Jour. Roy. Army Med. Corps, 1931, *56*, 241.
11.  Bruner.   Jour. Bact., 1946, *52*, 147.
12.  Bruner.   Cornell Vet., 1956, *46*, 11.
13.  Bruner and Edwards.   Ky. Agr. Exp. Sta. Bul. 404, 1940.
14.  Buxton.   Vet. Rec., 1957, *69*, 105.
15.  Callow.   Jour. Hyg. (London), 1959, *57*, 346.
16.  DeLay, Jackson, Jones, and Stover.   Am. Jour. Vet. Res., 1954, *15*, 122.
17.  DeLay, Jackson, Stover, Jones, and Worcester.   Jour. Am. Vet. Med. Assoc., 1955, *127*, 435.
18.  Edwards and Bruner.   Jour. Inf. Dis., 1940, *66*, 218.
19.  Edwards and Bruner.   Cornell Vet., 1946, *36*, 318.
20.  Edwards, Bruner, and Moran.   Ky. Agr. Exp. Sta. Bul. 525, 1948.
21.  Evans, Bruner, and Peckham.   Cornell Vet., 1955, *45*, 239.
22.  Ewing, McWhorter, Escobar, and Lubin.   Internatl. Bul. Bact. Nomencl. and Taxonom., 1965, *15*, 33.
23.  Galton, Harless, and Hardy.   Jour. Am. Vet. Med. Assoc., 1955, *126*, 57.
24.  Galton, Scatterday, and Hardy.   Jour. Inf. Dis., 1952, *91*, 1.
25.  Gärtner.   Correspond. d. Allgemein. Arztl. Verein Thüringen, 1888, *17*, 573.
26.  Good.   Am. Vet. Rev., 1911, *40*, 473.
27.  Good and Corbett.   Jour. Inf. Dis., 1913, *13*, 53.
28.  Good and Dimock.   Jour. Am. Vet. Med. Assoc., 1927, *71*, 31.
29.  Gordon and Tucker.   Brit. Vet. Jour., 1957, *113*, 99.
30.  Henning.   Onderstepoort Jour. Vet. Res., 1953, *26*, 3, 25, and 45.
31.  Hinshaw and McNeil.   Proc. U.S. Livestock Sanit. Assoc., 1943, *47*, 106.
32.  Hormaeche and Peluffo.   Arch. Urug. de Med., Cirug. y Espec., 1936, *9*, 673.
33.  Ibrahim.   Appl. Microbiol., 1969, *18*, 748.
34.  Jordan.   Brit. Vet. Jour., 1949, *110*, 387.
35.  Kauffmann.   Zeitschr. f. Hyg., 1930, *111*, 223.
36.  *Ibid.*, 1937, *119*, 356.
37.  Kauffmann.   Die Bakteriologie der Salmonella-gruppe. Ejnar Munksgaard, Copenhagen, 1941.
38.  Kauffmann.   Acta Path. et Microbiol. Scand., 1959, *45*, 406.
39.  Kauffmann and Edwards.   Jour. Lab. and Clin. Med., 1947, *32*, 548.
40.  Kerr and Brander.   Vet. Rec., 1964, *76*, 1105.
41.  Kilborne.   U.S. Dept. Agr., Bur. Anim. Indus. Bul. 3, 1893, p. 49.
42.  Klein.   Centrbl. f. Bakt., 1889, *5*, 689.
43.  Knox, Lewis, Hickie, and Johnston.   Jour. Hyg. (London), 1963, *61*, 175.
44.  Koon and Kelser.   Jour. Am. Vet. Med. Assoc., 1922, *62*, 193.
45.  Lilleengen.   Acta Path. et Microbiol. Scand., 1952, *30*, 194.
46.  Loeffler.   Centrbl. f. Bakt., 1892, *11*, 129.

47. Lovell.   Jour. Path. and Bact., 1931, *34*, 13.

48. McCullough and Eisele.   Jour. Inf. Dis., 1951, 88, 278; 89, 209 and 259.

49. Meyer and Boerner.   Jour. Med. Res., 1913, 29, 330.

50. Miura, Sato, and Miyamae.   Avian Dis., 1964, 8, 546.

51. Moore.   U.S. Dept. Agr., Bur. Anim. Indus. Bul. 8, 1895, p. 63.

52. Peckham.   Jour. Hyg. (London), 1923, *22*, 69.

53. Rettger.   Jour. Med. Res., 1909, *21*, 117.

54. Rettger and Scoville.   Jour. Bact., 1920, *26*, 217.

55. Reynolds, Smith, Smyser, and Miner.   Jour. Am. Vet. Med. Assoc., 1969, *155*, 1600.

56. Rokey and Erling.   *Ibid.*, 1960, *136*, 381.

57. Salmon and Smith.   Report on swine plague. U.S. Bur. Anim. Indus., 2d Ann. Rpt., 1885.

58. Sanders, Sweeney, Friedman, Boring, Randall, and Polk.   Jour. Am. Med. Assoc., 1963, *186*, 984.

59. Schermer and Ehrlich.   Berl. tierärztl. Wchnschr., 1921, 37, 469.

60. Schütze.   Jour. Hyg. (London), 1934, *34*, 344.

61. Shearer.   Vet. Rec., 1957, *69*, 693.

62. Sieburth.   Jour. Immunol., 1957, 78, 380.

63. Sieburth.   Am. Jour. Vet. Res., 1958, *19*, 729.

64. Smith.   U.S. Dept. Agr., Bur. Anim. Indus. Bul. 3, 1893, p. 53.

65. Smith.   Jour. Hyg. (London), 1956, *54*, 419.

66. Smith and Stewart.   Boston Soc. Med. Sci. Jour., 1897, *16*, 12.

67. Smyser and Van Roekel.   Avian Dis., 1958, 2, 428.

68. Solowey, McFarlane, Spaulding, and Chemerda.   Am. Jour. Pub. Health, 1947, *37*, 971.

69. Watkins, Glowers, and Grumbles.   Avian Dis., 1959, 3, 290.

70. Watson.   Vet. Rec., 1960, *72*, 62.

71. Weil and Felix.   Wien. klin. Wchnschr., 1918, *31*, 896.

72. Weil and Saxl.   *Ibid.*, 1917, *30*, 519.

73. White.   Med. Res. Council, Spec. Rpt. Ser. 103 (Brit.), 1926.

74. Williams.   Am. Jour. Vet. Res., 1953, *14*, 465.

75. Younie.   Canad. Jour. Comp. Med., 1941, 5, 164.

## THE GENUS *SHIGELLA*

This genus is named for Shiga, the Japanese bacteriologist who discovered the dysentery bacillus in 1898. It is made up of nonmotile rods, although some of the less-well-known species have been reported as motile. They produce acid but no gas from carbohydrates, except with some types of *Sh. flexneri*. It has been stated that true *Shigella* do not occur in animals other than primates, but they often cause bacillary dysentery in lower primates, particularly when the diet is inadequate. It now appears that dogs in highly endemic areas of shigellosis may be at least transient excreters of *Shigella* organisms. Whether they actually carry *Shigella* as they do *Salmonella* remains to be demonstrated (2). Within recent years a serological classification has evolved whereby the isolates from bacillary dysentery in man can be readily identified. The type species is *Shigella dysenteriae* (1).

The shigellae respond more favorably to chemotherapeutic agents than do the salmonellae. The sulfa drugs, nitrofuran compounds, and ampicillin trihydrate have been most effective in treating and controlling infections caused by the former bacteria.

### REFERENCES

1.  Edwards and Ewing.   Identification of enterobacteriaceae. Burgess Publishing Co., Minneapolis, Minn., 1955.
2.  Floyd.   Jour. Bact., 1955, 70, 621.

# XIV | The *Brucellaceae*

Within the family *Brucellaceae* are found small, coccoid to rod-shaped cells that may require blood, serum, or similar enrichment material in order to grow. They are parasites and pathogens which affect warm-blooded animals, including man. The important pathogenic genera are; *Pasteurella*, *Bordetella*, *Brucella*, *Hemophilus*, *Moraxella*, and *Actinobacillus*.

## THE GENUS *PASTEURELLA*

Microorganisms within this genus are sometimes divided into the hemorrhagic septicemia group which includes *Past. multocida*, *Past. hemolytica*, *Past. gallinarum*, and possibly *Past. pneumotropica* and *Past. ureae*. In addition other *Pasteurella* species possess similar cultural characteristics, but produce diseases of somewhat different type. One of them is *Past. anatipestifer*, the cause of a septicemic disease of ducks. Three others are the causative agents of diseases of rodents which are transmissible to man. *Past. pestis* produces bubonic plague of man. It has its natural reservoir in rats. *Past. tularensis* is the cause of tularemia. It occurs principally in wild rabbits. *Past. novicida* is a rodent type that resembles *Past. tularensis*. *Past. pseudotuberculosis* causes a disease of guinea pigs and other rodents.

### *Pasteurella multocida*

In 1880 Pasteur (39) described the organism that causes cholera in fowls. Later it was learned that the fowl cholera bacillus could not be differentiated culturally from the organisms of rabbit septicemia, of swine plague, and of certain pneumonias of cattle. The apparent identity of these organisms and the similarity of the diseases produced by them in the various animal species led Hueppe (22) in 1886 to group them under one name, *Bact. septicemiae hemorrhagicae*. Trevisan (47), the following year, proposed that the several disease-producing agents be recognized as separate species but that they be

173

grouped in a single genus, *Pasteurella*, named in honor of Pasteur. Lignières (28), in 1901, applied the name *pasteurelloses* to the group of diseases caused by these organisms, a name that has come into rather common use.

Although it had been recognized that the cultural and biochemic features of the *Pasteurella* organisms isolated from birds, cattle, swine, sheep, rabbits, reindeer, American bison, and other wild animals were essentially identical. Flügge's (12) classification, established in 1886, was followed for years. According to his system, *Past. aviseptica* caused fowl cholera, *Past. suiseptica* caused swine plague, *Past. lepiseptica* caused snuffles and pneumonia in rabbits, *Past. boviseptica* caused pneumonia and sometimes septicemia of cattle, and *Past. oviseptica* caused pneumonia in sheep.

Because these organisms cannot be differentiated from each other on any basis now known, including serological tests, Rosenbusch and Merchant (44) proposed, as Hueppe had many years before, that the hemorrhagic septicemia organisms of the various animals be recognized as a single species. Because Kitt (26) was the first to make the suggestion, they urged that the name of the species be *Past. multocida*, derived by eliminating the middle name of the trinomial *Bacterium bipolare multocidum* which Kitt proposed. This has been adopted here.

Many years ago Moore (32) found members of the hemorrhagic septicemia group present on the mucous membranes of the respiratory tract of apparently normal cattle, sheep, swine, dogs, and cats. These observations were confirmed by Jorgensen (24) in cattle. One of the strains isolated by Jorgensen was tested on a cow after it was found to be of unusual virulence for rabbits. It proved to be highly virulent for the animal, destroying it with typical *Pasteurella* pneumonia in 3 days following spraying of the culture into the nostrils. A majority of the strains isolated from mucous membranes of cattle were nonpathogenic, but this is not surprising because the majority of the strains derived from acute infections of cattle show little virulence for rabbits and other experimental animals.

**Morphology and Staining Reactions.** These are very small ovoid rods measuring about 0.3 microns wide by 0.4 to 0.5 microns long. When seen in carefully stained films from tissue, the ends of the rods are more deeply stained than the central portion, giving to them a distinct bipolar appearance. This characteristic is not so marked in bacilli from cultures, and in any case it may be easily obscured by overstaining. Wright's or Giemsa's stains are recommended for demonstrating it, although careful staining with methylene blue usually is satisfactory. In the fresh material, unstained, the bipolar appearance usually can be seen. Pasteur referred to the fowl cholera bacillus as his "figure-of-eight bacillus."

The *Pasteurella* are Gram-negative and nonsporeforming. Many strains form a capsular substance when freshly isolated, but usually this property is quickly lost.

**Cultural Features.** Organisms of this group are easily cultivated on ordinary infusion agar, although growth is never luxuriant. Media made from meat extract is not suitable unless enriched with a little blood of serum.

In infusion broth, growth is manifested by slight clouding and a viscid sediment. Growth in broth is greatly increased by the addition of a few drops of sterile serum. Excellent growth is obtained on blood agar plates. The blood is not altered except that some strains may exhibit a slight greenish haze around the deep colonies. Gelatin is not liquefied. Milk supports growth but is only slightly changed; the litmus usually turns from a blue to a violet color. Indol is produced. Glucose, mannitol, and sucrose are fermented with acid but no gas is produced. Lactose, maltose, and salicin are not attacked by most strains. Usually they are not soluble in ox bile; a few are easily dissolved. Toxins are not formed.

On agar, colonies of *Past. multocida* present a definite dissociation pattern showing for practical purposes three principal colonial variants: (*a*) mucoid colonies that are large, flowing, of moderate virulence for mice, and not typable by the usual serologic methods; (*b*) smooth or fluorescent colonies that are medium-sized and discrete (they are quite virulent for mice and typable); and (*c*) rough or blue colonies that are small and discrete, low in virulence for mice, and autoagglutinable.

The mucoid colonies as well as the smooth types contain capsular material, but serologic typing depends on the presence of type-specific soluble antigen associated with the capsules of the smooth or fluorescent forms. By using these forms, Roberts (42), Carter (7), and others have established four serologic types, which Roberts labeled I, II, III, and IV and Carter B, A, C, and D, respectively. In so doing they used precipitation, capsular swelling, and hemagglutination tests. Carter recommends the hemagglutination test for identification of the serotypes. He employs human erythrocytes that have been exposed to extracts of smooth *Pasteurella* and tests them with known antisera. According to Carter (7, 8), types A and B predominate in cattle. Type A strains are most frequently associated with pneumonia. Type B strains are usually recovered from animals with epizootic hemorrhagic septicemia. Type A strains predominate as the cause of fowl cholera. Only type C strains have been recovered from dogs and cats. Types A and D are most common in swine. Type D infections appear to be generally sporadic and have a wide host range, but most strains isolated from atrophic rhinitis of swine are either type D or mucoid. In 1963 Carter (9) added a fifth type, Type E, which came from cattle in Central Africa. Namioka and Bruner (34) studied 156 cultures by means of agglutination tests and found them to be divisible into ten O groups. By correlation with Carter's capsular Types A, B, C, and D, 12 serotypes were delineated. Further work showed that only certain serotypes within Carter's Type A were pathogenic for chickens and effective as bacterins (35). By 1967, Namioka (33) had described 15 serotypes. Among these 5: A and 9: A were pathogenic for fowl, while 1: A, 3: A, and 7: A were found to be less pathogenic for birds, but more likely to cause pneumonia in swine, sheep, and cattle.

**Resistance.** Cultures of *Pasteurella* die out quickly, and transplants must be made at least twice each month. Organisms dried on cover glasses in the air but protected from light usually die in less than 24 hours. Cultures are also easily and quickly killed with all ordinary disinfectants. Some authors have thought that these organisms lived widely as saprophytes. It is clear that many of them live on normal mucous membranes but it is doubtful if they thrive elsewhere.

**Pathogenicity.** Of the experimental animals, rabbits and mice are highly susceptible to inoculation. Guinea pigs and rats are resistant. The pathogenicity of different strains for these animals varies enormously. Certain strains injected subcutaneously will kill rabbits and mice overnight. In these animals the blood and tissues are teeming with bipolar bacilli. Other strains, even when freshly isolated, will cause only an edematous swelling at the point of inoculation, but after a few days the rabbit begins to emaciate and it dies after a week or more. In these instances the pleural cavity is filled with fluid and fibrinous material and the lungs are pneumonic, the affected portions being solid. In still other cases the edematous area may disappear after a few days, and the animals show no further effect of the inoculation. Strains from fowl cholera and swine plague usually are highly virulent; those from cattle and sheep are variable, a great many of them being practically avirulent for experimental animals. It appears that virulence is an attribute of serotypes plus colonial variation. Yaw *et al.* (52) tested the smooth and rough variants of types A, B, and C on mice and chickens. Mucoid variants were not used. They found that the smooth forms of all three serotypes were highly virulent for mice, but only the smooth variant of type A was virulent for chickens. The rough forms were much less virulent for mice.

The naturally occurring hemorrhagic septicemias seem to be diseases of devitalization. Presumably under conditions of lowered host vitality, organisms that are already being carried by the animals on their respiratory mucous membranes are unleashed and assume a pathogenicity which they formerly did not possess. Once the disease begins in a herd or flock, it is likely to spread rapidly.

Some of the conditons that are believed to be predisposing in the several pasteurelloses are: fowl cholera—poor sanitation, poor ventilation of pens, overcrowding; rabbit septicemia—poor sanitation and crowding, poor ventilation of hutches; swine plague—other diseases such as cholera and influenza, malnutrition due to poor feeds and intestinal parasites, insanitary crowded conditions; shipping pneumonia of cattle and sheep—exposure to cold, wet weather, shipping and driving long distances, crowding, and exhaustion. It is probable, too, that certain respiratory viruses are involved.

The naturally occurring diseases seldom spread to species other than the one in which they appear. That is to say, an outbreak in chickens seldom spreads to cattle or sheep, even though they may be in intimate contact with them, and the cattle disease will not spread to sheep or birds. If the strains of organisms concerned in outbreaks are isolated and injected into other species, however, they often prove capable of producing acute fatal septicemic diseases. Thus certain cultures isolated from birds are capable of causing rapidly fatal septicemia when inoculated intravenously into horses, cattle, sheep, rabbits, and white mice. Gouchenour (14) isolated an organism from an outbreak of hemorrhagic septicemia in American bison in Yellowstone National Park which proved highly pathogenic for nearly all species of animals in which its virulence was tried.

*Fowl cholera*, the pasteurellosis of birds, affects chickens principally, although ducks, geese, turkeys, swans, and other birds are susceptible. Wild birds frequently become infected and may, at times, be the source of infection for domestic flocks. In many cases the disease is peracute and manifested by an overwhelming bacteremia. Films of the blood or spleen pulp will then show large numbers of the minute, bipolar-staining organisms. Outbreaks generally begin in a few birds in apparently healthy flocks. The daily mortality in a flock usually rises sharply, the peak being reached as a rule within a few days (Alberts and Graham, 1). The fatalities vary from 10 to 75 percent.

The affected birds generally exhibit signs of depression, sleepiness, inappetence, and diarrhea. Death may occur within a few hours, or after 2 or 3 days. In some birds the course is much longer. Hendrickson and Hilbert (19) were able to cultivate the *Pasteurella* organism from the blood of chronically affected chickens, daily, for days and weeks. In one case this lasted as long as 49 days.

On the duck "ranches" of Long Island, cholera may take a heavy toll of the ducklings, which are raised in large numbers in very crowded, insanitary quarters. The autopsy findings usually consist of a few petechiae of the heart, a slightly swollen spleen, and perhaps a little reddening of the mucosa of the anterior part of the intestine.

The fowl cholera organism is frequently associated with chronic infections of the air sacs accompanied by accumulations of dry caseous material, with inflammatory processes in the wattles, especially of male birds, which frequently lead to necrosis, and with infections of the mucous membranes of the head, a condition commonly called *colds*. Also it is frequently found in the peritoneal cavity of young laying birds mixed with yolk material from ruptured ova. Whether the organism has anything to do with the rupture of the yolks, or is a secondary invader, is not known.

*Rabbit septicemia* may be very acute, with hardly any premonitory signs. The causative organism can easily be found in films of the blood or spleen pulp after death. A more common form of the disease is less acute, the affected animals being clearly ill for some days during which they have fever, a nasal discharge of a seropurulent nature, inappetence, and finally difficult breathing. These animals suffer from a fibrinous pneumonia, the greater part of the lungs often being hepatized and the pleura covered with a fibrinous deposit. If such animals do not die within a few days, they become emaciated and usually are worthless afterward. *Snuffles* is the common name applied to a milder respiratory infection caused by this organism. This initially involves only the upper respiratory tract. Affected animals exhibit a mucopurulent exudate, which partially occludes the nares and frequently also the conjunctiva. The animals have difficulty in breathing. The noises made by a colony of affected animals are characteristic and are responsible for the common name of the disease. Some cases end in fibrinous pneumonia and death.

The lesions are minimal in the peracute cases and generally are limited to a few petchiae on the heart and some of the serous membranes. In the chronic cases the lesions are limited, as a rule, to the organs of the thorax.

*Swine plague* usually consists of a fibrinous penumonia accompanied in some cases by septicemia. Peracute cases have been described but they rarely occur.

The pneumonias that accompany low-grade cholera virus infections, or cholera infections in partially immunized animals, are frequently of this type. The lungs present a characteristic appearance, similar to those seen in this disease in rabbits and cattle. The anterior lobes are most often involved and frequently the anterior portions of the diaphragmatic lobes as well. The lungs are firm and liverlike in consistency. The surface is covered with a serofibrinous exudate, and a turbid fluid containing flakes of fibrin is found in the thoracic cavity. The cut surface of the involved lung is firm and mottled in color, some lobules being dark red and others grayish. The lobules often are widely separated by the interlobular connective tissue which is distended by serofibrinous fluid.

Sautter, Pomeroy, and Fenstermacher (46) reported a case of pasteurellosis in a sow in which the lungs were not involved. The outstanding gross lesions were vegetative endocarditis and evidence of bacteremia.

A disease known as *atrophic rhinitis* (see p. 1358) is prevalent in swine in the Midwest and Canada. It is a contagious, chronic disease that affects young pigs and produces sneezing, nosebleed, stunted growth, and malformation of the turbinate bones. The etiology of this disease has been studied by a number of workers. In Canada, Gwatkin and co-workers (15) have presented evidence that nasal instillation of *Past. multocida* produces rhinitis in baby pigs and in rabbits. It now appears that *Past. multocida* is only a secondary invader in atrophic rhinitis of swine.

*Hemorrhagic septicemia* of cattle, goats, and sheep usually takes the pectoral or pneumonic form. The affected animals suffer from very high temperatures (106 to 108 F or higher). They breathe with great difficulty in the later stages of the infection, and the death rate is high. The disease often occurs after exposure or shipping. In cattle it is frequently called *shipping fever* or *shipping pneumonia*. It is not clear, however, that all cases known under these names are pasteurellosis, because there are reports of instances in which the *Pasteurella* organisms were not found and evidence to suggest that a virus was concerned (45). In fact an accumulation of evidence indicates that shipping fever of cattle is primarily a viral infection, the *Pasteurella* and other bacteria being secondary invaders which probably account for the severity of the disease and pneumonic complications (17, 20). The work of Reisinger *et al.* (41) on a paramyxovirus (SF-4) which was associated with shipping fever in cattle and which belongs to the parainfluenza group is interesting and probably significant (see p. 1071).

The lungs in typical cases have the appearance of those of swine suffering from *Pasteurella* infection, described above. The bipolar organisms can be seen in abundance in stained films made from the pneumonic tissue. They can readily be cultivated from these tissues, and they can be found in large numbers in stained sections in the exudate in the alveoli. The organism recovered from such cases often exhibits little virulence for rabbits. This is usually not true of *Pasteurella* organisms from other animals. That these organisms are the primary inciting agents of this disease seems doubtful, but it is quite probable that they play a dominant role in the production of the pneumonia that is the immediate cause of the deaths.

A few organisms can usually be recovered from the spleen and blood of cattle suffering from *Pasteurella* pneumonia. They are not found in large numbers, and the disease is not regarded as a bacteremia. Also, hemorrhages have never been a prominent finding. Hemorrhagic septicemia, therefore, is regarded as a misleading name for this disease in cattle. If an acute, bacteremic form of this disease occurs, it is very rare, apparently, in this country. The organism is found at times in the udders of cattle, where it causes mastitis. It has been isolated from sporadic cases (48) and from outbreaks (2).

It is not uncommon to find pure, or nearly pure, cultures of *Pasteurella* in respiratory infections of calves. In some the infection involves only the upper part of the tract. The animals suffer from fever, inappetence, and depression, and a mucopurulent exudate runs from their nostrils. The mortality from this disease may not be very great. Frequently however, in outbreaks of this disease in groups of calves, some develop pneumonia of the shipping fever type. They usually die.

In acute cases in sheep, inflammation in the abomasum and in portions of the small intestine may be evident. The liver may show evenly distributed small areas of necrosis. Rarely the infection localizes in the brain of sheep, producing symptoms characteristic of encephalitis. *Pasteurella* appear to be a common cause of severe ovine mastitis. (49). The condition is often called *bluebag* and it may occur sporadically or enzootically. Death may follow infection. In the surviving animal the udder is almost always useless.

*Infectious bovine rhinotracheitis* (see p. 968) occurs in all parts of the United States. Although this infection is caused by a virus, it has been stated that *Past. multocida* is consistently present in all typical cases (31). The organism has caused purulent leptomeningitis in a dog. The condition was accompanied by signs of depression, anorexia, vomition, incoordination, and marked muscular twitching of the head and neck (43). It was found in three horses, a pony, and a donkey in which death appeared to result from a *Pasteurella* septicemia (40).

**Other *Pasteurella* of the Hemorrhagic Septicemia Group.** Jones (23) in 1921 studied the organisms isolated from an outbreak of hemorrhagic septicemia in a large herd of cattle and found one that hemolyzed horse and cow blood cells. In other respects it was similar to *Past. multocida,* but the possession of this distinguishing feature led to the name *Past. hemolytica* (36). The organism does not produce indol. In addition to the sugars fermented by *Past. multocida,* lactose and maltose are fermented by *Past. hemolytica.* It appears that cultures of *Past. hemolytica* fall into one of two major serologic divisions and that there are a number of serotypes within the species (10). Furthermore, ovine strains may be the same type as bovine strains.

This organism occurs in pneumonia in cattle and sheep. Biberstein and Kennedy (4) have described field infections in lambs in California in which the predominant gross lesions were serosal hemorrhages, congestion, and edema of the lungs and lymph nodes. Distinct bacterial colonies were found constantly in the lungs, liver, spleen, and adrenal cortex, but no well-developed inflammatory reaction was associated with them. Experimental lambs that survived the first day following inoculation with a smooth variant of the organism developed such complications as arthritis, pericarditis, and meningitis. No pneumonia comparable to the field conditions associated with shipping fever was seen in the experimentally infected lambs.

In 1955 Hall *et al.* (16) studied a *Pasteurella* that they had isolated from chronic cholera in chickens. It did not produce indol, was nonhemolytic, and possessed low virulence. Because of these differences as well as some atypical serological and growth behavior, they named it *Pasteurella gallinarum.*

An organism, *Pasteurella pneumotropica,* was isolated by Olson and Meadows (38) from an infection of the soft tissues of the hand of a woman following a cat bite. Previously, it had been isolated from healthy and diseased mice and from sick rats, hamsters, and dogs. It has rarely infected man, and most cases have resulted from bites by cats and dogs. This bacterium differs mainly from *Past. multocida* in its ability to ferment maltose and split urea and an inability to ferment mannitol.

In 1966 Wang and Haiby (51) reported a case of human meningitis caused by *Pasteurella ureae.* They indicated that the organism was a variety of *Past. hemolytica,* that it formed a distinct serologic group, that it was characterized by a strong urease reaction, and that recently isolated strains have all been of human origin.

At this time it appears that *Past. hemolytica, Past. gallinarum, Past. pneumotoropica,* and *Past. ureae* may all be variants of *Past multocida.*

**Immunity to Pasteurella Infections.** It is of interest to note that the first bac-

terial vaccine was one used to combat fowl cholera. It was made by Pasteur
(39) in 1880, and its success was the basis of many other studies that laid the
foundations of our knowledge of artificial immunization against infectious diseases. The Pasteur vaccine consisted of living cultures of two grades of virulence. It was administered as a prophylactic measure in two doses, a few days
apart, the first being less virulent than the second. This type of vaccine is no
longer used.

1. *Bacterins.* These may be cultures of the specific organism killed with
heat or chemicals or a suspension of formalinized chicken embryo in which
the bacterium has been propagated. They may also consist of the antigens absorbed by aluminum hydroxide from formalin killed cultures. They are used
on cattle and sheep from 1 to 3 weeks before the animals are to be shipped in
order to allow antibodies to form by the time they are needed. On fowls they
should be used before an outbreak begins, if possible. According to Carter (6)
and Dougherty III (11), the bacterin made from formalinized chicken embryo
is the one of choice in immunizing fowl.

2. *Aggressin.* In 1924 Gouchenour isolated a *Pasteurella* from an American
bison that was unusually virulent for most of the domestic animals. By injecting a calf intrapleurally with this isolate, he produced an aggressin that was
quite popular for a time. It is no longer available. With regard to aggressins
it should be noted that they are antigenic, and temporarily they enhance susceptibility rather than immunity; hence they should always be given to animals that are normal and not under the stresses that seem to induce outbreaks.

3. *Immune serum.* Two kinds of immune serum are available for treating
animals that are believed to be in the early stages of the disease. One is made
from cattle, the other from horses. For use on cattle the homologous product
is always preferable because fewer serum reactions will be obtained following
its administration. Otherwise, so far as is known, one is as good as the other.
Large doses of antiserum are useful in treating the disease in its early stages.
If it is to be employed in a herd of cattle, it is advisable to take temperatures
of all animals and to use large doses of the antiserum on those in which pyrexia is found. Smaller doses may be given to exposed animals that have normal temperatures. It is probably useless to give serum to animals in which
pneumonia is fully developed.

**Evaluation of Biologic Products.** Since the work of Pasteur, bacterins and immune serums have been widely used as immunizing agents. They are employed to vaccinate sheep and cattle before shipping, especially during winter
months. Bacterins have been used not only to prevent pasteurellosis in fowl,
but also to cure it. In 1920, Van Es and Martin (50) were unable to find any
value in such products. On the other hand, Buckley and Gouchenour (5)
found that cattle and laboratory animals could be protected against inoculation with virulent organisms by means of vaccines, bacterins, and aggressin.
In 1966, Matsuoka *et al.* (30) recommended an inactivated vaccine including

parainfluenza-3 virus, *Past. multocida,* and *Past. hemolytica* as a means of protecting calves. They were vaccinated at 4 to 10 weeks of age and again at weaning time. Each of these views has numerous adherents; the treatment of pasturellosis with biologic products has been highly recommended by many and just as actively condemned by many others.

At the present time the value of these products in preventing the disease has not been satisfactorily assessed. The question is confused, in mammals at least, by etiological complications. Then the finding of serologic types by Little and Lyon (29) and subsequent studies by Carter (6, 7) and Namioka and Murata (35) have demonstrated the importance of selecting *Past. multocida* strains for bacterin and antiserum production on a serological or immunological basis rather than on zoological grounds. Apparently, immunization is attained only by contact with smooth forms of the serotypes, and it is effective only against homologous infection (52). In view of these findings, it seems evident that the production of effective biologics depends on the selection of the proper strains, and also that more extensive field trials should be conducted to establish the efficacy of these products.

**Chemotherapy.** Apparently the *Pasteurella* are much more sensitive to antibiotics and sulfa drugs than most Gram-negative organisms. Sulfamerazine (27) has merit in the treatment of pasteurellosis. Reports on the efficacy of antibiotics vary, but penicillin, aureomycin, neomycin, terramycin, polymyxin B, chloromycetin, and dihydrostreptomycin have been employed with success. Hawley (18) treated calves with a terramycin and antiserum combination and reported dramatic recoveries of the animals.

**Control Measures.** In 1923 Beach (3) stated that sanitary improvements, the reduction of overcrowding, and avoidance of concentrated feeding usually bring about a rapid disappearance of pasteurellosis in fowl. Present procedure utilizes biological products and antibiotics, mostly the latter, in controlling the disease.

Some preliminary results in the control and treatment of shipping fever in beef cattle were reported in 1955 by King *et al.* (25). Although no final conclusions were reached with regard to the results of the tests, it was stated that neither penicillin nor serum, when used prophylactically prior to shipment, gave satisfactory results. The recommendation was made that livestock disease-control and railroad officials study methods for improving the sanitation and the facilities in caring for cattle in transit, and it was inferred that this would greatly reduce the incidence of pasteurellosis in these animals. A report by Foley *et al.* (13) suggests pretreatment with a tranquilizing agent of cattle destined for shipment. They claim that treated animals are more easily handled, adapt more readily to feedlot environment, and show a lower incidence of infection.

**The Disease in Man.** In 1952 Olsen and Needham (37) reviewed 21 cases of human pasteurellosis and added a series of 37 cases that they had examined at the Mayo Clinic. Reports compiled by 1970 (21) list 316 cases in man.

Where no animal contact can be found, a reservoir of *Past. multocida* infection in man with interhuman transmission is postulated. Suppurative diseases of the respiratory tract were most common, but wound infections, meningitis, abscesses, and septicemia were also observed. Many of the patients came from rural areas and most cases of wound infection resulted from animal bites. Such lesions frequently are slow in healing and present a dirty, watery discharge.

## REFERENCES

1. Alberts and Graham.  North Am. Vet., 1948, *29*, 24.
2. Barnum.  Canad. Jour. Comp. Med. and Vet. Sci., 1954, *18*, 113.
3. Beach.  Poultry Sci., 1923, *1*, 186.
4. Biberstein and Kennedy.  Am. Jour. Vet. Res., 1959, *20*, 94.
5. Buckley and Gouchenour.  Jour. Am. Vet. Med. Assoc., 1924, *66*, 308.
6. Carter.  Am. Jour. Vet. Res., 1950, *11*, 252.
7. *Ibid.*, 1955, *16*, 481.
8. *Ibid.*, 1957, *18*, 437.
9. Carter.  Canad. Vet. Jour., 1963, *4*, 61.
10. *Ibid.*, 170.
11. Dougherty, III.  Cornell Vet., 1953, *43*, 421.
12. Flügge.  Die mikroorganismen.  F. C. W. Vogel, Leipzig, 1886.
13. Foley, McDonald, Robertson, and Siegrist.  Vet. Med., 1958, *53*, 515.
14. Gouchenour.  Jour. Am. Vet. Med. Assoc., 1924, *65*, 433.
15. Gwatkin, Dzenis, and Byrne.  Canad. Jour. Comp. Med. and Vet. Sci., 1953, *17*, 215.
16. Hall, Heddleston, Legenhausen, and Hughes.  Am. Jour. Vet. Res., 1955, *16*, 598.
17. Hamdy, Trapp, and Gale.  *Ibid.*, 1964, *25*, 128.
18. Hawley.  Jour. Am. Vet. Med. Assoc., 1952, *121*, 371.
19. Hendrickson and Hilbert.  Rpt. N.Y. State Vet. Coll. for 1930–31, p. 167.
20. Hetrick, Chang, Byrne, and Hansen.  Am. Jour. Vet. Res., 1963, *24*, 939.
21. Hubbert and Rosen.  Am. Jour. Pub. Health, 1970, *60*, 1103.
22. Hueppe.  Berl. klin. Wchnschr., 1886, *23*, 753, 776, and 794.
23. Jones.  Jour. Exp. Med., 1921, *34*, 561.
24. Jorgensen.  Cornell Vet., 1925, *15*, 205.
25. King, Edgington, Ferguson, Thomas, Pounden, and Klosterman.  Jour. Am. Vet. Med. Assoc., 1955, *127*, 320.
26. Kitt.  Sitzungsber.  Gesellsch. f. Morph. u. Phys. München, Bd. I, 1885, p. 240.
27. Larsen.  Vet. Med., 1948, *43*, 231.
28. Lignières.  Ann. l'Inst. Past., 1901, *15*, 734.
29. Little and Lyon.  Am. Jour. Vet. Res., 1943, *4*, 110.
30. Matsuoka, Gale, Ose, and Berkman.  Canad. Jour. Comp. Med. and Vet. Sci., 1966, *30*, 228.
31. Miller.  Jour. Am. Vet. Med. Assoc., 1955, *126*, 463
32. Moore.  U.S. Dept. of Agr., Bur. Anim. Indus. Bul. 3, 1895.
33. Namioka.  Jap. Agr. Res. Quart., 1967, *1*, 26.

34. Namioka and Bruner.  Cornell Vet., 1963, 53, 41.
35. Namioka and Murata.  *Ibid.*, 1964, 54, 520.
36. Newsom and Cross.  Jour. Am. Vet. Med. Assoc., 1932, 80, 711.
37. Olsen and Needham.  Am. Jour. Med. Sci., 1952, 224, 77.
38. Olson and Meadows.  Am. Jour. Clin. Path., 1969, 51, 709.
39. Pasteur.  Comp. rend. Acad. Sci., 1880, 90, 239, 952, and 1030.
40. Pavri and Apte.  Vet. Rec., 1967, 80, 437.
41. Reisinger, Heddleston, and Manthei.  Jour. Am. Vet. Med. Assoc., 1959, 135, 147.
42. Roberts.  Jour. Comp. Path. and Bact., 1947, 57, 261.
43. Rogers and Elder.  Austral. Vet. Jour., 1967, 43, 81.
44. Rosenbusch and Merchant.  Jour. Bact., 1939, 37, 69.
45. Ryff and Glenn.  Jour. Am. Vet. Med. Assoc., 1957, 131, 469.
46. Sautter, Pomeroy, and Fenstermacher.  *Ibid.*, 1946, 109, 369.
47. Trevisan.  Rendiconti. Reale Istituto Lombardo di Scienze e Lettere, Milan, 1887, p. 94.
48. Tucker.  Cornell Vet., 1953, 43, 378.
49. Tunnicliff.  Vet. Med., 1949, 44, 498.
50. Van Es and Martin.  Nebr. Agr. Exp. Sta. Res. Bul. 17, 1920.
51. Wang and Haiby.  Am. Jour. Clin. Path., 1966, 45, 562.
52. Yaw, Briefman, and Kakavas.  Am. Jour. Vet. Res., 1956, 17, 157.

### Pasteurella anatipestifer

This organism is believed to be the cause of a septicemic disease of ducks known as *infectious serositis, new duck disease* (3), or *antipestifer infection.* It has been described under the generic names of *Pfeifferella* (4) and *Moraxella* (2), but in the seventh edition of *Bergey's Manual,* it is placed in the genus *Pasteurella.* In morphology the organism is similar to *Past. multocida.* In cultural features it differs in that it is able to liquefy gelatin as well as co-agulated serum and egg. It does not ferment sugars. On primary isolation best growth is obtained if the infected material is seeded on medium that contains blood or serum and incubated under 10 percent $CO_2$.

Young ducks are most susceptible to infection and in field cases may show torticollis and extreme nervous signs. Tremors of the head and often loss of balance are seen. The mortality frequently is high. On postmortem examination infected ducks exhibit fibrinous pericarditis, perihepatitis with an enlarged liver, and splenitis. The air sac membranes usually are grossly thickened and opaque. Marshall *et al.* (5) have identified *Past. anatipestifer* in smears of exudate from infected ducks by the FA technic. Although it has been stated that ducks and sometimes geese are the hosts of this organism, in 1970 Bruner *et al.* (1) found it in pheasants and Munday *et al.* (6) in a black swan.

Consistent isolation of the organism from birds that show typical lesions is not always possible. Some of the isolates tend to lose virulence readily but others retain their ability to reproduce the disease experimentally for long periods. A bacterin made from embryonated eggs is being studied as a means of controlling the disease (7).

## REFERENCES

1. Bruner, Angstrom, and Price. Cornell Vet., 1970, *60*, 491.
2. Bruner and Fabricant. *Ibid.*, 1954, *44*, 461.
3. Dougherty, III, Saunders, and Parsons, Jr. Am. Jour. Path., 1955, *31*, 475.
4. Hendrickson and Hilbert. Cornell Vet., 1932, *22*, 239.
5. Marshall, Hansen, and Eveland. *Ibid.*, 1961, *51*, 24.
6. Munday, Corbould, Heddleston, and Harry. Austral. Vet. Jour., 1970, *46*, 322.
7. Price. Cornell Univ. Thesis, 1959.

### *Pasteurella pestis*

This organism is the cause of *plague* or *pest* of man. Time after time in past centuries plague spread over Europe from its endemic centers in Asia, destroying millions of people and spreading terror among the population. The disease became known as the *black death*. In warm climates the disease usually assumes the *bubonic* forms, so called from the swollen lymph nodes, known as *buboes*, which characterize it. In cold climates the disease is apt to take the pneumonic form, a much more fatal and contagious type.

Bubonic plague is not a disease of any of the domestic animals. It occurs naturally in rodents, especially in rats, in which it spreads rapidly at times. The disease in rats is quite similar to that in man and the mortality is about as great. The infection spreads from rat to rat, and from rat to man, through the agency of the rat flea (*Xenopsylla cheopis*). In recent times it has often been observed in plague centers that great human epidemics have been preceded by great rat epidemics.

In addition to rats, the disease also occurs naturally in marmots, ground squirrels, and other rodents. Unlike the rat, these creatures often live in areas sparsely inhabited by man. When plague spreads in such areas, it is known as the *sylvatic* form. In some of the wild animals that do not live in close association with man, plague has a much greater tendency to assume the more highly contagious pneumonic form than it does in the rat, and the disease contracted from them by man is also more likely to assume the pneumonic form.

Most cases of plague occur in the so-called *plague centers* of Asia (India, Burma, China, and Manchuria), but there are endemic foci in Africa, South and North America, and Hawaii. Western Europe has been practically free from the plague since the middle of the 18th century. It is believed that the first occurrence of this disease in the Western Hemisphere was a case in 1899 in Brazil. It appeared in San Francisco in 1900, probably brought in by oriental rats. After the epidemic of 1900, a second was reported in San Francisco in 1907. In 1914 plague struck the Gulf states (Texas, Louisiana, and Florida), and in 1924 it broke out in Los Angeles.

About 1908 it was discovered that plague infection existed in ground squirrels and other wild rodents in California. By 1960 it was known to be present in 17 of the western states as far east as North Dakota, Kansas, Oklahoma, and Texas. In this area, pockets of enzootic and epizootic plague have been found in 38 species of wild rodents. Of these, 11 rodent genera (including two of rabbits) are recognized to be of major importance in the ecology of sylvatic plague (4). Although this is an ever-present threat to man, only 67 human cases with 43 deaths have been traced to wild-rodent contact in these states in the last 40 years. During the years 1900–1951 there were 523 cases of plague in man and 340 deaths in the United States. These were found in 36 counties located in 12 states (Link, 8).

**Morphology and Staining Reactions.** The plague bacillus is a little larger than the organisms of hemorrhagic septicemia but otherwise resembles them very closely. Organisms in tissues usually measure about 0.5 microns by 1.5 microns. They may be readily stained with ordinary stains, and the bipolar appearance is easily demonstrated if diluted stains are used. The organism is Gram-negative and capsules are not ordinarily developed. In media containing 3 percent salt solution great pleomorphism is exhibited, and this characteristic is used for diagnostic purposes.

**Cultural Features.** The growth on most media resembles that of the hemorrhagic septicemia organisms but is a little more luxuriant. Colonies on agar become a little larger, and they develop a little more rapidly. Gelatin is not liquefied; milk is slightly acidified but not coagulated. Indol is not formed. Acid but no gas is formed from glucose, levulose, maltose, galactose, and mannitol. Lactose, sucrose, dulcitol, raffinose, and inulin are not attacked.

There are three physiological types. Type I does not ferment glycerol but reduces nitrate, type II ferments glycerol and reduces nitrate, and type III ferments glycerol and does not reduce nitrate. Type I is responsible for sylvatic or wild-rodent plague in the western United States (1).

The organism grows best at temperatures somewhat below that of the body. It grows poorly when the temperature is below 20 C and above 38 C. It is nonhemolytic and forms a toxin that appears to be intermediate between endotoxin and exotoxin. This toxicity is not associated with somatic complexes as in the enteric bacteria, and the toxin does not diffuse freely into the surrounding medium like diphtheria, tetanus, and botulinus toxins. It can be prepared in soluble form by phage lysis and differs from other endotoxins in that it is readily transformed into toxoid by formalin (1). The organism also produces a spreading factor and a coagulase (7).

According to Rockenmacher (9), catalase determinations can be used to distinguish between virulent and avirulent strains of *Past. pestis*, the former being able to decompose hydrogen peroxide more rapidly than the latter. Hudson *et al.* (5) claim that the FA technic is superior to animal inoculation in detecting *Past. pestis* in animal tissues.

**Resistance.** The plague organism does not exhibit any marked resistance to deleterious influence. Its life outside the animal body is precarious, and it seems to disappear speedily from soil, water, and buried cadavers. It can survive for months in the dried carcasses of small animals.

**Pathogenicity for Experimental Animals.** *Past. pestis* is pathogenic for rodents. The disease may be diagnosed by inoculating guinea pigs subcutaneously or, when specimens have undergone gross contamination and decomposition, by rubbing the material on the freshly shaven abdomen; the plague bacilli penetrate the minute abrasions while the contaminants do not. The animals die in 2 to 5 days; postmortem findings are characteristic and include subcutaneous and general congestion, congested spleen, granular liver, and pleural effusion. The bacilli may be found in spleen films and elsewhere, and cultured. For safety's sake it is important that the animal be freed of ectoparasites before inoculation.

According to Jawetz and Meyer (6), chick embryos of 12 to 14 days' incubation are highly susceptible to infection with virulent *Past. pestis* organisms, but newly hatched chicks are very resistant to plague infection, probably through the action of a cellular mechanism that is activated at hatching time. Hyperimmune plague antiserum of known protective value for mice is incapable of protecting chick embryos against an infective dose of *Past. pestis*. This is taken to indicate that a cellular defense mechanism must be present for antiserum to exert its protective action. In the absence of such a mechanism only the antitoxic, but not the anti-infectious, activity of antiserum becomes evident.

**Immunity.** Many vaccines have been used in preventing plague in man. The most widely used of these is Haffkine's vaccine in which virulent cultures are grown for several weeks and then killed with heat and phenol. This vaccine contains the products of autolysis of the organism as well as intact bacilli. It has been used very successfully in India as a prophylactic procedure. During World War II the United States Army used formalin-killed, virulent plague bacilli with apparent success. The use of living avirulent strains has been investigated with encouraging results by Grasset (3) in South Africa.

**Chemotherapy.** Sulfadiazine and streptomycin appear to be effective in treating plague (2). It has also been shown that aureomycin, chloromycetin, and terramycin are useful as therapeutic agents.

**Control Measures.** In dealing with plague, dependence is largely placed upon warfare on rats. Ratproofing of buildings, wharves, and ships has done much to keep the disease down and to prevent its spreading to parts of the world where it has not previously existed. Shipping from plague centers is subjected to cyanide fumigation before cargoes are discharged in plague-free areas in order to destroy the rats that may have found their way aboard. Modern steel ships also are so built as to be ratproof, or to offer few places for rats to hide.

**REFERENCES**

1. Burrows.  Textbook of microbiology. 17th ed. W. B. Saunders Co., Philadelphia, 1959.
2. Frobisher.  Fundamentals of microbiology. 8th ed. W. B. Saunders Co., Philadelphia, 1968.
3. Grasset.  Trans. Roy. Soc. Trop. Med. and Hyg., 1946, *40*, 275.
4. Hubbert, Goldenberg, Kartman, and Prince.  Jour. Am. Vet. Med. Assoc., 1966, *149*, 1651.
5. Hudson, Quan, and Kartman.  Jour. Hyg. (London), 1962, *60*, 443.
6. Jawetz and Meyer.  Am. Jour. Path., 1944, *20*, 457.
7. Jawetz and Meyer.  Jour. Immunol., 1944, *49*, 15.
8. Link.  U.S. Public Health Service Monograph no. 26, 1954.
9. Rockenmacher.  Proc. Soc. Exp. Biol. and Med., 1949, *71*, 99.

*Francisella* a ### *Pasteurella tularensis*

This organism is the cause of tularemia, otherwise known as *deer-fly fever*, *rabbit fever*, and *Ohara's disease*. The disease affects various rodents, especially the wild cottontail rabbit, water rats, and beaver, and occasionally certain birds and sheep. It has been reported in the dog and in the coyote (18). Man becomes infected from some of these animals either through direct contact with them or their carcasses or through the agency of ticks, lice (26), or bloodsucking flies.

The disease was first recognized in ground squirrels in California by McCoy (20) in 1911. These animals become fatally infected with the lesions resembling those of bubonic plague, with which tularemia was at first confused. McCoy and Chapin (21) in 1912 isolated and described the causative organism. In 1914 Wherry and Lamb (31) found tularemia infection in man and reported it as the first recognized case.

Some years later Francis identified the organism as the cause of a serious disease of man in Utah. Francis (10) gave the name *tularemia* to the disease, the name being derived from Tulare County, California, from whence came the ground squirrels with which McCoy was working when the disease was discovered. For some years it was thought that the disease was confined to the United States, but it is now known to exist in the Scandinavian countries, in Soviet Russia, and in Japan. In these countries, as well as in the United States, the disease has become of considerable importance as a human infection.

**Morphology and Staining Reactions.** This organism is much more pleomorphic than any of the others included in this group. In cultures bacillary forms up to 2 and even 3 microns in length may be seen. Coccoid forms usually are mixed with the bacillary types. Polar granules sometimes can be seen but these do not regularly occur. The organism is Gram-negative; it stains with the usual stains. It has neither capsules nor spores.

**Cultural Features.** *Past. tularensis* will not grow on ordinary agar or in plain bouillon. Media containing cystine is necessary (11). This may be supplied by adding egg yolk or salts containing cystine to ordinary types of culture media. Francis recommends a blood-glucose-cystine medium for the organism.

On suitable media *Past. tularensis* develops readily, forming a smooth, viscous, grayish-white growth. It does not liquefy gelatin and grows poorly in milk. It forms acid but no gas from glucose, levulose, and glycerol.

This organism differs considerably from other members of the *Pasteurella* group, and it is doubtful whether it should be included with them. It is included here for convenience rather than from conviction.

**Pathogenicity.** The guinea pig is easily infected with this organism, and therefore is frequently used in diagnostic work. A generalized, fatal disease develops in which the most striking lesions are multiple necrotic areas in the liver and spleen. Great care must be taken when working with this disease, for many laboratory workers have contracted the infection (16). Apparently the organism is capable of entering the unbroken skin.

Parker and Dade (24; 1929) have reported severe losses in lambs pastured on land in Montana that is heavily infected with woodticks, and have shown that it is this tick which carries the infection. The ticks become infected, of course, by feeding upon wild rodents in which the disease is enzootic. The disease has been reported in epizootics in sheep in Idaho (12) and in Wyoming (27), in pen-raised beavers in Oregon (2), and in rabbits in South Carolina (19). It has occurred in cats and dogs. It has also appeared in calves and domestic chickens. It can infect practically all rodents and has been isolated from beavers, foxes, skunks, coyotes, bobcats, deer, snakes, quail, prairie chickens, pheasants, shrikes, ducks, gulls, hawks, owls, muskrats (water rats), and monkeys (4).

The greatest reservoir of tularemia in the United States is in the wild-rabbit population, especially in many of midwestern states. It is from the handling of the carcasses of such rabbits that most of the human cases in this country originate. Of 266 authenticated cases of tularemia in California reported during the years 1927–1951, 81 percent were contracted from rabbits. Jack rabbits were involved more frequently than the cottontail. Cases are contracted from the bites of bloodsucking insects that have fed upon infected rabbits (13). Washburn and Tuohy (30) reported that tick-borne infection was almost twice as common in Arkansas as was rabbit-borne infection. Later it was shown by Calhoun (5) that the lone star tick (*Amblyomma americanum*) was the important carrier of *Past. tularensis* in Arkansas and by Hopla (14) that the bacterium multiplied in this arthropod. The argasid ticks (3) as well as members of the genus *Dermacentor* (1) also can transmit tularemia. In general, strains of *Past. tularensis* obtained from North American ticks, lagomorphs, and sheep are highly virulent and those from beaver, rodents, and water are less so (28).

The organism sometimes becomes prevalent in water holes and in small streams, being spread from the bodies of infected water animals such as water rats and beavers (8). Human cases have been reported from contact with such water (22).

**Immunity.** One attack of tularemia gives a very solid and lasting immunity. Individuals who have suffered from the disease develop agglutinins that persist for long periods—sometimes for many years after all symptoms have disappeared. These agglutinins will react with *Brucella abortus,* and *Brucella* agglutinins will react with the organism of tularemia. This is something that should be kept in mind when serological tests for diagnosis are utilized. The titer for the homologous organism is usually very much higher than it is for the heterologous; hence if both organisms are tested it is simple to judge which is specific.

Foshay, Hesselbrock, Wittenberg, and Rodenberg (9) prepared a vaccine from *Past. tularensis* by oxidizing the bacterial growth in the presence of aqueous sodium nitrite and acetic acid. After 4 hours' treatment the bacteria were washed free of the acid and salts, phenolized, and standardized. This vaccine proved valuable in protecting against tularemia. Live avirulent vaccines have also been recommended for use (6, 29).

**Chemotherapy.** It is reported that the sulfonamides and penicillin have little effect on the course of tularemia infection. Streptomycin is very effective in treating this disease (7, 15, 25). Woodward, Ravy, Eppes, Holbrook, and Hightower (32) indicate that aureomycin also is useful in curing tularemia and oxytetracycline has been used successfully by Frank and Meinershagen (12) in treating sheep. The probability of a patient dying from the disease is low, especially if he receives appropriate therapy.

### Pasteurella novicida

This is a new species described by Larson *et al.* (17). It was isolated from water. It is highly pathogenic for mice, hamsters, guinea pigs, and rabbits. In many cultural characteristics, in morphology, and in pathogenicity it closely resembles *Past. tularensis,* but it can be distinguished from this organism by fermentation studies and serologic tests (23).

### REFERENCES

1. Allred, Stagg, and Lavender.   Jour. Inf. Dis., 1956, 99, 143.
2. Bell, Owen, Jellison, Moore, and Buker.   Am. Jour. Vet. Res., 1962, 23, 884.
3. Burgdorfer and Owen.   Jour. Inf. Dis., 1956, 98, 67.
4. Burroughs, Holdenried, Longanecker, and Meyer.   Ibid., 1945, 76, 115.
5. Calhoun.   Am. Jour. Trop. Med. and Hyg., 1954, 3, 360.
6. Chamberlain.   Appl. Microbiol., 1965, 13, 232.
7. Chapman, Coriell, Kawol, Nelson, and Downs.   Jour. Bact., 1946, 51, 607.
8. Editorial.   Pub. Health Rpts. (U.S.), 1940, 55, 227.
9. Foshay, Hesselbrock, Wittenberg, and Rodenberg.   Am. Jour. Pub. Health, 1942, 32, 1131.
10. Francis.   Jour. Am. Med. Assoc., 1922, 78, 1015.

11.   Francis.   Pub. Health Rpts. (U.S.), 1923, *38*, 1396.
12.   Frank and Meinershagen.   Vet. Med., 1961, *56*, 374.
13.   Hillman and Morgan.   Jour. Am. Med. Assoc., 1937, *108*, 538.
14.   Hopla.   Am. Jour. Hyg., 1955, *61*, 371.
15.   Howe, Coriell, Bookwalter, and Ellingson.   Jour. Am. Med. Assoc., 1946, *132*, 195.
16.   Lake and Francis.   Pub. Health Rpts. (U.S.), 1922, 37, 392.
17.   Larson, Wicht, and Jellison.   *Ibid.*, 1955, *70*, 253.
18.   Lundgren, Marchette, and Smart.   Jour. Inf. Dis., 1957, *101*, 154.
19.   McCahan, Moody, and Hayes.   Am. Jour. Hyg., 1962, *75*, 335.
20.   McCoy.   U.S. Pub. Health Service Bul. 43, 1911.
21.   McCoy and Chapin.   Jour. Inf. Dis., 1912, *10*, 61.
22.   Nikanorov.   Abstract, Jour. Am. Med. Assoc., 1929, *93*, 696.
23.   Owen, Buker, Jellison, Lackman, and Bell.   Jour. Bact., 1964, *87*, 676.
24.   Parker and Dade.   Jour. Am. Vet. Med. Assoc., 1929, *75*, 173.
25.   Peterson and Parker.   Pub. Health Rpts. (U.S.), 1946, *61*, 1231.
26.   Price.   Am. Jour. Hyg., 1956, *63*, 186.
27.   Ryff, Michael, and Norton.   Jour. Am. Vet. Med. Assoc., 1961, *138*, 309.
28.   Thorpe, Sidwell, Johnson, Smart, and Parker.   Am. Jour. Trop. Med. and Hyg., 1965, *14*, 622.
29.   Tulis, Eigelsbach, and Hornick.   Proc. Soc. Exp. Biol. and Med., 1969, *132*, 893.
30.   Washburn and Tuohy.   South. Med. Jour., 1949, *42*, 60.
31.   Wherry and Lamb.   Jour. Inf. Dis., 1914, *15*, 331.
32.   Woodward, Ravy, Eppes, Holbrook, and Hightower.   Jour. Am. Med. Assoc., 1949, *139*, 830.

### Pasteurella pseudotuberculosis

SYNONYMS:   *Bacterium pseudotuberculosis rodentium,*
*Corynebacterium rodentium*

This organism is the cause of a plaguelike disease of guinea pigs, sometimes of rats, and occasionally of other rodents, which has been called *Pasteurella pseudotuberculosis*. The organism has little importance in animal pathology except in stocks of guinea pigs, although rare infections with it have been reported in cattle, sheep, goats, horses, pigs, foxes, mink, rabbits, chinchillas, birds, monkeys, and man. In 1940 it was found by Beaudette (1) in a blackbird, and in 1944 it was isolated by Rosenwald and Dickinson (12) from sick and dead turkeys. This organism resembles that of plague so closely, and the lesions in guinea pigs are so similar, that it is easy to confuse one with the other. In fact, an organism isolated from a rabbit in Alaska in 1965 and identified as *Past. pestis* was eventually established as a strain of *Past. pseudotuberculosis* (9).

**Morphology and Staining Reactions.** This organism varies from coccoid to bacillary forms 5 microns or more in length. They generally appear singly; occasionally they are in chains. Bipolar staining can sometimes be noted. This organism is somewhat larger than the hemorrhagic septicemia bacilli. It is Gram-negative, non-acid-fast, and not encapsulated.

**Cultural Features.** *Past. pseudotuberculosis* differs from others in the *Pasteurella* group by being motile. Motility, however, is seldom seen in strains grown at body temperature; young cultures grown at 18 to 26 C are most favorable for detecting it.

On plain agar good growth occurs without the addition of serum or other enrichment. Blood agar shows no evidence of hemolysis. The colonies are small, translucent, and granular. In old colonies the centers are raised and more opaque than the periphery, which frequently shows radial striations. The consistency is soft and butyrous.

Growth in broth is fairly good. There is moderate turbidity in 24 hours at 37 C, but later the growth sediments into a viscid mass. A surface ring usually appears. On potato there is a thin growth which is cream-colored at first, later becoming yellow, and then brown. Litmus milk slowly becomes alkaline. Indol is not formed. Acid but no gas is formed from glucose, maltose, mannitol, salicin, arabinose, xylose, rhamnose, and glycerol. Sucrose is sometimes fermented. Lactose, raffinose, dulcitol, and sorbitol are not attacked.

Based on O antigens, there are five somatic groups of organisms. The same H antigen is found in all strains with one exception. A common somatic antigen exists in Group II and the *Salmonella* Group B. Ransom (10) has indicated that the organism also shares two envelope and one somatic antigen with *Past. pestis*. According to Mair (5) the majority of strains prevalent in England and Europe belong in serologic type 1.

**Pathogenicity.** The disease is most often seen spontaneously in stocks of guinea pigs. The affected animals sicken, lose weight, develop diarrhea, and die in 3 to 4 weeks. In such animals the mesenteric lymph nodes are greatly swollen and caseous, and there may be nodular abscesses in the intestinal wall originating in follicles. Similar nodules usually stud the liver and spleen thickly. Outbreaks of pseudotuberculosis have been encountered in chinchilla colonies (4) and in mink (2), and the organism has been isolated from a bovine (6) and an ovine (17) fetus. In cattle it has also been associated with pneumonia as well as with abortion (3), and it has caused infection in cats, characterized by abdominal and urinary disturbances (7).

According to Thal (15), there are toxic and atoxic strains of *Past. pseudotuberculosis*, the toxic ones producing an exotoxin that is thermolabile and transferable into a toxoid that stimulates the production of antitoxin. The existence of the toxin explains certain differences in the susceptibility of laboratory animals. Guinea pigs succumb easily to infection with virulent strains, but mice are more resistant. For white rats only toxic strains are pathogenic.

**Mode of Transmission.** Natural infection is supposed to occur through ingestion of the causative organism because primary localizations appear in the intestinal wall and the mesenteric lymph nodes.

**Diagnosis.** *Past. pseudotuberculosis* resembles *Past. pestis* in cultural characteristics and in the disease it produces in guinea pigs. However, it can be differentiated from the latter by its avidity for urea and ability to grow well on desoxycholate citrate agar, while *Past. pestis* fails to attack urea and grows poorly on desoxycholate citrate agar. Phage typing and inability to cross-immunize also identify the species.

**Immunity.** Thal (15) has found a live avirulent culture that is capable of producing a solid immunity in guinea pigs against virulent strains. Intranasal instillation has produced satisfactory results (16).

**The Disease in Man.** Although the disease is rare in man, *Past. pseudotuberculosis* can produce severe and fatal infections (8). The symptoms and anatomical changes simulate those caused by enteric fever, tularemia, and tuberculosis (11). The organism is fairly resistant to penicillin and streptomycin, but is sensitive to sulfa drugs (14).

## REFERENCES

1. Beaudette.   Jour. Am. Vet. Med. Assoc., 1940, 97, 151.
2. Henriksson.   9th Nord. Vet. Cong., Copenhagen, 1962, p. 59.
3. Langford.   Canad. Vet. Jour., 1969, 10, 208.
4. Laughton, Till, and Noble.   Vet. Rec., 1963, 75, 835.
5. Mair.   Jour. Path. and Bact., 1965, 90, 275.
6. Mair and Harbourne.   Vet. Rec., 1963, 75, 559.
7. Mair, Harbourne, Greenwood, and White.   *Ibid.*, 1967, 81, 461.
8. Meyer.   Personal communication, 1957.
9. Quan, Knapp, Goldenberg, Hudson, Lawton, Chen, and Kartman.   Am. Jour. Trop. Med. and Hyg., 1965, 14, 424.
10. Ransom.   Proc. Soc. Exp. Biol. and Med., 1956, 93, 551.
11. Reimann.   Am. Jour. Hyg., 1932, 16, 206.
12. Rosenwald and Dickinson.   Am. Jour. Vet. Res., 1944, 5, 246.
13. Schütze.   A system of bacteriology in relation to medicine. Med. Res. Council (Brit.), 1929, vol. IV, p. 474.
14. Snyder and Vogel.   Northwest Med., 1943, 42, 14.
15. Thal.   Untersuchungen über *Pasteurella pseudotuberculosis* unter besonderer Berücksichtigung ihres immunologischen Verhaltens. Berlingska Boktryckeriet, Lund, 1954.
16. Thal, Hanko, and Knapp.   Acta Vet. Scand., 1964, 5, 179.
17. Watson and Hunter.   Vet. Rec., 1960, 72, 770.

## THE GENUS *BORDETELLA*

In this genus there are three species, *Bordetella pertussis*, etiologically associated with whooping cough in man and *Bordetella parapertussis* and occasionally *Bordetella bronchiseptica* connected with a whooping-cough-like disease. These organisms are Gram-negative coccobacilli that are hemolytic, inactive in carbohydrate media, and able to produce dermonecrotic toxin. Serologically they are very closely related (8), and *B. pertussis* antitoxin neutralizes the toxin of *B. parapertussis* and of *B. bronchiseptica*. Because only *B. bronchiseptica* has been associated with diseases of the lower animals it is considered here.

### *Bordetella bronchiseptica*

For years this organism was classified with the *Brucella* although it did not exactly fit the definition of this genus. In the seventh edition of *Bergey's Manual* it was placed in the genus *Bordetella*.

*B. bronchiseptica* was first described by Ferry (4, 5) in 1910. It was isolated from the upper respiratory tract of a dog suffering from distemper, and it was erroneously believed to be the cause of that condition.

**Morphology and Staining Reactions.** *B. bronchiseptica* is a small, Gram-negative bacillus that is motile by means of peritrichic flagella.

**Cultural Features.** The organism grows readily on ordinary laboratory media, but it does not ferment any of the carbohydrates. On litmus milk it will grow and intensify the alkaline reaction. It multiplies well on potato and produces a tan-colored growth that ages into brown. It is hemolytic for rabbit and guinea pig corpuscles and freshly isolated cultures will produce a rapidly fatal disease in guinea pigs upon intraperitoneal injection.

**Pathogenicity.** *B. bronchiseptica* is encountered frequently in bronchopneumonias and other respiratory infections in rodents (rabbits, guinea pigs, and rats) as well as in horses, swine, dogs, cats, and, occasionally, monkeys and man. In animal houses of research laboratories, epidemics of pneumonia produced by this organism frequently cause serious trouble (13). When guinea pigs are used in research work as a means of detecting *Brucella* of the abortion group, care must be taken not to confuse this organism, which may spontaneously appear, with the others. The cultural characters of *B. bronchiseptica* are sufficiently like those of *Brucella abortus* or *Brucella suis* to mislead even an experienced worker. Because *B. bronchiseptica* in young cultures is actively motile, whereas the others are nonmotile, a simple hanging drop often will clear up doubts.

Ferry (4), McGowan (9), and many others regarded this organism as the cause of the highly fatal and widespread disease of dogs known as *canine distemper*. Carré (1) and others contested this view, claiming that distemper was caused by a virus and that the bacterial agent of Ferry was only a secondary invader. The work of Laidlaw and Dunkin (7) finally settled the matter by showing that canine distemper is a virus disease and that it occurs in the complete absence of the bacterial agent. These findings relegate this organism to a minor position so far as canine distemper is concerned, but they do not prove that it is of no importance in canine pathology. It has been clearly shown to be pathogenic and to be capable of setting up serious respiratory infection in the dog in the absence of virus (15), but its greatest role undoubtedly is in producing complications in the virus disease, in particular the bronchopneumonia which so often is the immediate cause of death.

*B. bronchiseptica* has been recovered from the lungs of young pigs suffering from a respiratory disease. The infection is seen most commonly at 3 to 8 weeks of age. It produces few deaths in the acute stages, but many cases become chronic and result in severe stunting. The most striking lesion is an edema of the lungs (10). Whether *B. bronchiseptica* is a primary cause of a pneumonia in pigs or whether it is secondary to other agents such as viruses or pleuropneumonialike organisms remains to be established. Cross and Claflin (2) and Ross *et al.* (12) have indicated that the organism may also be important in producing atrophic rhinitis in swine. Injection of pure cultures resulted in mild to moderate turbinate atrophy. Harris and Switzer (6) have indicated that *Pasteurella multocida,* type D, will become established and persist only in the nasal cavities of swine after preconditioning of the nasal epithelium by *B. bronchiseptica* rhinitis. Although atrophy was not any more severe macroscopically, a concurrent infection by both organisms increased the intensity of the microscopic changes as compared with those in turbinates of pigs infected with *B. bronchiseptica* alone.

**Immunity.** *B. bronchiseptica* cross-agglutinates partially with the other *Brucella,* as was shown first by Evans (3). This should be remembered by the laboratory worker who runs blood tests on guinea pigs for detecting agglutinins for *Br. abortus* or *Br. suis.*

Mixed bacterins containing *B. bronchiseptica* and antibacterial sera containing antibodies for this organism are available commercially for treating dogs to prevent or alleviate the pneumonia which frequently occurs in distemper. These products obviously will not affect the primary virus infections, but they may be useful against the bacterial complications which frequently are the immediate cause of death. Some companies manufacture distemper antisera from dogs that are immunized against *B. bronchiseptica,* streptococci, *Pasteurella* types, and other organisms frequently found in clinical cases, as well as against the virus of canine distemper. A bacterin was used successfully in protecting rats (16).

**Chemotherapy.** Rosen *et al.* (11) in treating infected rats concluded that streptomycin temporarily checked the disease, that sulfonamides reduced the death rate but were not a cure, and that terramycin therapy was highly satisfactory. Switzer (14) has stated that pigs experimentally infected with nasal bordetellosis were successfully freed of the infection by treatment with sulfamethazine at the level of 100 g per ton of feed.

**REFERENCES**

1. Carré.   Bul. Soc. Cent. Med. Vet., 1905, 59, 335.
2. Cross and Claflin.   Jour. Am. Vet. Med. Assoc., 1962, *141,* 1467.
3. Evans.   Jour. Inf. Dis., 1916, *18,* 578.
4. Ferry.   Am. Vet. Rev., 1910, 37, 499.
5. Ferry.   Jour. Inf. Dis., 1911, 8, 399.
6. Harris and Switzer.   Am. Jour. Vet. Res., 1968, *29,* 777.
7. Laidlaw and Dunkin.   Jour. Comp. Path. and Therap., 1926, 39, 201, 203, and 222.
8. Leslie and Gardner.   Jour. Hyg. (London), 1931, *31,* 423.
9. McGowan.   Jour. Path. and Bact., 1911, *15,* 372.

10.  Ray.   Jour. Am. Vet. Med. Assoc., 1950, *116*, 51.
11.  Rosen, Hunt, and Benarde.   *Ibid.*, 1954, *124*, 300.
12.  Ross, Duncan, and Switzer.   Vet. Med., 1963, *58*, 566.
13.  Smith.   Jour. Med. Res., 1914, *24*, 291.
14.  Switzer.   Vet. Med., 1963, *58*, 571.
15.  Torrey and Rahe.   Jour. Med. Res., 1913, *22*, 291.
16.  Wickert, Rosen, Dawson, and Hunt.   Jour. Am. Vet. Med. Assoc., 1958, *133*, 363.

## THE GENUS *BRUCELLA*

Within this genus are three closely related species that have been recognized for many years. They are *Brucella abortus, Brucella suis,* and *Brucella melitensis.* Two more species that possess characteristics much like those of *Br. suis, Brucella canis,* and *Brucella neotomae,* have now been established, and a sixth, *Brucella ovis,* whose relationship is less clear, has been included. The diseases caused by these organisms are now generally known as *brucelloses.* Special names are given to the individual diseases in different animals and in man.

### Brucella abortus

SYNONYMS:   *Bacillus abortus,* Bang's bacillus

This organism is the cause of brucellosis of cattle, a widespread disease which is also known as *infectious abortion* and *Bang's disease.* Most cases of contagious or infectious abortion in cattle are caused by it.

Although *Br. abortus* is principally associated with cattle, it is found in other species. It has been reported in sheep (34). It has been isolated from the uterine contents of aborting mares and from an aborted human fetus (Carpenter and Boak, 10), but apparently it does not play an important role in abortions in either of these species. It has appeared infrequently in chickens and dogs, in rare cases causing canine abortion, and it has been isolated from the submaxillary lymph nodes of swine slaughtered in a packing plant (35). It has been described in bison, elk, and moose in Canada (11). It has been found in hygromas of the knees of cattle and in inflammations of the bursae located beneath the two attachments of the ligamentum nuchae in horses. In fact, Roderick *et al.* (44) have shown that the injection of either *Br. abortus* or *Br. suis* in combination with *Actinomyces bovis* results in the conditions generally known as *fistula of the withers* and *poll evil.* In man *Br. abortus* causes a disease known as *brucellosis* or *undulant fever,* but it is not the sole incitant of this malady because some cases are due to *Br. suis* and others to *Br. melitensis.* All three species produce the same clinical syndrome in man and it now appears that *Br. canis* must be included in this category.

*Br. abortus* produces a generalized disease when injected into guinea pigs, rabbits, mice, and rats. The organism was first described by Bang (1) in Denmark in 1897. It was first recognized in the United States by McNeal and Kerr (37) in 1910.

**Morphology and Staining Reactions.** *Br. abortus* is a small, Gram-negative, nonsporeforming rod. It is frequently so short as easily to be mistaken for a coccus. In exudates it is frequently found in clumps, but otherwise the characteristic arrangement is single. It sometimes grows intracellularly. It stains with the ordinary stains but with some difficulty.

**Cultural Features.** The organism was first cultivated by Bang and Stribolt in a mixture of agar and gelatin that contained serum. This mixture is not necessary; in fact the organism grows fairly well in ordinary infusion agar without enrichment. Glucose agar and glycerol agar are used by some in preference to ordinary agar. A little serum enhances the growth. Liver agar is regarded by some as an especially favorable medium.

Using the Liborius method, Bang and Stribolt discovered, after several days' incubation, a zone of colonies about 5 mm below the surface of the medium. No growth occurred on the surface nor deeper in the medium. After several transfers the organism finally acquired the property of growing on the surface and thereafter grew readily with no special attention on ordinary agar slants.

For a long time it was thought that the organism required a concentration of oxygen below that of the atmosphere. Being neither aerobic in the ordinary sense, nor anaerobic, it was classed as a microaerobic or microaerophilic organism. In 1921 Huddleson (24) showed that it was not the oxygen of the atmosphere that affected the growth but rather the carbon dioxide tension. If a closed vessel that contains the cultures is partially exhausted of air, and if $CO_2$ is introduced to a concentration of about 10 percent, luxuriant growth of the organism occurs irrespective of the amount of oxygen present, so long as the free oxygen is not completely eliminated.

Prior to the time of Huddleson's discovery, it had been the practice in most laboratories to "lower the oxygen tension" in containers in which *Br. abortus* was to be grown by connecting them with other containers in which *Bacillus subtilis* or other active aerobic bacteria were growing, a method introduced by Nowak in 1908 (39). Later it was discovered that a method advocated by Preisz in 1902 served practically as well. This consisted merely in using containers in which there was relatively little air space and sealing them hermetically. In both instances the $CO_2$ content rises because of the respiratory activities of the bacteria and of viable tissue cells that are usually introduced simultaneously with the bacteria in the inoculum. These methods are more haphazard than Huddleson's, and although they generally will succeed, the latter method is preferable.

The organism grows rather scantily in fluid media, producing a faint clouding. Carbohydrates are not fermented. Gelatin is not liquefied. The organism will multiply in milk but produces no visible changes in it. On blood agar there is no effect on the blood cells. Colonies on solid media are smooth, shiny, and translucent.

The *Brucella* Subcommittee on Bacterial Nomenclature recognizes nine biotypes of *Br. abortus*. This classification is based upon differences in virulence for experimental animals, in host reservoirs, and in biochemical activities.

**Resistance.** *Br. abortus* is not very resistant to disinfectants or to sunlight and drying. Putrefaction destroys it rather quickly. When protected from complete drying, it may retain its vitality for several months. It is destroyed by pasteurization. An experiment was conducted by Kuzdas and Morse (31) on the survival of *Br. abortus* in the spleens of infected guinea pig carcasses. During the cold months of January and February the organisms survived for 44 days in carcasses placed upon the ground and for 29 days in those buried at a depth of 2 feet. Survival time in June and August was 1 day. Counts of viable bacteria in desiccated *Br. abortus* Strain 19 vaccine decreased to an unsatisfactory level within 12 weeks at a temperature of 25 C and within 3 days at 37.5 C (33).

**Pathogenicity for Cattle.** The organism was first found by Bang in the uterochorionic space of a cow in which abortion was impending. A brownish, pasty, nonodorous exudate is to be found there. The organisms usually are present in pure culture. Many are enclosed in the protoplasm of epithelial

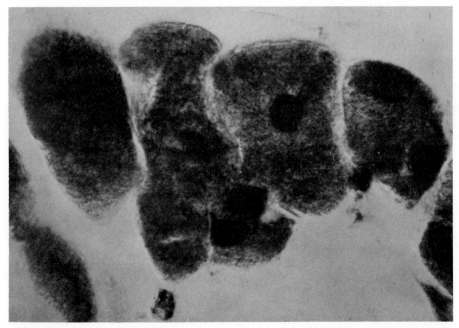

*Fig. 9.* Localization of *Brucella abortus* in the bovine placenta. Epithelial cells of the chorion are greatly swollen and packed with bacilli. The nuclei are pyknotic. (After Theobald Smith; courtesy *Jour. Exp. Med.*)

cells. Smith (47) has shown that these cells are derived from the outer fetal envelope, the chorion. The chorion presents dull, thickened, leatherlike areas, due to the multiplication of this organism. Generally this membrane is edematous.

It is apparent that the organism induces an inflammation of the membrane and that interference with the circulation of the fetus may explain why abortion occurs. The fetus usually shows a dropsical condition, a fact which also points toward a circulatory disturbance. The organism may also be found, generally in pure culture, in the alimentary tract and in the lungs of aborted fetuses. The other tissues of the fetus usually are sterile. The location of the organism suggests that it is taken into the fetus by the swallowing of the amniotic fluid rather than through the blood stream.

After calving or abortion the organism does not usually persist long in the uterus. It may be recognized for a few days but later it seems to disappear. It is thought by some that the fetal membranes represent the only medium on which the organism thrives; hence, when the membranes disappear, the organism disappears also. Another explanation for this behavior concerns a substance known as *erythritol,* a constituent of normal bovine fetal fluids, that appears to stimulate the growth of *Br. abortus* in bovine phagocytes (42).

Besides the pregnant uterus, the organism is frequently recognized in another organ, the udder. The lymph nodes adjacent to the udder and uterus are usually infected when these organs are involved. Occasionally the organism may be found in some of the other organs of the body, but lesions are not induced and it is probable that they harbor the bacilli only for a short time. *Br. abortus* has been isolated from hygromas of the·knee joints of cattle. In bulls, infection of the epididymis and testicle sometimes occurs. In these cases abscessation usually develops and the organs are destroyed. On the other hand, Rankin (43) has declared that bulls may become infected in calfhood and retain this condition into adult life, but are rarely responsible for the spread of disease to cows during natural service and that brucellosis is not an important cause of infertility in bulls.

A rather high percentage of involved animals develop infection of the udder, and it is in this organ that the disease maintains itself in the host from one gestation period to the next. The infected udders cannot be detected clinically, but the organism may be isolated by inoculating the milk into guinea pigs. Experience has shown that nonpregnant animals which have high agglutinin titers toward antigens made from *Br. abortus* usually have one or more infected quarters in their udders. Such animals usually are carriers for life, though a few are able to throw off the organism. Udder infection with members of the *Brucella* has considerable public health significance because organisms are discharged in the milk.

*Br. abortus* may occasionally be isolated from the lymph nodes of the digestive tract and from the spleens of cattle. No lesions may be recognized in these organs. It appears probable that the organism is located in these organs

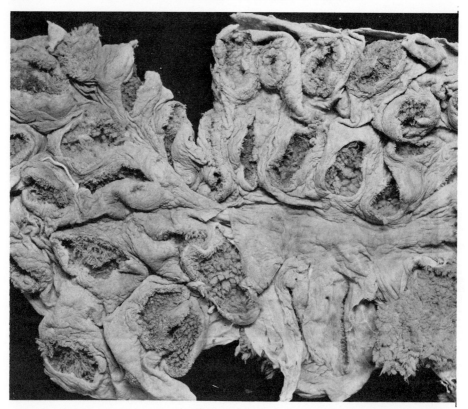

*Fig. 10.* Infection of the bovine placenta with *Brucella abortus*. The surface shown is that of the chorion. This membrane normally is thin and transparent. Here it is transformed into a thick, opaque, yellowish-white, leatherlike membrane covered with granular debris. The fetal cotyledons are necrotic, this being evidenced by the fact that they are yellowish in color and filled with granular exudate. In an earlier stage of its development the lesions of the chorion consist of edema and dull granular thickening of the surface epithelium. From these early lesions it is possible to demonstrate the bacilli-choked cells shown in figure 9. They cannot be found in such advanced lesions as the ones shown here.

transiently. It likewise may be isolated occasionally from the blood stream.

When calves are fed upon infected milk, the organism can be found in the lymph glands of the digestive canal but, within a few weeks after the infected milk is withdrawn, it generally disappears. Until sexual maturity is reached the genital organs seldom become involved. Calfhood infection usually does not result in permanent infection.

There is some evidence that *Brucella* organisms may lodge in the navicular bursa as well as in the proximal and terminal bursa of the ligamentum nuchae of the horse and that mild cases of brucellosis occur in this animal (12).

**Mode of Infection.** The disease in cattle probably results most often from the ingestion of discharges of aborting animals, although it has been shown experimentally that they can easily be infected through the mucous membranes of the eye, and this may be an important avenue of infection. Another possible entry of the organism that should not be overlooked is the skin, either through slight abrasions or through uninjured portions. Hardy has shown that laboratory animals may be infected through the uninjured skin.

Infections of cows may occur by way of the genital tract, either from the semen of diseased bulls or by contamination from sound bulls that have recently served infected cows. Bulls, likewise, are probably infected by serving cows that are discharging bacilli in their genital secretions. Transfer of the disease from one sex to the other by copulation is not a frequent occurrence but it is known to occur; consequently positively reacting bulls should never be used to breed negative cows. Bendixen and Blom (4) were able to demonstrate *Br. abortus* in the semen of 15 in a series of 58 blood-reacting bulls by culture and guinea pig inoculation. Abundant organisms were found in the semen in acute phases of vesiculitis, ampullitis, and epididymitis, and spread of the infection to inseminated cows was demonstrated in five cases. The use of infected bull semen in artificial insemination of cattle in Denmark resulted in serious damage.

Although the possibility of wild species acting as reservoirs of brucellosis in the United States has been considered it appears that their role is insignificant.

**Disease of Guinea Pigs Caused by Inoculation with *Br. abortus*.** The most reliable method of detecting *Br. abortus* in infected materials is by the inoculation of guinea pigs. The character of the disease in this animal assumes importance because of this fact.

Early workers claimed that the small laboratory animals could not be infected with *Br. abortus*. This idea was corrected by Smith and Fabyan (48) in 1912. These workers found that a chronic disease, somewhat resembling tuberculosis, occurred when injections of the organisms were made in pure culture or when milk naturally infected with the organism was used for inoculation. This work also solved a problem that Smith had studied in 1893 in which tuberclelike lesions occurred in guinea pigs which had been injected with market milk but in which the tubercle organism could not be found. A good description of the character of the lesions in guinea pigs is given by Fabyan (16; 1912).

The organisms are usually found in greatest numbers in the spleen of infected animals. This organ may remain normal in appearance and yet harbor numerous organisms; it may be nodular, or it may be enormously enlarged and engorged with blood. As was shown by Smillie (46; 1918), the number of organisms in the spleen reaches its height in about 3 to 4 weeks after injection, irrespective of the number of organisms in the inoculum. The lesions at this time are not yet fully developed, the greatest development being reached only after 6 weeks to 3 months. Organisms may be recovered from infected spleens months after inoculation although the number present may be rather small. Stinebring and Kessel (50) have demonstrated that mononuclear phagocytes obtained from the peritoneum of the guinea pig can be used success-fully to grow *Br. abortus*. Comparable growth could not be procured in mon-ocytes taken from a highly refractory animal such as the rat.

**The Diagnosis of Bang's Disease.** 1. *Clinical Means*. The presence of an infectious abortion may be determined by simple observation. Inasmuch as there are causes of abortion other than *Br. abortus*, it is not possible, without bacteriological or serological assistance, to be certain that this organism is the cause of the trouble.

2. *Recognition of* Br. abortus. This is often accomplished by direct culture. Liver agar medium is frequently used, and the cultures are incubated at 37 C under approximately 10 percent $CO_2$ tension. Gay and Damon (18) recom-mend direct injection of the yolk sacs of 3- to 5-day-old chick embryos for pri-mary isolation of *Brucella*, and Kuzdas and Morse (30) advocated the use of a selective medium in isolating these organisms from contaminated materials. Antibiotics such as polymyxin, actidione, bacitracin, and circulin as well as crystal violet inhibit other microorganisms in this medium. It is also possible to detect *Brucella* organisms by means of the FA technic (28).

(*a*) In the aborted fetus. Direct cultures will usually demonstrate *Br. abor-tus* in the stomach content, the intestinal content, or the lung tissue.

(*b*) In the placenta. Direct films from the outer surface of the chorion, es-pecially from the margins of the characteristic thickenings, will usually suffice to make a positive diagnosis without the necessity of recourse to cultural methods. The organism occurs free, also enclosed in epithelial cells. It is these cells choked with minute organisms which can be recognized with certainty, even though many other bacteria may have invaded the placenta in the meantime. For a description of these bacteria-choked cells, see Smith (47; 1919). The character of the placental lesions is so clear as to be nearly path-ognomonic without even a simple microscopic examination. See Hagan (22; 1926).

(*c*) In the uterine exudate. After abortion or calving, when the placenta has been infected, *Br. abortus* is present in the lochia and may be recognized by guinea pig inoculation. Within a few days, however, the organism seems to disappear and usually cannot be found in the uterus until the animal is again pregnant and reinfection of the organ occurs.

(*d*) In milk. When the udder is infected, *Br. abortus* can be readily de-tected by the intraperitoneal injection of milk into guinea pigs or by direct cultural means.

(*e*) In abscesses. Direct cultures from abscesses of the testicle and epidi-dymis usually give pure cultures of *Br. abortus,* and isolations have been made from hygromas in cattle and from infected bursae in horses.

3. *Serological Tests*. Both agglutination and complement-fixation tests have been used successfully for diagnosis. Because the former is as accurate as the latter and is much simpler, it is the method of choice. The agglutination test may be conducted with blood serum, whole blood, vaginal mucus, whey, or

milk. A ring test (MRT) using milk is also employed in a modified form of the agglutination test.

(*a*) Agglutination test. Two methods of conducting the test with blood serum are in common use. The tube or "slow" method is regarded as the standard procedure, but the plate or "rapid" method is accepted by many states in disease-control work. In competent hands the rapid test probably is as reliable as the standard method. The plate test gives results sooner than the tube test, but so far as the operator's time is concerned, it is doubtful whether the rapid test is more economical.

*The tube test.* Blood samples are obtained by bleeding the animals from the jugular vein. The blood is allowed to clot and the serum to separate. The serum is mixed, in small test tubes, with a suspension of a specially selected strain of *Br. abortus.*° This is supplied by the U.S. Department of Agriculture. Increasing dilutions of serum are placed in successive tubes beginning with a

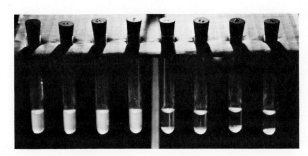

Fig. 11. The macroscopic or tube agglutination test for Bang's disease. Two tests are represented here. The four tubes on the left contain serum dilutions of 1:25, 1:50, 1:100, and 1:200. This serum is negative (devoid of agglutinins), indicated by the fact that the bacteria remain in suspension. The tubes on the right contain the same dilutions of a strongly positive serum, indicated by the fact that the bacteria have flocculated and settled to the bottom leaving the fluid perfectly clear.

dilution of 1:50 and doubling the dilution in each successive tube, viz.: 1:50, 1:100, 1:200. Complete agglutination in dilutions of 1:100 and higher may be considered as positive, and lack of agglutination in 1:50, as negative. Reactions in dilutions of 1:50 and no higher should be considered as suspicious, and judgment should be based upon the history of the animal and of the herd in which it has lived, or another test should be done 3 weeks later, in which case the status of the animal is usually cleared up.

The widespread practice in the United States of calfhood vaccination with Strain 19 has caused some modification of these interpretations. They are applicable only to animals that have been *officially* vaccinated between the ages of 3 and 8 months. Such animals usually become blood test reactors within 1 week after vaccination. They develop their highest titers in approximately 4 to 6 weeks and then generally begin to lose them steadily. In a very few animals these titers do not recede or recede so slowly that even after several years they are high enough to be considered positive in nonvaccinated ani-

° In the United States a phenolized antigen is supplied to all laboratories doing official testing in order that results may be as uniform as possible.

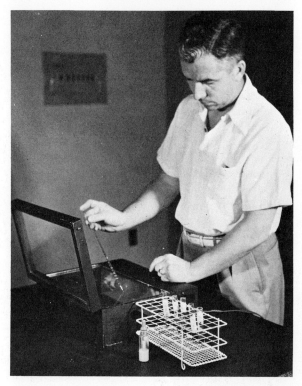

*Fig. 12.* The rapid or plate agglutination test. This test may be carried out on an ordinary microslide or a piece of window glass. If many are conducted, it is convenient to use a special box, such as the one depicted here. It is made of wood, painted black inside and out. A portion of the top consists of a glass plate, marked into squares. The serum and antigen dilutions are made on this plate. A hinged cover can be closed over the tests to reduce the evaporation of fluid from the serum-antigen mixtures. An electric lamp on one side of the interior of the box provides oblique illumination, which facilitates reading of the tests; it also provides warmth, which hastens the reactions.

mals. The blood test does not indicate whether or not such animals harbor virulent infection.

In the official eradication program sponsored by federal and state governments it has been the practice to ignore blood reactions in animals under 30 months of age but to regard titers of 1:100 or higher in older animals as evidence of active infection. This was changed in 1955 because statistical studies showed that, in about 98 percent of all cases, active infection in vaccinated animals caused titers of 1:200 or greater. In officially vaccinated animals, therefore, a titer of 1:100 is not considered as *positive,* as it is in other animals, but only as *suspicious.* When such animals are retested after an interval of 30 days or more and the titer is found to be receding, or stabilized, they are considered to be *negative.* They are listed as *positive* only when there is evidence that the titer is increasing.

Inasmuch as agglutinins pass from the blood to the milk, attempts have been made to use milk or whey titers as indicators of *Brucella* infection. In tube tests whey is less effective than serum in detecting infected animals. Cameron and Kendrick (9), however, have claimed that a whey plate test is highly efficient in diagnosing brucellois (see p. 206).

Vaginal mucus is collected by placing a gauze tampon in the vagina of the

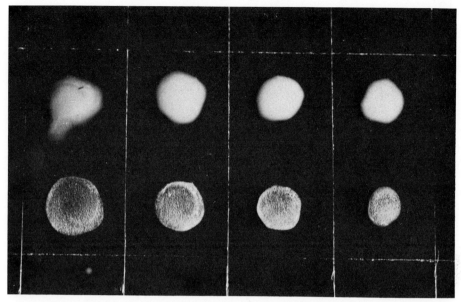

*Fig. 13.* The rapid or plate agglutination test for Bang's disease. Two tests are depicted, four dilutions of serum being tested in each case. These correspond to dilutions of 1:25, 1:50, 1:100, and 1:200, reading from left to right. The sample above is negative; the one below is positive in all dilutions.

animal. Dilutions, starting at 1:25, are made from the fluid pressed from the tampon and used in the test. It is claimed that the agglutination titer of the vaginal mucus is often higher than that of the blood, that it may be positive when the latter is negative, and the agglutinins may be evident in the mucus before they appear in the blood (29).

*The plate or rapid test.* The old slide test, used in many laboratories for identifying newly isolated cultures, has been adapted by Huddleson (25) for dealing with Bang's disease. The antigen is a very heavy suspension of specially selected strains of *Br. abortus* stained with gentian violet and brilliant green to make the tests more easily read. The preparation of this antigen requires great care in order that it may have the proper degree of sensitiveness. It is standardized so that it should give results comparable to those of the tube method. Serum, whole blood, or whey may be used in this test.

The test is done on a glass slide or plate. Special apparatus is not necessary although a simple box fitted with a plate-glass cover and containing a shielded electric lamp to supply illumination and warmth is desirable. The plate is marked off in squares for convenience. With a 0.2-ml pipette graduated to 0.01 ml, the following quantities of the undiluted serum under test are pipetted on the glass plate, each quantity into a different square: 0.08 ml, 0.04 ml, 0.02 ml, 0.01 ml, 0.005 ml. Immediately afterward one drop of the concentrated antigen is added to each lot of serum and mixed with it. The reactions can be read immediately in many cases, but it is advisable not to make the final reading until at least 8 minutes have elapsed, because some samples agglutinate rather slowly. If the antigen has been properly standardized, the dilutions used will give results comparable to those of 1:25, 1:50, 1:100, 1:200, and 1:400, respectively, in the standard tube test.

In 1955 Cameron and Kendrick (9) compared the efficiency of a whey plate test with the conventional blood test in diagnosing brucellosis. Their results indicate that the whey test is just as efficient as the blood test in detecting infection and that the whey test can be used to differentiate titers caused by virulent infection from those caused by vaccination.

Apparently a fair degree of accuracy can be obtained by using whole blood in this test instead of serum. The whole-blood method has been used for testing range cattle when it is desired to hold the animals in chutes until the results are known. A drop of blood is collected on a glass slide from an incision in the end of the tail. A drop of antigen is mixed with the blood and the results are obtained in a few minutes. This method cannot be expected to have the accuracy of the serum test because the presence of blood cells naturally interferes with the reading of the tests. In 1967 Nicoletti (40) recommended the utilization of the *card test* as a rapid, sensitive, and accurate means of screening for brucellosis, especially in range areas. This test utilizes disposable components and produces plasma quickly through the use of lectins (phytohemagglutinins) and an anticoagulant, uses one antigen-plasma (or serum) dilution, is read as negative or positive, and apparently reacts only with γG antibodies. The antigen is a stained buffered whole cell suspension of *Br. abortus* strain 1119–3.

*The ring test.* This is a modification of the agglutination test which is done with milk. It was introduced in Germany in 1937 by Fleischhauer (17), who called it the *ABR* (Abortus, Bang-Ring) *test*. This reaction is being used extensively in some of the Scandinavian countries (Bruhn, 7). It has been widely adopted in the United States, especially for survey purposes, and is now designated by the U.S. Department of Agriculture as the *Milk Ring Test* (MRT).

The test is a very simple one. The antigen most commonly used is a heavy suspension of *Br. abortus* stained with hematoxylin. It is mixed with fresh milk in a sterile tube in the proportion of one drop to each ml. The mixture is then incubated in a water bath at 37 C for a period of 30 to 60 minutes. The time interval used by different workers varies and apparently depends upon the characteristics of the antigen used. If the incubation lasts too long, nonspecific factors destroy the specificity of the test.

The test depends upon the fact that clumps of agglutinated organisms are carried to the surface by the rising fat globules, whereas the unagglutinated ones are not so affected. A negative test is indicated by a column of milk of a bluish color—approximately the same color as before incubation—capped by a cream layer that is uncolored. A strongly positive test is indicated by a decolorized milk column capped by a bluish-violet cream layer. Intermediate reactions are indicated by slightly colored cream layers with incomplete decolorization of the milk.

This test often fails in samples from individual cows, especially when the percentage of fat is low and when the milk is thickened by mastitis or by decreased glandular activity. It cannot be done with colostrum or with skimmed or homogenized milk. It is best adapted for composite or pooled milk samples. It can be used on can samples at milk-collecting stations in order to screen whole herds or areas quickly and economically. For this purpose it is more sensitive in detecting brucellosis than agglutination tests with whey, because the dilution factor does not affect it so much. Not all cows are in milk production at any given time and ring tests should be made at 6-month intervals or oftener. Herds showing evidence of brucellosis are then blood-tested to identify the individual reactors so that they can be removed.

Denmark recognizes the test in official accreditation of herds. In that country herds may be accredited as brucellosis-free on the basis of three consecutive negative rings tests on milk-can samples conducted at 4-month intervals and followed by one negative blood test, 3 to 6 months after the latest ring test, on all animals over 1 year of age.

Satisfactory hematoxylin-stained antigens for the MRT test are difficult to prepare. In 1950 Wood (51) added a sufficient quantity of an aqueous solution of 4,4'-bis(3,5-diphenyl-2-tetrazolinium)-biphenyl dichloride to a heavy suspension of living *Br. abortus* cells to make a final concentration of 1 to 16,000 and incubated the mixture at 37 C for 4 hours. The organisms reduced the compound to an intensely colored violet-blue formazan, apparently within the cells, and were stained by it without altering the antigenic specificity of their cell surfaces. After staining, the organisms were killed by heat and used as antigen. This product appears to be stable and uniform in color intensity, specificity, and sensitivity.

In 1953 Gregory (21) described his RMA (Rapid Milk Agglutination) test. In this test tetrazolinium antigen is placed in relatively fat-free milk, and after an incubation period of 50 minutes at 37 C and 30 additional minutes at room temperature agglutination is read as in regular tube tests. This technic eliminates the need for a cream line in the milk.

(*b*) The complement-fixation test. The technic of this test differs in different laboratories. When properly controlled, the test agrees in most instances with the agglutination test. The discrepancies that occur usually are with sera of low titer.

The conglutination complement-absorption test (CCAT) has also been used in the diagnosis of bovine brucellosis. Horse complement is used because bovine sera are less anticomplementary to horse than to guinea pig complement, and it is claimed that the CCAT occasionally detects antibody in bovine sera which are negative to agglutination and hemolytic CF tests (15).

(*c*) The dependability of serological tests. When properly conducted, the agglutination test is a highly accurate indication of infection with *Br. abortus*. The test is not perfect, however. Chronically infected cows have been found which did not develop a diagnostic titer. Recently infected cows gradually build up a diagnostic titer. Animals that contract infection in the last several weeks of the gestation period may abort when their blood titer is still below the diagnostic level. A retest 30 days later usually produces a positive result.

Vaccination with *Br. abortus*, Strain 19, a process now widely practiced, produces blood titers that cannot be distinguished, in any practicable way, from those caused by virulent infection. Vaccine titers in 90 percent or more of calves vaccinated when they are between 4 and 8 months of age will disappear or fall below the diagnostic level before the animals have reached 30 months of age. Animals vaccinated when older do not lose their titers so quickly, and some retain them indefinitely. Barner and colleagues (3) and others have devised ways of differentiating between vaccine and infection titers, but no reliable and practical method for field use has been found.

Nonspecific agglutinins for *Br. abortus* are sometimes encountered in cattle, especially after they have been vaccinated with biologic products containing some types of *Pasteurella* organisms. This appears to be caused by the possession of common antigens. Such reactions are rather fleeting and their nature can be clarified by a retest applied several weeks later. It is well to avoid blood-testing cattle, if possible, until a month or more has elapsed following vaccination with pasteurellae. Hess (23) has described another type of nonspecific sensitization that can be inactivated by heat treatment of 70 C for 10 minutes. Rose and Roepke (45) used pH values at about 4.0 on the plate test to inhibit nonspecific *Brucella* agglutination reactions. In evaluating serologic test procedures Nicoletti (41) recommended the use of a number of supplemental tests in order to provide more accurate methods for the eradication of brucellosis.

The prevalence of *Brucella* agglutinins in the serum of the horse suggests that it may be a reservoir of infection, but it is possible that the presence of these antibodies is the result of contact with organisms that share common antigens with the brucellae and that more precise tests are needed in order to establish this fact.

4. *Allergic Tests.* Many have attempted to diagnose *Br. abortus* infection in man and animals by means of skin tests. Reference to these tests for man will be made later. So far as animals are concerned, none has proved reliable. The test materials have consisted of suspensions of heat-killed bacilli, culture filtrates, and various extracts of the bacillary bodies. The term *abortin* was applied to some of the earlier extracts made for this purpose; of late they have been known under the general names of *brucellin* and *brucellergin*. These extracts generally have been administered intradermally; in some cases they have been introduced into the conjunctival sac.

**Natural Immunity.** Calves, infected *in utero* or from their surroundings after birth, remain infected ordinarily for only a short time unless they are raised on infected milk or kept in the presence of the infection. Within several weeks from the time they are removed from the presence of the infection, they usually free themselves of it and develop into uninfected cattle. There is evidence that calves infected with *Br. abortus* at 7 months of age may become infected permanently (38) but usually it is not until the animal reaches puberty, becomes pregnant, and the udder begins to function that danger of serious disease appears.

Adult animals that have never been in the presence of the organism are the most easily infected and the most likely to abort when infected. An animal that has aborted once or has been infected once as an adult, even though it may not have aborted, is not so readily infected a second time. A degree of immunity develops, therefore, as a result of the disease that has been overcome. This immunity frequently is not sufficient to prevent a second abortion, or even a third or a fourth. As a rule most animals, after one or two abortions, will thereafter carry their calves to full term even though they may remain infected.

There seems to be a considerable amount of variation in the resistance of individual cows to this disease. Some animals appear to be wholly resistant to natural and artificial infection even though their blood contains no antibodies, while others can be infected easily and repeatedly.

**Artificial Immunity.** (*a*) The use of bacterins or killed cultures. Cultures of *Br. abortus*, killed with heat or chemicals, have been extensively tried as a means of increasing the resistance of cattle to Bang's disease. The method is not harmful but the immunity produced is neither solid nor lasting. Usually the cultures are injected at intervals, beginning before the animals are bred and continuing throughout the gestation period. The method has practically been abandoned at the present time.

(*b*) The use of living virulent cultures. Live cultures of *Br. abortus* have long been used for artificially immunizing animals against Bang's disease. Earlier fully virulent cultures often were used, these usually being administered some time before the animals were bred, with the expectation that the organism would be eliminated before they became pregnant. These vaccines often caused udder infections and made permanent carriers, and it is claimed that breeding efficiency may be lowered by such treatment. However, when the abortion rate in herds is high, there is no doubt that the vaccines lower the rate appreciably. The use of virulent cultures for this purpose is no longer justified because certain attenuated cultures will accomplish as much as virulent ones without the dangers of the latter. Biologic manufacturers in the United States are no longer permitted to distribute virulent cultures for use as vaccines.

(*c*) The use of attenuated living cultures. The search for an attenuated strain of *Br. abortus* that would satisfactorily immunize cattle without having the undesirable effects of virulent strains has gone on for many years. The first success in this search came in 1930 when Buck (8) announced his *Strain*

*19*. A second was announced by McEwen and Priestley (36) in England when they described their *45/20 Strain*. A third is the *Mucoid Vaccine* of Huddleson (26).

*Strain 19* Brucella abortus *vaccine*. This vaccine has been subjected to very extensive field trials not only in the United States but also in many other countries. It consists of a viable culture of a strain that was discovered to have practically no virulence for guinea pigs and cattle but to possess excellent immunizing properties. The strain has great stability, since many deliberate attempts to increase or decrease its virulence have failed. It appears to have approximately the same properties now that it had in 1930.

Strain 19 is a smooth, agglutinogenic strain of *Br. abortus*. It is not entirely lacking in virulence. Guinea pigs can be infected with it, but the lesions are minimal or absent and the organism disappears from the tissues eventually, leaving no recognizable lesions. Pregnant cattle can be made to abort by inoculating them with large doses of Strain 19. In these cases the vaccine organism can usually be demonstrated without difficulty in the fetal membranes and the fetus itself. Susceptible cattle, associating with those that have aborted as a result of inoculation with the vaccine strain, do not become infected with it. A large volume of experience has been accumulated which shows that Strain 19 never is transmitted from one animal to another; that if any damage is done by the use of this vaccine, it is limited to the animal into which it is injected. Strain 19 is very rarely eliminated in the milk of vaccinated animals. It is capable of causing infections in man (2, 19, 49), though these usually are mild and result in recovery within a much shorter time than do infections with virulent strains. The vaccine, in view of its dangers for man, should be handled with due caution.

Strain 19 is furnished to manufacturers of biological products in the United States by the U.S. Department of Agriculture for the making of vaccine. This vaccine is the only one permitted to be used on cattle in the United States, except for experimental work. The commercial vaccine is furnished as a lyophilized product, consisting of organisms that have been frozen and dried in a sterile protective fluid such as skim milk. In sealed ampoules the product keeps very well. The dried organisms are suspended in sterile saline solution just before use.

The age limits for official vaccination of calves with Strain 19 were lowered September 1969 to 3 to 8 months (90 to 239 days) for dairy heifers and to 3 to 10 months (90 to 299 days) for beef heifers. The vaccine is administered as a single injection, subcutaneously. Intracaudal instead of subcutaneous vaccination has been recommended, and while it appears to be just as effective as the latter, Gregory (20) and Berman *et al.* (5) found little, if any, evidence to indicate that it is superior. This vaccine should not be used on the male calf because it may actually produce brucellosis and thereby affect the fertility of the animal (32).

With few exceptions the vaccine is well tolerated by calves. Agglutinins usually can be demonstrated after about 10 days, and these increase to a maximum in about 2 to 3 months, after which the blood titers usually decrease. In 90 percent of the animals the titers 12 months later will have receded to a point below the diagnostic level. Official vaccinates must be negative to the brucellosis test at the age of 20 months for dairy heifers and at the age of 24 months for beef heifers. Usually the former will be negative to the agglutination test by the time their first calves are born. The immunity conferred by vaccination is not absolute. It is great enough, however, to protect the greater number of young breeding animals through the period of their greatest susceptibility to the disease. Calfhood vaccination with Strain 19 is widely practiced in many parts of the world. This vaccine has done much to reduce the ravages of brucellosis in cattle.

The vaccination of adult cattle with Strain 19 is a matter over which there has been much controversy in the United States. It has been used widely enough to show that there is little danger in its use in adult animals. It should not be used on cattle in the later stages of pregnancy, although it seldom causes abortions. The principal objection to its use on adult stock is the fact that such animals usually develop more or less permanent agglutinin titers and that it is not possible, thereafter, to learn by the blood test whether or not the animal is infected with virulent organisms, because vaccinated and infected animals cannot be distinguished by serologic tests. The immunity conferred on adult animals is very good.

*The McEwen 45/20 vaccine.* McEwen and Priestley,.working in the British Isles, discovered a rough strain of *Br. abortus* that became progressively more pathogenic as it was passed in series in guinea pigs. The passage variant that served as a good immunizing agent, yet was not virulent enough to cause disease in cattle, was designated *45/20*. Being a rough type, it did not produce agglutinins in animals. In this respect it had an advantage over Strain 19. It was tested extensively in the field in Great Britain with apparent success. In 1944 the Ministry of Agriculture and Fisheries discontinued further use of this vaccine with the explanation that it did not immunize quite so well as Strain 19 and had a tendency to change in animal tissues, causing some animals to react. Strain 19 is now used for official vaccinating in the British Isles, but a killed 45/20 adjuvant vaccine (K 45/20 A) has been developed which promises to be an effective and economical method of reducing the "pool of infections" in areas where brucellosis is enzootic (13).

*The "M" vaccine of Huddleson.* In 1947 Huddleson reported that a mucoid, intermediate form of *Br. suis* served effectively to immunize guinea pigs against all three types of *Brucella*. In 1948 he reported (27) on the value of this vaccine for immunizing cattle. Agglutinins are produced by this strain only in low concentration and tend to disappear quickly. Furthermore, it appears that the immunity induced is not equal to that produced by Strain 19 (6, 14). For these reasons the use of this vaccine has been very limited, and it is not used in official work.

**Chemotherapy.** No practical chemotherapeutic methods for use in combating *Br. abortus* infections in cattle are known. Penicillin, streptomycin, aureomycin, and some of the other antibiotic agents have been tried without success.

**Control Measures.** *General procedure.* Many methods and combinations of methods have been used to control the ravages of brucellosis in cattle. The methods used depend upon local conditions, whether the animals are raised for dairy or beef purposes, how heavily infected the herds are, and preferences of the owners. Only two principles are involved: (*a*) the finding of the infected individuals and eliminating them from the herd, and (*b*) raising the resistance of the animals by vaccination to reduce spread of the disease.

In heavily infected herds, in which many valuable animals would have to be sacrificed if all diseased animals were to be removed, the so-called *test-and-slaughter* plan is not logical. In such herds it is best to advise systematic calfhood vaccination with Strain 19 between the ages of 3 to 8 months. If this is done for perhaps 5 years, clinical evidence of the disease generally disappears within 2 years, and at the end of the 5-year period natural attrition will have eliminated most of the chronically infected cows. Blood testing at this time usually will show few or no reactors, and these may then be eliminated. It is best in such groups to continue the calfhood vaccination plan as a means of retaining the herd immunity, so long as infected herds exist in the general area and exposure may occur.

In herds that are only lightly infected, blood testing and removal of reactors may be begun immediately. If there is any danger of exposure, it is well to conduct systematic calf vaccination as a protective measure.

To the surprise of many, it is found that numerous small herds in which no protective work has been done, are nevertheless free of brucellosis. Such groups may require no protective work, but unless they are thoroughly isolated and well protected it is best to advise calfhood vaccination.

*The control and eradication of Bovine Brucellosis in the United States.* A federal-state co-operative plan for the control and eradication of bovine brucellosis is now in progress in the United States. Since 1953 its operation has been greatly accelerated. *Certified* herds are those that have been found to be free of the disease, and *Modified-Certified Areas* are regions—townships, counties, groups of counties, or entire states—that as a result of complete testing are adjudged to have been nearly freed of the disease. When continued testing of such areas indicates that the disease has been completely eradicated, the term *Certified Brucellosis-free Area* will be used.

By 30 September 1970 there were 25 modified-certified and 20 certified-free states in the United States (see figure 14). This is in contrast to 31 December 1960 when only one state, New Hampshire, had achieved a Certified-Brucellosis Free status.

To hasten the work, reduce the cost, and check individual herds more frequently than can be done when each animal is blood-tested, the MRT test is used in dairy herds. This test may be employed in moderately infected areas

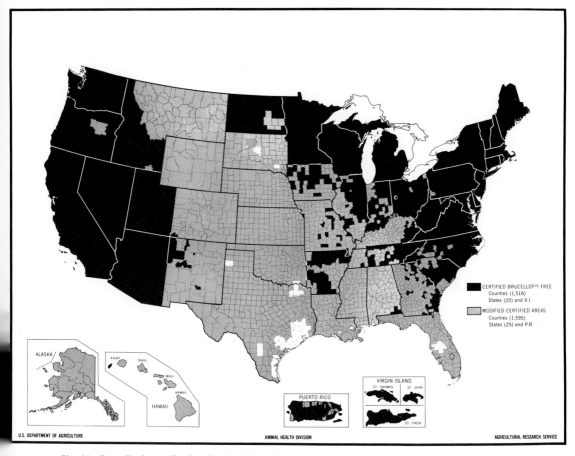

Fig. 14. Brucellosis eradication in the United States as of September 30, 1970. (Courtesy U.S. Department of Agriculture.)

for detecting diseased herds, and these are then subjected to blood testing of the individual animals. This technic is most useful, perhaps, in retesting areas that already have been certified, since it is possible to conduct several milk ring tests in less time and at less cost than a single blood test of all animals in any area.

The blood testing of beef animals on the open range is difficult and expensive. Fortunately it appears that the infection rate is not high in many areas. The MRT test is not useful for such cattle. The official plan at present permits modified certification of the individual range herd if at least 15 percent of the breeding cows going to or at slaughter centers are blood-tested during a 3-year period. The actual procedure involves tagging each animal to identify its state, county, and herd of origin. When reactors are found, they are traced to the herd of origin, and steps are taken to eliminate infection from the herd.

## REFERENCES

1.  Bang.   Jour. Comp. Path. and Therap., 1897, *10*, 125.
2.  Bardenwerper.   Jour. Am. Med. Assoc., 1954, *155*, 970.
3.  Barner, Oberst, and Atkeson.   Jour. Am. Vet. Med. Assoc., 1953, *122*, 302.
4.  Bendixen and Blom.   Vet. Jour., 1947, *103*, 337.
5.  Berman, Beach, and Irwin.   Am. Jour. Vet. Res., 1954, *15*, 406.
6.  Berman and Irwin.   Jour. Am. Vet. Med. Assoc., 1954, *125*, 401.
7.  Bruhn.   Am. Jour. Vet. Res., 1948, *9*, 360.
8.  Buck.   Jour. Agr. Res., 1930, *41*, 667.
9.  Cameron and Kendrick.   Proc. U.S. Livestock Sanit. Assoc., 1955, *59*, 138.
10. Carpenter and Boak.   Jour. Am. Med. Assoc., 1931, *96*, 1212.
11. Corner and Connell.   Canad. Jour. Comp. Med. and Vet. Sci., 1958, *22*, 9.
12. Cosgrove.   Vet. Rec., 1961, *73*, 1377.
13. Cunningham.   *Ibid.*, 1970, *86*, 2.
14. Edgington, King, and Frank.   Am. Jour. Vet. Res., 1952, *13*, 441.
15. Engelhard and Carlisle.   Proc. Soc. Exp. Biol. and Med., 1955, *88*, 670.
16. Fabyan.   Jour. Med. Res., 1912, *26*, 441.
17. Fleischhauer.   Berl. tierärztl. Wchnschr., 1937, *53*, 527.
18. Gay and Damon.   Pub. Health Rpts. (U.S.), 1951, *66*, 1204.
19. Gilman.   Cornell Vet., 1944, *34*, 193.
20. Gregory.   Austral. Vet. Jour., 1952, *28*, 265.
21. Gregory.   Jour. Comp. Path. and Therap., 1953, *63*, 171.
22. Hagan.   Cornell Vet., 1926, *16*, 274.
23. Hess.   Am. Jour. Vet. Res., 1953, *14*, 192.
24. Huddleson.   Cornell Vet., 1921, *11*, 210.
25. Huddleson.   Mich. Agr. Exp. Sta. Tech. Bul. 123, 1932.
26. Huddleson.   Am. Jour. Vet. Res., 1947, *8*, 374.
27. Huddleson.   Mich. Agr. Exp. Sta. Quart. Bul. 31, 1948.
28. Janney and Berman.   Am. Jour. Vet. Res., 1962, *23*, 596.
29. Jepsen and Vindekilde.   *Ibid.*, 1951, *12*, 97.
30. Kuzdas and Morse.   Jour. Bact., 1953, *66*, 502.
31. Kuzdas and Morse.   Cornell Vet., 1954, *44*, 216.
32. Lambert, Deyoe, and Painter.   Jour. Am. Vet. Med. Assoc., 1964, *145*, 909.
33. Love, Pietz, and Ranger.   *Ibid.*, 1966, *149*, 1177.
34. Luchsinger and Anderson.   *Ibid.*, 1967, *150*, 1017.
35. McCullough, Eisele, and Pavelchek.   Pub. Health Rpts. (U.S.), 1951, *66*, 205.
36. McEwen and Priestly.   Vet. Rec., 1938, *50*, 1097.
37. McNeal and Kerr.   Jour. Inf. Dis., 1910, *7*, 469.
38. Nagy and Hignett.   Res. Vet. Sci., 1967, *8*, 247.
39. Nowak.   Ann. l'Inst. Past., 1908, *22*, 541.
40. Nicoletti.   Jour. Am. Vet. Med. Assoc., 1967, *151*, 1778.
41. Nicoletti.   Am. Jour. Vet. Res., 1969, *30*, 1811.
42. Pearce, Williams, Harris-Smith, Fitzgeorge, and Smith.   Brit. Jour. Exp. Path., 1962, *43*, 31.
43. Rankin.   Vet. Rec., 1965, *77*, 132.
44. Roderick, Kimball, McLeod, and Frank.   Am. Jour. Vet. Res., 1948, *9*, 5.
45. Rose and Roepke.   *Ibid.*, 1957, *18*, 550.

46.  Smillie.  Jour. Exp. Med., 1918, *28*, 585.
47.  Smith.  *Ibid.*, 1919, *29*, 451.
48.  Smith and Fabyan.  Centrbl. f. Bakt., I Abt., Orig., 1912, *61*, 549.
49.  Spink and Thompson.  Jour. Am. Med. Assoc., 1953, *153*, 1162.
50.  Stinebring and Kessel.  Proc. Soc. Exp. Biol. and Med., 1959, *101*, 412.
51.  Wood.  Science, 1950, *112*, 86.

## Brucella suis

SYNONYM:  Porcine type of *Brucella*

In the report of the Chief of the Bureau of Animal Industry, U.S. Department of Agriculture, for 1914 (p. 30) there is a reference to the isolation of *Br. abortus* from a swine fetus. The person who made the isolation and identification was later identified as Jacob Traum.

For some years it was thought that this organism was identical with the one found in cattle, although several observers noted that the strain of porcine origin appeared to be more virulent for guinea pigs than the one commonly found in cattle. The lesions in guinea pigs caused by the bovine strain are proliferative in character, whereas those caused by infection with the porcine organism are both proliferative and degenerative, i.e., the swine organism commonly produces abscess formation and the bovine does not. The bovine organism usually will not destroy the guinea pig, or only after a number of months have elapsed, whereas the porcine variety will frequently cause death within 2 or 3 weeks. A common occurrence in guinea pigs inoculated with the porcine variety is the formation of abscesses behind the eyeball, causing the eye to be protruded from the socket. See Moulton and Meyer (19) for a discussion of the pathogenesis of *Br. suis* in guinea pigs.

It was noted by Traum, and the observation has been confirmed by all who have worked with the porcine type of *Brucella*, that the organism from the first generation will grow readily in ordinary atmosphere. In other words, the peculiar $CO_2$ requirements of bovine strains are not shared by those from swine.

*Br. suis* has been isolated from wild hares in Denmark (2). They were believed to be the carriers involved in four enzootics of brucellosis in swine. Pregnant cattle exposed to *Br. suis* by the intramammary route do not abort but develop severe mastitis, a high blood serum titer, and a bacteremia as indicated by recovery of the organisms from lymph nodes in widely scattered parts of the body (23).

**Morphology and Staining Reactions.** These are identical with those already described for *Br. abortus*. It is impossible to distinguish between the *Brucella* morphologically. At least three biotypes have been recognized.

**Pathogenicity.** Brucellosis of swine occurs in various parts of the United States, but it is not so widely distributed as the disease in cattle. There is very little of it in the eastern part of the United States. The main centers in this country seem to be in the north-central states, Iowa, Missouri, and Illinois (17), and in California (9, 11). The disease also occurs in several European countries, but it does not appear to be very prevalent in any of them (21).

When porcine infections were first recognized, and for a considerable time afterward, it was assumed that swine became infected through association with cattle or by drinking infected cows' milk. It is now known that *Br. abortus*, the bovine type, is not highly pathogenic for swine, but infections sometimes can be induced by feeding cows' milk contaminated with this organism (22). *Br. suis* is transmitted almost exclusively from pig to pig (6). However, it sometimes infects cows, and it may be eliminated in the milk of these animals.

In some herds of swine *Br. suis* causes severe losses from abortions. In others abortions are not frequent. Hutchings, Delez, and Donham (13) have shown experimentally that swine, after one contact with the infection, seldom will abort as a result of later contacts, although they are not immune and readily become reinfected. In many herds the disease exists without its being suspected. In infected herds orchitis is frequent in the boars, the testes becoming greatly swollen and necrotic. In most outbreaks some evidence of arthritis may be found. Infections that localize in the bodies of the vertebrae (spondylitis), especially of the lumbar and sacral regions, are not uncommon (Feldman and Olson, 8). These sometimes are unsuspected and are found only after slaughter, but more often symptoms of posterior paralysis caused by pressure from the necrotic tissue on the spinal cord are evidenced. According to Anderson and Davis (1), nodular splenitis in swine is associated with brucellosis and in the absence of other lesions justifies a presumptive diagnosis of this disease. Thomsen (21) claims that many cases show no symptoms and no gross lesions. In general, the disease in swine resembles that seen in brucellosis of man and the guinea pig rather than that caused by *Br. abortus* in cattle in that the infection is found frequently in many organs other than those of the genital system.

**Diagnosis.** Brucellosis in swine may be positively diagnosed by cultural methods and by the agglutination test (15). *Br. suis* can readily be isolated from the blood, spleen, uterus, lymph nodes, and other organs of many cases, in addition to the uterus and mammary gland of sows and the testes and semen of boars. The methods are the same as are used for *Br. abortus* except that it is not necessary to increase the $CO_2$ tension of the culture jar.

The agglutination test is not as reliable in swine as it is in cattle. Many actively infected animals fail to react to the test; hence it is impracticable to attempt to eradicate the disease from herds by testing and eliminating the reactors. Low-titer agglutination reactions also occur and are difficult to interpret. Hoerlein (10) claims that incubation of the tubes (Standard *Br. abortus* antigen is used) at 56 C for 16 hours will eliminate the nonspecific, but not the specific, reactions.

The agglutination test has value in determining whether or not infection exists in a herd. If it is present, the disease is handled on a herd basis.

**Immunity.** Both field and experimental evidence indicate that immunity of swine to brucellosis is very slight. It has been pointed out above that abortions usually do not occur after the first exposure, but most animals readily contract infection when re-exposed. Manthei (18) and Kernkamp and Roepke (16) have shown that *Br. abortus*, Strain 19, does not immunize swine and it does not protect cattle against *Br. suis* infection (24). No vaccines comparable to Strain 19 are in use to protect against swine brucellosis, but certain endotoxin-containing preparations of *Br. suis* are claimed to stimulate definite resistance to this organism (7).

**Chemotherapy.** Bunnell, Hutchings, and Donham (3) have shown that penicillin is useless for treating swine bruccellosis. Hutchings *et al.* (12) report streptomycin and sulfadiazine to be ineffective, but Cameron (5) has indicated that aureomycin is bactericidal for *Br. suis in vivo*.

**Control Measures.** In commercial swine herds the simplest way to eradicate the disease is to sell all stock for slaughter as they arrive at the proper age. When all stock has been eliminated in this way, the premises are thoroughly cleaned and disinfected. After they have been kept free of all swine for at

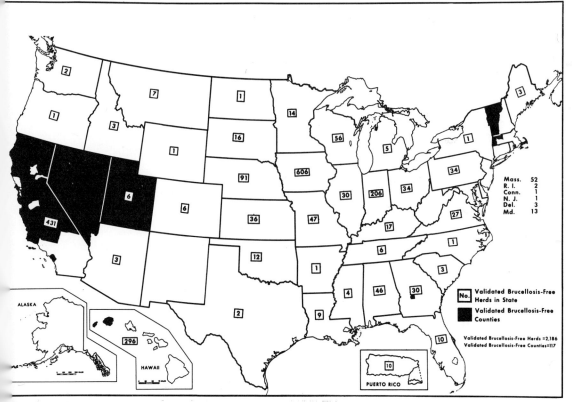

Fig. 15. Swine brucellosis eradication in the United States as of January 1966. (Courtesy U.S. Department of Agriculture.)

least 2 months (longer in winter), they may then be restocked from sources known to be brucellosis-free.

In breeding herds where blood lines must be preserved, Cameron (4) suggested a system which has been endorsed by Hutchings and Washko (14) and Spink *et al.* (20). Pigs are raised from the infected unit. They are weaned at 8 weeks of age and tested individually by the agglutination test. If negative, they are removed from the infected herd, placed on clean ground, and raised in isolation from the main herd. All pigs are tested periodically. Any reactors are immediately removed. When of breeding age, they are bred to noninfected boars. The original herd is disposed of as soon as the replacement unit has grown to sufficient size. This plan is usually successful.

The U.S. national goal calls for the eradicating of brucellosis from all species of livestock and it now appears that the disease can be wiped out in swine. The term used to designate swine free of brucellosis is "Validated Brucellosis-Free Herds." By 3 May 1966, three states had achieved this status.

### REFERENCES

1. Anderson and Davis. Jour. Am. Vet. Med. Assoc., 1957, *131*, 141.
2. Bendtsen, Christiansen, and Thomsen. Nord. Vetmed., 1956, 8, 1.
3. Bunnell, Hutchings, and Donham. Am. Jour. Vet. Res., 1947, 8, 367.
4. Cameron. *Ibid.*, 1946, 7, 21.
5. Cameron. Cornell Vet., 1951, *41*, 110.
6. Cotton and Buck. Jour. Am. Vet. Med. Assoc., 1932, *80*, 344.
7. Edens and Foster. Am. Jour. Vet. Res., 1966, *27*, 1327.
8. Feldman and Olson. Arch. Path., 1933, *16*, 195.
9. Hayes and Traum. North Am. Vet., 1920, *1*, 58.
10. Hoerlein. Cornell Vet., 1953, *43*, 28.
11. Howarth and Hayes. Jour. Am. Vet. Med. Assoc., 1931, 78, 830.
12. Hutchings, Bunnell, and Bay. Am. Jour. Vet. Res., 1950, *11*, 388.
13. Hutchings, Delez, and Donham. *Ibid.*, 1946, 7, 11.
14. Hutchings and Washko. Jour. Am. Vet. Med. Assoc., 1947, *110*, 171.
15. Johnson and Huddleson. *Ibid.*, 1931, 78, 849.
16. Kernkamp and Roepke. *Ibid.*, 1948, *113*, 564.
17. McNutt. Proc. U.S. Livestock Sanit. Assoc., 1938, *42*, 90.
18. Manthei. Am. Jour. Vet. Res., 1948, 9, 40.
19. Moulton and Meyer. Cornell Vet., 1958, *48*, 165.
20. Spink *et al.* Jour. Am. Med. Assoc., 1949, *141*, 326.
21. Thomsen. Brucella infection in swine. Levin and Munksgaard, Copenhagen, 1934.
22. Washko, Bay, Donham, and Hutchings. Am. Jour. Vet. Res., 1951, *12*, 320.
23. Washko and Hutchings. *Ibid.*, 1951, *12*, 165.
24. *Ibid.*, 1952, *13*, 24.

### *Brucella melitensis*

SYNONYMS: *Micrococcus melitensis, Bacterium melitensis,* caprine type of *Brucella*

This organism was first isolated by Bruce (4) in 1887 from the spleen of a resident of the Island of Malta who had died from a disease known as *Malta* or *Mediterranean fever*. In 1905 Zammit (16) discovered that the source of the infection was milk from infected goats. The disease in goats, and to a less extent in sheep, is prevalent in southern Europe (south of the 46th parallel), in Mexico, and in certain areas of the southwestern part of the United States, where it appears to have been imported from Mexico. An outbreak was recognized in southern Texas in 1911 and another in Arizona in 1922. It has been prevalent in mohair goats owned largely by Indian tribes in northern Arizona and southern Utah. In 1943 it was discovered in goat-milk cheese made in a small mountainous area on the Colorado–New Mexico state line. In 1946 Jordan and Borts (11) reported a number of human cases in Iowa in persons who had had no contact with goats or goat products. Shortly afterward Borts, McNutt, and Jordan (3) succeeded in isolating this type from swine on a farm on which a human infection had occurred. Since that time it has become evident that this type is well established in swine in the midwestern part of the United States. Experimental infection has been induced in this animal by Beal *et al.* (2), and studies by Hoerlein (9) have led to the conclusion that the pathogenesis of *Br. melitensis* for swine is similar to that of *Br. suis*.

Carpenter and Boak (5) reported the finding of three strains of *Br. melitensis* in cows' milk in the central part of New York in 1934. In 1947 Damon and Fagan (6) isolated this type from a human case in Indiana. The patient was a farmer who owned a small herd of cows. Eight of the nine animals were positive to the agglutination test, and one animal had recently aborted. *Br. melitensis* was found in the milk of one of these animals. It is apparent that this type of brucellosis has been encountered in many areas in the United States. It is of interest to note that Shaw (15) of the British Mediterranean Fever Commission isolated *Br. melitensis* from the milk of two blood-reacting cows on the Island of Malta in 1905. In 1952 it was found in wild hares shot in northern France (10). It was presumed that the infected animals contracted the disease from sheep and goats at pasture. In 1963 the organism was isolated from sheep in Argentina. It has been claimed that this was the first time *Br. melitensis* was actually proved to cause natural ovine brucellosis in the Western Hemisphere (13).

**Morphology and Staining Reactions.** *Br. melitensis* grows characteristically in the form of a small rod which is so short that it was mistaken for a coccus. In 1918 Evans (7) compared this organism with the one causing infectious abortion of cattle and discovered the close relationship between them. Meyer and Shaw (12) suggested that these two species be placed in a single genus, for which the name *Brucella* was proposed in honor of Bruce.

The staining characteristics of *Br. melitensis* are the same as those of the other *Brucella*. Morphologically these organisms are identical.

**Cultural Features.** It is not possible to differentiate *Br. melitensis* from the other types by any of the ordinary cultural features. *Br. abortus* differs from the other two in its special requirement for increased $CO_2$ tension for primary isolation. Three biotypes of *Br. melitensis* have been characterized. Special means of differentiating the *Brucella* are discussed below.

**Pathogenicity.** The disease in the goat appears to be quite like the corresponding infection in the cow. Abortions may occur. The udder becomes infected in a high percentage of cases, and these animals shed the organism in their milk. In many instances the effects upon the goat herd are so slight that the disease is not suspected until human infections are traced to it. Infections in sheep apparently are similar to those in goats. They are said to be common in southern Europe, but no cases have been reported in this species in North America.

**Diagnosis.** The diagnostic methods are the same as those used for brucellosis in other species. The agglutination test may be used, or the culture may be isolated by direct cultural means or through guinea pig inoculation.

**Immunity.** It has been claimed that strains of *Br. melitensis* have been used as a bacterin (killed adjuvant 53H38 vaccine) and as a vaccine (Rev. 1) in inducing a high degree of immunity in sheep (8) and in goats (1). Strain 19 vaccine was less effective.

**Chemotherapy.** Treatment of experimental *Br. melitensis* infection in mice with streptomycin combined with aureomycin, terramycin, or sulfadiazine resulted in the eradication of the organism from the spleen of 99 out of 100 animals. Therapy with single drugs was definitely inferior (14).

**REFERENCES**

1. Alton.   Jour. Comp. Path., 1966, *76*, 241.
2. Beal, Taylor, McCullough, Claflin, and Hutchings.   Am. Jour. Vet. Res., 1959, *20*, 634.
3. Borts, McNutt, and Jordan.   Jour. Am. Med. Assoc., 1946, *130*, 966.
4. Bruce.   Practitioner, 1887, *39*, 161; Ann. l'Inst. Past., 1893, 7, 289.
5. Carpenter and Boak.   Jour. Bact., 1934, *27*, 73.
6. Damon and Fagan.   Pub. Health Rpts. (U.S.), 1947, *62*, 1097.
7. Evans.   Jour. Inf. Dis., 1918, *22*, 580.
8. Ghosh, Sen, and Singh.   Jour. Comp. Path., 1968, *78*, 387.
9. Hoerlein.   Am. Jour. Vet. Res., 1952, *13*, 67.
10. Jacotot, Vallée, and Barrière.   Abstract in: North Am. Vet., 1952, *23*, 169.
11. Jordan and Borts.   Jour. Am. Med. Assoc., 1946, *130*, 72.
12. Meyer and Shaw.   Jour. Inf. Dis., 1920, *27*, 173.
13. Ossola, Szyfres, and Blood.   Am. Jour. Vet. Res., 1963, *24*, 446.
14. Shaffer, Kucera, and Spink.   Jour. Immunol., 1953, *70*, 31.
15. Shaw.   Rpt. Comm. appointed by the Admiralty, the War Office, and the Office of Civil Govt. of Malta for investigations on Mediterranean fever. London, 1907.
16. Zammit.   *Ibid.*

### Brucella neotomae

The organism was isolated from the desert wood rat, *Neotoma lepida*. According to Stoenner and Lackman (1, 2), it possesses most of the biochemical characteristics, antigenic composition, and colonial and cellular morphology of *Br. suis*. Fermentation of arabinose, galactose, glucose, levulose, and xylose, sensitivity to thionin and basic fuchsin, and greater infectivity for mice than for guinea pigs differentiate it from *Br. suis* as well as other *Brucella*.

In a survey of brucellosis in wildlife made in West Central Utah during the years 1954 to 1964, 15 isolations of *Br. neotomae* were made from desert wood rats (3).

### REFERENCES

1. Stoenner and Lackman.  Jour. Am. Vet. Med. Assoc., 1957, *130*, 411.
2. Stoenner and Lackman.  Am. Jour. Vet. Res., 1957, *18*, 947.
3. Thorpe, Sidwell, Bushman, Smart, and Moyes.  Jour. Am. Vet. Med. Assoc., 1965, *146*, 225.

### Brucella canis

SYNONYMS: Canine type of *Brucella*, *Br. suis*, type 5

In 1967 Taul *et al.* (8) reported outbreaks of canine abortion caused by a Gram-negative bacterium. This was soon followed by the observations of Carmichael and Kenney (2) on canine abortion caused by a *Brucella* species. The organism was characterized by Carmichael and Bruner (1) in 1968 and named *Brucella canis*. Although *Br. abortus* and *Br. suis* have been isolated from dogs (6) it appears that *Br. canis* is particularly adapted to the canine species and is widespread in breeding colonies in the United States. It will infect man, but does not transmit readily to other animals.

**Morphology and Staining Reactions.** The organism is a small rod-shaped bacillus similar to the other *Brucella* species in morphology and staining reactions.

**Cultural Features.** On agar slants it becomes quite mucoid. It most closely resembles *Br. suis* in growth characteristics, but analysis of culture extracts by electron capture detector chromatograms shows differences between the two organisms (1, 5) and *Br. canis* does not utilize erythritol (4).

**Pathogenicity.** Attention was focused on *Br. canis* because enzootics of canine abortions were occurring in dog-breeding colonies. Besides abortion, other clinical features of the disease were prolonged vaginal discharge after abortion, failure to conceive, and subcutaneous hemorrhage and edema of aborted fetuses (3). Persistent bacteremia is common and other characteristics of canine bruellosis are generalized lymphadenitis and splenitis and early undetectable embryonic deaths or abortions. In infected males epididymitis, dermatitis of the scrotum, and testicular atrophy (often unilateral) are common. Some males become sterile. Although most dogs are free of clinical signs many suffer reproductive failures and loss of vigor. Infected dogs may not have elevated tempeatures.

*Br. canis* will produce brucellosis in man. It has occurred in a laboratory technician and in an individual who assisted an infected whelping bitch. The domestic farm animals appear to be resistant to *Br. canis*, but foxes are susceptible.

**Diagnosis.** Clinical signs, direct culture, and agglutination tests have been utilized in diagnosing canine brucellosis. The organism cross-reacts with other *Brucella* species including *Br. ovis*, and also with *Bordetella bronchiseptica*, but the homologous titer indicates *Br. canis*.

**Control.** This has been accomplished by monthly monitoring of all animals for *Br. canis* infection using both blood culture and agglutination tests and removing all animals positive to either of these tests from the colony (3, 7).

**Chemotherapy.** None known to be successful.

## REFERENCES

1. Carmichael and Bruner.   Cornell Vet., 1968, 58, 579.
2. Carmichael and Kenney.   Jour. Am. Vet. Med. Assoc., 1968, 152, 605.
3. Hill, Van Hoosier, Jr., and McCormick.   Lab. Anim. Care, 1970, 20, 205.
4. Jones, Zanardi, Leong, and Wilson.   Jour. Bact., 1968, 95, 625.
5. Mitruka and Alexander.   Appl. Microbiol., 1970, 20, 649.
6. Moore.   Jour. Am. Vet. Med. Assoc., 1969, 155, 2034.
7. Moore, Gupta, and Conner.   *Ibid.*, 1968, 153, 523.
8. Taul, Powell, and Baker.   Vet. Med., 1967, 62, 543.

## Brucellosis (Undulant Fever) of Man

For more than a century a disease of man characterized by fever, chills, night sweats, and great weakness has been known in the Mediterranean countries of Europe. The causative agent of the disease was finally found in the blood of patients by David Bruce (2), a British military surgeon. The organism that was isolated was named *Micrococcus melitensis*. Because the work was done on the Island of Malta, the disease became known as *Malta fever*.

The source of the infection was not discovered for nearly 20 years, although it was realized that it was not directly contagious from man to man. A commission headed by Bruce discovered in 1904 that the blood of many of the milking goats on the Island of Malta contained agglutinins for the Malta fever organism. It was soon learned that infection was widespread in these goats and that the organism was secreted in the milk (Zammit, 23). The goats showed little evidence of disease, but their milk was very dangerous for persons who had not become immunized to the organism by drinking it from early life. Army and Navy personnel sent to the island from other parts of the world suffered greatly from the disease, whereas the natives seldom were affected.

The organism of Malta fever has been known since 1886, that of contagious abortion of cattle since 1897, and that of swine abortion since 1914. The relationship of swine abortion to that of cattle was seen from the beginning, but it was not until 1918 that it became known that these two organisms had any connection with Malta fever. In the first place, Bruce described the Malta fever organism as a coccus, and its relationship to caprine abortion was not appreciated. In the second place, most of the active work on bovine abortion was done in parts of the world where the Malta fever organism was not known; consequently there were few workers who had worked with both organisms.

In 1918 Alice Evans (5) showed for the first time that the three organisms were quite similar in morphology and in cultural reactions. The work of Evans was confirmed by Meyer and Shaw (18), and the suggestion was made that the Malta fever and the abortion-producing organisms be grouped together under the name *Brucella,* in honor of Bruce, who discovered the first member. This suggestion has met with general acceptance.

The discovery of the close relationship of the organisms of this new group immediately raised the question anew as to whether the abortion organisms might not at times be pathogenic for man. In 1924 Keefer (14), in Maryland, reported a case of Malta-fever-like disease occurring in a man who had not been exposed to Malta fever so far as could be established. Evans determined the organism isolated from this man to be *Br. abortus* rather than *Br. melitensis.* In 1926 Carpenter and Merriam (3) reported two human cases of brucellosis in a rural area of New York and supplied strong circumstantial evidence that the infections had been contracted by drinking infected raw cows' milk. Carpenter and others soon were able to demonstrate more cases of *Br. abortus* infection of man contracted from cattle. Since that time several thousand cases of undulant fever in man, caused by infections derived from cattle and swine rather than from goats, have been found in the United States and elsewhere; and the disease became known as brucellosis. It apparently had gone undiagnosed in past years, or was wrongly diagnosed as typhoid fever, paratyphoid fever, la grippe, and the like.

It is clear now that the undulant fever complex may be induced in man by any of these three types of *Brucella.* In the United States most cases are caused by *Br. abortus* and *Br. suis.* This is because these types are more prevalent than *Br. melitensis* in livestock. In the eastern part of the country human infections are mostly with *Br. abortus,* whereas in the north central part of the country (the swine belt) *Br. suis* infections probably outnumber those caused by *Br. abortus. Br. melitensis* infections are most common in Mexico and in certain small areas in the southwestern part of the United States. This type is also being found with considerable frequency in the midwestern states where the infection is apparently contracted from swine. In Alaska, clinical cases of brucellosis are appearing in the human population and there is evidence that the source of infection is the caribou (*Rangifer tar-*

*andus*). The identity of the *Brucella* strain has not been established. It may be a *Br. melitensis* type, a *Br. suis* type, or a new species (1).

Now that *Br. canis* has been added and is known to infect man, its role as a cause of human infection needs to be assessed.

The principal sources of human infections, so far as they are known, are as follows:

1. *Br. melitensis.* Most infections are contracted from the drinking of raw, infected goats' milk, or from eating certain cheeses made from such milk. Infections are also derived from direct contact with the infected secretions and excretions of goats and sheep. A few cases are known to have been contracted from swine and cattle. The organism produces a septicemia in pigs and it has been recovered from hams from such pigs 21 days after they were placed in cover pickle. No isolations were made after the hams were smoked (13).

2. *Br. abortus.* This type of infection is contracted by the drinking of raw, infected cows' milk. Reports from Italy have shown that the eating of certain cheeses made from unpasteurized cows' milk may result in infection. Apparently this rarely occurs and has not been reported in this country. Infection may be contracted by direct contact with infected fetuses, membranes, and discharges of aborting cows. In the United States the disease is a rural one. Its failure to occur in urban people is due to the fact that city people usually drink pasteurized milk and have no direct contacts with cattle. Most cases in city dwellers occur as a result of infections contracted during country vacation periods.

McCullough *et al.* (17) have recovered *Br. abortus* from the submaxillary lymph nodes of slaughtered hogs and state that they have observed human brucellosis due to *Br. abortus* in packing-house workers where exposure history implicated the hog as the source of infection.

3. *Br. suis.* Infections of man with this type occur usually in two occupational groups, farmers who raise swine and workers in slaughterhouses who handle swine carcasses.

**Brucellosis as an Occupational Hazard.** Brucellosis in man is very seldom if ever contracted from other men. Since the reservoir of infection is in infected animals, the disease in man will disappear when the animal reservoir is destroyed. As a matter of fact, there has been a great reduction in the number of human cases caused by *Br. abortus* during the last two decades in the United States and in other countries in which control and eradication campaigns in cattle have been pushed. Important in this respect are public awareness that human consumption of raw cows' milk is potentially dangerous and insistence that all milk, even that of the highest quality, be pasteurized. Milk is not damaged nutritionally by pasteurization, and its safety is increased. Human infections caused by *Br. suis* have not decreased so much in those areas of the United States where the organism has long been prevalent, probably because brucellosis in swine has not decreased so much as it has in cattle (9).

Although the susceptibility of the two sexes is about equal, at least two-thirds of the cases occurring in Iowa, according to Hardy, Jordan, Borts, and Hardy (7), were in men. These infections were partly *Br. abortus* and partly *Br. suis* infections. Iowa is largely a rural state and most of the cases were in farm families where the males usually were the caretakers of the livestock. Direct contact is apparently more hazardous than the drinking of infected milk, because male infections are more common even in areas where the predominating type is *Br. abortus*. Data collected in the United States and elsewhere agree that brucellosis, or undulant fever, may occur at all ages, but the greatest number of clinically recognized cases occur in the age group between 20 and 45 years (Hardy *et al.*, 7). Young infants, who consume a much larger volume of milk proportionally than adults, seldom become infected, although the disease has been recognized in children as young as 4 years of age.

Veterinarians in country practice face brucellosis as an occupational hazard because their work often requires them to come in contact with infected secretions. Blood-test surveys made before 1940 indicated that a comparatively large percentage of veterinarians reacted positively (10). Many of these had no clinical history of ever having had the disease. At that time infection in students in veterinary colleges was not uncommon. Since 1950 infection is less frequent in veterinarians and in veterinary students. This apparently is caused by the reduced incidence of infection in cattle and to the use of rubber gloves and sleeves in obstetrical work.

The high incidence of human cases in swine-slaughtering establishments in regions where swine infections are prevalent has pointed up the dangers in the handling of freshly slaughtered carcasses. As a rule, most cases in such plants occur in the personnel in the sticking and eviscerating rooms; those in the cutting and packing departments usually escape. This indicates that the greatest hazard comes from contact with the blood and internal organs of the carcasses. It should be remembered that in swine the *Brucella* organisms frequently occur in the blood; that the disease is more generalized than the corresponding one in cattle. It is true, also, that the *Br. suis* type is more highly pathogenic for man than *Br. abortus*. Both of these factors probably play a part in the difference between the hazards to man of handling swine and cattle carcasses. During an epidemic of brucellosis affecting 128 employees of a swine-slaughtering plant in Iowa, *Br. suis* was isolated from the air of the establishment (8). Although air-borne transmission of the disease is a possibility it does not appear that this is the usual route of infection.

*Br. suis* may retain its viability in fresh pork carcasses held at 40 F for as long as 3 weeks (12). In spite of this, no human cases have been traced to the handling of pork after it has been chilled. Perhaps this is caused by the fact that muscular tissue contains few organisms other than those in the blood vessels. Because carcasses are usually well bled out, market pork contains few organisms.

Human infections from contact with infected animal tissues and secretions probably occur through the unbroken skin. Hardy *et al.* (7) investigated this possibility, using guinea pigs as test animals. With cultures, infections were established in 18 percent of the animals by feeding, 80 percent by applying the culture to the unbroken skin where the hair had been clipped, 90 percent where the skin had been shaved, and 100 percent where the skin had been shaved and abraded. Cotton and Buck (4) conducted similar experiments on cattle. Using *Br. abortus,* they were able to show that infections could regularly be produced by dropping cultures on abraded areas of the skin, and in a number of cases on the undamaged skin, due precautions being taken in each case to see that the animals could not get the organisms in their mouths from licking the treated areas. Another possibility for the route of infection in human contact cases is suggested by their experiments on infecting cattle by dropping cultures into the uninjured conjunctival sac. Infections were regularly produced in this way.

**Diagnosis of Human Infections.** The diagnosis of human infections may be extraordinarily difficult because symptoms often are vague and atypical. The more acute forms are less difficult than the chronic cases. In the former the individual is acutely ill, suffers from great prostration and weakness, develops daily fever in the afternoon and evening, and suffers from chills and night sweats during which the fever disappears only to have the cycle recur on following days. The saw-tooth temperature chart is responsible for the name *undulant fever.* Such acute bouts usually ameliorate after a few days, but, following an interval of varying length during which the patient feels better, another period of acute symptoms may appear. There may be several such remissions. The symptoms are the same, no matter which types of *Brucella* is the infecting agent. Infections with *Br. melitensis* and *Br. suis* are usually more severe than those with *Br. abortus,* but this is not always the case. The mortality is low but recovery from infections often is very slow. Many persons never fully recover from the effects of the disease.

The symptoms of the chronic cases vary greatly. Usually the patient suffers from great debility, weakness, a low-grade remittent fever, joint pains, and other symptoms too numerous to mention. An osteoarticular complication of brucellosis is the *melitococcic spondylitis* of man reported in Italy. *Br. suis* has also been reported in septic arthritis of the hip. *Brucella* organisms have been implicated in cases of osteomyelitis (15) and in diseases of the nervous system (6). Perry (19) claims that calcific aortic stenosis is a residual lesion of brucellar endocarditis, chiefly caused by *Br. abortus* and Perry and Belter (20) have published a review on fatal brucellosis and heart disease.

Blood cultures, when positive, are diagnostic, but the isolation of the organism from the blood is usually difficult and often impossible, particularly when the offending organism is *Br. abortus.* Greater success is achieved in the acute than in the chronic cases, but repeated attempts often have to be made, even in the acute forms. The agglutination test may be used, but it must be interpreted with great caution because many infected individuals do not react and agglutinins, when present, may be the result of a previous unrecognized infection that may have had nothing to do with the current illness. According to Schuhardt and colleagues (21), the failure to react is caused in some cases by the presence of a *Brucella*-agglutinin-blocking antibody. This antibody is heat-labile and can be eliminated or markedly reduced by heating the serum at 56 C for 30 minutes.

The value of skin tests is controversial. Huddleson (11) recommends the use of a nucleoprotein fraction of *Br. abortus* for this purpose, but he was unable to differentiate between active cases of the disease and recovered or "sensitized" persons. Nonreactors to this test are considered as uninfected and probably susceptible to infection. Reactors may be actively infected or immune. It should be remembered that the skin test itself will sensitize normal individuals and make them agglutinin-positive.

In differentiating between actively infected and immune persons, Huddleson (11) has found a determination of opsonic activity toward the causative organism of value. The fresh blood of the patient is citrated (0.8 percent), mixed with a heavy suspension of *Br. abortus*, and incubated for 30 minutes, after which spreads are made on slides. These are stained and counts made of the numbers of bacteria ingested by the polymorphonuclear leukocytes. Normal opsonins are inhibited by the citrate, so that the blood of individuals who have had no contact with the infections shows practically no phagocytosis. The test is conducted as an adjunct to the skin test. When the skin test is positive and the phagocytic test positive, the individual is considered to be immune or at any rate recovering from infection. When the skin test is positive and the phagocytic test negative, the individual is considered to be suffering from an active infection.

**Immunity.** Various vaccines made from fractions of *Brucella* have been used in treating persons suffering from the chronic form of the disease, but in the United States no practicable means of immunizing persons who are exposed to the hazards of infection have been developed. In 1957 Zdrodowski, Vershilova, and Kotlarova (24) reported on large-scale immunization of human beings against melitensis brucellosis in Russia. Their vaccines consisted of live cultures of either *Br. abortus* (Strain 19) or *Br. abortus* (Russian strain), and they claimed that the morbidity rate among various classes of people living in endemic areas was reduced by 3.3 to 11.2 times following vaccination.

**Chemotherapy.** Brucellosis in man has been refractory to treatment with sulfonamides and antibiotics. Penicillin proved disappointing. Better success has been achieved with streptomycin, although the effects of this agent on the vestibular apparatus are frequently severe and some cases of total deafness have resulted from its use. Spink, Hall, Shaffer, and Braude (22) claim that the best results have been accomplished with aureomycin. They have also had gratifying results in many cases with a combination of dihydrostreptomycin (which is less toxic than streptomycin) and sulfadiazine. Killough *et al.* (16) treated 39 human patients using terramycin on 16, chloromycetin on

12, and aureomycin on 11. They stated that clinical response was excellent with each antibiotic, but a relapse rate of 69 percent indicated that these substances were not satifactory curative agents.

## REFERENCES

1.  Brody, Huntley, Overfield, and Maynard.   Jour. Inf. Dis., 1966, *116*, 263.
2.  Bruce.   Practitioner, 1887, *39*, 161.
3.  Carpenter and Merriam.   Jour. Am. Med. Assoc., 1926, *87*, 1269.
4.  Cotton and Buck.   Jour. Am. Vet. Med. Assoc., 1932, *80*, 342.
5.  Evans.   Jour. Inf. Dis., 1918, *22*, 580.
6.  Fincham, Sahs, and Joynt.   Jour. Am. Med. Assoc., 1963, *184*, 269.
7.  Hardy, Jordan, Borts, and Hardy.   Nat. Inst. Health Bul. 158, 1930.
8.  Harris, Hendricks, Gorman, and Held.   Pub. Health Rpts. (U.S.), 1962, *77*, 602.
9.  Hendricks and Borts.   *Ibid.*, 1964, *79*, 868.
10. Huddleson.   Brucellosis in man and animals.   The Commonwealth Fund, New York, 1939.
11. Huddleson, Johnson, and Hamann.   Am. Jour. Pub. Health, 1933, *23*, 917.
12. Hutchings, Bunnell, Donham, and Bay.   Proc. Am. Vet. Med. Assoc., 1950, p. 184.
13. Hutchings, McCullough, Donham, Eisele, and Bunnell.   Pub. Health Rpts. (U.S.), 1951, *66*, 1402.
14. Keefer.   Johns Hopkins Hosp. Bul., 1924, *35*, 6.
15. Kelly, Martin, Schirger, and Weed.   Jour. Am. Med. Assoc., 1960, *174*, 347.
16. Killough, Magill, and Smith.   *Ibid.*, 1951, *145*, 553.
17. McCullough, Eisele, and Pavelchek.   Pub. Health Rpts. (U.S.), 1951, *66*, 205.
18. Meyer and Shaw.   Jour. Inf. Dis., 1920, *27*, 173.
19. Perry.   Jour. Am. Med. Assoc., 1958, *166*, 1123.
20. Perry and Belter.   Am. Jour. Path., 1960, *36*, 673.
21. Schuhardt, Woodfin, and Knolle.   Jour. Bact., 1951, *61*, 299.
22. Spink, Hall, Shaffer, and Braude.   Jour. Am. Med. Assoc., 1949, *139*, 352.
23. Zammit.   Rpt. Comm. appointed by the Admiralty, the War Office, and the Office of Civil Govt. of Malta for investigations on Mediterranean fever. London, 1907.
24. Zdrodowski, Vershilova, and Kotlarova.   Jour. Inf. Dis., 1957, *101*, 1.

### Brucella ovis

Although there is some doubt regarding the placing of this organism in the genus *Brucella*, there appears to be none concerning its ability to cause a localized disease of the ovine genital tract. In the United States and Australia the disease has been confined mostly to males and is called *ram epididymitis* (2). In New Zealand late abortions associated with placental and fetal infections have been reported (16). The disease has also been observed in Czechoslovakia and in South America.

The organism was first isolated in 1953 by Buddle and Boyes (5) and described as *Br. ovis* (3) in 1956.

**Morphology and Staining Reactions.** *Br. ovis* is a Gram-negative cocco-bacillus, although it is somewhat acid-fast under certain conditions of staining (17). It is nonmotile, nonencapsulated, and nonsporulating.

**Cultural Features.** The organism requires enriched media and $CO_2$ for growth. It does not attack carhohydrates, change litmus milk, or reduce nitrates. It does not produce $H_2S$ or indol. It is catalase-positive (12). It is both oxidase- and urea-negative (10). It grows equally well on basic fuchsin and thionin media. On the basis of cross-reactions between its soluble antigens and those of *Br. melitensis,* Diaz *et al.* (7), believe that it belongs in the genus *Brucella.*

**Pathogenicity.** In the ram the earliest gross lesions are adhesions between the epididymis and the testis, usually in the distal portion of the organ. As the disease spreads, more and more of the epididymis becomes infected, and eventually the testis also becomes involved. Finally the palpable division between testis and epididymis is obliterated, and while the former atrophies, the latter acquires enormous size. The disease commonly affects one testicle, but bilateral lesions, usually at different stages of development, are frequently seen. Inapparent infection may occur, but in general, carriers eventually develop lesions.

According to Molello *et al.* (13) *Br. ovis* preferentially localizes in the inter-placentome of the pregnant ewe. In time an accumulation of exudate and bacteria may cause the placenta to become necrotic and separate from the caruncles, leading to fetal death. The bacteria are not highly pathogenic for pregnant sheep.

**Transmission.** The infection spreads rapidly from ram to ram, and venereal transmission has also been suggested. There is no evidence that the ewe harbors the infection from one season to the next or that the organism survives the winter on pasture.

**Diagnosis.** This is accomplished by palpation, culture of the semen, and demonstration of antibodies in the serum. A complement-fixation test employing the supernatant of a sonic-vibrated bacterial suspension as antigen has been recommended by Biberstein and McGowan (1) in detecting infected rams. Drimmelen *et al.* (8) claim that FA-treated semen films are useful in spotting the organism and Ris (14) employs an indirect hemagglutination test in which the erythrocytes are sensitized by antigens obtained through ultrasonic disintegration of *Br. ovis.* He states that palpation alone is not reliable and Hughes and Claxton (9) agree that clinical epididymitis is a most unreliable guide to the presence or absence of *Br. ovis* in individual rams.

In cases of abortion the organism can be cultured from the placental membranes and abomasal fluid of the fetus. The application of the FA techic to films from these sources also is helpful.

**Immunity.** In 1958 Buddle (4) advocated simultaneous vaccination with *Br. abortus,* Strain 19, and with a saline-in-oil adjuvant bacterin of formalinized *Br. ovis* in order to protect rams against the development of clinical epididymitis. In 1963 Buddle and co-workers (6) indicated that two doses of the adjuvant *Br. ovis* bacterin at an interval of 24 weeks was just as efficient as the Strain 19–*Br. ovis* combination. Kater and Hartly (11) have reported lameness in rams following vaccination by means of the simultaneous method. The ability of vaccines to provide immunity against naturally acquired infection has not been clearly established. There is evidence that agglutinin titers to *Br. abortus* antigen persist for several years in vaccinated rams (15).

**Chemotherapy.** *Br. ovis* is reported to be sensistive to penicillin and streptomycin. Experimental infection has been successfully treated with aureomycin and streptomycin, but the curing of chronic cases with antibiotics is doubtful.

## REFERENCES

1. Biberstein and McGowan. Cornell Vet., 1958, *48*, 31.
2. Biberstein, McKercher, and Wada. Jour. Am. Vet. Med. Assoc., 1959, *135*, 61.
3. Buddle. Jour. Hyg. (London), 1956, *54*, 351.
4. Buddle. New Zeal. Vet. Jour., 1958, *6*, 41.
5. Buddle and Boyes. Austral. Vet. Jour., 1953, *29*, 145.
6. Buddle, Calverley, and Boyes. New Zeal. Vet. Jour., 1963, *11*, 90.
7. Diaz, Jones, and Wilson. Jour. Bact., 1967, *93*, 1262.
8. Drimmelen, Botes, Claassen, Ross, and Viljoen. Jour. So. African Vet. Med. Assoc., 1963, *34*, 265.
9. Hughes and Claxton. Austral. Vet. Jour., 1968, *44*, 41.
10. Jones, Zanardi, Leong, and Wilson. Jour. Bact., 1968, *95*, 625.
11. Kater and Hartly. New Zeal. Vet. Jour., 1963, *11*, 65.
12. Kennedy, Frazier, and McGowan. Cornell Vet., 1956, *46*, 303.
13. Molello, Jensen, Flint, and Collier. Am. Jour. Vet. Res., 1963, *24*, 897.
14. Ris. New Zeal. Vet. Jour., 1964, *12*, 72.
15. *Ibid.*, 1967, *15*, 94.
16. Simmons and Hall. Austral. Vet. Jour., 1953, *29*, 33.
17. Stamp, McEwen, Watt, and Nisbet. Vet. Rec., 1950, *62*, 251.

## Differentiation of the Brucellae

Morphological and cultural features are not sufficiently characteristic to distinguish among *Br. abortus, Br. melitensis, Br. suis, Br. neotomae, Br. canis,* and *Br. ovis.* The host from which the organism is isolated cannot be relied upon entirely for identification, although each species has a principal one. Cattle and swine may be infected with the bovine, caprine, and porcine types. Sheep may be successfully inoculated with *Br. abortus,* and this infection may occur naturally, although *Br. melitensis* is the type usually found. The bovine, canine, caprine, and porcine types have been isolated from dogs. *Br. abortus* and *Br. suis* have been reported in horses. *Br. neotomae* has been confined mostly to rodents, *Br. canis* to dogs, and *Br. ovis* to sheep. Man suffers from the bovine, canine, caprine, and porcine types.

**Agglutinin Absorption.** This procedure was suggested by Meyer and Shaw (4) when straight agglutination tests were found to have little or no differential value. It appears that agglutinin absorption will not distinguish between the bovine and porcine types, and the caprine type cannot always be separated from the bovine. Morales and Lebron (6) prepared carbohydrate fractions from the bovine, caprine, and porcine types capable of distinguishing most *Br. melitensis* sera from *Br. abortus* and *Br. suis,* but were unable to separate *Br. abortus* and *Br. suis.* Straight agglutination will distinguish the canine type from the bovine, caprine, and porcine types, but not always from *Br. ovis.*

Other serologic tests concerned with the FA technic, bacteriophage typing, and gel-diffusion precipitation have not proved to be reliable in speciation studies within the genus *Brucella,* but Vivek (8) has indicated that the gel-diffusion method may be useful in identifying smooth strains of *Br. melitensis.*

**Gas Chromatographic Signatures.** Mitruka and Alexander (5) investigated a strain each of *Br. abortus, Br. melitensis, Br. suis, Br. ovis,* and *Br. canis* by gas chromatographic technics and concluded that they can be readily differentiated from one another by detecting the presence or absence of individual compounds.

**Urease Test.** *Br. suis* (7), *Br. canis,* and *Br. neotomae* are most active in urease production while *Br. ovis* is negative (3).

**Other Biochemical Reactions.** *Br. abortus, Br. suis* (2), and *Br. neotomae* usually produce $H_2S$, the other species do not. *Br. neotomae* and *Br. ovis* do not produce oxidase, the others do. *Br. ovis* is the only species that does not reduce nitrate.

**Dye Bacteriostasis.** Huddleson (1) in 1928 devised a system of differentiation by means of dyes that has been reasonably reliable. The dyes are added to a liver infusion agar. Basic fuchsin and thionin (certified dyes only) are used in final dilutions 1:50,000. On these dye media, the *Br. melitensis* and *Br. ovis* are not appreciably inhibited. *Br. suis, Br. canis,* and *Br. neotomae* grow more readily on the thionin medium and *Br. abortus* on the basic fuchsin. The scheme of separation is shown in table XIII.

*Table XIII.* GROWTH OF *BRUCELLA* TYPES IN DYE MEDIA

| Strain | Basic fuchsin | Thionin |
|---|---|---|
| *Br. abortus* | + | − |
| *Br. suis* | ± | + |
| *Br. canis* | ± | + |
| *Br. neotomae* | − | ± |
| *Br. melitensis* | + | + |
| *Br. ovis* | + | + |

$+$ = Good growth. $\pm$ = Slight growth.
$-$ = No growth.

**Gaseous Requirements.** Recently isolated strains of both *Br. abortus* and *Br. ovis* require an increased $CO_2$ tension for the initiation of growth. The other species do not have this requirement.

**Virulence for Guinea Pigs.** The porcine variety is the most virulent of all the species for this animal.

**Virulence of Man and Apes.** The bovine type is definitely less virulent than the porcine or caprine types. The canine type will infect man, but to date its degree of virulence has not been assessed. *Br. ovis* and *Br. neotomae* are not known to be pathogenic for man.

## REFERENCES

1.  Huddleson.   Mich. Agr. Exp. Sta. Tech. Bul. 100, 1929.
2.  Huddleson and Abell.   Jour. Bact., 1927, *13*, 13.
3.  Jones, Zanardi, Leong, and Wilson.   *Ibid.*, 1968, 95, 625.
4.  Meyer and Shaw.   Jour. Inf. Dis., 1920, 27, 173.
5.  Mitruka and Alexander.   Appl. Microbiol., 1970, *20*, 649.
6.  Morales and Lebron.   Proc. Soc. Exp. Biol. and Med., 1943, 52, 197.
7.  Pacheco and DeMello.   Jour. Bact., 1950, 59, 689.
8.  Vivek.   Cornell Univ. Thesis, 1961.

## THE GENUS *HEMOPHILUS*

Organisms of this group require blood, or certain substances in it, for satisfactory growth, especially when freshly isolated. One substance (X factor) now is recognized as a catalase of beef liver or the iron complex called *hemin*. Hemin probably is a necessary link in the synthesis of catalase. It can be replaced by cysteine, which reduces peroxide and makes catalase unnecessary. In addition, most of the species require for growth a substance (V factor) now recognized as Coenzyme I (Nicotinamide-adenine-dinucleotide—NAD, also called diphosphopyridine nucleotide—DPN), which is extractable from yeast, certain vegetable cells, and some bacteria, notably certain strains of staphylococci. The X factor withstands moderate autoclaving; the V factor is easily destroyed by heating. Fresh whole blood apparently contains both X and V factors in sufficient amounts for hemophilic growth.

The phenomenon of *satellitism,* or *satellite* formation, is often exhibited by organisms of this group when inoculated on media containing the X factor but lacking the V, as, for example, heated blood agar. Little or no growth will occur on such media except in the immediate neighborhood of colonies of other bacterial species, e.g., staphylococci, which produce the V factor and from which it diffuses into the surrounding medium.

The first organism of this group to be described is that which is now known as *Hemophilus influenzae*. This was described by Pfeiffer (22) in 1892. It was isolated from the upper respiratory tract of persons suffering from influenza and was believed to be the cause of that condition. In the great pandemic of human influenza in 1918–1919, however, it was discovered that Pfeiffer's bacillus was not invariably present in the disease, and it was shown by English and American workers that influenza was caused by a filterable virus. The influenza bacillus undoubtedly plays a secondary role in human influenza, and frequently has a part in the complications which so often develop, but true influenza can occur in its absence.

During the pandemic of human influenza in 1918, there appeared in the midwestern part of the United States a respiratory disease of swine that had not previously been seen. Koen, who worked with the disease in Iowa, was so impressed with its resemblance to the human disease that he dubbed it *swine flu* (8), and the disease soon became well known under that name. Only a few at that time believed that the swine disease had any connection with the human disease. Its probable relationship became known a dozen years later through the work of Shope (29).

Because a general description of the type species *Hemophilus influenzae* fits the various members of this group, it will be given here in detail and only special cultural characteristics will be listed in discussing other types.

**Morphology and Staining Reactions.** *H. influenzae* is Gram-negative, non-sporeforming, aerobic, and facultative. It is a nonmotile, tiny rod-shaped organism that may be quite pleomorphic. Some strains are encapsulated. In young cultures it usually appears as thin rods measuring about 0.2 microns in breadth and from 0.5 to 2.0 microns in length. Long thread forms frequently are seen. On some media these thread forms may predominate. Cultures older than 48 hours usually consist largely of coccoid elements, often arranged in large masses. Giant coccoids, club-shaped forms, and comma-shaped cells are frequently seen in old cultures. The organism stains rather poorly with ordinary stains. Old cultures are difficult to stain satisfactorily, no matter what stain is used.

**Cultural Features.** The organism is highly parasitic and sensitive to all but body conditions. No growth is obtained on plain or glycerol-containing agar, in broth, gelatin, milk, potato, or egg media, or on coagulated blood serum, unless the growth factors X and V are added, usually in the form of fresh blood or extracts of blood. Cultures must be incubated at about 37 C.

Agar slants to which 0.5 to 1.0 ml of defibrinated blood has been added may be used for isolation. There is no growth on the slant. The growth in the bloody fluid at the base of the slant is not evident until the fluid is examined microscopically. In such cultures the organism usually remains viable for about 2 weeks. On blood agar plates, well-established cultures grow feebly in the form of minute colonies, which have no observable effect upon the medium. When certain other bacteria appear on the plates, the influenza bacillus colonies near the contaminating colonies grow much more vigorously (a tendency known as *satellitism*). Good growth usually occurs in blood broth.

Another medium upon which this organism thrives is chocolate agar. It is made by adding defibrinated blood to agar at a temperature of 70 to 80 C. The surface colonies are circular in outline, grayish, flattened, semitransparent; they have sharp edges. Under the most favorable conditions the colonies do not become larger than about 1 mm in diameter. Best growth usually occurs around the margins of colonies of other bacteria.

Growth does not occur in litmus milk unless a little blood is added to it, and even then the growth is meager. The milk is not changed in appearance. These organisms do not, as a rule, ferment glucose, and they are not proteolytic. All strains reduce nitrates. Neither hydrogen sulfide nor indol is formed.

No attempt will be made to list all the members of this genus. Among the more common human strains are *H. influenzae*, which is concerned with respiratory diseases, meningitis, and conjunctivitis. It has been isolated from a case of appendicitis and from the infected incision (5). *H. ducreyi* appears in a disease known as *chancroid*. The animal types considered are *H. suis, H. hemoglobinophilus, H. gallinarum, H. ovis, H. agni,* and *H. parainfluenzae.*

### Hemophilus suis

SYNONYM:   *Hemophilus influenzae* var. *suis*

This organism was first described by Lewis and Shope (14) in 1931. In subsequent studies Shope (29) clearly demonstrated that, whereas *Hemophilus suis* was relatively harmless to pigs when inoculated alone, it became highly pathogenic for susceptible swine when inoculated with a filterable virus. The virus alone is also relatively harmless. Swine influenza is a disease produced only by the concerted action of the bacillus and the virus. The relationship between these two agents will be discussed more fully later under virus diseases (see p. 1026).

**Cultural Features.** *H. suis* resembles *H. influenzae* except that it is relatively inert biochemically and differs immunologically. Both X and V factors are required for growth.

**Pathogenicity.** *Hemophilus suis* is only slightly pathogenic for normal swine. After intranasal instillation a mild transitory illness sometimes occurs, but frequently there are no detectable symptoms. When illness is evident, the disease does not transmit to pen mates. When cultures are added to the virus of influenza, which alone will not cause serious illness in swine, typical influenza results and this disease will transmit naturally to pen mates.

The organism ordinarily is nonpathogenic for rabbits, guinea pigs, and white rats. It occasionally proves pathogenic for white mice.

In addition to the disease caused by the concerted action of *H. suis* and the swine influenza virus, it appears that pigs may be subject at times to pneumonia and pleurisy or meningoencephalitis caused by *H. parainfluenzae* and *H. parahemolyticus* (15, 16, 24). The last two organisms require factor V, but not X for growth.

Upon intratracheal inoculation *H. suis* is reported to cause Glasser's disease (polyserositis) in pigs without significant pulmonary involvement (18). Lesions caused by *H. suis* and by *Mycoplasma hyorhinis* are similar and cause much confusion in making a differential diagnosis between them.

**Immunity.** *H. suis* will not immunize swine against influenza. Although it is essential to the production of the disease, it is clear that the virus plays the important role.

### Hemophilus hemoglobinophilus

SYNONYM: *Hemophilus canis*

This organism is quite similar in morphology and cultural characteristics to the influenza bacillus. It was first isolated and described by Friedberger (11) in 1903 under the name *B. hemoglobinophilus canis*. Rivers (26), who studied this organism in 1922, reported that it formed acid from glucose, levulose, galactose, sucrose, xylose, and mannitol. Indol was produced and nitrates were reduced. The organism requires the X factor but can synthesize the V factor. It has been isolated by several workers from the preputial secretion of male dogs, where it seems to live a parasitic existence without doing much, if any, harm. It is nonpathogenic for laboratory animals.

### Hemophilus gallinarum

SYNONYM: *Bacillus hemoglobinophilus coryzae gallinarum*

The name *H. gallinarum* was proposed in 1934 by Eliot and Lewis (9) for an organism that had been described first by De Blieck (6) in Holland under the name given above as a synonym. The latter is invalid because it is not a binomial. It had also been previously studied by Nelson (19) in New Jersey; by Delaplane, Irwin, and Stuart (7) in Rhode Island; and by Pistor, Hoffman, Beach, and Schalm (23) and Schalm and Beach (28) in California. It is the cause of a serious and widespread disease of chickens known as *fowl coryza*. The organism is much like the influenza bacilli of man and swine, and the disease has some similarities, but unlike the other diseases this one seems not to be associated with a virus.

*H. gallinarum* is isolated with some difficulty. Nelson succeeded first by using rather coarse Berkefeld filters, which removed all ordinary bacteria but regularly passed this minute organism. Later he found that colonies could be obtained on blood agar plates seeded with nasal exudate, providing the plates were sealed with wax. De Blieck, also Eliot and Lewis, appear to have recovered it without sealing. This was confirmed by Bornstein and Samberg (3), who state that scanty growth and colonization were obtained on the surface of blood agar under aerobic conditions. However, incubation under an increased $CO_2$ tension of about 10 percent greatly enhanced the growth of the organism.

In culturing *H. gallinarum*, Bornstein and Samberg recommend the use of blood agar, incubated under increased $CO_2$ tension, or 7-day-old chicken embryos. The latter are inoculated in the yolk sac, and mortality results in 24 to 48 hours. The dead embryos are congested and present a heavy growth of the organism in both the yolk and the allantoic fluid. Here the organisms remain viable for 6 weeks under 5 C refrigeration as compared to 2 weeks in the case of blood agar. For isolation Bornstein and Samberg take material from facial swellings of cases of infectious coryza. The edematous area is swabbed with alcohol, the skin is pierced, and the fluid content is removed by pipette and streaked on blood agar.

**Cultural Features.** The organism is a facultative anaerobe that grows best on primary isolation when $CO_2$ is furnished. It appears that the V factor, but not the X factor, is required for growth (20). It is rather inactive biochemically. It does not produce indol or hydrogen sulfide. It does not change litmus or methylene blue milk or liquefy gelatin. It regularly ferments glucose and is irregular in fermenting mannose, galactose, levulose, maltose, sucrose, and dextrin (3).

**Pathogenicity.** The lesions produced in fowl by *H. gallinarum* are acute inflammation of the turbinates and sinus epithelium, disruption of the trachea without cellular infiltration, and acute air sacculitis characterized by swelling and heterophilic response (1). The exudate of natural cases of fowl coryza is highly infectious when introduced into the palatine cleft of susceptible birds. Filtrates of this material are not infectious except, as Nelson showed, when coarse Berkefeld candles are used for the filtration, and the filtrates are incubated for a time in the presence of fresh chicken blood. Pure cultures will reproduce the disease, and such cultures will retain their virulence for chickens after many generations in artificial media. Rabbits and guinea pigs are resistant to injections of pure cultures. Turkeys, pigeons, and many other species of birds are also refractory.

Raggi *et al.* (25) have found that concurrent deposition of infectious bronchitis virus and *H. gallinarum* into the nostrils of 6-week-old White Leghorns produces a shorter incubation period, higher mortality, and severe macro- and microscopic lesions than can be instituted in birds inoculated singly with similar amounts of either one of these agents.

**Immunity.** According to Page *et al.* (21) bacterins consisting of formalin-inactivated yolk-propagated cultures stimulate a high degree of immunity to the development of air-sac lesions and a limited, but significant resistance to upper respiratory-tract disease. There is evidence that recovered birds remain carriers of virulent bacilli, and it is in this manner that the disease appears to be propagated from year to year.

### Hemophilus of Bovine Origin

Watt (30) isolated from calf pneumonia a Gram-negative coccobacillus that belongs in the genus *Hemophilus*. The lesions in the calves were confined to the thoracic cavity. There was slight pleurisy, but the main changes occurred in the anterior and caudal lobes of the lungs, where purulent bronchitis was found.

The organism grew under aerobic, microaerophilic, or anaerobic conditions, but best under 10 percent $CO_2$ It required both X and V factors for growth, reduced nitrates, did not change litmus milk, and fermented only glucose.

When injected alone it did not produce calf pneumonia, but it did induce the typical disease in this animal when it was instilled intranasally in combination with a filterable agent that also came from pneumonic calf lung and had been passed serially in mice. The evidence suggests that some outbreaks of calf pneumonia have an etiology like that of influenza in man and swine.

Firehammer (10) isolated a member of the genus *Hemophilus* from an aborted bovine fetus. His organism required the V factor for growth but not the X factor. Kennedy *et al.* (12) studied an epizootic of bacterial meningoencephalitis in feedlot cattle caused by a *Hemophilus*like organism.

### *Hemophilus ovis*

*H. ovis* was described by Mitchell (17) in 1925. It occurred in a single flock of sheep in Canada, where it apparently was the active agent in a disease that caused acute illness and death in a number of animals. The symptoms and lesions of the natural disease were produced artificially by inoculating sheep with a pure culture.

In 1956 Roberts (27) isolated a pathogen from a ewe with mastitis. With this organism he was able to reproduce the disease. After studying its cultural characteristics, he proposed that it be named *H. ovis*.

Apparently the Mitchell and the Roberts strain were not compared, and it cannot be assumed that they are identical. They have, however, a number of similar characters.

**Cultural Features.** Mitchell's strain requires only the heat-stable (X) factor, although growth is more luxuriant when the blood is heated below the point at which the V factor is destroyed. Acid but no gas is formed from glucose, lactose, sucrose, maltose, mannose, mannitol, galactose, levulose, raffinose, and sorbitol. Rhamnose, arabinose, salicin, and inositol are not attacked.

Robert's strain did not grow in any media that did not contain either blood or cooked meat particles. Heating the blood to 80 C did not impair its effectiveness in promoting growth. $CO_2$ was required for growth on agar media. The organism produced acid but no gas from glucose, levulose, mannose, mannitol, sorbitol, and xylose. It did not ferment arabinose, dextrin, dulcitol, galactose, inositol, inulin, lactose, maltose, raffinose, rhamnose, trehalose, salicin, or sucrose.

**Pathogenicity.** With Mitchell's strain the onset of the disease was sudden and featured by great prostration, marked cyanosis, labored and distressed breathing, and fever in the early stages. Sixteen out of 17 naturally infected animals died within a few days. Some animals discharged a bloody fluid from the nostrils, and most of them discharged bloody feces. The lesions consisted of bronchopneumonia, which was always bilateral and involved the anterior lobes; intense congestion of the abdominal organs, especially the kidneys; petechiae on various organs; and a yellow, friable liver having a cooked appearance. The lesions were reproduced faithfully in a sheep that received culture intratracheally.

Pure cultures killed guinea pigs and rabbits but proved innocuous for chickens.

Robert's strain was isolated from the udder of a dead ewe. The left half of the gland was in a normal lactating state, but the right half was enlarged and turgid. When it was incised, brownish purulent fluid gushed out. Upon intradermal injection into a lamb, the isolate produced a diffuse abscess and death. When placed in one side of the udder of each of two dry ewes, it resulted in severe mastitis in the inoculated halves only, the other sides remaining normal.

**Immunity.** There is no information on this point. Mitchell failed to demonstrate toxin in culture filtrates.

### Hemophilus agni

This microorganism has been described as the cause of a rapidly fatal, but not directly contagious, disease of lambs (2, 13).

**Cultural Features.** *H. agni* requires hemoglobin or its derivatives for growth. Organisms from diseased tissues stain better with carbol fuchsin (1 :10 dilution) than with Gram's method.

**Pathogenicity.** The disease involves only lambs. An alert herdsman may note depression and stiffness in affected animals about 12 hours prior to death, but usually the first indication of disease is the presence of one or two dead lambs in the flock.

Gross lesions consist of hemorrhages, edema, and congestion. Individuals that survive for more than a day are affected with fibrinopurulent arthritis and eventually meningitis. Microscopically, multiple bacterial thrombosis, especially marked in the liver and voluntary muscles, is the most striking feature.

The disease can be reproduced by parenteral injection but does not spread by contact to control animals.

### Chemotherapy in Hemophilus Infections

Penicillin appears to have little effect against the members of the genus *Hemophilus*. The sulfonamides vary in effectiveness. Streptomycin, aureomycin, chloromycetin, and terramycin are reported to be most useful. Bornstein *et al.* (4) studied the therapeutic effect of streptomycin on infectious coryza of chickens and concluded that it was very effective in treating adult chickens, less so in young birds.

### REFERENCES

1.  Adler and Page.   Avian Dis., 1962, *6*, 1.
2.  Biberstein, McKercher, and Wada.   Jour. Am. Vet. Med. Assoc., 1959, *135*, 61.
3.  Bornstein and Samberg.   Am. Jour. Vet. Res., 1954, *15*, 612.
4.  Bornstein, Samberg, and Moses.   Jour. Am. Vet. Med. Assoc., 1955, *126*, 215.

5.  Branson.   Am. Jour. Clin. Path., 1967, *47*, 643.
6.  De Blieck.   Tijdsch. v. Diergeneensk., 1931, *58*, 310.
7.  Delaplane, Irwin, and Stuart.   R.I. State Coll., Agr. Exp. Sta. Bul. 244, 1934.
8.  Dorset, McBryde, and Niles.   Jour. Am. Vet. Med. Assoc., 1922, *62*, 162.
9.  Eliot and Lewis.   *Ibid.*, 1934, *84*, 878.
10. Firehammer.   *Ibid.*, 1959, *135*, 421.
11. Friedberger.   Centrbl. f. Bakt., I Abt., Orig., 1903, *33*, 401.
12. Kennedy, Biberstein, Howarth, Frazier, and Dungworth.   Am. Jour. Vet. Res., 1960, *21*, 403.
13. Kennedy, Frazier, Theilen, and Biberstein.   *Ibid.*, 1958, *19*, 645.
14. Lewis and Shope.   Jour. Exp. Med., 1931, *54*, 361.
15. Little.   Vet. Rec., 1970, *87*, 399.
16. Matthews and Pattison.   Jour. Comp. Path. and Therap., 1961, *71*, 44.
17. Mitchell.   Jour. Am. Vet. Med. Assoc., 1925, *68*, 8.
18. Neil, McKay, L'Ecuyer, and Corner.   Canad. Jour. Comp. Med., 1969, *33*, 187.
19. Nelson.   Proc. Soc. Exp. Biol. and Med., 1932, *30*, 306;   Jour. Exp. Med., 1933, *58*, 289 and 297.
20. Page.   Am. Jour. Vet. Res., 1962, *23*, 85.
21. Page, Rosenwald, and Price.   Avian Dis., 1963, *7*, 239.
22. Pfeiffer.   Deut. med. Wchnschr., 1892, *18*, 28.
23. Pistor, Hoffman, Beach, and Schalm.   Nulaid News, 1933, *11*, 7.
24. Radostits, Ruhnke, and Losos.   Canad. Vet. Jour., 1963, *4*, 265.
25. Raggi, Young, and Sharma.   Avian Dis., 1967, *11*, 308.
26. Rivers.   Jour. Bact., 1922, *7*, 579.
27. Roberts.   Austral. Vet. Jour., 1956, *33*, 330.
28. Schalm and Beach.   Science, 1934, *79*, 416.
29. Shope.   Jour. Exp. Med., 1931, *54*, 349 and 373.
30. Watt.   Jour. Comp. Path. and Therap., 1952, *62*, 102.

## THE GENUS *ACTINOBACILLUS*

There are at least six species in the genus *Actinobacillus*. *A. lignieresi* causes actinobacillosis in cattle, rarely in other animals. *A. actinomycetemcomitans* occurs in human cases of actinobacillosis either alone or mixed with the organisms causing actinomycosis. *A. equuli* is found in equulosis of foals. *A. actinoides* has been isolated from chronic pneumonia in calves. *A. seminis* has been implicated in genital disease in rams. *A* (*Malleomyces*) *mallei* is the cause of glanders, a disease primarily of solipeds.

### *Actinobacillus lignieresi*

This organism was first described by Lignières and Spitz (8, 9) in 1902. It had been isolated from Argentine cattle suffering from a disease which clinically resembled actinomycosis. Later this disease was recognized in Europe (2, 10), in the United States (19, 22), and in South Africa (13). It is quite common. It may be confused with actinomycosis.

**Morphology and Staining Reactions.** In the pus of the lesions of the disease the small rod-shaped organisms are encased in small cheeselike granules. These are quite similar to the "sulfur granules" of actinomycosis, but generally they are much smaller, measuring less than 1 mm in diameter. If these granules are picked out of the pus and crushed between slides, moderate magnification will show clublike bodies radiating out from the centers of the masses. Stains made from the crushed granules show small Gram-negative bacilli.

In cultures the organism exhibits considerable variation in morphology depending upon the medium used and whether surface or deep growth on solid media is examined. Diplococci and slender rods are seen in fluid cultures. Long curved forms are often seen in colonies growing in the depths of solid media. The bacilli are about 0.4 microns in width and from 1 to 15 microns in length. They are nonmotile, stain with the usual dyes, and are Gram-negative.

**Cultural Features.** This organism is quite serophilic, and little growth occurs in most media unless some serum or blood is present. It is rather strongly aerobic, to the extent that growth practically always fails under anaerobic conditions. On the other hand, primary cultures in fluid media or in stabs in solid media are more apt to succeed than surface cultures. Primary cultures succeed best when they are incubated in an atmosphere consisting of 10 percent carbon dioxide.

In serum agar, delicate, naillike growths appear along the length of the stab. Surface colonies are bluish white and very delicate. They are smooth, glistening, convex, and vary from 0.5 to 1 mm in diameter. There is good

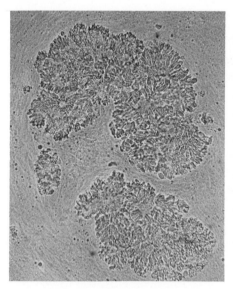 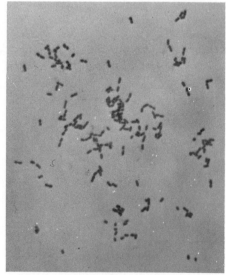

*Fig. 16* (left). *Actinobacillus lignieresi,* showing club-bearing rosettes in pus from a lymph node lesion. Unstained. X 360. (Courtesy L. R. Vawter.)

*Fig. 17* (right). *Actinobacillus lignieresi,* from a culture on serum agar incubated 24 hours at 37 C. X 1,000. (Courtesy L. R. Vawter.)

growth in serum gelatin but the medium is not liquefied. Glucose serum broth usually shows a characteristic growth consisting of small grayish granules, which adhere to the sides of the tube but are easily broken loose by shaking. The remainder of the broth is clear. Litmus milk usually remains unchanged. Sometimes it develops slight acidity. Excellent growth occurs on coagulated blood serum. The medium is not softened or liquefied. When dissolved in serum broth, glucose, lactose, sucrose, maltose, raffinose, and mannitol are regularly fermented. Xylose is fermented irregularly. Arabinose, dulcitol, salicin, and inulin are not attacked. Indol is formed in small amounts. Cultures must be transferred at frequent intervals; otherwise they lose viability. Tunnicliff (21) states that bovine and ovine strains appear to be similar, but that strains of either type may fail to agglutinate with a type serum. Magnusson found that all strains of this species isolated from cattle were serologically identical. Till and Palmer (20) after studying 26 strains by serologic tests stated that there are at least two types, with the majority belonging to one type.

**Pathogenicity.** This organism is only slightly pathogenic for guinea pigs and rabbits and not at all for rats and mice. In guinea pigs that have been inoculated intraperitoneally, a localized peritonitis in the scrotal sac may occur not unlike the Strauss reaction caused by the glanders bacillus.

The natural disease in cattle is manifested most commonly by slowly developing tumors, which may occur in any part of the body but are seen most frequently in the region of the lower jaws and neck. These are hard and often lobular. Sooner or later softened areas become evident, and these fluctuate upon pressure, indicating the presence of fluid, which is, in reality, a mucoid, nonodorous pus. This breaks through the skin, creating a deep ulcer which will not heal. In the meantime, the tumorous mass usually continues to enlarge and additional ulcers may form. A characteristic form of this disease is the so-called *wooden tongue* of cattle. In this disease the hard tumorous mass forms in the substance of the tongue, causing serious disability. Lesions in the internal organs, particularly of the lymphoid structures, the lungs, and the walls of the four compartments of the stomach, are not uncommon. Palotay (11) described three cases in cattle. One showed lesions in the subcutaneous tissue of the posterior limbs; in the submaxillary, internal iliac, and the prefemoral lymph glands; and in the ovaries. In another the tunics of the testicles were involved, and the third was evidenced by a large swelling in the middle posterior part of the thigh. Swarbrick (17) studied three atypical cases; one a circumscribed cutaneous lesion in the flank, one with urinary bladder involvement, and one a widespread infection in the head associated with multiple foreign bodies in the mouth. Hebeler *et al.* (5) reported an outbreak in a dairy herd with about 7 percent morbidity and a high incidence of lesions of the skin and related lymph nodes rather than tongue or alimentary tract involvement. Although the lesions of *A. lignieresi* tend to localize, generalized actinobacillosis has been observed in cattle (4).

This disease often is confused with actinomycosis. The true actinomycosis, which is caused by the "ray fungus," *Actinomyces bovis*, seldom occurs in the soft structures but is found mostly in the bone of the lower jaw.

Actinobacillosis is a relatively common disease of cattle in the western hemisphere. Usually it occurs as sporadic cases but occasionally small epizootics are seen. The mortality is not high, because the subcutaneous lesions yield readily to surgery if taken before they involve too much tissue. Cases of wooden tongue are more difficult to cure, and in some instances it may be desirable to slaughter rather than treat such animals.

Actinobacillosis occurs in sheep. According to Taylor (18), it is fairly common in this animal in Scotland. Reports (6) indicate that lesions of the disease often are found in the head region with involvement of the cheeks, nose, lips, and lymph glands. Abscesses are seen in the soft palate, pharynx, and lungs. Skin lesions have also been reported. The organism has been described as the cause of mastitis in the ewe (7).

Sautter *et al.* (15) have noted a case of actinobacillosis in a dog, and Fletcher (3) reported a case in the tongue of a dog. Their isolates did not

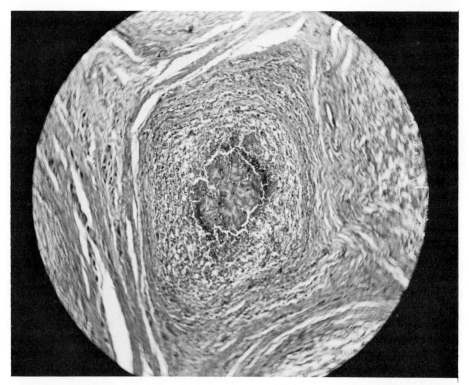

*Fig. 18.* Actinobacillosis, purulent focus in a case of "wooden tongue." The lesion consists principally of granulation tissue containing such foci as are depicted here. The rosette often is surrounded by a number of giant cells, epithelioid cells, and polymorphonuclear leukocytes. Stained with hematoxylin and eosin. X 600.

have all the characteristics of *A. lignieresi*. In 1969, Carb and Liu (1) found *A. lignieresi* to be the causative agent of a large, diffusely infiltrating granulomatous mass in the thigh of a 7.5-year-old Boston Terrier.

Several human infections with this organism have been reported. The pathogenicity for man apparently is not high (12).

**Immunity.** There is no evidence that animals may be successfully immunized to this disease, and no immunizing products are available.

**Chemotherapy.** The infection, like actinomycosis, is iodine-sensitive, and local lesions may be successfully treated by injecting them with an aqueous solution of iodine (Lugol's solution). Clinical experience has shown that NaI administered intravenously is highly successful in treating wooden tongue and other forms of actinobacillosis in which the lesions are inaccessible to local applications of iodine. *A. lignieresi* is very sensitive to the action of sulfonamides, particularly sulfapyridine, sulfamethazine, and sulfathiazole, and these substances may have value in treating the disease (16). It is also sensitive to aureomycin, terramycin, and chloromycetin (14).

## REFERENCES

1. Carb and Liu.   Jour. Am. Vet. Med. Assoc., 1969, *154*, 1062.
2. Davies and Torrance.   Jour. Comp. Path. and Therap., 1930, *43*, 216.
3. Fletcher.   Vet. Rec., 1956, *68*, 645.
4. Franco.   Vet. Med/SAC, 1970, *65*, 562.
5. Hebeler, Linton, and Osborne.   Vet. Rec., 1961, *73*, 517.
6. Johnson.   Austral. Vet. Jour., 1954, *30*, 105.
7. Laws and Elder.   *Ibid.*, 1969, *45*, 401.
8. Lignières and Spitz.   Bul. Soc. Cent. Méd. Vet., 1902, *20*, 487.
9. Lignières and Spitz.   Centrbl. f. Bakt., I Abt., Orig., 1903, *35*, 294.
10. Magnusson.   Acta Path. et Microbiol. Scand., 1928, *5*, 170.
11. Palotay.   Vet. Med., 1951, *46*, 52.
12. Pathak and Ristic.   Am. Jour. Vet. Res., 1962, *23*, 310.
13. Robinson.   Jour. So. African Vet. Med. Assoc., 1951, *22*, 85.
14. Sanders and Ristic.   Jour. Am. Vet. Med. Assoc., 1956, *129*, 478.
15. Sautter, Rowsell, and Hohn.   North Am. Vet., 1953, *34*, 341.
16. Smith.   Vet. Rec., 1951, *63*, 674.
17. Swarbrick.   Brit. Vet. Jour., 1967, *123*, 70.
18. Taylor.   Jour. Comp. Path. and Therap., 1944, *54*, 228.
19. Thompson.   Jour. Inf. Dis., 1933, *52*, 223.
20. Till and Palmer.   Vet. Rec., 1960, *72*, 527.
21. Tunnicliff.   Jour. Inf. Dis., 1941, *69*, 52.
22. Vawter.   Cornell Vet., 1933, *23*, 126.

### *Actinobacillus actinomycetemcomitans*

SYNONYM:   *Bacterium actinomycetemcomitans*

This organism was first described by Klinger (4) in 1912, who found it in a case of human actinomycosis in association with the ray fungus. Later Colebrook (2) in England and Bayne-Jones (1) in the United States found the same organism associated with human infection. Although human actinomycosis may be caused by the same organism that so commonly affects cattle, this organism has never been reported from cases of bovine disease. Its significance in human disease is not clear. King and Tatum (3) have pointed out the possibility of confusing *A. actinomycetemcomitans* with *Hemophilus aphrophilus,* an organism originally isolated from the blood and the heart valves of a case of human endocarditis. It has been claimed that, when metastatic lesions are present in a patient, *A. actinomycetemcomitans* can be found only in the primary lesions. It is present in the interior of the "sulfur granules" and may be demonstrated there by a simple microscopic examination of the crushed granules, as well as by cultural examinations.

**Morphology and Staining Reactions.** The organism occurs as coccobacilli or as rods 1.0 to 1.5 microns long by 0.6 to 0.8 micron broad. It is nonmotile and Gram-negative.

**Cultural Features.** On glucose agar small, smooth, slightly yellowish, adherent colonies are formed. Growth occurs in gelatin along the stab but the medium is not liquefied. When the gelatin is incubated at 37 C, a characteristic growth appears. Grayish-white granules form along the sides of the tube, and by fusion these eventually form a complete ring around the tube and a pellicle over the surface. A similar effect appears in broth cultures, but in this case the fluid finally becomes turbid. Growth does not occur in milk or on potato. Acid is formed from glucose and lactose but there is no gas formation. Growth in all media is enhanced by the addition of serum.

**Pathogenicity.** Except when very large doses are used, this organism is nonpathogenic for laboratory animals.

## REFERENCES

1. Bayne-Jones.   Jour. Bact., 1925, *10*, 569.
2. Colebrook.   Brit. Jour. Exp. Path., 1920, *1*, 197.
3. King and Tatum.   Jour. Inf. Dis., 1962, 3, 85.
4. Klinger.   Centrbl. f. Bakt., I Abt., Orig., 1912, *62*, 191.

### *Actinobacillus (Shigella) equuli*

SYNONYMS:   *Shigella equirulis, Bacillus nephritidis equi, Bacterium viscosum equi, Bacterium pyosepticus equi, Shigella equi, Shigella viscosa*

*A. equuli* is the causative agent in purulent infections of the joints and in kidney abscesses in very young foals. It has been found in adult horses. *A. equuli* was first described by Meyer (8), who found it in kidney abscesses in horses in South Africa and gave it the name *Bacillus nephritidis equi.* Magnusson (6), finding the organism in foals in Sweden and not recognizing it as the same as the organism described by Meyer, named it *Bacterium viscosum equi.* McFadyean and Edwards (5) recognized that the two organisms were identical.

Because this organism has been renamed each time a new classification has appeared and because the names that have been applied to the disease produced are no longer valid we propose that the infection be named *equulosis,* a designation based on the specific part of the binomial and more likely to remain fixed.

**Morphology and Staining Reactions.** This is a small rod-shaped organism. Short chains and filaments are often seen. Capsules have been described, but generally it is believed to be noncapsulated. It is nonmotile, stains easily with the ordinary stains, and is Gram-negative.

**Cultural Features.** *A. equuli* grows readily in ordinary media, producing rather abundant growth. Colonies on agar plates are smooth, rather dry in appearance, and tough. Dissociation readily occurs, especially when the medium is acid and the incubation temperature high, the product being small, smooth, glistening colonies, some of which are dwarf types. On agar slants the growth is diffuse, grayish white, and very mucoid. A ropy sediment forms in broth, and old cultures become very cloudy and mucoid. A grayish pellicle sometimes appears. Gelatin stabs show a filiform growth. There is no liquefaction. Litmus milk is slowly acidified and sometimes coagulated. The uncoagulated cultures generally are very slimy. Indol is not formed and the Voges-Proskauer test is negative. No toxins are generated. Blood is not hemolyzed. Acid but no gas is formed from glucose, lactose, sucrose, galactose, maltose, raffinose, xylose, and mannitol. Freshly isolated cultures must be transferred at weekly intervals to maintain viability unless especially prepared medium is used. (4).

**Pathogenicity.** In the past years approximately 30 percent of the foals lost each season in the Bluegrass area of Kentucky died of *A. equuli* infection (3). The use of antibiotics has now reduced losses from this infection by 50 percent.

About one-third of the foals that succumbed to equulosis died within the first 24 hours, and the majority succumbed prior to the 4th day following birth. In foals that died within the first 24 hours, the only visible lesion consisted of a severe enteritis. Rarely was there any evidence of nephritis. In foals which died at 2 or 3 days of age, the lesions observed at postmortem examination were more marked. These cases often exhibited a purulent nephritis, small abscesses being scattered throughout the cortex of the kidney. Many times the joints of the legs were affected. The joint lesions ranged from a slight increase in synovial fluid and congestion of the joint capsule to a purulent arthritis involving the joint cavity and tendon sheaths, with a great accumulation of fluid and extreme swelling. A few foals showed a severe purulent pleuropneumonia. The diagnosis was made by isolating the causative microorganism from the infected organs and joints of the diseased foal.

The fact that this infection was found in aborted fetuses definitely indicates a prenatal origin, but much of the evidence gained from postmortem studies of foals points to a postnatal origin of the infection. Apparently both types of infection occur in the foal.

Organisms closely related to if not identical with A. *equuli* have been iso-lated from endocarditis, septicemia, metritis, and arthritis in swine (2, 10), from joints of rabbits (1), and from outbreaks of calf diarrhea (9). The exact relationship of these bacteria to A. *equuli* and to A. *lignieresi* and the possi-bility that swine or other species of animals may act as carriers of the former needs further study.

**Mode of Infection.** A. *equuli* is an inhabitant of the intestinal canal of many horses, where it is apparently harmless. Dimock demonstrated it in cultures taken from the tonsillar region in 10 out of 12 horses that had died of causes unrelated to this disease, and others have had similar success. He also noted that the common verminous aneurysms of the mesenteric arteries often are in-fected with this organism, even when it cannot be demonstrated elsewhere. He believed that the larvae of *Strongylus vulgaris*, migrating from the intes-tinal lumen into the arteries, carry A. *equuli* with them and in this way set up infections in young susceptible animals. In prenatal infection it is possible that invasion of the fetal circulation by strongyle larvae of the dam may be a contributing factor.

A. *equuli* is not pathogenic for man. Unless very large doses are given, it is not pathogenic even for small laboratory animals.

**Immunity.** Specific treatment of foals with an antiserum prepared from A. *equuli* has been attempted but without encouraging results. After symptoms become evident, the prognosis is not good. Maguire (7) claims that he obtains satisfactory protection by vaccinating pregnant mares.

**Chemotherapy.** Streptomycin has been employed with very good results in treating equulosis in foals.

**REFERENCES**

1.   Arseculeratne.   Jour. Comp. Path. and Therap., 1962, 72, 33.
2.   Ashford and Shirlaw.   Vet. Rec., 1962, 74, 1417.
3.   Dimock, Edwards, and Bruner.   Ky. Agr. Exp. Sta. Bul. 509, 1947.
4.   McCollum and Doll.   Cornell Vet., 1951, 41, II.
5.   McFadyean and Edwards.   Jour. Comp. Path. and Therap., 1919, 32, 42.
6.   Magnusson.   Svensk. Veterinartijdskr., 1917, p. 81; Jour. Comp. Path. and Therap., 1919, 32, 143.
7.   Maguire.   Vet. Rec., 1958, 70, 989.
8.   Meyer.   Transvaal Dept. of Agr., Rpt. Govt. Bact., 1908–09, p. 122.
9.   Osbaldiston and Walker.   Cornell Vet., 1972, 62, 364.
10.   Wetmore, Thiel, Herman, and Harr.   Jour. Inf. Dis., 1963, 113, 186.

### *Actinobacillus actinoides*

SYNONYMS:   *Bacillus actinoides, Actionomyces actinoides*

This very peculiar organism was found by Smith (3) in cases of calf pneu-monia in 1917. It was described more fully in 1921 (4). It appears that Jones (1), in 1922, found a similar, if not identical, organism in a type of pneumonia commonly seen in old white laboratory rats and that Jones *et al.* (2), in 1964, isolated *A. actinoides* from the genitalia of two bulls affected with seminal vesiculitis.

**Morphology and Staining Reactions.** In tissues this organism usually appears as a slender rod. In cultures it may be bacillary or coccoid. Growing on media containing serum, the organisms usually are embedded in a nonstainable material resembling capsular substance. Long filaments and coccoid elements may be found in such masses. When growing on blood agar, the capsular material is not formed and the organisms appear in the earlier stages as long granular rods. Later the rods disappear and only coccoid elements are seen. The organism is nonmotile and Gram-negative.

**Cultural Features.** This organism is cultivated with difficulty and strains quickly die out. Smith and Jones found coagulated horse serum slants, to which calf serum water had been added, the most suitable medium. When bits of the affected lung tissue were rubbed over the slant and then deposited in the serum water at its base, growth was obtained. The slants had to be sealed airtight with sealing wax and incubation had to be at 37 C. The first evidence of growth was seen as scintillating flakes in the serum water after 3 or 4 days. These gradually enlarged, becoming mulberrylike masses in which crystals were embedded. When these granules were crushed on a slide, magnification showed delicate filaments with clublike bodies not unlike those of *Actinobacillus lignieresi*.

Growth on the surface of the slants does not occur at first, but after several generations of growth some strains develop tiny translucent colonies. Smith did not succeed in obtaining growth in broth, gelatin, milk, or potato.

**Pathogenicity.** Smith felt that his organism was the primary etiological agent in a certain type of pneumonia of calves, and Jones believed his first isolate to be the cause of rat pneumonia. The strains isolated by Jones *et al.* (2) came from two bulls and the authors have stated that two other animals held in the same bull-rearing unit showed similar clinical symptoms of seminal vesiculitis, but did not yield the bacterium on culture.

Smith injected cultures of *A. actinoides* into the trachea of calves and produced circumscribed areas of lung necrosis. When he injected the organism subcutaneously he induced the formation of an indurated lesion that later became necrotic.

In calves the pneumonic process becomes clinically evident when the animals are from 2 to 3 months of age, although it is obvious that the process is slow-moving and begins much earlier. By the time pneumonic symptoms are evident, the lungs usually are filled with abscesses from which pus-forming organisms, especially *Corynebacterium pyogenes,* may be isolated. From such lesions it is impossible to isolate the organism which Smith believed to be the primary pathogenic agent.

**Immunity.** Nothing is known about immunity to this organism.

## REFERENCES

1. Jones.   Jour. Exp. Med., 1922, *35*, 361.
2. Jones, Osborne, and Ashdown.   Vet. Rec., 1964, *76*, 24.
3. Smith.   Jour. Exp. Med., 1918, *28*, 333.
4. *Ibid.*, 1921, *33*, 441.

### *Actinobacillus seminis*

In 1960 Baynes and Simmons (1) described cases of ovine epididymitis in Australia from which they isolated an *Actinobacillus*. Because their isolate differed slightly in cultural chacteristics from *A. lignieresi* they named it *A. seminis*. Four years later Livingston and Hardy (2) found a similar organism in ovine epididymitis in Texas. Since then the disease has been described in rams in South Africa (4), in New Zealand, California, and probably is widespread in its distribution. It is apparent that actinobacilli may cause epididymitis in rams and it is possible that lesions produced by these bacteria have been confused with *Brucella ovis* infection.

**Morphology and Staining Reactions.** *A. seminis* is a pleomorphic Gramnegative, nonmotile, nonsporulating bacillus with individual organisms varying from coccoid forms to rods up to 4 $\mu$ in length.

**Cultural Features.** Sugars are not fermented, indol is not produced, urea or sodium citrate is not split, nitrate is not reduced, and coagulated blood serum is not lysed. Catalase is produced.

**Pathogenicity.** Mice and guinea pigs are resistant to inoculation. The natural disease appears to be limited to rams in which it produces enlarged testes and epididymides with the organism present in the semen.

**Diagnosis.** Isolation of *A. seminis* from the semen is the prescribed procedure. The organism is morphologically and serologically different from *Br. ovis*. Complement-fixation tests have been used, but will not detect all infected rams (3).

**Control.** This is a problem because the exact mode of transmission is not known. The high incidence of disease in unmated rams suggests a method of spread other than by venereal transmission. Ewe-to-ram transmission is possible, but apparently the former does not become infected. The disease is not controlled by removal of infected sheep or the isolation of mated from unmated rams (3).

**Chemotherapy.** According to Baynes and Simmons (1) their organism was sensitive to penicillin, the broad-spectrum antibiotics, sulfonamides, and novobiocin.

## REFERENCES

1. Baynes and Simmons.   Austral. Vet. Jour., 1960, *36*, 454.
2. Livingston and Hardy.   Am. Jour. Vet. Res., 1964, *25*, 660.

3.   Simmons, Baynes, and Ludford.    Austral. Vet. Jour., 1966, *42*, 183.
4.   Worthington and Bosman.    Jour. So. African Vet. Med. Assoc., 1968, 39(2), 81.

### *Actinobacillus (Malleomyces) mallei*

SYNONYMS: *Bacterium mallei, Bacillus mallei, Pfeifferella meallei, Loefflerella mallei, Corynebacterium mallei, Mycobacterium mallei*

A.° *mallei* is the cause of glanders, a disease primarily of solipeds (horses and the horse family). It also affects man and occasionally other kinds of animals, especially members of the cat family which have fed on infected horse meat. The disease is one of the oldest known and was described by the ancient Greeks and Romans. As early as the 17th century it was recognized as contagious, but there were dissenters from this belief as late as the middle of the 19th century. The infectious nature was proved by inoculation tests long before the causative agent was found. The organism was isolated and shown to be the etiological agent by Loeffler and Schütz (12) in 1882.

**Morphology and Staining Reactions.** In young cultures the cells are long, slender rods. Older cultures often are quite pleomorphic, the bacilli varying in size and shape from coccoid elements to long, slender filaments. The longer rods usually are distinctively beaded; the shorter may be bipolar because of granules lying in each end of the cell. The width is from 0.3 to 0.5 micron and the length from 0.7 to 5.0 microns. The cells are always Gram-negative. With the weaker dyes the organism stains rather poorly. Spores are not formed; there are no capsules and no flagella.

**Cultural Features.** A. *mallei* grows well but rather slowly upon ordinary laboratory media. Growth on such media generally is enhanced by the addition of glycerol. The organism is rather insensitive to acidity and will grow well on media that are too acid for most pathogenic bacteria.

After a few days' incubation of 37 C, the surface of glycerol agar slants becomes covered with a confluent growth, slightly cream-colored, smooth, moist, and viscid. Continued incubation causes the blanket of growth to increase in thickness and the color to darken until it is dark brown. It is now so viscid as to make it difficult to remove bits of growth with the inoculating loop. Upon plain agar the growth is much less luxuriant.

Very characteristic is the growth upon glycerol potato. Old potato cultures generally become exceedingly luxuriant, the blanket of growth being slimy and then viscid, light tan in the beginning and a mahogany brown finally.

---

° The proper name for the genus in which the glanders bacillus belongs is a matter of considerable uncertainty. Buchanan in 1916 proposed that it represent the type species of a new genus for which he proposed the name *Pfeifferella*. Inasmuch as Pfeiffer had had nothing to do with the organism, the appropriateness of the name was questioned and this brought from Buchanan the admission that the name was the result of a clerical error and that he had intended to propose the name *Loefflerella* in honor of Loeffler, who had first described it. Because the new generic name, inappropriate as it might be, had been published and therefore was valid, Buchanan, in order to avoid further confusion, did not attempt to correct the error. More recent generic names proposed have been *Loefferella* and *Malleomyces*. The latest is *Actinobacillus*, which appears in *Bergey's Manual*.

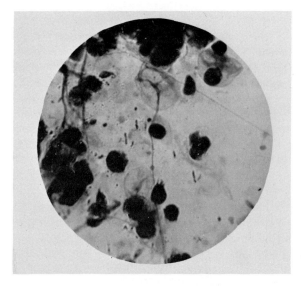

*Fig. 19. Actinobacillus mallei, a film from exudate in the scrotal sac of a guinea pig infected by intraperitoneal inoculation of a pure culture. X 1,000.*

In glycerol broth a viscid sediment forms, and if the cultures are not disturbed a heavy, slimy pellicle forms from which stalactites stretch in the medium toward the bottom of the tube or flask. The broth gradually darkens. Cultures several weeks old become coffee-colored.

The growth on gelatin usually is poor, and ordinarily there is no liquefaction, although some authors have described strains that caused slow liquefaction. Litmus milk is slightly acidified and coagulation may occur after long incubation. Carbohydrates usually are not fermented, but glucose media may be slightly acidified.

Indol is not produced, nitrates are not reduced, and blood is not hemolyzed.

According to Cravitz and Miller (3), strains of A. *mallei* can be separated into at least three serologic groups. Furthermore, a strong relationship exists between the serotypes in one of their groups and *Pseudomonas pseudomallei*. In fact they were unsuccessful in preparing a complement-fixation antigen that would differentiate between the two species.

**Resistance.** The organism possesses only slight powers of resistance to drying, heat, and chemicals. Outside the body it probably cannot, under the most favorable of conditions, exist longer than 2 or 3 months.

**Pathogenicity.** The organism is highly pathogenic for horses, mules, and asses. It is less so for cats (wild and tame), dogs, goats, and man. Sheep, swine, and cattle are highly resistant. Guinea pigs are easily infected artificially, rabbits less easily. The disease occurs almost entirely in the horse species and in carnivora that have consumed infected meat. Man is infected only occasionally when handling animals.

The infection in horses may be either acute or chronic. The latter is by far the more common form. In mules and asses the acute form is more frequent than it is in horses.

The mode of infection is a disputed question; however, it appears probable that ingestion is more important than inhalation. Infection of wounds of the skin occurs, though probably rather rarely. According to the work of Nocard (20) and of McFadyean (15), infection can easily be produced by feeding infected materials. In some cases lesions occur in the mesenteric lymph glands, but many times the lesions appear in the lungs and the mucosa of the upper air passages without evidence of disease processes in the intestine where the infection took place. The intestinal tract therefore probably has a considerable degree of organ immunity. The lungs appear very susceptible, because they are nearly always involved irrespective of the port of entry.

The lung lesions may take the form of nodules or of a diffuse, pneumonic process. The nodules have a characteristic histologic structure by which they may be recognized (4, 15). This structure is not unlike that of a tubercle. Through the rupture of lung nodules into bronchi and the carrying of infective material upward, the upper air passages frequently become the seat of characteristic lesions. Apparently, these lesions can also occur in animals by direct metastasis from the portal of entry, for sometimes well-marked lesions are found in the upper air passages when few or none exist in the lungs. The lesions in the nasal passages begin as submucosal nodules, which quickly rupture forming shallow, craterlike ulcers that exude a thick, sticky purulent material. This is discharged from the nostrils, constituting a highly dangerous exudate.

Glanders nodules may be found in other organs, especially in the liver and spleen. Frequently nodules form under the skin, particularly of the legs. These occur in the lymph channels, the infection localizing here and there and forming chains of nodules connected by indurated cords. The nodules usually break down forming craterlike ulcers that discharge a sticky, honeylike exudate containing the glanders bacillus. This form of glanders is known as *farcy*. Farcy can be a manifestation of local wound infection, but usually it is accompanied by lesions in the internal organs. McFadyean (15), who had much experience with glanders in London, stated, "No case of glanders with lesions elsewhere than in the lungs and with those organs healthy, has ever been recorded."

**Distribution and Mode of Infection.** Infection is contracted in most instances through ingestion, according to McFadyean (15), although it probably can occur through inhalation and through wound infection. Glanders has always, until recently, been the scourge of army horses. From ancient to modern times, wars have always caused the disease to flourish, and the distribution of army animals in civilian service afterward has served to spread the disease far and wide. The American Civil War caused the disease to extend over the eastern parts of the United States. It flourished mostly in the cities, where there were great concentrations of horses in the days of the horsecar and the

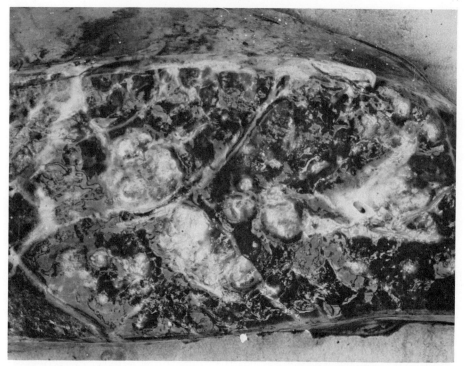

Fig. 20. Lesions of glanders in the lung of a horse. The lung is extensively involved. Not only are there nodules, but the hemorrhages indicate that there is a diffuse involvement with glanderous pneumonia.

great livery and delivery stables, but it was by no means unknown in rural districts. During the early part of the present century, after excellent diagnostic tests had been developed, the disease was rapidly brought under control, and the advent of the motor car and the motor truck, which diminished the horse populations of all cities, helped greatly in stamping out the disease. It has practically been eliminated from the United States and the countries of western Europe. It continued to exist in the Balkan states and in Russia, however, until very recent years and was reintroduced into Germany at the end of World War II by horses returning from those regions.

Infections are contracted mostly from the highly infectious nasal discharges which contaminate the surroundings, especially harnesses, feeding troughs, and the old-fashioned watering troughs. Carnivorous animals usually are infected by the eating of meat of glanderous horses. A number of serious outbreaks have occurred in zoological parks from the practice of feeding horse meat to members of the cat family (10). Human infections occur principally among persons whose work brings them into close association with diseased horses. Infections may also occur through wounds while conducting autopsies

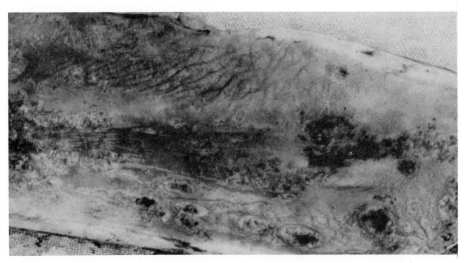

*Fig. 21.* Lesions of glanders in the nasal septum of a horse. Shown are ecchymotic hemor-rhages and the superficial ulcers from which a sticky discharge exudes.

or while handling meat from glanderous animals, but this danger apparently is not so great as was once supposed, because McFadyean (16) reports that cases among the personnel of horse-slaughtering establishments in London which handled thousands of diseased carcasses were very rare. A large num-ber of laboratory infections have been reported, a rather surprising fact in view of the comparatively slight infectivity of glanderous carcasses for man.

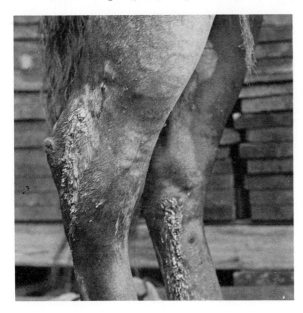

*Fig. 22.* Skin glanders or farcy of the horse.

**Diagnosis of Glanders.** There are a number of ways by which this disease can be definitely diagnosed. The most important of these are:

1. Physical examination and postmortem lesions. Well-developed clinical cases of glanders are generally easily diagnosed by the symptoms, and the lesions are easily recognized at autopsy in the majority of cases. Unfortunately such diagnoses can be made only after the animals are well advanced in the disease and have become dangerous spreaders of the infection.

2. Detection of the organism. *A. mallei* may be readily cultivated from closed lesions on plain or glycerol potato, or upon glycerol agar (preferably acid in reaction). When the lesion is open and other organisms are present, it is surer to inoculate several guinea pigs rather than to depend on cultures. If male guinea pigs are inoculated intraperitoneally with not too great a number of *A. mallei* organisms, a localized peritonitis involving the scrotal sac usually (not always) develops. As a result the scrotal sac becomes enlarged and painful. Usually the process requires several days to reach its height. The testicle itself becomes involved in a short time, and the whole organ is reduced to a mass of caseous pus which will break through the skin and discharge to the surface. This is known as the *Strauss reaction* (6). A similar reaction sometimes occurs owing to other organisms, e.g., *Pseudomonas*, *Corynebacterium*, *Brucella*, and *Actinobacillus* species; thus it is not diagnostic of glanders. If too many glanders organisms are injected, the guinea pig will develop a generalized peritonitis and die in a day or two without showing the scrotal changes. If the injection is made subcutaneously instead of intraperitoneally, an ulcer usually forms at the site of injection and the animal will die after 4 or 5 weeks with nodules in many of the internal organs.

3. Serological tests. (*a*) *Complement fixation*. This test has proved to be the most accurate of the serological methods of diagnosing glanders. It was first applied to the disease by the Germans about 1909 and soon afterward was introduced into this country as a diagnostic procedure by Mohler and Eichhorn (17).

(*b*) *Agglutination*. This was first used by McFadyean (13) in 1896. It is generally admitted to be not so accurate as the previous test. The New York City Health Department (1) reported it as about 84 percent accurate. The failures were in the chronic cases. Normal agglutinins exist in a concentration as high as 1 : 500 in many horses. Infected animals usually react in dilutions of 1 : 1,000 and higher (19).

(*c*) *Precipitation*. This test is performed with the serum of the animal suspected of being glandered and with an extract of the *A. mallei*. In the hands of some the test has been quite successful, although it probably is no more reliable than the agglutination test. A positive precipitation test is definitely indicative of glanders; a negative test does not exclude glanders.

(*d*) *Hemagglutination*. The use of the hemagglutination test has been proposed for the diagnosis of glanders (8). An HA titer above 1:640 is considered to be positive and it was claimed that this test is more sensitive than the mallein test.

4. Mallein tests. Mallein is a product in every way analogous to tuberculin. In the early days it was made by extracting, with glycerolated water, the glanders bacillus which had been grown on potato. Later the crude mallein was produced by growing the organism on glycerol broth. A slimy, slowly developing film appears on the surface, the broth is clouded, and a gummy sediment forms. The medium gradually darkens. After several months' incubation the culture is killed by steaming, and the organisms are removed by filtration. The filtrate constitutes the crude mallein. For special purposes this mallein is concentrated by evaporation, or is precipitated by alcohol in the form of a white powder.

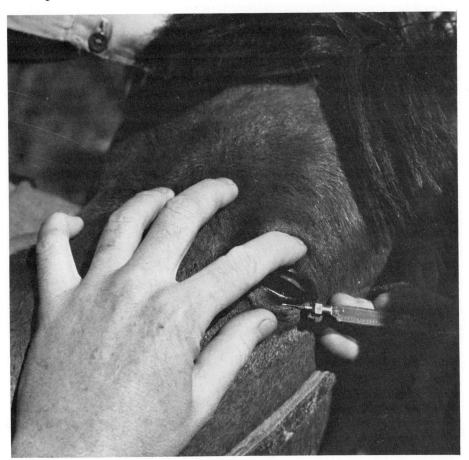

*Fig. 23.* Injection of mallein in the intrapalpebral test for the detection of glanders. (Courtesy Col. W. E. Jennings, Veterinary Corps, U.S. Army.)

Mallein, for normal animals, is an inert or, at the most, only a slightly toxic substance. Animals affected with glanders, however, are hypersensitive to it, and symptoms of intoxication occur when it is injected into them. It is, accordingly, a valuable diagnostic agent. Mallein has been used by some for treating glanders. The value as a curative agent is doubtful.

Mallein is used in three ways: (a) subcutaneous test, (b) ophthalmic test, (c) intrapalpebral test. When injected subcutaneously it gives rise to fever, which appears and subsides again within 24 hours after the injection. There is usually a marked swelling at the point of injection. Normal horses may show some swelling at this point, but the temperature curve is absent. The ophthalmic test consists of instilling some concentrated mallein into the eye (conjunctival sac). A pus-forming inflammation of the eye occurs within a few hours when the animal is glanderous. The intrapalpebral test consists of injecting a small amount of concentrated mallein into the skin of the lower eyelid. A local swelling and a pus-forming inflammation of the eye occur. The intrapalpebral test is more accurate than the ophthalmic and accordingly is more often used.

**Immunity.** It has been generally believed that animals never recover from glanders. Recovery certainly is not usual, but there have been many reports of horses which, after showing symptoms of the disease and after reacting to diagnostic tests, have made clinical recoveries and have become negative to the laboratory tests. It appears, then, that recoveries do occur (14).

Many attempts have been made to protect animals against glanders by the use of a variety of biological products, but not one has proved successful (18).

**Control Measures.** Control of the disease has been accomplished wholly by methods which involve early diagnosis and elimination of the reacting animals. Clinical examinations at frequent intervals, the use of mallein and the serological tests, and the destruction of animals that give evidence of infection by any of these tests have proved adequate. These methods have practically eliminated the disease from the United States and from many European countries. It should be noted that serologic tests are not entirely reliable in diagnosing glanders in areas where melioidosis also exists because of the common somatic antigens possessed by the causative organism (3).

**Glanders in Man.** Man is not highly susceptible to glanders; yet numerous infections have occurred in persons caring for glanderous animals, especially stablemen and veterinarians (2). The disease is characterized by swelling and pain at the point of infection (usually the hand, the lip, or the eye), which comes on in from 3 to 5 days, swelling of the neighboring lymph glands, development of nasal and mouth ulcers (in about half the cases), development of abscesses and pustules in the skin, joint inflammations, and general symptoms accompanied by fever. The cases usually end fatally in from 2 to 4 weeks. A few cases of glanders in man occurred in Russia during World War I. Chronic glanders in man has been vividly described by Gaiger (7), a British veterinarian who contracted the disease in India.

**Chemotherapy.** According to Howe and Miller (11), the sulfonamides are quite effective in treating glanders in man and in laboratory animals. Tyrothricin, streptomycin, chloromycetin, and aureomycin are effective *in vitro* but are ineffective in treating infected guinea pigs (9).

## REFERENCES

1. Anthony and Grund. Collected Studies from the Bureau of Laboratories, Dept. of Health, City of New York, 1912–13, 7, 291.
2. Coleman and Ewing. Jour. Med. Res., 1903, 4, 223.
3. Cravitz and Miller. Jour. Inf. Dis., 1950, 86, 46 and 52.
4. Duval and White. Jour. Exp. Med., 1907, 9, 352.
5. Fletcher. A system of bacteriology in relation to medicine. Med. Res. Council (Brit.), 1929, vol. V, p. 56.
6. Frothingham. Jour. Med. Res., 1901, 1, 331.
7. Gaiger. Jour. Comp. Path. and Therap., 1913, 26, 233; 1916, 29, 26.
8. Gangulee, Sen, and Sharma. Indian Vet. Jour., 1966, 43, 386.
9. Giolitti. Arch. Vet. Ital., 1951, 2, 15.
10. Hart. Jour. Am. Vet. Med. Assoc., 1916, 49, 659.
11. Howe and Miller. Ann. Int. Med., 1947, 26, 93.
12. Loeffler and Schütz. Deut. med. Wchnschr., 1882, 8, 707.
13. McFadyean. Jour. Comp. Path. and Therap., 1896, 9, 322.
14. *Ibid.*, 1900, 13, 55.
15. *Ibid.*, 1904, 17, 295.
16. *Ibid.*, 1905, 18, 23.
17. Mohler and Eichhorn. U.S. Dept. Agr., Bur. Anim. Indus. Bul. 136, 1911.
18. Mohler and Eichhorn. Proc. Am. Vet. Med. Assoc., 1913, p. 650.
19. Moore and Taylor. Jour. Inf. Dis., 1907, Sup. 3, 85.
20. Nocard. Bul. Soc. Cent. Med. Vet., 1894, 48, 225 and 367.

## THE GENUS *MORAXELLA*

Within the genus are small, short, rod-shaped cells which occur usually as diplobacilli. They are nonmotile, Gram-negative, and do not require factors V or X (see p. 232) for growth, but the addition of serum or ascitic fluid certainly stimulates them. Usually they do not attack carbohydrates, but they are actively proteolytic, oxidase-positive, and aerobic. *Bergey's Manual* lists three species; *M. lacunata*, *M. liquefaciens*, and *M. bovis*, with the first one designated the type species. *M. bovis* is our main concern because of its presence in pinkeye of cattle. A brief description of this species follows.

### *Moraxella (Hemophilus) bovis*

This organism, called *Hemophilus bovis*, has been isolated on numerous occasions from infectious keratitis or pinkeye of cattle, in which the primary lesions are confined to the cornea and conjunctiva. Because the characteristics of the organism do not fit those of the genus *Hemophilus* in that it predominantly occurs as a diplobacillus instead of in single forms, liquefies coagulated blood serum, does not reduce nitrates, and is less fastidious in its growth requirements, it now is listed in *Bergey's Manual* with other similar types in the genus *Moraxella*. Allen (1), Little and Jones (11), and Baldwin (2) have indicated that this microorganism is the cause of infectious keratitis of cattle, but Farley, Kliewer, Pearson, and Foote (5) state that *M. bovis* has not definitely been established as the cause of the disease even though it usually is present in acute cases. Inability to agree on the role of *M. bovis* in infectious keratitis may be due to lack of uniformity in the types studied. It is possible that the differences may be accounted for by bacterial variation. Jackson's (10) findings seem to support this theory. He has stated that *M. bovis* is the specific cause of infectious keratoconjunctivitis of cattle in Texas; that it is very exacting in its growth requirements on primary isolation and must have both the X and V factors for maximum growth; and that it is not stable, but dissociates readily from the smooth virulent type to a rough aviru- lent form. In 1961 Henson and Grumbles (6) demonstrated a labile hemolytic toxin in *M. bovis* cultures and a thermostable dermonecrotic toxin (endo- toxin) in the cell wall of the organism. They claim that they were able to pro- duce clinical infectious bovine keratoconjunctivitis by injecting their cultures intracorneally into rabbits and calves. Pugh *et al.* (12) indicated that sheep and mice develop keratoconjunctivitis when exposed to *M. bovis* by conjunc- tival instillation. Hughes *et al.* (9) found that a mercury sunlamp enhances the effect of *M. bovis* infection of the bovine eye. They concluded that ultra- violet radiation has a primary etiologic role in the disease. This was sup- ported by Hubbert and Hermann (7) who stated that a winter epizootic of infectious bovine keratoconjunctivitis (IBK) was caused by *M. bovis* com- bined with the effects of increased ultraviolet radiation of the cornea as a re- sult of reflection from fresh snow. Pugh *et al.* (13) have also claimed that infectious bovine rhinotracheitis virus, although not a primary etiologic agent of IBK, has the ability to increase the pathogenic effects of *M. bovis* by creat- ing a more suitable environment for the organism.

Infectious keratitis is a common ailment of cattle, especially in the range country of the western states, where it causes much damage. It is seen most often in Hereford cattle in hot, dusty periods of the year. Beginning with pho- tophobia and simple conjunctivitis, the inflammation later becomes purulent. Opacity of the cornea of the affected eyes usually develops, and frequently the inflammatory process invades the orbit and permanent blindness ensues. In the purulent discharge various pyogenic organisms may be found, particu- larly *Corynebacterium pyogenes*. These are, most likely, purely secondary in- vaders. The primary infecting agent is believed to be transmitted by direct contact, by flies, and possibly by infected dust. The disease often becomes ep- izootic, with thousands of animals becoming infected. Obviously further work on the etiology of this disease is needed.

A nonhemolytic diplobacillus, closely resembling *M. bovis*, has been iso- lated from the eyes of horses which had signs of conjunctivitis and erosion of their eyelid margins (8). Experimentally it could be established in equine, but not in bovine eyes.

**Chemotherapy.** The broad-spectrum antibiotics are effective in treating pink-eye in cattle. Scott (15) claims that cortisone acetate used in conjunction with antibiotic powder produces rapid recoveries with minimal scarring of the cornea. Ellis and Barnes (4) recommended the use of tylosin tartrate solution at a concentration of 50 mg per ml and Cooper (3) finds 0.5 percent ethidium bromide eye ointment to be efficacious. Schrimsher (14) used a combination of methylprednisolone, penicillin, and dihydrostreptomycin in the treatment of pinkeye in cattle and in nonspecific keratitis in horses and claimed that in each case only one application was required.

## REFERENCES

1. Allen.   Jour. Am. Vet. Med. Assoc., 1918, *54*, 307.
2. Baldwin.   Am. Jour. Vet. Res., 1945, *6*, 180.
3. Cooper.   Vet. Rec., 1960, *72*, 589.
4. Ellis and Barnes.   Vet. Med., 1961, *56*, 197.
5. Farley, Kliewer, Pearson, and Foote.   Am. Jour. Vet. Res., 1950, *11*, 17.
6. Henson and Grumbles.   Cornell Vet., 1961, *51*, 267.
7. Hubbert and Hermann.   Jour. Am. Vet. Med. Assoc., 1970, *157*, 452.
8. Hughes and Pugh.   Am. Jour. Vet. Res., 1970, *31*, 457.
9. Hughes, Pugh, and McDonald.   *Ibid.*, 1965, *26*, 1331.
10. Jackson.   *Ibid.*, 1953, *14*, 19.
11. Little and Jones.   Jour. Exp. Med., 1923, 38, 139; 1924, 39, 803.
12. Pugh, Hughes, and McDonald.   Am. Jour. Vet. Res., 1968, *29*, 2057.
13. Pugh, Hughes, and Packer.   *Ibid.*, 1970, *31*, 653.
14. Schrimsher.   Vet. Med., 1970, *65*, 169.
15. Scott.   Jour. Am. Vet. Med. Assoc., 1957, *130*, 257.

## THE GENERA *MIMA* AND *HERELLEA*

Mitchell and Burrell (4) have indicated that the *Mima, Herellea*, and *Moraxella* organisms are all related if not identical. *Mima polymorpha* and *Herellea vaginicola* are recognized species, but do not appear in the seventh edition of *Bergey's Manual*. Both are Gram-negative, aerobic, nonmotile pleomorphic diplococci. They are catalase-positive, oxidase-negative, and do not reduce nitrates. *M. polymorpha* does not ferment glucose. It is citrate-negative. *H. vaginicola* produces acid but no gas from glucose. It utilizes citrate.

Both *Mima* and *Herellea* bacteria have been found in the normal vagina, in cases of conjunctivitis, in cases of mimal endocarditis (5), and on the skin of normal human males (6). They are found frequently in clinical specimens from various animals, including the blood of sick dogs and the stomach contents of equine and bovine fetuses (1).

In 1960, Lindqvist (2) isolated a hemolytic species, that most likely belonged in the *Moraxella-Mima-Herellea* group, from sheep suffering from infectious keratoconjunctivitis. In 1965, Livingston *et al.* (3) isolated an agent from ovine pinkeye which they grew in cell culture and used to reproduce the disease. They claimed that Gram-negative cocci isolated from infected eyes did not produce signs of disease or enhance the virulence of their agent.

It is claimed that mimae organisms frequently are resistant to penicillin and streptomycin.

### REFERENCES

1.  Carter, Isoun, and Keahey.   Jour. Am. Vet. Med. Assoc., 1970, *156*, 1313.
2.  Lindqvist.   Jour. Inf. Dis., 1960, *106*, 162.
3.  Livingston, Moore, and Hardy.   Am. Jour. Vet. Res., 1965, *26*, 295.
4.  Mitchell and Burrell.   Bact. Proc., 1963, p. 64.
5.  Shea and Phillips.   Am. Jour. Med. Sci., 1966, *252*, 201.
6.  Taplin, Rebell, and Zaias.   Jour. Am. Med. Assoc., 1963, *186*, 952.

# XV | The *Bacteroidaceae*

Our knowledge of the nonsporebearing obligate anaerobes is fragmentary, and their classification is confused and certain to be changed as more information about them is acquired. A number of anaerobic streptococci have been described, usually from disease processes. The organism of true actinomycosis of cattle and man is at least partially anaerobic. Many spirochetes are anaerobic and nonsporebearing. Gram-negative, nonsporebearing bacteria are present in the intestinal tracts and mucous membranes of many warmblooded animals, particularly the herbivora. Omnivora are sometimes affected; carnivora seldom or never. They are normally strict anaerobes, but occasionally microaerophilic species occur. Some are pathogenic. Such organisms are now classified in the family *Bacteroidaceae* and five genera are listed.

Genus 1. *Bacteroides*—Found in the alimentary and urogenital tracts of man and other animals; some species are pathogenic.

Genus 2. *Fusobacterium*—Found in the buccal cavity and in various infections in man.

Genus 3. *Dialister*—Found, associated with influenza, in the respiratory tract of man.

Genus 4. *Spherophorus*—Found in the alimentary and urogenital tracts of man and other animals; also in various necrotic lesions.

Genus 5. *Streptobacillus*—Commonly found as an inhabitant of the nasopharynx of rats. Parasitic to pathogenic for rats, mice, man, and other animals.

The genus *Spherophorus* is the one most often involved in infections of domestic animals and is considered in detail. Others discussed are *Streptobacillus* and *Fusiformis*. The latter is not listed in the seventh edition of *Bergey's Manual*, but it is the generic name applied to an organism that is concerned in foot-rot in sheep, and for want of a better designation we shall employ it here. We mention *Bacteroides melaninogenicus* because of its relatively high incidence in cats where it is typically associated with purulent processes and occurs almost invariably in association with other organisms. Its presence in suppurative conditions in cats and other domestic animals suggests, at least, a contributory role in pathogenesis (4).

In 1959 Peckham (22) isolated an anaerobe from the blood and livers of quail and from the livers of chickens that were suffering from ulcerative enteritis (*quail disease*). Transmission experiments indicated that his isolate may be the cause of the disease. Its classification was not established.

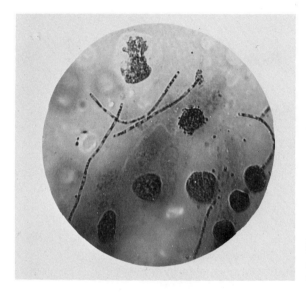

Fig. 24. Spherophorus necrophorus in a lung abscess in a calf. The long filaments with irregular distribution of chromatic material are characteristic. X 1,000.

*Tyzzer's disease* was described in 1917. It has been reported in mice, rats, rabbits, monkeys, and gerbils. Characteristic lesions occur in the large intestines accompanied by focal necrosis of the liver. Diarrhea, weakness, and death are frequently seen in infected animals. There are similarities among Tyzzer's disease of laboratory animals, Errington's disease of muskrats, spontaneous ileitis of rats, and ulcerative enteritis of quail and chickens (31). The causative agent is believed to be a bacterium that has been called *Bacillus piliformis*, *Actinobacillus piliformis*, and *Fusiformis piliformis*. Swellings that occur on the bacillus appear to be spores and it is possible that it may belong in the family *Bacillaceae* rather than in the *Bacteroidaceae*.

### Spherophorus necrophorus

SYNONYMS:   *Bacillus diphtheriae vitulorum, Streptothrix cuniculi, Corynebacterium necrophorum, Cladothrix cuniculi, Bacterium necrophorum, Actinomyces necrophorus, Fusiformis necrophorus,* calf diphtheria bacillus, necrosis bacillus.

This organism is found in necrotic lesions in warm-blooded animals. It produces the diseases commonly known under the collective name of *necrobacilloses*.

**Morphology and Staining Reactions.** In infected tissues this organism is ordinarily seen in the form of long filaments, but shorter elements and even coccoid forms occur. The rods are about 1 micron in width and may be in excess of 100 microns in length. In some cultures swollen rods are seen which may be nearly twice as thick as the usual forms. Freshly isolated strains growing in cooked-meat medium usually show a predominance of long filaments. The sides of these filaments are parallel and regular, and are either straight or form-sweeping curves. After prolonged artificial culture the predominating forms usually are short. Very young cultures stain uniformly as a rule, but the filaments in cultures older than 24 hours usually are vacuolated, that is, the stained portions are separated by sections that are almost or quite free of stain. The irregular distribution of cytoplasm along the filaments can easily be seen in unstained preparations. Some early authors have described branching, but most of those who have studied this organism agree that it does not branch. Flagella have not been demonstrated and motility is absent. Ordinary dyes stain young cultures readily. The organism is always Gram-negative.

**Cultural Features.** The necrosis bacillus is very sensitive to oxygen and under usual procedures growth does not occur unless good anaerobic conditions are obtained (12). Beveridge (2) claims, however, that growth occurs readily when the organism is placed in association with staphylococci, and that surface colonies on solid media which are well started anaerobically will continue to increase in size when incubated aerobically. It is difficult to obtain primary growths on solid media incubated in anaerobic jars because exposure to air damages the cells so that they frequently will not grow, the damage occurring before anaerobic conditions are established.

Growth in ordinary media is poor and frequently fails entirely. Plain agar, gelatin, and broth, for instance, are not suitable media for this organism. When enriched with serum or blood, they become suitable, but cultures quickly die out. Growth in litmus milk usually fails unless peptone or serum is added. Cooked-meat or liver-brain medium are very favorable and are recommended for isolations. Thioglycollate medium, without enrichment, works well in maintaining stock cultures. Even in these media cultures die out in most cases within 1 or 2 weeks, although occasionally a strain will remain viable for several months. Tunnicliff (30) reports that a liver-brain medium to which calcium carbonate is added will retain viability for a year or more. Under favorable conditions acid and gas are formed from glucose, lactose, sucrose, maltose, and salicin. The amount of acid formed is not great and gas formation is limited. In cooked-meat medium covered with a vaspar seal (petrolatum and paraffin in equal parts), a large bubble of gas is regularly formed. Hemolysis of horse blood occurs. Serum gelatin is not liquefied and coagulated serum is not digested. In clear, solid media, colonies are fuzzy when the medium is fairly soft and dense when it is more solid. Serologic studies have indicated that there are a number of types within the species (Walker and Dack, 32).

**Natural Habitat.** This organism has been found in the cecum of apparently normal swine (1), and it exists in the alimentary canals of other species of animals. Infections in animals generally occur when they are kept in filthy surroundings, especially when there are accumulations of manure under foot. It does not seem likely that the organism could multiply outside the body, but it undoubtedly remains viable in soil for short periods of time. Marsh and Tunnicliff (18) were able to demonstrate the organism in a wet pasture 10 months after sheep affected with foot-rot had run on it, but they could not demonstrate it after a second 10-month period. Under these conditions, which apparently were unusually favorable, the organism was able to survive through one winter in the rigorous climate of Montana.

**Pathogenicity.** *For experimental animals.* Progressive disease is produced in rabbits and white mice by subcutaneous injection of pure cultures. Guinea pigs are more resistant, but local lesions may develop. The rabbit is the most satisfactory animal for diagnostic use. If the material injected is contaminated with many other bacteria, as it is when taken from an intestinal ulcer, for example, it is best to introduce a bit of dry material from the depths of the lesions into a small subcutaneous pocket, rather than to inject it ground up and suspended in a fluid. Injection with considerable fluid seems to favor the contaminating organisms, whereas the necrosis bacillus thrives better when it is not unduly exposed to air, as in grinding, and the dryness seems to retard the other pathogens present. At the point of inoculation a spreading subcutaneous necrosis occurs, and the rabbit rapidly loses weight. It usually dies in from 4 to 7 days in a greatly emaciated condition. The autopsy examination in these cases commonly reveals no lesions in the internal organs. Extending for a considerable distance from the inoculation point, a pasty, whitish, necrotic material is seen. At its lower points there usually is considerable edema. Bits of this material smeared on slides and stained with dilute fuchsin generally show many filamentous forms, mixed with any other organisms that may have been present in the inoculum. Pure cultures can seldom be obtained from the local lesions when badly contaminated material has been used for inoculation, but, if cultures are made from the heart blood, liver, spleen, and kidneys in cooked-meat medium, quite often one or two of the cultures will prove to be pure. Some strains are less virulent for rabbits, and the animals may live for 2 weeks or longer. In these cases, necrotic areas usually are found in some of the internal organs and in the heart muscle, the lungs, liver, or kidneys, and pure cultures are readily obtained from them. Intravenous inoculation of cultures usually kills in from a few days to 2 or 3 weeks, depending upon the dosage and the virulence of the strain. Multiple necrotic areas are then found in the internal organs. Sometimes a fibrinous pleuritis or pericarditis is found. Inflammation of one or more joints is observed occasionally.

Intraportal injection of S. *necrophorus* into 33 cattle, 20 sheep, and 6 swine produced liver abscesses in 70 percent of the cattle and in 90 percent of the sheep. No abscesses were produced in the swine (Jensen *et al.*, 15).

*Natural infections.* S. *necrophorus* is found in association with a wide variety of lesions in horses, cattle, sheep, swine, and some birds. It has been found also in many wild animals such as reindeer, antelopes, buffaloes, monkeys, and even in several species of cold-blooded animals. It has been reported a number of times in man but there is some question about the identity of the human cultures and the necrosis bacillus of animals. Carnivorous animals appear to be highly resistant.

The role of this organism in many of the pathological processes with which it is associated, and of which it has been regarded in the past as the etiological agent, is not clear. At one time this organism was believed to be the cause of necrotic enteritis of swine, but Murray, Biester, Purwin, and McNutt (21) have demonstrated that S. *necrophorus,* although practically always present in the lesions, is not capable alone of producing the disease, which can be reproduced regularly by feeding cultures of *Salmonella cholerasuis.* In the experimentally induced cases the typical ulcers were produced and S. *necrophorus* was present in them, proving that the latter existed in the intestine as a saprophyte and took part in the ulcerating process only when another organism had initiated it. S. *necrophorus* has long been regarded as the causative agent of foot-rot in sheep, a contagious disease causing heavy losses in some sheep-raising countries. Beveridge (3) working in Australia has challenged this idea and has brought forth convincing evidence that the necrosis bacillus is not the primary agent. It has long been known that S. *necrophorus* often appears in the ulcers following the rupture of the vesicles of foot-and-mouth disease in cattle and of contagious ecthyma of sheep. The evidence indicates that this organism has little or no ability to invade normal mucous membranes or the skin but that it frequently thrives in wounds of the surfaces produced by mechanical injury or bacterial action. On the other hand, such lesions as the characteristic liver abscesses of cattle usually present pure cultures of S. *necrophorus,* and the organism may be seen in numbers at the margins of the necrotic areas; hence it can hardly be looked upon as a purely saprophytic type. The studies of Smith (29) indicate that there is a definite relationship between ulcers of the rumen and abscesses of the liver in beef cattle.

Necrobacillosis of horses usually takes the form of a gangrenous dermatitis of the feet and lower parts of the legs and occasionally as a necrotic pneumonia.

In cattle the lesions may be found in various parts. The common "foot-rot" or "fouls" has been thought to be caused by it, but experimentally cultures of the organism will not reproduce the disease (11). Infection of the mouth and pharynx of calves (calf diptheria) is an especially malignant form of the disease. Lesions are often found in the liver as firm, dry, sharply circumscribed areas of a light-yellow color, and sometimes as well-encapsulated abscesses.

In the latter instances, other bacteria as well as the necrosis bacillus usually are present; in the former type, it is generally present in pure culture. In calf diphtheria necrobacillosis of the brain sometimes occurs. Recently, Prchal (23) reported a cerebral abscess in a heifer caused by S. *necrophorus*. Lesions frequently appear on the skin, especially of the udder and teats of cattle. Uterine infections are not uncommon, and ulceration of the mucosa of the abomasum is often ascribed to this bacillus. The organism has been encountered in bovine mastitis (28) and in rumenitis of calves reared on an early-weaning feeding system (20).

In sheep S. *necrophorus* has been associated with the diseases known as *lip and leg ulceration* and *foot-rot*. The disease labeled *infective bulbar necrosis* (heel-abscess) of sheep, which occurs most often in the hind feet of ewes lambing under cool wet conditions, is attributed by Roberts *et al.* (24) to the penetration of the interdigital dermis and digital cushion by S. *necrophorus* and the proliferation of *Corynebacterium pyogenes* in the resulting necrotic mass.

In swine it appears to be involved in producing the common disease known as *ulcerative stomatitis* (sore mouth) and the condition known as *bullnose,* in which there is an infection of the subcutaneous tissues of the face, frequently originating in the wound made by the placing of a ring in the nose. It is also associated with necrosis of the epithelium and deeper structures of the intestines, a condition known as *necrotic enteritis.*

The organism also has been reported as a secondary invader in the virus disease of chickens known as *avian diphtheria* (fowlpox). Emmel (7) reported the occurrence of S. *necrophorus* infection in a flock of 400 six-week-old chickens. Lesions were located on various parts of the head. About 5 percent of the birds were involved.

Internal lesions caused by pure infections with this organism usually are firm, yellowish-white, tumorlike nodules consisting of tissues that have undergone caseation necrosis. The cut surface is dry and very firm. Around the younger lesions there may be inflammatory zones. In sections made of these lesions the specific organisms frequently can be seen as long filaments lying in parallel bundles and radiating outward from the center. They are practically never encapsulated. The organisms cannot always be demonstrated microscopically in the older lesions but cultures usually succeed. When the infection occurs on the surface of the skin or mucous membranes, the lesions are characterized by dry whitish patches, consisting of necrotic material, which extend deep into the underlying tissues. Usually a foul odor is present. Often abscesses are found in the internal organs, in which the necrosis bacillus is associated with other bacteria. In these instances the pus may be fluid or thick, but always malodorous. Such lesions usually have a thick fibrous capsule around them.

**Toxin Formation.** The fact that rabbits usually die after great emaciation when the only lesion is a comparatively small subcutaneous area of necrosis has led most workers to conclude that this organism produces an exotoxin. Filtrates of cultures, however, exhibit very little toxicity. A mild inflammatory lesion may be produced in rabbits by subcutaneous injection of filtrates, and it appears that the poisonous property is endotoxic in nature. That endotoxins exist in the bacilli cannot be doubted, because heat-killed cells will cause inflammation and necrosis when injected intradermally into rabbits. The endotoxic substance is strongly heat-stable.

**Immunity.** All attempts to produce immunity to this organism have failed. Cultures killed by heat, phenol, or formalin may prolong the life of treated rabbits for a day or two, but doses of cultures that kill the controls will also kill the treated animals. Antibodies in low titer may be produced by injecting repeated doses of killed culture. According to Feldman, Hester, and Wherry (9), there is no evidence to indicate that different animal species suffer from distinct strains of this organism. These workers found that agglutinins were present for S. *necrophorus* in the blood serum of a large percentage of normal-appearing horses, cattle, sheep, and swine, but that they were absent from the sera of calves, lambs, rabbits, and human beings. They conclude that the agglutination test for the detection of obscure lesions of necrobacillosis in mature horses, cattle, sheep, and swine is useless.

**Chemotherapy.** Reports on the use of the sulfonamides in the treatment of the necrobacilloses have indicated that certain members of this group of drugs are quite effective in treating these infections. Farquharson (8) reported marked success in treating calf diphtheria with sulfapyridine, and Hayes and Wright (14) found sulfamethazine to be exceptionally effective in treating an outbreak of this infection in 2,785 calves and feeder cattle. Forman (10) reported that sulfapyridine is specific for all types of foot-rot in cattle, and Lebovit (16) showed that sulfathiazole injected intravenously produced very satisfactory results when used early in the course of the disease or in chronic cases. Roberts, Kiesel, and Lewis (25) in a report on the results obtained in a small controlled experiment on foot-rot in cattle concluded that this disease is self-limiting and that about 80 percent of the infected animals will recover if no treatment except rest is given. They did not believe that sulfonamide therapy was as useful in this disease as others had claimed. Leventhal and Easterbrooks (17) treated foot-rot in cattle with a combination of a multiple enzyme preparation. (streptokinase, streptodornase, and human plasminogen) and tetracycline. They claimed marked success. Aureomycin has been recommended as effective in preventing the formation of liver abscesses in cattle (19).

**Human Infections.** A number of cases of human infections ascribed to the necrosis bacillus have appeared in the literature. The earlier reports dealt with local infections some of which were in persons working with the animal disease (Schmorl, 26). Later ones were cases of purulent pneumonia (27), deep-spreading abscesses (5), ulcerative colitis (6), and infections of the uterus (13). The cultural features of the organisms indicate that they are closely related to, if not identical with, S. *necrophorus*.

## REFERENCES

1. Bang.   Abstract, Centrbl. f. Bakt., 1893, *13*, 201.
2. Beveridge.   Jour. Path. and Bact., 1934, *38*, 467.
3. Beveridge.   Austral. Council Sci. and Indus. Res. Bul. 140, 1941.
4. Biberstein, Knight, and England.   Jour. Am. Vet. Med. Assoc., 1968, *153*, 1045.
5. Cunningham.   Arch. Path., 1930, 9, 843.
6. Dack, Heinz, and Dragstedt.   Arch. Surg., 1935, *31*, 225.
7. Emmel.   Jour. Am. Vet. Med. Assoc., 1948, *113*, 169.
8. Farquharson.   *Ibid.*, 1942, *101*, 88.
9. Feldman, Hester, and Wherry.   Jour. Inf. Dis., 1936, *59*, 159.
10. Foreman.   Jour. Am. Vet. Med. Assoc., 1946, *109*, 126.
11. Gupta, Fincher, and Bruner.   Cornell Vet., 1964, *54*, 66.
12. Hagan.   Jour. Inf. Dis., 1924, *35*, 390.
13. Harris and Brown.   Johns Hopkins Hosp. Bul., 1927, *40*, 203.
14. Hayes and Wright.   Jour. Am. Vet. Med. Assoc., 1949, *114*, 80.
15. Jensen, Flint, and Griner.   Am. Jour. Vet. Res., 1954, *15*, 5.
16. Lebovit.   Jour. Am. Vet. Med. Assoc., 1948, *112*, 453.
17. Leventhal and Easterbrooks.   *Ibid.*, 1956, *129*, 422.
18. Marsh and Tunnicliff.   Mont. Agr. Exp. Sta. Bul. 285, 1934.
19. Matsushima, Dowe, and Adams.   Proc. Soc. Exp. Biol. and Med., 1954, *85*, 18.
20. Mullen.   Vet. Rec., 1970, *86*, 587.
21. Murray, Biester, Purwin, and McNutt.   Jour. Am. Vet. Med. Assoc., 1927, 72, 34; 1928, 72, 1003.
22. Peckham.   Avian Dis., 1959, *3*, 471.
23. Prchal.   Jour. Am. Vet. Med. Assoc., 1956, *128*, 79.
24. Roberts, Graham, and Egerton.   Jour. Comp. Path., 1968, *78*, 1.
25. Roberts, Kiesel, and Lewis.   Cornell Vet., 1948, 38, 122.
26. Schmorl.   Deut. Zeitschr. f. Tiermed., 1891, *18*, 375.
27. Shaw and Bigger.   Jour. Am. Med. Assoc., 1934, *102*, 688.
28. Simon and McCoy.   Jour. Am. Vet. Med. Assoc., 1958, *133*, 165.
29. Smith.   Am. Jour. Vet. Res., 1944, 5, 234.
30. Tunnicliff.   Jour. Inf. Dis., 1938, *63*, 113.
31. Van Kruiningen and Blodgett.   Jour. Am. Vet. Med. Assoc., 1971, *158*, 1205.
32. Walker and Dack.   *Ibid.*, 1939, *65*, 285.

## *Fusiformis nodosus*

SYNONYM: *Actinomyces nodosus*

This organism was described by Beveridge (2) in 1941. He regards it as the cause of foot-rot in sheep. The work was done in Australia but he also examined material in the United States and found that the conditions in the two countries were the same. The organisms isolated in Australia were serologically related to a strain isolated in the United States.

According to Beveridge, two organisms usually predominate over all others in cases of foot-rot. One is a spiral organism that had previously been found

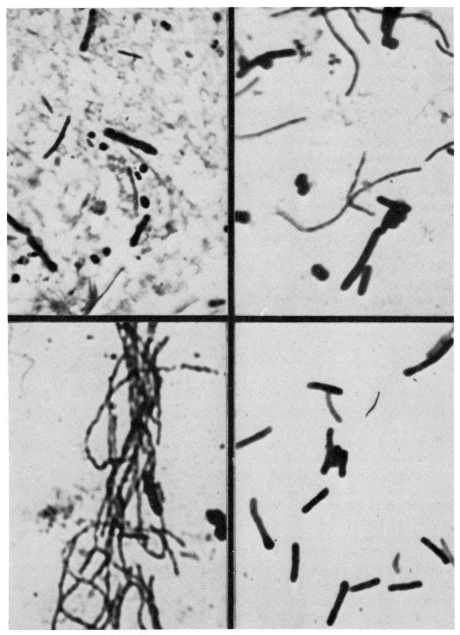

Fig. 25. (*Upper left*) *Fusiformis nodosus* in a smear from a foot-rot lesion. Carbol fuchsin. X 2,600 (*Upper right*) Spirochetelike organism in a smear from a foot-rot lesion. Krajian silver stain. X 2,500. (*Lower left*) Mass of spirochetelike organisms in a smear from a foot-rot lesion. Krajian silver stain. X 2,500. (*Lower right*) *Fusiformis nodosus* from a 3-day-old colony on agar. Carbol fuchsin. X 2,500. (Courtesy H. Marsh and K. D. Claus, *Cornell Vet.*)

and described by him in 1936 (1) and the other is a motile, fusiform bacillus. Both of these organisms were obtained in pure culture, and with them attempts were made to reproduce the disease by introducing them into scarified areas on the feet of sheep. Foot-rot was not produced in this way. Less abundant in the foot-rot lesions but usually present was *Spherophorus necrophorus*. Many attempts to produce foot-rot with this organism also failed. Rather scarce in stained films of the lesions was a fourth organism, a large, Gram-negative, nonmotile bacillus with clubbed ends. With pure cultures of this organism rather mild cases of foot rot were produced by inoculation. Typical foot-rot was readily produced when animals were inoculated with the large nonmotile bacillus and the spirochete. The nonmotile bacillus (*Fusiformis nodosus*) therefore is regarded as the primary cause of the disease with the spirochete (*Spirocheta penortha*) an accessory factor. The role of the motile, fusiform bacillus in the lesions is not clearly understood.

**Morphology and Staining Reactions.** The organism is a large, rod-shaped bacterium characterized by the presence of terminal enlargements, usually at both ends. These enlargements are more pronounced in organisms seen in tissue smears than in those developing in culture. The rods usually are straight but may be slightly curved. They are from 0.6 to 0.8 microns in diameter and from 3 to 10 microns in length, although few are more than 6 microns long. In cultures the organisms tend to be shorter and in old cultures they may even be coccoid in form. They are nonmotile and do not form spores or capsules. They stain readily with all ordinary dyes. They are Gram-negative and non-acid-fast. Organisms stained with methylene blue often show one or several metachromatic granules, usually located at the ends of the rod.

**Cultural Features.** The organism is an obligate anaerobe. Growth is enhanced when 5 percent or more of carbon dioxide is introduced into the anaerobic culture jar. Growth occurs best at 37 C. At room temperature very slow growth occurs. Cultures grow best in neutral or alkaline media.

Practically no growth is obtained on any of the ordinary media unless horse serum is added to them in a proportion of 10 percent. Not all lots of horse serum prove satisfactory, and sheep serum not only failed to promote growth but actually inhibited it in the presence of horse serum. Rabbit and cow serum were not satisfactory.

Best growth was obtained on "V-F" agar, which is a peptic digest of beef muscle and liver. Veal infusion media were not very favorable even when horse serum had been added. Growth did not occur on inspissated horse serum or egg medium. Growth was never luxuriant in any fluid media, and ordinary types even with serum added often failed to promote growth. A simple medium recommended for the isolation of *F. nodosus* consists of pulverized, suspended sheep horn in an anaerobic medium with 10 percent $CO_2$ (15). A liquid medium used by Thomas (16) contained hydrolyzed sheep hoof as a basic ingredient.

On "V-F" agar plates containing horse serum and 0.1 cystein hydrochloride as a reducing agent, surface colonies are obtained. These are generally of a smooth surface, develop up to a diameter of 1 mm, and usually lie in small "etched" depressions in the agar surface. If blood is added to the medium instead of serum, no hemolysis is observed. Heavy inocula will often cause the curdling of milk after several days' incubation without change in reaction, and later the curd is digested. In cooked-meat media the fragments are partially digested. In old cultures tyrosine crystals are formed. None of the ordinary carbohydrates is fermented. Nitrates are not reduced but hydrogen sulfide is formed.

**Natural Habitat.** *F. nodosus* has been found only in the lesions of foot-rot of sheep. Because it has been shown that foot-rot agent will remain virulent in pastures, even when continually moist, for only a few days, it is unlikely that the organism can survive long in nature away from animal tissue. Beveridge claims that apparently recovered sheep often harbor small, inconspicuous lesions in which the organism will remain viable for months and believes that the disease is kept alive in flocks of such animals.

**Pathogenicity.** Subcutaneous inoculation of sheep, rabbits, guinea pigs, and mice with large doses of the pure cultures of this organism produced nothing more than transitory local lesions. When *Sp. penortha* was added to the inoculum, the effect was not materially changed. Only by inoculating the scarified skin around the margins of the claws of sheep were any significant lesions produced. Although Beveridge (2) has indicated that *Sp. penortha* is the accessory factor in producing foot-rot in sheep, Roberts and Egerton (12) have concluded that spirochetes and motile fusiforms are probably not essential to the pathogenesis of this disease, but are derived from the environment. They believe that the synergistic association of *F. nodosus*, the transmitting agent, with *S. necrophorus*, a normal inhabitant of the ovine environment, results in foot-rot, the initial establishment of these two fastidious anaerobes being facilitated by the metabolism of *Corynebacterium pyogenes* and other aerobic diphtheroid bacteria found at the surface of the lesion.

Egerton and Parsonson (6) have distinguished two clinical forms of foot-rot. The virulent form is characterized by extensive separation of hoof horn and the benign form by interdigital dermatitis (scald). *F. nodosus* is the primary cause of both forms, but the resulting lesion depends upon the virulence of the bacterium.

*For cattle.* True foot-rot is an acute or chronic infection of the foot characterized by necrosis of tissues of the interdigital space and often complicated by coffin or pastern joint suppurative arthritis. Foot-rot varies in character from mild interdigital lesions to severe phlegmon that involves a high percentage of the herd. Dermatitis is often present and is a major factor in the cause of the disease. Monlux *et al.* (10) found mange (*Chorioptes bovis*) to be the etiological factor in a type of foot-rot in cattle. It is possible that various agents and environmental conditions account for different forms of the disease. In 1964 Gupta *et al.* (7) studied foot-rot in cattle. In many cases a direct examination of infected tissues revealed a Gram-negative bacillus, which re-sembled *F. nodosus,* and also a spirochete. Although neither the Gram-nega-tive bacillus nor the spirochete was isolated in pure culture, transmission experiments supported the premise that the former was able to initiate mild foot-rot in cattle.

In 1966, Egerton and Parsonson (5) investigated an outbreak of foot infec-tion in cattle and noted that necrotic material from interdigital lesions con-tained organisms that resembled *F. nodosus.* When such material was scari-fied into the interdigital skin a condition that mimicked foot-rot was induced in both cattle and sheep. An organism was then isolated from one of the in-fected sheep that had the properties of typical ovine strains of *F. nodosus.* It was pathogenic for both sheep and cattle.

**Toxin Formation.** No evidence of an exotoxin was observed.

**Immunity.** Agglutinin were readily produced by rabbit immunization. Anti-sera prepared with an American and an Australian strain cross-agglutinated but not completely. Sheep affected with foot-rot failed to agglutinate these antigens even in low dilution. This is ascribed to the rather superficial char-acter of the lesions of the disease.

The naturally occurring disease confers little immunity. An animal with one or two infected feet of long standing can be artificially infected on another foot. Attempts by Beveridge to immunize sheep by vaccines of several kinds containing heat-killed cultures were not successful, but subsequent studies by Egerton and Merritt (4) demonstrated that the serum of normal sheep was bactericidal *in vitro* for *F. nodosus* and that this activity increased upon vac-cination.

The disease is satisfactorily controlled in Australia by carefully examining the feet of all sheep at the beginning of the dry season, when the disease does not spread, and eliminating all those that show evidences of the disease.

**Chemotherapy.** Formalin and chloromycetin have been used rather widely in attempting to control foot-rot in sheep. Either substance must be applied lo-cally to the infected feet. If this is done properly, relapses will not be entirely prevented but the disease can be effectively controlled (9, 11, 13, 14). Harriss (8) recommends the use of an ointment containing 5 mg terramycin and 10,-000 units of polymyxin B sulfate per gram. Details on treatment and control of this disease have been published by Carter and Henderson (3).

## REFERENCES

1. Beveridge.   Austral. Jour. Exp. Biol. Med. Sci., 1936, *14*, 307.
2. Beveridge.   Austral. Council Sci. and Indus. Res. Bul. 140, 1941.
3. Carter and Henderson.   Canad. Jour. Comp. Med. and Vet. Sci., 1955, *19*, 26.
4. Egerton and Merritt.   Jour. Comp. Path., 1970. *80*, 369.
5. Egerton and Parsonson.   Austral. Vet. Jour., 1966, *42*, 425.
6. *Ibid.,* 1969, *45*, 345.
7. Gupta, Fincher, and Bruner.   Cornell Vet., 1964, *54*, 66.
8. Harriss.   Brit. Vet. Jour., 1955, *111*, 212.
9. Littlejohn.   Vet. Rec., 1955, *67*, 599.

10. Monlux, Raun, Diesch, and Hunt.  Jour. Am. Vet. Med. Assoc., 1961, *138*, 379.
11. Penny.  Brit. Vet. Jour., 1955, *111*, 125.
12. Roberts and Egerton.  Jour. Comp. Path., 1969, 79, 217.
13. Sambrook.  Vet. Rec., 1955, 67, 74.
14. Stewart.  Austral. Vet. Jour., 1954, *30*, 380.
15. Thomas.  *Ibid.*, 1958, *34*, 411.
16. Thomas.  *Ibid.*, 1963, 39, 434.

### Streptobacillus moniliformis

SYNONYMS:  *Streptothrix muris ratti, Actinomyces muris ratti, Haverhillia multiformis, Haverhillia moniliformis.*

This is a pleomorphic bacillus that varies from short rods to long, interwoven filaments which may fragment. Under certain conditions *Monilia*-like swellings occur along the filaments. The organism requires media enriched with ascitic fluid or blood serum for good growth. Anaerobic conditions sometimes favor growth on primary isolation.

S. *moniliformis* is pathogenic for mice and probably only parasitic for rats. Although it has not been established that this organism is the cause of Haverhill fever (3) or rat-bite fever (4, 6) of man, similar organisms which many have regarded as identical with S. *moniliformis* have been isolated from individuals suffering from these diseases.

An outbreak of tendon-sheath infection in turkeys caused by an organism very closely related to, if not identical with, S. *moniliformis* was described by Boyer *et al.* (1). Ten percent of the breeder toms in a flock were infected. They developed sore and swollen hocks, following which they became recumbent and eventually died. The organism was isolated from joint and bursal lesions of turkeys and also from a rat by Yamamoto and Clark (7). They pointed to the rat as a likely source of infection in the original epornitic.

In 1961 Ditchfield *et al.* (2) reported a case of S. *moniliformis* infection in a dog. The illness was characterized by acute gastroenteritis, arthritis, skin rash, and endocarditis. Treatment was of no benefit, and the dog died on the 17th day of illness. The authors stated that this was the first report of such an infection in domestic animals and that it closely resembled Haverhill fever in man. An outbreak of the disease that resulted in arrested pregnancy and abortion in mice was recorded in 1962 by Sawicki *et al.* (5). It has been isolated from chickens and from monkeys.

### REFERENCES

1. Boyer, Bruner, and Brown.  Avian Dis., 1958, 2, 418.
2. Ditchfield, Lord, and McKay.  Canad. Vet. Jour., 1961, 2, 457.
3. Parker and Hudson.  Am. Jour. Path., 1926, 2, 357.
4. van Rooyen.  Jour. Path. and Bact., 1936, 43, 455.
5. Sawicki, Bruce, and Andrewes.  Brit. Jour. Exp. Path., 1962, 43, 194.
6. Steen.  Acta Path. et Microbiol. Scand., 1951, 28, 17.
7. Yamamoto and Clark.  Vet. Rec., 1966, 79, 95.

# XVI | The *Micrococcaceae*

In many places in nature—in soil, water, air, and on the surfaces of plants and animals—are found organisms known as the *micrococci*. Among the genera recognized in the *Micrococcaceae* are *Micrococcus, Staphylococcus, Gaffkya, Sarcina, Methanococcus,* and *Peptococcus*. Most of these organisms apparently live a purely saprophytic existence, but some undoubtedly are capable of causing disease of man and animals. The important pathogens for animals are the staphylococci and only these organisms will be discussed.

The most frequent pus-forming organism of man belongs to this group. Several of the earliest bacteriologists recognized it in suppurative processes. Rosenbach (46) in 1884 clearly showed its relationship to pus formation in man and gave it the name *Staphylococcus pyogenes aureus*. The binomial *Staphylococcus aureus* will be used here. A less virulent variant that lacks the orange pigment is often designated as *Staphylococcus albus (epidermidis)*.

### Staphylococcus aureus and Staphylococcus albus

These organisms are not uncommon in animal infections and they occur frequently in diseases in man. When present in suppurative processes in animals, they are often associated with other species and their specific role is not so clear as in man. There is ample evidence that transmission between man and the lower animals occurs. Some of the strains that produce disease in animals are identical with those that infect man. They possess the same toxins and belong to the same phage groups. Other strains differ in toxin production and in resistance to phage lysis.

**Morphology and Staining Reactions.** The pathogenic staphylococci appear as perfectly spherical organisms of uniform size (about 0.8 microns in diameter). In pus the organisms frequently are grouped in irregular masses that remind one of a bunch of grapes. This appearance caused Ogsten (42) to adopt the generic name for the group (*staphylo* [Gr.] = "bunch of grapes"). In fluid

274

media the organisms usually appear singly or in small groups. They are non-motile, do not form spores, and usually do not possess capsular substance. The ordinary stains are readily taken, and young cultures always are Gram-positive. Older cultures lose part of their Gram-retaining ability. The acid-fast stain is not retained.

**Cultural Features.** Colonies of pathogenic staphylococci are porcelain white or yellowish orange when growing on solid media. The orange pigment is best seen on media that are rather dry, as on coagulated blood serum or on solid media that contain starch. The orange-colored cultures are the most active biochemically and their pathogenicity usually is greater. Their cultural features show quantitative rather than qualitative differences; hence they will be described together.

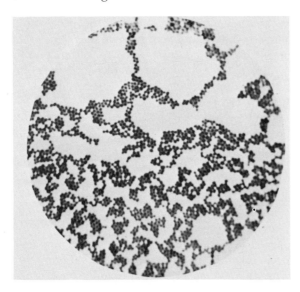

Fig. 26. *Staphylococcus aureus*, a stained film from a 24-hour-old culture on slant agar, showing typical arrangement in grapelike masses. X 900.

Broth is uniformly and rather heavily clouded. A moderate amount of rather viscid sediment forms in the bottom of the tube. The growth on agar is quite profuse, semitransparent, moist, and glistening. Gelatin is rapidly lique-fied by freshly isolated strains of *Staph. aureus*, but the property is easily lost upon continued cultivation. *Staph. albus* usually will not liquefy gelatin even when freshly isolated.

Some strains are strongly hemolytic; others have no action on blood. This matter will be referred to later. Litmus milk is reddened but frequently not coagulated. Acid but no gas is formed from glucose, lactose, sucrose, and mannitol by most cultures. In this group there is considerable variation in fermenting ability. Unlike many of the saprophytic micrococci, the pyogenic types are unable to utilize ammonium salts as a sole source of nitrogen. Nitrates usually are reduced. Certain strains of *Staph. aureus* produce bacteriocin (staphylococcin) an antibiotic that inhibits some Gram-negative, but not Gram-positive bacteria (25).

**Resistance.** Staphylococci are among the most resistant of non-spore-bearing organisms. Most strains are capable of resisting dehydration for long periods, they are relatively heat-resistant, and they tolerate the ordinary disinfectants better than the vegetative forms of most organisms. The use of staphylococci as indicators of swimming pool pollution has been suggested. They are more chlorine resistant than intestinal bacteria and their absence implies the lack of the enteric forms (22). There is evidence that vacuum packaging of sliced cold meats will inhibit the growth of, *Staph. aureus* (11).

**Staphylococcus Toxins.** The pathogenic staphylococci, particularly those of the *Staph. aureus* variety, produce one or several toxins. The hemolytic activity is due to *hemotoxins* (*staphylolysins*), a *leukocidin* is destructive to leukocytes, and a *necrotizing* toxin (*dermonecrotoxin*) causes tissue destruction around the point of injection in the skin. Some recognize a so-called *lethal toxin,* which kills rabbits when it is injected intravenously, although this probably is the same as the necrotoxin. An *enterotoxin* or enteric toxin is produced by some strains. Actually there appear to be four distinct immunological types of this toxin, designated A, B, C, and D (10).

Enterotoxins are responsible for many cases of food poisoning of man, most of which appear in the form of outbreaks because more than one person usually eats of the poisonous food. In these instances the staphylococci have been given the opportunity to multiply in food materials that have been prepared a considerable time before consumption and have not been properly refrigerated while being held (Dack *et al.,* 15; Jordan, 32). This is one of the most common forms of food poisoning in this country. In the past the public usually has referred to such illnesses as "ptomaine poisoning."

Various starchy foods, spray-dried milk (2, 3), meat food products, and cold meats, especially ham, have been involved in staphylococcic food-poisoning outbreaks. Staphylococci will form toxin when incubated in milk. That a high percentage of isolates from the bovine mammary gland produce enterotoxin was demonstrated by Bell and Veliz (4); hence it is possible that some food poisoning of man may be caused by the consumption of milk from cattle that are suffering from staphylococcic mastitis. Minett (40) and Crabtree and Litterer (14) suggest that this has occasionally happened. Except for very young kittens and suckling pigs that can be poisoned experimentally, domestic animals seem not to be susceptible to the enterotoxin. That rhesus monkeys will develop gastroenteritis when exposed to enterotoxin B was demonstrated by Kent (34).

Besides the toxins listed above many of the pathogenic staphylococci possess the enzymes coagulase, fibrinolysin (*staphylokinase*), and hyaluronidase. A chemotactic factor (*cytotaxin*) which attracts polymorphonuclear leukocytes may also be demonstrated (55).

In 1935 Glenny and Stevens (26) showed that two antigenically different hemolysins (hemotoxins) occur in staphylococci. They were designated *Alpha-lysin* and *Beta-lysin*. Within the next 5 years Smith and Price (49) reported the presence of *Gamma-lysin,* Williams and Harper (58) added *Delta-lysin,* and Elek and Levy (20) found *Epsilon-lysin.*

Alpha-, Beta-, and Delta-lysin are commonly associated with coagulase-positive strains of staphylococci. One of these lysins is present—either alone or in combination—in all coagulase-positive strains. Alpha- and Delta-lysin occur very frequently, and usually together, in staphylococcic cultures of human origin, while Beta-lysin, mostly in combination with the other two, is characteristic of animal strains and uncommon in human strains. Fraser (24) claims that staphylococci associated with disease conditions in dogs differ from human and other animal strains in that they seldom form a golden pigment or appreciable amounts of Alpha-lysin. Their most frequent hemolytic pattern appears to be the Beta-lysin–Delta-lysin variety.

Coagulase-negative strains produce none of these hemotoxins, but a high proportion will lyse red blood cells and this hemolysin is the Epsilon-lysin. The identity of the Gamma-lysin has not been clearly established. It probably is a combination of Alpha- and Delta-lysin activity.

The Alpha-lysin (39) is characterized by its ability to hemolyze both sheep and rabbit erythrocytes, by its ability to produce necrosis in the skin of guinea pigs, and by its lethality to white mice when injected intraperitoneally. The Beta-lysin does not hemolyze rabbit cells, does not produce necrosis, and is not lethal to mice. The Beta-lysin may show some hemolysis of sheep cells in the water bath, but usually there is none. When the tubes are cooled after incubation, however, hemolysis will occur (hot-cold hemolysis). The Delta-lysin is dermonecrotic and immunologically specific; it will hemolyze human, rabbit, sheep, guinea pig, and horse erythrocytes. The Epsilon-lysin readily hemolyzes both sheep and rabbit red blood cells. It is not neutralized by antisera for the other lysins.

Whether the ability to destroy leukocytes, produce necrosis and death, and cause gastroenteritis actually means that toxins other than the hemotoxins are involved remains to be answered. There is evidence that purified Alpha-lysin also possesses dermonecrotic, lethal, and leukocidal activities (35). It has frequently been pointed out that the enterotoxin differs from the others in being heat-resistant. Singer (48) has found that all the toxins of staphylococci are heat-resistant and thus refutes this concept. Strains from both animals and man that exhibit the hemolytic toxins also show evidence of the necrotoxin and the lethal toxin. Many strains from animals and man possess a weak enterotoxin. It is probable that all toxin-bearing staphylococci produce enterotoxin, but only a compartively few strains have sufficient potency to produce effective concentrations. The means available for testing for enterotoxin are not reliable; hence this question cannot be definitely answered at the present time. It does appear that the presence of coagulase and heat-stable deoxyribonuclease correlate well with enterotoxin production (54).

In ordinary laboratory media few strains of staphylococci produce potent toxins. The most successful method requires highly buffered media incubated at 37 C in an atmosphere of 20 percent carbon dioxide and 80 percent air (50). Reiser and Weiss (45) have supplied data on the production of staphylococcal enterotoxins A, B, and C, and Casman and Bennett (9) have submitted methods for the detection of trace amounts of enterotoxins A and B in foods.

The importance of the toxins of staphylococci in infections is not entirely clear. Strains from malignant suppurative processes often show toxins of less potency than strains isolated from the skin and other sources where there is no evidence of pathogenicity.

**Bacteriophage Typing of Staphylococci.** A number of workers have investigated phage typing of staphylococci (6, 18, 52). It is apparent that a multiplicity of phage types occur. Although strains derived from animals usually resist the human-strain typing phages, some are readily lysed. Those that resist initially can be lysed by propagating the phage on the particular strain, thereby producing phage adaptation (13).

Serological typing of staphylococci has been accomplished by gel-precipitation reactions (31) and by the FA technic (12).

**Pathogenicity for Experimental Animals.** Minute doses of staphylococci from pathologic conditions administered intravenously to rabbits usually will cause death within 48 hours. Cloudy swelling of the organs and bloody extravasations in the body cavities are found. Smaller doses or less virulent cultures will cause emaciation and death after some days or even 1 or 2 weeks. In these cases multiple abscesses will be found in the kidneys, the myocardium, and sometimes the lungs, bones, and joints. In acute cases the organism can readily be isolated from the blood, in chronic cases from the localized lesions.

Intradermal or subcutaneous injections will lead to the formation of abscesses. Some of the earlier workers found that severe furunculosis could be produced by rubbing cultures into the human skin.

Guinea pigs and mice may be infected experimentally, but these animals are more resistant than rabbits.

**Pathogenicity for Domestic Animals.** *Horse.* Undoubtedly streptococci play a more important role in pyogenic infections of horses than the staphylococci. The latter are found frequently in miscellaneous infections, often in association with other organisms. *Staph. aureus* is usually found in pure culture in the peculiar disease known as *botryomycosis.* At one time this disease was thought to be caused by infection with an organism belonging to the higher fungi, but this idea has now been discarded. Botryomycosis usually begins, after castration of male animals, in the stump of the spermatic cord. The infected cord becomes greatly enlarged and sclerotic. Small pockets of pus are found here and there in the mass of newformed tissue, and in the pus small granules resembling those of actinomycosis are found. When these granules are crushed, they yield masses of staphylococci embedded in a capsular material probably furnished by the host. Botryomycosis sometimes generalizes, in which case there is usually a fatal ending (McFadyean, 36).

*Cattle.* Staphylococci often are found in suppurative processes in cattle, frequently but not always in association with other organisms. Minett, Stableforth, and Edwards (41) stated that cases of mastitis caused by these organisms frequently were very acute, the animals exhibiting marked toxic symptoms, and that a considerable proportion died within a few days. Ferguson (23) studied eight such cases, in six of which the animals were critically ill, and of these, three resulted in death. Apparently in past years staphylococcic mastitis was just as common as today, but only the more severe cases were recognized. At present the incidence of this infection is probably no higher than formerly, but in some areas the emphasis has shifted from streptococci to staphylococci because effective antibiotic treatment within those regions has almost eliminated the former organism as a cause of mastitis. Streptococci yield readily to penicillin treatment, whereas staphylococci tend to become resistant to this antibiotic. Edwards and Rippon (19) studied 395 strains of staphylococci pathogenic for the bovine udder. By phage typing, 381 of these strains fell into five main types. They were coagulase-positive and many were resistant to penicillin.

Occasionally staphylococci cause botryomycosis of the bovine udder (5). This is a granulomatous lesion of a chronic nature and clinically is sometimes diagnosed as actinomycosis.

*Other animals.* Birds usually are regarded as quite resistant to *Staphylococcus* infections; however, Madsen (37) reports serious losses in turkeys from a purulent synovitis caused by organisms of this group. Earlier Jungherr and Plastridge (33) described a similar disease in young cockerels and recently Carnaghan (8) claimed that *Staph. aureus* isolated from the vertebrae of chickens was the cause of spondylitis and spinal-cord compression.

Dogs, cats, and swine are fairly resistant to *Staph. aureus* infections, but staphylococci septicemia has been reported in dogs (57), and although the incidence of staphylococcal dermatitis is low in the dog and cat the organism is nearly always present (29, 30). Magnusson (38) found that 41 percent of the lesions in the udder of swine which were diagnosed clinically as actinomycosis were in reality caused by staphylococci. It has also been incriminated in abortion in swine (51). It has been reported by Hardy and Price (28) as the cause of dermatitis in range sheep and as an infection of tick-infested lambs in England (56). It also causes mastitis in this animal as well as in goats (17). It is a significant cause of neonatal infection of lambs in Western Australia (16). It has produced arthritis in the white-tailed deer (47) and mastitis in mink (53).

**Immunity.** Repeated injections of heat-killed staphylococci will protect rabbits against otherwise fatal doses of *Staph. aureus*. Bacterins, expecially autogenous bacterins, frequently appear to be of value in combating chronic infections in man. They are sometimes used on animals, although the results are not clear-cut. Immune serum has been used with apparently favorable results in some cases and with none in others. Bacteriophage has been advocated for dealing with chronic infections, but the evidence suggests that it is useless because the phage is rapidly inactivated when introduced parenterally. Local dressings of phage, in which case inactivation by tissue fluids is retarded, may have some value.

*Staphylococcus* toxoid is easily made by treating filtrates with 0.3 percent formalin for a few hours. These preparations stimulate antitoxin formation very promptly and appear to have value in treating some chronic infections. Special efforts have been made to vaccinate dairy cattle with toxoids, bacterins, and combinations of toxoid-bacterin in the hope of preventing staphylococcic mastitis. These attempts have not been very successful.

Immunity in *Staphylococcus* infections probably depends in part upon stimulation of phagocytosis (opsonic) and in part upon antitoxin.

**Chemotherapy.** The sulfonamides have not been especially effective against *Staphylococcus* infections. Penicillin is useful in treating certain types of this infection, but strains of staphylococci tend to become drug-fast, or resistant. These organisms show a marked tendency in this direction, and antibiotic-resistant strains soon appear in animals, hospitals, or localities where much antibiotic therapy is used. Many cases of staphylococcic mastitis do not respond to antibiotic treatment. According to Platonow and Blobel (43) this may be due in part to the protection afforded the organism by barriers of fibrosed tissue. Of the antibacterial products now known, aureomycin, terramycin, erythromycin (ilotycin), oleandomycin, chlorquinaldol, cetyl-pyridinium chloride, methicillin, gentamicin, cephalothin, cephaloridine, cephalexin, triacetyl-oleandomycin, tetracycline-oleandomycin, novobiocin-penicillin, novobiocin-tetracycline, and nitrofurazone-penicillin appear to be most effective in treating infections caused by staphylococci.

A bactericidal spray whose active ingredient is 2-chloro-4-phenyl-phenol, is reported to be extremely effective against these cocci (1).

**The Disease in Man.** In man staphylococci cause boils, furuncles, infections of the mucous membranes, osteomyelitis, impetigo, pustular acne, gastroenteritis, septicemia, and mastitis. They are frequently involved in other processes. They have caused staphylococcal sepsis in mothers and newborn babies, broncho-pneumonia, and pulmonary bacterial pseudomycosis (botryomycosis, 27).

Boe and Vogelsang (7) have shown that the incidence of penicillin-resistant pathogenic staphylococci has increased in persons who have been treated with this antibiotic. Fairlie and Kendall (21) reported three fatal cases of *Staphylococcus* enteritis that occurred after prophylactic use of penicillin and dihydrostreptomycin. They recommended prompt discontinuance of such treatment in patients that develop fever and diarrhea. Some cases of staphylococcic enteritis show marked improvement after erythromycin (ilotycin) is given. It is apparent that the use of antibiotics tends to build up drug-resisting staphylococci. This occurs frequently in hospitals, and hospital-acquired staphylococcal disease has become a formidable cause of illness and death (44). Aseptic technics and sanitary measures must be combined with the rational use of antibiotics in controlling this organism because there is no known cure-all.

## REFERENCES

1. Andersen.   Appl. Microbiol., 1963, *11*, 239.
2. Anderson and Stone.   Jour. Hyg. (London), 1955, *53*, 387.
3. Armijo, Henderson, Timothée, and Robinson.   Am. Jour. Pub. Health, 1957, *47*, 1093.
4. Bell and Veliz.   Vet. Med., 1952, *47*, 321.
5. Blackburn.   Brit. Vet. Jour., 1959, *115*, 311.
6. Blair and Carr.   Jour. Inf. Dis., 1953, *93*, 1.
7. Boe and Vogelsang.   Acta Path. et Microbiol., Scand., 1951, *29*, 368.
8. Carnaghan.   Jour. Comp. Path., 1966, *76*, 9.
9. Casman and Bennett.   Appl. Microbiol., 1965, *13*, 181.
10. Casman, Bennett, Dorsey, and Issa.   Jour. Bact., 1967, *94*, 1875.
11. Christiansen and Foster.   Appl. Microbiol., 1965, *13*, 1023.
12. Cohen and Oeding.   Jour. Bact., 1962, *84*, 735.
13. Coles and Eisenstark.   Am. Jour. Vet. Res., 1959, *78*, 832.
14. Crabtree and Litterer.   Am. Jour. Pub. Health, 1934, *24*, 1116.
15. Dack, Cary, Woolpert, and Wiggers.   Jour. Prev. Med., 1930, *4*, 167.
16. Dennis.   Vet. Rec., 1966, *79*, 38.
17. Derbyshire.   Jour. Comp. Path. and Therap., 1958, *68*, 232.
18. Edds and Saunders.   Am. Jour. Vet. Res., 1966, *27*, 951.
19. Edwards and Rippon.   Jour. Comp. Path. and Therap., 1957, *67*, 111.
20. Elek and Levy.   Jour. Path. and Bact., 1950, *62*, 541.
21. Fairlie and Kendall.   Jour. Am. Med. Assoc., 1953, *153*, 90.
22. Favero, Drake, and Randall.   Pub. Health Rpts. (U.S.), 1964, *79*, 61.
23. Ferguson.   Cornell Vet., 1940, *30*, 299.
24. Fraser.   Res. Vet. Sci., 1964, *5*, 365.
25. Gagliano and Hinsdill.   Jour. Bact., 1970, *104*, 117.
26. Glenny and Stevens.   Jour. Path. and Bact., 1935, *40*, 201.
27. Greenblatt, Heredia, Rubenstein, and Alpert.   Am. Jour. Clin. Path., 1964, *41*, 188.
28. Hardy and Price.   Jour. Am. Vet. Med. Assoc., 1951, *119*, 445.
29. Hearst.   Vet. Med., 1967, *62*, 475.
30. Ibid., 1967, *62*, 541.
31. Jensen.   Acta Path. et Microbiol. Scand., 1961, *52*, 175.
32. Jordan.   Jour. Am. Med. Assoc., 1930, *94*, 1648.
33. Jungherr and Plastridge.   Jour. Am. Vet. Med. Assoc., 1941, *98*, 27.
34. Kent.   Am. Jour. Path., 1966, *48*, 387.
35. Kumar, Loken, Kenyon, and Lindorfer.   Jour. Exp. Med., 1962, *115*, 1107.
36. McFadyean.   Jour. Comp. Path. and Therap., 1919, *32*, 73.
37. Madsen.   The Turkey World, 1942, *17*, no. 2.
38. Magnusson.   Acta Path. et Microbiol. Scand., 1928, *5*, 588.
39. Marks and Vaughan.   Jour. Path. and Bact., 1950, *62*, 597.
40. Minett.   Jour. Hyg. (London), 1938, *38*, 623.
41. Minett, Stableforth, and Edwards.   Jour. Comp. Path. and Therap., 1929, *42*, 213.

42.  Ogsten.   Arch. f. klin. Chirurg., 1880, *25*, 588.

43.  Platonow and Blobel.   Jour. Am. Vet. Med. Assoc., 1963, *142*, 1097.

44.  Ravenholt and Ravenholt.   Am. Jour. Pub. Health, 1958, *48*, 277.

45.  Reiser and Weiss.   Appl. Microbiol., 1969, *18*, 1041.

46.  Rosenbach.   Mikroorganismen bei den Wundinfektionskrankheiten des Men schen. J. F. Bergmann, Wiesbaden, 1884.

47.  Sikes, Hayes, and Prestwood.   Canad. Jour. Comp. Med. and Vet. Sci., 1968, *32*, 388.

48.  Singer.   Cornell Univ. Thesis, 1941.

49.  Smith and Price.   Jour. Path. and Bact., 1938, *47*, 379.

50.  Surgalla, Kadavy, Bergdoll, and Dack.   Jour. Inf. Dis., 1951, *89*, 180.

51.  Thorne and Nilsson.   Acta Vet. Scand., 1961, *2*, 311.

52.  Torheim.   Acta Path. et Microbiol. Scand., 1960, *49*, 397.

53.  Trautwein and Helmboldt.   Jour. Am. Vet. Med. Assoc., 1966, *149*, 924.

54.  Victor, Lachica, Weiss, and Deibel.   Appl. Microbiol., 1969, *18*, 126.

55.  Walker, Barlet, and Kurtz.   Jour. Bact., 1969, 97, 1005.

56.  Watson.   Vet. Rec., 1964, *76*, 743.

57.  Wells.   *Ibid.*, 1953, *65*, 607.

58.  Williams and Harper.   Jour. Path. and Bact., 1947, *59*, 69.

# XVII | The *Lactobacillaceae*

The family *Lactobacillaceae* contains both the lactic acid cocci and the lactic acid rods. Only two of the genera are sufficiently important to be considered here. Both contain spherical forms and are listed as *Diplococcus* and *Streptococcus*.

## THE GENUS *DIPLOCOCCUS*

The genus contains the organisms known as the pneumococci, usually parasites of man. They generally occur in pairs but may appear in chains. They are soluble in 10 percent bile, whereas streptococci are not soluble in bile solutions. On blood agar they may produce slight hemolysis, but usually show methemoglobin formation with green zones around the colonies. At present over 70 serological types designated by Roman numerals are recognized. These are analogous to the Lancefield groups of streptococci and are differentiated chiefly on the basis of the Neufeld *Quellung* reaction (swelling of the capsules) as induced by type-specific antisera.

Pneumococci cause pneumonia in man. Their habitat is the normal mouth and throat of man. They have been isolated occasionally from the upper respiratory tract of apparently healthy animals (2) but have not been considered to be an important cause of disease in these animals. Dhanda and Sekariah (1) have reported the isolation of pneumococci Types III, XXVIII, and XXVIIIA from cases of pneumonia and sudden death in sheep and goats, and Smith and Stables (5) and MacLachlan *et al.* (4) have described outbreaks of mastitis in cattle both caused by Type III pneumococci.

Studies by Kislak *et al.* (3) have indicated that penicillin G is the drug of choice in treating man, except in patients who are allergic to it. These should receive erythromycin.

## REFERENCES

1. Dhanda and Sekariah.    Indian Vet. Jour., 1958, 35, 473.
2. Finland.    Medicine, 1942, 21, 307.
3. Kislak, Razavi, Daly, and Finland.    Am. Jour. Med. Sci., 1965, 250, 261.
4. MacLachlan, Wilson, and Stuart.    Vet. Rec., 1958, 70, 987.
5. Smith and Stables.    Vet. Rec., 1958, 70, 986.

## THE GENUS *STREPTOCOCCUS*

Streptococci cause a variety of diseases of man and the lower animals besides appearing as saprophytes in milk and milk products. As early as 1880 Rosenbach observed these organisms in suppurative inflammatory conditions. In addition to the virulent forms, it is now known that relatively harmless parasitic streptococci are frequently present in the throat and intestinal tract of animals. Some of these cocci may assume a pathogenic role when normal resistance is markedly reduced.

### GENERAL CHARACTERISTICS

**Morphology and Staining Properties.** The group of cocci that characteristically develop into chains resembling strings of beads are known as *streptococci*. The chains may be short (diplococci) or they may be very long. Chain length depends upon species differences and upon the medium on which the culture is growing. Typical chain formation is best seen in fluid media; on solid media the chains become so entangled that their demonstration is impossible.

The individual cells of streptococci are seldom perfectly spherical, and frequently there is considerable variation in the size and shape of the elements in a single culture. Sometimes the cells are flattened from side to side; more often they are elongated. In fact, certain animal strains of streptococci may be so pleomorphic on primary isolation that they can readily be mistaken for short rods. Usually a few transfers on artificial media will bring forth the typical coccus form. Spores are never formed. With rare exceptions they are nonmotile. A number of species form definite capsules when developing in tissues or in culture media containing blood serum. Such strains show the mucoid or the matt types of colony formation rather than the smooth (glossy) or the rough forms usually produced. Most streptococci are Gram-positive. In old cultures many Gram-negative forms are commonly found. They are easily stained with all the usual dyes. They are never acid-fast.

**Cultural Features.** The streptococci are among the more fastidious bacteria with respect to nutritive requirements. They usually will not grow on meat extract media, and growth ordinarily is poor even on infusion media unless it is enriched by the addition of blood, ascitic fluid, or similar substances. However, horse meat infusion agar, without enrichment, has proved to be an excellent medium for the isolation of animal strains of streptococci (Bruner, 7).

All streptococci produce small, delicate, translucent colonies of a diameter of about 1 mm on solid media. Heavy inoculations give confluent growths that are nearly transparent. The surface of the growth is smooth and glistening, and the margins of individual colonies are perfectly circular. Deep colonies in agar usually are lenticular in shape. In softer media they may be globular. In size they may be hardly large enough to be easily visible with the naked eye. Usually there is no growth on potato. When growth is obtained on gelatin, it consists of a string of delicate beads along the line of the stab, with little or no growth on the surface, and in most cases without evidence of liquefaction.

In fluid media, growth usually is a little more abundant than in solids. In broth there may be a faint cloudiness or the medium may remain perfectly clear except for a fluffy sediment in the bottom of the tube. The appearance usually gives an accurate clue as to whether the coccus is growing in short or long chains; the short-chain type causes uniform clouding, whereas the long-chain type quickly sediments. All streptococci grow well in milk. With few exceptions the milk is soured through the formation of lactic acid from the milk sugar. Most streptococci grow readily under aerobic as well as anaerobic conditions. There are some strains, however, that grow only under anaerobic conditions. They are catalase-negative.

Sugars are fermented by all streptococci. The end product is largely lactic acid. Gas is produced by only a few streptococci and by none of the types that are of importance in pathology.

**Physiological Characteristics.** The growth range of streptococci varies from below 10 C to above 45 C. The pathogenic types have a much narrower range than this.

The resistance of streptococci to heat is not great. The pathogenic types are usually killed by temperatures well below those used for pasteurization (ca. 63 C for 30 minutes). It is well known, however, that the milk-souring types are not wholly destroyed by pasteurization, and some of the intestinal types have rather unusual resistance. One of the thermophilic types grows at 50 C. Likewise, the resistance to drying and to chemical disinfection is not very great as a rule. However, when cultures are rapidly and completely dried, they often remain viable for very long periods of time; hence it is possible that streptococci withstand drying better than is generally supposed.

**Habitat.** The streptococci are found on the mucous membranes of men and animals, in various suppurative processes in these hosts, and in milk and milk products. It is frequently said that these organisms exist principally as animal parasites. Stark and Sherman have found *Str. lactis* on growing vegetation and enterococci have been isolated from plants in a wild environment. This raises the question of whether these organisms may not occur more commonly on plants than has been hitherto supposed. In general, the increased growth on media enriched by blood or tissue extracts suggests that the streptococci are adapted for parasitic rather than saprophytic existence.

## DIFFERENTIATION OF THE STREPTOCOCCI

Since 1884, when Rosenbach (56) described *Str. pyogenes,* the importance of certain streptococci in pyogenic processes of man has been known. For many years adequate means of differentiating and identifying the numerous species of streptococci were not available. Morphological features were early recognized as inadequate. Differences in fermentative characteristics proved confusing until other means of establishing primary groupings were found. Not all of these problems have been solved, but great progress was made in 1903 when Schottmüller (58) introduced the method of primary grouping according to action upon blood cells. Additional methods, described below, now make it possible to identify most species.

**Action of Streptococci on Red Blood Cells.** According to their action upon erythrocytes of animals, all streptococci may be placed in one of the following classes:

1. *The Hemolytic Group* includes those forming a soluble hemolysin that causes the freeing of hemoglobin from erythrocytes.

2. *The Viridans Group* includes those causing an alteration of the hemoglobin, without freeing it from the cells, in the course of which its color is changed through various shades of green to greenish black.

3. *The Anhemolytic Group* includes those causing no noticeable change in erythrocytes.

Smith and Brown (63) pointed out that under certain conditions streptococci belonging to the viridans group cause hemolysis of blood cells; they therefore thought it best to rename the groups and suggested the use of the first three letters of the Greek alphabet as designations. Their *Alpha group* is the viridans group of Schottmüller; the *Beta* is the hemolytic group, and *Gamma* designates the anhemolytic group. Both systems of nomenclature are used.

*The blood agar plate:* Identification of the grouping is generally done on a blood agar plate. From 5 to 10 percent of sterile, defibrinated horse blood is added to the melted and cooled nutrient agar just before it is poured into the plate. The use of horse blood is particularly important. It is well known that the red corpuscles of different animal species vary widely in their resistance to different streptococcic hemolysins. At times it may be desirable to use the red cells of some particular species in observing the action of streptococcal hemolysin; but, if the results are to be used for purposes of identification or classification, they should always be controlled by parallel tests with horse erythrocytes. Streak plates often are used, but it is better to use poured plates and to base the classification upon the deep rather than the surface colonies.

Colonies of the *Alpha* or *viridans* group at the end of 18 to 24 hours' incubation at 37 C show a slight or marked discoloration of a narrow zone of blood cells immediately surrounding the colony. The discoloration is easily seen with the naked eye. Under the microscope it can be seen that the ery-

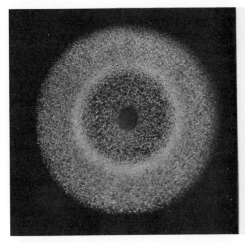 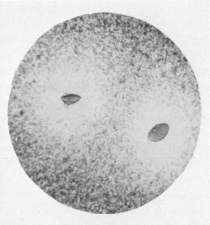

*Fig. 27 (left).* *Streptococcus* of the Alpha type on a blood agar plate. This plate had been incubated 48 hours at 37 C. The colony appears in the center, surrounded by a wide zone in which the blood cells are discolored but intact. The color of this zone is greenish. Beyond the greenish zone is a narrow zone of partially hemolyzed cells. X 7.

*Fig. 28 (right).* *Streptococcus* of the Beta type on a blood agar plate. This plate had been incubated about 36 hours at 37 C. The two colonies are surrounded by zones in which the red blood cells have apparently disappeared. To the naked eye the hemolyzed zones appear much sharper than they do in the photograph. X 7.

throcytes in the discolored zone are intact. If the incubation is carried on for a longer period, and especially if the incubation continues at room temperature or lower, a clear zone appears outside the greenish area. Under the microscope it may be seen that the blood cells have dissolved. The cells of the discolored zone remain intact, however, no matter how long the incubation is continued.

Colonies of the *Beta* or *hemolytic* group show no discolored zone under any circumstances. As soon as they begin to develop, a solution of the blood cells about the colonies appears. After 18 to 24 hours' incubation, the minute colonies have developed clear, transparent zones about them from 1 to 3 mm in breadth. Under the microscope these zones appear perfectly clear; no intact blood cells can be found in them.

Solution of the erythrocytes occurs because of a soluble hemolytic substance (*streptolysin*) produced by the organisms in greatest abundance during the period of logarithmic increase. It may be demonstrated by adding a washed blood cell suspension to a broth culture from 4 to 15 hours old; the cells are lysed within a few minutes. Older cultures show reduced or no activity. The hemolysis produced by organisms of the Alpha or viridans group is not of this character. In this case it is probable that it is due, in part at least, to hemolyzing concentrations of acid.

The terms *hemolytic* and *nonhemolytic* continue to be used in connection with streptococci, but not without considerable confusion. Most authors consider all streptococci, except those of the Beta group, as nonhemolytic. This usage will be followed here. Certain nonhemolytic organisms of the Alpha type produce little discoloration, especially if the basic agar medium contains little fermentable sugar or if the plates are incubated at a temperature below 37 C. In these instances the secondary solution of corpuscles always exhibited by Alpha-type organisms may closely simulate the Beta type of hemolysis. The cleared zones in these instances are not usually so clear as those of Beta organisms, however, and young broth cultures contain no hemolytic substance.

**Limiting Hydrogen-Ion Concentration (for Hemolytic Streptococci).** Avery and Cullen (2) early called attention to the fact that hemolytic streptococci of human origin growing in the presence of fermentable sugar will seldom carry the pH beyond 5.0, whereas the majority of strains of bovine origin will carry it to pH 4.5 or 4.3.

**Hydrolysis of Sodium Hippurate (for Hemolytic Streptococci).** Ayers and Rupp (3) pointed out that hemolytic streptococci of bovine origin would break down sodium hippurate, whereas those of human origin would not. It appears to be true that cultures of human origin never attack this substance, but Edwards (23) has shown that some bovine strains do not either. As a matter of fact, this test is practically specific for certain streptococci associated with bovine mastitis (*Str. agalactiae* and *Str. uberis*).

**The Fibrinolytic Test (for Hemolytic Streptococci).** Tillett and Garner (66; 1933) described a reaction that appears to be valuable in differentiating hemolytic streptococci that are human pathogens. Young cultures in broth (or filtrates) are mixed with oxalated human plasma. A clot is then formed by the addition of calcium chloride. Most organisms belonging to Lancefield's Group A will liquefy this clot in a very short time, usually within 10 minutes in a water bath at 37 C. With some exceptions, streptococci of other groups will not liquefy the clot at all, or only after a long incubation period.

**Lancefield's Serological Method (for Hemolytic Streptococci).** In 1933 Lancefield (36) described her method of differentiating hemolytic streptococci. It utilizes the precipitation test. The antigens are extracts of cultures prepared with hot, dilute hydrochloric acid. The antigen is carbohydrate in nature, similar to the "residue antigens" or "specific soluble substances" (SSS) that give immunological specificity to the types of pneumococci. In her first study, Lancefield differentiated five types of streptococci, which she designated as Groups A, B, C, D, and E. In recent years, nine additional groups, F, G, H, K, L, M, N, O, and P, have been recognized. Not all strains now placed in the Lancefield groups are hemolytic; a few nonhemolytic types have been fitted into the classification. Furthermore, not all strains of streptococci that hemolyze horse blood can be typed. According to Feller and Stevens (24), hemolysis on sheep blood agar is a more reliable indication that a culture can be placed in the Lancefield system than is hemolysis of horse blood.

*Group A.* This group contains the strains causing scarlet fever, septic sore throat, empyema, puerperal sepsis, and many other diseases in human beings. It includes the highly pathogenic human-type streptococci that are of great concern to public health workers. (For differential characters see table XIV.)

*Group B.* These streptococci usually are of bovine origin. They may or may not produce Beta hemolysis in blood agar plates. They hydrolyze sodium hippurate. (See table XIV.)

*Group C.* Members of this group frequently have been isolated from suppurative and acute inflammatory lesions in horses, cattle, guinea pigs, and other animals. They also have been isolated from human infections, but their pathogenicity for man appears to be lower than that of Group A types. (For differential characters see table XIV.)

*Group D.* These streptococci are members of the group of enterococci. They differ markedly from cocci of Groups A, B, and C in a number of cultural features, as shown in table XIV. The motile strains of streptococci that have been described fall in this group (28).

*Group F.* The strains that belong to this group have been derived from minor infections of the respiratory tract in man and from the normal human throat. They do not produce a fibrinolysin active on human fibrin. They induce Beta hemolysis on blood agar plates but are not known to secrete a filterable hemolysin. They form a final acidity in glucose broth of pH 4.8 to 5.2. They do not hydrolyze sodium hippurate, reduce methylene blue milk, or grow on 40 percent bile agar. They ferment lactose, salicin, and usually trehalose, but not sorbitol.

*Group G.* The streptococci of this group are certainly pathogenic. They have been isolated from tonsillitis, endocarditis, and urinary infections in man, from pneumonia in the monkey, from mastitis in cattle, and from otitis in the dog. They have also been isolated from the normal human throat. Available evidence suggests that Group G, like Group C strains, have a definitely lower virulence for man than has *Str. pyogenes*. Group G strains produce a fibrinolysin acting on human fibrin. They are Beta-hemolytic. They do not grow on 40 percent bile agar, hydrolyze sodium hippurate, or reduce methylene blue. They ferment trehalose and lactose, but not sorbitol, and are variable in attacking salicin.

*Groups E, H, and K.* Group E strains have been isolated from milk and from swine. Snoeyenbos and colleagues (64) have found these organisms in abscesses in the lymph glands of swine, and Collier (13) has shown them to be the cause of lymphadenitis of the pharyngeal region of this animal. The differential characters of this group are given in table XIV. Groups H and K strains are found in the nose and throat of normal persons, and their ability to produce disease is open to question. Because of their action on blood agar they are considered to be hemolytic types, but they do not produce a soluble hemolysin. Group H types do not digest fibrin but mimic Group A strains in most fermentative characters. Group K streptococci are similar to Group H types but rarely ferment trehalose.

*Groups L, M, and N.* Organisms belonging to Groups L and M appear to be pathogenic for certain animals, especially the dog. Group L types have been isolated from the skin and pharynx of man. In Norway (50) they have been recovered from the skin and from the mucous membranes of the pharynx and vagina of swine. It is believed there that the transmission of these types from swine to cattle results in mastitis. Group N strains are apparently non-pathogenic. *Str. lactis* is placed in Group N, and the differential characters are given in table XIV. Groups L and M contain Beta-hemolytic types that produce soluble hemolysins. They do not grow on bile agar. Group L strains ferment trehalose, usually lactose, but not salicin or sorbitol. They may or may not hydrolyze sodium hippurate. Group M strains ferment lactose, but not trehalose, salicin, or sorbitol.

*Group O.* Boissard and Wormald (6) described this group in 1950. A great majority of their strains were found in routine swabbings of perfectly healthy human throats, but some were involved in tonsillitis and gingivitis. The organisms are Beta-hemolytic and possess the common group antigen O. They are sodium-hippurate- and sorbitol-negative. They vary in their action on trehalose and grow on 10 percent, but not on 40 percent, bile agar.

*Group P.* This group was proposed by Moberg and Thal (43) in 1954. It contains strains of Beta-hemolytic streptococci that were isolated from diseased swine and a hen and represented a serological entity. These organisms attack esculin, salicin, sorbitol, and trehalose. They do not utilize sodium hippurate.

Modifications of the original procedure of Lancefield for the identification of streptococci have been developed and are being used to group these organisms and to subdivide them into types within the groups. The Ouchterlong's agar gel diffusion technic has been employed and the identification of specific antigens has been accomplished by separating electrophoretic fractions by means of column chromatography and exposing them to antiserums (30). It appears that the use of these methods will produce alterations in the Lancefield classification, but until the changes are more clearly delineated we will hold to the streptococcic groupings as presented above.

**Fermentation of Carbohydrates.** Many carbohydrates have been used by workers in attempts to differentiate streptococci. Little progress was made, however, until fermentation tests were relegated to a secondary role. Their value appears to be in differentiating between organisms that are grouped together on the basis of other characteristics. Thus, a certain fermentation may have great value in differentiating between closely related hemolytic organisms but have none at all when applied to organisms of another group.

In the differentiation of mastitis streptococci from others frequently found in milk, the fermentation of esculin has been very useful. The organisms of mastitis do not attack this substance, whereas most other streptococci likely to be found in milk do. Edwards recommends the medium of Harrison and Vanderlek, which is a 2 percent peptone solution in which 0.5 g each of esculin and iron citrate scales are dissolved. The splitting of esculin is indicated by a blackening of the medium.

Organisms of Lancefield's Group C come from man and animals. In 1932 Edwards (23) demonstrated that the human types fermented trehalose but not sorbitol. The animal types, with the exception of *Str. equi,* fermented sorbitol but not trehalose. *Str. equi* fermented neither trehalose nor sorbitol.

**Tolerance Tests.** Sherman and his students (60; 1937) found that, in general, the streptococci of the "enterococcus" group are much more resistant to various influences than organisms, otherwise similar, that belong to the pyogenic class. The enterococci, for example, will grow at temperatures as low as 10 C and as high as 45 C; they will grow in media that contain 6.5 percent sodium chloride; they will grow in exceedingly alkaline media (pH 9.6); they will grow in milk containing as much as 0.1 percent methylene blue; and they generally will survive heating to 60 C for 30 minutes, whereas the majority of other streptococci are unable to endure these conditions.

**Miscellaneous Tests.** Other tests for the differentiation of streptococci are (*a*) production of ammonia from peptone, (*b*) liquefaction of gelatin, (*c*) hydrolyzation of starch, (*d*) growth in the presence of 10 to 40 percent bile, (*e*) curdling and reducing power in milk, and (*f*) virulence for animals, especially rabbits.

Sherman (60) classified streptococci upon the basis of a series of physiological tests. Table XIV is a composite from several tables given in this paper. This table includes a number of groups and species which quite certainly are not pathogenic, but they are nevertheless included here because they are often encountered when pathogenic forms are sought. It will be noted that all hemolytic organisms fall into the first group, except two types, which are placed in the enterococcus group. Because a soluble hemotoxin cannot be demonstrated in fluid cultures for the last mentioned, although a definite hemolysis occurs on blood plates, the question may be raised whether they really belong to the Beta group of Schottmüller. On the other hand, the hemolytic strength of *Str. agalactiae* usually is weak and often wholly absent, and the question can be raised in this instance whether the organism really belongs to the Beta group. The classification, however, undoubtedly will be useful until increasing knowledge causes a realignment of the groups. In this classification most of the forms pathogenic for man and animals are included in the first (pyogenic) group.

## THE HEMOLYTIC STREPTOCOCCI

### *Streptococcus pyogenes*

This organism is generally regarded as the type species of this group. It was isolated and described by Rosenbach (56) in 1884. It has long been recognized as the cause of a series of malignant suppurative infections in man which frequently terminate in septicemia.

Table XIV. DIFFERENTIATION OF THE STREPTOCOCCI *

| Division | Hemolysis | Lancefield serological group | Fibrinolysis | Sodium hippurate | Growth at 10 C | Growth at 45 C | 6.5% NaCl | pH 9.6 | 0.1% methylene blue | Survival at 60 C for 30 minutes | Gelatin liquefaction | NH₃ from peptone | Milk curdled | Lactose | Trehalose | Sorbitol | Group or species |
|---|---|---|---|---|---|---|---|---|---|---|---|---|---|---|---|---|---|
| Pyogenic | + | A | + | − | − | − | − | − | − | − | − | + | − | + | + | − | Str. pyogenes |
|  | ± | B | − | + | − | − | − | − | − | − | − | + | + | + | + | − | Str. agalactiae |
|  | + | C | − | − | − | − | − | − | − | − | − | − | − | − | − | − | Str. equi |
|  | + | C | − | − | − | − | − | − | − | − | − | + | − | +,± | − | + | "Animal pyogenes" |
|  | + | C | ± | − | − | − | − | − | − | − | − | + | ± | ±,+ | + | − | Human C |
|  | + | E | − | − | − | − | − | − | − | − | − | + | − | + | + | + | Group E |
| Viridans | − |  |  |  | − | ± | − | − | − | − | − | − | ± | + | ± | − | Str. salivarius |
|  | − |  |  |  | − | + | − | − | − | ± | − | − | − | − | + | − | Str. equinus |
|  | − |  |  |  | − | + | − | − | − | + | − | − | + | + | ± | ± | Str. bovis |
|  |  |  |  |  | − | + | − | − | − | + | − | − | + | + | − | − | Str. thermophilus |
| Lactic | − | N |  |  | + | − | − | − | ++ | + | − | + | + | + | + | − | Str. lactis |
|  | − | N |  |  | + | − | − | − | + | ± | − | − | + | + | − | − | Str. cremoris |
| Enterococci | − | D |  |  | + | + | + | + | + | + | − | + | + | + | + | + | Str. fecalis |
|  | − | D |  | ± | + | + | + | + | + | + | + | + | + | + | + | + | Str. liquefaciens |
|  | + | D |  | ± | + | + | + | + | + | + | ± | + | + | + | + | + | Str. zymogenes |
|  | + | D |  |  | + | + | + | + | + | + | − | + | + | + | ± | − | Str. durans |

* Adapted from Sherman.

*Streptococcus pyogenes* is the specific name for a group of organisms not wholly identical but having in common the Group A carbohydrate of Lancefield. Griffiths has demonstrated at least 23 types within the group, and Lancefield has shown that distinctions are made on the basis of two type-specific antigens. One of these, the "M" antigen, is a nucleoprotein located apparently very superficially in the cell wall. The other, designated the "T" antigen, also appears to be a protein that is closely associated with M. These antigens are independent and may occur in various combinations. Besides, distinctly different M and T substances occur and either one may be lacking in a strain of the streptococci.

As a means of rapid identification of Group A streptococci in throat cultures the fluorescent antibody (FA) technic may be employed (54). All members of this group are Beta-hemolytic and produce soluble hemolysins. These are known as *streptolysin* S and *streptolysin* O. The latter appears to be more important to the virulence of hemolytic streptococci and is cardiotoxic. It is also believed to have *leukocidin* activity. All Group A streptococci produce, in varying degree, a toxin that causes inflammation when injected into the human skin (*erythrogenic toxin.*) They also produce *streptokinase*, the plasmin activator that initiates the fibrinolytic dissolution of fibrin clots, and *streptodornase*, a deoxyribonuclease unrelated to virulence. A combination of streptokinase and streptodornase sometimes is used for clinical application in the enzymatic debridement of necrotic tissue and dissolution of fibrous exudates. Certain types of Group A streptococci secrete the spreading factor (*hyaluronidase*) of Duran-Reynals. Strains are found in the throat and nasopharynx of a considerable percentage of apparently normal people. They are also found in tonsillitis, sore throat, otitis media, puerperal fever, scarlet fever, erysipelas, bronchopneumonia, wound infections, and other conditions of man. Large-scale food-borne epidemics of streptococcal pharyngitis have been reported (20) and the observation has been made (53) that a single strain of hemolytic streptococci almost exclusively predominates in patients with streptococcal infections and in the carrier state.

In epidemics of sore throat caused by this organism, some individuals may exhibit the skin rash characteristic of scarlet fever, whereas many others do not. In other outbreaks, practically all may exhibit the rash. This probably depends upon individual susceptibility in the first instance and upon especially virulent strains possessed of an unusually strong erythrogenic toxin in the second. When the skin manifestations are prominent, the cases are diagnosed as scarlet fever; when the skin manifestations are absent, the condition is termed septic sore throat. Not uncommonly a Beta-hemolytic *Streptococcus* infection is followed by endocarditis and sometimes arthritis. These conditions, especially the former, may terminate in so-called *rheumatic fever*. It is interesting to note that in tropical Africa, where the incidence of rheumatic fever is very low, the carrier rate of Beta-hemolytic streptoccocci is also low (32).

So far as is known, *Str. pyogenes* plays only a small role in infections of domestic animals. Many of the supposed infections with this organism that have been described in the past are now known to be caused by other types of hemolytic streptococci belonging to the Lancefield Group C. *Str. pyogenes* occasionally invades the udder of cattle, as a result of contact with human beings (generally milkers) who are suffering from sore throat or have the infections on their hands. In the milk cistern of the udder the organism is capable of multiplication, as a result of which inflammation (garget or mastitis) is produced. The milk from such cattle sometimes causes serious outbreaks of scarlet fever or septic sore throat, if it is marketed in the raw state. Bovine mastitis commonly is caused by *Str. agalactiae* (Lancefield's Group B), an organism that has generally been considered to be nonpathogenic for man, but is now known to occur in the human female genital tract, to cause neonatal infection, and meningitis (35, 39).

### Streptococcus agalactiae

SYNONYM:  *Streptococcus mastitidis*

*Str. agalactiae* belongs to Lancefield's Group B. It occurs in inflamed udders of cattle the world over. It causes a majority of the cases of bovine mastitis. Some workers have claimed that *Str. agalactiae* exists in normal udders. This is not true. What consitutes a "normal" udder depends upon the clinical acuity of the observer. It is true that milk from infected udders may be so little changed as to pass for normal, and infected udders sometimes are so little altered that the abnormality escapes detection.

**Morphology and Staining Reactions.** In secretions from infected udders, *Str. agalactiae* usually appears in the form of long chains. In some samples these are numerous and easily found in stained films; in other cases, even though the milk may be markedly altered in appearance, the organisms may be so scarce as to be found with great difficulty. The organism is Gram-positive and is readily stained by all the ordinary stains

**Cultural Features.** It will be noted in table XIV that this organism resembles *Str. pyogenes* quite closely. In morphology and in its growth characteristics on ordinary culture media the organism cannot be distinguished from it. On blood agar, however, the hemolytic power of *Str. agalactiae* is much more limited and variable. The most actively hemolytic strains produce hemolytic zones not more than 1 mm broad. Many strains produce only a suggestion of hemolysis on blood agar plates, and others produce none whatsoever. Some strains produce a suggestion of greenish discoloration without hemolysis on blood agar plates.

Growth in serum broth is granular or flocculent, the growth appearing in the bottoms of the tubes, the rest of the broth remaining clear. Litmus milk, incubated at 37 C, is acidified and coagulated within 48 hours. There is slight reduction of the litmus at the bottoms of the tubes. At 10 C there is no observable growth in 5 days. Methylene blue milk is not reduced. In glucose

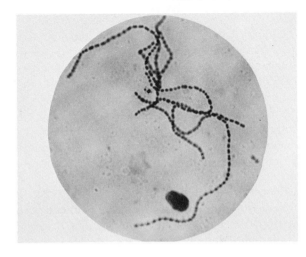

Fig. 29. *Streptococcus agalac-tiae*, from a stained film made from a sample of mastitis milk which had been incubated overnight at 37 C. Similar chains are often found in the fresh udder secretion. Note that the chains consist of a series of paired organisms. This is characteristic but not diagnostic. X 1,000.

broth the final hydrogen-ion concentration is from pH 4.4 to 4.7. Sodium hippurate is hydrolyzed. Glucose, lactose, sucrose, and maltose are regularly fermented; salicin is usually but not always. Inulin, mannitol, and raffinose are never attacked. Esculin is not broken down. Gelatin is not hydrolyzed. Many but not all strains of *Str. agalactiae* produce a brick-reddish growth on solid media, especially when the medium contains starch.

According to Gochnauer and Wilson (26), about 90 percent of *Str. agalactiae* strains tested produced hyaluronidase, and it appears that the enzyme formed by this organism is serologically distinct from that liberated by Group A streptococci (72).

*The CAMP phenomenon.* In 1944 Christie, Atkins, and Munch-Petersen (12) reported the finding of a lytic phenomenon produced by about 96 percent (47) of the streptococci belonging to Lancefield's serological group B. This phenomenon is now referred to as the CAMP phenomenon. It was shown that the culturing of certain milk on cow blood agar plates yielded colonies of strongly hemolytic streptococci which, when subcultured, failed to show hemolysis. Re-examination of the original plates revealed the presence of many staphylococci of the Alpha-Beta type; that is, their colonies were in the center of a clear zone, which in turn was surrounded by a large darkened area where the staphylococcal Beta toxin had altered, but not lysed, the cow red cells. Wherever there were colonies of the *Streptococcus* within these zones of darkening, the colonies were surrounded by an area of complete hemolysis, but elsewhere on the plates they produced no distinct hemolysis.

**Resistance.** Resistance to heat, drying, and chemicals is not great. Most strains will withstand 50 C but not 60 C moist heat for 30 minutes. The organism is readily destroyed by pasteurization.

**Pathogenicity.** This organism is the cause of a large portion of all cases of chronic catarrhal mastitis in dairy cattle. The disease is to be distinguished from acute mastitis in which the udder becomes greatly swollen, reddened, and painful and in which the animal usually develops a fever and may die. The disease caused by *Str. agalactiae* usually begins insidiously and develops gradually. The milk, or udder secretion, becomes altered in varying degrees, sometimes showing little or no abnormality and sometimes showing flakes, stringy masses of fibrin, blood, and thick purulent material. In many cases the degree of alteration of the milk varies from time to time, being thick and purulent at one time and practically normal at another. The inflammation in the udder causes the formation of new interstitial tissue, and thus fibrosis changes the normal soft consistency of the gland to hardness, generally in the form of indurated masses that may not be seen but may be palpated.

Normal milk has a pH slightly on the acid side of neutrality, whereas blood serum is slightly alkaline. In inflamed udders the milk secretion is mixed with inflammatory exudate derived from the blood serum. The alkaline exudate causes the pH to shift to the alkaline side, and this fact is the basis of the color tests for mastitis. Unfortunately it happens that in the early and late stages of the lactation period, milk is more alkaline than normal; hence the color tests are not safely used as the sole criterion of the existence of mastitis.

As would be expected, the number of leukocytes in milk coming from inflamed udders is much greater than the number found in normal milk. Frequently leukocyte counts are made as an aid in diagnosis. The modified Whiteside test as described by Murphy and Hanson (45) is often used for this purpose. It is performed by mixing 5 drops of foremilk and 1 drop of N NaOH solution on a glass slide. After 20 seconds a positive test is indicated by the presence of a precipitate. The amount and character of the precipitate can be correlated with the number of leukocytes present in the milk. Schalm and Noorlander (57) developed a similar test which they have designated the California mastitis test (CMT). They combine equal amounts of milk and an anionic surface-active agent consisting of a 3- to 5-percent concentration of alkyl arylsulfonate (pH 7.0) plus bromcresol purple indicator. Depending on the leukocyte count of the milk, the reaction varies from slight precipitation of amorphous material, which tends to disappear, to immediate development of a viscid gel. The bromcresol purple reveals abnormal alkalinity or acidity of the milk and provides a contrasting color.

The streptococci in most cases are difficult to demonstrate by direct methods, although frequently they can be found in the centrifuged sediment of the milk. To detect the organism it is best to culture the milk by streaking blood agar plates. Typical colonies are tested by the FA technic (69), the CAMP test, and subjected to biochemical studies.

**Transmission.** *Str. agalactiae* passes from infected to noninfected cows by way of the hands of the milkers or the cups of the milking machines. This is clearly shown by the fact that the disease does not ordinarily spread rapidly but gradually extends from one animal to another with relation to the milking sequence. This observation led to the practice of transferring cows with abnormal udders to the end of the milking line, a procedure not usually followed today because it is difficult to disinfect the vacated stall completely and it therefore remains a potential source of danger to the next occupant.

If a milking machine is used, animals with abnormal udders are best milked last, and by hand. A milking machine is safe if the equipment receives proper care and is not used upon diseased udders. If it is impractical to restrict the use to normal cows, the milking cups should be cleansed after each cow is milked. A method that seems effective is first to rinse them in a pail of clear water and then in a chlorine solution. In hand milking it has been found profitable to have all milkers wash their hands with soap and water and dry them on a sterile towel after milking one animal and before beginning with the next, as a means of reducing the chance of carrying the infection from one animal to another. It appears to be helpful also to dip the ends of the teats of all animals, immediately after milking, into a dilute solution of chlorine.

Badly diseased animals not only are a menace to other animals in the herd but usually are unprofitable to the owner because of the reduced milk yield caused by the disease. It is best to dispose of such animals. Campbell and Norcross (11) used complement-fixation and agar gel diffusion tests to detect antibodies against cellular antigens of *Str. agalactiae* in the colostrum of 20 first-calf heifers. None of the udders was infected with the organism at the time of sampling. This would indicate contact with *Str. agalactiae* at an early age even though there was no evidence of established infection.

**Immunity.** Vaccines of various kinds have been used for the treatment of bovine streptococcic mastitis. The reports are somewhat conflicting but it may safely be said that such products have been of little service. Fortunately it happens that the disease can rather readily be brought under control in any herd by hygienic means.

According to Smith (62), agglutinins for hematoxylin-stained *Str. agalactiae* antigen can be detected in infected cows by means of a milk ring test.

**Chemotherapy.** Many drugs and antibiotics have used singly or in combination to treat the inflamed bovine udder. These agents appear to be much more effective against the infections caused by *Str. agalactiae* than they are against those caused by other microorganisms (38). A large number of substances have met with varying measures of success in the therapy of streptococci mastitis, but of them all penicillin appears to be most effective. It is usually administered in infusions, although intramuscular injections are also recommended (46). Combinations of penicillin and polyvinylpyrrolidone (40) and penicillin and furacin (33) are credited with additive effects against *Str. agalactiae*. One of the problems of intramammary treatment of clinical mastitis has been the persistence of antibacterial agents in the milk. Various tests are now in use to detect the presence of such substances and determine when the milk is marketable (21, 31).

### Streptococcus dysgalactiae

This organism differs from *Str. agalactiae* only in minor cultural particulars, but the disease produced is quite different. It belongs to Lancefield's Group C. The chains usually are short or medium in length. The colonies are usually nonhemolytic, and they often show a distinct greenish discoloration. Litmus milk is not always coagulated in 48 hours at 37 C. Methylene blue milk, however, is regularly reduced. The final pH in glucose broth varies between 5.3 and 5.0. It never goes below 5.0. Sodium hippurate is not hydrolyzed. This is perhaps the best single test for differentiating this species from *Str. agalactiae*. **Pathogenesis.** Unlike *Str. agalactiae*, this species does not appear to spread gradually and insidiously. The infection is sporadic but apparently rather widespread. The onset of the disease usually is acute, and the disease is severe, though it often disappears after a time, frequently leaving a nonsecreting mammary gland in its wake. Unlike the *Str. agalactiae* type of infection, the disease cannot be eradicated from herds by careful hygienic procedures. The history of some of these cases indicates that the infection began in an injured teat.

### Streptococcus uberis

This organism differs from the previous one principally in the following details: It is nonhemolytic but may produce slight greening on blood agar; it is salicin- and esculin-positive and hippurate-positive. According to Seeley (59), a group antigen of *Str. uberis* has not been identified, and the organism is allied to the streptococci of the "viridans" division in this respect. *Str. uberis*, however, grows to some extent at 10 C, and all strains tested hydrolyze arginine; these reactions are unlike those of the "viridans" division, the defined members of which are largely negative on both counts.

The organism is less frequently encountered than the two species previously described and as a rule produces acute cases of mastitis that end in recovery after a short time.

The habitat of the organism is highly speculative. Cullen and Little (15) have isolated it from the rumen, lips, and rectum of cows and from soil samples from the field grazed by these animals. Gullen (29) found the skin of cows to be the most important reservoir of *Str. uberis*, the abdomen and lips being most heavily involved. Sweeney (65) stated that the coccus was an obligatory parasite of the udder surface and that this site serves as the most important reservoir for infections of the mammary gland parenchyma.

### Other Streptococci that Cause Mastitis

Streptococci of other types are sometimes encountered as causative agents in cases of bovine mastitis, although these are a small minority of the total number. It has already been mentioned that *Str. pyogenes* sometimes infects an udder, producing an acute mastitis that may be the source of severe and widespread outbreaks of scarlet fever and septic sore throat in people. Occasionally organisms belonging to Lancefield's Group C and classed among the "animal pyogenes" types appear in milk. These have a remarkable resemblance to the human type, and before the Lancefield typing method was introduced, such organisms caused milk "scares." Outbreaks of mastitis caused by hemolytic streptococci belonging to Lancefield's Group G have been reported in the United States and in Canada (4) and by members of Group E in Norway (50).

It should be stressed that many cases of bovine mastitis are caused by microorganisms other than streptococci. These are considered in their respective categories, as well as the presence of mastitis in animals other than the cow. The National Mastitis Council, Inc. (48), has prepared a guide *Microbiological procedures for the diagnosis of bovine mastitis* and the Mastitis Subcommittee of the Technical Development Committee (42) has presented information on its control.

**Chemotherapy.** Sensitivity tests should be used in order to select the most effective agent. Although penicillin usually is successful in treating streptococcic mastitis, the tests may show that other antibiotics such as tyrothrycin, terramycin, or aureomycin would be even more efficacious. In some cases combinations of penicillin and a sulfonamide, penicillin and nitrofurazone (5-nitro-2-furaldehyde semicarbazone), or other mixtures may be indicated.

### *Streptococcus equi*

This organism is regarded as the causative factor of a disease of young horses known as *strangles*. It is also found in suppurations in horses not clearly identified with strangles. It has been isolated from the abdominal lymph glands of burros where the clinical syndrome and lesions differed from those seen in strangles (73).

**Morphology and Staining Reactions.** *Str. equi* occurs in exudates and in fluid cultures in the form of long chains, exceptionally in short chains. Sometimes the chains are surrounded by definite capsular material. The organism is readily stained with the usual dyes and is Gram-positive when cultures are young. Old cultures retain the Gram stain poorly.

**Cultural Features.** This organism has a strong hemolytic toxin that causes it to show wide zones of Beta-type hemolysis around colonies on blood plates and to hemolyze blood cells suspended in broth cultures. Acid is formed from glucose, sucrose, maltose, and galactose. *Str. equi* does not ferment lactose and sorbitol, nor will it acidify milk. In these respects it differs from *Str. pyogenes*, on the one hand, and from the "animal pyogenes" types, on the other. Sodium hippurate is not hydrolyzed. It falls into Lancefield's Group C.

**Resistance.** *Str. equi* is said to be somewhat more resistant than most streptococci. Even though this may be, it is certain that it is rather easily destroyed by chemical disinfectants, by heat, and by drying.

**Pathogenicity.** *Str. equi* does not affect any of the domesticated animals, ex-

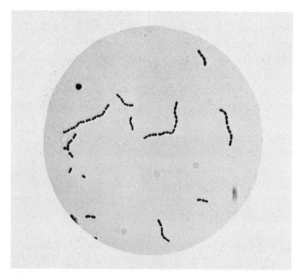

Fig. 30. Streptococcus equi, a stained film from a 24-hour-old serum broth culture. X 1,000.

cept members of the horse family, and it is nonpathogenic for man. When injected subcutaneously, recently isolated strains will kill white mice within a day or two with septicemia, and large doses may kill rabbits and guinea pigs. Older strains may produce pyemia in mice, with deaths after a week or more. When injected subcutaneously into horses, abscesses usually are produced. When inoculated intranasally with broth cultures in the log phase of growth typical strangles can be induced in horses (Bryans et al., 10).

In the natural disease, young animals usually are the victims. The disease begins with a respiratory infection, followed by swelling and abscessation of the lymph glands of the head and neck. Sometimes the infection spreads through the lymphatics to the forelegs and trunk, causing multiple abscesses. Occasionally abscessation of some of the internal lymph glands occurs, in which case the animal usually dies.

**Immunity.** Unlike most *Streptococcus* infections, one attack of strangles usually leaves the animal permanently immune. Bazeley (5) was the first to show that the 4- to 5-hour-old culture of a recently isolated strain of *Str. equi* is highly virulent and immunogenic. In this vigorously growing stage the organism has a large capsule, a high negative surface charge, and generally a diplococcal form. An older culture is deficient in these properties. Vaccination with organisms killed in the virulent phase produces a response identical to that conferred by a natural attack. Anti-*Streptococcus* serum, when administered early, often appears to lessen the severity of infections.

**Chemotherapy.** After the strangles abscesses have drained, clinical signs disappear. For this reason some authors feel that the use of antibiotics or sulfonamides, especially in well developed cases, to suppress or retard abscessation may be contraindicated (22).

## Other Hemolytic Streptococci of Animals

Hemolytic streptococci of Lancefield's Groups B, C, F, G, and O are also found in infections of man. In diseases of animals, members of Group C are common and organisms of Groups E, L, M, and P occur. Krantz and Dunne (34) obtained all of Lancefield's groups, except H from cattle, and B from swine. Cultures from domestic animals yielded hemolytic as well as nonhemolytic streptococci.

Group C contains strains that are of both human (*Str. equisimilis*) and animal origin (*Str. zooepidemicus* or Sherman's "animal pyogenes type" and *Str. equi*, an equine-adapted type). The members of this group are distinguished by their biochemical behavior (see table XIV, p. 292).

Dimock and Edwards (18) studied a large series of hemolytic streptococci of animal origin in 1933. Exclusive of *Str. equi*, 96 percent of their strains were indistinguishable from each other. These strains originated in infections of horses, cows, chickens, foxes, rabbits, and guinea pigs. They were remarkably like *Str. pyogenes* and undoubtedly have been mistaken for this species in the past. It was shown that these organisms fermented sorbitol and failed to ferment trehalose, whereas *Str. pyogenes* and *Str. equisimilis* did the reverse. Apparently the animal-type organisms of Group C are harmless to man. How dangerous they are to animals is not fully known. One organism belonging to this subgroup is *Str. genitalium*, which produces metritis and cervicitis in breeding mares and causes many mares to become barren and others to abort. According to Dimock, Edwards, and Bruner (19), this organism accounted for 17 percent of the equine abortions in Kentucky as well as for 25 percent of the deaths of foals. Of all the bacteria causing infections encountered in a study of the breeding problems of the equine species, this microorganism occupies the most prominent place. Anaerobic streptococci and a motile *Streptococcus* (8) of Lancefield's Group D were involved in equine abortions on rare occasions.

It has been established that *Str. equisimilis* will infect swine, producing bone lesions (55); that *Str. zooepidemicus* will cause mastitis in this species, and that Group E streptococci (1, 17, 74) are especially common in swine cervical abscesses (lymphadenitis, jowl abscess).

Another organism of the *Str. zooepidemicus* subgroup, which sometimes causes acute, fatal septicemia in chickens, is known as *Str. gallinarum*. The disease is called *apoplectiform septicemia*. An outbreak of this infection in a flock of White Rock chickens was reported by Peckham (51) in 1966.

Hemolytic streptococci are often found in virus infections of the upper respiratory tract of chicks and adult birds. These presumably belong to the "animal pyogenes" type, although Edwards studied one such organism that conformed to the human rather than the animal type. We have encountered *Str. agalactiae*, *Str. dysgalactiae*, and *Str. uberis* among bacterial isolates from chickens.

## THE NONHEMOLYTIC STREPTOCOCCI OF ANIMALS

A great many organisms of rather diverse characteristics are included under this heading. About the only things that they have in common are a similarity in morphology, a low degree or an absence of pathogenic power, and an inability to produce a soluble hemolysin. It has already been pointed out that many members of this group are capable of causing a slight hemolysis on blood plates because of acid production. Some of them (viridans group) induce chemical changes in blood cells which cause them to take on a greenish discoloration. This phenomenon is usually more marked in cooked blood media than in those in which fresh blood is used, and, in many instances, the phenomenon is seen only when the blood has been cooked.

According to Lancefield, most nonhemolytic streptociocci do not contain polysaccharide group antigens such as have been found in the hemolytic streptococci. However, it is possible to classify some of these nonhemolytic types with the Beta types on the basis of antigenic analysis. Certain others, lacking the polysaccharide group antigens of the hemolytic streptococci, can be recognized as specific serological types that fit within their own species. Sherman, Niven, and Smiley (61), using the precipitation technic, found that strains of Str. salivarius (Alpha type) fall into two main types and an unknown number of other types.

Organisms belonging in the nonhemolytic group are found on many normal mucous membranes, on the skin, in many animal products, and occasionally elsewhere. They are frequently found in inflammatory conditions in all species of animals, including man. Most of these processes cannot be inititated by inoculation with pure cultures. It is assumed, therefore, that in most instances these organisms are playing a secondary role. However, Van Dorssen (70) isolated an Alpha Streptococcus from cases of spontaneous metritis in mink and with it induced abortion of pregnant guinea pigs, and Friedlander et al. (25) demonstrated that organisms of the Alpha type caused a high incidence rate of polyarthritis in albino rats and mice when injected intravenously. Brunson, Fehr, and Davis (9) studied cardiac lesions in rabbits caused by Streptococcus viridans. In an outbreak of infectious arthritis in calves, Van Pelt et al. (71) found the most frequent isolate from the suppurative synovial fluid to be an Alpha-type Streptococcus.

### Streptococcus salivarius

This organism, of which there are numerous varieties, is found as a normal inhabitant of the human mouth. It may also be found in human feces, probably as a survivor from the oral cavity. Apparently a large percentage of the viridans type of streptococci found in human infections belong to this group. Many strains give a strong Alpha reaction on blood media; others are weak or give no reaction. These organisms form a large amount of acid from glucose, and acidulate and coagulate milk promptly. Most strains ferment raffinose and some, inulin. Esculin frequently is attacked. *Streptococcus mitis* of many authors is closely related to, or is a variety of, this organism.

### Streptococcus bovis

This organism is always present in the mouths and intestinal tracts of cattle and, because of fecal contamination, is usually present in milk, where it may be mistaken for *Str. agalactiae*. So far as is known, this species has no pathogenicity for cattle. An organism very closely related to *Str. bovis* has been found in the intestinal tract of man, and some have thought that it played an etiological role in ulcerative colitis. This species is able to grow at relatively high temperatures and has unusual thermal resistance. Like *Str. salivarius*, it usually ferments raffinose and inulin. Most strains actively hydrolyze starch, an unusual characteristic of streptococci. It does not hydrolyze sodium hippurate but does attack esculin, characteristics that differentiate it from the streptococci of bovine mastitis.

### Streptococcus equinus

This organism is always abundantly present in the feces of horses. It was first isolated from air, undoubtedly because of the presence of dried horse manure, a situation which was formerly common enough in most cities. A striking characteristic of this organism is its inability to ferment lactose. It will be remembered that this also is true of *Str. equi*. It does not grow well in milk and does not cause coagulation. It does not grow at temperatures lower than 20 C. *Str. equinus* is not known to be pathogenic for animals.

### Streptococcus lactis

This organism has no pathogenic properties, but because of its omnipresence in milk and milk products pathologists should be able to recognize it and differentiate it from other organisms that may be responsible for disease. *Str. lactis* is the common milk-souring organism. In sour milk it usually occurs in short chains, whereas most pathogenic streptococci form long chains. This is a fact that is of considerable differential value; however, it is not always a safe rule to follow. In culture media, particularly those that contain serum, this organism often forms long chains. A characteristic that has long been recognized is its rapid growth in milk. If litmus or other reducible dyes are present, the dye is reduced before coagulation occurs. The milk-souring *Streptococcus* grows at relatively low temperatures, and also at relatively high temperatures. Reduction and coagulation of litmus milk will occur at temperatures as low as 10 C. Esculin is almost always attacked.

The normal habitat of *Str. lactis* long has been a mystery. Many workers have shown that it is not found in milk drawn aseptically from the udder; neither is it found in the mouths or intestines of cattle. Stark and Sherman have succeeded in isolating typical strains from certain plants. Perhaps it is from such sources that initial invasion of dairies occurs. Once established in a dairy or milk plant, it flourishes and, being quite heat resistant, maintains itself on the utensils and equipment.

### Streptococcus cremoris

This organism is closely related to *Str. lactis*. It usually forms longer chains, produces less acid, and is less heat-resistant than the usual milk-souring organism. It is sometimes used in commercial "starters" either alone or with *Str. lactis*. It has not been identified elsewhere than in milk and milk products.

### The Enterococci

The term enterococcus has long been used by French workers to designate a group of streptococci that normally occurs in the intestine of man. They have been employed as indicator organisms of fecal contamination, but their isolation from plants (44) and grass silage (37) has undermined their value for this purpose. The most important of these organisms is *Str. fecalis*. It is known to occur in the intestines of several of the domestic animals as well as of man. There is some disagreement as to the exact classification of the types of enterococci. At present we will consider *Str. liquefaciens* to be a variant of *Str. fecalis* that liquefies gelatin, and *Str. zymogenes* and *Str. durans* to be Beta-hemolytic variants of *Str. fecalis*. Deibel (16) considers *Str. fecalis* to be made up of two species, *Str. fecalis* and *Str. faecium* with *Str. durans* classed as a variety of the latter.

Enterococci are characterized by great hardiness. Sherman separated them from other streptococci on the basis of their ability to grow in the presence of high concentrations of salt (6.5 percent NaCl) and in very alkaline media (pH 9.6). They grow through a wide temperature range (10 to 45 C) and thrive in the presence of 0.1 percent methylene blue. All enterococci belong to Lancefield's Group D. In addition the presence of this antigen has been demonstrated in *Str. bovis* and *Str. equinus*, but they are considered to be separate entities because they give opposite reactions to the biochemical tests listed above. Motile streptococci are usually considered to be a rarity, but Graudal (27) states that they are not uncommon among the enterococci.

Enterococci generally are regarded as harmless for man and animals but have been found in pathogenic processes, especially in subacute bacterial endocarditis (60). A member of this group was reported to be associated with both local and generalized infections in nutria (52).

In 1967, Nowlan and Deibel (49) described the Group Q streptococci. These organisms have unique serological and physiological characteristics, but possess the Group D antigen. They differ from established enterococcal species in failing to hydrolyze arginine or to initiate growth in 0.1 percent methylene blue milk. They are less active in fermenting carbohydrates. The species name *Streptococcus avium* was suggested to indicate their characteristic occurrence in chicken fecal specimens.

## IMMUNITY TO *STREPTOCOCCUS* INFECTIONS

As a general rule, recovery from *Streptococcus* infections does not confer immunity. Various workers have found it difficult to immunize animals effectively with heat-killed cultures; likewise there was little encouragement in the earlier work in which culture filtrates were used. In 1924, however, the Dicks demonstrated that the scarlet fever *Streptococcus* produced a potent toxin that could be neutralized with specific antitoxin, and this finding led to new interest in the subject. Antitoxic sera for use against those streptococci that produce soluble toxins (*Str. pyogenes* group) apparently have value when given to patients in very early stages of the infection, but they have not proved wholly satisfactory. Against the streptococci that do not form soluble toxins, immune sera are of very doubtful value. What value they may have is probably measured by their opsonic content.

Massell *et al.* (41) have presented evidence that the use of type 3 streptococcal M protein in vaccinating healthy siblings of human patients with rheumatic fever may induce rather than prevent the disease. Heat-killed and living cultures of *Str. agalactiae* have been used both for prophylaxis and cure of bovine streptococcic mastitis. There are conflicting reports on the efficacy of these products, but it is quite certain that their value is very limited. The *Str. equi* bacterin of Bazeley (5) described under that organism has merit, and the administration of streptococcal bacterin to pregnant sows may help in controlling abscess formation of piglets (14).

## CHEMOTHERAPY OF *STREPTOCOCCUS* INFECTIONS

It is firmly established that sulfanilamide is highly successful in treating human hemolytic *Streptococcus* infections. Many antibiotic substances have been tried in treating these infections and have proved to be highly successful. Where possible, sensitivity tests should be used in selecting the most effective chemotherapeutic agent. Among the agents recommended in treating streptococcic infections are penicillin, bacitracin, aureomycin, terramycin, and erythromycin.

Combinations of penicillin and the sulfonamides have proved effective in treating certain infections caused by streptococci. Penicillin and sulfamethazine are used in treating streptococcic metritis in mares, and penicillin combined with streptomycin has produced good results in eliminating mixed infections caused by streptococci and Gram-negative bacteria. The enterococci appear to be more resistant to the action of the antibiotics and sulfa compounds than do the other streptococci. There are reports (67) indicating that ampicillin, penicillin G, and vancomycin are the most effective agents against the enterococci and that synergistic action is obtained by combining streptomycin with ampicillin or with vancomycin.

## REFERENCES

1. Armstrong, Boehm, and Ellis.   Am. Jour. Vet. Res., 1970, *31*, 823.
2. Avery and Cullen.   Jour. Exp. Med., 1919, *29*, 215.
3. Ayers and Rupp.   Jour. Inf. Dis., 1922, *30*, 388.
4. Barnum and Fuller.   Canad. Jour. Comp. Med. and Vet. Sci., 1953, *17*, 465.
5. Bazeley.   Austral. Vet. Jour., 1943, *19*, 62.
6. Boissard and Wormald.   Jour. Path. and Bact., 1950, *62*, 37.
7. Bruner.   North Am. Vet., 1949, *30*, 243.
8. Bruner, Edwards, Doll, and Moran.   Cornell Vet., 1948, *38*, 313.
9. Brunson, Fehr, and Davis.   Am. Jour. Path., 1957, *33*, 977.
10. Bryans, Doll, and Shephard.   Cornell Vet., 1964, *54*, 198.
11. Campbell and Norcross.   Am. Jour. Vet. Res., 1964, *25*, 993.
12. Christie, Atkins, and Munch-Petersen.   Austral. Jour. Exp. Biol. and Med. Sci., 1944, *22*, 197.
13. Collier.   Jour. Am. Vet. Med. Assoc., 1956, *129*, 543.
14. Conner, Hoefer, and Ellis.   *Ibid.*, 1965, *147*, 479.
15. Cullen and Little.   Vet. Rec., 1969, *84*, 115.
16. Deibel.   Bact. Rev., 1964, *28*, 330.
17. Deibel, Yao, Jacobs, and Niven, Jr.   Jour. Inf. Dis., 1964, *114*, 327.
18. Dimock and Edwards.   Ky. Agr. Exp. Sta. Bul. 338, 1933.
19. Dimock, Edwards, and Bruner.   Cornell Vet., 1947, *37*, 89.
20. Dudding, Dillon, Wannamaker, Kilton, Chapman, and Anthony.   Jour. Inf. Dis., 1969, *120*, 225.
21. Eberhart, Watrous, Hokanson, and Burch.   Jour. Am. Vet. Med. Assoc., 1963, *143*, 390.
22. Ebert.   Vet. Med., 1969, *64*, 71.
23. Edwards.   Jour. Bact., 1932, *23*, 259.
24. Feller and Stevens.   Jour. Lab. and Clin. Med., 1952, *39*, 484.
25. Friedlander, Habermann, and Parr.   Jour. Inf. Dis., 1951, *88*, 298.
26. Gochnauer and Wilson.   Jour. Bact., 1951, *62*, 405.
27. Graudal.   Acta Path. et Microbiol. Scand., 1952, *31*, 46.
28. *Ibid.*, 1957, *41*, 397.
29. Gullen.   Brit. Vet. Jour., 1966, *122*, 333.
30. Halbert and Auerbach.   Jour. Exp. Med., 1961, *113*, 131.
31. Hokanson, Watrous, Burch, and Eberhart.   Jour. Am. Vet. Med. Assoc., 1963, *143*, 395.
32. Jelliffe and Reed.   Jour. Trop. Med. and Hyg. (London), 1953, *56*, 33.
33. Kakavas, Roberts, de Courcy, and Ewing.   Jour. Am. Vet. Med. Assoc., 1951, *119*, 203.
34. Krantz and Dunne.   Am. Jour. Vet. Res., 1965, *26*, 951.
35. Kvittingen.   Acta Path. et Microbiol. Scand., 1968, *74*, 143.
36. Lancefield.   Jour. Exp. Med., 1933, *57*, 571.
37. Langston, Gutierrez, and Bouma.   Jour. Bact., 1960, *80*, 714.
38. Little and Plastridge.   Bovine mastitis. McGraw-Hill Book Co., New York and London, 1946.
39. MacKnight, Ellis, Jensen, and Franz.   Appl. Microbiol., 1969, *17*, 926.
40. McAuliff, Phillips, and Steele.   Jour. Am. Vet. Med. Assoc., 1958, *133*, 169.

41. Massell, Honikman, and Amezcua. Jour. Am. Med. Assoc., 1969, *207*, 1115.
42. Mastitis Subcommittee of the Technical Development Committee. Vet. Rec., 1965, *77*, 612.
43. Moeberg and Thal. Nord. Vetmed., 1954, *6*, 69.
44. Mundt. Appl. Microbiol., 1963, *11*, 141.
45. Murphy and Hanson. Cornell Vet., 1941, *31*, 47.
46. Murphy and Stuart. *Ibid.*, 1954, *44*, 139.
47. Murphy, Stuart, and Reed. Vet. Rec., 1952, *64*, 133.
48. National Mastitis Council, Inc. Microbiological procedures for the diagnosis of Bovine mastitis. Washington: The Author, 1969.
49. Nowlan and Deibel. Jour. Bact., 1967, *94*, 291.
50. Olsen. Jour. Am. Vet. Med. Assoc., 1957, *130*, 338.
51. Peckham. Avian Dis., 1966, *10*, 413.
52. Pridham and Thackeray. Canad. Jour. Comp. Med. and Vet. Sci., 1959, *23*, 81.
53. Quinn and Lowry. Appl. Microbiol., 1969, *17*, 412.
54. Redys, Parzick, and Borman. Pub. Health Rpts. (U.S.), 1963, *78*, 222.
55. Roberts, Ramsey, Switzer, and Layton. Am. Jour. Vet. Res., 1967, *28*, 1677.
56. Rosenbach. Mikroorganismen bei den Wundinfektionskrankheiten des Menschen. J. F. Bergmann, Wiesbaden, 1884.
57. Schalm and Noorlander. Jour. Am. Vet. Med. Assoc., 1957, *130*, 199.
58. Schottmüller. Münch. med. Wchnschr., 1903, *50*, 849.
59. Seeley. Jour. Bact., 1951, *62*, 107.
60. Sherman. Bact. Rev., 1937, *1*, 1.
61. Sherman, Niven, and Smiley. Jour. Bact., 1943, *45*, 249.
62. Smith. Jour. Comp. Path. and Therap., 1954, *64*, 1.
63. Smith and Brown. Jour. Med. Res., 1915, *31*, 455.
64. Snoeyenbos, Bachman, and Wilson. Jour. Am. Vet. Med. Assoc., 1952, *120*, 134.
65. Sweeney. Res. Vet. Sci., 1964, *5*, 483.
66. Tillett and Garner. Jour. Exp. Med., 1933, *58*, 485.
67. Toala, McDonald, Wilcox, and Finland. Am. Jour. Med. Sci., 1969, *258*, 416.
68. Topley and Wilson. Principles of bacteriology and immunity. 3d ed. Williams and Wilkins Co., Baltimore, 1946.
69. Tuomi and Nurmi. Acta Vet. Scand., 1964, *5*, 50.
70. Van Dorssen. Jour. Comp. Path. and Therap., 1954, *64*, 94.
71. Van Pelt, Langham, and Sleight. Jour. Am. Vet. Med. Assoc., 1966, *149*, 303.
72. Wenner, Gibson, and Jaques. Proc. Soc. Exp. Biol. and Med., 1951, *76*, 585.
73. Wisecup, Schroder, and Page. Jour. Am. Vet. Med. Assoc., 1967, *150*, 303.
74. Yae, Jacobs, Deibel, and Niven, Jr. Jour. Inf. Dis., 1964, *114*, 333.

# XVIII | The *Corynebacteriaceae*

The members of the family *Corynebacteriaceae* that are important as animal pathogens fall in three genera—*Corynebacterium, Listeria,* and *Erysipelothrix.* They are Gram-positive, pleomorphic rods.

## THE GENUS *CORYNEBACTERIUM*

Within the genus *Corynebacterium* we find a large number of species, frequently referred to as the *diptheroid bacilli* because their morphology is similar to that of *Corynebacterium diptheriae,* the cause of human diphtheria and the type species of the group.

All diptheroid bacilli are Gram-positive, at least when the cells are young, and they show a rather high degree of pleomorphism. Pathogenic members of the genus *Corynebacterium* are nonmotile, but certain apparently harmless species found in the soil are motile (6). When stained with polychrome dyes or methylene blue, most species show granules and beading. The cells often are definitely clublike in form, i.e., they are swollen at one or both ends. In both tissues and cultures they tend to form masses in which the cells are arranged in parallel or palisade formation, an arrangement that is not common in any other type of bacteria except the acid-fast organisms. The cells of many species resemble some of the acid-fast bacteria in morphology as well, but diphtheroid organisms are never acid-fast. It is true that organisms in the genera *Corynebacterium, Mycobacterium,* and *Nocardia* possess a common type of cell-wall structure (8).

### *Corynebacterium pyogenes*

This organism is the most frequent pus-forming organism in cattle, swine, and sheep. It has been found in other animals occasionally. It rarely affects man.

308

**Morphology and Staining Reactions.** *C. pyogenes* most often occurs as small slender rods, which frequently are slightly curved and often clubbed at one end. The individual elements are usually short, and some strains form chains that are hard to distinguish from streptococci. There is great variation in morphology between different strains, and between individual cells of a single strain. The organism is nonmotile and never forms a capsule. It is Gram-positive.

**Cultural Features.** Ordinarily there is no growth on plain agar or in plain broth unless a considerable amount of blood, tissue, or tissue debris is carried over in the inoculum. It grows readily in milk, which is coagulated within 48 hours. The curd slowly dissolves although the medium remains acid. Growth occurs readily on coagulated serum slants. Along the line of growth a trough of liquefaction develops.

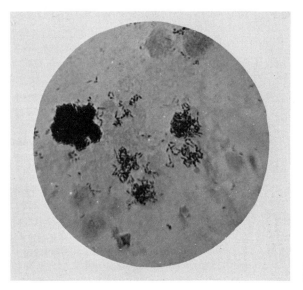

*Fig. 31. Corynebacterium py-ogenes,* a film from vegetations on the heart valve of a calf. X 1,000.

A few drops of blood or blood serum make all of the usual laboratory media favorable for the growth of this organism. In fluid media the growth is granular and sinks to the bottom of the tube. In blood broth a layer of brownish-red pigmentation appears above the layer of sedimented blood cells. This is caused by the liberation of hemoglobin as a result of the hemolytic activity of the organism.

On blood agar plates the organism behaves very characteristically. Even after several days' incubation the colonies are very small and translucent. After 18 hours' incubation at 37 C they may easily be overlooked, for at that time there is no evidence of hemolysis. At about 24 hours, hemolysis of the Beta type begins to be evident, and this makes them conspicuous. These zones are exceedingly clear but always narrow, seldom exceeding 2 mm in diameter.

In suitable basic media, glucose, lactose, sucrose, maltose, galactose, and xylose are fermented; mannitol, raffinose, salicin, and inulin are not attacked. Gas is never formed.

Growth occurs best at body temperature. The minimum temperature of growth is about 24 C. The organism is aerobic and facultative anaerobic. Indol, hydrogen sulfide, and nitrites are not produced. Gelatin is liquefied. An excellent description is that of Brown and Orcutt, 1920 (4).

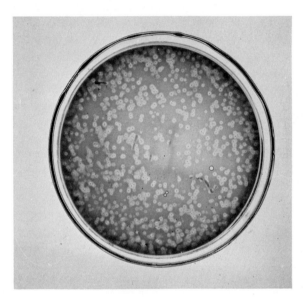

Fig. 32. *Corynebacterium pyogenes,* a blood agar plate incubated for 36 hours at 37 C. The colonies may be discerned as minute points surrounded by narrow zones of Beta-type hemolysis. Blood plates incubated overnight may have numerous colonies on them, but they are likely to be overlooked unless they are inspected with great care because the hemolytic zones at that time have not appeared. At about 24 hours' incubation the hemolytic zones begin to appear, but they are not well developed until about 36 hours.

Ryff and Browne (14) have claimed that the adaption of *C. pyogenes* to growth on unenriched media reduces its ability to digest coagulated blood serum and gelatin but enhances its fermentative activity. They also indicated that the various strains of this organism show a close serological relationship. Afnan (1) described a strain derived from bovine mastitis that appeared to be *C. pyogenes,* but a subsequent examination revealed that it produced catalase, reduced nitrate, and showed a CAMPlike phenomenon, properties not possessed by typical cultures of *C. pyogenes.*

**Resistance.** *C. pyogenes* is a very delicate organism. It is easily destroyed by heat, drying, and ordinary disinfectants.

**Pathogenicity for Experimental Animals.** Guinea pigs, rats, and mice are quite resistant to infection. Subcutaneous injections of cultures result in the formation of abscesses, which usually develop slowly and become well encapsulated.

Rabbits are most susceptible. After intravenous injection no immediate effects are seen, but in 2 or 3 weeks the animals begin to lose weight and may become lame or paralyzed. Abscesses may develop in the kidneys, lymph nodes, or the muscular tissue, but more often they are found in the bones or joints. Paralysis usually is caused by the formation of an abscess in the vertebral column, which brings pressure to bear on the spinal cord.

According to Gwatkin (10), the superficial injection of a pure culture into the tongue of a calf resulted in the formation of a hard lump in the tissue beneath the inoculated area. This was accompanied by erosion of the mucous membrane and extrusion of pus. Rubbing the organisms on the tongue produced no lesions.

**The Natural Disease.** *In cattle.* C. *pyogenes* can be found in a great variety of suppurative conditions in cattle. Abscesses caused by this organism usually develop slowly and often have heavy fibrotic capsules. The pus may be thick, greenish white, and nonodorous, or it may be thin and fetid, especially when other organisms are associated with C. *pyogenes*. Cardiac valvular vegetations are frequently associated with this organism. Some lesions develop as granulomatous tumors that resemble, and often are diagnosed as, actinomycosis. See Magnusson (12), Vawter (15), and Davies (9).

This organism is nearly always found in necrotic and suppurating pneumonias in cattle, presumably as a secondary invader in most cases. It may cause generalized disease in cattle (7). It often causes destructive arthritis in calves. It causes sporadic cases of mastitis, some of which are acute and are followed by recovery, while others become chronic and lead to much tissue destruction and even sloughing of large portions of the gland. In many European countries the disease is seen most often during the summer months in dry cows and heifers on pasture and is therefore called *summer mastitis* (Bean, Miller, and Heishman, 3). In 1954 Weaver (16) surveyed the so-called *summer mastitis* in England and concluded that it was impossible to distinguish clinically between the disease caused by C. *pyogenes* and other forms of acute mastitis.

In the United States the infection is seen at all times of the year and more often in lactating than in dry cows. The organism sometimes causes much damage to the immature udders of young calves that are kept together and develop a habit of suckling each other. In these animals secondary infections of the joints frequently result in suppurative arthritis, which usually leads to death of the animals. Umbilical infections often occur in calves, usually leading to death.

C. *pyogenes* is very frequently found in purulent metritis in cattle, usually in association with staphylococci.

*In swine.* The character and location of the lesions in swine are much like those in cattle. Generally in association with other pyogenic organisms, it is commonly found in suppurative pneumonias and, in fact, in nearly all suppurative conditions. Multiple joint involvement not infrequently occurs as a part of these infections. This often appears after farrowing, which probably means that uterine infections are the primary localizations. Stiffness of gait, lameness, progressive cachexia, pneumonia, and paralysis of the hindquarters are often seen.

*In sheep and goats.* Chronic purulent pneumonia and joint infections of sheep resulting in acute lameness are frequently caused by this organism. It is associated with much connective tissue formation and with pleurisy, accompanied by an ill-smelling pleural exudate. Abroad this condition is often called *pyobacillosis*. See Jowett (11).

Cameron and Britton (5) have described a type of *C. pyogenes* infection in sheep fed upon large amounts of grain, especially barley, in which bilateral deep-seated chronic abscesses developed in the larynx. It was believed to be caused by abrasions due to the gulping of the grain. Affected lambs breathe with great difficulty and the mortality rate is high.

The organism also affects goats where it is most often seen in cases of mastitis, in fact it may be considered to be one of the most common causes of mastitis in this species of animal.

*In other animals.* Zaki and Farrag (17) have reported *C. pyogenes* to be a rare cause of metritis in the horse and of pyometritis in the dog. It is commonly associated with pneumonia in the camel and has been isolated from traumatic reticulitis in the buffalo and from septicemias as well as from suppurative lesions in birds held in captivity.

**Mode of Transmission.** It is presumed that this organism is a natural inhabitant of normal mucous membranes. Ochi and Zaizen (13) found organisms very similar to *C. pyogenes* on many of the mucous membranes of normal cattle and guinea pigs, but these organisms were less proteolytic and less hemolytic than those found in infectious processes; hence they gave them the name of *C. pseudo-pyogenes*. Certainly, typical cultures of *C. pyogenes* can be found in superficial inflammations of the mucosae of the intestinal and genitourinary tracts of both cattle and swine, an indication that the organism is commonly present at such sites.

**Diagnosis.** The presence of *C. pyogenes* in inflammatory exudates can best be demonstrated by making cultures on blood agar plates. These should be incubated not less than 36 hours at 37 C unless other organisms threaten to overrun the plate. The minute colonies, surrounded by sharp, clear, narrow zones of hemolysis, are quite distinctive. Such colonies should be picked and transferred to blood agar slants. The subcultures can be identified by their action on litmus milk and especially by their ability to liquefy solidified blood serum slants.

**Immunity.** Little is known about immunity to this organism. There are no biological products available for use against it.

**Chemotherapy.** Although *C. pyogenes* is quite sensitive to penicillin and some of the other antibiotics *in vitro*, it usually will not respond *in vivo*. This is probably due to the tissue reaction, which walls off the organism and makes it inaccessible to antibiotics.

**The Disease in Man.** Ballard *et al.* (2) described a case of *C. pyogenes* infection in man in which the organism invaded tissue already weakened and damaged by frostbite. According to their article, this was the second reported case of human infection caused by this organism.

## REFERENCES

1. Afnan.   Vet. Rec., 1970, *86*, 229.
2. Ballard, Upsher, and Seely.   Am. Jour. Clin. Path., 1947, *17*, 209.
3. Bean, Miller, and Heishman.   Jour. Am. Vet. Med. Assoc., 1943, *103*, 200.
4. Brown and Orcutt.   Jour. Exp. Med., 1920, *32*, 219.
5. Cameron and Britton.   Cornell Vet., 1943, *33*, 265.
6. Clark and Carr.   Jour. Bact., 1951, *62*, 1.
7. Cowie.   Vet. Rec., 1962, *74*, 258.
8. Cummins.   Am. Rev. Resp. Dis., 1965, *92*(II), 63.
9. Davies.   Jour. Comp. Path. and Therap., 1930, *43*, 147.
10. Gwatkin.   Canad. Jour. Comp. Med. and Vet. Sci., 1952, *16*, 422.
11. Jowett.   Jour. Comp. Path. and Therap., 1930, *43*, 109.
12. Magnusson.   Acta Path. et Microbiol. Scand., 1928, *5*, 170.
13. Ochi and Zaizen.   Jour. Jap. Soc. Vet. Sci., 1936, *15*, 13; 1937, *16*, 8.
14. Ryff and Browne.   Am. Jour. Vet. Res., 1954, *15*, 617.
15. Vawter.   Cornell Vet., 1933, *23*, 126.
16. Weaver.   Vet. Rec., 1955, *67*, 735.
17. Zaki and Farrag.   Vet. Med., 1955, *50*, 219.

### *Corynebacterium renale*

SYNONYMS:   *Bacillus renalis bovis, Bacillus pyelonephritidis bovis*

This organism is found principally in cattle, but it also has been seen in horses and sheep, and one case has been described in a dog (11). Female animals are affected much more commonly than males (2). It has been found only in the urinary tract, where it produces a diphtheritic inflammation of the urinary bladder, or the ureters, of the kidney pelvis, and frequently of the kidney tissue itself (4). The lesions are characteristic and are quite alike in the several species affected. The disease is known under several different names: bacillary pyelonephritis of cattle, specific pyelonephritis of cattle, infectious pyelonephritis of cattle.

**Morphology and Staining Reactions.** *C. renale* is a rather large diphtheroid bacillus. Individual organisms do not vary greatly in morphology, all being rather short stumpy rods that usually are a little thicker at one end than at the other. In exudates and in cultures the organisms are found in clumps varying from a few cells to many hundreds. It is nonmotile, non-sporebearing, and nonencapsulated. It is strongly Gram-positive and stains readily with the usual stains. Bars and granules are sometimes seen when stained with methylene blue.

**Cultural Features.** Growth occurs in all of the ordinary laboratory media, but it is greatly favored by a little blood or serum. For isolation purposes blood plates are most convenient. After 24 hours' incubation at 37 C, *C. renale* colonies may be seen as minute opaque bodies. After 48 hours the colonies become larger than those of streptococci, but smaller than those of staphylococci. The older colonies are opaque and ivory-colored, and the margins are uneven. Their surfaces are quite dull in appearance. There is no action upon the blood cells.

In broth and other liquid media there may be slight clouding, but most of the growth appears in the form of a granular sediment. A quite characteristic reaction is seen in litmus milk. It begins with the reduction of the litmus in the bottom of the tube, followed by the formation of a soft curd, which is slowly digested. The medium is alkaline at all times. Finally the medium is reduced to a fluid with a Burgundy wine color and a heavy sediment in the bottom.

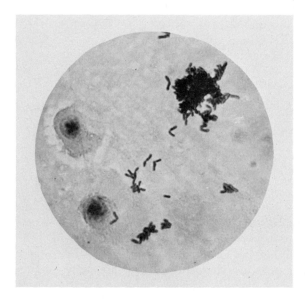

Fig. 33. Corynebacterium renale, a film from urine of a naturally infected cow. X 1,000.

Lovell (8) has called attention to a characteristic reaction of *C. renale* when it is grown on agar in plates to which 10 percent sterilized skim milk has been added. The colonies develop with a cream-to-yellow pigmentation, and after 48 hours each colony is surrounded by a wide halo or zone of translucency. Later these zones become indistinct, so they should be examined at the proper time. Apparently they are caused by digestion of the suspended casein molecules. The reaction is not diagnostic, but it is given by most strains of *C. renale* and seldom by other diphtheroids; hence it has diagnostic value.

Coagulated blood serum and gelatin support good growth of this organism, but neither medium is softened or liquefied. Growth on potato is fairly abundant. At first the color is dull and grayish; later it is somewhat cream-colored and dry in appearance.

Of the usual carbohydrates employed for differential purposes, only glucose is fermented by most strains. There is no gas formation. In media devoid of fermentable sugar considerable alkali is produced. Good growth occurs in sterile bovine urine, and the reaction becomes strongly alkaline because of the production of ammonia from urea. It has long been known that this organism is a powerful urea splitter and that the urine of infected animals is always strongly alkaline for this reason. It is quite certain that at least part of the bladder irritation seen in this disease is caused by the ammoniacal fermentation of the urine in the bladder. Christensen's urea medium, commonly used by bacteriologists studying the enteric organisms to differentiate the organisms belonging to the *Proteus* group, is useful in testing strains of this organism for ability to split urea.

Feenstra, Thorp, and Clark (6) studied 19 strains of diphtheroid organisms from cases of pyelonephritis in cattle. Thirteen of these strains conformed to the descriptions of *C. renale*, but six differed in several particulars. They concluded, "It seems likely that there are two distinct species of corynebacteria involved as etiological agents in infectious bovine pyelonephritis, although heretofore only one has been described." This may have been true, but it did not accord with the experience of most other workers. The strains were isolated from tissues and urine of infected animals. It is possible that the atypical strains were not the etiological agents of the disease processes with which they were associated. That more than one serotype exists was confirmed by Yanagawa *et al.* (12), in 1967. They extracted antigenic fractions from cells of *C. renale* and divided 78 strains into three types; all isolates from cattle falling in type III.

**Resistance.** No records of resistance tests have been found. Laboratory strains die out quite easily, however, so it is safe to say that its resistance to physical and chemical factors is not great.

**Pathogenicity for Experimental Animals.** *C. renale* is only slightly virulent for laboratory animals. Enderlen (3) produced pyelonephritis in two rabbits by injecting large doses of bacterial suspensions intravenously after ligating the ureters. He, and many others, failed to induce infections in this species and in guinea pigs by other methods. Lovell and Cotchin (9) were successful in infecting some of a series of white mice by intravenous injection. Attempts to produce the disease in cattle have usually failed when the organisms have been given by routes other than the urinogenital tract. When cultures are injected into the urinary bladder by way of the urethra, success is not always attained but the disease unquestionably has been established in this way by several groups of workers, such as Jones and Little (7) and Feenstra, Clark, and Thorp (5). Earlier there was controversy over the question of whether the disease was hematogenous in origin or strictly localized in the urinary tract, which was invaded through the urethra. It is now agreed by most students that the evidence strongly favors the second hypothesis. The fact that the disease is much more common in cows than in bulls is in accord with this conception, the shorter and wider urethra of the cow favoring the entrance of the infecting organism from the outside.

**The Natural Disease.** In natural infections the urinary bladder is always involved, one or both ureters in most cases, and usually one or both kidneys (1). The walls of affected bladders are thickened and the mucosa is superficially ulcerated and covered with a slimy secretion mixed with shreds of tissue and fibrin. Petechiae and larger hemorrhages are usually present in the bladder wall, and small clots of blood often are found in the bladder content. The affected ureters become enormously distended, and the mucosa usually contains necrotic areas, or is necrotic in its entirety. The kidneys often are greatly enlarged, and in extreme cases most of the kidney substance may undergo necrosis. More often the kidney pelvis is found to be enlarged, the papillae are necrotic, and abscesses occur throughout the kidney structure. The content of the affected pelvis consists of a grayish, slimy, nonodorous exudate, mixed with fibrin, small blood clots, necrotic tissue, and calcareous material.

Great numbers of the characteristic diphtheroid bacilli may be found both free and bound in the fragments of necrotic tissue in this exudate. These generally occur in clumps, arranged in palisade and radiating fashion. Quite often streptococci are found in this exudate also.

The urine, which is voided in small amounts at frequent intervals because of the bladder irritation, contains much albumin, leukocytes, fibrin, epithelial debris, and usually small bright-red blood clots.

**Mode of Transmission.** Jones and Little (7) and others have reported the finding of *C. renale* in many young and adult cattle that were apparently normal. These findings are more numerous in herds where clinical cases have been recognized, but they have often been found in herds in which the disease has never been recognized. This strongly suggests that this organism is more widespread than had been thought earlier. The sporadic distribution of cases is perhaps caused by unknown factors rather than by the presence of the specific organism alone. The available evidence indicates that the bacterium is spread from animal to animal by contamination of the urinogenital orifices with urine from diseased or carrier animals. In herds in which the adult cows are stanchioned, it is not unusual to find several neighboring cows infected. It is supposed that this is caused by the switching of tails contaminated with infected urine.

**Diagnosis.** The symptoms of this disease are quite characteristic in most cases. For laboratory confirmation, a sample of urine should be collected in a sterile bottle. If, as is generally the case, it contains blood clots or bits of necrotic tissue, films may be made from these on slides and stained with the Gram technic. The finding of the characteristic clumps of short, stubby organisms that retain the Gram stain is presumptive evidence. If clumps are not present, the sample may be centrifuged and the sediment examined microscopically. For final confirmation, the sediment should be streaked on an agar plate, with or without enrichment, and after 24 to 36 hours' incubation at 37 C a search for characteristic colonies should be made. If transplants from these show the typical morphology and staining reactions, if haloes are formed on 10 percent milk agar, if the litmus milk reaction is typical, if urea is split forming ammonia, and if only glucose is fermented, the diagnosis may be considered as established.

Diagnosticians must be on their guard against confusing morphologically similar organisms with *C. renale*. It is well known that diphtheroid organisms are often present on skin and mucous membranes. Jones and Little (7), in their study of the bladder and urethra of young calves, found five types of diphtheroids in apparently normal organs. Most of these occurred in the sheaths of bull calves. Four of these species differed culturally and serologically from *C. renale*; the fifth apparently was identical with it.

**Immunity.** Little is known about immunity to this disease. Without treatment, recoveries probably never occur after the disease is well established. There are no biological products of value in this disease.

**Chemotherapy.** Until the appearance of antibiotic therapy there were no forms of treatment that materially affected the course of the disease. Unless the animals are unusually valuable and unless the diagnosis is not established until emaciation has occurred, it is best to advise slaughter for beef. *C. renale* is sensitive *in vitro* and *in vivo* to penicillin, and there are many reports of apparent cures with large doses of this substance. In some cases such animals have relapsed after a few weeks or months; in other cases the cure appears to have been complete (Morse, 10).

**Control Measures.** As soon as cases are recognized, the animals should be segregated from other susceptible stock, treated with penicillin, or slaughtered. Treated animals should be carefully watched for a year or more for a return of the symptoms.

**The Disease in Man.** No cases of this disease have been recognized in man. So far as is known, this organism is not pathogenic for man.

**REFERENCES**

1. Boyd.   Cornell Vet., 1918, 8, 120.
2. Boyd and Bishop.   Jour. Am. Vet. Med. Assoc., 1937, 90, 154.
3. Enderlen.   Deut. Zeitschr. f. Tiermed, 1891, 17, 325.
4. Ernst.   Centrbl. f. Bakt., I Abt., Orig., 1905, 39, 549; 1906, 40, 79.
5. Feenstra, Clark, and Thorp.   Mich. State Coll. Vet., 1945, 5, 147.
6. Feenstra, Thorp, and Clark.   Jour. Bact., 1945, 50, 497.
7. Jones and Little.   Jour. Exp. Med., 1925, 42, 593; 1926, 43, 11; 1930, 51, 909.
8. Lovell.   Jour. Comp. Path. and Therap., 1946, 56, 196.
9. Lovell and Cotchin.   Ibid., 205.
10. Morse.   Cornell Vet., 1948, 38, 273.
11. Olafson.   Ibid., 1930, 20, 69.
12. Yanagawa, Basri, and Otsuki.   Jap. Jour. Vet. Res., 1967, 15, 111.

### *Corynebacterium pseudotuberculosis*

SYNONYMS: The Preisz-Nocard bacillus, *Corynebacterium ovis*

This organism is the cause of caseous lymphadenitis of sheep, sometimes called pseudotuberculosis, of ulcerative lymphangitis of horses, and of a form of suppurative lymphangitis in cattle (14).

**Morphology and Staining Reactions.** The organism is a pleomorphic rod. Frequently it is so short that it may easily be mistaken for a coccus. In the caseous pus from lymph nodes it sometimes occurs as rod forms that resemble quite closely the organism of human diphtheria. It forms no spores and is nonmotile. It retains the Gram stain but is not acid-fast.

**Cultural Features.** The organism will grow on all the ordinary media, although not luxuriantly. The colonies on agar are quite characteristic. They grow slowly and do not reach maximum size for several days when incubated at the optimum temperature (37 C). When fully developed they have papilliform centers surrounded by concentric rings that parallel the irregular margin. The color is grayish or yellowish and the surfaces are dull and dry. When touched with the needle, they fragment easily. Entire smaller colonies may be pushed around the surface of the medium like flakes of paraffin.

On blood agar plates the colonies are slightly hemolytic (2). The organism grows well on Loeffler's blood serum but does not liquefy it. The colonies on this medium are moist and orange yellow in color. Growth occurs in milk but there is little change in the appearance of the medium. On broth a fragile pellicle is formed. Glucose and maltose are fermented without gas formation. Lactose, sucrose, raffinose, dextrin, and inulin are not attacked.

According to Hall and Stone (4), this organism produces a true toxin in various culture media which is similar to, but not so potent as, that of the human diphtheria bacillus (*C. diphtheriae*). They claimed that this toxin was partially neutralized by diphtheria antitoxin. Mitchell and Walker (13) confirmed the production of a soluble toxin but could find no relation between it and that of the diphtheria organism. Results obtained by Lovell and Zaki (10) were in accord with the findings of Mitchell and Walker and Jolly's (7) experiments indicating that the exotoxin acts primarily on the local vascular bed of the victim.

**Pathogenicity for Experimental Animals.** By inoculation *C. pseudotuberculosis* is pathogenic for horses, cattle, sheep, goats, rabbits, and guinea pigs. Fowls are refractory.

In guinea pigs, intraperitoneal injection of large doses produces rapid intoxication and death from peritonitis. Smaller doses or less virulent strains have a tendency to localize in the scrotal sac, thus producing a condition indistinguishable from that caused by the glanders bacillus (the Strauss reaction). Because ulcerative lymphangitis of horses caused by this organism simulates glanders or farcy, this fact should be kept in mind when guinea pig inoculation is used for the diagnosis of glanders.

**The Natural Disease.** *In horses.* Ulcerative lymphangitis in horses resembles cutaneous glanders (farcy) quite closely. Nodules appear on the legs and these break down to form ulcers, which exude a thick greenish pus usually mixed with blood. They are located most often around the fetlock. These lesions fill with cicatricial tissue and heal after a time, but others appear nearby. Some cases heal spontaneously within a few weeks, but most of them progress slowly for months and even years.

According to Hughes and Biberstein (6), *C. pseudotuberculosis* causes an enzootic form of chronic abscesses during the late summer and fall months in horses located in the coastal and central valley area of California.

*In sheep.* The disease in sheep is known as *caseous lymphadenitis.* It occurs with great frequency in certain areas of the midwestern parts of the United States and Canada, particularly between the Rocky Mountains and the Cascade chain. It is not seen in the eastern half of this country except in sheep which have been imported from the West, and it does not seem to spread except in the area mentioned. It is prevalent in many other parts of the world.

The disease affects the lymph nodes, especially those of the chest. Eventually the infected glands become converted into large encapsulated abscesses. In the younger lesions the pus is butyrous; in old ones it becomes dry and granular. Calcification is not common. The color of the pus is a greenish yellow. It is nonodorous. Frequently the abscesses become several times as large as the lymph nodes in which they originate. Nodules are often found in the lungs. The old lung and lymph node lesions have a characteristic appearance on cross section. The inspissated pus is arranged in concentric layers resembling an onion. Nodules are not usually found in the liver, spleen, or kidneys.

Old sheep, apparently quite normal, are often found at slaughter to be rather badly affected. Eventually, if the animals are allowed to live long enough, they become emaciated and weak, and will die.

*In cattle.* From the paucity of reports, it is probable that the disease does not often occur in cattle. Kitt (8) found it in a case of bronchopneumonia in a cow. It was reported by Hall and Stone (4) in a calf. It is reported that a considerable number of cases of the so-called "skin-lesion tuberculosis" in Utah contain this organism (3). See "Acid-fast Bacilli Associated with Ulcerative Lymphangitis in Cattle," page 462.

**Mode of Transmission.** The manner in which infections with this organism are spread is not known. It is suspected to be related to soil contaminations. It seems probable that most infections are contracted through skin abrasions. The location of the lesions in the fetlock region of the horse suggests this. In sheep, infections may occur through docking, castration, and shearing wounds, though this is largely speculation. Infection by inhalation of dust is a possibility in sheep.

**Diagnosis.** The appearance of the lesions in sheep is quite characteristic, and the organism usually can be isolated from the abscesses without difficulty.

The dry, scaly colonies, which cause hemolysis on blood agar plates, are easily recognized. The disease in horses must be differentiated from skin glanders (farcy). This can easily be done by isolation of the causative organism and by applying the mallein test. The complement-fixation test may also be used to exclude the presence of glanders. A new *in vitro* test (antihemolysin-inhibition) has been described by Zaki (15), the reaction depending on the ability of *C. pseudotuberculosis* antiserum to neutralize the inhibitory action of the organism upon staphylococcal Beta-lysin. In 1960 Awad (1) described an agglutination test which he claims is diagnostic for caseous lymphadenitis in sheep. A titer above 1:64 is considered to be significant.

**Immunity.** Hard (5) used mice to demonstrate an adoptive transfer of immunity to *C. pseudotuberculosis.* This was accomplished by intraperitoneal injections of sensitized, viable, macrophagelike and lymphoid peritoneal cells.

No biological agents are available for the prevention or treatment of diseases caused by *C. pseudotuberculosis* (12).

**Chemotherapy.** Although there are antibiotics effective against *C. pseudotuberculosis,* the lesions caused by it, especially in sheep, are so encapsulated that these medicaments could hardly be expected to penetrate and kill all organisms except in very slight infections (11). In treating chronic abscesses in horses it is recommended (6) that ichthyol ointment be applied to hasten maturation. When mature, the abscess is incised, drained, and flushed with an antiseptic. This procedure usually brings prompt recovery.

**Control Measures.** No practicable control measures have been developed.

**The Disease in Man.** In 1966, Lopez *et al.* (9) reported the first case of *C. pseudotuberculosis* in man. The clinical picture consisted of fatigue, muscular aches, tenderness and enlargement of the liver, and localized lymphadenopathy. Conclusive bacteriologic identification of the microorganism was established in specimens obtained by lymph node aspiration and surgical excision of the involved lymph node. Examination of the node revealed a pathologic process manifested by focal areas of chronic inflammation. There were nests of epithelioid cells surrounded by fibroblastic reaction and a chronic sclerosing lymphadenitis.

## REFERENCES

1. Awad.　Am. Jour. Vet. Res., 1960, *81*, 251.
2. Carne.　Jour. Path. and Bact., 1939, *49*, 313.
3. Daines and Austin.　Jour. Am. Vet. Med. Assoc., 1932, *80*, 414.
4. Hall and Stone.　Jour. Inf. Dis., 1916, *18*, 195.
5. Hard.　Jour. Comp. Path., 1970, *80*, 329.
6. Hughes and Biberstein.　Jour. Am. Vet. Med. Assoc., 1959, *135*, 559.
7. Jolly.　Jour. Comp. Path., 1965, *75*, 417.
8. Kitt.　Monatshefte f. prakt. Tierheilk., 1890, *1*, 145.
9. Lopez, Wong, and Quesada.　Am. Jour. Clin. Path., 1966, *46*, 562.
10. Lovell and Zaki.　Res. Vet. Sci., 1966, 7, 302.
11. Maddy.　Jour. Am. Vet. Med. Assoc., 1953, *122*, 257.

12.   Minett.   Jour. Comp. Path. and Therap., 1922, 35, 71.
13.   Mitchell and Walker.   Canad. Jour. Comp. Med., 1944, 8, 3.
14.   Norgaard and Mohler.   16th Ann. Rpt., U.S. Dept. Agr., Washington, 1899.
15.   Zaki.   Res. Vet. Sci., 1968, 9, 489.

### Corynebacterium equi

This organism was first described and named by Magnusson (12) in southern Sweden in 1923 as the causative agent of a purulent pneumonia in foals which frequently was associated with pyemia. In 1936 Holth and Amundsen (10) described tuberculosislike lesions in the cervical lymph modes of swine which they attributed to a coccobacillus. Bendixen and Jepsen (1) in 1938 first recognized the identity of the swine and the foal organisms, and because the organism occurred much more commonly in swine than in horses, Plum (13) proposed that it be rechristened *Corynebacterium magnusson-holth.* This suggestion is not likely to be accepted generally. Dimock and Edwards (7) and others have found *C. equi* in this country in foals, and Karlson, Moses, and Feldman (11) have isolated it from many swine lymph nodes. One case has been reported of its isolation from an aborting carabao in India (3) and another from a sheep in Australia that was affected with chronic pneumonia and pleurisy (14).

**Morphology and Staining Reactions.** *C. equi* is a rather large organism that shows considerable pleomorphism ranging from coccoid forms to bacillary forms. On solid media the form usually is coccoid; in fluids it usually is bacillary. Sometimes short chains are found in fluid media. Metachromatic granules can usually be demonstrated, especially in cultures grown in milk.

The gross appearance of the growth of this organism suggests that it is a capsule former, and a number of the authors state that capsules are formed. Karlson, Moses, and Feldman, however, were unable to convince themselves that capsules were present.

This organism is Gram-positive and it stains readily with other dyes. A number of authors claim that acid-fast forms are demonstrable in old cultures, but several other workers have been unable to confirm this. Spores are not formed.

**Cultural Features.** Good growth occurs on all the ordinary media. After 2 days' incubation, colonies on the surface of agar plates measure nearly 1 cm in diameter and are raised, moist, translucent, and regular in outline. At first they are white, but a rose-pink color soon appears. Old cultures are distinctly pinkish, especially those that are developing on potato. There is a rather poor growth in milk, without coagulation or other evidence of change in the chemical composition. Carbohydrates are not fermented, blood cells are not attacked, and neither gelatin nor blood serum is digested. Several serological types in this species can be demonstrated by agglutination tests. By complement fixation, however, it can be demonstrated that there is a species-specific antigen as well (3). The cultures studied by Bruner and Edwards (4) fell into four serologic groups and cultures from the genital tract of mares, from aborted equine fetuses, from pneumonia of foals, and from the submaxillary lymph gland of hogs belonged to the same serologic group.

**Resistance.** *C. equi* does not appear to be especially resistant to ordinary physical and chemical agents, but it does have a surprising resistance to acids. Cotchin (6) found that it would successfully resist the action of 2.5 percent oxalic acid for 1 hour and made use of this property for its isolation from tissues contaminated with other bacteria.

**Pathogenicity for Experimental Animals.** The pathogenicity of *C. equi* is low. Cotchin found that local abscesses could be produced by subcutaneous inoculation of laboratory animals and swine with large doses of culture. Karlson, Moses, and Feldman (11) failed in an attempt to produce lymph node lesions in swine by the feeding of large doses of culture.

**Natural Infections.** *In horses.* Magnusson found this organism in 23 of a series of 78 cases of suppurative pneumonia in young foals. In these cases the thoracic lymph nodes were greatly enlarged and suppurative. In none of these cases were any lesions found in the lymph nodes of the head, a feature by which this disease can be differentiated from strangles. Chronic pneumonia with secondary enteritis and subacute pneumonia with secondary arthritis have been observed in foals (5). In the former there was abscessation in the lungs and intestines, and in the latter there were abscesses in the lungs and a seropurulent arthritis. Abscesses in the liver are rarely found and they have not been observed in the spleen or kidneys. This disease has been seen in Kentucky by Dimock, Edwards, and Bruner (8) and in California by Britton (2).

This organism has been isolated by the Kentucky group from the uterine discharge of a number of aborting mares and is suspected of being the causative factor of this condition in some cases.

*In swine.* The infection in swine occurs in the lymph nodes and particularly in those of the cervical region. It was the belief of Holth and Amundsen (8), who first found the organism in swine, that it caused a tuberclelike disease, and this view was taken also by other Scandinavian workers, notably Plum (13), who confirmed the Norwegian findings. Karlson, Moses, and Feldman (11), in the United States, do not accept this view because they were able to demonstrate the organism in approximately as many apparently normal as diseased lymph nodes. They believe the acid-fast organisms that the European workers describe as acid-fast forms of *C. equi* are, in reality, tubercle bacilli with which the organism is developing concurrently. They believe, on the basis of their findings, that the organism is relatively if not wholly nonpathogenic, and that when gross lesions are evident it is because tubercle bacilli are present as well as *C. equi.* The lymph nodes cultured by these workers contained other bacteria as a rule, but *C. equi* was readily isolated in pure culture because of the fact that it resisted treatment with oxalic acid, which destroyed practically all other bacteria except tubercle bacilli.

**Mode of Transmission.** There is no information on the mode of transmission of this organism. Magnusson expressed the belief that it lives in the soil, but no proof was provided that this is the case.

**Diagnosis.** In neither horses nor swine can the presence of this organism be more than suspected before a bacteriological examination with isolation of the organism is made. Sippel *et al.* (15) have recovered three species of the genus *Corynebacterium* from the lungs of foals: *C. equi, C. pseudotuberculosis,* and *C. pyogenes.* They claim that the clinical appearance of these infections is quite similar and that the three diseases are difficult to distinguish on this basis.

**Immunity.** No practicable methods of immunizing against this organism have been developed. Magnusson encountered difficulty in producing high titers in experimental animals.

**Chemotherapy.** There is little information on this subject. Britton reported failure in treating an infected foal with sulfanilamide and sulfaquinoxaline. Doll and Dimock (9) in a study of penicillin dosage and blood levels for horses reported that the penicillin resistance of *C. equi* is so great that dosage for maintaining effective blood levels is impractical.

**Control Measures.** There are no known methods of preventing infections with *C. equi* except general sanitary measures, which may minimize but will not eliminate them.

**The Disease in Man.** So far as is known this organism is not pathogenic for man.

## REFERENCES

1. Bendixen and Jepsen. Medlemsblad f. d. Danske Dyrlaegeforning, 1938, *21,* 401.
2. Britton. Cornell Vet., 1945, *35,* 370.
3. Bruner, Dimock, and Edwards. Jour. Inf. Dis., 1939, *65,* 92.
4. Bruner and Edwards. Ky. Agr. Exp. Sta. Bul. 414, 1941.
5. Burrows. Jour. Am. Vet. Med. Assoc., 1968, *152,* 1119.
6. Cotchin. Jour. Comp. Path. and Therap., 1943, *53,* 298.
7. Dimock and Edwards. Ky. Agr. Exp. Sta. Bul. 333, 1932.
8. Dimock, Edwards, and Bruner. *Ibid.,* 509, 1947.
9. Doll and Dimock. Jour. Am. Vet. Med. Assoc., 1946, *108,* 209.
10. Holth and Amundsen. Norsk Vet.-Tidsskr., 1936, *48,* 2.
11. Karlson, Moses, and Feldman. Jour. Inf. Dis., 1940, *67,* 243.
12. Magnusson. Arch. f. Tierheilk., 1923, *50,* 22.
13. Plum. Cornell Vet., 1940, *30,* 14.
14. Roberts. Austral. Vet., Jour., 1957, *33,* 21.
15. Sippel, Keahey, and Bullard. Jour. Am. Vet. Med. Assoc., 1968, *153,* 1610.

## THE GENUS *LISTERIA*

In 1927 Pirie (50) in South Africa isolated an organism from a plaguelike disease of the gerbille (a rodent) for which he created a new genus called

*Listerella.* Inasmuch as it was pointed out to him later that this name had been utilized for a genus of slime molds, he proposed in 1940 that the name be changed to *Listeria* (51), a suggestion that will be followed here in spite of the fact that this name also appears to have been pre-empted.

Generally believed to be identical with Pirie's organism are several others: one which Murray of England (40) first found in stock rabbits and which produces a mononucleosis; one which Gill first found in sheep in New Zealand which produces "circling disease" of sheep and cattle; one which TenBroeck found in a chicken in New Jersey which produces necrotic myocarditis and pericarditis; and one which Schultz in California and Burn in Connecticut found in cases of fatal meningoencephalitis of man. The name *Listeria monocytogenes* has been applied to the organism and it appears listeric infections are rather common in domestic animals and in man (27).

### Listeria monocytogenes

SYNONYM:   *Listerella monocytogenes*

**Morphology and Staining Reactions.** This organism occurs in the form of small rods, 1 to 2 microns in length, which frequently show slight clubbing and therefore appear like diphtheroids. Coccoid elements are commonly found. Young cultures are motile. This fact can readily be demonstrated by inoculation into the semisolid agar recommended by Edwards and Bruner (14). Spores are not produced. It is Gram-positive and non-acid-fast. Gram-negative cells can usually be found in young cultures, and old cultures often are nearly wholly Gram-negative.

**Culture Features.** Growth occurs on most of the ordinary laboratory media, although it is never abundant. In general, the gross features of cultures resemble those of streptococci.

Methods for the isolation of *L. monoctyogenes* have been published by Olson *et al.* (44) and by March (39). We prefer to use blood plates. The colonies may be seen after 24 hours' incubation at 37 C as minute points (deep colonies) and as small, flat, bluish-white, transparent surface colonies. The deep colonies are surrounded by narrow zones of hemolysis of the Beta type, and this characteristic makes them conspicuous. The surface colonies seldom if ever exceed 1 mm in diameter.

Broth is faintly and uniformly clouded. Growth is favored by the presence of a little sterile serum or defibrinated blood. When blood cells are present, hemoglobin, released from them, diffuses upward from the layer of sedimented cells. Glucose greatly favors growth.

Stab cultures in gelatin appear as a line of discrete colonies along the stab. Seastone (57) says that an especially characteristic growth may be seen in semisolid agar containing glucose. Stab cultures in this medium usually show a cloud of minute colonies surrounding the line of the stab.

Acid without gas is formed from glucose, rhamnose, and salicin within 48 hours. Sucrose and dextrin are fermented, but more slowly. Results are in con-

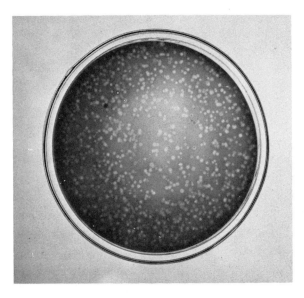

Fig. 34. Listeria monocytogenes, a blood agar plate incubated at 37 C for 24 hours. The
colonies are not discernible in
the photograph. They are very
minute, each being surrounded
by a sharply defined but narrow
zone of Beta-type hemolysis.

stant with maltose, lactose, and glycerol. These substances usually are fermented slightly and slowly.

Litmus milk supports growth, but there is little change in the appearance of
the medium as a rule. Sometimes it is slightly acidified. There is no growth on
potato. Hydrogen sulfide and indol are not formed, and nitrates are not reduced.

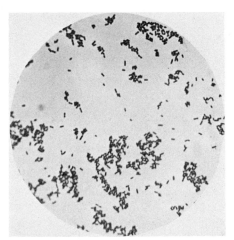

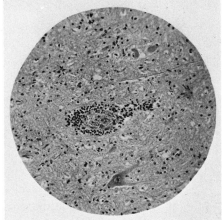

Fig. 35 (left). Listeria monocytogenes, a culture from a serum-agar slant incubated for 18
hours at 37 C. X 750.

Fig. 36 (right). Listeriosis in the brain of a cow. The cells infiltrating the brain substance
are both mononuclears and polymorphonuclears. There is marked perivascular cuffing. X 55.
(Courtesy S. H. McNutt.)

**Resistance** *L. monocytogenes* is readily killed by pasteurization, but will survive for 67 to 200 days in soil, depending on its type and moisture content (63).

**Pathogenicity.** *For rodents.* Large doses given intravenously to rabbits cause a marked mononuclear leukocytosis of the myeloid type, focal necrosis of the liver, necrotic areas in the myocardium, and extensive involvement of the meninges. These lesions are also found in the guinea pig and other rodents. The natural disease in the gerbille, known as the *Tiger River disease*, described by Pirie (50), presented similar lesions.

At the end of 2 weeks' gestation organisms instilled in the eyes of rabbits not only caused conjunctivitis, but also produced abortion (28). The addition of *L. monocytogenes* to the drinking water usually produced abortions and sometimes death in pregnant rabbits, while nonpregnant and male rabbits apparently were not affected (28).

*For cattle and sheep.* Infection in sheep was first described by Gill (21) of New Zealand in 1931. He gave the illness the name of "circling disease" because of the characteristic actions of affected animals. In the United States the infection was first diagnosed in cattle by Jones and Little (34) in New Jersey in 1934, by Fincher (18) in New York cattle in 1935, and by Olafson (42) in 1936 in New York sheep. It now appears that the disease is scattered throughout the United States because it has been reported in cattle and sheep from all sections of the country. In these animals the organism usually causes an encephalitis, although it has been associated with neonatal septicemia in calves (32) and with valvular endocarditis in sheep (46). It has been reported as the cause of an outbreak of visceral and cerebral listeriosis in sheep (23). The ewes developed nervous symptoms, while the lambs appeared dull, some were scouring, and all were losing weight. Postmortem examinations revealed typical lesions of cerebral listeriosis in the ewes and numerous foci of necrosis in the liver, spleens, and gastrohepatic lymph nodes of the lambs. In the latter *L. monocytogenes* was isolated from all internal organs, but not from the brain. Listeric myelitis has also been observed in lambs (20). It was characterized by paralysis of one or more limbs. There were no lesions in the brain and the bacteria were isolated only from the spinal cord.

In the encephalomyelitic form the cerebrospinal fluid may be cloudy because of an increased globulin and leukocyte content. There may be some congestion of the meninges. Usually the visceral organs show little or no evidence of disease. Sections of the brain of such animals show polymorphonuclear and mononuclear foci in the white matter of the cerebrum and cerebellum and perivascular cuffing with mononuclear cells. The causative organism can readily be isolated from these brains, but the organisms often appear to be present in small numbers; hence it is well to inoculate the cultures liberally. Affected sheep show signs of depression, weakness, incoordination of movement, fever, walking in circles, pushing against objects, progressive paralysis, and death within 2 or 3 days. The symptoms in cattle are similar.

Graham, Hester, and Levine (24) isolated this organism from the stomach content of an aborted bovine fetus, and from the liver and brain of a rabbit that was inoculated with the same material. There was no history of listeriosis in the herd from which the cow came. It had been slaughtered immediately after aborting and was not available for study. Since this report *L. monocytogenes* has been definitely established as an infrequent cause of bovine abortion (17, 59, 60). It has also been found in cases of abortion in sheep.

*For chickens.* TenBroeck, whose observations were recorded by Seastone (57) in 1935, isolated this organism from a case of necrotic myocarditis in a chicken in 1932. Patterson (48) recorded the disease in four flocks in England in 1937. The latter found only one case of necrotic myocarditis in 17 fowls studied; hence it appears that this is not a common finding. The affected birds suffered from emaciation and general weakness. The lesions consisted of edematous tissues, fluid in the body cavity and in the pericardial sac, and focal necrosis of the liver. The organism was readily isolated from all birds by culturing the liver. Gray (25) has reviewed listeriosis in fowl. He concludes that there are no pathognomonic symptoms or lesions for the infection because the bacterium is often associated with some other disorder in the bird. Our findings confirm Gray's observations in that we obtain one to two cultures each year from chickens presented for postmortem, but there has been no definite disease syndrome connected with the isolates.

*For swine.* Biester and Schwarte (6) have seen several outbreaks of listeriosis in swine in Iowa. Young animals were affected more commonly than old. The symptoms were vague but suggestive of disturbances of consciousness. The lesions in the central nervous system were not marked, but were similar to those seen in sheep. It was the belief of these authors that diagnosis of this condition in swine could be made with certainty only by recovering the causative organism. Postmortem reports of the New York State Veterinary College include a case of visceral listeriosis in a pig in which focal necrosis of the liver and peritonitis were the chief lesions; there was no involvement of the central nervous system. Also included is a case of encephalitis in a pig. Hale (29) isolated *L. monocytogenes* from the internal organs of two baby pigs that died after showing clinical symptoms of diarrhea, weakness, and stiffness.

*For horses.* Svenkerud (61) reported the occurrence of *Listeria* infection in a horse. The animal suddenly became ill and showed nervous symptoms consisting of paralysis of the jaw and throat muscles as well as incoordination of gait. The organism was isolated from the liver and muscular tissues of the animal. Emerson and Jarvis (15) described listeriosis in ponies characterized clinically by signs of elevated temperature, restlessness, mild colic, depression, inappetence, jaundice, and reddish urine.

*For other animals.* Experimentally, listeriosis has been induced in mice, hamsters, and turkeys (9, 37). The organism has been isolated from the brain of a moose (1) that showed symptoms similar to the so-called *moose sickness*, from the brains of foxes suspected of having rabies (55), and Pittman and

Cherry (52) have claimed tha *L. monocytogenes* occurred frequently in Georgia among feral animals which had abnormal behavior but which were rabies-negative. Their results indicated also that *Listeria* can usually be isolated from the brains of such animals only after cold enrichment. In 1968, Carroll *et al.* (11) diagnosed listeriosis in a dog that developed cellular brain lesions consistent with those found in the disease.

*For man.* Burn (10) found an organism in four human infections that he concluded was identical with strains isolated from cattle by Jones and Little (34). Three of these cases were newborn infants who died within a short time. All showed focal necrosis of the liver and meningitis with a thick green exudate in the subarachnoid space covering the medulla, pons, and parietal lobes. In one case a pneumococcus was isolated in addition to the *Listeria;* in the other two the organism was in pure culture. A fourth case was of a 53-year-old man suffering from bilateral otitis media followed by meningitis. A Type-2 pneumococcus and *Listeria* were isolated from the brain at autopsy. The lesions resembled those seen in the infants. Schultz, Terry, Brice, and Gebhart (56) and Berry (5) saw cases of meningitis similar to those described by Burn. Numerous cases of *Listeria* meningitis have since been reported (3, 13, 22, 30) and instances where *L. monocytogenes* has been incriminated in rheumatic valvular heart disease, granulomatous involvement of the spleen, and placental infection have been recorded (2, 31, 49). It has caused persistent infection in a surgical incision (62) and it has been isolated from an aortic aneurysm (41).

The finding of antibody titers in apparently healthy people and in patients of different categories indicates that *L. monocytogenes* is a frequent invader of man (65).

Pons and Julianelle (53) isolated a culture of *Listeria* from the blood of a girl suffering from a disease that was diagnosed as infectious mononucleosis (a disease probably caused by a virus). The patient showed fever, angina, enlarged axillary and cervical glands, a palpable spleen, and a leukocytosis varying from 11,000 to 17,000 per mm³ with 40 percent monocytes. These authors (35) observed that young cultures, when applied to the conjunctiva of rabbits, guinea pigs, or rats, caused a distinct, purulent conjunctivitis, which developed in from 1 to 5 days. When the swollen lids were forced apart, a thick, heavy exudate composed largely of mononuclear cells was expelled. The conjunctiva was acutely inflamed, the cornea became opaque and pitted, and the blood vessels pushed out to the pupillary margin. The reaction subsided in from 5 to 10 days, and the lesion healed in from 1 to 3 weeks. Pons and Julianelle thought this test valuable for diagnosis. Graham and co-workers found that strains isolated from sheep and cattle gave this reaction in the rabbit's eye. The FA technic has also been employed in identifying *L. monocytogenes* (58), and an intradermal test with *listerin* (a tuberculinlike product from *Listeria*) has been recommended by Eveleth *et al.* (16).

**Mode of Transmission.** It has been suggested that ensilage is a factor in pro-

ducing listeriosis and that the nasal route is the portal of entry. Obtaining experimental infections by feeding ensilage or by intranasal inoculations usually
is not possible, but Gray (26) isolated the same serotype from range cattle
that had become infected after eating oat silage and from mice that were fed
this silage. Reports by Blenden *et al.* (7), Darie (12), and Welshimer (54) indicate that *L. monocytogenes* will grow in corn silage extract medium, that it
is present in silage, and that it can be isolated from vegetation which has
died and remained in the fields over the winter.

Olson and Segre (45) claim that they isolated a nonbacterial listeriosis-en-
hancing agent from a sheep kept on the premises where an outbreak of listeriosis had occurred. Intranasal exposure of sheep to *Listeria* and this agent
produced clinical symptoms of listeriosis in 18 to 22 days and subsequent
death.

Although listeriosis does occur in human infants there is evidence that the
gravid female does not carry *L. monocytogenes* in her reproductive tract (54).

A new species, *Listeria grayi*, was reported by Blenden and Szatalowicz
(8), in 1967. Characterization of this organism is not adequate for assigning it
species status or evaluating its role in human disease. Certainly listeriosis in
man must be regarded as a common source-type infection whose status as a
zoonotic disease remains unproved.

**Immunity.** Julianelle and Pons (36) found that eight strains which they studied
fell into two agglutinative groups. Their Type I was composed of two rabbit
and two human strains, and Type II contained one cow, one goat, one sheep,
and one human strain. Seastone had previously noted that a rabbit strain agglutinated differently than did strains from other animals. It was suggested
that possibly it would be found that Type I was essentially a rodent type
(rabbit, gerbille) and Type II a ruminant type (sheep, cattle). The organism
found by Graham *et al.* (24) in a bovine fetus was tested with type serum
from Julianelle and found to fall into the rodent group. Two additional serological types have been added making a total, at present, of four. In man, in
the United States, organisms belonging in Type IV are the most common (38).

Olafson (42) showed that it was possible to build up a partial defense
mechanism in susceptible sheep against *Listeria* infection through subcutaneous and intravenous injection of the inciting organism. Whereas intracerebral inoculation of untreated sheep with *Listeria* cultures produced a rapidly
fatal encephalitis, intracerebral inoculations of the vaccinated sheep sometimes resulted in acute disease and death, but more often in a chronic form of
the disease or in no disease at all.

Attempts to vaccinate sheep during an outbreak of listeriosis were not successful according to Olson *et al.* (43), but Osbold, Njoku-Obi, and Abare (47)
claim that sheep can be immunized successfully by vaccinating subcutaneously with virulent live cultures. As a rule the disease is so sporadic that
immunizing procedures are not of great service.

**Chemotherapy.** Olafson (34) reported some success in treating circling disease of ruminants with the sulfonamides. Jensen and Mackey (33) stated that the results of treating cattle with penicillin and sulfanilamide were good when the drugs were administered before prostration developed. Foley, Epstein, and Lee (19) found that *Listeria* strains isolated from animals were quite resistant to penicillin *in vitro*. Bennett and colleagues (4) reported that terramycin and aureomycin were effective when used early in the treatment of this infection.

## REFERENCES

1.　Archibald.　Canad. Vet. Jour., 1960, *1*, 225.
2.　Baker, Felton, and Muchmore.　Am. Jour. Med. Sci., 1961, *241*, 739.
3.　Barrow and Pugh.　Jour. Path. and Bact., 1958, 75, 9.
4.　Bennett, Russell, and Derivaux.　Antibiotics and Chemother., 1952, 2, 142.
5.　Berry.　Med. Jour., 1950, *1*, 894.
6.　Biester and Schwarte.　Proc. U.S. Livestock Sanit. Assoc., 1940, *44*, 42.
7.　Blenden, Gates, and Khan.　Am. Jour. Vet. Res., 1968, 29, 2237.
8.　Blenden and Szatalowicz.　Jour. Am. Vet. Med. Assoc., 1967, *151*, 1761.
9.　Bolin and Eveleth.　Avian Dis., 1961, 5, 229.
10.　Burn.　Jour. Bact., 1935, *30*, 573. Am. Jour. Path., 1936, *12*, 341.
11.　Carroll, Jasmin, and Baucom.　Am. Jour. Vet. Clin. Path., 1968, 2, 133.
12.　Darie.　Lucr. Inst. Cerc. Vet. Bioprep. (Pasteur), 1967, *6*, 60.
13.　Dedrick.　Am. Jour. Med. Sci., 1957, *233*, 617.
14.　Edwards and Bruner.　Ky. Agr. Exp. Sta. Cir. 54, 1942, p. 19.
15.　Emerson and Jarvis.　Jour. Am. Vet. Med. Assoc., 1968, *152*, 1645.
16.　Eveleth, Bolin, and Turn.　Farm Res., 1961, *21*, 14.
17.　Ferguson, Bohl, and Ingalls.　Jour. Am. Vet. Med. Assoc., 1951, *118*, 10.
18.　Fincher.　Cornell Vet., 1935, *25*, 61.
19.　Foley, Epstein, and Lee.　Jour. Bact., 1944, *47*, 110.
20.　Gates, Blenden, and Kintner.　Jour. Am. Vet. Med. Assoc., 1967, *150*, 200.
21.　Gill.　Vet. Jour., 1931, *87*, 60; 1933, 89, 258.
22.　Girard and Gavin.　Jour. Path. and Bact., 1957, *74*, 93.
23.　Gitter and Terlecki.　Vet. Rec., 1965, 77, 11.
24.　Graham, Hester, and Levine.　Science, 1939, *90*, 336.
25.　Gray.　Avian Dis., 1958, 2, 296.
26.　Gray.　Jour. Am. Vet. Med. Assoc., 1960, *136*, 205.
27.　Gray.　Am. Jour. Pub. Health, 1963, *53*, 554.
28.　Gray, Singh, and Thorp, Jr.　Proc. Soc. Exp. Biol. and Med., 1955, 89, 163 and 169.
29.　Hale.　Jour. Am. Vet. Med. Assoc., 1959, *135*, 324.
30.　Hood.　Am. Jour. Clin. Path., 1957, *28*, 18.
31.　Inhorn, Smits, and Christenson.　*Ibid.*, 1960, *33*, 330.
32.　Jack.　Vet. Rec., 1961, 73, 826.
33.　Jensen and Mackey.　Jour. Am. Vet. Med. Assoc., 1949, *114*, 420.
34.　Jones and Little.　Arch. Path., 1934, *18*, 580.
35.　Julianelle and Pons.　Proc. Soc. Exp. Biol. and Med., 1939, *40*, 362.
36.　*Ibid.*, 364.
37.　Kautter, Silverman, Roessler, and Drawdy.　Jour. Inf. Dis., 1963, *112*, 167.

38. King and Seeliger. Jour. Bact., 1959, 77, 122.
39. March. Cornell Vet., 1956, 46, 274.
40. Murray, Webb, and Swann. Jour. Path. and Bact., 1926, 29, 407.
41. Navarrete-Reyna, Rosenstein, and Sonnenwirth. Am. Jour. Clin. Path., 1965, 43, 438.
42. Olafson. Cornell Vet., 1940, 30, 141.
43. Olson, Cook, and Bagdonas. Am. Jour. Vet. Res., 1951, 12, 306.
44. Olson, Dunn, and Rollins. *Ibid.*, 1953, 14, 82.
45. Olson and Segre. *Ibid.*, 1956, 17, 235.
46. Osebold and Cordy. Jour. Am. Vet. Med. Assoc., 1963, 143, 990.
47. Osebold, Njoku-Obi, and Abare. Am. Jour. Vet. Res., 1959, 20, 966.
48. Patterson. Vet. Rec., 1937, 49, 49.
49. Philipson. Acta Path. et Microbiol. Scand., 1960, 48, 24.
50. Pirie. Pub. So. African Inst. Med. Res., 1927, 3, 163.
51. Pirie. Science, 1940, 91, 383.
52. Pittman and Cherry. Am. Jour. Vet. Res., 1967, 28, 779.
53. Pons and Julianelle. Proc. Soc. Exp. Biol. and Med., 1939, 40, 360.
54. Quarles, Jr. and Pittman. Jour. Bact., 1966, 91, 2112.
55. Scholtens and Brim. Jour. Am. Vet. Med. Assoc., 1964, 145, 466.
56. Schultz, Terry, Brice, and Gebhart. Proc. Soc. Exp. Biol. and Med., 1934, 31, 1021.
57. Seastone. Jour. Exp. Med., 1935, 62, 203.
58. Smith, Marshall, and Eveland. Proc. Soc. Exp. Biol. and Med., 1960, 103, 842.
59. Smith, Reynolds, and Bennett. Jour. Am. Vet. Med. Assoc., 1955, 126, 106.
60. Stockton, Neu, Carpenter, and Gray. *Ibid.*, 1954, 124, 102.
61. Svenkerud. Norsk Vet.-Tidsskr., 1948, 60, 321.
62. Torregrosa. Am. Jour. Clin. Path., 1968, 50, 689.
63. Welshimer. Jour. Bact., 1960, 80, 316.
64. *Ibid.*, 1968, 95, 300.
65. Winblad and Borglin. Acta Path. et Microbiol. Scand., 1963, 58, 133.

## THE GENUS *ERYSIPELOTHRIX*

Two species were formerly recognized, the "mouse septicemia bacillus" described by Koch (26) and the "swine erysipelas bacillus" described by Loeffler (28). The first was isolated from putrid mouse blood, the second from pigs suffering from a disease now known as *swine erysipelas*. For many years Koch's organism was given the specific name *murisepticae* and Loeffler's *rhusiopathiae*. There is no longer any reason to regard these as different species. Apparently they are only variants, principally in pathogenicity, of a single species which now is known as *Erysipelothrix insidiosa*.

In addition to the original sources, *E. insidiosa* has been found in lambs suffering from polyarthritis, in calves suffering from a similar disease, in turkeys and ducks suffering from acute, septicemic infections, in wild and laboratory-bred mice suffering acute outbreaks, in the tonsils and on mucous membranes of apparently normal swine, in various decaying plant and animal tissues, in the slime on the bodies of both fresh- and salt-water fish, and in suppurative lesions in man, a disease which is known as *erysipeloid*.

### Erysipelothrix insidiosa

SYNONYMS:    *Bacillus rhusiopathiae suis,*
*Bacterium erysipelatos suum, Bacterium rhusiopathiae,*
*Erysipelothrix rhusiopathiae,* swine rotlauf bacillus

This organism is the cause of swine erysipelas, long recognized as the most destructive disease of young pigs in many parts of continental Europe. For many years it was believed not to exist in this country although Moore (34) isolated a culture thought to be *E. insidiosa* as early as 1892. In 1920 Ten-Broeck (55) obtained the organism from the tonsils of 5 of 16 pigs affected with hog cholera in New Jersey. In 1921 Creech (9) succeeded in isolating it from the skin lesions of the "diamond skin disease," a condition that had been recognized for years as similar to the mildest form of European swine erysipelas. This finding removed all doubt as to the presence of the disease in this country. In 1922 Ward (63) called attention to the fact that a form of polyarthritis in swine in this country is caused by this organism. In 1931 acute swine erysipelas with serious losses occurred in some isolated areas in South Dakota. Since that time it has been found in many areas of the United States. In some parts of the swine belt (South Dakota, Nebraska, Iowa) the disease has developed into one of the major problems of the industry, as it has been for many years in continental Europe.

**Morphology and Staining Reactions.** The organism usually occurs as a small, slim rod that is straight or slightly curved. In cultures made from rough colonies long filaments are commonly found. These often are beaded and exhibit

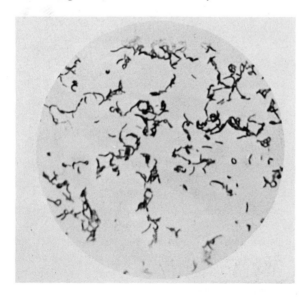

Fig. 37. Erysipelothrix insidiosa, a culture on serum agar, incubated for 24 hours at 37 C. X 1,000.

swollen areas. It stains readily with ordinary stains and is Gram-positive. It is nonmotile and does not form spores.

**Cultural Features.** On agar and coagulated blood serum small, delicate colonies, so fine that they may readily be overlooked, are formed. On gelatin the colonies are very small and have a fuzzy appearance. When magnified this is seen to be due to filaments that radiate from the central core. Gelatin stabs are particularly characteristic. Beadlike colonies form along the line of stab and finally coalesce to form a spike from which fine filaments push outward into the medium at right angles, giving the whole growth the appearance of an inverted, delicate test-tube brush. The gelatin is not liquefied. Broth is slightly clouded, and a flaky sediment collects in the bottom of the tube. There is no growth on potato. Milk is not usually altered, but occasionally it is slightly acidified. Narrow discolored zones appear around deep colonies on blood agar plates. Hydrogen sulfide is produced and nitrates reduced. Indol is not formed. Fermentation reactions differ according to strain. Some strains apparently do not ferment any carbohydrates but most ferment glucose, lactose, and levulose. According to Gledhill (16), *Erysipelothrix* strains are qualitatively homogeneous as regards their antigens, the difference between serological groups arising from differences in the quantitative distribution of the antigens. Truszczynski (57) has demonstrated the presence of type-specific and species-specific antigens by means of the gel-diffusion precipitation test; the former occurred in acid extracts, broth cultures, and bacterial fractions, and the latter in broth cultures and bacterial fractions.

**Resistance.** The organism is rather resistant to drying and to such procedures as smoking, pickling, and salting. The remarkable life span of the erysipelas bacterium is shown by the fact that a 22-year-old erysipelas broth culture, not kept at low temperatures but exposed to the temperature variations of the seasons, was still able to kill mice and to produce in swine, percutaneously, a local skin reaction leading to immunization. (65).

Once infected with the disease, farms usually experience recurrences of it from year to year. Doyle (12) has stated that there is little evidence to support the view that *E. insidiosa* remains viable for many months in the soil. A strong case can be made for the healthy carrier pig as the principal source of infection. The bacterium survives for relatively long periods in putrefying flesh and in water. It is not resistant to heat. Cultures are destroyed by exposure to moist heat at 55 C for 10 minutes. The organism is quite resistant to phenol, a fact that can be used in isolating it from contaminated tissues.

**Pathogenicity.** *For laboratory animals.* White mice and pigeons are very susceptible to infection by inoculation and are commonly used in diagnostic work. After subcutaneous inoculation they usually die in from 18 hours to 4 days. Rabbits are not highly susceptible. Usually a local reaction occurs and the animal may die after 6 or 7 days. Guinea pigs are quite resistant. Inoculated mice usually show evidence of conjunctivitis, first serous and later purulent, which glues their eyelids together. They sit with arched backs and roughened hair and do not eat. The lesions consist of enlargement of the spleen, discrete grayish foci in the liver, and occasionally congestion of the lungs. The blood and spleen contain large numbers of organisms, many of which have been taken up by phagocytes. Pigeons that have been inoculated in the breast muscles show swelling and hemorrhagic inflammation around the point of inoculation. The spleen is swollen and the liver may show focal necrosis. The organism is abundant in the blood and tissues. Wayson (64) has given a good account of a natural outbreak of this disease in wild mice, and Balfour-Jones (2) has described an outbreak in a stock of laboratory mice. Experiments by Shuman and Lee (50) have shown that the intraperitoneal injection of a virulent culture into the hamster causes the animal to die within about 8 to 12 days. It is possible to establish a chronic infection in rats.

*For swine.* The disease has been reproduced by oral, intravenous, intramuscular, subcutaneous, or intraperitoneal injection of cultures, but such results are usually not obtained with any degree of regularity. However, in 1951 Shuman (48) experimented extensively with the percutaneous (skin scarification) method of Fortner and Dinter and concluded that through the use of this procedure, or by intradermal injection, swine erysipelas with its systemic and cutaneous manifestations can be consistently induced in susceptible animals.

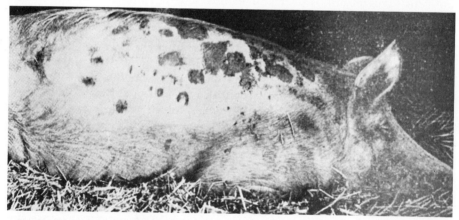

*Fig. 38.* Diamond skin disease of the pig. Characteristic lesions of one type of swine erysipelas are visible. (Courtesy R. A. McIntosh.)

Several forms of swine erysipelas are recognized. The acute form of the disease is a septicemia. The spleen and lymph nodes are enlarged and reddened, and the mucosa of the stomach and small intestine is acutely inflamed, hemorrhagic, and sometimes ulcerated. The kidneys generally show cloudy swelling and are often petechiated. Red patches commonly occur on the skin, particularly of the ears, abdomen, and insides of the legs. The mortality from this form of the disease is very high.

The chronic form of the disease nearly always takes the form of a vegeta-

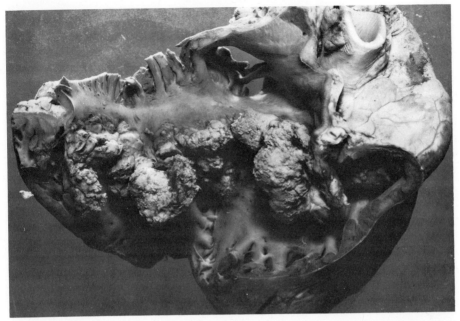

*Fig. 39.* Subacute bacterial endocarditis (porcine). *Erysipelothrix insidiosa* was isolated from the lesion. (Courtesy W. L. Boyd and H. C. H. Kernkamp.)

tive endocarditis. The heart valves, particularly the mitral, are eroded and become so covered with fibrin deposits that their functioning is seriously impaired. Affected animals invariably die from this condition sooner or later, and often suddenly.

The arthritic form of the disease generally occurs in older animals, although arthritis may be part of the picture in the more acute forms of the disease. The joints become enlarged and painful, the animals are reluctant to move, the gait is stilted, and they become stunted in growth.

The urticarial, or skin, form of the disease often is found in association with internal lesions, or it may occur without evident involvement of the viscera. The lesions consist, in the beginning, of reddish or purplish rhomboidal blotches on the skin, several cm in diameter and are found principally on the abdomen. The shape of these blotches is like that of a diamond and has given the disease its common name, "diamond skin disease." The urticarial areas later become necrotic; the affected skin dries into dense scabs, which finally peel off, leaving a bleeding area if removed too soon.

*For sheep.* Poels (40) in 1913 described a polyarthritis in sheep caused by the swine erysipelas organism. The disease was first recognized in this country by Ray (42) in 1930 and by Marsh (32), working independently. It has been described in Europe, Australia (67), and New Zealand.

The condition is seen in lambs, beginning when they are from 2 to 3 months of age. It is thought that the disease is contracted through umbilical infection, but apparently this has not been proved. The affected animals develop a stiff gait. They eat well but do not thrive. Advanced cases often get down and find difficulty in arising. Affected animals seldom die from the disease. Lesions are not present in the visceral organs; in fact they are found nowhere except in some of the joints of the legs. One joint or several of them may be affected. The involved joint usually is swollen and the joint capsule is thickened. Granulation tissue occurs on the inner surface of the capsule. The fluid is generally thin but pus cells are present in smears. The specific organism usually cannot be found in smears, but cultures are easily obtained. The organism is in every way typical.

*For cattle.* In 1953 Moulton *et al.* (36) reported an outbreak of arthritis in 6 out of 20 calves in a herd. The tibiotarsal, stifle, and carpal joints were involved. *E. insidiosa* was isolated from one of the infected joints. A case of bovine encephalomeningitis has been attributed to this organism (66).

*For birds.* According to Van Es and McGrath (59), the swine erysipelas organism is pathogenic for turkeys, chickens, geese, ducks, mud hens, pigeons, parrots, quail, and many small wild birds and larger species often found in zoological parks. In this country the species most often and most seriously affected is the turkey. The first outbreak of this kind was recognized by Beaudette and Hudson (3) in 1936. In 1938 Van Roekel, Bullis, and Clarke (60) described three outbreaks occurring in Massachusetts, Vermont, and New York. Madsen (31), shortly before, described an outbreak in Utah. The disease is an important one economically both in this country and abroad.

Affected turkeys usually are adult, or nearing adult age. They exhibit a cyanotic skin that is most obvious as a "blue comb." The birds become droopy, develop diarrhea, and die. Frequently the male birds show the highest mortality. The lesions consist of massive hemorrhages and petechiae in the muscles of the breast and legs, also large hemorrhages on the various serous membranes, particularly those of the heart. Hemorrhages occur in the mucosa of the gizzard and of the small intestine, and the content of the intestine often is bloody. The liver and spleen are ordinarily congested and enlarged. The causative organism can easily be isolated from any of the tissues. In several reports on outbreaks in turkeys it was noted that the first cases appeared within a few weeks after the birds came in contact with sheep or a sheep range.

Noting the size of the spleen may help in the differential diagnosis of erysipelas in turkeys. In erysipelas it is usually enlarged, but in pasteurellosis it remains about normal.

Graham, Levine, and Hester (18) described an outbreak of erysipelas infection in a large flock of ducks in which between 10,000 and 12,000 ducklings about 10 weeks of age were lost. The disease has been found in ducks on Long Island (11). Other reports (13, 22, 41, 58, 61) point to the occurrence of this organism in chickens, pheasants, and other fowl. It has caused outbreaks in broiler-breeder poultry flocks (4) and in starlings (14).

*For other animals. E. insidiosa* (23) has been isolated from spleen and liver tissue of the caiman (*Caiman crocodilus*) and the American crocodile (*Crocodilus acutus*). It has produced an epizootic of erysipelas septicemia in captive bottle-nosed dolphins (15).

*For man.* Many cases of wound infection of the hands have been reported. In Europe most of the human cases have been attributed to the handling of infected swine and pork, but some have occurred in fishermen and fish dealers who have had no contact with swine. According to Klauder, Righter, and Harkins (25), the disease is fairly common among fish handlers along the entire Atlantic seaboard of the United States. Most marine animals appear

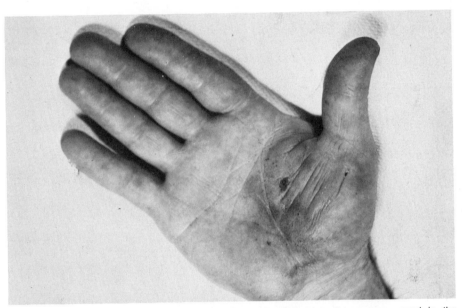

Fig. 40. The hand of a butcher affected with erysipeloid. A small puncture wound in the palm had been made by a sharp bone splinter from a pig carcass. Note the small wound and the large erythematous area surrounding it. (Courtesy J. V. Klauder.)

not to be infected with this organism but merely carry it as a saprophyte on their surface slime; however, septicemia (47) and cutaneous lesions (52) have been reported in porpoises.

Human infections with this organism were well discussed by Klauder (24) in 1938. More than half of the cases recognized in the region of Philadelphia were in slaughter-house employees, who, presumably, were infected from pork and pork products.

Klauder studied a number of cases among veterinary students who apparently had contracted infection from horse carcasses in the dissecting room. Morrill (35) has also reported on student infections contracted in this way. In this instance the specific organism was isolated from one of the horse car-casses on which one of the infected students had been working.

Evans and Narotsky (13) reported two field cases of *E. insidiosa* infection in chickens and stated that the senior author became infected in the left index finger while performing an autopsy on one of the birds.

The infection in man is known as *erysipeloid* to distinguish it from human erysipelas, which is caused by a hemolytic *Streptococcus*. The disease is rarely manifested by septicemia, which is likely to be fatal. The usual type is disclosed by a local lesion developing from an abrasion of the skin where the infection enters. The lesion usually is on one of the fingers. The intensity of the inflammation varies. The infected finger swells, and often the swelling ex-tends throughout the entire hand. There is no suppuration and no pitting on pressure. A throbbing and burning pain that usually prevents sleep is a con-spicuous symptom. There is marked erythema of the infected region, some-times local arthritis. In the majority of cases the infection runs a course of about 3 weeks; a few heal in a shorter period and some require much longer. Local treatment of the wound and the use of sulfonamides is of little value. The efficacy of specific antiserum in the treatment of erysipeloid is open to question. However, it is reported that penicillin treatment is followed by rapid recovery. The disease in man usually is self-limiting and will heal spon-taneously within a month in most instances. That it does sometimes cause septicemia and terminate in endocarditis and death is attested by Schiffman and Black (45) and by McCarty and Bornstein (29).

In Scandinavian countries a disease called *sealer's finger* or *speckfinger* (*blubber finger*) attacks only persons engaged in catching seals or stripping the sealskin of blubber (54). The cause of this lesion has not been fully deter-mined, but its marked resemblance to erysipeloid and the fact that a disease of the same category as swine erysipelas occurs in seals has led to much work in attempts to establish its etiology.

**Source of Infection.** In the acute septicemic form of the disease in swine, the erysipelas organism may be found in the intestinal content in large numbers, and it occurs in the urine. The infection is spread through the discharges of such animals and the contamination of food materials thereby. Carrier ani-mals exist, and such animals probably serve to spread the disease. In fact, apparently healthy pigs have been found to carry virulent organisms in their tonsils, gall bladders, and the flask-shaped glands that occur on their ileo-cecal valves.

The organism has been isolated from a diseased rat caught at a dump (Stiles, 53). Community saleyards and stockyards frequently are sources of infection. Pork trimmings in garbage probably account for many sporadic cases. It should be remembered that this organism is unusually resistant to smoking and salting, hence pickled and smoked products often are capable of causing infections. It has been suspected also that fish products, often used as protein supplements in animal foods, may be responsible for introducing infections. The erysipelas bacillus has been isolated repeatedly from samples of commercial ground fish meal, indicating that such material is not always heated enough to destroy this organism. Anti-hog-cholera serum and virus sometimes are contaminated with the erysipelas organism. All serum produced under federal license in the United States must be pasteurized; hence dissemination of erysipelas infection in this way is avoided. Hog cholera virus sold for field use is examined bacteriologically and by pigeon inoculation for erysipelas contamination before it is released.

**Diagnosis.** The differentiation in the field of acute swine erysipelas from hog cholera offers considerable difficulty, and even clinicians with great experience sometimes mistake one for the other. It should be remembered that, in the United States, hog cholera is the most important disease of swine, and failure to recognize it is always a costly error. When in doubt, it is best always to administer anti-hog-cholera serum, because this will forestall disastrous experiences if the disease proves to be cholera, and, furthermore, anti-hog-cholera serum often has a very favorable effect upon erysipelas infections. The reason for this is not known. Possibly erysipelas antibodies occur in anti-hog-cholera serum, or perhaps it is a wholly nonspecific phenomenon.

In acute hog cholera the affected animals are always sick for several days before they die; in acute erysipelas infection deaths often occur within a few hours after the first symptoms are noted. In cholera the disease is progressive and there are few recoveries; in erysipelas the sick animals often recover after a few days. In cholera the outbreak reaches a crisis rather slowly; in erysipelas the crisis is apt to develop quickly. In cholera the affected animals are usually lethargic; in erysipelas they are usually bright and alert until shortly before death. Lameness is not common in cholera; it is frequent in erysipelas. Cholera-affected hogs usually will not eat for several days before death; erysipelas-affected animals frequently will continue to eat after hyperthermia and other symptoms are exhibited. Diarrhea is not as common in erysipelas as it is in cholera. The lesions often are not of great help in the differential diagnosis between these diseases. In erysipelas the spleen usually is slightly enlarged, tense, and bluish red in color, whereas in cholera it is usually unchanged, or it may present one or more wedge-shaped infarcts along its margin. In erysipelas the mucosa of the stomach is often highly inflamed, showing a dark bluish-red discoloration; this is not often found in cholera. The lymph nodes may or may not be congested, whereas they usually are hemorrhagic in cholera. Petechiation of the epiglottis, trachea, kidneys, and urinary bladder may be found in both diseases.

Schoening, Creech, and Grey (46) introduced a rapid, whole-blood agglutination test that may be used in the field to detect subacute and chronic cases of erysipelas. It is of no value in dealing with acute outbreaks because recently infected animals have not had time to develop agglutinins. A heavy suspension of *E. insidiosa*, consisting of smooth forms of the organism only, is mixed on a slide with a drop of freshly drawn blood, in the proportion of two drops of the antigen to one of blood. Clumping of the organisms within 2 minutes is indicative of infection. Unfortunately this antigen is not stable. It must be prepared and standardized with great care, and it must be checked frequently to insure its accuracy. McNutt and Leith (30) found this test useful in eliminating the chronically infected animals from a herd. Because of the instability of the antigen, this material is not available commercially.

The use of a hemagglutination test in the diagnosis of swine erysipelas has been suggested. Sheep erythrocytes sensitized with *E. insidiosa* protein would serve as antigen. Hemocultures are sometimes useful as a diagnostic aid in swine erysipelas. Five to 10 ml of blood are drawn aseptically and placed in 70 ml of sterile tryptose broth for cultivation of the organism (21). Wood (68) recommends the use of a selective liquid medium that consists of tryptose broth base, horse serum, kanamycin, vancomycin, and novobiocin for the isolation of *E. insidiosa* from inoculums containing small numbers of viable cells. The fluorescent antibody technic (10, 33) is useful in identifying *E. insidiosa*, and triple sugar iron agar (62) aids in the recognition of cultures.

**Immunity.** Biological products available for immunization are antiserum, vaccine, bacterin, and culture-antiserum (simultaneous treatment).

*Antiserum.* Immune serum is of value both for prophylaxis and for treatment. For treatment, 10 to 30 ml of serum are injected as early in the course of the disease as possible. Losses may occur in spite of such procedure. For prophylaxis the serum is very successful, the principal disadvantage being that the immunity is short-lived. It can be depended upon to protect for not more than 15 days. For animals weighing less than 100 pounds, 5 ml of the serum are sufficient. For large animals, 1 ml additional is allowed for each 20 pounds in excess of 100 pounds of body weight.

*Vaccine.* This is the oldest method of immunization to this disease. A vaccine was developed and successfully used by Pasteur and Thuillier (39) in 1883, and their method is still employed.

Attenuation of the culture for swine was accomplished by passing it through rabbits. In the course of time such cultures acquire great virulence for rabbits, but simultaneously they lose virulence for swine. Two strains are used, the most attenuated being injected first and the second about a week later. The procedure usually immunizes safely for periods of 8 months to 1 year, which ordinarily is as long as is necessary because the life span of swine is not much longer than that. Breeding stock may require reimmunization after 1 year. This method is not wholly safe because vaccination erysipelas often occurs. For this reason it is not used in the United States.

In past years many avirulent strains of *E. insidiosa* have been used as vaccines, mostly with indifferent success. Continued search for cultures that lack virulence but are strongly immunogenic has produced some more promising vaccines. One of these is the erysipelas vaccine avirulent (EVA) of Gray and Norden, Jr. (19). It has been specially licensed by the U.S. Department of Agriculture and is available to veterinarians. EVA is a lyophilized single strain of *E. insidiosa*. According to the authors, it is a live culture that is entirely avirulent to mice, guinea pigs, pigeons, swine, turkeys, and man. The product may be used with or without the simultaneous administration of antiserum, and it induces a high level of immunity. Avirulent erysipelas vaccines have been employed by the oral route in vaccinating swine (27, 44). It is claimed that this method is safe for pigs, does not produce the carrier state, and induces immunity in about 80 percent of the pigs for periods over 6 months.

*Bacterin.* These agents were not highly successful in immunizing against erysipelas until 1947 when Traub (56) and Dinter, independently of each other, prepared adsorbed *E. insidiosa* bacterin. By their procedure the organisms are grown in a fluid medium, killed with formalin, and adsorbed by aluminum hydroxide (7). A similar bacterin has been produced in this country from three of the highly antigenic isolates of Dinter, and field trials with swine and turkeys have indicated that this product is highly satisfactory as an immunizing agent (6, 8, 17).

*Simultaneous treatment.* This is employed for prophylactic immunization only in certain states where erysipelas is common and disease control officials have authorized its use. Restrictions on indiscriminate sale of the culture have been imposed in the belief that it is unwise to distribute virulent organisms in areas where swine erysipelas is not prevalent.

The culture-antiserum method is used preferably on weanling pigs. The young animal is given from 5 to 20 ml of antiserum subcutaneously in one site and from 0.25 to 0.5 ml of culture in another. The serum dose should be carefully graded, because overdoses of serum reduce the firmness and duration of the resultant immunity. Some like to repeat the procedure in about 14 days. Others give a second dose of culture alone in about 14 days. The immunity induced is generally solid and lasting.

**Evaluation of Biological Products.** Until it was demonstrated that the percutaneous method of injection was highly consistent in inducing experimental swine erysipelas infection, there was no good test for indicating the immunity or susceptibility of swine to this disease. By means of the percutaneous test Shuman and Schoening (51) have shown that culture-antiserum vaccination of baby pigs 2 to 5 days after farrowing is of no value in protecting them up to market age and of limited value in protecting them as weanlings. The vaccination of weanling pigs (average age, 58 days) produced worth-while protection through the usual marketable age of 5 to 7 months.

Other workers (6, 17) have tested the adsorbed erysipelas bacterin and indicate that a single 5-ml dose given to weanling pigs (about 8 weeks old) produces more satisfactory results than the simultaneous treatment. Ray (43) has stated that a second dose of bacterin, given 2 to 4 weeks after the first, materially increases the titer of the animal and markedly prolongs the immunity. When two doses are given, the first is sometimes administered before the baby pig is weaned. The EVA induces a high level of immunity, and avirulent erysipelas strains are as effective as oral erysipelas vaccines (38). It has

been stated that the feeding of antibiotics does not interfere with oral vaccination.

Neher *et al.* (37) concluded that vaccination will not prevent arthritis.

According to Doyle (12) either an absorbed bacterin or a living avirulent
strain can be safely used. The avirulent vaccine is cheaper to produce, the
dose is smaller, and it probably gives a longer protection. Four to 5 months is
about the maximum duration of protection from one dose of bacterin or vaccine. Breeding-stock should be vaccinated twice a year. There is evidence
that pigs farrowed by immune sows should not be vaccinated until they are 3
months old (49).

**Chemotherapy.** Reports on the use of sulfonamides in treating *Erysipelothrix*
infection indicate that they are of little value (Woodbine, 69). Streptomycin
and aureomycin appear to be more effective than the sulfonamides but less
active than penicillin against these bacteria. Penicillin seems to be very effective in treating the infection in mice (Harvey, Libby, and Waller, 20), in turkeys (Brown, Doll, Bruner, and Kinkaid, 5), and in swine (Aitken, 1),

## REFERENCES

1.  Aitken.   North Am. Vet., 1949, *30,* 25.
2.  Balfour-Jones.   Brit. Jour. Exp. Path., 1935, *16,* 236.
3.  Beaudette and Hudson.   Jour. Am. Vet. Med. Assoc., 1936, *88, 475.*
4.  Borland.   Vet. Rec., 1970, *86,* 564.
5.  Brown, Doll, Bruner, and Kinkaid.   Jour. Am. Vet. Med. Assoc., 1949, *114,* 438.
6.  Calloway, Clark, Price, and Vezey.   Vet. Med., 1955, *50,* 39.
7.  Cooper, Personeus, and Choman.   Canad. Jour. Comp. Med. and Vet. Sci., 1954, *18,* 83.
8.  Cooper, Personeus, Harvey, and Percival.   Am. Jour. Vet. Res., 1954, *15,* 594.
9.  Creech.   Jour. Am. Vet. Med. Assoc., 1921, *59,* 139.
10.  Dacres and Groth.   Jour. Bact., 1959, *78,* 298.
11.  Dougherty, III, and Bruner.   Cornell Vet., 1954, *44,* 209.
12.  Doyle.   Vet. Rev. and Annot., 1960, *6,* 95.
13.  Evans and Narotsky.   Cornell Vet., 1954, *44,* 32.
14.  Faddoul, Fellows, and Baird.   Avian Dis., 1968, *12,* 61.
15.  Geraci, Sauer, and Medway.   Am. Jour. Vet. Res., 1966, *27,* 597.
16.  Gledhill.   Jour. Path. and Bact., 1945, *57,* 179.
17.  Gouge, Bolton, and Alson.   Am. Jour. Vet. Res., 1956, *27,* 135.
18.  Graham, Levine, and Hester.   Jour. Am. Vet. Med. Assoc., 1939, *95,* 211.
19.  Gray and Norden, Jr.   *Ibid.,* 1955, *127,* 506.
20.  Harvey, Libby, and Waller.   Proc. Soc. Exp. Biol. and Med., 1945, *60,* 307.
21.  Hubbard.   Jour. Am. Vet. Med. Assoc., 1952, *120,* 291.
22.  Hudson, Black, Bivins, and Tudor.   *Ibid.,* 1952, *121,* 278.
23.  Jasmin and Baucom.   Am. Jour. Vet. Clin. Path., 1967, *1,* 173.
24.  Klauder.   Jour. Am. Med. Assoc., 1938, *111,* 1345.
25.  Klauder, Righter, and Harkins.   Arch. Dermatol. and Syphilol., 1926, *14,* 662.

26. Koch. Investigations into the etiology of traumatic infective diseases. New Sydenham Society, London, 1880.

27. Lawson, Pepevnak, Walker, and Crawley. Canad. Vet. Jour., 1966, 7, 13.

28. Loeffler. Arb. kaiserl. Gesundhsamte, 1886, *1*, 46.

29. McCarty and Bornstein. Am. Jour. Clin. Path., 1960, *33, 39.*

30. McNutt and Leith. Mich. State Coll. Vet., 1945, 5, 97.

31. Madsen. Jour. Am. Vet. Med. Assoc., 1937, *91*, 206.

32. Marsh. *Ibid.*, 1931, *78*, 57.

33. Marshall, Eveland, and Smith. Am. Jour. Vet. Res., 1959, *2J*, 1077.

34. Moore. Jour. Comp. Med. and Vet. Arch., 1892, *13*, 333.

35. Morrill. Jour. Inf. Dis., 1939, *65*, 322.

36. Moulton, Rhode, and Wheat. Jour. Am. Vet. Med. Assoc., 1953, *123*, 335.

37. Neher, Swenson, Doyle, and Sikes. Am. Jour. Vet. Res., 1958, *19*, 5.

38. Ose, Barnes, and Berkman. Jour. Am. Vet. Med. Assoc., 1963, *143*, 1084.

39. Pasteur and Thuillier. Comp. rend. Acad. Sci., 1883, 97, 1163.

40. Poels. Folia Microbiologica, 1913, 2, I.

41. Raines and Winkel. Jour. Am. Vet. Med. Assoc., 1956, *129*, 399.

42. Ray. *Ibid.*, 1930, 77, 107.

43. *Ibid.*, 1958, *132*, 365.

44. Sampson, Sauter, Wilkins, and Driesens. *Ibid.*, 1965, *147*, 484.

45. Schiffman and Black. N. Eng. Jour. Med., 1956, *255*, 1148.

46. Schoening, Creech, and Grey. North Am. Vet., 1932, *13*, 19.

47. Seibold and Neal. Jour. Am. Vet. Med. Assoc., 1956, *128*, 537.

48. Shuman. Proc. Am. Vet. Med. Assoc., 1951, p. 153.

49. Shuman. Jour. Am. Vet. Med. Assoc., 1961, *139*, 777.

50. Shuman and Lee. Jour. Bact., 1950, *60*, 677.

51. Shuman and Schoening. Jour. Am. Vet. Med. Assoc., 1953, *123*, 301, 304, and 307.

52. Simpson, Wood, and Young. *Ibid.*, 1958, *133*, 558.

53. Stiles. Am. Jour. Vet. Res., 1944, 5, 243.

54. Svenkerud, Rosted, and Thorshaug. Nord. Vet. Med., 1951, 3, 147.

55. TenBroeck. Jour. Exp. Med., 1920, *32*, 331.

56. Traub. Monatsh f. Vetmed., 1947, *10*, 165.

57. Truszczynski. Am. Jour. Vet. Res., 1961, *22*, 846.

58. Vance and Whenham. Canad. Jour. Comp. Med. and Vet Sci., 1958, *22*, 86.

59. Van Es and McGrath. Nebr. Agr. Exp. Sta. Res. Bul. 84, 1936.

60. Van Roekel, Bullis, and Clarke. Jour. Am. Vet. Med. Assoc., 1938, *92*, 403.

61. Vickers and Bierer. *Ibid.*, 1958, *133*, 223.

62. *Ibid.*, 543.

63. Ward. *Ibid.*, 1922, *61*, 155.

64. Wayson. Pub. Health Rpts. (U.S.), 1927, *42*, 1489.

65. Wellmann. Jour. Am. Vet. Med. Assoc., 1955, *127*, 331.

66. Whaley, Robinson, Newberre, and Sippel. Vet. Med., 1958, *53*, 475.

67. Whitten. Austral. Vet. Jour., 1952, *28*, 6.

68. Wood. Am. Jour. Vet. Res., 1965, *26*, 1303.

69. Woodbine. Vet. Jour., 1946, *102*, 88.

# XIX | The *Bacillaceae*

Within the family *Bacillaceae* are two genera—*Bacillus* and *Clostridium*. Both are capable of producing endospores. The former contains aerobic species while the latter is made up of anaerobic types.

## THE GENUS *BACILLUS*

Although there are numerous species in the genus, *Bacillus anthracis* is unique in that it is the only truly pathogenic aerobic sporulating species.

### Bacillus anthracis

*B. anthracis* causes the disease known as *anthrax* (Ger. *milzbrand;* Fr. *charbon*). The herbivorous animals, especially cattle and sheep, are affected by it. Horses, deer, buffalo, and other wild herbivora, guinea pigs, and mice are very susceptible to infection. Swine are not so susceptible and the disease frequently runs a chronic course. Dogs, cats, rats, and most birds are relatively insusceptible but can be infected artificially. Cold-blooded animals are not affected. The disease often produces death in man, but he is not so susceptible as the herbivorous animals.

**Morphology and Staining Reactions.** The anthrax bacillus is a large, straight, square-ended rod usually about 1 micron in diameter and from 3 to 6 microns long. In cultures it forms long chains which, unstained, appear as solid filaments because the square ends of the individual cells fit very closely together. In tissues long filaments are never seen. Here the elements occur either individually or in short chains of two to five or six organisms. In tissues the organism is regularly encapsulated, a single capsule enclosing as many organisms as remain in a chain. The capsules are well marked and can be stained rather readily. Spores are formed in abundance when the organism is growing in the presence of air. Becuase of lack of sufficient oxygen, spores are not formed in the blood and internal organs. It is Gram-positive and stains easily with all the usual dyes. It is not acid-fast.

**Cultural Features.** The anthrax organism grows readily upon the simplest of organic infusions. Best growth occurs on solid media exposed to the air. Anaerobically, growth will appear but it is meager. Even in a fluid medium in a tube with the surface exposed to the air, in which the dissolved oxygen is short of saturation, the growth of the anthrax organism is not luxuriant.

On agar plates the anthrax organism develops into characteristic "ground-glass" surface colonies. The margins of these colonies are irregular and resemble, under low magnification, locks of wavy hair. It is for this reason that they are sometimes described as "Medusa-head" colonies, after the mythological maiden whose flowing locks were changed to serpents. Both the ground-glass and the Medusa-head appearance are caused by the fact that in such colonies the organism grows in the form of long filaments which lie in parallel wavy bundles like locks of a well-combed coiffure. Deep colonies are small, ragged, and stringy. It happens that there are many aerobic spore-forming bacilli that form surface colonies resembling those of anthrax. In differentiating the anthrax bacillus from most of these, the deep colonies will be found to be more useful than the more conspicuous surface ones. Most of these organisms, other than the anthrax organism, either fail to develop in the depths of the agar medium, or if they do develop, the colonies are small and compact.

On gelatin plates the characteristic Medusa-head colonies appear, but the gelatin soon liquefies and this spoils further colony development. Each colony sinks into a liquefied pool, and continued growth is virtually in a liquid medium.

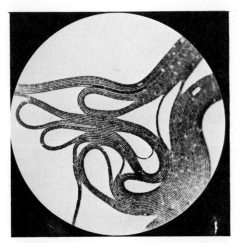 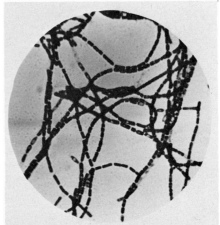

*Fig. 41 (left). Bacillus anthracis*, an impression preparation from a colony on a gelatin plate. The habit of the bacilli of forming long filamentous chains that lie parallel accounts for the "Medusa-head" appearance of the colonies. X 150.

*Fig. 42 (right). Bacillus anthracis*, a stained preparation from a 24-hour-old culture on solid media, showing arrangement of cells in long chains and the development of spores in many of the organisms. X 725.

Milk is rendered slightly acid and a soft curd usually is formed, but this quickly undergoes digestion by a rennetlike enzyme. In liquid media a fluffy growth usually begins near the surface, but after a few hours of incubation this gravitates to the bottom of the tube. The fluid usually remains clear except for this delicate filamentous mass at the bottom of the tube. Usually a dull whitish ring appears on the wall of the tube at the level of the fluid surface.

The anthrax bacillus grows readily on the cut surface of many boiled vegetables, such as potatoes, beets, and carrots, on the pod of a string bean, or on the cut surface of a banana. On all of these media the growth is spreading, dull, dry, mealy, and grayish white in color. Sporulation occurs early and profusely on these substances.

Acid but no gas is produced in glucose, sucrose, maltose, and salicin.

**Resistance.** In the growing or bacillary form, the anthrax bacillus is possessed of only slight resistance. It is killed by pasteurization, is easily destroyed by ordinary disinfectants, and quickly succumbs to the action of putrefactive bacteria.

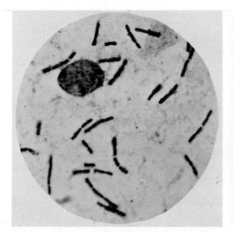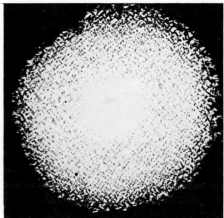

Fig. 43 (left). *Bacillus anthracis* in a bovine spleen. In tissues anthrax bacilli occur in short chains surrounded by a common capsule. The capsular material shows indistinctly in the illustration. It is responsible for the lack of sharpness of outline of the organisms. X 700.

Fig. 44 (right). *Bacillus anthracis,* a surface colony on agar photographed by transmitted light showing the "ground-glass" appearance. X 6.

The spores are readily formed providing the organism is under aerobic conditions. In the organs of animals dead of anthrax the oxygen supply is insufficient for spore formation; consequently they are killed within a few days by the putrefactive process. If the carcass is opened, the tissues are exposed to air, the organisms then are able to sporulate, and their resistance is greatly enhanced. The spores resist drying for long periods of time. There are many records of spores having survived for 10 or more years. Umeno and Nobata (36) reported the finding of viable spores which developed into virulent cultures in the spring of 1938 from threads that had been impregnated with anthrax spores from a potato culture in 1879. Anthrax spores are not so resistant to heat as is commonly supposed, a 10-minute exposure to boiling water being enough to destroy some strains. At 120 C, dry heat, it is necessary to expose anthrax spores for 1 hour in order to kill all the spores. An abrupt change in

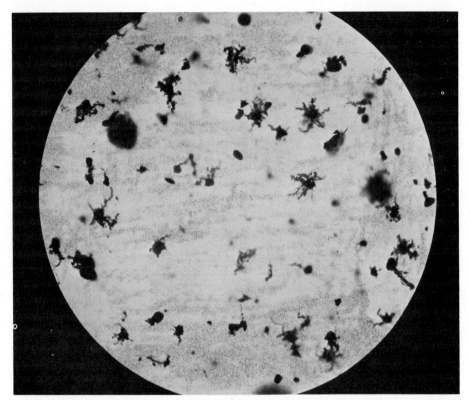

Fig. 45. *Bacillus anthracis,* deep colonies in an agar plate. The photograph was taken by transmitted light with slight magnification. The irregular colonies are characteristic. Many common aerobic sporebearing bacteria have surface colonies that resemble those of the anthrax organism, but most of these produce small dense colonies in the depths of the medium.

resistance occurs at 160 C. Spores are killed much more rapidly above than below this point. Sanitizing burlap feed bags contaminated with anthrax spores can be accomplished by exposing them to dielectric heat at 112.7 C for 30 minutes (Bryan, 6).

Laboratory workers should remember that the time needed to fix a spore film at any given temperature is much less than that required to kill the spores.

**Sources of Infection.** The anthrax bacillus is not usually transmitted directly from one individual to another. The organism swarms in the tissues of affected animals and is eliminated in the secretions and excretions a short time before death. If animals dying of anthrax are autopsied, or if the carcasses are left to be devoured by birds or animals of prey, the organism may be widely scattered on the soil. It is scattered further by floods. The bacillus is able to maintain itself for long periods in soil. Grasses growing in lowlands become infected, and the disease may be contracted in midwinter by animals feeding upon hay grown on such lands. Animals pastured on infected areas must be artificially immunized or heavy losses from the disease will occur. In hot climates where flies are abundant, the disease is transmitted by the bloodsucking varieties, notably by the large horseflies of the genus *Tabanus*.

Anthrax infection frequently is carried long distances. In the past, tanneries often have been responsible for introducing anthrax into regions where it had not previously existed. Dried hides from anthrax-infected animals from parts of South America, Manchuria, or the infected areas of North America, when soaked in the tannery, leave anthrax spores in the soaking liquids. If these are discharged, without disinfection, into streams, the latter during flood periods may cause more or less permanent infection of low-lying pastures. In the United States human anthrax has resulted from handling imported hair and wool. Carpet wools originating in Asia, North Africa, and possibly southern Europe, and goat hair and skins coming from Asia have been incriminated (Wolff and Heimann, 37). In 1960 Albrink *et al.* (1) reported an outbreak of human inhalation anthrax in which there were three fatal cases. The epidemic, the first in modern times, occurred in a New Hampshire goat hair processing mill in millworkers.

In England imported feeding stuffs, particularly protein concentrates, often are infected with anthrax spores (16). The situation in Great Britain is quite different from that which prevails in this country inasmuch as we produce practically all of our animal feeds, and essentially all of it comes from anthrax-free districts, whereas Great Britain is forced to import her foodstuffs largely from South America, where anthrax is much more prevalent than here. Anthrax may get into animal feed in the United States on rare occasions. In 1952 a series of outbreaks of anthrax occurred in swine in this country. These were traced to feed supplements which contained raw bone meal of foreign origin (9).

According to Hanson (14), Kercheval, a physician who lived in Bardstown, Kentucky, was the first to describe anthrax in man and cattle in North America. This occurred in 1824. It is postulated that anthrax was introduced into the Ohio Valley in the early days of westward migration and has persisted there to the present.

In 1955 Stein and Van Ness (31) reported the results of a 10-year survey of anthrax in the United States. From 1945–1954 losses among cattle, horses, mules, swine, and sheep were reported to be 17,604. These cases appeared in

3,447 outbreaks in 39 states. States reporting no cases were Arizona, Connect-icut, Delaware, Idaho, Maine, New Hampshire, Rhode Island, Vermont, and West Virginia. States reporting 100 or more outbreaks were California (271), Illinois (205), Indiana (222), Iowa (133), Kansas (368), Louisiana (413), Missouri (267), New Jersey (114), Ohio (317), South Dakota (150), Tennessee (142), and Texas (288). During this period there were 483 cases in man, 8 of which occurred in veterinarians. In 1950 there were 61 outbreaks in 12 states with 595 losses of animals. In 1952 these numbers jumped to 1,644; 32; and 3,451, respectively. Most of the deaths that occurred were in cattle and swine. By 1955 the respective figures had dropped to 122, 20, and 264. Apparently, the high incidence rate in 1952 was caused by contaminated feed. The source of infection for the 1962 and 1963 outbreaks that occurred in bison in the Northwest Territories of Canada is less clear. The disease was introduced into the Hook Lake area in 1962 and spread across the Slave River to the Grand Detour region, a distance of 40 miles, by 1963. Carrion eaters were the suspected transporting agents (8).

Infection may occur in three ways: (*a*) through the alimentary tract; (*b*) through the skin; (*c*) through inhalation. It is much easier to infect animals through the injured skin and by way of the respiratory tract than by the alimentary tract; nevertheless it is thought that the majority of natural infections occur through the ingestion of infected food materials.

**Pathogenicity.** The manifestations of the disease depend upon the manner of infection. When it occurs through the internal organs (no visible evidence of a localization), its principal character is the sudden onset and rapidly fatal course. The peracute form that sometimes occurs in herbivora may terminate fatally in 1 or 2 hours; the acute form in less than 24 hours. The animals have a high fever and usually show bleeding from the body openings. The organism can be found in the excretions or in the blood in large numbers at the time of death, and its identification in stained films constitutes the simplest and most certain way of making an accurate diagnosis.

Localized anthrax is seen when infection has occurred through a wound in the skin. This form occurs naturally more often in man than in any of the domestic animals. Cutaneous anthrax takes the form of a swelling of an edematous nature which is hot and painful at first but later becomes cold and painless. In man this type of anthrax lesion is called *malignant carbuncle,* because in its earlier stages it resembles a developing furuncle or carbuncle caused by *Staphylococcus aureus.* Recoveries in both animals and man are more frequent when the disease is localized than when it is septicemic. Localized infections often become generalized, however.

Anthrax in *cattle, sheep,* and *horses* usually appears in the spring and summer months, and most infections result from grazing on infected pastures. The cases usually are acute or peracute and most of them are fatal.

In *swine* and *dogs* anthrax generally assumes a localized form. These animals are infected only by ingesting heavily contaminated feed, either the raw meat of other animals which have died of anthrax or, in the case of swine, infected bone or meat meal given as a feed supplement. In these cases the organism apparently enters the tissues from the upper part of the digestive tract, probably through the tonsils, and the disease is manifested by an inflammatory edema of the tissues of the head and neck. Often these regions become greatly distorted and swollen, and suffocation may occur through severe edema of the glottis. In these animals the infection occasionally localizes in the intestinal wall, the mesenteric lymph nodes, and the spleen.

A number of outbreaks of anthrax have occurred in *mink*, in which the mortality frequently is very heavy. The disease in this species is generally peracute and generalized. It occurs only when fresh meat from an infected carcass has been fed.

Generalized anthrax may easily be induced in susceptible animals by the inhalation of spores. In man, infections of this type occur among employees of plants in which hides, wool, and hair are processed, the spores being thrown into the air from the infected materials handled. The human form is a rapidly fatal malady known as *woolsorter's disease*.

**Bacteriological Diagnosis.** Diagnosis of the disease by means of recognition of the organism or its products may be made in a number of ways. The most important of these are:

1. Direct microscopic examination of tissues and fluids. This method is simple and certain when the animal has just died and putrefaction has not set in. The organism can be found in the blood stream or in films from practically any organ when the disease has assumed the septicemic form. In the local forms the local lesion must, of course, be examined. The organism is a relatively short, thick, Gram-positive rod, usually arranged in pairs or in chains of three, four, or five bacilli. Spores are not seen. With proper staining it may be observed that the chain of organisms is surrounded by a common capsule.

If putrefaction has begun, it is not always an easy matter to make an accurate diagnosis by the direct film method. Many of the anaerobic bacteria of decomposition resemble the anthrax bacillus quite closely. Usually these organisms are somewhat longer, and are arranged in chains longer than are formed by the anthrax bacillus in tissues. When many extraneous bacteria are present, it is better not to depend upon the direct microscopic method for making a diagnosis.

2. Cultural methods. When the tissues and blood are fresh, there is no difficulty in cultivating the causative organism. If the tissues are decomposing, difficulties arise from two angles: first, the anthrax organism rapidly dies off and there may be few or no viable bacteria remaining and, second, other organisms that resemble the anthrax bacillus very closely may be present.

The characteristic "ground-glass" type of colony is searched for on plate cultures made from the organs or blood when the tissues are not absolutely fresh. Examination of the peripheries of these colonies under moderate magnification should show no motile organisms when the plates are from 18 to 24 hours old, and the other characteristics of anthrax colonies should be carefully looked for. If the organism is in pure culture, look for deep colonies. If it is the anthrax organism, these will be loose and ragged. Most other organisms that are anthraxlike produce small compact colonies in the depths of the medium.

When animal feeds or other suspected substances are cultured, pasteurization may be employed first in order to eliminate contaminating non-spore-bearing organisms. Then the material may be plated in dilutions or injected into test animals. Pearce and Powell have developed a selective medium for isolating *B. anthracis* from soil samples (22), Burdon (7) has published methods for the positive identification of virulent strains without the use of motility or animal virulence tests, and Kinsely (20) has employed phenethyl alcohol and chloral hydrate in selective media to differentiate *B. anthracis* from *B. cereus*. The latter is a member of the genus *Bacillus* and is similar to the anthrax organism, but lacks its pathogenic powers.

3. Animal inoculation. Guinea pig inoculation is usually relied upon to decide between anthrax, and anthraxlike, colonies. Direct inoculation of guinea pigs with tissues, exudates, etc., is a reliable method of diagnosing the disease providing the material does not contain other organisms that destroy the experimental animal before the anthrax organism can be expected to make itself evident. Organisms of the malignant edema group (anaerobes) frequently do this. If viable anthrax organisms are present and if the animal does not die from other causes earlier, it will usually die from anthrax in from 36 to 48 hours after subcutaneous injection. Occasionally death is as late as the 5th day after injection. The tissues of the guinea pig will be found swarming with the organism, and there will be a gelatinous infiltration under the skin at the point of inoculation.

4. Serodiagnosis. The thermo-precipitation test (Ascoli test) is used very successfully in Europe for the detection of anthrax-infected hides. It may also be used with other tissues.

For the Ascoli test a precipitating serum of high titer is needed. Very few animals produce a serum satisfactory for this work; hence it is rather expensive. The bit of hide or other tissue is extracted with water, either by boiling or with the aid of chloroform. In this way a clear fluid is obtained which should contain anthrax protein if the organism is present in the tissues. This is known as *precipitinogen*. The fluid is layered in a very narrow tube with some of the precipitating serum (precipitin). The formation of a whitish ring at the line of juncture of the two fluids constitutes a positive reaction. The agar gel precipitin technic has proved to be useful in anthrax antibody determinations (26). In this test an extract of the anthrax organism is used as an antigen.

**Immunity.** Because toxic properties were not demonstrated in cultures for many years the cause of death in anthrax was a much debated question. At one time the mechanical hypothesis, i.e., that the bacteria multiplied until the capillaries were choked, was seriously considered. The hypothesis was abandoned. In 1939 Peter (24) suggested that capillary damage resulted from hyalinization of vessel walls and the formation of thrombi. Death was caused principally by thrombosis of the capillaries. In 1955 Smith *et al.* (29) reported that *B. anthracis* produces a toxin *in vivo* which is responsible for the death of the host. In guinea pigs dying of anthrax this toxin is found mainly in the plasma. It produces edema and the lethal effect when injected intravenously. Both actions are specifically neutralized by anthrax antiserum. The cause of death in the guinea pig is secondary shock resulting from vascular damage accompanied by oligemia and renal failure (uremia). Klein *et al.* (21) studied toxin production in the rhesus monkey and found it to be present in the blood at the terminal stage of anthrax and also present in increasing amounts in the lymph as death approached. It is now known that this toxicity can be produced *in vitro* in mediums containing large amounts of serum (15) and that it can be neutralized by specific antiserum. Remmele *et al.* (27) injected anthrax toxin into the cerebrospinal fluid of the monkey and demonstrated that death resulted from a terminal anoxia mediated by the central nervous system.

Resistance can easily be built up in susceptible animals by the injection of living attenuated cultures. Dead cultures and culture filtrates are generally considered useless for this purpose; however, formalin-killed cultures recently have been advocated for immunization. It is difficult or impossible to produce absolute immunity to anthrax infection. Vaccines will induce sufficient immunity to protect against natural infection, and thus are of practical value.

*Pasteur vaccine.* The first vaccine for anthrax was made by Pasteur in 1879. Attempting to use the method that had succeeded in weakening the virulence of the fowl cholera organism, he found that it did not succeed with the anthrax organism because of its habit of forming spores, which then resisted attenuation. Success was finally achieved when it was discovered that incubation at 42 to 43 C inhibited sporulation and attenuated the vegetative forms.

The vaccine strains are produced by cultivating the organism at 42 to 43 C continuously, with daily transfers to fresh medium. At this temperature the virulence of the organism is gradually lost. Two vaccines are used, the first consisting of a strain that has been cultivated longer at the abnormal incubation temperature, and consequently has less virulence, than the second vaccine. The degree of immunity obtained appears to be directly related to the virulence of the vaccine strains used; consequently the first and weaker vaccine is to prepare the animal for the more virulent second.

The vaccine is a bouillon culture of the attenuated strain. Vaccine no. 1 has been so attenuated that it will produce anthrax in mice and sometimes in young guinea pigs but not in older guinea pigs or rabbits. Vaccine no. 2 has been attenuated to the point where it will not ordinarily kill rabbits, but it should kill guinea pigs. Vaccine no. 2 is given about 10 to 12 days after no. 1.

The vaccine prepared by Pasteur has been extremely successful in many parts of the world where anthrax is a menace. In many areas the disease has been practically eliminated by systematic vaccination. Animals sometimes do not receive sufficient protection, and in some other cases the vaccine proves too powerful and animals die from the treatment. *Owners of animals should always be warned that the anthrax vaccine is occasionally responsible for anthrax. The vaccine should never be used except when a definite diagnosis of anthrax has been made on the premises.*

A distinct disadvantage of this vaccine is that it does not keep well. The organisms are supplied in the form of a bouillon culture to which preservatives cannot be added and in which sporulation does not occur readily; hence the organisms tend to die out rather rapidly. This disadvantage is overcome in the spore vaccine.

Neither the Pasteur nor the other vaccines for anthrax can be depended upon to give sufficient immunity to protect the animals for a period longer than 1 year. In especially bad districts it is sometimes necessary to vaccinate more often than once a year, but usually if the animals are vaccinated early in the spring before being turned on pasture or range, sufficient protection is given.

*Spore vaccine.* In order to avoid the uncertainty occasioned by deterioration of the Pasteur vaccine, spore vaccines became popular. The anthrax cultures are attenuated as for the Pasteur vaccine. They are then grown on a peptone-free agar for 4 to 7 days at 37 C, at the end of which time the majority of the bacilli have sporulated. The cultures are washed down with sterile physiological salt solution. The resultant suspension is heated at 60 C for 30 minutes to destroy all vegetative forms. The number of spores in the suspension is determined by plating measured quantities. The suspensions are now usually diluted until each ml contains one million spores. One ml of such a suspension constitutes a normal dose for cattle and horses; about 0.25 ml for sheep. Each lot of spore vaccine should be tested for pathogenicity on guinea pigs and rabbits.

*Special vaccines.* Besides the vaccines of standard degrees of virulence, as described under the heading of Pasteur vaccine, a number of vaccines of other grades of virulence are available and are used for special conditions. In some districts especially virulent strains of the anthrax organism abound and the ordinary vaccines will not fully protect. A no. 3 and even a no. 4 vaccine, consisting of cultures less attenuated than the no. 2 Pasteur, are used. Obviously the danger of vaccination troubles is greater when these more virulent vaccines are used; hence they should not be used unless it is known that the weaker vaccines will not protect. When these highly virulent cultures are employed to vaccinate dairy cattle, the milk from any cow showing a vaccination reaction (swelling at the site of injection and a rise in body temperature) should not be used until such animal returns to normal (30).

A special vaccine that apparently has advantages over the ordinary ones is that of Mazzucchi; it has been named *Carbozoo.* This is a no. 2 spore vaccine suspended in a solution of saponin. The saponin acts as a local irritant inducing a rapidly forming gelatinous infiltration at the point of injection which walls off the spores from the lymph vessels and delays their absorption. It is claimed that this vaccine immunizes more solidly and more safely than the usual ones. Fully virulent bacilli usually prove innocuous when introduced in this way, according to the proponents of the method. Manufacturers of biologics have found that the immunizing value of many antigens is improved when they are incorporated in adjuvants that act as local irritants, or which retard absorption in any way, and this principle undoubtedly is the one upon which the success of this special vaccine depends.

*Avirulent anthrax vaccine.* When virulent anthrax strains are grown on 50 percent serum agar in an atmosphere of 10 to 30 percent carbon dioxide, smooth mucoid colonies and rough nonencapsulated dissociants appear (Sterne, 32). In many instances these rough variants prove to be avirulent and can be used successfully to immunize guinea pigs and sheep against large doses of virulent anthrax bacilli. In 1946 Sterne (33) reported that more than 30 million doses of anthrax vaccine made as described above had been successfully used in South Africa. The same vaccine is employed for all domestic animals. Recently, in the United States, Personeus and colleagues (23) studied a vaccine made from a nonencapsulated variant of *B. anthracis* obtained from Onderstepoort and reported it to be excellent for protecting sheep and goats against anthrax.

*Anthrax bacterin.* Killed anthrax organisms appear to have very little immunizing ability and are seldom used in infected districts. However, because of fear of the introduction of living strains, even though attenuated, and the fact that some workers have found a little value in them, this product is the only one permitted in some states of this country by livestock disease-control officials. It was thought that such products were safe and could do no harm even if little good was accomplished. This idea was rudely shattered some years ago by the occurrence of numerous cases of anthrax which were traced to such a commercial product. The bacterin had been made from a virulent strain, and, quite evidently, the product had not been sterilized in the course of manufacture.

*Anthrax aggressin.* Bail in 1904 showed that rabbits and sheep might be protected against otherwise fatal doses of anthrax bacilli by injecting them with filter-sterilized fluid from the edematous tissue of local anthrax lesions. The immunizing substance in this material is termed *aggressin* because when mixed with virulent anthrax cultures it has the effect of increasing their virulence. The nature of this substance is unknown, but apparently it acts by inhibiting phagocytosis. When injected alone, an antagonistic substance, an *antiaggressin,* is supposed to be produced and to be responsible for the heightened resistance.

Anthrax aggressin has been made on a commercial scale, but the immunity produced is not always sufficiently strong to protect, and the cost of production is fairly high. The product is seldom used at the present time.

Substances that may be listed as artificial aggressins have been prepared and used by a number of workers in vaccinating against anthrax. Boor and Tresselt (5) made a cell-free filtrate from an anthrax culture and then concentrated the metabolic products in the filtrate to obtain an immunizing agent for sheep. Belton and Strange (4) described a semisynthetic medium in which virulent and nonvirulent strains of *B. anthracis* will produce a protective antigen that can be concentrated by lyophilization or by alum precipitation to yield a nontoxic immunizing product. According to Strange and Thorne (34), the purified antigen has the physical and chemical properties of a protein. An artificial aggressin for immunization of man has been prepared by adsorbing protective antigen, from filtrates of anaerobic cultures of *B. anthracis,* on an aluminum hydroxide gel (25). This product was claimed to be highly protective for the lower animals and man and to be well tolerated in man.

*Antianthrax serum.* This may be produced from horses, cattle, or sheep. Horses and sheep produce the more potent sera. Horses are generally used because of the greater ease of immunization, i.e., they are less likely to die of anthrax during the immunization procedure and will yield much more serum.

Horses are first given the simultaneous treatment (serum and culture) for anthrax, followed by injections of small quantities of virulent cultures. Beginning with a 0.005-ml loopful, the dose is gradually increased at intervals of 3 or 4 weeks until finally whole-agar-slant cultures and even mass cultures of young virulent strains are used. All injections are given subcutaneously since there seems to be no advantage in intravenous injections.

In the past, antianthrax serum was used in treating herds where anthrax infection existed. All animals not showing fever or other signs of infection were given a 50-ml dose. Those showing a fever but no other symptoms were given from 100 to 300 ml. Animals severely infected with anthrax, if treated at all, were given larger doses. Frequently the administration of serum markedly alleviated symptoms in a few minutes. On the 2nd and 3rd day after treatment relapses sometimes occurred, in which case another dose of serum was administered. Animals that were severely infected and even showed bacilli in the blood sometimes recovered with serum treatment.

Within recent years some of the biological supply houses have announced the discontinuance of antianthrax serum because of its uncertain value and its expense and because of the superiority of certain chemotherapeutic agents as curative agents.

**Local Immunity in Anthrax.** Local immunity has already been discussed on page 27). Here we shall merely call attention to the phenomenon. Besredka in 1919 made the claim that the skin was the only organ susceptible to anthrax infection, that this organ was the only one capable of building up a protective mechanism, that the process could be developed without the formation of demonstrable antibodies in the body fluids, and that whatever antibodies were developed were of minor importance so far as protection of the host was concerned. All of these facts have been contested, and it is doubtful that they can be sustained. Nevertheless it appears fairly certain from the results obtained by a considerable number of European workers that immunization to anthrax can be obtained more readily by intradermal than by subcutaneous injection. Very small quantities of vaccine are used, but the protection given is more rapidly produced, and more certain, than when the materials are injected in the ordinary way.

**Comparative Efficiency of Anthrax Biologics.** A study of the comparative value of the various products for producing immunity in previously unexposed animals was made by the United States Department of Agriculture (12). The findings indicated that spore vaccines, particularly when they are injected intradermally rather than subcutaneously, are the most effective agents for producing active immunity to anthrax. Well-marked immunity was also obtained with anthrax bacterin (washed culture) and anthrax spore vaccine in saponin. Aggressin was found to be inferior to the products named above, and bacterin made from whole culture (broth) had practically no value. Antianthrax serum immunized quickly and satisfactorily, but the duration of the immunity naturally was short. Because the South African avirulent anthrax vaccine is of more recent development, it was not included in this study, but results obtained from its use in South Africa and from trials in this country indicate it to be quite safe and very effective. Tests with the alum-precipitated protective antigens have indicated that they are effective in immunizing cattle, sheep, and man (17, 25, 28). For the best results two injections are recommended.

**Chemotherapy in Anthrax.** Antibiotics such as penicillin, terramycin, and tetracycline are all effective in treating anthrax (2, 3, 18, 35), but Jones, Jr. *et al.* (19) have indicated that penicillin and dihydrostreptomycin are the best. Results are most satisfactory in those species (swine, dogs, man) in which the disease runs a less acute course. The earlier that treatment is begun, the better. In the herbivorous animals, the course often is too rapid, they are not recognized to be ill until near death, and treatment is ineffective. Recoveries have been effected in these species, however, as a result of antibiotic treatment even when bacteremia has developed.

**Control Measures.** In the infected areas of the United States vaccines are used in the control of anthrax. In certain regions the spore vaccine is injected intradermally, and in other sections subcutaneous inoculation of this vaccine combined with an adjuvant is preferred. Combinations of these methods sometimes are used, and, in the areas of great anthrax virulence, original vaccination may be followed by a second, or even third, dose of special, highly virulent vaccine. Favorable results have also been reported from areas where the South African variant vaccine and other recently developed immunizing materials have been used.

In the infected areas vaccination usually is carried out in the spring, on horses, mules, cattle, sheep, and sometimes swine. A certain percentage of the animals will show severe or even fatal reactions to the vaccine. This is especially true among sheep. Such animals may be treated with penicillin, terramycin, tetracycline, antiserum, or combinations of these substances.

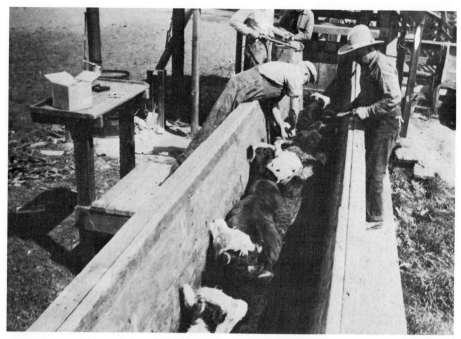

*Fig. 46.* Vaccinating range cattle against anthrax. The use of such chutes for restraining semiwild range cattle is common practice. (Courtesy Jen-Sal Laboratories, Inc.)

The carcasses of animals that die of anthrax should be completely burned or buried very deeply. Carcasses that are opened and the parts scattered provide an opportunity for sporulation of the anthrax bacillus, and the spores remain viable in a contaminated area for years.

**Treatment of Anthrax in Man.** Anthrax in man may assume any of four forms, viz.: (*a*) the skin or cutaneous type (malignant carbuncle), (*b*) the pulmonary form (woolsorter's disease), (*c*) the intestinal form, or (*d*) the acute meningitis syndrome (Haight, 13). The pulmonary and intestinal forms of the disease are usually quickly fatal. The fourth type was in the same category until penicillin was introduced.

Ordinarily serum has been used to treat human anthrax. It has been useful in curing the cutaneous form, but usually has not been administered quickly enough in the pulmonary or intestinal form to prevent fatalities. Furthermore, large doses of antianthrax serum given intravenously often cause serum sickness. According to Gold (11), neoarsphenamine was not effective against anthrax, but sulfathiazole was very effective and is considered the best remedy among the sulfonamides. A report by Ellingson, Kadull, Bookwalter, and Howe (10) indicates that penicillin has marked therapeutic value in curing anthrax infection. More recent reports substantiate their findings and also show that combinations of penicillin and sulfathiazole produce excellent results. Streptomycin, aureomycin, and terramycin have been used singly in a few cases and are reported to be effective.

## REFERENCES

1.  Albrink, Brooks, Biron, and Kopel.   Am. Jour. Path., 1960, *36*, 457.
2.  Bailey.   Jour. Am. Vet. Med. Assoc., 1953, *122*, 305.
3.  *Ibid.*, 1954, *124*, 296.
4.  Belton and Strange.   Brit. Jour. Exp. Path., 1954, *35*, 144.
5.  Boor and Tresselt.   Am. Jour. Vet. Res., 1955, *16*, 425.
6.  Bryan.   *Ibid.*, 1953, *14*, 328.
7.  Burdon.   Jour. Bact., 1956, *25*, 71.
8.  Cousineau and McClenaghan.   Canad. Vet. Jour., 1965, *6*, 22.
9.  Editorial.   North Am. Vet., 1952, *33*, 450.
10. Ellingson, Kadull, Bookwalter, and Howe.   Jour. Am. Med. Assoc., 1946, *131*, 1105.
11. Gold.   Arch. Int. Med., 1942, *70*, 785.
12. Gouchenour, Schoening, Stein, and Mohler.   U.S. Dept. Agr. Tech. Bul. 468, 1935.
13. Haight.   Am. Jour. Med. Sci., 1952, *224*, 57.
14. Hanson.   Jour. Am. Vet. Med. Assoc., 1959, *135*, 463.
15. Harris-Smith, Smith, and Keppie.   Jour. Gen. Microbiol., 1958, *19*, 91.
16. Jackson.   Jour. Comp. Path. and Therap., 1930, *43*, 95.
17. Jackson, Wright, and Armstrong.   Am. Jour. Vet. Res., 1957, *18*, 771.
18. Johnson and Percival.   Jour. Am. Vet. Med. Assoc., 1955, *127*, 142.
19. Jones, Jr., Klein, Lincoln, Walker, Mahlandt, and Dobbs.   Jour. Bact., 1967, *94*, 609.
20. Kinsely.   *Ibid.*, 1965, *90*, 1778.
21. Klein, Hodges, Mahlandt, Jones, Haines, and Lincoln.   Science, 1962, *138*, 1331.
22. McGoughey and St. George.   Vet. Rec., 1955, *67*, 132.
23. Personeus, Cooper, and Percival.   Am. Jour. Vet. Res., 1956, *27*, 153.
24. Peter.   Centrbl. f. Bakt., I Abt., Orig., 1939, *144*, 463.
25. Puziss and Wright.   Jour. Bact., 1963, *85*, 230.
26. Ray, Jr., and Kadull.   Appl. Microbiol., 1964, *12*, 349.
27. Remmele, Klein, Vick, Walker, Mahlandt, and Lincoln.   Jour. Inf. Dis., 1968, *118*, 104.
28. Schlingman, Devlin, Wright, Maine, and Manning.   Am. Jour. Vet. Res., 1956, *17*, 256.
29. Smith, Keppie, and Stanley.   Brit. Jour. Exp. Path., 1955, *36*, 460.
30. Stein.   North Am. Vet., 1952, *33*, 420.
31. Stein and Van Ness.   Vet. Med., 1955, *50*, 579.
32. Sterne.   Onderstepoort Jour. Vet. Sci. and An. Ind., 1937, *9*, 49.
33. *Ibid.*, 1946, *21*, 41.
34. Strange and Thorne.   Jour. Bact., 1958, *76*, 192.
35. Sugg.   Jour. Am. Vet. Med. Assoc., 1948, *113*, 467.
36. Umeno and Nobata.   Jour. Jap. Soc. Vet. Sci., 1938, *17*, 87.
37. Wolff and Heimann.   Am. Jour. Hyg., 1951, *53*, 80.

## THE GENUS *CLOSTRIDIUM*

The anaerobic sporebearing organisms that are classed together under the generic name *Clostridium* are quite similar in morphology and staining qualities. All are rather large, rod-shaped, and Gram-positive when young. The rods usually are straight. Some species commonly appear in tissue fluids singly or in pairs, whereas others usually are found in long chains. The spores in most species are oval, are located somewhat centrally in the rod, and often are greater in diameter than the rod itself. Because of their great similarity in form, it is usually not possible to be certain of the identity of these organisms without studying their cultural and serological characteristics. In many instances the symptoms and lesions of the diseases produced by them are sufficiently characteristic to enable a reliable diagnosis to be made.

The application of the usual serologic, including FA, tests to the intact clostridial cells has not been especially rewarding, because antigens common to the bacilli and their spores produce many cross-reactions. Ellner and Green (8), however, used soluble antigens from 10 species of pathogenic clostridia to divide these organisms into groups based upon the presence or absence of precipitin lines in agar-gel tests.

These organisms may be divided into two groups on the basis of their disease-producing mechanisms. The first consists of those species that have little or no power to invade and multiply in living tissues. Such organisms owe their pathogenicity to their power of forming powerful toxins, which are produced in localized areas or outside the body. The damage in these instances is almost or wholly caused by the absorption of the poison. The organisms of this group which will be described are *Cl. tetani* and *Cl. botulinum*. The second and larger group consists of species that have the power to invade and multiply in tissues. These organisms in most cases also produce toxins, but the toxins are much less potent than those of the first group and the damages to the tissues are not caused wholly by them. These organisms are sometimes referred to as the *gas gangrene* group because many of them are concerned in wound infections of the gas gangrene type in man. Wounds of animals sometimes become infected with pathogenic anaerobes, in which case the condition is similar to that of man. A number of these organisms, however, find their way into animal tissues through the digestive tract, and thus we have rapidly developing, highly fatal infections without the existence of wounds of the skin.

The number of species which has been found in these gangrenous infections of animals is large. The ones most frequently encountered are the only ones that will be considered here. These are:

*Clostridium chauvoei.*     The cause of blackleg in cattle and sheep.
*Clostridium septicum.*     The cause of braxy in sheep and of malignant edema infections in other species.

| | |
|---|---|
| *Clostridium perfringens.* | The cause of lamb dysentery, "struck," and "pulpy kidney disease" of sheep, and occasionally of malignant edema infections of other species. |
| *Clostridium novyi.* | The cause of "black disease" of sheep and occasionally of malignant edema infections of other species. |
| *Clostridium hemolyticum.* | The cause of bacterial icterohemoglobinuria or "red water" of cattle. |

The nonpathogen *Clostridium sporogenes* is also found in a considerable proportion of gas gangrene cases, but its contribution to the pathology of the disease is uncertain. Although *Clostridium bifermentans* (*sordelli*) produces a very potent toxin, it is encountered only sporadically in gangrenous infections of animals. Two outbreaks of *Cl. sordelli* infection in Rambouillet rams that occurred in Montana in 1962 were described by Smith *et al.* (33).

The sporebearing anaerobic bacteria cause animal diseases that are infectious without being contagious, that is to say, the diseases seldom if ever are transmitted from one animal to another. Most of these organisms have their habitat in the soil, and it is from soil, or vegetation, that the infections are derived. Epizootics seldom occur, although it is possible for them to happen when conditions become favorable for a large number of animals to become infected from the same source simultaneously.

## THE TOXIN-FORMING, NONINVASIVE GROUP

### *Clostridium tetani*

SYNONYM: *Bacillus tetani*

The causative agent of tetanus is the best known of all anaerobic, sporebearing bacilli, principally because the symptoms of the disease are so well known and characteristic that it has not been confused with any other of the anaerobic infections. The organism was isolated in impure culture by Nicolaier (24) in 1884 from white mice that had been inoculated with garden soil. In 1889 Kitasato (16) obtained pure cultures by heating mixed cultures from infected wounds, thus destroying the ordinary bacteria of suppuration but leaving the heat-resistant tetanus spores. In the following year (1890) Von Behring and Kitasato (2) published their classical work announcing the discovery of bacterial toxins, of which the first was that of *Cl. tetani*.

**Morphology and Staining Reactions.** *Cl. tetani* is a straight, slender rod from 0.4 to 0.6 microns in width and from 2 to 5 microns in length. In both tissues and cultures it most often occurs singly, but sometimes chains of organisms forming long filaments are seen. In old cultures the rods and threads disappear leaving the spherical spores. These spores are formed after 24 to 48 hours' incubation and appear in the ends of the rods, swelling them so they have the appearance of badminton rackets or drumsticks. In some media

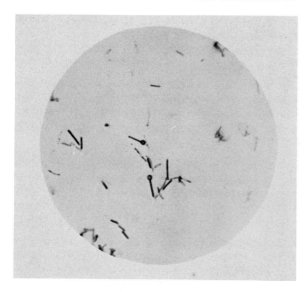

Fig. 47. *Clostridium tetani*, a stained preparation of a 48-hour-old culture in a meat-piece medium. The terminal spherical spores are characteristic. X 1,000.

spores are formed in abundance; in others even after prolonged incubation they are few in number. Cultures are Gram-positive when young but after a few days most of the cells become Gram-negative. Young cultures are actively motile by means of peritrichic flagella.

**Cultural Features.** The tetanus organism grows on all the ordinary media of the laboratory provided only that fairly good anaerobic conditions are maintained. It will grow in aerobic cultures in association with other aerobic organisms. Deep agar colonies are fluffy, cottony spheres. When blood is present, hemolysis occurs. Broth becomes slightly clouded but clears by sedimentation. Gelatin stabs first develop a spike of growth along the stab, next cottony filaments extend from the stab at a right angle into the medium, giving a brushlike effect, then liquefaction and blackening of the medium occur, and gas bubbles are formed. Litmus milk is not usually changed. A soft clot may be formed. Coagulated blood serum is softened and in old cultures may be blackened but it is not liquefied. Cooked-meat medium and brain medium are not digested but become turbid and give off a very foul odor. Carbohydrates are not fermented, but glucose greatly favors growth in the simpler types of media. Growth occurs best at 37 C, but slow growth occurs at 20 C. Serological types have been described by Gunnison (13). According to Smith (32), there are 10 serotypes, which are differentiated on the basis of H antigens, except for type IV, which is nonmotile. All strains share a common somatic antigen but possess others in addition to it.

**Resistance.** *Cl. tetani* spores are highly resistant and when protected from light and heat remain viable for years. Theobald Smith found a number of strains that resisted steaming at 100 C for 40 to 60 minutes. Five percent phenol is said to destroy tetanus spores in 10 to 12 hours; the addition of 0.5 percent hydrochloric acid may reduce the time to 2 hours.

**Natural Habitat.** The organism of tetanus was found originally by Nicolaier (24) in garden soils, 12 out of 18 samples being positive. Fildes (11), in England, examined 70 soil samples, including both cultivated and uncultivated, and found 33 positive. Sanada and Nishida (30) have indicated that the higher the temperature applied to soil specimens the weaker the toxigenicity of *Cl. tetani* cultures isolated from them and that the properties of atoxic strains were indistinguishable from those of *Clostridium tetanomorphum*.

A number of workers have found the organism to be commonly present in horse manure. Some have found it in the feces of cows, sheep, dogs, chickens, rats, and guinea pigs, whereas others have failed to find it in some of these species, a fact which suggests that these animals may only be transitory hosts for the organism. Noble (26), for example, found it in 11 out of 61 samples of horses' feces, but failed to find it in 21 samples from cows. Human feces also are sometimes infected with tetanus bacilli. The experiences of various workers on this subject have differed widely, some being unable to find the organism in large series of cases, others finding it in a relatively large proportion. TenBroeck and Bauer (35) demonstrated tetanus bacilli in the stools of 27 of 78 individuals living in Peking, China, and concluded that the organism must be living in the intestinal canal because certain individuals who had lived on

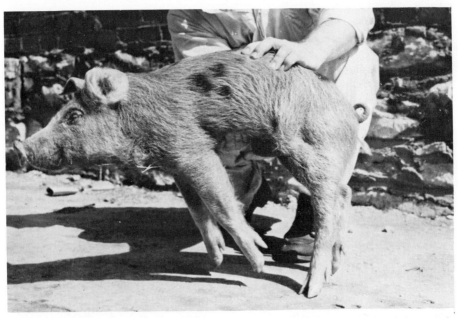

*Fig. 48.* Tetanus in a pig. Tetanic spasms of the muscles manifested by rigidity of the parts is characteristic of tetanus in all animals. (Courtesy Jen-Sal Laboratories, Inc.)

an almost sterile diet for more than a month continued to yield several million tetanus spores per stool.

**Pathogenicity.** Infections in all animals and man occur as a result of wound contamination. Clean wounds rarely result in tetanus. It is the dirty wound containing foreign material, particularly soil, that is most dangerous. Deep penetrating wounds are much more dangerous than superficial ones. During the World War of 1914–1918, the study of tetanus was greatly stimulated by the large number of human cases that developed in troops fighting on the cultivated fields of Flanders. It had been known previously that tetanus spores, washed free from toxin, did not oridinarily produce tetanus when injected into animals; that the spores in such cases did not germinate but were taken up by phagocytes and ultimately destroyed. It was learned that tetanus spores would not germinate in living tissues, probably because of the presence of too much oxygen, and that germination occurred only when the spores lodged in destroyed tissues. Cultures of the tetanus organism will produce tetanus upon inoculation because the toxin present is a local tissue destroyer and thus a suitable environment is provided. When soil or foreign materials of other kinds accompany tetanus spores into a wound, they pave the way for the germination of the spores and the setting up of an infection. Tulloch (36) showed that when washed spores were introduced with the toxins of some of the organisms causing gas gangrene, tetanus resulted with regularity. It was also observed by other English workers that the injection of washed tetanus spores suspended in a dilute solution of calcium chloride produced tetanus, and that infections regularly occurred in animals receiving washed spore suspensions by inoculation into areas of the skin into which calcium salts had previously been injected. When spores were injected intravenously and a calcium solution subcutaneously, tetanus resulted through local multiplication of the tetanus organism at the site of the injection of the salt. Calcium salts seem to alter tissues in a manner that makes them more favorable for germination of the tetanus spore.

Of the domesticated animals, the horse is by far the most often affected with tetanus. Sheep are rather frequently affected, cattle and swine occasionally, carnivorous animals rarely, and birds never. The occurrence of the naturally acquired disease seems to correspond fairly closely to the susceptibility of the animals to tetanus toxin. The amount of toxin needed per gram of body weight to kill a chicken is about 350,000 times as great as it is for the horse. For the dog it is about 600 times as great.

In tetanus infections the bacilli do not multiply in any part of the body other than the local area where the infection occurs. As soon as toxin forms, it and pyogenic bacteria, which are also usually present in the wound, prepare a nidus where conditions are favorable for the tetanus organism, and it is here that the organisms multiply and the toxin is generated. The local effects of tetanus are negligible; the principal agent in the production of the disease is the toxin, which is one of the most poisonous substances known. Pillemer,

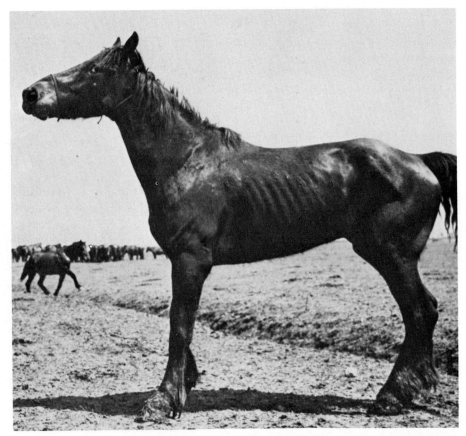

*Fig. 49.* Tetanus in a horse showing rigidity of the muscles. The membrana nictitans is visible. (Courtesy Sgt. V. W. Loomis, 2604 Veterinary Station Hospital, Veterinary Corps, U.S. Army.)

Wittler, and Grossberg (28) in 1946 succeeded in preparing a purified tetanus toxin in crystalline form. This material contained between 50 and 75 million mouse MLD's per mg of nitrogen. It appears that tetanus toxin contains two poisons: *tetanospasmin,* the portion that affects the nervous tissue, and *tetano- lysin,* a hemolysin. The former is by far the more important.

There is considerable controversy about the manner by which tetanus toxin reaches the central nervous system, where its principal effects are produced. If a fatal dose of tetanus toxin is injected into the foot of a susceptible animal, the onset of the disease may be greatly delayed by severing the principal motor nerve trunks of that leg (19) or by infiltrating the nerve trunk with an- titoxin (22). Fatal tetanus may be produced by injecting into one of the pe- ripheral nerve trunks a dose of toxin which is not great enough to cause death when injected intravenously. These and many other similar experiments seem to indicate that the tetanus toxin is absorbed by the peripheral nerves and that most of it passes through the nerves centripetally until it reaches the motor cells of the anterior horn of the cord, at which time general symptoms of the disease make their appearance. Abel and his co-workers (1) in a series of publications beginning in 1934 have maintained that the toxin exhibits both a central and peripheral action, each of which may be demonstrated independently of the other. The peripheral effect is caused by direct absorption of the toxin by the motor end organs, but the central effect results from poisoning of the motor nerve centers by toxin carried there by way of the arterial circulation. On the other hand, Friedemann, Hollander, and Tarlov (12) have presented experimental data in support of the axis-cylinder pathway of toxin transfer to the central nervous system. In a fatal case of tetanus in the dog, toxin was found in the blood stream, but whether or not it reached the nervous system by this route is unknown (25). Miyasaki *et al.* (23) studied the mode of action of tetanus toxin in rabbits. They stated that no toxin was recovered from the central nervous system when it was injected intramuscularly into rabbits, although it was recovered from the serum, local muscles, and peripheral nerves innervating these muscles. They claimed that tetanus toxin has two pharmacologic actions, spastic and paralytic, according to the site of its injection or to the target where it is made to act. Spastic signs of tetanus do not develop in rabbits unless the toxin enters and remains for some time in the general circulation.

The symptoms of tetanus are similar in all animals. They consist of chronic or tetanic spasms of the muscles. Sometimes these begin in one part of the body, where the infected wound is located, but generally the disease extends to all parts. The frequency with which the facial muscles are affected, thus making it difficult for the victim to open his mouth, is responsible for the name *lockjaw*, by which the disease is commonly known.

Infections in horses occur most often as a result of nail wounds in the foot. In sheep the infection is seen most often after lambs are castrated or docked. In cattle it may be a puerperal infection following calving, or it may follow dehorning, castration, and nose ringing of bulls. Herd and Riches (14) and Wallis (37) have reported outbreaks of idiopathic tetanus in groups of heifers and have suggested that this condition was caused by an autointoxication resulting from massive multiplication of *Cl. tetani* in the forestomachs under certain unspecified conditions. In swine it is most frequently seen as a result of castration wound infection. The disease appears in dogs and cats, usually following wound infection (20). In all animals it may occur as a result of infection of otherwise trivial wounds, and even when no wounds can be found. Umbilical infections of newborn animals often occur.

**Natural Immunity.** Birds and other animals that are naturally resistant to tetanus have no antibodies in their tissues. The brain tissue of such animals, however seems to have no affinity for the toxin, as was first demonstrated by Metchnikoff (21). The blood of most cattle contains neutralizing antibodies, and small amounts are found in the blood of sheep and goats. It has been suggested that perhaps this comes about from the activity of tetanus bacilli in the forestomachs of these ruminants. The blood of horses, dogs, pigs, and men does not normally contain antitoxin. The brain tissue of all susceptible animals possesses the power of uniting with tetanus toxin *in vitro* and thereby neutralizing it.

**Passive Immunity.** Effective means of rendering susceptible animals immune prophylactically are available. This may be accomplished either actively or passively. When an animal has suffered a wound from which it is feared tetanus may develop, it is necessary to use a method by which resistance can be conferred quickly. In this situation *tetanus antitoxin* is indicated. Usually 1,500 units are adequate to give complete protection for a period of several weeks, which ordinarily is long enough. If another wound is incurred a few months later, another dose of antitoxin is needed. Repeated doses of antitoxin may result in anaphylactic shocks in all animals except the horse, for which the serum is homologous.

When symptoms of tetanus have appeared, the efficacy of the antitoxin is not so great as when it is used prophylatically. In animals already suffering from the disease, the antitoxin is adminstered as soon as possible and is given preferably in a single dose of from 100,000 to 200,000 units. In addition, adequate treatment includes large doses of penicillin and sedation. Animals frequently die in spite of such treatment. On the other hand, when the infected wound is thoroughly cleaned surgically and treated with antiseptics, and the animals are kept quiet in a darkened room, one-third or more of them will recover without treatment with antitoxin. The therapeutic effectiveness of tetanus antitoxin is markedly reduced by simultaneous administration of cortisone (5).

Records kept for a 15-year period on the treatment of human cases of tetanus by the Cook County Hospital in Chicago show that 84 percent mortality occurred in tetanus patients with an incubation period of less than 10 days and 25 percent mortality in those with an incubation period of 14 to 25 days. These figures held in spite of increased use of antitoxin.

**Active Immunity.** Active immunization of horses against tetanus was introduced by Ramon and Lemetayer (29) of the Pasteur Institute in Paris and has proved to be a thoroughly practical procedure. The immunizing substance is *tetanus toxoid* or *anatoxin*. This is made by incubating highly potent toxin with 0.4 percent formalin until the toxicity has been completely destroyed. This requires several weeks. The solution may be used as it is, but an improved product results from precipitating the toxoid from solution with alum (potassium aluminum sulfate). The precipitate contains the active principle freed from extraneous material. After it has been washed, it is suspended in saline solution. A single injection of this material will produce an appreciable degree of immunity, but experience has shown that it is best to give a second and a third dose at about 3-week intervals. Such animals will have sufficient antitoxin in their blood to protect them from natural infection for at least a year. Fessler (10) recommends that horses should be given two toxoid injections 6 to 8 weeks apart, followed by a booster dose 6 to 12 months later and then by annual booster injections. A similar regimen will be effective for other domestic animals. If dangerous wounds are contracted later, it is best to administer another dose at once. This will cause an immediate increase in antibodies. If the animal has not already had toxoid, the latter is useless in an emergency because the initial production of antitoxin is too slow. It has been established that a simultaneous injection of tetanus antitoxin and toxoid will-not significantly reduce the efficacy of the former, but will markedly decrease the ability of the latter to produce active immunity.

According to Skudder and McCarroll (31) there is no substitute for the prophylactic immunization of man with tetanus toxoid prior to injury. This treatment proved to be very effective in World War II. Three doses are usually given, each dose containing about 10,000 detoxified guinea pig MLD per ml. Originally it was recommended that a booster injection be given at 3- to 4-year intervals, but subsequent findings have indicated that this period should be no less than 5 years and in 1967 Edsall *et al.* (7) reported that booster doses of tetanus toxoid are being given to man with unnecessary and indeed excessive frequency and this practice has produced allergic (Arthus-type) reactions in the recipients. They recommend that annual routine toxoid boosters of all kinds be discontinued, that routine boosters in individuals known to have had primary immunization including a reinforcing dose be given only at 10-year intervals, and that emergency boosters be given no closer than 1 year apart.

**Chemotherapy.** Many drugs have been used in the symptomatic treatment of tetanus. Karitzky (15) claimed that acidosis is the main cause of death in tetanus infection and that the treatment of acidosis markedly reduces the mortality rate in man. Couvy (6) reported success in treating tetanus of man by administering antiserum and urotropine. Sedatives, such as mephenesin (3) and *d*-tubocurarine choloride (4), are recommended, and the tranquilizing drug chlorpromazine hydrochloride (18, 27) is also prescribed. In testing antibiotics on mice infected with tetanus, Taylor and Novak (34) concluded that aureomycin, penicillin, and terramycin reduced mortalities. Chloromycetin was of some value, antitoxin of little value, and polymyxin B ineffective. The tranquilizers, diazepam (7-chloro-1,3-dihydro-1-methyl-5-phenyl-2H-1,4-benzo-diazephin-2-one) and chlor diazepoxide (7-chloro-2-methyl-amino-5-phenyl-3H-1,4-benzodiazepine 4-oxide) are highly recommended in treating tetanus (9, 17), and an evaluation of serologic and antimicrobial therapy in the treatment of tetanus in the United States has been published by Young *et al.* (38).

## REFERENCES

1.  Abel.  Johns Hopkins Hosp. Bul., 1938, *63*, 373.
2.  Von Behring and Kitasato.  Deut. med. Wchnschr., 1890, *16*, 1113.
3.  Boles and Smith.  Jour. Am. Med. Assoc., 1951, *146*, 1296.

4. Booth and Pierson. Jour. Am. Vet. Med. Assoc., 1956, *128*, 257.
5. Chang and Weinstein. Proc. Soc. Exp. Biol. and Med., 1957, *94*, 431.
6. Couvy. Vet. Bul., 1948, *18*, 469.
7. Edsall, Elliott, Peebles, Levine, and Eldred. Jour. Am. Med. Assoc., 1967, *202*, 17.
8. Ellner and Green. Jour. Bact., 1963, *86*, 1098.
9. Femi-Pearse and Fleming. Jour. Trop. Med. and Hyg. (London), 1965, *68*, 305.
10. Fessler. Jour. Am. Vet. Med. Assoc., 1966, *148*, 399.
11. Fildes. Brit. Jour. Exp. Path., 1925, *6*, 62.
12. Friedemann, Hollander, and Tarlov. Jour. Immunol., 1941, *40*, 325.
13. Gunnison. *Ibid.*, 1937, *32*, 63.
14. Herd and Riches. Austral. Vet. Jour., 1964, *40*, 356.
15. Karitzky. Arch. Klin. Chir., 1947, *260*, 1.
16. Kitasato. Zeitschr. f. Hyg., 1889, *7*, 225.
17. Lowenthal and Lavalette. Jour. Trop. Med. and Hyg. (London), 1966, *69*, 157.
18. Lundvall. Jour. Am. Vet. Med. Assoc., 1958, *132*, 254.
19. Marie. Ann. l'Inst. Past., 1897, *11*, 591.
20. Mason. Jour. So. African Vet. Med. Assoc., 1964, *35*, 209.
21. Metchnikoff. Ann. l'Inst. Past., 1898, *12*, 81.
22. Meyer and Ransom. Arch. Path. and Pharm., 1903, *49*, 369.
23. Miyasaki, Okada, Muto, Itokazu, Matsui, Ebisawa, Kagabe, and Kimuro. Jap. Jour. Exp. Med., 1967, *37*, 217.
24. Nicolaier. Deut. med. Wchnschr., 1884, *10*, 842.
25. Nielsen and Rowsell. Jour. Am. Vet. Med. Assoc., 1956, *128*, 59.
26. Noble. Jour. Inf. Dis., 1915, *16*, 132.
27. Owen, Leam, and Nestel. Vet. Rec., 1959, *71*, 61.
28. Pillemer, Wittler, and Grossberg. Science, 1946, *103*, 615.
29. Ramon and Lemetayer. Comp. rend. Soc. Biol. (Paris), 1931, *106*, 21.
30. Sanada and Nishida. Jour. Bact., 1965, *89*, 626.
31. Skudder and McCarroll. Jour. Am. Med. Assoc., 1964, *188*, 625.
32. Smith. Introduction to pathogenic anaerobes. Univ. of Chicago Press, Chicago, 1954.
33. Smith, Safford, and Hawkins. Cornell Vet., 1962, *52*, 62.
34. Taylor and Novak. Antibiotics and Chemother., 1952, *2*, 517.
35. TenBroeck and Bauer. Jour. Exp. Med., 1922, *36*, 261.
36. Tulloch. Jour. Hyg. (London), 1919–20, *18*, 103.
37. Wallis. Vet. Rec., 1963, 75, 188.
38. Young, LaForce, and Bennett. Jour. Inf. Dis., 1969, *120*, 153.

### Clostridium botulinum

SYNONYM: *Bacillus botulinus*

As a disease of man botulism has been known for many years. The disease was given its name by Müller (51) in 1870. The causative agent was found in 1897 by Van Ermengem (19), who studied an outbreak occurring in Ellezelles, Belgium, in a group of persons who ate an imperfectly preserved smoked ham at a dinner. The organism was found in the ham and the tissues of one of the persons who died of the disease. The toxicogenic properties of the organism were recognized by Van Ermengem, also the fact that the toxin wrought its damage by attacking portions of the nervous system.

In Europe numerous outbreaks of the disease have occurred, the greater number being traced to hams, sausages, and other meat products. Beginning about 1919, a series of outbreaks have been recognized in the United States, but these have been traced, with but few exceptions, to canned vegetables. It has been shown by Meyer and Dubovsky (46) that the organism is commonly present in the soil in all parts of the world. Botulism is caused, therefore, by food materials that have been contaminated with soil, imperfectly sterilized, and then allowed to stand, with the air excluded, sufficiently long to allow the organism to generate its powerful toxin. The disease is an intoxication, almost never a bacterial infection, although there are a few reports of wound infection in man (12, 30). In one of these cases which terminated fatally the clinical course was strikingly similar to botulism and *Cl. botulinum* type A was isolated. The organism has little or no ability to generate toxin in the alimentary tract of mammals, but it is reported to do so in the crops of birds (13).

In the United States botulism in horses was studied by Buckley and Shippen (8) and Graham and associates (24). Hart (31) described an outbreak in a large flock of chickens, and Hall and Stiles (29) reported an outbreak in captive mink. Dogs (35) may be poisoned with the toxin, but reports of natural cases in this species are rare. Sporadic cases of botulism in animals frequently are diagnosed on a purely clinical basis in this country, but it is likely that most of these diagnoses are incorrect. *Lamziekte,* a disease of cattle in South Africa, *loin disease* of cattle in parts of Texas, and *alkali disease* of ducks in the United States apparently are botulism. Seddon (55) has described botulism in cattle in Tasmania, and Bennetts and Hall (6) have described it in sheep in western Australia.

Organisms causing botulism can be divided into proteolytic and nonproteolytic groups. The former is often designated *Cl. parabotulinum* and the latter *Cl. botulinum.* However, the serological specificity of the toxin is not always related to the proteolytic activity of the organism producing it. Strains that produce Type B toxin occur in both the ovolytic and nonovolytic groups. Because the type of toxin is of greater practical importance than proteolytic power, all toxicogenic strains are designated as *Cl. botulinum.*

**Morphology and Staining Reactions.** The types within the species cannot be distinguished on a morphological basis. All are relatively large rods which usually occur singly but may form short chains. They measure from 0.5 to 0.8 microns in width and from 3 to 6 microns in length. Motility occurs in young cultures, the cells being provided with peritrichic flagella. Spores form readily and abundantly. They are oval, are located centrally and excentrically, and cause slight bulging of the cells. The organism is Gram-positive but in old cultures the cells usually decolorize.

**Cultural Features.** Colonies in deep agar are fluffy. Better growths occur in media made from liver than in those made from muscle tissue. Gelatin is rapidly liquefied. Acid and gas are produced from glucose, levulose, and maltose. The fermentation of other sugars is variable from strain to strain and from type to type.

The nonproteolytic types (*Cl. botulinum*) acidify but do not coagulate milk. They do not liquefy coagulated blood serum or coagulated egg albumen, nor do they digest brain or meat medium.

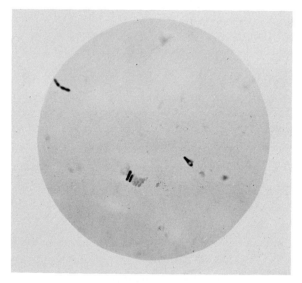

Fig. 50. *Clostridium botulinum,* a culture in meat-piece medium incubated 48 hours at 37 C. X 1,000.

The proteolytic types (*Cl. parabotulinum*) slowly curdle milk and partially digest and darken the curd. When inoculated on coagulated blood serum or egg albumen, they digest and blacken these media and produce a putrefactive odor. They also digest and blacken brain or meat medium and emit putrefactive odors.

All organisms included in these species are strict anaerobes but are not fastidious, otherwise, in their growth requirements. They grow best at temperatures around 30 C but are capable of growing in a wide range of temperatures up to that of the body. The strains that are not proteolytic nevertheless give off a strong odor, which is suggestive of putrefaction but is not so powerful as that produced by the protein-liquifying types.

It appears that the species is rather heterogeneous serologically. According to Mandia (42), there are at least six serotypes of *Cl. botulinum* in his Group II of proteolytic clostridia, and antigens are shared by some strains with *Cl. sporogenes* (43).

**Resistance of the Organism.** The spores are highly resistant and withstand boiling for 30 minutes to several hours and autoclaving at 120 C for as long as

20 minutes. Krabbenhoft *et al.* (38) have added viable *Cl. botulinum* Type A spores to ground meat and inactivated them by exposure to gamma radiation. Botulism toxin is inactivated by ordinary cooking procedures, but certain un-cooked foods may develop toxin, even when stored at 2 to 4 C, and the titer produced may remain constant for 2 to 4 years before declining rapidly (26).

**The Cultural and Toxicogenic Types.** In 1919 Burke (9) found that the strains in her possession, which had been isolated from California products, were not alike toxicologically although agreeing in cultural features. The toxins of all strains produced practically the same effects on animals, but antitoxins that would neutralize the toxins of one group of organisms would not neutralize those of another, and vice versa. On the basis of her experiments she differen-tiated two types and designated them as Types A and B. The Type A organism appears to be the one occurring most commonly in soils of the United States and is the one that was found in most of the outbreaks of botulism originating in canned goods packed by commercial firms in California between 1919 and 1925. The Type B organism also seems to be widely distributed, but is en-countered more frequently in the middle west and eastern parts of the coun-try. It also occurs in Europe.

In 1922 Bengston (4) described another type, which she had isolated from fly larvae. This organism differs from those previously described in certain cultural features and in the toxin produced. She designated the organism as Type C. In 1922 Seddon (55) isolated an anaerobe from botulism in cattle in Australia which proved to be a variant of Type C. In 1927 Theiler and Robin-son (60) found that two mules which had died after eating out of the same manger had been poisoned by botulinus toxin which came from a decompos-ing rat carcass in the hay. Robinson (54) in 1930 showed this organism to be toxicologically identical with Type C.

At present Type C is split into two groups, designated $C_a$ and $C_b$. Type $C_a$ is associated with fly larvae and usually affects only birds, whereas Type $C_b$ affects birds and other animals. The toxins of these subtypes are related in that $C_a$ antitoxin protects against both $C_a$ and $C_b$ toxin, while $C_b$ antitoxin protects against $C_b$ toxin but not $C_a$ toxin.

In 1929 Meyer and Gunnison (47) studied the organism causing the South African *lamziekte*, found it to be different from those previously described, and designated it as Type D.

In 1936 Type E was isolated (27) in Russia from fish, consumption of which resulted in human botulism. It also has been found as a cause of human bot-ulism in the United States (32). The Type E toxin is not neutralized by an-titoxins of the other four types. Toxins produced by different strains of Type E vary in pathogenicity for the common laboratory animals but are neutral-ized reciprocally by their antitoxins.

Still another type, Type F, was isolated from an outbreak of human botu-lism on the Danish Island of Langeland in 1958 by Möller and Scheibel (50). According to Dolman and Murakami (14) this prototype F strain resembles

Type A and American Type B strains in its proteolytic and saccharolytic properties. Antitoxin prepared from Type F did not neutralize other types of botulinus toxins, but Type E antitoxin showed slight cross-neutralization with Type F toxin.

In 1924 Bengston (5) studied all available strains of the organism of botulism in a comparative way and suggested that they be divided into proteolytic (*Cl. parabotulinum*) and nonproteolytic (*Cl. botulinum*) groups. Bengston's original division has been modified by later findings, and at present the proteolytic group includes Type A, Type F, and some strains of Type B (American strains are usually proteolytic, whereas many of the European are not). The nonproteolytic group includes some strains of Type B and Types C, D, and E. It is probable that Van Ermengem's original strain was a nonproteolytic variant of Type B.

Certain characteristic differences, aside from properties of the toxins and proteolytic activity, may be noted among the several known types of the organism of botulism. The Type A organism produces spores that are extraordinarily resistant to heat. For organisms of this type Esty (20) and Meyer have reported maximum resistances up to 5.5 hours at 100 C. Organisms of the other types show much less resistance, most of them being destroyed by boiling for a very short time. Undoubtedly this difference in heat resistance explains why there has been so much difficulty in controlling botulism in canned goods where soil contamination may be a factor.

The Type A organism usually possesses the most virulent toxin; in fact, no more poisonous substance has ever been found than the toxin of certain strains of this type. Lamanna, McElroy, and Eklund (40) succeeded in purifying this toxin in 1946. The product was far more potent than tetanus toxin (about 25×) measured in terms of its nitrogen content. Although Wentzel *et al.* (61) have stated that an ammonium sulfate precipitated toxin of one of their Type D strains was 20,000 times more toxic for mice than a similar preparation of Type A toxin, most reports have indicated that the crystalline form of the latter is the most potent of all botulism toxins.

The toxins of both A and B types affect a great variety of animals, both vertebrate and invertebrate. Earthworms, snails, tadpoles, frogs, fish, birds, dogs, cats, mink, ferrets, muskrats, horses, monkeys, and man have been poisoned. Cattle may be poisoned, but apparently they are somewhat less susceptible than most other mammals, and swine are quite resistant.

By using properly graded doses of toxin from unknown strains, Graham and Schwarze (25) were able to make a rapid differentiation between the A and B types by the inoculation of chickens and dogs. These species are relatively resistant to the B type of toxin while very susceptible to the A type; thus, unless excessive doses are used, they will remain free of symptoms in the presence of the B type but show typical botulism in the presence of the A type.

Bengston found Type C originally in the larvae of a blowfly, *Lucilia caesar*, which obtained it from putrefying carcasses upon which they had fed.

When these larvae were fed to chickens, a characteristic disease that had long been recognized as a disease entity, *limber neck*, was produced. The birds exhibit sleepiness and finally are unable to hold up their heads because of a flaccid paralysis of the neck muscles. Such birds usually die.

An outbreak in pheasants caused by Type C was described by Dinter and Kull (13). The toxin-containing food proved to be the larvae of flies (*Caliphora* and *Lucilia*) which had fed on carcasses of wild rabbits. The toxin titer was relatively low in the larvae before they were eaten, but it increased considerably in the crops of the birds. This indicated that the larvae contained not only toxin but also organisms and that the crop acted as an incubator. The disease has been reported in pheasants in Canada (21).

Kalmbach and Gunderson (37) proved that a devastating disease in wild ducks and other water birds in an area centering around Great Salt Lake in Utah was caused by botulism, the organism belonging to Type C. In shallow, stagnant water in pools that dry up during the hot months, decaying vegetation provides a favorable medium for the growth of this organism and the generation of its toxin. Many thousands of ducks, feeding upon such vegetation on the bottom of the water holes, die each year. The disease has long been known as the *western duck sickness* or as the *alkali disease* since it was believed that it was caused by salt poisoning. In 1949 Quortrup and Gorham (52) isolated strains of Type C from the stomachs of ducks obtained from the Bear River marshes in Utah. Toxin from these strains proved to be much more pathogenic for mink and ferrets than those of Type A or Type B. Type C is the most common cause of food poisoning in mink in Sweden (49). Further reports indicate that the same is true in other countries (2, 23, 28). Type C intoxication has been diagnosed in domestic ducks (53) and in pigs (3).

The organism isolated by Theiler and Robinson from a rat carcass and described as the cause of botulism in mules originally was designated as Type E, but Robinson later showed it to be Type C. Seddon's *Tasmanian Midland* disease and botulism of sheep in western Australia are caused by Type C. These animals become intoxicated through ingestion of rabbit carrion, which is the most common source of the toxin (6).

Bengston's original strain appears to have been Type $C_a$. It is considered to be pathogenic only for fowl. Seddon's Type $C_b$ is pathogenic for cattle, sheep, horses, swine, and mules. It probably was the cause of the human case of Type C poisoning reported by Meyer (16). The subtype of Type C that is responsible for botulism in mink and ferrets has not been established for all outbreaks, but in the one described by Avery *et al.* (2) it was claimed to be Type $C_b$.

The Type D organism has been found only in a disease of cattle of South Africa known as *lamziekte*, or the lame sickness. The etiology of this disease was finally cleared up by Theiler and his co-workers (59) in 1926. It occurs only in certain restricted areas in cattle on the range. In these areas the cattle have the habit of bone chewing, which, it was shown, is caused by a phosphorus deficiency that creates the abnormal appetite. The bones of animals dying on the veld (range) were eagerly sought and chewed. Some of these bones were in advanced stages of decomposition, and in them the botulinum toxin often was present. A disease evidently the same as lamziekte occurs in certain parts of the Texas plains, where phosphorus deficiency exists and bone chewing is common. The symptoms are the same as those of the South African disease. *Cl. botulinum* Type D has been found in mud samples taken from lakes in the Zululand game parks of Africa (45).

Gunnison, Cummings, and Meyer proposed that a strain isolated from spoiled fish in Russia be designated as Type E. In 1957 three Indian women died on the northern British Columbian Coast after eating raw salmon eggs that contained Type E botulinus toxin. One year later, a similar fatality occurred in the same region, but Type B toxin was found in the fish eggs (15). Strains of Type E have been found in botulism in man in the United States and in 1963 the eating of canned tuna fish that contained Type E toxin proved to be the cause (36). The organism also was found in smoked fish. Since 1969 it has been isolated from salmon and other marine fish in the Pacific Northwest, from home-canned gefilte fish, from fish taken from the Great Lakes, and from bottom and shoreline sediments of Green Bay of Lake Michigan.

Although the pathogenicity of the toxins of Type E strains vary, this type can affect birds, monkeys, man, and laboratory animals. Skulberg and Valland (56) indicated that mink were substantially less susceptible to Type E than to Type C toxin when the toxins were given by mouth and that outbreaks of botulism in mink caused by *Cl. botulinum* Type E may be regarded as questionable.

Apparently Type F is widely distributed in the United States and has been reported in Argentina. While the prototype strain was proteolytic some of the more recently isolated strains were not. Isolations of Type F cultures have been made from crabs (*Collinectes sapidus*) in Virginia (63), from a salmon in the Columbia River (11), and from marine sediments from the coasts of Oregon and California (17). Outbreaks of intoxication caused by this type have been limited to man.

**Pathogenicity.** The toxin of the organism of botulism enters the body through the intestinal tract, but the damages caused by it are almost wholly in the nervous system. Histological changes have not been found in the nervous system, however; hence there is much doubt as to the manner by which damage is caused. It has been suggested that the damage is to the peripheral nerves rather than to the central nervous system.

The symptoms are essentially those of paralysis. Disturbances in vision occur, there is difficulty in locomotion, the tongue often becomes paralyzed, swallowing becomes impossible because of pharyngeal paralysis, and respiratory paralysis finally terminates the disease.

**Sources of Infection for Animals.** Man is susceptible to Types A, B, C, E, and

F; mink to A, B, and C; birds to A, sometimes B, and C; and ruminants primarily to C and D. Most cases of botulism of man occur, as has been stated earlier, from the eating of preserved food, especially canned vegetables. These are not ordinarily eaten by animals, but several large outbreaks have been caused by feeding spoiled canned goods to chickens. It is difficult to see how conditions favorable for the generation of botulinum toxin can develop in the food of the herbivorous animals, as they are ordinarily maintained. In moldy hay and grain that have been damp or wet for a time, it is possible for the toxin to develop. We believe that most reported cases of botulism in horses and cattle are the result of erroneous diagnoses.

Although convenience (plastic-packaged, requiring little or no heat prior to consumption) foods have been suspect as a cause of outbreaks in man, surveys have shown that the incidence of *Cl. botulinum* organisms in these substances is extremely low (34, 58).

**Diagnosis.** The bacteriologic diagnosis of botulism in animals is difficult, and there are many clinical diagnoses that cannot be sustained bacteriologically. The finding of the organism in the intestinal tract of the affected animal or the fact of its presence in food materials is not sufficient to prove its connection with the disease. It must be remembered that organisms of this group are widespread in nature and are likely to be encountered in any foodstuffs that may be contaminated by soil (dust). To prove that a food is guilty it must be shown that it actually contains toxin in an amount sufficient to cause poisoning.

Lamanna (39) was the first to use hemagglutination-inhibition (HI) tests in identifying botulism toxin. He found that Type A toxin agglutinated chicken, guinea pig, rabbit, sheep, and human erythrocytes. Hemagglutination was specifically prevented by Type A antitoxin but not by Types B or C. It is now known that HI tests can be used to distinguish Types A, B, and C. However, hemagglutination by Type D toxin can be inhibited by either Type C or Type D antiserum (57). This indicates a closer relationship between Types C and D than between Types A, B, and C. It also shows that the lethal toxins and hemagglutinins of Types C and D are not the same thing, for the lethal toxins are neutralized only by the homologous antitoxins. It has also been shown that Type E antitoxin may neutralize Type F toxin, but the reverse is not true (18).

Immunofluorescence has been used to identify *Cl. botulinum* Types A, B, C, and E (33, 48), and Cone and Lechowich (10) employed pyrolysis-gas-liquid chromatography to differentiate among Types A, B, and E.

**Immunity.** Homologous antitoxins protect animals very well against botulism. In practice they are of little use because the disease does not appear frequently enough in any one herd to warrant prophylactic immunization, and for curative purposes antitoxins are of little value. Polyvalent antitoxins (Types A, B, and C) are made commercially and are available. If given very early in the disease, it is thought that they have some curative effect. It is believed that antitoxin (Type C) has some value in treating wild ducks exposed to botulism.

Formalinized, alum-precipitated toxoids have been used successfully in immunizing mink (1), horses (62), cattle, sheep, pheasants, and ducks (7). In some areas polyvalent toxoids are used for this purpose. In Australia nonimmune cattle and sheep are usually given a series of two injections and from then on a refresher dose each year (6, 41).

Pentavalent toxoids absorbed on aluminum phosphate have been used on human volunteers with apparent success (22) but the disease appears so rarely that vaccination is not practical. It is noteworthy that Marty (44) was able to reactivate partially a fomalin-inactivated *Cl. botulinum* Type C toxin by adding sodium bisulfite to neutralize the formalin.

## REFERENCES

1. Appleton and White.   Am. Jour. Vet. Res., 1959, *20,* 166.
2. Avery, Dolman, Stovell, and Wood.   Canad. Jour. Comp. Med. and Vet. Sci., 1959, *23,* 203.
3. Beiers and Simmons.   Austral. Vet. Jour., 1967, *43,* 270.
4. Bengston.   Pub. Health Rpts. (U.S.), 1922, *37,* 164.
5. Bengston.   U.S. Pub. Health Serv., Hyg. Lab. Bul. 136, 1924.
6. Bennetts and Hall.   Jour. Agr. (West Austral.), 1937, *14,* 381.
7. Boroff and Reilly.   Jour. Bact., 1959, *77,* 142.
8. Buckley and Shippen.   Jour. Am. Vet. Med. Assoc., 1917, *50,* 809.
9. Burke.   Jour. Bact., 1919, *4,* 555.
10. Cone and Lechowich.   Appl. Microbiol., 1970, *19,* 138.
11. Craig and Pilcher.   Science, 1966, *153,* 311.
12. Davis, Mattman, and Wiley.   Jour. Am. Med. Assoc., 1951, *146,* 646.
13. Dinter and Kull.   Nord. Vetmed., 1954, *6,* 866.
14. Dolman and Murakami.   Jour. Inf. Dis., 1961, *109,* 107.
15. Dolman, Tomsich, Campbell, and Laing.   *Ibid.,* 1960, *106,* 5.
16. Editorial.   Vet. Med., 1954, *49,* 132.
17. Eklund and Poysky.   Science, 1965, *149,* 306.
18. Eklund, Poysky, and Wieler.   Appl. Microbiol., 1967, *15,* 1316.
19. Van Ermengem.   Zeitschr. f. Hyg., 1897, *26,* 1.
20. Esty.   Jour. Am. Pub. Health Assoc., 1923, *13,* 108.
21. Fish, Mitchell, and Barnum.   Canad. Vet. Jour., 1967, *8,* 10.
22. Flock, Cardella, and Gearinger.   Jour. Immunol., 1963, *90,* 697.
23. Gitter.   Vet. Rec., 1959, *71,* 868.
24. Graham and Brueckner.   Jour. Bact., 1919, *4,* 1.
25. Graham and Schwarze.   Jour. Am. Med. Assoc., 1922, *76,* 1743.
26. Grecz, Wagenaar, and Dack.   Appl. Microbiol., 1965, *13,* 1014.
27. Gunnison, Cummings, and Meyer.   Proc. Soc. Exp. Biol. and Med., 1936, *35,* 278.
28. Gustavsen, Hauge, Loftsgård, Oftebro, Rossebø, Tjaberg, and Aaneland. Canad. Vet. Jour., 1969, *10,* 244.
29. Hall and Stiles.   Jour. Bact., 1938, *36,* 282.

30. Hampson. *Ibid.*, 1951, *61*, 647.
31. Hart. Jour. Am. Vet. Med. Assoc., 1920, *57*, 75.
32. Hazen. Science, 1938, *87*, 413.
33. Hunter and Rosen. Avian Dis., 1967, *11*, 345.
34. Insalata, Witzeman, Fredericks, and Sunga. Appl. Microbiol., 1969, *17*, 542.
35. Jackson. Vet. Med., 1953, *48*, 509.
36. Johnston, Feldman, and Sullivan. Pub. Health Rpts. (U.S.), 1963, *78*, 561.
37. Kalmbach and Gunderson. U.S. Dept. Agr. Tech. Bul. 411, 1934.
38. Krabbenhoft, Corlett, Anderson, and Elliker. Appl. Microbiol., 1964, *12*, 424.
39. Lamanna. Proc. Soc. Exp. Biol. and Med., 1948, *69*, 332.
40. Lamanna, McElroy, and Eklund. Science, 1946, *103*, 613.
41. Larsen, Nicholes, and Gebhardt. Am. Jour. Vet. Res., 1955, *26*, 573.
42. Mandia. Jour. Immunol., 1951, *67*, 49.
43. Mandia and Bruner. *Ibid.*, 1951, *66*, 497.
44. Marty. Am. Jour. Vet. Res., 1961, *22*, 770.
45. Mason. Jour. So. African Vet. Med. Assoc., 1968, *39*, 37.
46. Meyer and Dubovsky. Jour. Inf. Dis., 1922, *31*, 559.
47. Meyer and Gunnison. *Ibid.*, 1929, *45*, 96.
48. Midura, Inouye, and Bodily. Pub. Health Rpts. (U.S.), 1967, *82*, 275.
49. Moberg. 15th Internatl. Vet. Cong., Stockholm, 1953, *1*, 1.
50. Möller and Scheibel. Acta Path. et Microbiol. Scand., 1960, *48*, 80.
51. Müller. Deut. Klin., 1870, *22*, 27.
52. Quortrup and Gorham. Am. Jour. Vet. Res., 1949, *10*, 268.
53. Richardson, Brewer, and Holdeman. Jour. Am. Vet. Med. Assoc., 1965, *146*, 737.
54. Robinson. Rpt. Dir. Vet. Service and Anim. Indus., Union So. Africa, 1930, *16*, 107.
55. Seddon. Jour. Comp. Path. and Therap., 1922, *35*, 147.
56. Skulberg and Valland. Acta Vet. Scand., 1969, *10*, 137.
57. Sterne. Science, 1954, *119*, 440.
58. Taclindo, Jr., Midura, Nygaard, and Bodily. Appl. Microbiol., 1967, *15*, 426.
59. Theiler *et al.* 11th and 12th Ann. Rpts., Dir. Vet. Ed. and Res., Union So. Africa, 1927, *2*, 821.
60. Theiler and Robinson. Zeitschr. f. Infektionskr. Haustiere, 1927, *31*, 165.
61. Wentzel, Sterne, and Polson. Nature, 1950, *166*, 739.
62. White and Appleton. Jour. Am. Vet. Med. Assoc., 1960, *137*, 652.
63. Williams-Walls. Science, 1968, *162*, 375.

## THE TISSUE-INVADING GROUP

### *Clostridium chauvoei*

SYNONYMS: *Bacillus chauvoei, Bacillus carbonis, Bacillus anthracis symptomatici, Clostridium feseri, Clostridium chauvei*

This organism affects cattle principally, sometimes sheep, goats, and deer. Guinea pigs may readily be infected by inoculation. Although it is generally stated that other domestic animals and man are immune, Sterne and Edwards

(21) claim to have isolated *Cl. chauvoei* from two cases of blackleg in pigs, Clay (5) has reported an incident of black quarter in the pig, and Langford (12) recorded a feed-borne outbreak in mink that were fed infected beef liver. About 25 percent of the involved mink kits died. Apparently, the disease is very rare in the pig because it possesses a high order of natural immunity. In cattle the disease is known as *blackleg, black quarter, quarter ill,* or *symptomatic anthrax.* In England it is reported that the disease is common in certain areas, where it usually is seen as a postparturient infection in sheep. The infection is widespread in large areas of the range country of the United States, where the losses are principally in cattle. In this species the disease occurs without any evident portal of entry.

**Morphology and Staining Reactions.** This organism is seen in tissues and cultures as a straight, round-ended rod about 0.6 microns in width and from 3 to 8 microns long. It usually appears singly or in chains of three to five organisms in the peritoneal exudate of inoculated guinea pigs, and this fact is useful in distinguishing it from *Cl. septicum* and other anaerobic bacilli which frequently occur in materials suspected of blackleg. The latter organisms usually occur in long chains. Spores are oval and appear excentrically, swelling the rods into lemon-shaped structures. Very young cultures are motile by means of peritrichic flagella. The cells stain somewhat unevenly. The Gram stain is positive when the cultures are young but erratic after they are a few days old.

**Cultural Features.** *Cl. chauvoei* is a little more exacting in its cultural requirements than are most of the organisms in this group. It is strictly anaerobic and will not grow on ordinary glucose agar except when tissues are carried over in the inoculum. The addition of blood or tissue makes ordinary broth and agar favorable for it. It will grow luxuriantly on all media made with a liver infusion base, without enrichment.

Deep colonies on agar are delicate and compact, being irregularly spherical. When blood is present, there is evidence of slight hemolysis, but definite

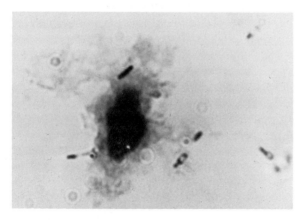

Fig. 51. *Clostridium chauvoei,* a film from a brain-liver medium culture incubated 48 hours at 37 C. X 1,500.

zones are not formed around surface colonies. In plain broth there is usually no growth unless blood or tissue has been carried over with the inoculum. In liver broth the fluid becomes moderately clouded. Gelatin containing a little serum is slowly liquefied, and a few gas bubbles are formed. Growth on coagulated blood serum and coagulated egg is poor, and there is no liquefaction. Cooked-meat medium becomes pinkish, and the fluid is slightly clouded. Liver-brain medium gives excellent growth and is a good medium on which to maintain cultures. It is not digested. Acid and gas are formed from glucose, levulose, galactose, maltose, lactose, and sucrose, Inulin, salicin, mannitol, glycerol, and dextrin are not fermented. Cultures of this organism give off a characteristic odor by which experienced workers frequently can identify the species. It is not putrefactive but is rather butyric. Although Kerrin (9) was able to demonstrate only weak exotoxin production, Jayaraman *et al.* (8) obtained a much higher yield. According to Moussa (15), all but two of the 37 strains of *Cl. chauvoei* that he studied possessed a single O antigen and could be divided into two groups based on H antigens which, like the single O, were distinct from those of *Cl. septicum.* The two nonconforming strains showed no antigenic relationship to other *Cl. chauvoei* strains, but possessed antigens occurring in some *Cl. septicum* strains. All strains of *Cl. chauvoei* and *Cl. septicum* that Moussa examined had a common spore antigen.

**Normal Habitat and Mode of Infection.** The organism of blackleg exists in the soil. Whether it multiplies there, or whether it merely lives there in the spore form and multiplies in the intestinal canal of animals, is not known. In any case it is known that when pastures or grazing grounds once become infected, the disease will reappear regularly in susceptible animals year after year. In sheep, the disease often seems to be a wound infection, occurring after lambing, docking, and shearing (14). In cattle, wounds are seldom found and it is believed that infections occur mostly through the digestive tract. In Montana infection has been reported in ewes soon after they were shorn while pregnant. The organism was recovered from edematous fetuses in these ewes (4).

The studies of Kerry (10) may help to throw some light on this matter. He was able to find *Cl. chauvoei* in the livers and spleens of 20 percent of normal healthy cattle whose organs were removed immediately after slaughter. This suggests that idiopathic infections may be the result of dissemination from such reservoirs. Cobb and McKay (6) in a bacteriological survey of the livers of normal dogs of Ontario found *Cl. chauvoei* to be the most common bacterium encountered in the adult animal. The organism did not appear to settle in the liver until the middle of the dog's first year of life.

**Pathogenicity.** Guinea pigs are easily infected by inoculation and are the best animals for diagnostic work. Mice can sometimes be infected and also rabbits. Experimental animals usually die in about 48 hours. The muscles in the region of the point of inoculation are hemorrhagic and darkened, and there may be a little edema but no gas present. The abdominal cavity usually is moist, and the liver may have a semicooked appearance. Films from the liver surface show numerous typical bacilli arranged singly, in pairs, or in very short chains. Pure cultures are easily obtained from the peritoneal fluid, and usually from the heart blood.

Bovine infections occur mostly in young animals, from 4 months to 2 years old. Lameness is the first manifestation. A diffuse swelling usually appears in the region of the shoulder or of the rump, and the animal shows fever and great depression. If the swollen region is palpated, it is found to be soft and when pressed a crackling sound is heard because of the gas in the muscular tissue. The affected animals usually die within a day or two. The lesions consist of blackened muscular tissue where the swelling existed. The tissues are quite dry, and gas bubbles are found throughout. They give off a characteristic rancid odor. Cases of blackleg occur in which muscular lesions are not found, or the lesions may be small and located in such obscure muscles as the psoas group or those of the diaphragm. In addition to the characteristic muscle lesions, the liver may be swollen and show collections of small gas bubbles, especially if some hours have elapsed since death occurred. In calves, vegetative lesions may be found on the heart valves, the heart muscle is often pale and friable, and there may be fluid and fibrin in both chest and abdominal cavities.

The disease is prevalent in the states of the Mississippi Valley and in the range regions beyond. It also exists in many small areas in nearly all parts of the world where cattle are kept.

**Immunity.** The few animals that recover from an attack of this disease appear to be permanently immune. In regions where the disease is common, young cattle are regularly immunized in order to prevent losses. The immunization is ordinarily done in late winter or early spring because the infections are contracted on the range or pasture during the grazing season. Several methods for successfully immunizing animals are available. For many years vaccines were used. Later they were largely replaced in the United States by tissue or culture filtrates (aggressins). These were better but were much more expensive to manufacture. In recent years the blackleg bacterin has been used to the exclusion of all former methods. Bacterins are very satisfactory and cheaper than filtrates. Immune sera have been prepared. These will protect when administered prophylactically, but they are expensive and the duration of the immunity is too short for practical use. When they are given in large amounts and very early in the course of the disease, infected animals may sometimes be saved.

*Vaccines.* A number of different vaccines have been used more or less successfully for the prevention of blackleg. The two best known are those of Arloing, Cornevin, and Thomas (2)—known generally as the Lyon vaccine, since the workers were at the Veterinary School at Lyon, France—and the Kitt (11) vaccine, which is, essentially, a modification of the Lyon vaccine. In both of these vaccines, the diseased muscular tissue is used as a basis. By a process of drying and heating, the vegetative forms of the blackleg bacilli in the muscular tissue are killed and the spores are attenuated until they no longer have sufficient virulence to be dangerous. The original Lyon vaccine consisted of two vaccines, one weaker and intended for use first, and another stronger, intended for use about 10 days after the first. The Kitt vaccine consisted of only a single injection of material that had been attenuated. For many years a modification of the Kitt vaccine was made and distributed by the United States Department of Agriculture (17) free of cost to the cattlemen of the midwest. This vaccine gave reasonably good results and certainly prevented heavy losses from the disease. The vaccine consisted of blackleg muscle which was ground up, spread upon plates or shallow pans, and heated for 6 hours at 94 to 95 C. The dry scale was afterward scraped off, ground to a brownish powder, and stored until needed. When it was to be used, weighed amounts were soaked in water, the material was filtered, and the filtrate was used. Insignificant reactions to the vaccine usually resulted. Occasionally a few losses from blackleg occurred from this vaccine, and sometimes animals appeared to lack proper protection after its use. This vaccine is no longer made because better products are now available. At the time the manufacture of the vaccine was discontinued, approximately 50,000,000 doses had been distributed.

*Aggressin.* It has been shown by several workers that filtrates of the blackleg tumor fluids possess immunizing properties. Schoenleber, Haslam, and Franklin (19; 1917) applied the method of field practice and found it very successful. The aggressin, when properly prepared, gives a strong immunity and is perfectly safe. The immunity is active. It persists longer than that conferred by the older vaccines.

*Germ-free filtrate (artificial aggressin).* Nitta (16), of Japan, observed that filtrates of blackleg cultures grown in the presence of meat fragments had immunizing properties that were nearly as great as those of true aggressin. These substances do not appear in ordinary cultures. The method of production is to cultivate the organism in flasks that contain a meat-piece medium, to squeeze the juice out after growth is completed, and to free the juice of the organisms by filtration. This product can be made more cheaply than the true aggressin, which necessitates the sacrifice of calves in its production.

*Blackleg bacterin: blackleg anaculture.* Following the discovery that formalin had the power of destroying the poisonous properties of toxins while preserving their antigenic value, Leclainche and Vallee (13) tried the procedure on cultures of the blackleg organism and discovered that formolized whole cultures constituted a safe and effective immunizing product. About the same time, or perhaps earlier, the same procedure had been discovered by the research staff of an American commercial company. The product has been extensively used in this country and is unquestionably a safe, reliable immunizing agent for cattle. The immunizing substance resides in the bacterial cells; hence the cultures are concentrated by sedimentation before the formolization is carried out. Some companies add alum to the finished product to delay absorption and enhance the antigenicity of the bacterin. The material can be produced more cheaply than either naturally or artificially produced aggressin, for the reason that Berkefeld filtration is eliminated, and this is the most expensive procedure in aggressin manufacture. Because the product does not depend upon a detoxified toxin, or antitoxin, for its immunizing properties, but rather upon the antigenic proteins of the killed bacterial cells, the term *anaculture* has been proposed for it.

*The combined chauvoei-septicum bacterin.* In some areas losses formerly occurred from what was thought to be blackleg after the calves had been vaccinated against that disease. Breed (3) showed that many of these cases were not true blackleg but infections with *Clostridium septicum.* In such areas he advocated the use of a mixed bacterin made by adding the latter to the blackleg culture before formalinization. This product is made commercially and used widely with apparent success. Some commercial companies have gone a step further and have added *Pasteurella multocida* to the *chauvoei-septicum* combination making a triple-antigen bacterin. In fact it has been demonstrated that sheep respond to individual components of a combined bacterin more favorably than to single bacterins (20). Sheep sometimes develop local reactions following injection of bacterins and in New Zealand the side of the upper neck is recommended as the optimal site for vaccination (7).

False blackleg may be caused by *Cl. novyi* and occasionally by *Cl. perfringens.* Anacultures of these types are also effective prophylactics.

*Blackleg serum.* By immunizing horses with washed cultures of the blackleg organism, a highly potent serum can be obtained that is useful, if used in large amounts, in protecting valuable calves when blackleg is present in a herd and in treating cases which have already developed.

**Chemotherapy.** Chemotherapeutic agents had little effect on blackleg infection until the advent of penicillin. Aitken (1) reports that this antibiotic is quite effective in treating blackleg in cattle if it is administered sufficiently early, and Butler and Marsh (4) describe similar results for sheep. Percival and colleagues (18) have demonstrated the usefulness of aureomycin in this disease.

**REFERENCES**

1. Aitken.   North Am. Vet., 1949, *30*, 441.
2. Arloing, Cornevin, and Thomas.   Le charbon symptomatique du boeuf. Asselin et Houzeau, Paris, 1887.
3. Breed.   Jour. Am. Vet. Med. Assoc., 1937, *90*, 521.
4. Butler and Marsh.   *Ibid.*, 1956, *128*, 401.
5. Clay.   Vet. Rec., 1960, *72*, 265.
6. Cobb and McKay.   Jour. Comp. Path. and Therap., 1962, *72*, 92.
7. Cooper and Jull.   New Zeal. Vet. Jour., 1966, *14*, 171.
8. Jayaraman, Lal, and Dhanda.   Indian Vet. Jour., 1962, *39*, 481.

 9.  Kerrin.   Jour. Path. and Bact., 1934, *38*, 219.
10.  Kerry.   Vet. Rec., 1964, *76*, 396.
11.  Kitt.   Centrbl. f. Bakt., 1888, *3*, 572.
12.  Langford.   Canad. Vet. Jour., 1970, *11*, 170.
13.  Leclainche and Vallee.   Rev. gén. méd. vét., 1925, *34*, 293; Comp. rend. Soc. Biol. (Paris), 1925, *92*, 1273.
14.  March.   Jour. Am. Vet. Med. Assoc., 1919, *56*, 319; 1922, *62*, 217.
15.  Moussa.   Jour. Path. and Bact., 1959, 77, 341.
16.  Nitta.   Jour. Am. Vet. Med. Assoc., 1918, *53*, 466.
17.  Norgaard (Mohler).   U.S. Dept. Agr., Bur. Anim. Indus. Cir. 31, 1911.
18.  Percival, Leaming, Martini, and Tonelli.   Cornell Vet., 1953, *43*, 92.
19.  Schoenleber, Haslam, and Franklin.   Kan. Agr. Exp. Sta. Cir. 59, 1917.
20.  Sterne, Batty, Thomson, and Robertson.   Vet. Rec., 1962, *74*, 909.
21.  Sterne and Edwards.   *Ibid.*, 1955, *67*, 314.

### *Clostridium septicum*

SYNONYMS:  *Vibrion septique, Bacillus septicus;* probably Ghon-Sachs bacillus; also erroneously, *Bacillus edematis-maligni, Bacillus edematis*

This organism was first identified by Pasteur and Joubert (8) in 1877 from carcasses of animals thought to have died from anthrax. About this time Koch (6) isolated his *malignant edema bacillus* from animals that had been inoculated with soil. Koch regarded the two organisms as identical, but, since this organism was strongly proteolytic and Pasteur's was not, it is evident that they were not identical. Koch's organism has been lost; hence it is not possible to know precisely what organism he had. His cultures may have contained *Cl. septicum* contaminated by a proteolytic anaerobe such as *Clostridium sporogenes. Cl. septicum* is generally called the *malignant edema bacillus* and the condition produced in animals is termed *malignant edema,* but it is not the malignant edema bacillus first described by Koch.

**Morphology and Staining Reactions.** *Cl. septicum* is a rather large rod of the shape and size of the blackleg organism. It is from 0.6 to 0.8 micron wide and 3 to 8 microns long. Usually it is straight and the ends are rounded. In cultures it often occurs singly or in short chains, but in animal exudates it appears in long chains. It has already been pointed out that the tendency of this organism to form long chains on the surface of the liver of inoculated guinea pigs is a feature by which it may be distinguished from *Cl. chauvoei,* which occurs singly or in very short chains. Young cultures show active motility because of peritrichic flagella. The spores are oval, occur excentrically, and swell the cells in which they are formed. It is Gram-positive, but, like most of the other organisms of this group, old cultures usually decolorize. It stains readily with all the usual stains.

**Cultural Features.** This organism grows readily in all ordinary media so long as good anaerobic conditions prevail. In its growth vigor it differs from the blackleg organism with which it is often confused, the latter being much more fastidious in its requirements than *Cl. septicum.*

Colonies in deep agar usually are cottony and filamentous. In blood agar plates the colonies are surrounded by hemolytic zones. Gelatin is liquefied and a few gas bubbles are formed in it. Plain infusion broth is lightly clouded. Litmus milk is coagulated and some gas may be formed in the curd. The curd is not digested. Coagulated blood serum and coagulated egg albumen are not digested. There is good growth in meat medium and in brain-liver medium, but there is no digestion or darkening. Acid and gas are formed from glucose, levulose, galactose, maltose, lactose, and salicin. Sucrose and mannitol are not fermented.

The organism produces a toxin. The lethal part of this toxin is called *alpha toxin* and is also hemolytic (12). Cultures of *Cl. septicum* agglutinate red blood cells. This hemagglutination can be neutralized by specific antisera. Furthermore, the agglutinating factor is associated with the bacterial cell, but not with the toxins. It is thermolabile and is not destroyed by 0.5 percent formalin, 0.5 percent phenol, or absolute alcohol (2).

Strains of *Cl. septicum* are serologically heterogeneous. By antigenic analysis of their somatic and flagellar agglutinogens they can be divided into six groups defined by two O and five H antigens (7). The possession of common antigens renders the straight agglutination test useless as a means of distinguishing between *Cl. septicum* and *Cl. chauvoei*, but their toxins are specific. Protection against infection with *Cl. septicum* is afforded, for the most part, by immunization directed against the somatic antigens.

**Natural Habitat and Mode of Infection.** *Cl. septicum* exists in all fertile soils and in the intestinal tracts of herbivorous animals. As in the case of *Cl. chau-*

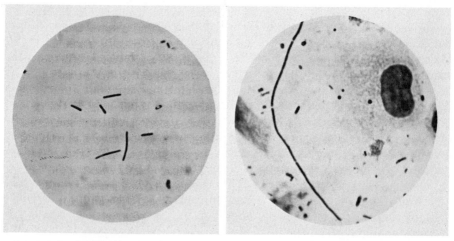

*Fig. 52 (left).* Clostridium septicum, a culture in meat-piece medium incubated for 48 hours at 37 C. One sporulated bacillus is seen in the photograph. X 700.

*Fig. 53 (right).* Clostridium septicum, a stained film from the surface of the liver of a guinea pig inoculated with a pure culture. The long filaments are characteristic. They are helpful in differentiating this organism from Clostridium chauvoei, which never forms such filaments. X 700.

*voei*, it is not known whether it multiples in the soil or whether it merely exists in the form of spores formed by organisms present in animal excrement.

Infections occur through wounds in many cases but not all can be accounted for in this way. The disease of sheep known as *bradsot* or *braxy*, which occurs in Norway, Iceland, and Scotland, is caused by *Cl. septicum*, the lesions being internal. It is supposed that the infection occurs through the digestive tract.

**Pathogenicity.** Pure cultures will kill guinea pigs, which are highly susceptible also to *Cl. chauvoei*, and rabbits, mice, and pigeons, which are resistant to the blackleg organism. The lesions in guinea pigs cannot be distinguished from those of blackleg. A blood-tinged gelatinous exudate is found beneath the skin at the point of inoculation, and the muscular tissue is dark red in color. Gas is not usually present in the tissues. The peritoneal cavity often is moist and may have a little more fluid in it than normal. The liver is lighter than normal, having a semicooked appearance. Stained films from the liver surface show long, jointed chains of cells.

Wound infections in animals are known under the general name of *malignant edema*. Such infections are characterized by rapidly extending swellings, which are soft and pit on pressure. The diseased animals show fever and other signs of intoxication, and most of them die within a few hours or in 1 or 2 days. The affected tissues are infiltrated with large quantities of gelatinous exudate most of which is in the subcutaneous and intermuscular connective tissue. The muscular tissue is dark red but, unlike blackleg, contains little or no gas. Infections in cattle sometimes resemble blackleg very closely. In recognition of this, the organism is referred to in German literature as the *parablackleg bacillus*. It is believed that in many cases cattle and sheep suffer from a mixed infection with blackleg and other anaerobic organisms, and that the organism of blackleg in such cases often is overlooked because it grows more delicately than the others and is crowded out of cultures (1).

*Cl. septicum* causes infections not only in cattle and sheep, which are also susceptible to blackleg, but also in horses and man, who are not susceptible to blackleg, and in swine which are only slightly susceptible. Clostridial infections are generally considered to be of little significance in poultry, but *Cl. septicum* infection does occur in chickens (5, 10). In a broiler flock infected with this organism the birds showed varying degrees of depression, incoordination, inappetence, and ataxia. The mortality was about 1 percent. The feed was formulated commercially, delivered in bulk, and fed manually from a storage bin. In another instance *Cl. septicum* along with *Clostridium perfringens* Type A, staphylococci, and coliforms caused a subcutaneous infection of growing chickens. It was characterized by sudden onset and accompanied by gangrenous cellulitis that involved the subcutis and underlying muscles of the legs and lateroventral abdominal wall.

Braxy or bradsot destroys large numbers of sheep each year in northwestern Europe, principally in Norway, Scotland, the Faroe Islands, and Iceland

(4). The disease is apparently caused by *Cl. septicum,* by ingestion, although experimenters have had little success in producing the disease in that way. It is thought that some accessory factors, as yet unrecognized, are responsible for the infections. Affected animals die very suddenly without previously showing symptoms, or after only a few hours of symptoms. The walls of the abomasum and the first part of the small intestine are edematous, hemorrhagic, and sometimes necrotic. The internal organs show only degenerative changes.

**Immunity.** *Cl. septicum* produces a toxin of moderate potency. Usually 0.5 to 1.0 ml of a filtrate of a culture will kill guinea pigs within a few minutes. According to Dalling (3), an antitoxin can be prepared by inoculating animals with the toxin, but the toxin always is highly irritating and produces necrosis at the point of injection. Animals may be immunized by injecting them with formolized whole cultures of *Cl. septicum.* This usually produces lifelong immunity (Smith, 11). It appears that immunity against this organism is primarily antibacterial rather than antitoxic.

High titer *Cl. septicum* antitoxin has been produced in horses, but has been of little practical value in treating infection in animals.

**Chemotherapy.** Reed and Orr (9) reported that sulfathiazole was effective in controlling *Cl. septicum* infection in experimentally infected wounds of animals if the drug was administered locally and before the infection became well established. Both narrow- and broad-spectrum antibiotics are recommended as therapeutic agents. The tetracyclines have been very effective in treating chickens (10).

## REFERENCES

1.  Breed.   Jour. Am. Vet. Med. Assoc., 1937, *90*, 521.
2.  Dafaalla and Soltys.   Brit. Jour. Exp. Path., 1952, *32*, 510.
3.  Dalling.   Jour. Comp. Path. and Therap., 1926, *39*, 148.
4.  Gordon.   Vet. Rec., 1934, *14*, 1 and 1016.
5.  Helfer, Dickinson, and Smith.   Avian Dis., 1969, *13*, 231.
6.  Koch.   Mitt. a. d. kaiserl. Gesundheitsamte, 1881, *1*, 54.
7.  Moussa.   Jour. Path. and Bact., 1959, 77, 341.
8.  Pasteur and Joubert.   Bul. Acad. Med., II Ser., 1877, *6*, 781.
9.  Reed and Orr.   Am. Jour. Med. Sci., 1943, *206*, 379.
10.  Saunders and Bickford.   Avian Dis., 1965, 9, 317.
11.  Smith. Introduction to pathogenic anaerobes. Univ. of Chicago Press, Chicago, 1954, p. 147.
12.  Warrack, Bidwell, and Oakley. Jour. Path. and Bact., 1951, *63*, 293.

### *Clostridium novyi*

SYNONYMS: Novy's *B. edematis maligni II, Clostridium edematiens*

This organism was first described by Novy (6), in 1894, who isolated it from a guinea pig that had been inoculated with unsterilized milk protein. It was lost sight of for many years until Weinberg and Séguin (14) rediscovered it in gas gangrene infections of man in 1915. They gave it the name *Cl. edematiens,* and this name is still used by most English and French workers. It is quite similar to *Cl. septicum* in its cultural features and in pathenogenicity.

**Morphology and Staining Reactions.** This is one of the largest of anaerobic bacilli. It measures 0.8 to 1.0 micron in breadth and is from 3 to 10 microns long. The rods usually are quite straight and the ends rounded. The spores generally are present in abundance. They are located subterminally and are oval. Young cultures are motile by peritrichic flagella. Young cultures are Gram-positive; older cultures usually lose this property.

**Cultural Features.** This organism is more strictly anaerobic than most of the other disease producers. To obtain surface growths, the anaerobic apparatus must be in good working order. In deep agar cultures the colonies grow well, especially when glucose is present. The colonies vary in form, some being compact and of a yellowish tinge, others loose and woolly. The medium is disrupted by gas formation. On blood agar the colonies are surrounded by hemolytic zones. Gelatin is liquefied. Broth supports a poor growth, most of which sediments to the bottom. Litmus milk is reduced but not coagulated. Coagulated blood serum and egg albumen are not liquefied. There is good growth in cooked-meat medium. The meat fragments become reddish in color and a rancid smell is emitted. Acid and gas are formed from glucose, levulose, maltose, xylose, starch, and glycerol. Lactose, sucrose, mannitol, dulcitol, inulin, and salicin are not fermented. A toxin that is more potent than those of most of the tissue-invading anaerobes is formed. According to Oakley, Warrack, and Clarke (7), this toxin possesses six components, which they designate by small Greek letters, the alpha component being the classic lethal part of the toxin. Three immunologic types of *Cl. novyi* have been defined by Scott, Turner, and Vawter (8) and designated Type A, Type B, and Type C. None of these types produces a toxin containing all the six components demonstrated by Oakley, Warrack, and Clarke.

**Pathogenicity.** *Cl. novyi* is pathogenic, by inoculation, for a wide variety of animals, and naturally occurring cases have been found in many species. The horse, cow, sheep, goat, pig, dog, cat, guinea pig, rabbit, white rat, white mouse, fowls, and man are susceptible. Guinea pigs inoculated subcutaneously die in from 24 to 48 hours. At the injection spot there is edema extending into the intermuscular connective tissue. The muscles are dark red in color. A little gas may be present. In the abdominal cavity there is usually considerable clear fluid, which coagulates upon exposure to air.

This organism is occasionally found as the cause of maligant edema in cattle and sheep. The condition begins in a wound and cannot be distinguished from that caused by *Cl. septicum* without a bacteriological examination. In Australia two peculiar diseases of sheep are attributed to this organism. One is known as *swelled head* or *big head,* a condition seen in young Merino rams, rarely in older males or females of any age (3). It is believed to be caused by infection of head wounds obtained in fighting. An infiltration of the tissues of the head and often the neck and brisket with a gelatinous, nongaseous fluid occurs. Death results in practically all cases. The other disease has been given the name of *black disease,* and this has been reported from Europe as well as Australia. The most characteristic lesion in this disease is necrosis of the liver. The extensive hemorrhages seen on the inner surfaces of the hides gave origin to the name. Affected animals almost always die, usually within a few hours after showing the first symptoms. Turner (11) established that this disease developed only in regions where the liver fluke abounded, and that the organism multiplies in parts of the liver damaged by the fluke. Wardle (13) reports that excellent progress in bringing the disease under control has been achieved by campaigns aimed at eradicating the fluke through destruction of the snail which is the intermediate host.

Black disease has been found in a number of countries other than Australia, including New Zealand, Germany, Romania, France, Chile, and the United States. The organism is found in the soil (5) and the disease probably is seen wherever the sheep liver fluke occurs.

Black disease has also been reported in cattle in Australia. There the disease has been nearly eliminated from sheep, but continues to appear in cattle (12). A case was recognized in Tasmania in a horse, and it was postulated that the infection was carried by *Strongylus* larvae instead of flukes (12).

Byrne and Armstrong (4) reported two outbreaks of an alimentary tract infection of cattle caused by *Cl. novyi.* These outbreaks occurred in Canadian cattle. They presented atypical symptoms of blackleg infection. In the first outbreak 21 of 47 animals died. In the second outbreak prompt diagnosis and the use of a bacterin containing *Cl. novyi* is given credit for limiting deaths to 2 in a herd of 50 cattle. Bourne and Kerry (2) have described cases of sudden death in sows from which *Cl. novyi* was isolated. The clinical signs and postmortem lesions resembled those seen in anthrax.

Batty *et al.* (1) have used the FA technic in detecting *Cl. novyi* infection in cases of rapid death in sheep, cattle, and swine.

**Immunity.** It is possible to prepare highly potent antitoxin by immunizing animals against culture filtrates, and such antitoxins have been used prophylactically in dealing with lacerated wounds of man in which there is great danger of gas gangrene infection. Such serums are of little value in animals because the disease progresses too rapidly to make any kind of specific treatment possible.

Turner (11) had very good results in prophylactically immunizing sheep in black-disease districts with formolized whole broth cultures. Several doses are needed to give the necessary degree of immunity. Tunnicliff and Marsh (10) used an alum-precipitated toxoid given in a single dose of 5 ml and found that it protected sheep against toxin and against the natural disease that occurs in the Bitter Root Valley in Montana.

**Chemotherapy.** According to Taylor and Novak (9), infections in mice were effectively controlled, prophylactically, by the local administration of terramycin, aureomycin, penicillin, and chloromycetin, in that order.

## REFERENCES

1. Batty, Buntain, and Walker.  Vet. Rec., 1964, 76, 1115.
2. Bourne and Kerry.  *Ibid.*, 1965, 77, 1463.
3. Bull.  Jour. Comp. Path. and Therap., 1935, 48, 21.
4. Byrne and Armstrong.  Canad. Jour. Comp. Med., 1948, 12, 155.
5. Nishida and Nakagawara.  Jour. Bact., 1964, 88, 1636.
6. Novy.  Zeitschr. f. Hyg., 1894, 17, 209.
7. Oakley, Warrack, and Clarke.  Jour. Gen. Microbiol., 1947, 1, 91.
8. Scott, Turner, and Vawter.  Proc. 12th Int. Vet. Cong., 1934, p. 168.
9. Taylor and Novak.  Antibiotics and Chemother., 1952, 2, 639.
10. Tunnicliff and Marsh.  Jour. Am. Vet. Med. Assoc., 1939, 94, 98.
11. Turner.  Austral. Council Sci. and Indus. Res. Bul. 46, 1930.
12. Turner.  Vet. Rec., 1956, 68, 425.
13. Wardle.  Austral. Vet. Jour., 1936, 12, 189.
14. Weinberg and Séguin.  Comp. rend. Soc. Biol. (Paris), 1915, 78, 507.

### *Clostridium perfringens*

SYNONYMS:  *Clostridium welchii, Bacillus aerogenes capsulatus, Bacillus phlegmonis emphysematosae*, Welch Bacillus, gas bacillus

The organism was first isolated and described by Welch and Nuttall (38) from a decomposing human cadaver in which the tissues were gaseous. It was named by them *Bacillus aerogenes capsulatus*, a term that does not conform to accepted rules of nomenclature and therefore is invalid. The name *Bacillus perfringens* was given the organism by Veillon and Zuber (37) in 1898. In 1900 Migula termed it *Bacillus welchii*, the name by which it is best known to American workers; however, Veillon and Zuber's name seems clearly to have precedence, and it has been used in recent editions of *Bergey's Manual;* hence it will be used here. The term "Welch bacillus" will probably remain in use even if the formal name is divorced from Welch's name.

*Cl. perfringens* is widespread in the soil and is found in the alimentary tract of nearly all species of warm-blooded animals. It has been stated that a culture made from any shoe sole will yield *Cl. perfringens*. Canada and Strong (5) indicated that the livers of 12 percent of the newly slaughtered bovine animals examined by them contained this organism and that the livers of apparently healthy dogs may harbor it. It is frequently found as a postmortem invader from the alimentary tract in the tissues of bloating cadavers of man and animals. For this reason some caution is necessary in drawing conclusions based upon the presence of the organism in the tissues collected after death. It is found more often in the so-called gas gangrene infections of man than any other organism, although it generally is associated with other species of anaerobes in these processes. It is found also in malignant edemalike infections of animals, particularly sheep. Toxicogenic varieties of the organism are concerned in fatal toxemias in sheep, calves, young pigs, and man. These are discussed below.

**Morphology and Staining Reactions.** *Cl. perfringens* occurs as thick, straight-sided rods, either singly or in pairs, seldom in chains. The individual cells are about 1.0 micron wide and from 4 to 8 microns long. The spores are oval and small enough not to cause much swelling of the rods. Spores do not form in highly acid media; hence they are not apt to be found in media that contain fermentable carbohydrate. Strains vary in their ability to sporulate; in some cases it is difficult to find spores no matter what the nature of the culture medium. In old cultures many queer forms may be found: clubbed types, ballooned cells, and filaments. Capsules are formed in tissues and in some types of culture media. There are no flagella; the organism is therefore nonmotile. Young cultures retain the Gram stain; older ones frequently decolorize.

**Cultural Features.** In deep agar, colonies are small and biconvex. If fermentable sugar is present, the medium will be fragmented and even blown out of the tube by the abundance of gas formed. If blood is present, it will be hemolyzed. Sharp hemolytic zones are formed around colonies on plates. In broth there is excellent growth, the fluid becoming greatly clouded. Gelatin is rapidly liquefied. In semisolid medium the avidity of *Cl. perfringens* for gelatin results in a type of growth that presents the illusion of motility. Coagulated egg medium and Loeffler's blood serum are not liquefied. There is good growth in cooked-meat medium, with considerable gas formation. The meat fragments are pinkish and not digested. A sour odor is emitted. A very characteristic reaction occurs in litmus milk—the "stormy" fermentation. The milk quickly coagulates and the curd is fragmented by active gas formation. Acid and gas are formed from glucose, levulose, galactose, mannose, maltose, lactose, sucrose, xylose, trehalose, raffinose, starch, glycogen, and inositol. Some strains attack glycerol and inulin.

Although isolates of *Cl. perfringens* show no consistent differences as far as cultural characteristics are concerned, there are at least five toxicogenic types which have been designated A, B, C, D, and E (35, 40). A sixth, Type F, was described in 1949 (42). Although some workers believe it to be a variant of Type C, this point is not clearly established and we will treat it in this discussion as a sixth type (Type F). With relationship to the diseases produced, these types are distributed as follows:

*Type A.* This is the classical *Cl. perfringens* that is found in human infections. Type A strains are occasionally responsible for infected traumatic wounds of animals and have been reported to be the cause of outbreaks in calves, suckling lambs, and goats.

*Type B.* This type is usually found in the disease known as *lamb dysentery.* It is also known as the LD bacillus or as *B. agni.* It has been reported in necrotic enterotoxemia in calves and lambs.

*Type C.* A disease of adult sheep in England known as *struck* or *strike* is caused by this type. The organism is sometimes called *B. paludis.* Type C strains also appear in hemorrhagic enterotoxemia of lambs, calves, and baby pigs.

*Type D.* This type is found in a common and destructive disease of sheep, described in Australia, New Zealand, Wales, and the United States. It is known as *enterotoxemia, pulpy kidney disease,* and *overeating.* The organism is also known under the name of *B. ovitoxicus.* It is believed by some to cause a similar equine disease known as *grass sickness.* It is also believed to cause enterotoxemia in goats and calves. It has been isolated on at least one occasion from a case of gas gangrene in man (25).

*Type E.* This type contains strains that cause dysentery or enterotoxemia in lambs and calves.

*Type F.* This type causes enteritis necroticans, an enterotoxemic disease of man carrying a mortality rate of about 40 percent.

These organisms produce 12 toxic substances (35) which are demonstrated by their activity on lecithin and hyaluronic and deoxyribonucleic acids, and by their ability to cause lysis of erythrocytes, necrosis following intracutaneous injection, and death following intravenous inoculation. The alpha toxin is lethal, hemolytic, and necrotizing. It has the ability to split lecithin or lecithin-protein complexes. This toxin is found in all six types. The beta toxin is lethal and necrotizing and is found in Types B, C, and F. The gamma toxin is lethal, but not hemolytic or necrotizing, and it is found in Types B, C, and F. The delta toxin is lethal and hemolytic. It is found in Types B and C. The epsilon toxin, produced by strains of Types B and D, appears early in the growth of culture as a prototoxin and is converted about 5 to 7 days after it is produced into a highly lethal toxin by the action of proteolytic enzymes of the organisms. Trypsin will also activate this prototoxin. The eta toxin is lethal. It is rarely produced and only by strains of Type A. The theta toxin is lethal, hemolytic, and oxygen-labile. It is found in some Type A strains and in Types B, C, D, and E. The iota toxin is formed as a prototoxin. It is lethal and is produced only by Type E strains. The kappa toxin is collagenase. It is lethal and is found in Types A, C, and E, and sometimes in Type D. The lambda toxin is a nonlethal proteinase that is found in Types B and E and sometimes in Type D. The mu toxin is nonlethal hyaluronidase. It occurs in Type B and is variable in its occurrence in Types A and D. The nu toxin is nonlethal deoxyribonuclease and it is found in all six types.

Identification of these types is based on toxin neutralization and determination of enzymatic activity. Type A antitoxin will neutralize only the homologous toxin. Type B antitoxin will neutralize the toxins of Types A, B, C, D, and F. Type C antitoxin will neutralize the toxins of Types A, C, and F. Type D antitoxin will neutralize the toxins of Types A and D and Type E that of A and E. It should be noted that either Type C or Type D antitoxin may neutralize the toxicity of Type B filtrate. Type C antitoxin will neutralize the filtrate of a young culture (about 6 to 8 hours) of Type B. At this time the beta, gamma, and delta toxins are formed while epsilon prototoxin is in its nontoxic state. The toxicity of the filtrate of the same culture, after 5 to 7 days of incubation, will be inhibited by Type D antitoxin, for the beta, gamma, and delta toxins will have become spontaneously inactivated, and the epsilon prototoxin will have become activated by the proteolytic enzymes of the organism. The exact neutralizing ability of toxin F is not clear, but it can be tentatively identified by its lack of production of theta and delta toxin and greater resistance to heat. A routine procedure for the typing of *Cl. perfringens* strains has been described by Oakley and Warrack (30).

Studies on serological relationships have indicated considerable heterogeneity within the species. Cross reactions due to common capsular antigens have been found, and the use of the Quellung reaction and agar gel diffusion technics have demonstrated the sharing of common antigens among the six toxicogenic types.

**Resistance of the Organism.** In accepted methods of cooking, especially stuffed fowl, *Cl. perfringens* may survive and create a hazard if subsequent storage is at a temperature range permitting multiplication (ca. 18 to 37 C).

**Pathogenicity.** *Cl. perfringens* may be found either alone or mixed with other bacteria, in diseases of animals. Different strains vary greatly in pathogenicity. Most will kill white mice, guinea pigs, and pigeons by inoculation. Rabbits are more resistant. The lesions in inoculated animals are similar to those produced by *Cl. septicum*. It has been established that germ-free guinea pigs will die with signs and lesions of acute enterotoxemia following oral ingestion of *Cl. perfringens* Types B, C, D, and E, but Type A is innocuous when administered by this route (18).

*For sheep. Cl. perfringens,* Type A, has been reported in California to be the cause of a disease in nursing lambs that is characterized by severe hemolytic anemia, icterus, and hemoglobinuria (23).

*Lamb dysentery* is a disease that destroys many lambs during the first 2 weeks of life. In most cases symptoms appear within a few hours after birth. It is prevalent in the border country of England and Scotland, where it was first described by Gaiger and Dalling (9). An infection that apparently is the same was described in Montana by Tunnicliff (36) in 1933. The disease consists of an enteritis. In some cases there may be extensive ulcerations. *Cl. perfringens,* Type B, is found in the diarrheal discharges and intestinal contents. Here it produces a powerful toxin, and although the organism does not ordinarily invade the tissues absorption of the toxin accounts for the disease. Affected lambs usually die within a few hours. The LD bacillus of Dalling and his associates differs from the classical Welch bacillus in that it liquefies coagulated serum and clots an alkaline egg medium. Tunnicliff's strain did not show these characteristics.

*Struck* and *strike* are local names for a disease of sheep which occurs in England and in Wales (22). Adult sheep are affected. The stricken animals die so suddenly that the only symptoms are the death convulsions. The mortality is very high. If carcasses are examined immediately after death, the only lesions are severe enteritis and peritonitis. If the examination is postponed for a few hours, the muscles present the appearance of gas gangrene.

The Type C organism found in this disease is much more toxic than the other types.

Griner and Johnson (13) reported an outbreak of enterotoxemia of lambs in which the disease was characterized by sudden onset, early death, and, at necropsy, a severe hemorrhagic enteritis. The apparent cause was *Cl. perfringens* Type C.

*Enterotoxemia* of sheep is another disease associated with a highly toxic intestinal content. The condition is like lamb dysentery except that the latter occurs only in very young lambs whereas this disease is seen in older animals and is primarily a true toxemia. There is no enteritis, probably because the organism does not produce beta, gamma, or delta toxins. The disease is accompanied by marked decomposition of the kidneys, a condition described by Gill (10) in New Zealand as *pulpy kidney disease* and now believed to be a postmortem change associated with enterotoxemia. Enterotoxemia was described first by Bennetts (2) in western Australia but has been seen since in other countries including the United States. Newsom and Thorp (29) say that this disease causes greater losses among feed-lot lambs in Colorado than all other diseases combined. These authors call the disease *overeating*. It appears when the diet is changed suddenly and large quantities of highly concentrated feed such as corn, barley, peas, and cane are eaten. In these circumstances, the rumen flora cannot adapt itself quickly to the changed environment, and large amounts of undigested or partly digested food escapes into the small intestine. This provides an ideal substrate for *Cl. perfringens*, Type D, a normal inhabitant of the intestine, to grow rapidly and produce a high concentration of toxin. This poison is absorbed and the sheep dies of acute enterotoxemia (4). Filtrates of the intestinal contents will kill laboratory animals and lambs when injected parenterally, and such animals can be protected from the filtrates by administering antitoxin of Type B as well as Type D.

*For calves. Cl. perfringens* sometimes causes a severe form of infection in calves. The animals develop hemorrhagic enteritis and usually die within a few hours after the first symptoms of weakness and prostration are observed. Diarrhea is not a common symptom. Except for the hemorrhagic lesions in the intestines, probably caused in most cases by beta toxin, the disease resembles enterotoxemia rather than lamb dysentery. The findings of Griner and Bracken (12) have shown that Type C causes enterotoxemia in calves. This type is probably the most common cause, but Schofield (34) reported an outbreak due to Type A, Hepple (15) and Frank (8) cases due to Type B, and Griner *et al.* (11) cases due to Type D.

It has been stated that enterotoxemia caused by *Cl. perfringens* may be a more common factor in sudden death of cattle than is indicated by the paucity of reports in the literature and that Type A may be isolated frequently from infected cattle, although its significance is not clear.

*For pigs.* Field and Gibson (7) described an outbreak in piglets in which the mortality was very heavy during the first 72 hours of life. Severe enteritis accompanied by hemmorrhage was noted mainly in the jejunum of the dead pigs and the infection was shown to be caused by *Cl. perfringens,* Type C. Reports from Canada (24) and from Scandinavia (17) have listed Type C as the cause of enterotoxemia in the newborn pig and the incitant of necrotizing enteritis in piglets.

*For fowl. Cl. perfringens* has been isolated from necrotic enteritis infection in fowl and used to induce experimental infection in healthy birds (31). The disease apparently is not common in birds although it is possible that ulcerative enteritis (see p. 262) may be caused by a similar anaerobe.

*For man.* Type A is important in wound infections, combining with other organisms to produce gas gangrene. Although the outbreaks of food poisoning caused by this organism usually are mild (16), fatalities have been reported (16, 20). Foodborne disease surveillance records (27, 41) in the United States have shown that *Cl. perfringens* ranks second in producing outbreaks with either *Salmonella* or staphylococci ranking first or third—this varies from year to year. The vehicle most often responsible in the food-poisoning cases resulting from *Cl. perfringens* was beef. The incubation period is usually about 8 to 22 hours and the symptoms are diarrhea and abdominal pain without vomiting or a rise in temperature. It has been postulated (28) that *Cl. perfringens* food-poisoning is caused neither by infection nor bacterial exotoxin but by phosphorylcholine produced by hydrolysis of lecithin in the food by bacterial lecithinase.

As an aid in the diagnosis of *Cl. perfringens* food-poisoning, Harmon and Kautter (14) recommend a method which utilizes the hemolytic and lecithinase activities of the alpha toxin.

A single case of gas gangrene, caused by Type D, was reported by Morinaga *et al.* (25).

*Enteritis necroticans* was described by Zeissler and Rassfeld-Sternberg (42) in 1949 in Germany. It is a disease of man caused by Type F. The onset is acute with severe pain, vomiting, and profuse diarrhea. Lesions consist primarily of a necrotic inflammation of the small intestine, particularly the jejunum. This type is an excellent producer of beta toxin, which probably accounts for the severe intestinal lesions.

**Immunity.** Dalling (6) has reported good results with two methods for controlling lamb dysentery. One method is to immunize the ewes before lambing time with a toxin-antitoxin mixture or with formolized cultures. Antibodies are then secreted in the first milk (colostrum), and these give adequate protection. The second method is to inject antitoxin into the lambs as soon as they are born.

For preventing "struck," McEwen (21) advises immunization with toxoid.

Enterotoxemia can be prevented, or outbreaks halted, in older lambs by restriction of feed. The addition of sulfur to the ration has proved to be successful because it tends to reduce food intake. Active immunization of older lambs or ewes for the protection of young lambs succeeds, but vaccination of the young lambs themselves is not satisfactory.

In vaccinating against this disease Bennetts (3) and Whitlock and Fabricant (39) recommend the use of formolized whole culture (anaculture). It is also advisable to give a second injection to sheep when vaccinating against enterotoxemia for the first time (19). A single dose may provide only transitory protection. The epsilon toxin seems to be the major one concerned. It is antigenic as a prototoxin but produces a much higher level of immunity when changed to the active toxin and then detoxified by the addition of formalin. The use of such toxoid after adsorption on alum has been recommended (10, 26), but Percival *et al.* (32) state that the presence of alum in *Cl. perfringens* Type D vaccine increases the severity and persistence of local reactions following vaccination. According to them, the toxoid without the alum is just as effective. Baldwin and colleagues (1) claim the *Cl. perfringens* Type D antitoxin may be used to stop losses.

**Chemotherapy.** Reed and Orr (33) reported that the local application of sulfathiazole or sulfadiazine aided in the control of *Cl. perfringens* infection. Penicillin is reported to be effective against this bacillus.

## REFERENCES

1. Baldwin, Frederick, and Ray. Am. Jour. Vet. Res., 1948, 9, 296.
2. Bennetts. Austral. Council Sci. and Indus. Res. Bul. 57, 1932.
3. Bennetts. Austral. Vet. Jour., 1936, 12, 196.
4. Bullen and Battey. Vet. Rec., 1957, 69, 1268.
5. Canada and Strong. Jour. Bact., 1965, 89, 1623.
6. Dalling. Vet. Rec., 1928, 8, 841.
7. Field and Gibson. *Ibid.*, 1954, 67, 31.
8. Frank. Am. Jour. Vet. Res., 1956, 17, 492.
9. Gaiger and Dalling. Jour. Comp. Path. and Therap., 1921, 34, 79.
10. Gill. New Zealand Jour. Agr., 1932, 45, 332.
11. Griner, Aichelman, and Brown. Jour. Am. Vet. Med. Assoc., 1956, 129, 375.
12. Griner and Bracken. *Ibid.*, 1953, 122, 99.
13. Griner and Johnson. *Ibid.*, 1954, 125, 125.
14. Harmon and Kautter. Appl. Microbiol., 1970, 20, 913.
15. Hepple. Vet. Rec., 1952, 64, 633.
16. Hobbs, Smith, Oakley, Warrack, and Cruickshank. Jour. Hyg. (London), 1953, 51, 75.
17. Høgh. Acta Vet. Scand., 1967, 8, 301.
18. Horton, Madden, and McCullough. Appl. Microbiol., 1970, 19, 314.
19. Jansen, Visser, and Knoetze. Jour. So. African Vet. Med. Assoc., 1965, 36, 365.
20. Kellert and Meeler. Am. Jour. Clin. Path., 1953, 23, 1234.
21. McEwen. Jour. Comp. Path. and Therap., 1930, 43, 1; 1933, 46, 108.
22. McEwen and Roberts. *Ibid.*, 1931, 44, 26.
23. McGowan, Moulton, and Rood. Jour. Am. Vet. Med. Assoc., 1958, 133, 219.
24. Moon and Bergeland. Canad. Vet. Jour., 1965, 6, 159.

25.  Morinaga, Nakamura, Yoshizawa, and Nishida.   Jour. Bact., 1965, *90*, 826.
26.  Muth.   Am. Jour. Vet. Res., 1946, *7*, 355.
27.  National CDC Foodborne Outbreaks.   Jour. Am. Vet. Med. Assoc., 1969, *155*, 1390.
28.  Nelson, Ager, Marks, and Emanuel.   Am. Jour. Epidemiol., 1966, *83*, 86.
29.  Newsom and Thorp.   Jour. Am. Vet. Med. Assoc., 1938, *93*, 165.
30.  Oakley and Warrack.   Jour. Hyg. (London), 1953, *51*, 102.
31.  Parish.   Jour. Comp. Path. and Therap., 1961, *71*, 405.
32.  Percival, Burkhart, Cooper, and Martini.   Am. Jour. Vet. Res., 1954, *15*, 574.
33.  Reed and Orr.   Am. Jour. Med. Sci., 1943, *206*, 379.
34.  Schofield.   Jour. Am. Vet. Med. Assoc., 1955, *126*, 192.
35.  Smith.   Introduction to pathogenic anaerobes. Univ. of Chicago Press, Chicago, 1954.
36.  Tunnicliff.   Jour. Inf. Dis., 1933, *52*, 407.
37.  Veillon and Zuber.   Arch. Med. Exp., 1898, *10*, 517.
38.  Welch and Nuttall.   Johns Hopkins Hosp. Bul. 1892, *3*, 81.
39.  Whitlock and Fabricant.   Cornell Vet., 1947, *37*, 211.
40.  Wilsdon.   2d Ann. Rpt., Dir. Inst. An. Path., Cambridge, 1931, p. 53.
41.  Woodward, Gangarosa, Brachman, and Curlin.   Am. Jour. Pub. Health, 1970, *60*, 130.
42.  Zeissler and Rassfeld-Sternberg.   Brit. Med. Jour., 1949, *1*, 267.

### *Clostridium hemolyticum*

SYNONYMS:   *Clostridium hemolyticus bovis, Bacillus hemolyticus*

This organism is the cause of a disease of cattle, occasionally of sheep, commonly known as *red water disease*. It is also known as *hemorrhagic disease* and *infectious icterohemoglobinuria*. One case in a hog has been described by Records and Huber (7).

So far as is known the disease occurs only in rather restricted districts, especially in the poorly drained mountain and valley pastures of the Sierra Nevada, Cascade, and Rocky Mountains in the western part of the United States. It has been reported also in the delta parishes of Louisiana, along the Gulf of Mexico, in Florida (3), and in central Mexico. It occurs in cattle in New Zealand (5). A closely related organism has been isolated from a similar disease in Chile (10). The organism shows a predilection for alkaline water, and the disease is associated with pastures that contain swampy areas which continually maintain a pH of 8.0 or higher. In the United States the disease occurs principally during the summer and early fall months. The organism was described by Vawter and Records (12) in 1926. The disease was first reported by Meyer (6) in 1916, later by Mack and Records (4) and by Records and Vawter (8). As a result of the earlier studies it was believed that the disease was caused by *Cl. perfringens*, but it is now known that this organism is merely a secondary or agonal invader.

**Morphology and Staining Reactions.** This organism is somewhat larger than most of the other tissue-invading anaerobic bacilli. It measures from 1.0 to 1.3

microns in breadth and from 3.0 to 5.6 microns in length. It has straight sides and rounded ends. It occurs singly, as a rule, but may form short chains in tissues and cultures. The spores are oval and are located subterminally. They cause bulging of the cells in which they lie. The cells are actively motile when young. Young cells are Gram-positive, but when they are more than 24 hours old they rapidly lose their ability to retain this stain.

**Cultural Features.** Deep agar colonies are lenticular at first, later becoming woolly. Little or no gas is formed unless fermentable sugar is added to the medium. When blood is present it is rapidly hemolyzed. Gelatin is liquefied in from 2 to 4 days. Coagulated serum and egg media are not softened or liquefied. Cooked-meat media and brain media support good growth, but there is no digestion of the solids and no blackening unless iron salts are added. Even in the presence of an abundance of iron salts the blackening is but slight. Milk is not changed. Glucose and levulose are the only carbohydrates fermented. These are actively destroyed with the evolution of both acid and gas. Hydrogen sulfide is formed in large amounts in liver media and in media containing proteose-peptone. The methyl-red and Voges-Proskauer tests are negative, and nitrates are not reduced. Indol is formed in large amounts.

This organism is rather exacting in its cultural requirements. Good anaerobic conditions are necessary, and the media must contain tryptophan for optimum growth and toxin formation. Vawter and Records depend principally upon a peptic, liver-digest medium in their work.

A striking feature of this organism is the powerful hemolytic toxin it forms. This toxin is the principal reason for the great pathogenicity of the organism. The hemolytic toxin is rather unstable and reaches its greatest concentration in cultures within 16 hours, after which it rapidly disappears. It appears to be lecithinase. It is serologically related to, if not identical with, the beta toxin of *Cl. novyi* but is not related serologically to the alpha toxin of *Cl. perfringens*. A second toxin having necrotizing properties is present in cultures. This substance is present in young cultures but is most marked in older ones. Serologic studies by Vawter and Records (14) indicate that all strains of *Cl. hemolyticum*, with one exception, are uniform in composition.

**Pathogenicity.** *The natural disease.* The disease presents quite a uniform picture, which is readily recognized by those who have had experience with it. Appetite, rumination, lactation, and bowel movement suddenly cease, and the afflicted animal stands apart from the rest of the herd, presenting a picture of acute illness. The back is arched, the abdomen is tucked up, and it is difficult to make the animal move. Breathing is shallow, and there is grunting with each step. The temperature varies from 104 to 106 F in the early stages but becomes subnormal before death. The feces become deeply bile-stained or bloody. The urine is a dark-red or port-wine color, clear but foamy. The color is due to large amounts of hemoglobin. There are no intact erythrocytes in the urine. Sugar is absent but albumin tests are strongly positive.

At the time when hemoglobinuria appears, as much as 40 to 50 percent of

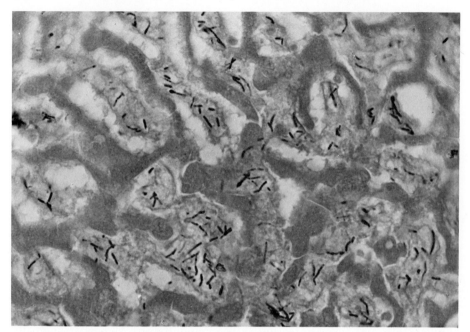

*Fig. 54. Clostridium hemolyticum* in the characteristic liver infarct. A few of the organisms are beginning to form spores. X 700 (Courtesy Edward Records.)

all of the erythrocytes of the body have been destroyed. The red cell count at this time may not be greater than 2,000,000 per mm³ and the hemoglobin readings may be as low as 3.5 g per 100 ml of blood. The leukocyte count increases, sometimes to as high as 30,000 per mm.³ Death is caused by anoxemia because of the wholesale destruction of erythrocytes. The mortality is high, varying from 90 to 95 percent in untreated animals.

The most characteristic lesion is the large infarct that is always found in the liver. This is a mass of necrotic tissue, varying from 5 to 20 cm in diameter, often mottled, and usually lighter in color than the normal liver tissue. This lesion may be located in any part of the organ. It is formed as a result of an occluding thrombosis of one of the branches of the portal vein. The tissue has undergone coagulation necrosis. In the sinusoids of these areas great numbers of large rod-shaped bacteria containing subterminal or terminal spores may be seen.

Extensive hemorrhages are found on the serous membranes, in the subcutaneous connective tissue, and in the substance of the visceral organs. Acute degenerative changes occur in the organs, and the peritoneal and pleural cavities usually contain large quantities of hemoglobin-stained transudates. Besides the subserous hemorrhages that regularly occur in the intestinal wall, there is a severe hemorrhagic enteritis, the mucous membrane often being almost wholly undermined with extensive hemorrhage.

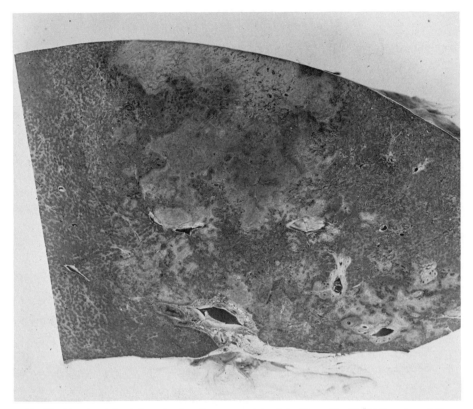

*Fig. 55.* Massive infarct in a bovine liver caused by infection with *Clostridium hemolyticum*. This lesion is characteristic of the red water disease of cattle. (Courtesy Edward Records.)

*The experimental disease.* Vawter and Records (13) readily killed cattle by inoculating them with pure cultures of *Cl. hemolyticum*, the animals dying with typical symptoms within 36 hours. The lesions in such animals are typical except that the liver infarcts are absent. Repeated attempts to produce the disease by feeding large amounts of pure cultures have failed. Records and Vawter (9) fed encysted cercariae of the liver fluke to young cattle and followed the feedings with large amounts of pure culture of *Cl. hemolyticum*, thinking that fluke invasion might pave the way for the entrance of the organism, but the experiments failed even though the flukes invaded the liver tissue of all the experimental animals. The mode of natural transmission of this disease is unknown. That apparently normal cattle may act as carriers in infected areas has been demonstrated by Smith and Jasmin (11), who isolated *Cl. hemolyticum* from livers of such animals.

Rabbits, guinea pigs, and mice may be readily killed by toxin-containing cultures. Subcutaneous injection leads to the formation of a hemorrhagic, edematous area at the point of inoculation with little or no gas formation. Intravenous inoculation of rabbits usually leads to death in from 2 to 4 hours with great blood destruction and hemoglobinuria.

**Immunity.** Records and Vawter (13) developed an immune serum that proved highly effective in protecting animals against artificial inoculation of otherwise fatal doses of culture. This serum also exhibited considerable curative power when given in large doses to animals that were just beginning to show hemoglobinuria before the temperature receded to subnormal. The same workers developed a phenolized whole-culture vaccine, also a glycerolated vaccine that served to protect quite well. An improved, formolized bacterin, adsorbed on aluminum hydroxide, has been advocated. It protects for a full pasture season and often for a full year. A mineral oil adjuvant bacterin also is highly recommended (1). On the other hand, Claus and Macheak (2) have suggested that *Cl. hemolyticum* bacterins which have been completely detoxified do not stimulate the formation of antitoxin.

## REFERENCES

1.  Claus.  Am. Jour. Vet. Res. 1964, *25*, 699.
2.  Claus and Macheak.  *Ibid.*, 1965, *26*, 353.
3.  McCain.  *Ibid.*, 1967, *28*, 878.
4.  Mack and Records.  Jour. Am. Vet. Med. Assoc., 1917, *52*, 143.
5.  Marshall.  New Zeal. Vet. Jour., 1959, *7*, 115.
6.  Meyer.  Jour. Am. Vet. Med. Assoc., 1916, *48*, 552.
7.  Records and Huber.  *Ibid.*, 1931, *78*, 863.
8.  Records and Vawter.  *Ibid.*, 1921, *60*, 155.

*Table XV.*  CHARACTERISTICS OF TISSUE-INVADING SPOREBEARING ANAEROBES

| Morphological and biochemical tests | *Cl. chauvoei* | *Cl. septicum* | *Cl. perfringens* | *Cl. novyi* | *Cl. hemolyticum* |
|---|---|---|---|---|---|
| Spores | S.T. | S.T. | Cent. | S.T. | S.T. |
| Motility | + | + | − | + | + |
| Deep agar colonies | Pin point | Fluffy lenticular | Lenticular | Lenticular | Lenticular |
| Brain medium | o | o | o | o | o |
| Coagulated albumin | o | o | o | o | o |
| Milk | Coagulation | Coagulation | Stormy ferm. | o | Coagulation |
| Gelatin | Gas liq. | Gas liq. | Gas liq., black | Gas liq., black | Gas liq. |
| Glucose agar | No growth | Growth | Growth | Growth | Growth |
| Glucose | + | + | + | + | + |
| Lactose | + | + | + | − | − |
| Sucrose | + | − | + | − | − |
| Maltose | + | + | + | + | − |
| Galactose | + | + | + | + | − |
| Salicin | − | + | − | − | − |
| Pathogenic | + | + | + | + | + |
| Toxin formed | ± | + | + | + | + |
| Liver surface smear | Single | Single and filaments | Single and short chains | Single and chains | ? |

S.T. = Subterminal.   Cent. = Central.   o = No change.

9.  Records and Vawter.  Ann. Rpt. Nev. Agr. Exp. Sta., 1931, p. 19.
10. Smith.  Introduction to pathogenic anaerobes. Univ. of Chicago Press, Chicago, 1954, p. 147.
11. Smith and Jasmin.  Jour. Am. Vet. Med. Assoc., 1956, *129*, 68.
12. Vawter and Records.  *Ibid.*, 1926, *68*, 494.
13. *Ibid.*, 1929, *75*, 201.
14. Vawter and Records.  Jour. Inf. Dis., 1931, *48*, 581.

## DIFFERENTIATION OF THE TISSUE-INVADING SPOREBEARING ANAEROBES

The sporebearing anaerobic bacteria which produce phlegmonous conditions in animals are not always easily identified, because they are similar in their morphology, cultural features, and often pathogenicity. In addition to those which have been described and which are the most important ones, a great many other species have been reported and are often encountered in animal infections. Table XV gives the more important cultural characteristics of the anaerobic bacteria that commonly infect animals.

# XX | The *Mycobacteriaceae*

The family *Mycobacteriaceae* consists of two genera, *Mycobacterium* and *Mycococcus*. They contain bacterial cells that are spherical to rod-shaped, and may show branching under proper conditions. They are aerobic, Gram-positive, mesophilic, and do not produce conidia. They are found in soil, dairy products, and as parasites of animals, including man. The genus *Mycobacterium* embraces the acid-fast organisms, the species within the family that are most important to animal health.

## THE GENUS *MYCOBACTERIUM*

The property of acid-fastness is possessed by a large group of rod-shaped organisms. A great many species of these organisms are found in the soil where they live a saprophytic existence. A few species are wholly parasitic and pathogenic in the sense that they cause transmissible diseases. In another sense all acid-fast organisms are at least mildly pathogenic, for all of them contain irritating lipoids and proteins and when inoculated into tissues of living animals they cause the formation of granulomatous lesions that are called *tubercles*. Tubercles may be produced by inoculating heat-killed cultures, certain extracts of cultures, or living organisms. Sabin (85), working with chemical fractions prepared by Anderson, showed that tubercles are produced by tissue stimulation with a constituent of the phospholipid fraction of the bacillary bodies, a substance that proved to be a saturated fatty acid to which the name *phthioic acid* was given. It appears that the principal difference between the pathogenic and the nonpathogenic species of this group is that the former possess the power of multiplication in the tissues whereas the latter do not. The similarity of the chemical composition of some well-known acid-fast organisms is indicated in table XVI, which is taken from Chargoff, Pangborn, and Anderson (12).

The simple rod-shaped, acid-fast organisms referred to above belong to the genus *Mycobacterium*. Besides the mycobacteria, the property of acid-fastness is possessed in variable degree by certain higher bacteria, actinomycetes, and molds. Some have claimed to have induced acid-fastness in bacteria that normally do not have this character by cultivating them on media of high fat content. Bruner (10) was unable to accomplish this and decided that such results are artifacts. On the other hand, organisms that are normally acid-fast are often found in a non-acid-fast form, and many of them can be induced to develop in this form by cultivating them in media in which there is little available carbon. Often it is impossible to demonstrate acid-fast organisms in films and sections of diseased tissue, but cultures are readily obtained. Some have thought that the acid-fast form is but one stage in a cycle in which other stages are non-acid-fast, but there is little to support such hypothesis. When acid-fast organisms cannot be demonstrated microscopically, it means, in most cases at least, that the numbers present are very few, but it may be that in some cases the organisms present are starved, as in carbon-free media, and exist temporarily in a non-acid-fast form.

Table XVI.   THE CHEMICAL COMPOSITION OF SEVERAL
TYPICAL ACID-FAST ORGANISMS

| Substances present | Myco. tuberculosis | | | Myco. phlei |
| --- | --- | --- | --- | --- |
| | Human type | Bovine type | Avian type | (Timothy bacillus) |
| Phosphatid | 6.54 | 1.53 | 2.26 | 0.59 |
| Acetone-soluble wax | 6.20 | 3.34 | 2.19 | 2.75 |
| Chloroform-soluble wax | 11.30 | 8.52 | 1.79 | 4.98 |
| Total lipoids | 23.78 | 13.40 | 15.26 | 8.37 |
| Polysaccharide | 0.78 | 1.09 | 1.02 | 3.90 |
| Dried bacterial residue | 75.01 | 85.50 | 83.71 | 87.70 |

## Mycobacterium tuberculosis

SYNONYMS:   *Bacillus tuberculosis, Bacterium tuberculosis,* tubercle bacillus

The disease caused by this organism was described over 2,000 years ago, and bone lesions found in Egyptian mummies proved that it existed among people long before that. Quite naturally there was much confusion between tuberculosis and other diseases of man in ancient and medieval times, and this confusion lasted until after the middle of the 19th century. Many early writers claimed the disease to be infectious, but others regarded it as a form of malignant tumor and noninfectious until after the causative agent had been found and experimentation had removed all doubt as to its nature. Although he was not the first to claim infectiousness, Villemin (103) demonstrated, in 1865, that tuberculous tissue from man and cattle produced the disease in rabbits by inoculation.

The tubercle bacillus probably was first seen in tissues by Baumgarten (5)

in 1882. In the same year Koch (50) succeeded in demonstrating the organisms in diseased tissues by staining them with alkaline methylene blue and counterstaining with Bismarck brown (vesuvin). With this method the tubercle bacilli remained blue while all other organisms and tissues lost the blue and took on the brown color of the counterstain. Koch also found that the organism could be cultivated in pure culture on a medium consisting of coagulated bovine serum. With such cultures he readily reproduced the disease in experimental animals and thus removed all doubt as to its etiological relationship. His final report on this work was published in 1884 (51).

**Morphology and Staining Features.** *Mycobacterium tuberculosis* in both tissues and cultures is a slender rod-shaped organism. It shows considerable pleomorphism. Were it not for its acid-fastness it might be classed in the diphtheroid group. Granules are often evident in stained preparations. Reference will be made below to the several types of tubercle bacilli. In general,

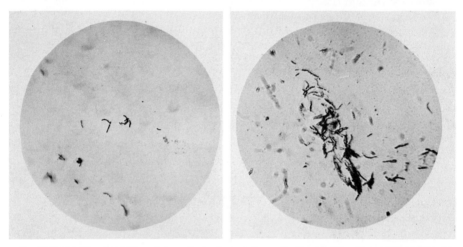

Fig. 56 (left). Mycobacterium tuberculosis, human type, in the sputum of a consumptive patient. X 700.

Fig. 57 (right). Mycobacterium tuberculosis, human type, from a culture on glycerol-egg medium incubated 6 weeks at 37 C. X 700.

the *human* type is more apt to be beaded and the cells are usually longer than the *bovine* type. The latter usually is rather short, relatively plump, and solid staining. The *avian* type is more variable than either of the mammalian types, sometimes appearing in the form of long beaded rods and at other times as very short, solid-staining forms. The difference in morphology is not a sufficient basis upon which to differentiate one type from another.

All forms are strongly acid- and alcohol-fast, and they are Gram-positive. The acid-fast characteristic aids in finding tubercle bacilli in tissues and exudates since it is possible to stain them differently from other bacteria, tissue cells, and tissue debris.

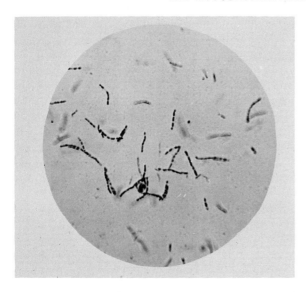

Fig. 58. Mycobacterium tuber-culosis, bovine type, from a cul-ture on Dorset's egg medium in-cubated 6 weeks at 37 C. These long beaded forms are seen only in cultures. In tissues this type or-dinarily is solid-staining and shorter than the other types. X 1,000.

**Cultural Features.** Koch first cultivated tubercle bacilli on bovine blood serum that had been coagulated with heat. He was not able to induce the or-ganism to grow on any of the media commonly employed in the laboratory. In 1902 Dorset (16) introduced the use of coagulated egg medium. Many modifications of the original formula have been made, and these continue to be our best media for isolating tubercle bacilli from infected tissues. Excellent media may be made by adding yolk material to basic media solidified with agar. Many of the egg media contain dyes which act as inhibiting agents for other bacteria that frequently are associated with tubercle bacilli in the mate-rials cultured. Glycerol in egg media favors the growth of the human but not of the bovine type of bacilli.

In 1887 Nocard and Roux (68) reported that cultures could be successfully propagated on ordinary infusion agar fortified with from 5 to 8 percent glyc-erol. Glycerol agar is not satisfactory for isolating mammalian tubercle ba-cilli from tissues, but it usually succeeds in the case of the avian type. After mammalian types have become accustomed to growth on richer culture media, they can be adapted to grow on the glycerol agar without difficulty.

Dubos (19) has shown that agar has an inhibiting influence on the growth of mammalian tubercle bacilli because of the presence of long-chain fatty acids that cannot easily be removed. Avian bacilli are not greatly inhibited by these substances in the concentrations in which they occur in commercial agar. The influence of these fatty acids can be neutralized by the addition of a small amount of serum albumin. Mammalian bacilli from pathological le-sions can be isolated on such medium. Other agar media recommended for their economy, simplicity of preparation, and ability to grow tubercle bacilli from small inocula easily, recognizably, and in a short period of time are oleic agar (20, 79), blood agar (79, 98), and charcoal agar (42, 79).

On solid media, tubercle bacilli multiply slowly. The avian type multiplies much faster than either of the mammalian, and, of the mammalian, the human develops much more readily and much faster than the bovine. English workers have used the terms *eugonic* and *dysgonic* in referring to the ease with which mammalian bacilli can be cultivated, the first term being equivalent in general to the human and the latter to the bovine type.

All tubercle bacilli are aerobic in nature. Growth does not occur under anaerobic conditions, and it is inhibited even when the culture tubes are sealed so the amount of available air is limited. Growth occurs only at temperatures close to that of the body.

On solid media it is not possible to differentiate between the human and bovine type of cultures by the gross appearance of the growth. Primary cultures usually require from 3 to 4 weeks' incubation at 37 C before colonies can be detected with the naked eye. As has been said above, human cultures usually develop a little faster than the bovine. The colonies appear first as minute dull flakes, which gradually thicken into dry, irregular masses that stand high above the surface of the medium. The color is slightly yellowish, but if exposed to light it gradually changes through shades of deep yellow to a brick red. When cultures have become accustomed to growing on media, confluent growth that covers the entire surface develops. These have the appearance of rough, waxy blankets, which after several weeks' incubation become thick and wrinkled. Where this blanket reaches the margin of the surface of the medium, it often crowds up the side of the glass container for an

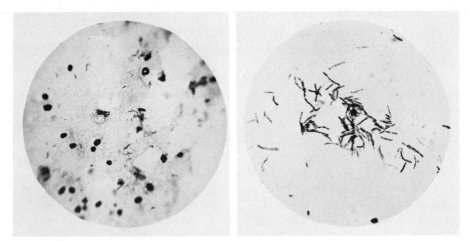

Fig. 59 (left). *Mycobacterium tuberculosis*, avian type, a film from a liver lesion of a naturally infected chicken. X 325.

Fig. 60 (right). *Mycobacterium tuberculosis*, avian type, from a culture on Dorset's egg medium which had been incubated 6 weeks at 37 C. X 700.

appreciable distance. Old, isolated colonies on solid media become so firm and so loosely attached to the medium that they may be caused to skate around with the inoculating loop, or, if the tubes are shaken vigorously, the dry growth often breaks loose and emits a rattling noise.

The avian-type tubercle bacillus presents a different appearance. The primary colonies are smooth and shiny. They develop much more rapidly than the mammalian types and are not so fastidious in their nutritive requirements. Colonies usually may be detected within less than a week and are well developed in 2 weeks. The colonies are soft in consistency. They cannot be pushed around the surface nor shaken loose as can the other types. When heavily inoculated, the surface blanket is moist, soft, and not wrinkled greatly. The color is a light cream but, like the mammalian types, it becomes yellowish, pinkish, and even dull reddish if incubated in the presence of light.

Theobald Smith (92) early pointed out a growth character by which the mammalian types generally may be differentiated from each other. This depends upon the fact that the human type utilizes glycerol very actively whereas its utilization by the bovine type is limited. When cultivated upon a broth containing 3 percent glycerol, human types produce enough acid to maintain a terminal acidity, whereas bovine types leave the medium alkaline. Smith tested his fully developed cultures with phenolphthalein. If the reaction is acid, there is a strong probability that the strain belongs to the human type; if alkaline, that it is of the bovine type. If the original glycerol content of the medium is below 1 percent, both types will produce an alkaline terminal reaction. This reaction generally holds true, but the method is cumbersome and slow because the strains must be trained to grow well on fluid media before the differentiation can be made. More rapid *in vitro* tests have been used by Harrington and Karlson (38). They found that the human type produced niacin and nicotinamidase and reduced nitrate to nitrite, whereas the bovine type did not. The growth of the human type was inhibited by nicotinamide, but not by the thiophene-2-carboxylic acid hydrazide, whereas the opposite was true for the bovine type.

On fluid media, except in those in which special wetting agents are included, growth is restricted to the surface. To obtain successful cultures one must very carefully transfer small dry flakes of growth to the surface of the medium. If this is successfully done, a thin, waxy pellicle grows from the original flakes and finally it covers the entire surface. The pellicle then thickens and becomes a heavy, wrinkled blanket of growth. Along the edges where the fluid surface meets the glass wall of the container, the blanket pushes up from the top of the medium for as much as a centimeter. The mammalian types present a very dry, rough surface; the avian is much softer, moister, and less wrinkled. Beneath the pellicle, mammalian cultures usually show a perfectly clear medium with little or no sediment; the avian cultures generally show considerable mucoid sediment, and stalactites of a slimy nature often extend downward from the pellicle when the cultures become old. When exposed to light, all types of tubercle bacilli gradually change from a creamy color, through shades of tan, to a reddish tan.

In 1945 Dubos (18) described a method by which diffuse growths of all types may be obtained in liquid media. The method hastens multiplication, and it is sufficiently adequate for primary isolations from infected tissues to be made with it. It is based upon the discovery that certain complex lipids have the property of stimulating tubercle bacilli remarkably, and that at the same time they serve as wetting agents which coat the bacterial cells, causing them to break apart and become dispersed in the fluid instead of adhering to each other in waxy masses that float on the surface. The agent that Dubos found best adapted for this use is a synthetic, nonionic compound consisting of esters of long-chain fatty acids and of polyhydric alcohols, manufactured commercially and sold under the trade name of Tween. There are several Tweens, the one best adapted for this use being known as *Tween 80*. Dubos and Middlebrook (20) showed that Tween 80 had toxic as well as stimulating properties, especially for mammalian types. This property was shown to occur because of small amounts of unesterified fatty acids that exist as impurities in the product. This toxic action can be neutralized by adding a serum albumin fraction, which also served as a growth stimulant. Several fluid media for cultivating tubercle bacilli were developed by these authors.

The discovery that traces of free fatty acids are inhibitory to the growth of mammalian tubercle bacilli suggested an answer to the question of why many media will support growth of these organisms when the inoculum is large but will not do so when it is small. Obviously, a good medium for isolating these organisms from tissues where they are present, usually in relatively small numbers, is one that contains all the necessary nutrients and at the same time is relatively free of inhibiting substances. Cummings, Drummond, and Lewis (14) have shown that heating increases the ether-soluble material in several kinds of egg media. About twice as much is present when these media are coagulated in the autoclave at 100 C as when they are inspissated at 85 C. The latter, therefore, makes a much better medium than the former.

Moore (66) and Fite and Olson (29) have shown that all three types of tubercle bacilli can be cultivated on the chorioallantoic membrane of the developing chick embryo. Characteristic lesions are produced, and these are associated with rapid multiplication of the bacilli. There are some differences in the appearance of the lesions depending upon the type of the infection, but these are not sufficiently distinctive to enable differentiation to be made. Moore also produced similar lesions with acid-fast organisms other than tubercle bacilli.

**The Types of Tubercle Bacilli.** Villemin (103) showed that tuberculosis could be produced in rabbits by inoculating them either with sputum from human cases or with tissue from nodules that occur on the chest wall of tuberculous cattle. He believed, therefore, that the diseases of man and cattle were identical and caused by a single virulent agent. This belief was also held at first by

Koch because, after demonstrating tubercle bacilli in human tissues, he found what appeared to be the same organism in tissues of tuberculous cattle. Rivolta (83), however, in 1889 showed that the organism that affects birds was not identical with those affecting mammals, and Smith (91) in 1898 pointed out certain differences in cultural characteristics and pathogenicity between the types ordinarily found in man and those usually found in cattle.

Three types of tubercle bacilli are now recognized as being responsible for tuberculosis in warm-blooded animals.* These are the human type, the bovine type, and the avian type. Of these, the mammalian types (human and bovine) are very closely related, the differences between them being quantitative rather than qualitative. The avian type differs from the mammalian types in many respects. In *Bergey's Manual* these three have been elevated to species rank and bear the names *Myco. tuberculosis*, *Myco. bovis*, and *Myco. avium*. We prefer to regard them as types of *Myco. tuberculosis*.

It is true that classification has always been a problem, especially so when dealing with the mycobacteria isolated from man. The concept that the so-called *atypical* or *unclassified* acid-fast bacteria originate from pathogenic organisms is reasonable. In fact Reimann and Pik-Chun-Ma (80) have indicated that aged cultures of a strain of *Myco. tuberculosis* gave rise to progeny that had the characteristics of Group III mycobacteria; some formed pigment like Group II types; and one resembled Group IV strains (see below—Runyon's groups). The variants did not have the features of Group I mycobacteria. Within these groups the irregular types most commonly associated with pulmonary disease in man have been *Myco. kansasi*, *Myco. xenopei*, and the "Battey" bacillus. It is possible that some atypical strains are host-adapted forms. The horse modifies the bovine type. Pigeons, ducks, and crows attenuate the avian type. The vole probably changed a bovine type to produce the vole bacillus. *Myco. kansasi* has been derived from the bovine animal and a scotochromogenic strain of the avian type has been isolated from a trumpeter swan. It is believed by some that the bovine type may change to the human type in man. It may also be possible that saprophytic strains, under certain conditions, turn into virulent ones. Runyon placed the unclassified strains in four groups. His designations with some modifications follow:

Group I contains the *photochromogens* commonly associated with tuberculosislike disease. In it have been placed such organisms as *Myco. ulcerans* and *Myco. marinum (balnei)*, producers of skin ulcers, and *Myco. kansasi*, an acid-fast bacillus related to the human type and capable of causing pulmonary disease in man.

Group II is made up of the yellow-orange-red *scotochromogens*. These are the organisms that frequently occur in adenitis in children, rarely are found

---

* Actually, if we include the vole bacillus, there are four types of tubercle bacilli known to be infective for warm-blooded animals. See page 442. Because the vole bacillus differs in many respects from the others and is virtually nonpathogenic for man and the domesticated animal species, it is considered separately.

as independent agents of pulmonary disease, and usually are considered to be saprophytes.

Group III contains the "Battey" bacilli which are *nonphotochromogens*. These bacteria are highly pleomorphic and produce *Nocardia* like filaments. They cause pulmonary disease and seem to be more closely related to the avian than to the other types of tubercle bacilli. Another organism that has been associated with progressive pulmonary disease in man is *Myco. xenopei* (17). Actually it does not quite fit in any group, but Runyon has placed it in group III even though it is pigmented.

Group IV is reserved for the *rapid growers*. Most of these belong to *Myco. fortuitum*, organisms that will not grow at 45 C, and to the *Myco. phlei* and *Myco. smegmatis* subgroups. *Myco. fortuitum* is pathogenic for man and the lower animals. It has been implicated in a serious epizootic of bovine mastitis in a large Oregon dairy herd (72).

Hobby *et al.* (44) studied 391 mycobacterial strains isolated from patients in veterans administration hospitals. Of these cultures, 240 belonged in Group I, 3 to Group II, 114 to Group III, and 19 to Group IV. Only 15 cultures failed to fit into one of these groups and they appeared to fall intermediate between Groups II and III.

The Group I cultures were susceptible to isoniazid, usually sensitive to ethionamide, cycloserine, streptomycin, and viomycin. The Group II strains were susceptible to streptomycin, viomycin, ethionamide, kanamycin, and PAS (see *Chemotherapy*). The Group III and Group IV strains showed little sensitivity to any of these substances.

**Differentiation of the Types of Tubercle Bacilli.** Identification of the types of tubercle bacilli cannot be based upon the host from which they are isolated, for, as will be shown below, the host relationship is far from a fixed one. Some idea of the type may be gained by microscopic examination of the organisms, but this is uncertain because there is considerable variation in the size and shape of each type. Cultural features generally will serve to differentiate the avian from the mammalian, but distinguishing between the two mammalian types on cultural grounds is quite uncertain. The most satisfactory method is based upon pathogenesis for experimental animals, although this sometimes fails too, because some strains exhibit properties that partake of more than one type. This is especially true of strains that have grown in unusual hosts, their pathogenicity apparently being modified by them.

*Relative virulence for laboratory animals of the types of tubercle bacilli.* The avian type of the tubercle bacillus usually is highly pathogenic for chickens and rabbits. It is nonpathogenic for guinea pigs as a rule. Local lesions are frequently produced in this species of animal but only rarely does the disease become gereralized. The mammalian types are almost wholly non-pathogenic for chickens, but most strains will produce progressive infections in guinea pigs leading to their death from generalized tuberculosis. These features serve to distinguish the avian-type bacillus from the mammalian types.

The differentiation of the mammalian types from each other is more difficult. On the whole, the bovine type is perhaps a little more virulent for guinea pigs than the human, as measured by the rapidity of the development of the lesions and the time of death of the animals, but this difference is too slight to make it useful in differentiating the types. In the rabbit, however, there is generally an appreciable difference in the virulence of the two types, as was first pointed out by Smith (91). When this animal is given a small dose of bovine-type tubercle bacilli of normal virulence, a progressive disease is set up which leads to its death in from 3 weeks to 3 months. A dose of the same size of human-type bacilli of normal virulence usually produces only local lesions, from which the animal recovers. At the end of 3 months rabbits that have been inoculated with human material usually not only are living but have taken on weight and appear to be thriving. A clear presentation of the value of the rabbit test for differentiating human-type tubercle bacilli from bovine type may be found in the papers of Park and Krumwiede (70), who used the method extensively.

When it is desired to determine the type of tubercle bacilli present in tissues, the best available procedure involves the experimental inoculation of guinea pigs, rabbits, and chickens. Care must be taken to be sure that the experimental animals are not naturally infected. There is comparatively little chance of this happening in rabbits and guinea pigs, but there is real danger of mistakes with chickens if there is no proof that they came from a tuberculosis-free flock. The safest procedure in all cases is to inject mammalian tuberculin intradermally into the mammals and avian tuberculin into the chickens before they are used. Negative reactions indicate that it is safe to use the animals.

It is best always to isolate the organism in pure culture, because in this way the dosage may be better regulated. A small bit of the culture is scraped from the surface of the solid medium and weighed. It is then placed in a small mortar and ground until the larger clumps are broken up. Broth or saline solution is added to make a smooth emulsion of the bacilli, and this is diluted until there is about 0.1 mg of tubercle bacilli per ml of fluid. About 0.1 ml of this fluid is injected into each of the experimental animals, making a dose of about 0.01 mg. After a little experience it is possible to judge with sufficient accuracy the amount of material that need be scraped from the culture, thereby eliminating the laborious weighing process on each sample.

*Table XVII.* RELATIVE VIRULENCE FOR LABORATORY ANIMALS OF THE TYPES OF TUBERCLE BACILLI

| Type | Guinea pig | Rabbit | Chicken |
|------|-----------|--------|---------|
| Human | + | ± | o |
| Bovine | + | + | o |
| Avian | ± | + | + |

The guinea pigs should be injected subcutaneously in one of the thighs or into the muscular tissue. The rabbits are injected in the ear vein, and the chickens in the brachial vein where it crosses the second joint on the under-surface of the wing.

If the strain is a typical avian type, the chickens and rabbits will gradually lose weight and usually will die after several weeks but the guinea pigs will remain well. If it is a bovine type, the rabbits and guinea pigs will sicken and die but the chickens will remain well. If it is a human type, the guinea pigs will die but the rabbits and chickens will remain well. All animals that remain alive after 8 to 10 weeks should be destroyed and autopsied.

**Resistance.** Tubercle bacilli do not form spores and they exhibit only moderate resistance to heat. They are destroyed by pasteurization. Resistance to desiccation is fairly great. Direct sunlight is rapidly fatal to them. To most disinfectants the resistance is somewhat greater than that exhibited by non-sporing organisms. This is especially true of resistance to acids and alkalies. This property is often used in isolating tubercle bacilli from sputum or exudates contaminated by other bacteria. In moist soils, manure heaps, and old strawstacks, tubercle bacilli may remain alive for very long periods. Schalk, Roderick, Foust, and Harshfield (88) were able to show that avian-type tubercle bacilli would remain viable in heavily infected plots of ground for periods as long as 4 years, and in buried fowl carcasses for more than 2 years. These facts are of great importance in practical control measures against tuberculosis in animals.

**The Pathogenesis of Tuberculosis.** The name of this disease is derived from the Latin word *tuberculum,* which means a small lump or nodule. It is an apt name for tuberculosis because the disease is characterized by the formation of small masses of inflammatory tissue, or tubercles, in the organs where the bacilli lodge and multiply. By whatever route they enter the body, tubercle bacilli encounter phagocytic cells which engulf and carry them into the lymphatic vessels of the region. The initial, or primary, lesions may develop where invasion of tissue first occurred, or in the lymph nodes which drain that area. The bacilli are always arrested for a time by these nodes, and tubercles are formed in them. In the more resistant species and individuals, the lesions may be confined for long periods, even for the life of the individual, in these nodes. The disease is then said to be localized or arrested. In the more susceptible, the disease progresses by the escape of bacilli through the lymphatics to the next series of nodes, where secondary foci develop. If the disease continues to progress, the organisms eventually reach the blood stream, by which they are scattered to all parts of the body. Such individuals are said to be suffering from generalized tuberculosis.

Tubercles have a characteristic microscopic structure by which they may be tentatively identified. In the very early stages they consist of small nests of cells derived by stimulation of the histiocytes of the organ in which the bacilli have lodged. These surround the nidus of multiplying organisms—it is clearly

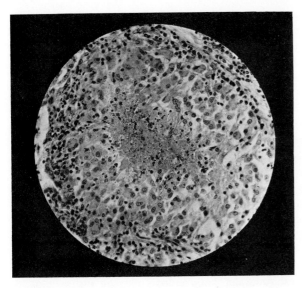

*Fig. 61.* A very early tubercle in the lung of a rabbit caused by *Mycobacterium tuberculosis*, avian type. The structure is typical of all primary tubercles irrespective of the type of bacillus concerned. The central area of necrosis is surrounded by a layer of epithelioid cells which make up the greater part of the field. The periphery of the lesion consists of fibroblasts and lymphocytes. Giant cells appear a little later near the margin of the necrotic area. X 110.

a defense mechanism of the body. These cells are usually known as *epithelioid cells*, because they have large vesicular nuclei and a generous amount of cytoplasm. They are produced by multiplication *in situ* and probably also by infiltration from the blood. A few granulocytic leukocytes generally are found in the center of these early cell nests, and lymphocytic cells tend to collect about their peripheries. Stimulated by the tubercle bacilli in their centers, these tubercles continue to enlarge. Shortly they may be seen with the naked eye as translucent, pearly structures like small grains of tapioca. As growth of the tubercles continues, necrosis begins in their centers, and the pearllike appearance gives way to yellowish-white opaqueness. Generally about this time another type of cell appears in the lesion—giant cells of the Langhans type. These are formed from epithelioid cells, either by fusion or by continued growth and multiplication of nuclei without division of cytoplasm. They become quite large and conspicuous. Their cytoplasm is clear, and their nuclei, numbering from two or three to ten or more, are arranged in the form of a crescent, or half-circle, around the periphery of one side of the cell. Tubercle bacilli frequently can be seen lying within the cytoplasm of these cells. As the tuberculous mass grows and the necrotic center becomes larger and larger, epithelioid and giant cells can generally be found just outside the advancing necrotic front.

Old tuberculous masses may be of very large size. They may involve entire lung lobes and large areas of the liver and spleen. They may cause lymph nodes to become 20 times as large as normal. The central parts of such lesions usually consist of very dry, cheesy material in which calcium deposits often appear, so that a gritty sound is given off when they are incised. Such lesions often become heavily encapsulated by dense connective tissue.

When tuberculous necrosis occurs in the lungs, the process often causes perforation of the bronchi and bronchioles, in which case the caseous material escapes into the air passages and is coughed up. The sputum thus becomes purulent and it contains tubercle bacilli, often in large numbers. Such individuals are called *open cases,* because they discharge bacilli in air droplets during coughing, and the sputum is highly infectious. Man often expectorates, thus grossly contaminating his environment. Animals swallow such sputum, but the organisms escape with the fecal material and thus infect their surroundings. Frequently in man but rarely in animals, the discharge of tuberculous pus from lung abscesses leaves large cavities. Because the yellow elastic tissue of the arteries is more resistant to necrosis than other tissues, it frequently happens that large vessels are exposed. These often rupture into the cavities, and the blood then escapes into the air passages. *Hemoptysis,* or bleeding into the air passages, may be so severe in man as to lead to death; and moderate hemoptysis, with bloody sputum, is a common symptom of advanced pulmonary tuberculosis. This condition is unusual in animals because cavitation rarely occurs even when the lesions become very large.

**Pathogenicity for Experimental Animals.** Tuberculosis can be induced in almost any animal by injecting a sufficiently large dose of the avian, bovine, or human type of tubercle bacilli. Even garter snakes can be killed with the avian type. Actually, mammalian bacilli have little pathogenicity for birds, but avian organisms are pathogenic for many mammals. The specific susceptibilities of farm animals and man to the different types of tubercle bacilli will be discussed later. The animals used most commonly for diagnostic purposes are monkeys, guinea pigs, rabbits, hamsters, white mice, and chickens. The type of disease produced in experimental animals depends greatly upon the manner in which infection is accomplished. Experimental animals are usually infected by intravenous, subcutaneous, intramuscular, and oral administration of cultures or infectious materials.

1. *By intravenous inoculation.* When tubercle bacilli are injected intravenously in animals in large doses, the host usually sickens quickly and may die within a few days, even when the virulence of the culture is not particularly high. The lesions in such animals usually are not visible, microscopically, but tubercle bacilli may be demonstrated in large numbers in films from the spleen and liver. If the dose is smaller, the inoculated animal will live longer, exhibit fever, inappetence, and weight loss. The spleen and liver of such animals may be swollen and filled with myriads of minute, translucent bodies. These are young tubercles, and this form of the disease, resulting from countless localizations in the tissues, is known as *miliary* tuberculosis. If the dose is still smaller, the effects upon the animal are less severe, it will live longer, and, if the virulence of the culture is low or the resistance of the species especially high, the animal may eventually recover. If the animal dies, however, a greatly enlarged spleen and liver containing few or many areas of necrosis usually are found. The lungs in these cases are also involved, the lesions vary-

ing from many small, translucent tubercles embedded in the parenchyma to large confluent necrotic areas involving as much as whole lobes. Generally there is no pleuritis, but excess fluid may be found in the pleural cavity. Lesions are only rarely found in the kidneys. In chickens the bone marrow is frequently involved.

2. *By subcutaneous or intramuscular inoculation.* The first lesions found in animals inoculated in these ways are at the site of inoculation and in the lymph nodes that drain the area. There is first local swelling, followed by necrosis at the point of inoculation, particularly when the dose of organisms is large. Often the necrosis extends to the skin, and a tuberculous ulcer appears. The local lymph nodes swell and become hard and rather painful. Caseation necrosis develops in them. A little later the infection will be found to have progressed by way of the lymphatics to the next set of lymph nodes and eventually, if the organism has sufficient pathogenicity, to the thoracic duct and thence into the blood stream. Because of hematogenous distribution the autopsy picture now becomes similar to that seen when moderate doses of the same culture are injected intravenously.

3. *By oral administration.* Susceptible animals infected by mouth usually show swelling and caseation necrosis of the lymph nodes of the alimentary canal (parotid, submaxillary, retropharyngeal, mesenteric) and ulcers may appear in the intestinal mucosa. Later, lesions in the spleen, liver, and lungs may be found. If the dose is given by capsule, infection of the lymph nodes of the head will be avoided and the initial lesions will be found in the mesenteric lymph nodes. There is evidence to indicate that alimentary infection can occur with the primary lesions appearing in the lungs, especially if the infecting organisms are fed with butter or other fatty materials, but this certainly is exceptional rather than frequent.

**Tuberculosis in Animals, including Man.** *In cattle.* In adult cattle, the lesions of tuberculosis usually are found in the lungs and the lymph nodes of the head and thorax. Most infections seem to be contracted by inhalation, but undoubtedly some occur through ingestion of the organism. In recently infected animals, the bronchial, mediastinal, submaxillary, and retropharyngeal nodes more often exhibit visible lesions than the lungs, but this may well be because small pulmonary lesions are not readily found. The lung lesions usually take the form of caseocalcareous masses located in the anterior lobes. The sizes vary from ones that can easily be overlooked to those that involve entire lobes. Active lesions may show hyperemia around the periphery of the caseous masses. Old, inactive lesions may become very calcareous and heavily encapsulated. Tubercle bacilli often are difficult to demonstrate by microscopic means, especially in the older lesions, but cultural methods and guinea pig inoculation usually succeed.

Relatively common where tuberculosis of cattle is prevalent is the so-called *pearl disease*, a form of tuberculous pleuritis or peritonitis. In this form of the disease large masses of smooth, grapelike bodies are found covering the ser-

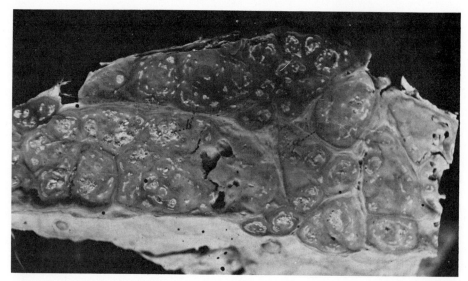

Fig. 62. Advanced tuberculosis in the lung of a cow. The entire diaphragmatic lobe is involved in the tuberculous process. There is extensive necrosis and fibrosis. The necrotic tissue contains large amounts of calcareous material.

ous surfaces. Adhesions usually are absent, or few in number. Often the lung tissue itself is not so seriously involved as its serous surface. In a majority of cases of lung tuberculosis in cattle, however, the disease causes massive adhesions of the lungs to the chest wall, the fibrous tissue being so strong that the lungs cannot be removed from the cavity except by the use of a cutting instrument.

Less often involved in adult cattle are the liver, the spleen, and the mesenteric lymph nodes. In less than 1 percent of all cases, even when fairly advanced, is udder infection found. In these cases the lesions resemble those found elsewhere. They may be nodular, or they may involve large areas of tissue. In the latter, discharge of bacilli occurs into the milk channels and the milk from such animals may contain large numbers of organisms. This milk is very dangerous for man, especially children, and for other animals when it is consumed in a raw state. Bovine-type tubercle bacilli frequently escape in milk of tuberculous cows when there are no detectable lesions in the udder. These organisms generally are fewer in number and less dangerous for this reason. Tubercle bacilli can also enter milk from contamination with fecal material. No matter how they enter the milk and no matter whether numerous or scanty, such organisms are dangerous to human health.

Calves fed on milk containing tubercle bacilli usually show primary lesions in the abdominal cavity rather than the thorax. In these cases the mesenteric lymph nodes may become greatly enlarged and hardened. When incised they show nodular lesions of a typical character. In these cases the liver and portal lymph nodes usually are involved. Lung lesions, if present, are secondary. Calves may also be infected by inhalation, in which cases the distribution of lesions is like that of most adults. A good description of the lesions of tuberculosis in cattle is given by Stamp (94).

Avian-type tubercle bacilli have frequently been found in bovine lesions in the north-central part of the United States where tuberculosis in poultry is prevalent. These organisms are picked up from the soil, which is polluted by infected chickens. The lesions, as a rule, are insignificant. They are usually found in the lymph nodes that drain the alimentary canal. They have no effect on the health of the animals but are important in that such animals will regularly react to avian tuberculin and johnin and thus may be mistaken for cases of paratuberculosis or Johne's disease. Such animals also occasionally react to mammalian tuberculin.

In Denmark, Plum (73), Bang (3), and others have found cases of infectious abortion in cattle apparently caused by avian-type tubercle bacilli. In these instances tuberculous lesions are found in the uterine wall and in the placenta. The diagnosis of such cases can readily be made by examining the placenta, or the uterine discharge following abortion. The lesions may remain in the uterine wall from one gestation period to the next, and such animals become chronic aborters. The organisms are not usually found in any other body organs or tissues, except occasionally in the mesenteric lymph nodes, a fact which suggests that the disease may be contracted through the digestive tract. Plum succeeded in producing abortion in one animal by injecting avian tubercle bacilli into the jugular vein. Although avian tuberculosis is common in some parts of the United States where there are also many dairy herds, this form of the disease has been reported only on one occasion (Fincher, Evans, and Saunders, 27).

Mitchell and Duthie (64) caused infection of the udder of one cow by injecting avian tubercle bacilli into the jugular vein. Apparently naturally occurring cases are rare, but one was reported by Stuart and Marshall (97) in 1952. Clinically the cow showed evidence of mastitis and on postmortem examination revealed visible lesions of tuberculosis. Acid-fast bacilli which proved to be the avian type were isolated. In the same year Thordal-Christensen (99) reported a case of generalized avian tuberculosis in a cow. Avian tubercle bacilli were recovered from mammary gland secretion and from pus obtained from the esophagus. There were lesions in the mammary gland, uterine wall, and lungs and in the bronchial, inguinal, and supramammary lymph glands. The processes were of a productive character without caseation and contained few bacilli except for those in the uterus, which carried many. In 1958 Pearson and McGowan (71) described a case of avian tuberculosis in a cow in which the infection was confined to the left lung and was not found elsewhere in the animal. In 1967, Lesslie and Birn (55) reported 18 cases in cows that were eliminating the avian type in their milk. None was classified as a positive reactor to the single intradermal tuberculin test.

*In Swine.* Swine are subject to infection with all three types of tubercle ba-cilli. The incidence of these types in hogs depends upon the locality in which the animals live and the character of their feed. The human-type infection, for example, almost always occurs in swine that are fed on garbage. Uncooked garbage from hospitals and sanitoria should never be fed to swine. Where tuberculosis is prevalent in cattle, most of the tubercle infections in swine come from that source. In the corn belt of the United States, which might also be called the swine belt, the vast majority of cases are of the avian type, the reason being that tuberculosis in chickens in this area is prevalent, whereas bovine tuberculosis is almost nonexistent. For an account of this situation, see Feldman (21).

Generally speaking, the bovine-type organism is capable of causing a more serious form of the disease than either of the other two types. Infections with the bovine organism generally are progressive and will lead to death of the animal eventually. It should be remembered that the life span of most swine, in the United States at least, is not over 8 to 9 months, by which time they are sent for slaughter. Such animals do not live long enough to become active spreaders of the disease; hence swine-to-swine transmission probably seldom occurs. Tuberculosis of swine is a disease contracted more from environment than from other swine.

Lesions of tuberculosis, irrespective of type, are found more often in the ab-dominal cavity of hogs than is the case in cattle. Infections are contracted most commonly by ingestion; thus the primary lesions are found in the lymph nodes of the head and of the abdominal cavity (*tuberculous adenitis*). In hu-man-type infections the lesions are seldom found in any other locations and they are usually of minimal size. In avian-type infections, the majority show only adenitis but a few cases may exhibit lesions in the liver, spleen, and lungs. The bovine type more often involves the visceral organs. Extensive lung lesions resembling those of cattle are not uncommon, and liver and spleen lesions are relatively frequent. A peculiar type of tuberculous lesion is frequently seen in the spleen of pigs infected with the bovine type of organ-ism. These are tumorlike bodies, more or less spherical in shape and varying in size up to about 5 cm in diameter. They stand up prominently as yellow-ish-white masses with dense, glistening capsules. The larger ones often have a smooth, shallow, craterlike depression on top. When they are incised, they are found to consist of firm but soft tissue, and each contains a cavity, half as large in diameter as the entire nodule, filled with clear, limpid fluid. There is no evidence of calcification in these lesions.

*In horses.* Horses are relatively susceptible to infection with bovine-type tubercle bacilli, but cases are infrequently encountered except when they live in very intimate association with tuberculous cattle.

The lesions of equine tuberculosis are most frequent in the lymph nodes of the pharyngeal region and in those of the mesentery, but lung, liver, and spleen lesions are not rare. In some cases the lesions appear very much like

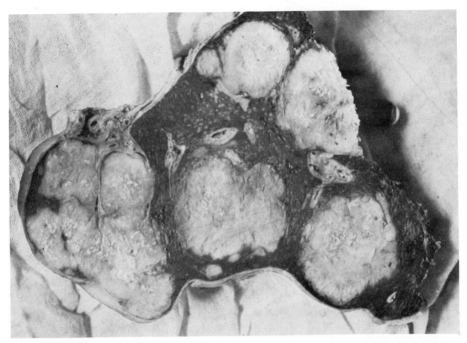

*Fig. 63.* Tuberculosis of the spleen in a horse. Lesions in horses often resemble tumors, being white or gray in color, uniform in consistency, and lacking obvious gross evidence of necrosis.

those in cattle, there being both caseation necrosis and calcification in the older lesions. In many instances, however, they do not have the usual appearance but consist of yellowish-white masses of rather soft tissue which have the appearance of a tumor. Necrosis is not obvious to the naked eye, nor is there any calcification.

Many strains of tubercle bacilli isolated from horses are subvirulent for experimental animals, and some are nearly avirulent. Reports on avian-type tuberculosis in the horse are rare, but Lesslie and Davis (56) described a case in which this type produced lesions in the lymph glands, lungs, and skin.

*In sheep and goats.* This disease is rather rare in sheep and goats (58). In sheep most of the infections that have been typed abroad were found to be of the bovine type, but in the United States most have proved to be avian in origin. These cases have been found in areas of the country where avian tuberculosis is common, but bovine tuberculosis is rare. Harshfield, Roderick, and Hawn (39) described 19 cases of tuberculosis in sheep, all of which proved to be infections of the avian type. In the report of the Chief of the Bureau of Animal Industry, U.S. Department of Agriculture, for 1940, it is stated that eight cases of tuberculosis in sheep had been investigated in that year, seven of which proved to have been caused by the avian- and one by the bovine-type bacillus. Lesions of the lungs and thoracic lymph nodes were found in all these cases, a majority showed liver tubercles, and the spleen was involved in about one-half of the cases.

The data on tuberculosis in goats is very meager, a fact that bears out the impression that the goat is relatively resistant to infection. Soliman *et al.* (93) described an outbreak in goats in 1953 in England. Out of 41 animals examined in a flock, 32 showed macroscopic lesions. The lesions were mainly intestinal and the disease was of a progressive nature only in young kids. The type

Table XVIII.   TYPES OF TUBERCLE BACILLI
AFFECTING DOGS AND CATS
(NATURALLY OCCURRING CASES)

| Animal species | Type of tubercle bacilli | | | | | |
|---|---|---|---|---|---|---|
| | Human | | Bovine | | Avian | |
| | No. | % | No. | % | No. | % |
| Dogs | 389 | 65.7 | 189 | 32.0 | 2* | 0.3 |
| Cats | 6 | 4.6 | 125 | 95.4 | 0 | 0.0 |

* One of these cases was credited to an author who denies having reported such a case; therefore it must be regarded as an error.

of the organism causing the infection was not determined. A brief review of tuberculosis in goats was given, and although it appears that the bovine type has been concerned in most known cases of tuberculosis in this animal, the avian type has caused some.

*In Dogs and Cats.* Cases of tuberculosis in dogs (69) and cats are not common in the United States but appear to be more common elsewhere. Dogs are susceptible to both human- and bovine-type infections, but the majority of cases have been shown to be caused by the human type. Many cases have been reported in which small lap dogs have obviously been infected by their tuberculous masters. Cats, on the other hand, appear to be very resistant to human-type infections and seldom are infected by tuberculous owners. They are quite susceptible to bovine-type infections, however, and usually contract the disease by drinking milk from tuberculous cows. Hix *et al.* (43) have reported a case of avian-type infection in the cat, and Wilkinson (107) described a granuloma associated with the human type.

In dogs, the disease usually involves the thoracic organs primarily. Lesions elsewhere are infrequent. In cats, the primary lesions are usually in the abdominal organs but the lungs often become involved secondarily.

Verge and Senthille (102) reviewed all reported cases of dog and cat tuberculosis from all parts of the world in which the infecting organism had been typed. Their findings are reported in table XVIII.

*In chickens.* Chickens are not susceptible to mammalian tubercle bacilli; all cases are caused by avian-type organisms. Infections are contracted by ingestion of bacilli from infected soil and water. The organism is sometimes found in eggs laid by tuberculous hens, and this may occasionally account for

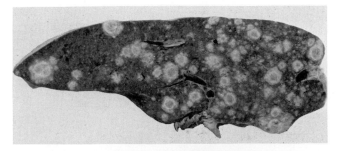

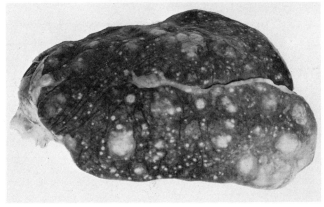

*Fig. 64.* Tuberculosis of the liver in a chicken. (*Upper*) Gross lesions in cut section. (*Lower*) Lesions as seen from the surface.

the way the disease enters previously uninfected flocks. On page 412 it has been pointed out that avian-type tubercle bacilli have remarkable ability to maintain themselves for long periods on infected premises.

Unlike mammals, birds seldom suffer from tuberculosis of the lungs. The lesions occur in the intestinal tract in the form of ulcers in the liver and spleen and frequently in the bones and joints. Other lesions are rare.

The intestinal ulcers may be found in any part of the intestine. They are readily found as tumorlike masses on the outside of the gut up to 4 or 5 cm in diameter. When incised they are found to be filled with caseous material, which is discharged through a relatively small ulcerated passage into the lumen of the intestine. Great masses of bacilli are ordinarily demonstrated with ease in this material, and it is these bacilli, discharged with the feces, which cause the soil contamination. There may be 1 or 2 or 20 or more such ulcers in the intestine of a single bird.

Liver lesions are always found in such infected birds. These appear as caseous areas, varying in size, distributed throughout all parts of the greatly enlarged organ. The consistency is unchanged, because the tuberculous tissue is only slightly firmer than the normal hepatic tissue. There is no calcification. In some cases the tuberculous areas are few and the lesions relatively large. In others numerous minute lesions are seen. Occasionally myriads of tubercle

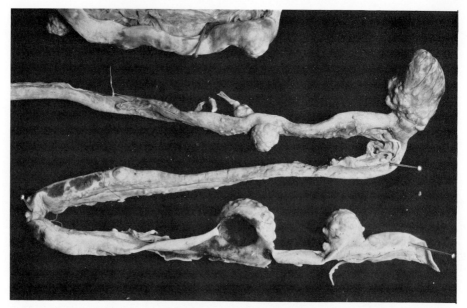

*Fig. 65.* Tuberculosis of the intestine in a chicken. Intestinal ulcers are common in avian tuberculosis. These ulcers gradually become very deep, the tissues of the intestinal wall forming saclike structures that appear on the serous surface like tumors. The centers are filled with dry, caseous material, which gradually discharges into the intestinal lumen.

bacilli are found in livers that are dark greenish in color but exhibit no lesions visible to the naked eye. The spleen is generally enlarged, showing moderate to marked hypertrophy. Instead of the normal, smooth surface, tuberculous spleens usually become nodular. When incised a few large caseous masses may be seen or large numbers of very minute foci.

Infected joints are swollen and contain caseous material. Tubercle bacilli may be found in abundance in this material and, in fact, in all tuberculous lesions in birds.

Tuberculosis in birds develops rather slowly. Well-developed lesions seldom are found in birds of less than 1 year of age, and such birds seldom become spreaders during the first few months of the course of the infection. The disease is manifested by loss of body weight, and listlessness, weakness, and paleness of the tissue toward the end of its course. The owners frequently refer to the disease as "going light." Lameness, caused by bone and joint lesions, is frequent.

*In birds other than chickens.* Tuberculosis occurs in turkeys, pigeons, pheasants, ducks, and geese, as well as in many wild birds. The disease in these species is essentially like that in chickens. Ducks and geese are not infected as often as chickens, pheasants, and turkeys. In 1966, Bickford *et al.* (8) investigated the epizootiology of tuberculosis in starlings on a farm in Indiana where there was a high incidence of avian tubercle bacilli in the swine.

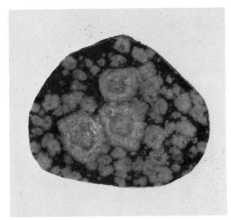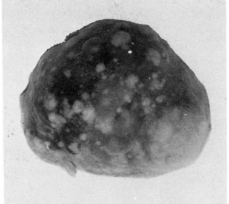

*Fig. 66.* Tuberculosis of the spleen in a chicken. (*Right*) Lesions as seen on the spleen surface. (*Left*) Lesions seen in cut section. (Courtesy E. L. Brunett.)

Of 125 starlings examined, 7 had gross tubercles in the liver, and 1 also had lesions in the spleen and intestines.

*In wild animals.* Tuberculosis in wild animals is not common except when they are in captivity. The disease has been found on several occasions in wild birds (6, 63) living a natural life. It has been described in free living African (Cape) buffalo (36), and there have been a considerable number of reports of the disease in wild deer. Cases in deer are caused in almost all instances by the bovine-type bacillus, and infection results from association with cattle on pasture or by browsing on land that is used for pasturage of cattle. It is not unlikely that some of the "breaks" in tuberculosis-free herds are caused by the introduction of the disease by infected wild deer.

Tuberculosis has always been one of the major problems of zoological parks. The most severe losses have been among birds, but extreme care is necessary to control decrement among members of the monkey family. The human type causes losses among apes and the bovine type among reindeer and other ruminants. The latter has been found in an outbreak in mink on a fur-raising farm (76), but avian-type tuberculosis also occurs in this animal (37, 108). Both bovine- and avian-type tuberculosis have been reported in captive kangaroos (100). The human-type bacillus has caused tuberculosis in a captive rhinoceros (74) and the disease has been described in the elephant (90). Tubercle bacilli of the cold-blooded type, to which reference will be made later, cause serious losses among reptiles and amphibia.

Tuberculosis among wild field mice (voles) occurs in England. The vole bacillus is different from the types previously described. It is discussed on page 442.

*Human tuberculosis.* The most common form of tuberculosis of man is that known as *phthisis* or *pulmonary consumption*. This disease affects primarily the lungs and pleura and the associated lymph nodes. In many individuals the disease becomes arrested early and no symptoms are induced. Such individuals will, however, react to tuberculin, and x-rays may show one or several small encapsulated and calcareous lesions. In others, unfortunately, the disease spreads from the original focus and causes large exudative and destructive lesions. The victim suffers from a low-grade, intermittent fever, weakness, shortness of breath, a hacking cough, loss of weight, and finally great emaciation. Large amounts of purulent sputum are raised, and this often is very rich in tubercle bacilli. Frequently there are severe and often fatal hemmorrhages from large blood vessels that have been damaged by the necrotizing process. This type of tuberculosis is caused by tubercle bacilli of the human type in most cases. The disease is transmitted from man to man, animal infections playing little part in it except in cases in which the bovine-type bacillus is involved. Griffith (33) in England and workers in the Scandinavian countries, where bovine tuberculosis formerly was prevalent, showed that from 1 to 6 percent of human pulmonary infections were caused by the bovine type. This situation does not exist in the United States, where bovine tubercle infection is now comparatively rare.

Extrapulmonary tuberculosis of man is often caused by tubercle bacilli of the bovine type. These infections occur more often in children than in adults and are caused by the drinking of infected cows' milk. They involve the lymph nodes of the pharyngeal region and the abdominal organs instead of the organs of the thorax. Bovine tubercle bacilli are often found in infections of the bones and joints, of the skin (*lupus*), and in tuberculous meningitis. All these forms of tuberculosis are caused more often by bacilli of the human type than by those of the bovine type except, possibly, the infections of the neck glands (*scrofula*), in which the bovine type may be more frequent than the human type. Because bovine tuberculosis has been reduced in incidence in the United States, and because a large part of all milk consumed is pasteurized, it has been noted by surgeons that those forms of tuberculosis in which the bovine-type bacillus frequently occurs are becoming rare. Whereas in the early part of the century scrofula among children was not uncommon in many parts of this country, it has now become a rare disease (96).

*Table XIX.* TYPES OF TUBERCLE BACILLI ISOLATED FROM CASES OF HUMAN TUBERCULOSIS

| Type of disease | Age groups of patients | | | | | |
| --- | --- | --- | --- | --- | --- | --- |
| | 16 years and older | | 5 to 16 years | | Under 5 years | |
| | Human | Bovine | Human | Bovine | Human | Bovine |
| Pulmonary tuberculosis | 497 | 3 | 6 | 0 | 28 | 1 |
| Cervical adenitis (scrofula) | 27 | 1 | 17 | 14 | 9 | 11 |
| Abdominal | 15 | 4 | 7 | 8 | 9 | 11 |
| Generalized | 33 | 1 | 7 | 5 | 72 | 16 |
| Total of all kinds | 625 | 14 | 85 | 37 | 201 | 51 |

That tubercle infection of children with bacilli of the bovine type was an important matter earlier in this century in the United States and elsewhere is clearly shown by statistics collected by Park and Krumwiede (70), which were published in 1912. Some of the more significant of their findings are shown in table XIX. Nearly half the cases included were studied by the authors in and around New York City. It can be noted in this table that the bovine-type infections were largely in young children and that they were largely extrapulmonary forms of the disease.

It has been generally believed that human beings are not susceptible to infection with the avian-type tubercle bacillus. This matter was critically reviewed in 1947 by Feldman (21), who concluded that the evidence indicated that a few authentic cases had occurred. Feldman, Hutchinson, Schwarting, and Karlson (24) have recently added another case in which the evidence seems to be quite clear. In this instance a child showed extensive lung lesions. Some of the previously described cases also were of a serious nature. It must be accepted that, although the avian tubercle bacillus ordinarily has little virulence for man, infections do occur and a study that was made in 1957–1964 by Kubin *et al.* (54) in Czechoslovakia on nine cases revealed the seriousness of the disease's clinical course.

**Infectivity of the Several Types of *Mycobacterium Tuberculosis* for the Domesticated Animals and Man.** Whereas the three types of tubercle bacilli are in their native hosts when they are found in man, cattle, and birds, all of them appear in other hosts, and they often produce serious diseases in the foreign hosts. Some species of animals are susceptible to infection with only one type, but others may be infected with two or all three. This makes a rather confusing situation. To clarify the matter, the pathogenicity of each type of organism for each of the domestic animals and man will be reviewed. Table XX, taken from Griffith (33), who studied this matter for many years in England, is

*Table XX.* TOTAL NUMBER OF CASES OF NATURAL TUBERCULOSIS IN DIFFERENT ANIMALS IN WHICH THE TYPE OF TUBERCLE BACILLUS HAS BEEN DETERMINED

| Species of animal | Number of cases | Types of tubercle bacilli found | | |
|---|---|---|---|---|
| | | Bovine | Human | Avian |
| Horse | 25 | 24 | — | 1 |
| Pig | 163 | 118* | 5 | 43 |
| Cat | 20 | 20 | — | — |
| Dog | 4 | 1 | 3 | — |
| Goat | 1 | 1 | — | — |
| Sheep | 4 | 2 | — | 2 |
| Cattle | 52 | 50 | 1 | 1 |
| Fowl | 13 | — | — | 13 |
| Guinea pig | 6 | 5 | 1 | — |
| Rabbit | 8 | 4 | — | 4 |

* Three cases showed mixed types of tubercle bacilli.

included although it must be remembered that the incidence of the different types varies in the British Isles from that in the United States and else where in the world. The table does, however, show the susceptibilities of the several species of animals.

In general, it may be pointed out that the human-type bacillus is capable of invading a number of species of animals but produces progressive disease only in the dog and rarely in the cat. The avian type is more cosmopolitan because it is capable of causing serious infections not only in birds but in swine and sheep, and rarely in man. The bovine type is the most cosmopolitan because it can produce serious disease in all domesticated animals, except birds, and in man.

I. Pathogenicity of the Bovine Type of *Myco. tuberculosis.*
    a. For cattle. Causes a progressive and destructive disease.
    b. For horses. Causes a progressive disease.
    c. For swine. Highly infective. The disease is progressive and fairly frequent where swine associate with tuberculous cattle.
    d. For sheep and goats. Progressive infections occur but are relatively rare.
    e. For dogs. Causes progressive infections, but this type is not so common in dogs as in man.
    f. For cats. Causes a progressive disease. Most common type in cats.
    g. For birds. Not infective. Naturally occurring cases unknown.
    h. For man. Causes a progressive disease in man, especially in children. Most cases involve the lymph nodes and abdominal organs rather than lungs, but pulmonary cases are not rare.

II. Pathogenicity of the Human Type of *Myco. tuberculosis.*
    a. For cattle. Causes only miminal lesions in the lymph nodes. Of no importance except animals will react to tuberculin. Careless caretakers suffering from pulmonary tuberculosis may cause many animals to become sensitized to tuberculin.
    b. For horses. No cases reported but it is probable that horses would react like cattle.
    c. For swine. Lesions confined to lymph nodes of the alimentary tracts. Minimal in nature and not important.
    d. For sheep and goats. No cases reported.
    e. For dogs. Progressive tuberculosis produced. Mostly respiratory infection contracted from tuberculous owners.
    f. For cats. Apparently highly resistant, but a few cases on record.
    g. For birds. All birds, except members of the *Psittacidae* (parrot family), are resistant. Cases reported in parrots that associated with tuberculous owners.

III. Pathogenicity of the Avian Type of *Myco. tuberculosis.*
    a. For birds. All birds thought to be susceptible. Disease occurs mostly in domesticated birds and wild birds kept in captivity.

b. For cattle. Persistent uterine infections which result in abortions. Minimal lymph node lesions, of little importance except that animals react to tests made with avian tuberculin and johnin when paratuberculosis or Johne's disease are searched for.

c. For horses. Cases have been reported. Of little importance.

d. For swine. Lesions usually but not always confined to lymph nodes. This is by far the most common type of tubercle infection of swine in the United States.

e. For sheep. May produce progressive disease. Lesions occur in lungs as well as lymph nodes. Most cases of tuberculosis in sheep in this country in recent years have been caused by this type. Not a common disease, however, because sheep do not usually associate with tuberculous chickens.

f. For goats. Rare cases reported. May produce progressive disease.

g. For dogs and cats. Table XX shows no cases, but rare ones occur.

h. For man. Infectivity is low but a few cases of progressive tuberculosis have been shown to be due to this type.

**Routes of Infection in Tuberculosis.** The localization of the lesions in tuberculosis and the character of the disease depend in considerable degree upon the manner in which the infection enters the body. It is clear that there are several routes that may be followed.

1. *Inhalation.* The fact that tubercle lesions in adult human beings and cattle occur more frequently in the chest cavity than elsewhere suggests that infection commonly occurs through inhalation. Experimentally it has been shown by McFadyean (60) and others that infections can easily be produced in guinea pigs by spraying them with tubercle bacilli. This fact, coupled with the knowledge that in pulmonary tuberculosis both man and cow cough into the air droplets of secretion containing tubercle bacilli that can readily be inhaled by others near them, is rather convincing evidence. On the other hand, it is more difficult to produce infections, even in highly susceptible animals, with moderate doses of tubercle bacilli fed in gelatin capsules, and when infections are induced in this way, lesions are almost invariably found in the mesenteric lymph nodes. Because these nodes often are free of lesions when the chest organs are severely infected, it does not seem likely that the organism generally enters by the intestinal route. On the other hand, Ravenel (77) many years ago showed that tubercle bacilli suspended in butter could be found in the lacteals shortly after feeding; hence it appears to be possible for these organisms to reach the lungs, in some cases at least, without leaving lesions in the digestive tract. Lung infection can also be produced experimentally by causing susceptible animals to inhale tubercle bacilli suspended in dust.

2. *Ingestion.* Ingestion of tubercle bacilli in considerable numbers in infected milk readily produces tuberculosis in young animals. In these cases lesions usually occur in the lymph nodes of the alimentary canal, tuberculous

ulcers frequently are found in the intestine, and lesions occur in the liver and spleen more frequently than in the organs of the chest. Before pasteurization of skim milk and whey became the general practice, many calves and pigs were infected with tuberculosis from these products brought back to the farm from the creamery or milk station. Human beings and animals affected primarily with pulmonary tuberculosis often develop intestinal lesions from the swallowing of quantities of infective sputum. Infection in birds is nearly always the result of ingestion of organisms picked up with the feed from the ground. Intestinal ulcers and liver and spleen lesions are commonly found in avian tuberculosis.

3. *Wound infection.* Certain lesions of the skin of man, known as *sarcoids,* have been thought to be due to the activities of tubercle bacilli. These are fleshy, tumorlike growths, usually not associated with necrosis. Acid-fast organisms resembling avian-type tubercle bacilli have been isolated from some sarcoids, but the basic question still remains, are patients with clearly defined sarcoidosis suffering from some type of mycobacterial infection?

Tuberculosis of the skin, or *lupus,* occasionally occurs in man but is very rare in animals. In man the disease has been called *pathologists' warts* or *prosector's wart* because it often begins in skin wounds apparently contaminated with tubercle bacilli while handling infected tissues. The lesion may be caused by human or bovine tubercle bacilli, which usually are of attenuated virulence from residence in the skin (34).

An ulcerous skin lesion that sometimes occurs on the lower extremities of man is also caused by an acid-fast microorganism known as *Myco. ulcerans.* This organism prefers to grow at temperatures lower than 37 C and is antigenically distinct from other pathogenic species of *Mycobacterium.* Experimentally it produces ulcerative skin lesions in rats, mice, and calves (25, 101). It has caused udder infection in dairy cattle.

Another acid-fast organism concerned in producing skin lesions was named *Myco. balnei* (26). Restudy of this strain has indicated that it is identical with *Myco. marinum,* a previously established type (32). In Uganda, an acid-fast bacillus that caused extensive skin ulcers mainly among children has been described under the name *Myco. buruli* (13).

Tuberclelike skin lesions of cattle are quite common. It is a form of lymphangitis, associated with acid-fast bacteria. (See page 462.) Although many have referred to these lesions as *skin tuberculosis,* most workers have failed to isolate tubercle bacilli from them or to infect experimental animals. Their tuberculous nature has not been proved, and epidemiological evidence suggests that the causative agent is not the tubercle bacillus.

4. *Congenital tuberculosis.* A few instances have been described in which newborn calves were infected with generalized tuberculosis. In these instances a tuberculous lesion has developed in the placenta, and this has eroded into the fetal blood vessels, thus showering the fetal tissues with organisms. Such animals die shortly after birth.

Congenital tuberculosis should be carefully distinguished from hereditary tuberculosis, of which much may be heard but which is, in reality, fictitious. Neither this nor any other infectious disease is inherited. Any known disease-producing agent, if carried in the germ plasm, would destroy that heredity-carrying bit of protoplasm. Young animals born into an environment where tuberculosis is rampant naturally are apt to acquire the disease from their surroundings. The "tuberculous taint" which people and animals were supposed to carry in their family trees is, in reality, merely familial infections as a result of intimate association in the same environment.

**Diagnosis.** The diagnosis of tuberculosis in animals after death is seldom difficult because the lesions present a characteristic appearance. In cases of doubt the causative organism can be demonstrated in stained films, in cultures, or in experimental animals. Diagnosis during life is more difficult. Because of their short life span, the disease does not reach advanced development in most animals. When it does, the victim usually loses weight, and mammals frequently develop a dry cough when the lungs are extensively involved. Milking cows give a reduced amount of milk, and hens cease to lay eggs. The disease may be suspected, but other than clinical means are usually required to make a positive diagnosis. Bacteriologic examinations during life are possible, but difficult, in animals. In tuberculous cattle careful examination or culture of milk after it has been subjected to centrifugation may be employed in diagnosing udder infection (61). Aids in detecting and identifying tubercle bacilli now being used are the FA technic (31); the use of para-aminobenzoic acid medium (45); guinea pig inoculation, a procedure believed to be superior to culture; microscopic examination of cultures (84); and specific bacteriophages (4, 78).

In man sputum frequently is a good source of material for direct examination, culture, or animal inoculation. A technic of rapid slide cultivation of tubercle bacilli has been developed (7). It is not as accurate as routine culture methods but often leads to a much quicker diagnosis. Roentgenograms are not so useful in animals as in man because of their cost and the difficulty in obtaining them, and, in the larger animals, because of the thickness of the thorax.

*Serological tests for tuberculosis.* Attempts to apply the complement-fixation and other serological tests to the problem of diagnosis have been made in cattle. These have failed because of nonspecificity of the reactions. Tuberculous animals usually will react, but a considerable number of apparently noninfected animals also react. It is probable that cattle are often sensitized by acid-fast organisms other than tubercle bacilli, and that this negates the value of the test. A test based on the hemolysis of sheep erythrocytes, coated with an extract of the human-type tubercle bacillus, which occurs if appropriate antibodies and guinea pig complement are present, is sometimes used along with the tuberculin tests (28). This hemolytic test is supposed to give fewer false positive reactions in tuberculosis-free herds, but like the other serological tests it is nonspecific.

Moses, Feldman, and Mann (67) found it possible to prepare an agglutinating antigen with cultures of avian tubercle bacilli with which they conducted rapid or plate tests with sera of infected birds. In a series of infected chickens they found that this test compared favorably with the results of the tuberculin test. A group of naturally infected pigeons failed to react, however. Schaefer (87) has employed agglutination tests in classifying strains of avian tubercle bacilli, *Myco. kansasi*, *Myco. balnei*, and bacteria of the "Battey" and scoto-chromogenic types, while Stanford and Beck (95) used double-diffusion pre-cipitation tests to establish individual patterns for *Myco. fortuitum*, *Myco. kansasi*, *Myco. phlei*, *Myco. smegmatis*, and human tubercle bacilli.

*The tuberculin tests.* For the diagnosis of tubercle infection in animals, principal dependence is placed on tuberculin tests. These tests are used extensively on cattle, swine, and chickens, and occasionally on other species. When testing for the mammalian types of tuberculosis, tuberculin made from either human- or bovine-type tubercle bacilli can be used. When testing for the avian type of tuberculosis, tuberculin made from bacilli of that type must be used. Animals may be tested with both types, simultaneously, when the in-tradermal method is used.

*Tuberculin.* Tuberculin is a protein, or protein-derivative, produced by tu-bercle bacilli during growth. It is contained in any aqueous extract of the or-ganisms and is present in any medium upon which tubercle bacilli have grown. Until recently the tuberculin of commerce was made from cultures grown on glycerol broth. Most of it is now made from cultures grown on syn-thetic media.

The nature of tuberculin remained obscure from the time it was discovered

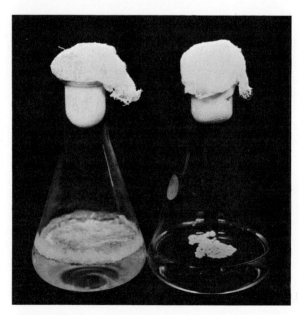

Fig. 67. *Mycobacterium tuber-culosis*, bovine type, a growth on glycerol broth. In the right-hand flask the culture is about 2 weeks old; in the left it is about 2 months old. Growth appears as a dull-grayish-white pellicle, which finally covers the surface of the fluid medium, becomes thick, opaque, and folded into creases, and pushes up on the sides of the flask at the margins. The fluid re-mains perfectly clear.

by Koch in 1890 (52) until Long and Seibert (57) finally obtained it in a purified form in 1926. It was long believed to be a protein, but chemical analysis was impossible so long as the organism was cultivated on a medium containing protein. By growing the organism on a synthetic, protein-free medium, Long and Seibert were able to precipitate from the filtrate a crystalline protein that apparently is the active principle.

So long as impure tuberculins were used, their concentrations were expressed in terms of Koch's OT (Old Tuberculin). OT is a glycerol broth filtrate that has been evaporated to one-tenth of its original volume. Different lots vary in potency, although, when standardized conditions of production are adhered to, the variation is not great. Because the active principle can now be obtained in relatively pure form (Purified Protein Derivative-PPD), the concentration can be accurately measured in terms of this principle.

All tuberculin used on cattle in the United States is supplied by the U.S. Department of Agriculture. It is made from three strains of the human type which are grown in a synthetic medium, in flasks. Equal numbers of cultures, which have grown until maximum growth has occurred, are assembled and steamed for 3 hours to destroy the organisms and aid in their extraction. The masses of dead organisms are filtered out, the filtrate is concentrated by evaporation to 20 percent of the original volume, and this is diluted with an equal volume of 1 percent phenol solution and enough glycerol is added to make a final concentration of 0.3 percent. After a final filtration through Berkefeld filters it is ready to be bottled.

It was first discovered by Koch that tuberculin was highly toxic for the tuberculous but nearly innocuous for normal animals. When tuberculin is injected into animals harboring one or more tubercles, a *general reaction* manifested by fever and constitutional symptoms occurs if the dose is sufficiently large. If the animal is destroyed while at the height of the reaction, it will be found that an inflammatory reaction has occurred around the tubercles present in the organs. This is termed the *focal reaction*. When sufficient tuberculin is used, tuberculous animals sometimes react so violently as to die. If the tuberculin is injected into a tissue from whence it is not quickly disseminated, such as the dense layers of the skin, *a local reaction* at the point of injection becomes manifest.

**Application of Tuberculin Tests in Animals.** The tuberculins used on animals are relatively concentrated. Those used on man are greatly diluted because it is considered unwise to incite constitutional reactions for fear of stimulating the progress of the disease itself. Because reacting animals are ordinarily destroyed when they are found to be reactors to the tests, there is no reason to fear severe reactions. Concentrated tuberculin will give reactions in some cases when weaker solutions fail.

There are three basic methods of applying tuberculin as a diagnostic agent: the method of subcutaneous administration, sometimes called the *thermal test;* the method of applying the tuberculin to the mucous membranes of the eye, the *ophthalmic method;* and the *intradermal* or intracutaneous method. A thermal intravenous test has been used rarely and without marked success to supplement the intradermal tuberculin test.

1. *The thermal test.* This was formerly the standard method of testing cattle for tuberculosis. In later years it has been largely replaced by tests that require less time. The tuberculin (10 percent Koch's OT, 2 ml or more) is injected subcutaneously after several temperatures have been taken at 2-hour intervals to make certain that the animal is not suffering a fever from some other cause. After 8 hours, temperatures are again taken at 2-hour intervals through the 16th or 18th hour after the injection. A typical reaction consists of a rise in temperature of at least 2 degrees F, which appears some time between the 8th and 18th hours and subsides within 24 hours.

As has been explained above, this form of test is not used on human beings because of the danger from the constitutional reaction.

2. *The ophthalmic test.* This test is sometimes used on cattle. A concentrated tuberculin (Koch's OT) is instilled into the conjunctival sac with a camel's-hair brush or with a medicine dropper. A positive reaction is indicated by an inflammation of the conjunctiva during the course of which pus is formed and appears at the inner canthus. One instillation of tuberculin serves to render the eye more sensitive to another; hence it is common practice to sensitize the eye by one treatment and to repeat the treatment 2 or 3 days later, the reaction being observed and judged after the second instillation. The inflammation and appearance of the exudate are prompt. The test is usually read from 4 to 6 hours after the application of the second dose of tuberculin.

3. *The intradermal test.* This test is now extensively used on cattle, swine, chickens, and man. The tuberculin used on animals is more concentrated than that used for the thermal test. A small quantity, usually not more than 0.1 ml, is injected into the deeper layers of the skin (dermis) with a fine hypodermic needle introduced nearly parallel to the skin surface. In routine work in the United States the site of injection usually is the thin, hairless skin on the undersurface of the tail near its base. In swine the skin of one of the ears usually is injected and in chickens the margin of one of the wattles. Positive reactions are indicated by firm, warm swellings at the point of injection. The reactions in cattle are judged on the 3rd day, sometimes a little later. The same period is used for tests in swine, but reactions in chickens are best judged in about 48 hours.

In England it has long been customary to inject tuberculin into the thick skin of one side of the neck, the area having been shaved previously. The reaction is judged by the increase in skin thickness as determined by calipers. This method has not become popular in this country because it requires more time to conduct, but recent work by Johnson and co-workers indicates that this skin area may be more sensitive and thus better adapted as the site of injection than is the tail fold.

A modification of the intradermal tuberculin test for cattle is the *Stormont test*. This was developed by Kerr, Lamont, and McGirr (48) in Ireland. It involves two injections of tuberculin into the same skin site, 7 days apart. The tests are read within 24 hours after the second injection. The authors claim that initial sensitization of the skin by the primary injection gives a sharper reaction to the second. The results of comparative tests—the single intradermal method measured against the double method—were analyzed statistically by Priestley (75). It was claimed that, in measuring the results against the finding of lesions in the slaughtered animals, the Stormont test had an error of only 1.8 percent, whereas the single injection method showed 18.9 percent error on a group of over 300 animals. Although this procedure was employed in England for a time, it has now been discontinued.

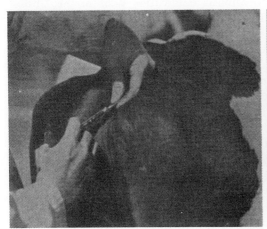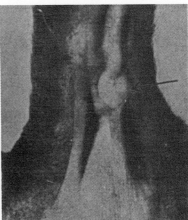

*Fig. 68.* The intradermal tuberculin test in cattle. (*Left*) Making the intradermal injection into the right tail fold. (*Right*) Typical swelling at the point of injection 72 hours later. (Courtesy E. T. Faulder.)

Tuberculin testing of dogs and cats has not been widely practiced in the United States. Granting that the intradermal method is helpful, the BCG vaccine provides an additional diagnostic aid (40). This vaccine is injected subcutaneously and the dog or cat that produces an early reaction at the site of inoculation should be regarded as a tuberculous suspect.

In tuberculin testing in man, 0.000,05 to 0.005 mg of PPD are rubbed in the scarified skin (Von Pirquet test) or injected intradermally (Mantoux test), or thin filter paper is impregnated with tuberculin about four times as strong as OT, dried, and taped on the cleansed skin (Vollmer's patch test). Positive tests are indicated by local inflammatory reactions. A test that is coming into wide usage is the tuberculin tine test, a multiple-puncture intradermal skin test (2). It is claimed that the disk, which contains four tines impregnated with four times standard strength OT, is a sterile, self-sufficient, and disposable unit that is easily administered and read. A jet injector gun has been described as a rapid, inexpensive, and reasonably reliable method of mass tuberculin skin testing (41).

**The Reliability of Tuberculin Tests on Animals.** Tuberculin is regarded as a highly accurate diagnostic agent when it is properly used and the results are properly interpreted. It is not infallible, however, particularly in cattle. No matter how carefully it is used some errors occur. When lesions of tuberculosis are extensive, the tissues often are so saturated with tuberculoprotein as to make them insensitive to tuberculin; hence in advanced cases of the disease, the tuberculin test often is falsely negative. On the other hand, a certain number of animals that give positive reactions to tuberculin fail to show lesions at autopsy. In the millions of tuberculin tests that have been applied to cattle in connection with the tuberculosis eradication plan in the United States, these animals have amounted to a small fraction of 1 percent of the total. Of the number that have reacted to tuberculin, however, they have amounted to from 10 to more than 50 percent. This percentage has gradually risen as the disease has been reduced, a fact that was foreseen in the beginning since a few spurious reactions amounted to a small fraction of the total when many tuberculous cattle were being slaughtered, but a much larger fraction when the actual tuberculosis cases have been reduced. Presumably, when the last tuberculous cow has been slaughtered, there will still be a small percentage of cattle that will react to tuberculin.

Cattle that have reacted to tuberculin but fail to show lesions of tuberculosis at autopsy are called NVL (No Visible Lesion) or NGL (No Gross Lesion) cases. The cause of these reactions has never been determined but several plausible hypotheses have been offered:

1. That many such animals are in the early stages of the disease, at which time reactions to tuberculin will occur though there are no visible lesions.

2. That many animals have small lesions that may be located in parts of the carcass not ordinarily examined in routine meat inspection work.

3. That animals which have been in contact with avian tubercle bacilli will ordinarily exhibit slight or no visible lesions but some of these will react to tuberculin. Also, cattle may be sensitized to tuberculin by contact with human tubercle bacilli. It is possible to produce tuberculin sensitivity in guinea pigs by oral administration of killed *Myco. tuberculosis* (106) and this leads to speculation over the likelihood of similar reactivity appearing in other animals.

4. That some, perhaps many, animals come in contact with acid-fast organisms other than tubercle bacilli which are able to sensitize them to tuberculin. For instance, experiments in calves have shown that *Nocardia farcinica* may sensitize these animals to avian or mammalian tuberculin or both (1). Certainly the potential role of scotochromes in producing skin sensitivity in man to the tine test deserves further investigation.

**Mechanism of the Tuberculin Reaction.** Despite the fact that the tuberculin reaction is the best known and most studied of the allergic reactions, its mechanism is still largely unknown. In guinea pigs age is a factor in inducing sensitization to tubercle bacilli. Those less than 4 weeks old usually fail to develop an allergic state and it is possible that this serologic unresponsiveness may reflect a form of specific immune suppression (47). In adult guinea pigs the reaction can be elicited by the injection of living or dead tubercle bacilli or of tuberculoproteins. High-grade allergic sensitization can be produced most easily by the use of living cultures, less easily with dead cultures, and with considerable difficulty with the extracts of cultures. Apparently specific humoral (circulating) antibodies are not necessary for the allergic reaction, but in all cases it seems to be clear that tubercles must have formed, or at any rate that the granulomatous tissue reactions characteristic of infections with acid-fast organisms must be present. Accordingly, cellular hypersensitivity appears to be a typical immunological phenomenon in which macrophages and lymphocytes of the host become sensitive to tuberculin. The reactions are quite specific in that the tuberculins must be made from the type of organism that is responsible for the infection if reactions are to be obtained consistently. It is true that a certain amount of cross-reacting occurs, that is, animals affected with avian tuberculosis occasionally will give reactions with mammalian tuberculin and vice versa.

After an intradermal or intracutaneous injection of tuberculin an early polymorphonuclear and eosinophilic cell infiltration occurs at the point of injection, but these cells are soon replaced by histiocytic and mononuclear cells. Histamine apparently plays only a minor, if any, role in the tuberculin reaction.

Edema appears early and lasts for 5 to 7 days. Changes occur in the arteries of the region resulting in thrombosis of the vessels. These changes are those that occur in cattle, according to the studies of Feldman and Fitch (22).

In tuberculous rabbits the intravenous injection of tuberculin results in a destruction of erythrocytes accompanied by significant changes in mean corpuscular volume. Like changes occur in rabbits during the course of ultimately fatal infections without the injection of tuberculin. It may be that such effects are due to the liberation of tuberculin from foci of infection. It is possible that erythrocyte destruction occurs in human tuberculosis (86). There is evidence that individuals who are highly sensitive to tuberculin PPD develop a statistically significant elevation in serum alph-1 globulin during their response to the skin test (49).

**Immunity in Tuberculosis.** The waxy substance present in tubercle and other acid-fast bacilli serves to protect them against the antagonistic influences of the body. Even in naturally nonsusceptible species of animals, tubercle bacilli usually are destroyed only after a long time. In the sensitized animal a cellular immunity resides in the activated macrophages, enabling them to consume bacteria. Frequently the immune response in such species consists of a walling-off reaction in which the nidus of bacilli is surrounded by a dense wall of tissue that keeps the organisms more or less dormant.

That a form of immunity does occur in the course of tubercle infection was first shown in the so-called *phenomenon of Koch*. It was observed by Koch (53) that guinea pigs which were already infected with a low-grade tubercle infection reacted differently to a second inoculation of a culture of high virulence than animals which had not suffered the primary infection. The animals that were already infected proved to be refractory to the second dose. Whereas the previously normal animal developed an acute, progressively fatal disease, the previously infected developed only a swelling at the point of inoculation. This became a local abscess, which opened to the surface and sloughed away the necrotic tissue and the virulent bacilli without involvement of the neighboring lymph nodes. Much later Calmette and Guerin (11), using a dose of virulent tubercle bacilli intravenously which produced acute, fatal, miliary tuberculosis in normal cattle, found that tuberculin-reacting cattle (infected) could not be so killed. These animals showed an immediate reaction from which they rapidly recovered, and then they continued on their course of life as if nothing had happened. These experiments show that a new, more acute infection cannot be superimposed upon one already established; that a chronic disease is a protection from a more acute form.

These altered reactions are manifestations of a state of allergy. The relation of allergy to immunity is a question over which there has been a great deal of controversy. Some believe that allergy and immunity are identical; others think that they are different properties that have no relationship to each other. The allergic condition evidently has an important role to play in the course of the disease. When small infective doses of tubercle bacilli reach individuals of the susceptible species that have not previously encountered infection (initial infection), there is a marked tendency of the tissues to wall off the infection and to reduce it to a latent state. In allergic individuals, on the other hand, there is a tendency for the tissues to react with an acute, inflammatory reaction when tubercle bacilli, escaping from a primary lesion, find themselves deposited in a new location. These lesions do not tend to heal but rather to spread and to destroy large amounts of tissue. Some believe that one or two latent tubercles in the lungs of adult persons derived from old childhood infections render them somewhat resistent to serious reinfection later in life. Others think that the latent infections, because of the state of allergy produced, favor a spreading destructive disease when reinfections occur. Studies made by the U.S. Public Health Service support the former view. Their observations show that the degree of postvaccinal tuberculin sensitivity in guinea pigs is parallel with the degree of acquired resistance. Dannenberg, Jr. (15) claims that delayed hypersensitivity in tuberculosis is both beneficial and detrimental. In low concentrations, tuberculin stimulates the development of immunity in macrophages. Therefore, the presence of hypersensitivity is an asset in preventing pulmonary tuberculosis, for only small units of one to three bacilli reach the alveolar spaces where the infection begins. In high concentrations, tuberculin kills macrophages and thus is responsible for caseation and much of the tissue injury accompanying the disease.

**Artificial Immunization.** Because of its great importance, it is likely that more attempts have been made to find immunization methods for tuberculosis than for any other disease of man or animals. Unfortunately these methods have not met with a large measure of success. The earlier attempts at immunization have been reviewed by Mohler and Schroeder (65). The matter will not be discussed in detail here, but a few of the products that have been tried will be described briefly.

1. Tuberculin. This name has been given to a variety of aqueous extracts of tubercle bacilli. Tuberculin was first made by Koch (52) in the hope that it would have immunizing value, but these hopes have not been realized. In the course of the work of testing it on patients, its diagnostic value was discovered and it is for this purpose that it is used today.

2. Killed tubercle bacilli. When large numbers of tubercle bacilli, killed by heat or chemicals, are deposited in tissues, tuberculous tissue is produced around the deposit and abscessation is likely to occur. When used as vaccines, therefore, the dosage must be kept small. There is evidence that such vaccines enhance the resisting power of experimental animals somewhat, but the products have never been of service in practical work.

3. Living cultures. Numerous experiments with attenuated tubercle bacilli and with acid-fast organisms other than tubercle bacilli as vaccines for enhancing the resistance of animals to tuberculosis have been tried but with little success until recently. Perhaps the best known of these vaccines that have now been discarded was the *bovovaccine* of Von Behring, a vaccine which was widely heralded for protecting cattle. The nature of the vaccine was not disclosed for a long time but finally it became known that it consisted of a virulent strain of human tubercle bacilli. The vaccine will, indeed, confer a rather strong resistance on cattle, and with little damage to them, but the method was given up when it was learned that some of the vaccinated cattle were eliminating human tubercle bacilli in their milk.

Another highly publicized vaccine was that of Friedman, who came to the United States in the early part of the century with a "turtle serum" treatment for tuberculosis. Later it developed that the product was a suspension of living acid-fast bacilli that had been isolated from a turtle suffering from "cold-blood" tuberculosis. This vaccine proved worthless except as a means of enriching the pocket of the vendor.

*BCG vaccine.* The letters by which this vaccine is designated stand for the *bacillus of Calmette and Guerin* (11). These French workers cultured a bovine-type tubercle bacillus continuously on a bile-saturated medium for 13 years, during which the culture was renewed 70 times. Under these conditions it gradually changed in physical characteristics and lost in virulence until, at the end of the period, it had completely lost its tuberculogenic properties. For many years this culture has been used as a vaccine on many kinds of animals, monkeys, and man. It has proved to be quite harmless, and it confers an appreciable, but not absolute, resistance to tuberculosis on the part of individuals into which it has been injected.

To be effective it must be given before virulent tubercle infection has occurred. This means that it must be given very early in life, in most instances. It can be given to very young calves in areas in which bovine tuberculosis is prevalent, to reduce their susceptibility to tuberculous infection. It has not been employed for this purpose in the United States, because the eradication program has made it unnecessary. It is used rather widely on human infants born into tuberculous environments, largely in Europe but to some extent in the United States. Such infants usually successfully resist infection that destroys many not so protected (Holm, 46). It is also used on adult persons, negative to the tuberculin test, whose work brings them into close contact with patients suffering with tuberculosis. Since the incidence of tuberculous infection has fallen to a low figure in this country, it is obvious that our population is becoming more and more susceptible to infection as a result of the lack of early immunizing exposures. The need for a vaccine to protect young doctors, nurses, research workers, and hospital attendants is becoming more apparent. According to Holm, BCG vaccination of all children has been compulsory in Denmark since 1940, and the results have been excellent.

Calmette terms this method of immunization in which a mild, harmless infection is instituted to protect against a more virulent one, *premunizing*, and the result, a state of *premunition*. It is thought that the immunity conferred by the vaccine is transient, lasting only as long as the vaccine organisms persist in the tissues, a matter of not longer than a few months. Virulent infection, contracted during this period, is successfully resisted, and the lesions are walled off and arrested. These lesions constitute a protecting mechanism thereafter.

*The vole bacillus vaccine.* This organism was isolated by Wells (104) from voles or field mice in England in 1937. It is described on page 442. Wells and Brooke (105) found that, although this organism had relatively low virulence for guinea pigs, it had appreciable immunizing properties against both human and bovine types of tubercle bacilli. In comparison with BCG, they concluded that the vole bacillus gave the stronger protection. Birkhaug (9) in 1946 confirmed the work insofar as immunizing properties were concerned but did not find it any better than BCG, and he considered the latter somewhat safer for vaccine purposes because of its lower virulence. Griffith and Dalling (35) found that the vole bacillus considerably enhanced the resistance of calves against inoculation with virulent bovine tubercle cultures. This was manifested by the fact that the vaccinated calves lived considerably longer than the control animals. Nine calves, after vaccination, were given virulent tubercle cultures by mouth. Two control animals showed extensive glandular lesions when destroyed. Four of the vaccinated animals showed no lesions, and five only trivial glandular lesions. Living, virulent cultures were found in the tissues of the calves that showed no lesions, and it was felt that had the animals been allowed to live longer, tuberculosis probably would have developed after the influence of the vole bacillus had disappeared.

**Chemotherapy.** A large number of substances have been tried in the hope of finding a chemical agent that would destroy or restrain the development of tubercle bacilli in animal tissues and that would at the same time be tolerated by the host. For many years there were no hopeful results. In 1938 Rich and Follis (82) reported that sulfanilamide inhibited the development of experimental tuberculosis in the guinea pig. In 1942 Feldman, Hinshaw, and Moses (23) reported on the efficacy of a new drug, a sulfone compound known as *promin*. These results were encouraging, but the compounds had serious toxic properties that made their general application impossible.

According to a report to the Council on Pharmacy and Chemistry of the American Medical Association it now appears that streptomycin, *p*-aminosalicylic acid (PAS), and isoniazid constitute the major chemotherapeutic agents used in the treatment of tuberculosis in man. To this may now be added the combination of rifampin-isoniazid, which upon oral administration has proved effective and less toxic than the best regimen previously available. The use of terramycin is indicated when streptomycin resistance develops. Viomycin is limited in efficacy and is toxic. Amithiozone (tibione) is relatively ineffective. Pyrazinamide (aldinamide), although possessing immediate therapeutic effect, soon produces toxic manifestations in the patient. Synthesized modifications of isoniazid appear to be no more than secondary weapons—substitutes for streptomycin and isoniazid when tubercle bacilli become resistant to these drugs. Neomycin exerts too toxic an effect on the kidney and the auditory branch of the eighth cranial nerve. Mycomycin and erythromycin are ineffective *in vivo* (81). The report indicates that the treatment of tuberculosis has been advanced by the use of certain drugs, but much more effective ones must be found before we can rely on chemotherapy to cure tuberculosis. McDermott (59) published a review of the chemotherapy of tuberculosis in 1962. It appears that the resistance of *Myco. tuberculosis* to drug therapy is increasing. Gerszten *et al.* (30) state that patients with records of prior treatment develop chronic disease or die more frequently than patients without prior therapy.

Chemotherapeutic agents for tuberculosis probably will find little application in animals in this country, except possibly in poultry. In countries where bovine tuberculosis is still a serious problem, such agents may be used. To prevent the development of tuberculosis in calves exposed to heavily infected cattle Seelemann *et al.* (89) recommend the feeding of "Ferroteben" (a complex iron salt of *o*-oxybenzal-isonicotinic acid-hydrazid) at the rate of 10 mg per kg of body weight. Merkal and Thurston (62) found benzalkonium chloride to be bactericidal for saprophytic mycobacteria.

**Control Measures.** *In cattle.* BCG vaccination is used abroad to a limited extent to reduce the ravages of tuberculosis, but principal dependence everywhere is placed on the tuberculin test and the elimination of reactors for controlling this disease. In the United States and Canada the tuberculin test is being used systematically and country-wide with the object not only of controlling but of eradicating the disease. The method has been used in Great Britain for the same purpose.

The Federal-State Co-operative Plan for the Eradication of Bovine Tuberculosis was launched in the United States in 1917. This plan involved cooperation of the states with the federal government in a uniform approach to the solution of the problem. It became known as *The Accredited Herd Plan of Bovine Tuberculosis Eradication.* In outline the project was simple; in practice the agencies concerned had to meet many serious obstacles, not the least of which was strenuous opposition from a small portion of livestock owners. The plan was that every bovine animal in the country was to be subjected to tuberculin tests and those that reacted were to be removed and slaughtered. All slaughtered animals were subjected to veterinary meat inspection examinations to determine the extent of the development of the disease in each case and to ascertain whether or not any portions of the carcasses might be salvaged for human food. Before condemned animals were slaughtered, their market value was determined by experienced appraisers and the owners were

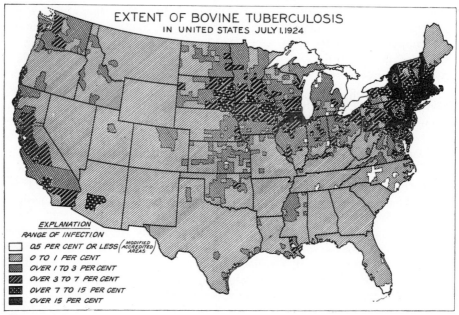

EXTENT OF BOVINE TUBERCULOSIS
IN UNITED STATES JULY 1, 1924

*EXPLANATION*
*RANGE OF INFECTION*

- 0.5 PER CENT OR LESS (MODIFIED ACCREDITED AREAS)
- 0 TO 1 PER CENT
- OVER 1 TO 3 PER CENT
- OVER 3 TO 7 PER CENT
- OVER 7 TO 15 PER CENT
- OVER 15 PER CENT

*Fig. 69.* This map showing the extent of bovine tuberculosis in the United States in 1924 conveys a good idea of the distribution of the disease before much progress had been made in the work of eradication.

reimbursed for their losses from the public treasuries of the federal and state governments.

The Accredited Herd Plan has met with excellent success. Whereas it was estimated in 1922 that about 4.0 percent of all cattle in the country were infected with tuberculosis, by 1940 the estimated number had been reduced to about 0.46 percent. The incidence of this disease had been reduced in less than 20 years by more than 85 percent. The great war, and the dislocations which occurred during and afterward, greatly decreased the efforts that could be put into this work, and there was little progress during the decade from 1940 to 1950, but the ground that had been gained earlier was not lost.

The eradication work has progressed steadily since normal conditions were restored following World War II. In January 1965 New Hampshire became the first state to attain an Accredited Tuberculosis-Free status. Maine achieved this goal in October 1967. Bovine tuberculosis has ceased to be an important public health or economic problem in this country, but the disease has not been eradicated, and it is clear that efforts will have to be continued for a considerable time before this objective is reached. Systematic testing of all cattle must continue in order that all centers of infection may be detected and stamped out. We now have a highly susceptible bovine population in which the disease could spread quickly if it got started.

Instructions for the *TB Manual* of the USDA, dated 11 Dec 1968 state: "When the presence of *M. bovis* has been confirmed by culture on any premises, liquidation of the herd remains the procedure of choice. Otherwise, the herd shall remain in quarantine until it has passed two negative tuberculin tests at intervals of at least 60 days and an additional two negative tuberculin tests at intervals of 6 months, the total quarantine period to be not less than 16 months after the last reactor has been disclosed. The entire herd must be included in three of the four required tests."

*In poultry.* The stamping out of tuberculosis in poultry is in many ways more difficult than in cattle because of widespread soil contamination. In the United States the disease occurs largely in the north-central states, although many other smaller infected areas exist. The disease is no longer a serious problem to commercial poultry raisers, largely because of their general practice of selling off all old birds annually and using as laying birds only those that were hatched the previous spring. Because tuberculosis develops slowly, very few birds less than 1 year old will develop "open" cases. Where this practice is used consistently, the disease tends to disappear from infected premises. The disease is serious principally in the barnyard flocks where poultry raising is incidental and not the principal business of the farmer. Such birds often range over the entire farm and are allowed to live for several years. Under such conditions advanced cases of the disease occur, and the premises are constantly reinfected.

The tuberculin test is useful in detecting infected flocks as well as infected birds. The removal of such birds will not eliminate the disease from the flock, because it is impossible to disinfect the soil, which continues for many months to cause new infections. If only a few affected birds are found, it is advisable to remove them and to retest the flock repeatedly at intervals of 1 or 2 months. If the percentage of reactors is high, it is best to advise slaughter of all birds and to start a new flock in new or thoroughly disinfected buildings located on soil that has not previously been occupied by birds. If old runs must be used, they should be plowed and cropped, and new birds should not be allowed on them for at least 1 year. The owners should be advised to eliminate the old flock annually and replace it with young birds.

*In man.* The elimination of tuberculosis from cattle has removed the hazard of bovine-type infection of man in the United States. Tuberculosis of the human type has been greatly reduced by education, early diagnosis, and hospitalization. The family continues to be the most important epidemiologic unit in the development of tuberculosis, and the adult members of the family are the most significant segment, both as sources of infection and as victims. The incidence of tuberculosis among employees and nurses at sanitoria remains high, and cases among medical students are more numerous than those in young adults in general. Control of the disease must be aimed at reducing infection of these classes. BCG vaccination has some value, but isolation, sanitation, and other factors must also be utilized.

*In other animals.* Because the three principal reservoirs of tubercle infection are in man, cattle, and poultry, the disease will disappear in other species as soon as these reservoirs are drained.

### Mycobacterium microti (The Vole Bacillus)

This organism might be termed a third type of mammalian tubercle organism. It was isolated by Wells (104) from wild voles (*Microtus agrestis*) caught in various parts of England. The disease closely resembles tuberculosis. The caseous lesions contain masses of acid-fast organisms that are different from previously known tubercle types. The disease itself is of little importance, but the causative agent serves to immunize animals against tuberculosis, and there is considerable interest in it for use as a practicable vaccine for both man and animals.

**Morphology and Staining Features.** The vole bacillus is much longer and more slender than human tubercle bacilli. Some organisms show granules and vacuolization along their entire length. Many cells assume S-shaped forms. Others are sickle-shaped, or rather spiral. Branched forms have not been seen. It is strongly Gram-positive and acid-fast. Like tubercle bacilli, it does not stain well with ordinary stains.

**Cultural Features.** Cultures grow very slowly. On the best media colonies are not usually seen until after a month's incubation at 37 C. They will not grow at room temperature. Nonglycerolated egg media is good for isolation. The colonies appear as pearly white conical or granular masses. The organism grows very well on potato after becoming adapted to growth on artificial media, but it will not grow on glycerol-egg or glycerol-agar media. It will grow as small filmy flakes on the surface of tryptinized broth but not on plain broth. A fine deposit forms in the depths of the fluid.

**Pathogenicity for Experimental Animals.** Relatively large doses (0.1 to 1.0 mg) injected intravenously in rabbits cause death from acute miliary tuberculosis. Small intravenous doses, or doses given subcutaneously, generally produce only trivial local lesions in which the bacilli gradually perish. Relatively large doses injected intraperitoneally in guinea pigs cause a generalized disease resembling acute tuberculosis. If the dose is not too large, the lesions in the organs tend to retrogress and the bacilli die out. When 1 to 5 mg of vole bacilli are injected intraperitoneally in white rats, lung lesions similar to those produced by other tubercle bacilli are produced. The rats usually do not die, and the organism has been found in the spleen of such animals for as long as 493 days. Noncaseous lesions resembling tubercles are found in the liver, spleen, and lymph nodes of golden hamsters inoculated subcutaneously. Fowls show no ill effects from inoculation with large doses of vole organisms, but the organism can be found as long as 4 months later in the spleen.

The immunizing properties of this organism are discussed on page 438.

## REFERENCES

1. Awad. Jour. Comp. Path. and Therap., 1958, 68, 324.
2. Badger, Breitwieser, and Muench. Am. Rev. Resp. Dis., 1963, 87, 338.
3. Bang. Maanedskr. f. Dyrlaeger, 1920, 31, 415.
4. Bates and Fitzhugh. Am. Rev. Resp. Dis., 1967, 96, 7.
5. Baumgarten. Centrbl. med. Wissenschr., 1882, 20, 257 and 337.
6. Beaudette and Hudson. Jour. Am. Vet. Med. Assoc., 1936, 89, 215.
7. Berry and Lowry. Jour. Am. Med. Assoc., 1953, 151, 1199.
8. Bickford, Ellis, and Moses. Jour. Am. Vet. Med. Assoc., 1966, 149, 312.
9. Birkhaug. Am. Rev. Tuberc., 1946, 53, 411.
10. Bruner. Jour. Inf. Dis., 1934, 55, 26.
11. Calmette and Guerin. Ann. l'Inst. Past., 1924, 38, 371; 1926, 40, 89.
12. Chargoff, Pangborn, and Anderson. Jour. Biol. Chem., 1931, 90, 45.
13. Clancey. Jour. Path. and Bact., 1964, 88, 175.
14. Cummings, Drummond, and Lewis. Pub. Health Rpts. (U.S.), 1948, 63, 1305.
15. Dannenberg, Jr. Bact. Rev., 1968, 32, 85.
16. Dorset. Am. Med., 1902, 3, 555.
17. Doyle, Evander, and Gruft. Am. Rev. Resp. Dis., 1968, 97, 919.
18. Dubos. Proc. Soc. Exp. Biol. and Med., 1945, 58, 361.
19. *Ibid.*, 1946, 63, 56.
20. Dubos and Middlebrook. Am. Rev. Tuberc., 1947, 56, 334.
21. Feldman. Ann. N.Y. Acad. Sci., 1947, 48, 469.
22. Feldman and Fitch. Arch. Path., 1937, 24, 599.
23. Feldman, Hinshaw, and Moses. Am. Rev. Tuberc., 1942, 45, 303.
24. Feldman, Hutchinson, Schwarting, and Karlson. Am. Jour. Path., 1949, 25, 1183.

25.  Feldman and Karlson.   Am. Rev. Tuberc., 1957, 75, 266.
26.  Fenner.   *Ibid.*, 1956, 73, 650.
27.  Fincher, Evans, and Saunders.   Cornell Vet., 1954, 44, 240.
28.  Fisher and Gregory.   Austral. Vet. Jour., 1951, 27, 25.
29.  Fite and Olson.   Pub. Health Rpts. (U.S.), 1944, 59, 1423.
30.  Gerszten, Brummer, Allison, and Hench.   Jour. Am. Med. Assoc., 1963, 185, 6.
31.  Gilkerson and Kanner.   Jour. Bact., 1963, 86, 890.
32.  Gordon and Mihm.   Jour. Gen. Microbiol., 1959, 21, 736.
33.  Griffith.   Jour. Comp. Path. and Therap., 1928, 41, 122.
34.  Griffith.   Jour. Hyg. (London), 1957, 55, 1.
35.  Griffith and Dalling.   *Ibid.*, 1940, 40, 673.
36.  Guilbridge, Rollinson, McAnulty, Alley, and Wells.   Jour. Comp. Path. and Therap., 1963, 73, 337.
37.  Hall and Winkel.   Jour. Am. Vet. Med. Assoc., 1957, 131, 49.
38.  Harrington and Karlson.   Am. Jour. Vet. Res., 1966, 27, 1193.
39.  Harshfield, Roderick, and Hawn.   Jour. Am. Vet. Med. Assoc., 1937, 91, 323.
40.  Hawthorne and Lauder.   Am. Rev. Resp. Dis., 1962, 85, 858.
41.  Hendrix, Jr., Nichols, and Hursh.   Am. Jour. Pub. Health, 1966, 56, 818.
42.  Hirsch.   Am. Rev. Tuberc., 1954, 70, 955.
43.  Hix, Jones, and Karlson.   Jour. Am. Vet. Med. Assoc., 1961, 138, 641.
44.  Hobby, Redmond, Runyon, Schaffer, Wayne, and Wichelhausen.   Am. Rev. Resp. Dis., 1967, 95, 954.
45.  Hok, Seng, Yen, and San.   *Ibid.*, 1966, 94, 620.
46.  Holm.   Pub. Health Rpts. (U.S.), 1946, 61, 1298.
47.  Janicki and Aron.   Jour. Immunol., 1968, 101, 121.
48.  Kerr, Lamont, and McGirr.   Vet. Rec., 1946, 58, 443 and 451.
49.  Klein and Patnode.   Proc. Soc. Exp. Biol. and Med., 1963, 113, 627.
50.  Koch.   Berl. klin. Wchnschr., 1882, 19, 221.
51.  Koch.   Mittheilung. Gesundheitsamte, 1884, 2, 1.
52.  Koch.   Centrbl. f. Bakt., 1890, 8, 563.
53.  Koch.   Deut. med. Wchnschr., 1891, 17, 101.
54.  Kubin, Krumi, Horak, Lukavsky, and Vanek.   Am. Rev. Resp. Dis., 1966, 94, 20.
55.  Lesslie and Birn.   Vet. Rec., 1967, 80, 559.
56.  Lesslie and Davies.   *Ibid.*, 1958, 70, 82.
57.  Long and Seibert.   Trans. Nat. Tuberc. Assoc., 1926, p. 270.
58.  Luke.   Vet. Rec., 1958, 70, 529.
59.  McDermott.   Am. Rev. Resp. Dis., 1962, 86, 323.
60.  McFadyean.   Jour. Comp. Path. and Therap., 1910, 23, 239.
61.  Maitland.   Jour. Hyg. (London), 1950, 48, 397.
62.  Merkal and Thurston.   Am. Jour. Vet. Res., 1968, 29, 757.
63.  Mitchell and Duthie.   Am. Rev. Tuberc., 1929, 19, 134.
64.  Mitchell and Duthie.   Canad. Jour. Res., 1930, 2, 406.
65.  Mohler and Schroeder.   Proc. Am. Vet. Med. Assoc., 1909, p. 252.
66.  Moore.   Am. Jour. Path., 1942, 18, 827.
67.  Moses, Feldman, and Mann.   Am. Jour. Vet. Res., 1943, 4, 390.
68.  Nocard and Roux.   Ann. l'Inst. Past., 1887, 1, 19.
69.  Olsson.   Cornell Vet., 1957, 47, 193.

70. Park and Krumwiede. Jour. Med. Res., 1911, *20*, 313; 1912, *22*, 109.
71. Pearson and McGowan. Brit. Vet. Jour., 1958, *114*, 477.
72. Peterson. Jour. Am. Vet. Med. Assoc., 1965, *147*, 1600.
73. Plum. Acta Path. et Microbiol. Scand., 1938, Sup. 37, 438.
74. Powers and Price. Jour. Am. Vet. Med. Assoc., 1967, *151*, 890.
75. Priestley. Vet. Rec. 1946, *58*, 455.
76. Pulling. Jour. Am. Vet. Med. Assoc., 1952, *121*, 389.
77. Ravenel and Reichel. Jour. Med. Res., 1908, *13*, 1.
78. Redmond and Cater. Am. Rev. Resp. Dis., 1960, *82*, 781.
79. Reed and Morgante. Am. Jour. Med. Sci., 1956, *231*, 320.
80. Reimann and Pik-Chun-Ma. Am. Rev. Resp. Dis., 1965, *92*, 193.
81. Rpt. to the Council on Pharmacy and Chemistry. Jour. Am. Med. Assoc., 1954, *154*, 52.
82. Rich and Follis. Johns Hopkins Hosp. Bul., 1938, *62*, 77.
83. Rivolta. Gior. di anat. e fisol., 1889, *1*, 122.
84. Runyon. Am. Jour. Clin. Path., 1970, *54*, 578.
85. Sabin. Jour. Exp. Med., 1930, 52, Sup. 3.
86. Sandage, Brandt, and Birkeland. Jour. Inf. Dis., 1951, *88*, 9.
87. Schaefer. Am. Rev. Resp. Dis., 1965, *92*, 85.
88. Schalk, Roderick, Foust, and Harshfield. N. Dak. Agr. Exp. Sta. Tech. Bul. 279, 1935.
89. Seelemann, Buschkiel, and Rackow. Centrbl. f. Vet-Med., 1957, *4*, 80.
90. Seneviratna, Wettimuny, and Seneviratna. Vet. Med., 1966, *61*, 129.
91. Smith. Jour. Exp. Med., 1898, *3*, 451.
92. Smith. Jour. Med. Res., 1905, 7, 253; 1905, *8*, 405.
93. Soliman, Rollinson, Barron, and Spratling. Vet. Rec., 1953, *65*, 421.
94. Stamp. *Ibid.*, 1944, *56*, 443.
95. Stanford and Beck. Jour. Path. and Bact., 1968, *95*, 131.
96. Steele. Jour. Am. Vet. Med. Assoc., 1954, *125*, 280.
97. Stuart and Marshall. Vet. Rec., 1952, *64*, 309.
98. Tarshia and Frisch. Am. Jour. Clin. Path., 1951, *21*, 101.
99. Thordal-Christensen. Nord. Vetmed., 1952, *4*, 577.
100. Tilden and Williamson. Jour. Am. Vet. Med. Assoc., 1957, *131*, 526.
101. Tolhurst, Buckle, and Wellington. Jour. Hyg. (London), 1959, *57*, 47.
102. Verge and Senthille. Rec. Med. Vet., 1942, *118*, 49.
103. Villemin. Comp. rend. Acad. Sci., 1865, *61*, 1012.
104. Wells. Brit. Jour. Exp. Path., 1938, *19*, 324.
105. Wells and Brooke. *Ibid.*, 1940, *21*, 104.
106. Whitehead and Corson. Cornell Vet., 1962, *52*, 36.
107. Wilkinson. Vet. Rec., 1964, *76*, 777.
108. Wilton and Vance. Canad. Jour. Comp. Med. and Vet. Sci., 1959, *23*, 256.

## *Mycobacterium paratuberculosis*

SYNONYMS: *Mycobacterium johnei, Mycobacterium enteritidis,* Johne's bacillus, bacillus of Johne's disease

This organism causes disease in cattle, sheep, goats, llamas, and some wild ruminants. It has been reported in the European red deer (80). It has been described in horses and a donkey (Larsen *et al.* Am. Jour. Vet. Res., 1972,

33, 2185). In English-speaking countries it is usually known as *Johne's disease*. It is also known as *paratuberculosis, chronic bacterial enteritis, chronic hypertrophic enteritis,* and a number of colloquial names. The causative organism was first recognized in Germany by Johne and Frothingham (28) in 1895, who saw it in the tissues of diseased cattle. These workers mistook the organisms for avian tubercle bacilli and thought they were dealing with an isolated case of a peculiar nature. Later it was recognized that many cases of this disease occurred. They were regarded as atypical tuberculosis until 1905, when Bang (2) in Denmark showed that it could readily be transmitted to other cattle and that the disease was not a form of tuberculosis but a separate entity. *Mycobacterium paratuberculosis* was first isolated and grown in artificial media by Twort (76) in 1911. Many others have isolated the organism from cattle since that time by using a special technic developed by Twort.

Howarth (26), Dunkin (10), McEwen (45), and others who have worked with sheep and goats have failed in their attempts to isolate *Myco. paratuberculosis* from these species using the technic that generally succeeds with cattle material. In 1945 Taylor (71) claimed to have cultivated the organism in 4 out of 15 attempts. All four animals from which cultures were derived came from a single farm. McEwen (45), Hagan (19), and Levi (42) found no difficulty in infecting sheep with material from cattle, and all were able to recover the organisms in culture. Taylor's original successes may have been with a strain of this type. Later Taylor (74) isolated a strain from sheep in Iceland and two from sheep in Scotland. One of the Scottish strains was considered to be the classical bovine type and the other was a highly pigmented strain. The Icelandic strain was similar to the classic variety. Taylor stated that growth of the Icelandic and pigmented strains, hitherto said to be resistant to artificial cultivation, was obtained on media that contained 60 percent egg yolk and that both were probably varieties of the classical type. He also showed that these two strains were capable of producing clinical Johne's disease in cattle and that they retained their cultural characteristics after one passage through cattle (75). It seems reasonable to conclude that the same species of organism is found in cattle, sheep, and goats, but that unrecognized host factors render cultivation from sheep and goats more difficult than from cattle. In 1965, Stuart (70) recovered a pigmented variant of *Myco. paratuberculosis* from an experimentally infected cow. It differed from the pigmented sheep strains only in some cultural characteristics.

**Morphology and Staining Reactions.** *Myco. paratuberculosis* appears in both tissues and cultures as a short, thick rod measuring about 0.5 by 1.0 micron. It is considerably smaller than any of the tubercle bacilli. In tissues and feces it commonly appears in clumps, some containing a great many organisms. This arrangement is an aid in its identification. It is strongly acid- and alcohol-fast and Gram-positive. It has neither spores nor capsules. In tissues it develops intracellularly in the epithelioid and giant cells which appear at the site of localization.

**Cultural Features.** The causative agent of Johne's disease was first obtained in artificial culture by Twort (76) in 1911. This worker succeeded in obtaining growth after earlier workers had failed by the expedient of incorporating in his media a suspension of heat-killed acid-fast organisms of other species. This was done after he had experienced repeated failures to obtain growth of this organism on a variety of media that are suitable for tubercle bacilli. It occurred to Twort that perhaps some essential substance for growth of the Johne bacillus was absent from his media and that possibly whatever was needed might exist in the substance of other acid-fast organisms. Having proved the correctness of this hypothesis, he sought to isolate this "essential substance" by extracting the cultures and by using extracts of many other substances. It was found that both water and fat solvents were capable of removing the necessary substance from several species of acid-fast organisms, but extracts of other bacteria and of plant and animal tissues did not contain it. All of this work was described in detail by Twort and Ingram (77) in 1913. Little more was learned of the nature of this "essential substance" until the work of Wooley and McCarter (81) appeared in 1940. These authors showed that "phthiocol," which Newman, Crowder, and Anderson (51) had isolated from the human tubercle bacillus in 1934, had the qualities of the necessary factor. Almquist and Klose (1) in 1939 had shown that phthiocol possessed the antihemorrhagic qualities of vitamin K; therefore Wooley and McCarter tried the synthetic vitamin K (2-methyl naphthoquinone) and found it also to be effective. However, their cultures did not thrive quite so well with the extracts as with suspensions of acid-fast bacteria.

In 1953 Francis et al. (13) isolated from *Myco. phlei* a substance which they named *mycobactin*. They claimed that this material occurred in relatively high concentration (1 percent of dry weight) in this organism and that it possessed most if not all of the "essential substance" of Twort. They succeeded in isolating their factor as a crystalline aluminium complex and also in an amorphous metal-free form. They indicated that it is not phthiocol, that it is a hitherto-undescribed compound, and that it bears the probable empirical formula of $C_{47}H_{75}O_{10}N_5$. More recent findings on mycobactins, iron-chelating growth factors from mycobacteria, were published by Snow (67) in 1970.

Primary cultures of the Johne organism grow very slowly on all media, much more slowly than tubercle bacilli. On Dorset's egg medium, fortified with about 5 percent, by weight, of the moist cells of one of the rapidly growing saprophytic acid-fast organisms added before sterilization and coagulation, the organism can be grown without great difficulty from infected lymph nodes, where it often exists in the absence of other bacteria. The cultures must be incubated at 37 C for about 6 weeks before evidences of growth appear. During the period of incubation the tubes must be partially closed so that evaporation will not cause dehydration of the media. Growth appears in the form of very small, dry, irregular colonies, not unlike primary cultures of mammalian tubercle bacilli. When these are subcultured on fresh media of the same type, a confluent growth is obtained. This usually is visible after 2 or 3 weeks' incubation but reaches its maximum only after 5 or 6 weeks.

Other media recommended for the primary culture of the Johne bacillus are Taylor's modification of Finlayson's egg medium (73) and Smith's modified Dubos' solid and liquid media (65). For primary cultivation of *Myco. paratuberculosis*, Merkal *et al.* (49) advocate the use of benzalkonium chloride as a decontaminant followed by inoculation onto modified Herrold's medium (an egg-yolk agar plus mycobactin). A lymph-node-egg-yolk medium proved to be less satisfactory. Organisms accustomed to growth in the laboratory are dry and flaky and of a cream color. Even after many years of artificial culture, the organism will give little or no growth on most of the media that serve for tubercle bacilli if the essential supplement is not added. Meager growths may occur, but, if so, they will fail after two or three transplants on the same unfortified medium.

It is usually difficult to train this organism to grow on fluid media. On ordinary glycerol broth to which the "essential substance" has been added in the form of the killed cells of *Myco. phlei*, growth is always poor. After several months' incubation, small floating islands of growth may develop, and there may be considerable sediment in the bottom of the flasks, but complete pellicles are rarely formed. Synthetic media, especially those of Long (43) and Dorset, Henley, and Moskey (6), and Smith's modified Dubos' liquid medium are much more successful. It is generally necessary to add "essential substance" to these media in the beginning, but after a few generations many strains can be induced to grow without it. Strains adapted to such media often grow profusely and heavily. These growths resemble those of mammalian tubercle bacilli, being dry, rough, folded pellicles with clear underlying medium.

**Resistance.** The organism of Johne's disease has about the same degree of resistance to deleterious influences as tubercle bacilli. It is resistant to acids and alkalies and to antiformin. These substances are used to treat contaminated tissues and fecal material in order to eliminate other bacteria when cultures are made. Lovell, Levi, and Francis (44) found that cultures remained viable in sterilized water for more than 9 months. Cultures were recovered from intestinal scrapings suspended in unsterilized river water for 163 days. Bacilli stored first at $-14$ C for 5 months, then at 4 C for 5 months, and finally at 38 C for 8 months were still viable (38).

Naturally infected feces showed viable bacilli when exposed to atmospheric conditions but kept moist for as long as 245 days. The organism is highly resistant to penicillin; in fact, this antibiotic is sometimes added to culture media to prevent growth of other contaminating bacteria (65).

**Pathogenicity for Experimental Animals.** None of the small laboratory animals are very susceptible to infection with *Myco. paratuberculosis*. Large doses injected into local tissues, or into the body cavities, will cause necrosis and pro-

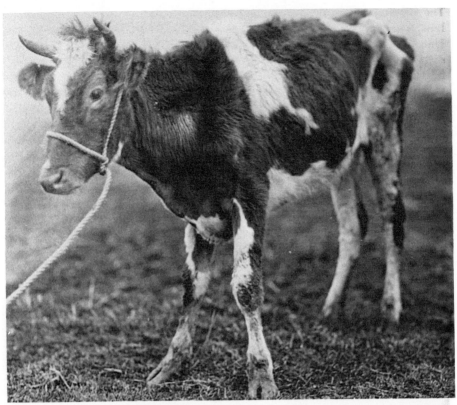

*Fig.70.* An advanced case of Johne's disease. The animal is emaciated, has a rough dry coat, a harsh skin, is constantly scouring, and is so weak that it must brace its legs to keep from falling. This animal had been artificially infected slightly more than 1 year previously by being fed material that contained the organism.

liferation of tissue. In the peritoneum tuberclelike masses of tissue appear around clumps of the infected organisms. These are not evidence of infection, but merely the reactions to lipoids contained in the bacterial cells. The cells do not multiply, and the lesions gradually disappear. Francis (12), in England, has reported apparent success in infecting very young mice (13 to 14 days old) and young hamsters by feeding them with massive doses of cultures of *Myco. paratuberculosis*. Chandler (5) has also infected mice, and Gilmour *et al.* (16) have studied the pathogenesis of Johne's disease in orally dosed hamsters. It appears that the use of such animals in diagnostic work is limited, especially in cases where relatively small numbers of organisms are encountered.

Experimental infections have been established in calves (17), sheep (33), and pigs (32) by oral administration of large doses of Johne's bacilli. The disease has been induced in colts by intravenous inoculation (Larsen *et al.* Am. Jour. Vet. Res., 1972, 33, 2185).

**The Natural Disease.** Johne's disease is prevalent in France, Belgium, Holland, Denmark, and the British Isles. The disease occurs throughout the United States and Canada, but it does not appear to be a serious problem in many areas. It is probable that the disease is more prevalent than is now believed. Taylor (72) cultured the ileocecal lymph nodes of 243 adult cattle slaughtered routinely in the Berkshire abattoir in England for Johne's bacilli. He succeeded in isolating cultures from 37 animals, an incidence of 15 percent. He concludes that this high percentage indicates that the infection is much more prevalent in England than clinical cases would suggest. Rankin (54) recovered *Myco. paratuberculosis* from lymph nodes of 6 and 7.5 percent of two groups of apparently normal English cattle. The corresponding figure for cattle from Ireland slaughtered in England was 0.8 percent. He also identified a culture of this species taken from a mesenteric lymph gland of a horse that had shown no clinical signs of illness (55). In all the countries mentioned, the infection is best known in cattle, but it also occurs in sheep. We have even less information about its distribution in sheep than we have in cattle. It has been identified in both sheep and goats in the United States.

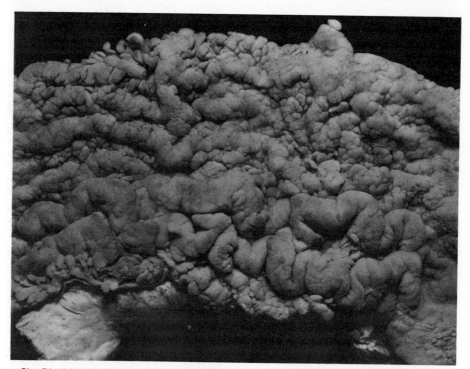

*Fig. 71.* Johne's disease, showing the mucous membrane of a portion of the ileum. The wall is greatly thickened by large deposits of epithelioid cells in the subepithelial tissue of the mucosa. The irregular folds and plaques are characteristic. There is a complete absence of ulcers and necrosis.

It is a disease of young animals. Cattle seldom develop symptoms after 5 years of age, and most cases appear in 2- and 3-year-old females. The disease most often becomes apparent in the early part of the first or second lactation period. The greatest losses occur among high-producing animals. The strain of lactation breaks down the resistance of the animal to an infection that previously had been latent. The organism lodges in the intestinal canal and the lymph nodes of the mesentery. The lower end of the small intestine, the cecum, and the beginning of the colon are the parts most often involved, but advanced cases may show lesions in all parts of the alimentary canal from the stomach to the anus. The lesions in the intestinal wall take the form of a thickening that may be very obvious or very slight. This thickening is caused by the proliferation of great masses of epithelioid cells in the lower layers of the mucosa and the submucosa. Unlike tubercle infections, there are no tubercles and no necrosis. The epithelium always remains intact, but it is often thrown into deep folds that cannot be flattened by stretching of the gut wall. The mesenteric lymph nodes never show great enlargement or necrosis, but they are often slightly enlarged. Sometimes the lymphatics on the serous surface of the affected bowel become filled with epithelioid cells which convert the usually inconspicuous channels into glassy, tortuous cords along the mesenteric attachment. Great numbers of small acid-fast organisms usually can be easily demonstrated in films made from scrapings from the cut surface of the thickened portion of the intestinal wall, or from that of the lymph nodes which drain the affected areas. The organisms are usually found in clumps,

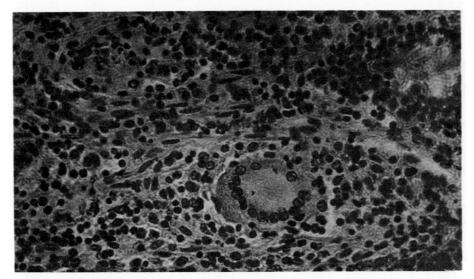

*Fig. 72.* Johne's disease, a section through the subepithelial tissue of the mucosa of the small intestine of an acute case, showing the epithelioid cells that infiltrate this tissue and cause thickening of the mucosa. A typical giant cell is shown. X 600.

and many of them are located intracellularly. In sections, most of the organisms are present in the epithelioid cells. Large giant cells, of the type seen in tubercles, are usually conspicuous in sections.

Lesions in other organs are rare. Organisms sometimes can be demonstrated in the liver but lesions are absent. Although reports of uterine infection in cattle are few Pearson (52) records two cases in cattle in England in which infection occurred in the uterine mucosa, and in one of these a congenital infection of the fetus was found, the organism being isolated from the ileocecal lymph nodes and bowel of the fetus, and in 1967, Kopecky et al. (34) found 18 cases of uterine infection among 148 culls of a 1,000-cow dairy herd in which paratuberculosis was a problem. Fourteen of these 18 positive specimens came from cows that presented no clinical evidence of Johne's disease. It is possible that transuterine infection is not as uncommon as originally believed. Doyle (8) examined the udder tissue of 34 cows clinically affected with Johne's disease and obtained positive cultures from the udders of two. He concluded that the excretion of Johne's bacilli in the milk is rare and probably occurs only in the fulminating type of infection. In old cases of Johne's disease, calcareous plaques often can be found in the large blood ves-

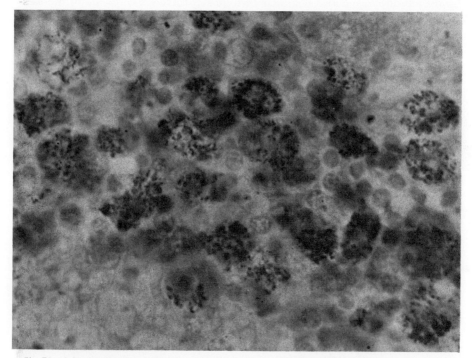

Fig. 73. Johne's disease, showing epithelioid cells in the mucous membrane of a rapidly progressive case of the disease. The cells are packed with masses of *Mycobacterium paratuberculosis*. This preparation had been stained with the Ziehl-Neelsen technic for acid-fast bacteria. In preparations stained with hematoxylin and eosin these cells appear quite normal. X 1,000.

sels near the heart (Hagan, 19; Gifford, Eveleth, and Gifford, 14). Organisms cannot be demonstrated in these lesions, which are believed to be caused by metabolic disturbances occasioned by the disease.

Larsen and Kopecky (36) examined the genital organs of six bulls having clinical signs of paratuberculosis and found Johne's bacilli in these organs from all six animals.

Stewart, McCallum, and Taylor (69) studied the blood picture in cases of Johne's disease in cattle and sheep. A lowered hemoglobin was found, also a reduced content of calcium and magnesium. Because hemoglobin and calcium are often low in emaciated animals, whatever the cause, they regarded these levels of little significance. The lowered magnesium level, however, is unusual, and the authors considered it of some diagnostic value. As a result of their study of sheep, they determined the normal level of this element to be $2.65 \pm 0.21$ mg percent, whereas the average level of 19 cases of Johne's disease was 1.98. In cattle, the normal blood level was considered to be $2.98 \pm 0.28$, whereas the average of 15 cases of Johne's disease was 2.20.

The symptoms of Johne's disease are quite variable. It is clear that many animals harbor the disease and probably are spreaders of infection, without showing any definite evidence of malfunction. It is clear, also, that many infected animals recover from the disease. Allergic tests indicate that in infected herds there usually are many infected animals that never show evidence of the disease. The usual history of an infected herd is that losses are never heavy at any one time, but new cases continue to appear from time to time and the losses over a period of years may be considerable. Evidence indicates that factors other than the organism itself are responsible for the clinical cases. Smythe (66) in England has pointed out that, although the infection may exist in herds that are raised on alkaline soils, high in lime, the disease does not usually seriously affect them. When such animals are moved to acid soils, they often develop clinical symptoms shortly thereafter. Jansen (27) has pointed out the same thing in Holland, it has been observed in France, and there is similar evidence in the United States. It seems likely that some soil deficiencies may have an important effect upon the development of the disease. In line with this thought, of course, is the old observation that the disease, which has been latent in young heifers, often appears suddenly during the early part of the lactation period—a time when the mineral balance of the animal is suffering strain.

The initial symptoms are vague. One of the earliest is edema of the intermandibular space. General unthriftiness quickly becomes evident. The hair coat becomes dry, and the skin loses its normal pliability. A diarrhea begins and frequently is very profuse. The body temperature at this time is normal. The gluteal muscles begin to shrink, and the tail and hind legs become soiled with the liquid feces. If the scouring continues, dehydration occurs and general emaciation develops. The postorbital fat disappears and the eyes sink into their sockets. The animal stands listlessly and cannot be induced to eat for many days. Death may occur within a week from the time the diarrhea begins. On the other hand, many animals after scouring for a few days will cease to do so, their appetite will return, and there may be much improvement in condition. This may last only a short time and be followed by a second attack of scouring, or it may be permanent. Some cases will apparently recover completely only to break down during the early part of the next lactation period the following year (Hagan and Zeissig, 21).

The foregoing description has dealt with the disease in cattle. In sheep and goats the symptoms and lesions are similar. The disease apparently may be more acute in these animals than in cattle. The lesions frequently are not conspicuous. Instead of great bowel-wall thickening, often there may be no observable thickening but petechial hemorrhages may be seen. In some cases, however, the thickening is marked and similar to that seen in cattle. A study by Stamp and Watt (68) of the pathology of Johne's disease in sheep as it occurs in Scotland also indicates that the lesions vary from insignificant to characteristic masses of epithelioid and giant cells which may undergo encapsulation, necrosis, caseation, and calcification. They suggest that the pigmented variety of *Myco. paratuberculosis* is more virulent for sheep than is the classical strain. Nakamatsu *et al.* (50) conducted a histopathological study on 45 naturally infected goats and determined that the lesions were located mainly in the intestines and regional lymph nodes. They concluded that certain remote lesions occurring in the kidneys, walls of capillaries, and connective tissues were of an allergic nature rather than the result of direct contact with *Myco. paratuberculosis*.

**Mode of Transmission.** Experimentally it is easy to produce infections in young calves by drenching them with infected materials. Very large doses will usually produce clinical symptoms in from 6 to 18 months when the animal is infected before it is 1 year old. Older animals can be readily infected by mouth with large doses of material, but they do not usually develop clinical symptoms and they often throw off the infection completely. Factors other than the virulence of cultures determine whether or not the clinically obvious disease will be produced.

Although it would appear that the natural route of infection is by the way of the mouth it is evident that transuterine infection must be considered and there is also the possibility that the infected bull may be the agent that transmits the disease to the cow (34, 36, 52).

Vallee and Rinjard (78) showed that subcutaneous injection of this organism never produces the disease. A local lesion develops which is gradually absorbed. Rankin (57) injected 3-year-old cattle intravenously with *Myco. paratuberculosis* and, although he could recover the organism from the lymphatic systems of his animals 4 years after inoculation, none developed clinical Johne's disease within this period. Exposure of calves to an environment naturally contaminated with *Myco. paratuberculosis* usually leads to the development of infected animals, whereas exposure of adult cattle to the same conditions seldom does (58, 59).

**Diagnosis.** Several methods are available for detecting the presence of this disease in animals. The principal ones are as follows:

1. *Clinical methods.* Animals that persistently scour and emaciate should be looked upon with suspicion. If such animals die or are slaughtered, a portion of the lower end of the small intestine should be sent to a laboratory to be examined.

2. *Examination of Feces.* Positive diagnoses may be made in many cases by staining fecal samples. Small shreds of mucus should be sought and spread on new, chemically cleaned slides, which are stained with the Ziehl-Neelson technic. The specific organism is quite small and has a tendency to occur in clumps. It must be distinguished from larger acid-fast organisms, which are common in cattle feces. Levi (41) has shown that it is possible to cultivate the organism from many samples of feces which are only suspicious on microscopic examination or microscopically negative. This is a laborious task hardly applicable to general use but it may be of some value in especially important cases. Harding (25) has used fluorescent microscopy to detect *Myco. paratuberculosis* in sections of tissues. It should be possible to use this technic in fecal examinations.

Various methods for concentrating the organisms present in intestinal mucosa and in feces are in use. The thorough mixing of infective material, distilled water, and white gasoline followed by centrifugation is effective in drawing acid-fast bacteria into the interface of the treated specimen. Trypsin digestion of tissue also facilitates the demonstration of small numbers of bacilli (37).

In clinical Johne's disease in the cow an examination of the milk may reveal the organism, but negative results are not a reliable means of diagnosis.

3. *Scrapings from the rectal mucous membrane.* In a certain number of advanced cases, probably not more than one-fourth of all of them, the disease spreads to the lower bowel and even the rectum. In such cases the thickened rectal mucosa may be recognized by palpation. If no thickening is recognized, a bit of the mucosa may be obtained for microscopic examination. The fragment should be well rinsed with clean water, placed on a slide, and crushed. Films made from the crushed fragment then are stained for acid-fast organisms. It should be kept in mind that acid-fast bacteria occur in the feces of all cows and that these must be differentiated from the bacillus of Johne's disease. The Johne bacillus is smaller than most of the saprophytic forms, and it occurs in characteristic clumps. An experienced observer usually can be sure of the identification of the organisms seen.

4. *The allergic tests.* In 1909, before the bacillus of Johne's disease had been cultivated artificially, Oluf Bang (3) called attention to the fact that many infected animals would react to avian tuberculin administered subcutaneously. This test was used by many workers with fairly satisfactory results. One of Twort's first efforts after obtaining pure cultures of the organism causing Johne's disease was to make a product analogous to tuberculin for use in diagnosis. Twort's cultures grew rather poorly, however, and the products

which he was able to make were not successful, although it was demonstrated that reactions could be obtained in some animals. Beach and Hastings (4), in this country, were the first to use johnin, or paratuberculin, intravenously. Their work, and that of others (35), has demonstrated that this method of administration is more effective than is subcutaneous injection. It has not been demonstrated, however, that johnin is any more effective, or has any advantages over, avian tuberculin when used intravenously.

The physiological reaction following the intravenous injection of johnin and avian tuberculin is the same. Normal animals, if not overdosed, show little or no reaction. Diseased animals, however, usually begin to show signs of discomfort within an hour or so. There is depression, the animal ceases to eat, the head is held low, the hair coat stands on end, and the animal may shiver. Some animals begin to scour profusely and this may last for several days. The fever curve begins from the 3rd to the 5th hour after injection of the test material and reaches its height from the 5th to the 8th hour, depending upon the size of the dose and the potency of the test fluid. After the peak has been reached, the temperature usually falls quickly to normal by the 10th or 12th hour (Hagan and Zeissig, 22).

The potency of the early johnins was low. When it was learned how to cultivate *Myco. paratuberculosis* in synthetic media without the addition of extracts of other acid-fast organisms, and when profuse growths were produced, much better allergic products were obtained. With such products attention was turned to the application of the intradermal test. Johnson (29) and Johnson and Cox (30) in the United States, McIntosh and Konst (46) in Canada, and a number of English workers have produced potent johnin and have devised methods of obtaining standardized products. Undoubtedly these are more potent and more specific than the earlier products used, and, according to Sikes (64), the intradermal johnin test when properly applied is a highly efficient biological test for sensitivity to *Myco. paratuberculosis* infection in cattle. He cautions against repeated tests in the same site, claiming that such procedure results in negative tests in infected animals. A new site for each test is best; otherwise let 20 weeks elapse between tests.

Unfortunately, all johnins fail to elicit reactions in some cases of the disease. Also, they cause reactions in cattle that appear to be noninfected, but on this score the fault, in many cases at least, is that there are no methods to confirm the presence of the disease at autopsy. In some cases the lesions are so slight or so inconspicuous that great difficulty is experienced in finding them. In herds in which occasional clinical cases are occurring, it is not uncommon to find a considerable number of reacting animals. Many of these animals, if not destroyed as a result of the test, live their normal life spans without exhibiting symptoms and frequently fail to react on tests administered later. This is part of the evidence that adult animals often harbor the infection without showing it, and that they often free themselves of it spontaneously.

Allergic tests are of value in determining the existence of the disease in herds, and, if the number of reactors is small, it may be eliminated, in some cases at least, by destroying the reactors.

5. *Serological tests*. Hagan and Zeissig (23) found that the complement-fixation test could be used for the diagnosis of Johne's disease in cattle. The antigens were made from tubercle bacilli and therefore were nonspecific. They would be of little value in animals sensitized by any other acid-fast organisms, including tubercle bacilli. In their experimentally infected cattle, the test became positive as soon as the allergic tests, and long before clinical symptoms appeared, and it remained positive in animals so debilitated from the disease that they would no longer react to allergic tests. It was in such cases that the test was believed to have its principal value. It was obvious, however, that many animals that probably were not infected with Johne's disease reacted, presumably because of sensitization with heterologous antigens. Sirgurdsson, Vigfusson, and Theodors (63), working with sheep in Iceland, also found the test of value. Their antigen was made by extracting the affected intestinal mucosa of animals suffering from the disease and may be regarded as specific. It is of interest to note that this antigen had to be separated from an "inhibitor," a substance that inhibited complement fixation. The inhibitor was also present in the intestinal mucosa of infected sheep; it appeared to be a product of the pathogenic process and possibly influenced the pathogenesis of the disease (60).

Sigurdsson *et al*. examined a flock of 55 sheep of which 31 were proved at autopsy to have been infected. Of these, 30 had reacted strongly to the test. Four others which had been strongly positive serologically did not show lesions. Of 118 sheep from a noninfected area which were tested, only 4 reacted, and these rather weakly. Only about 50 percent of 39 infected animals in their experimental flock reacted to intradermal tests with a johnin PPD (Purified Protein Derivative). As a result they were inclined to regard the serological test as much more reliable in sheep than the allergic one.

Larsen *et al*. (39) sensitized sheep erythrocytes with johnin (PPD) and used these cells in hemagglutination tests. They found that the test was not specific; that animals sensitized with Johne's bacilli as well as with other species within the genus *Mycobacterium* reacted. FA and gel-diffusion-precipitin tests have also been used in efforts to diagnose Johne's disease, but it appears that cultural examination of fecal specimens is of more value than serologic procedures in detecting paratuberculous cattle before they develop clinical signs of the disease.

**Immunity.** Animals that develop clinical evidence of Johne's disease seldom recover fully. Often they improve temporarily and seem to be fully recovered only to suffer a recurrence after days, weeks, or months. One animal observed (Hagan and Zeissig, 24) remained well for 5 years after having suffered severely from the disease during its first and second lactation periods. Minimal lesions were found at autopsy. It has already been pointed out that many more animals react to allergic tests than ever show symptoms and that in these asymptomatic animals the disease develops only to a limited extent and then is often thrown off.

A definite age immunity exists in this disease (Hagan, 20). Artificial infection by drenching with massive doses of infective material succeeds readily in calves but usually fails to produce clinical disease in older animals. Calves that are introduced into infected surroundings after they are 6 months of age seldom develop into clinical cases, though they may become allergic reactors, indicating that they harbor infection. Rankin (56) has estimated that the intravenous dose of *Myco. paratuberculosis* necessary to produce disease in a 1-month-old calf is about 5 mg of cultivated organisms weighed wet.

Based on the ability of intravenously-administered johnin or treatment with methotrexate, antihistamines, or histadine decarboxylase inhibitor to desensitize cattle clinically ill with paratuberculosis, Merkal *et al.* (48), postulated that the immunologic mechanisms involved are related to an antigen-antibody reaction of immediate hypersensitivity, which mediates diarrhea, and to a delayed hypersensitivity (involving antigen and competent lymphocytes), which releases cytotoxin and pyrogen and mediates the febrile responses, emaciation, and anemia.

Vallee and Rinjard (78) in 1926 began a series of experiments in France to determine whether the bacillus of Johne might be used as a vaccine to protect cattle. It was found that subcutaneous injection of these organisms mixed with mineral oil and pumice produced dense tumors at the point of inoculation and these remained for many months. Large doses injected without oil usually ulcerate and discharge fairly promptly. In a report published in 1934 (79), these authors state that over 12,000 animals had been vaccinated, that the vaccine had had no untoward effects, and that it was believed to have given an appreciable protection against the disease. Doyle (7) tested the method in England in 1945 and in 1964 (9) found it to be highly efficient against natural infection under field conditions. Sigurdsson (61) vaccinated lambs with heat-killed *Myco. paratuberculosis* suspended in mineral oil and concluded that the bacterin provoked a satisfactory resistance to subsequent infection. By 1960 about 450,000 sheep had been vaccinated by this method and excellent protection obtained (62).

In a small experiment conducted in this country (Hagan, 18) it was shown that vaccination did not prevent infection but the vaccinated calves withstood the disease better than the controls. The method has not been tried on commercial herds in this country. It deserves consideration, because there is evidence that virulent strains used as whole heat-killed or as methanol-treated bacterins produce a high degree of hypersensitivity and immunity (15). The principal objection is that, because of cross-sensitization, some of these animals would react to mammalian tuberculin. See Johnson, Milligan, and Cox (31).

**Chemotherapy.** Numerous chemotherapeutic agents have been tried in the treatment of Johne's disease. So far none has influenced the course of the disease to any marked degree, although streptomycin, viomycin, and isoniazid are effective *in vitro* against the organism (11, 40, 53).

**The Disease in Man.** There are no reports of human infections.

**Control Measures.** The control of Johne's disease is an unsolved problem. It spreads insidiously through exchange of cattle and sheep in which the disease is latent. Before animals are imported into uninfected regions, johnin testing is advised, since most animals in the latent stages of the disease will react. It is obvious that the disease is far more widespread than the clinical cases suggest, because in many regions the disease is largely a latent one. The relationship to soil conditions has been discussed. It is possible that when the specific deficiencies are known, they may be remedied by inclusion of these elements in the feed.

Because it is clear that most clinical cases, which undoubtedly are the most serious spreaders of infection, are infected in early calfhood, protection of the young calves is indicated. These should be removed from their dams as soon as possible and raised separately, in different barns and on different pastures. Marsh (47) states that the infection can be eliminated from a farm where there has been an outbreak in sheep by disposing of all the sheep and leaving the area free from sheep or cattle for 1 year before restocking. The success reported by Sigurdsson (62) in the vaccination of lambs warrants the use of bacterin, especially in areas where the disease is prevalent.

The testing with avian tuberculin or johnin, with elimination of reactors, is obviously a wasteful procedure because many reactors will never develop the disease. If they are few in number, this method may be tried, and sometimes it succeeds. In other herds, new reactors will continue to be encountered on each of many successive tests. Furthermore, clinical cases frequently develop in such herds between tests, an indication that some cases are missed by the tests.

## REFERENCES

1. Almquist and Klose. Jour. Am. Chem. Soc., 1939, *61*, 1611.
2. Bang. Berl. tierärztl. Wchnschr., 1906, p. 759.
3. Bang. Centrbl. f. Bakt., I Abt., Orig., 1909, *51*, 450.
4. Beach and Hastings. Jour. Inf. Dis., 1922, *30*, 68.
5. Chandler. Jour. Comp. Path. and Therap., 1962, *72*, 198.
6. Dorset, Henley, and Moskey. Jour. Am. Vet. Med. Assoc., 1926, *70*, 373.
7. Doyle. Vet. Rec., 1945, *57*, 385.
8. Doyle. Brit. Vet. Jour., 1954, *110*, 215.
9. Doyle. Vet. Rec., 1964, *76*, 73.
10. Dunkin. Jour. Comp. Path. and Therap., 1935, *48*, 236.
11. Ford. Brit. Vet. Jour., 1952, *108*, 411.
12. Francis. *Ibid.*, 1943, *53*, 140.
13. Francis, Macturk, Madinaveitia, and Snow. Biochem. Jour., 1953, *55*, 596.
14. Gifford, Eveleth, and Gifford. Vet. Med., 1942, *37*, 416.

15. Gilmour and Brotherston. Jour. Comp. Path., 1966, *76*, 341.
16. Gilmour, Campbell, and Brotherston. Jour. Comp. Path. and Therap., 1963, *73*, 98.
17. Gilmour, Nisbet, and Brotherston. Jour. Comp. Path., 1965, *75*, 281.
18. Hagan. Cornell Vet., 1935, *25*, 345.
19. Hagan. Symposium series, Am. Assoc. Adv. Sci., 1937, vol. *I*, p. 69.
20. Hagan. Cornell Vet., 1938, *28*, 34.
21. Hagan and Zeissig. Rpt. N.Y. State Vet. Coll. for 1927–28, p. 150.
22. Hagan and Zeissig. Jour. Am. Vet. Med. Assoc., 1929, *74*, 985.
23. *Ibid.*, 1933, *82*, 391.
24. *Ibid.*, 1935, *87*, 199.
25. Harding. Jour. Comp. Path. and Therap., 1957, *67*, 180.
26. Howarth. Jour. Am. Vet. Med. Assoc., 1932, *81*, 383.
27. Jansen. *Ibid.*, 1948, *112*, 52.
28. Johne and Frothingham. Deut. Zeitschr. f. Tiermed., 1895, *21*, 438.
29. Johnson. Am. Jour. Vet. Res., 1944, *5*, 320.
30. Johnson and Cox. *Ibid.*, 1942, *3*, 131.
31. Johnson, Milligan, and Cox. *Ibid.*, 1941, *9*, 115.
32. Jørgensen. Acta Vet. Scand., 1969, *10*, 275.
33. Kluge, Merkal, Monlux, Larsen, Kopecky, Ramsey, and Lehmann. Am. Jour. Vet. Res., 1968, *29*, 953.
34. Kopecky, Larsen, and Merkal. *Ibid.*, 1967, *28*, 1043.
35. Larsen and Kopecky. *Ibid.*, 1965, *26*, 673.
36. *Ibid.*, 1970, *31*, 255.
37. Larsen and Merkal. *Ibid.*, 1961, *22*, 1074.
38. Larsen, Merkal, and Vardaman. *Ibid.*, 1956, *17*, 549.
39. Larsen, Porter, and Vardaman. *Ibid.*, 1953, *14*, 362.
40. Larsen and Vardaman. *Ibid.*, 1952, *13*, 466.
41. Levi. Vet. Rec., 1948, *60*, 336.
42. Levi. Jour. Comp. Path. and Therap., 1948, *58*, 38.
43. Long and Seibert. Trans. Nat. Tuberc. Assoc., 1926, p. 270.
44. Lovell, Levi, and Francis. Jour. Comp. Path. and Therap., 1944, *54*, 120.
45. McEwen. *Ibid.*, 1939, *52*, 69.
46. McIntosh and Konst. Canad. Jour. Pub. Health, 1943, *34*, 557.
47. Marsh. Jour. Am. Vet. Med. Assoc., 1952, *120*, 20.
48. Merkal, Kopecky, Larsen, and Ness. Am. Jour. Vet. Res., 1970, *31*, 475.
49. Merkal, Kopecky, Larsen, and Thurston. *Ibid.*, 1964, *25*, 1290.
50. Nakamatsu, Fujimoto, and Satoh. Jap. Jour. Vet. Res., 1968, *16*, 103.
51. Newman, Crowder, and Anderson. Jour. Biol. Chem., 1934, *105*, 279.
52. Pearson. Vet. Rec., 1955, *67*, 615.
53. Rankin. *Ibid.*, 1953, *65*, 649.
54. *Ibid.*, 1954, *66*, 550.
55. Rankin. Jour. Path. and Bact., 1956, *72*, 689.
56. *Ibid.*, 1959, *77*, 638.
57. *Ibid.*, 1961, *71*, 6.
58. *Ibid.*, 10.
59. *Ibid.*, 1962, *72*, 113.
60. Sigurdsson. Jour. Immunol., 1947, *57*, 11.

61.  *Ibid.*, 1952, *68*, 559.
62.  Sigurdsson.   Am. Jour. Vet. Res., 1960, *80*, 54.
63.  Sigurdsson, Vigfusson, and Theodors.   Jour. Comp. Path. and Therap., 1945, *55*, 45.
64.  Sikes.   Am. Jour. Vet. Res., 1953, *14*, 12.
65.  Smith.   Jour. Path. and Bact., 1953, *66*, 375.
66.  Smythe.   Vet. Rec., 1935, *15*, 85.
67.  Snow.   Bact. Rev., 1970, *34*, 99.
68.  Stamp and Watt.   Jour. Comp. Path. and Therap., 1954, *64*, 26.
69.  Stewart, McCallum, and Taylor.   *Ibid.*, 1945, *55*, 45.
70.  Stuart.   Brit. Vet. Jour., 1965, *121*, 332.
71.  Taylor.   Jour. Comp. Path. and Therap., 1945, *55*, 41.
72.  Taylor.   Vet. Rec., 1949, *61*, 539.
73.  Taylor.   Jour. Path. and Bact., 1950, *62*, 647.
74.  *Ibid.*, 1951, *63*, 323.
75.  Taylor.   Jour. Comp. Path. and Therap., 1953, *63*, 368.
76.  Twort.   Proc. Roy. Soc. Med., 1911, Series B, *83*, 158.
77.  Twort and Ingram.   Johne's disease. Baillière, Tindall and Cox, London, 1913.
78.  Vallee and Rinjard.   Rev. gén. méd., vét., 1926, 35, 1.
79.  Vallee, Rinjard, and Vallee.   *Ibid.*, 1934, *43*, 50.
80.  Vance.   Canad. Vet. Jour., 1961, *2*, 305.
81.  Wooley and McCarter.   Proc. Soc. Exp. Biol. and Med., 1940, *45*, 357.

## *Mycobacterium lepraemurium* (The Acid-Fast Organism of Rat Leprosy)

In a rat-destruction campaign waged in Odessa in 1901 Stephansky (5) found about 5 percent of the animals to be suffering from a disease which resembles human leprosy, particularly in the fact that the lesions contain large numbers of acid-fast organisms. The disease has been seen in other parts of the world (3), but usually only a fraction of 1 percent of the population is involved. In some cases there is enlargement of the lymph nodes, particularly those of the axillary and inguinal regions. The glands become enlarged and hardened but do not suppurate. Myriads of acid-fast bacilli, usually located intracellularly in large cells which probably are epithelioid in nature, can be found in such glands. In other cases the disease affects the skin and subcutaneous tissue and sometimes the underlying muscle. The hair is lost from such areas, and sometimes ulcers are formed from which a thick discharge, rich in bacilli, exudes. In the granulation tissue which forms beneath the skin, bacilli are plentiful. Lesions in the internal organs are rare, except that nephritis usually exists, in which cases bacilli cannot be demonstrated in the kidneys.

Although lesions were induced in rats by injecting infected tissues, isolated cultures failed to reproduce the disease and apparently the bacillus of rat leprosy was not cultured on artificial media for many years. In 1962, Rees and Tee (4) succeeded in cultivating *Myco. lepraemurium* in rat fibroblasts and studied the mycobacterial antigens of the bacilli. In 1966, Kato and Gozsy (1) achieved limited multiplication of the rat leprosy bacillus by employing an alkaline (pH 8.4) galactomannan-containing medium alone or in parabiosis with a feeder strain (*Torula minuta*). Hyperosmolarity (NaCl, 2 percent) enhanced multiplication in both cases.

The rat leprosy organism probably has no relation to that of human leprosy, inasmuch as rats are resistant to inoculation with leprous tissue from man. Although it has been believed that the disease is not transmissible to other domestic animals, Lawrence and Wickham (2) have described cat leprosy and have stated that the acid-fast bacilli which they obtained from this animal had the properties of *Myco. lepraemurium* and produced typical infection in rats.

### REFERENCES

1. Kato and Gozsy. Jour. Bact., 1966, *91*, 1859.
2. Lawrence and Wickham. Aust. Vet. Jour., 1963, *39*, 391.
3. Rabinowitsch. Centrbl. f. Bakt., I Abt., Orig., 1903, *33*, 577.
4. Rees and Tee. Brit. Jour. Exp. Path., 1962, *43*, 480.
5. Stephansky. Centrbl. f. Bakt., I Abt., Orig., 1903, *33*, 481.

### Acid-Fast Bacilli Associated with Ulcerative Lymphangitis in Cattle

In the course of the work of eradicating bovine tuberculosis in the United States, much attention has been given to a condition that occurs in many parts of the country to which the name *skin lesion tuberculosis* was early attached. Traum (12) appears to have been the first to call attention to the fact that these lesions sometimes caused cattle to react to the tuberculin test. Ani-

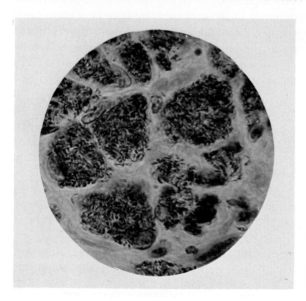

*Fig. 74.* The acid-fast organism of rat leprosy. Large epithelioid-type cells are located in the granulomatous lesion of the subcutaneous tissue and packed with the acid-fast lepra bacilli. X 1,000.

mals in some areas are more often affected with these lesions than those in others, and the distribution of cases does not correspond to the distribution of orthodox tuberculosis. It is now fairly certain that the condition is not caused by tubercle bacilli.

The lesions usually occur in the skin of the lower parts of the legs. They first appear as nodules that seem to be attached to the skin but are actually located in the subcutaneous tissue. In the course of time these nodules usually soften and ulcerate through the skin. In the meantime, other nodules often appear along the course of the lymphatics. It is not uncommon to see animals having from 4 to 5 to as many as 25 nodules, many of which have broken through the skin. After discharging their contents, the lesions usually heal. In some cases, instead of discharging, the lesions coalesce forming large dense masses consisting largely of connective tissue in which areas of suppuration occur. The pus may be fluid, pasty, or dry, inspissated, and calcareous. The neighboring lymph nodes usually do not become involved, unlike the situation which invariably occurs in the presence of true tubercle infection.

The histological structure of these nodules resembles that of tuberculous tissue. Acid-fast bacilli that cannot be distinguished morphologically from bovine tubercle bacilli can be found in most cases, although usually they are not numerous. Many workers (1, 2, 3, 5, 6, 10, 12) have studied these lesions, but none has succeeded either in obtaining cultures of the acid-fast organism or in causing infections in laboratory animals. Although many have tried to transmit this condition, the only successful effort appears to be that of Hedström (4). He used finely dispersed tissue material taken from skin lesions in their early stage of development. Animals were injected, either intra- or subcutaneously into several places on the lateral surface of the neck and on the lateral sides of the forelimb. Six weeks after the inoculations the skin where the intracutaneous injections were made showed small, solid swellings, which gradually increased, later became node-forming, and finally reached the size of a hazelnut about 6 months after the inoculation. Where the tissue material was injected subcutaneously no reaction was observed.

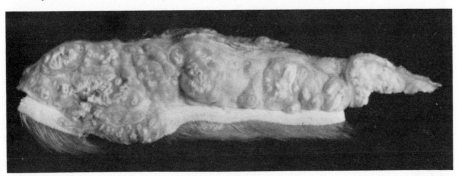

*Fig. 75.* Acid-fast lymphangitis, cross section of gross lesions in the subcutaneous tissue of a cow. Note ulceration through skin. Reduced one-half.

Several workers have occasionally isolated cultures of acid-fast bacilli, but the strains isolated have the characteristics of saprophytes, i.e., they have been incapable of producing more than an abscess at the point of inoculation (12).

Animals affected with these lesions do not always react to tuberculin, and when reactions occur they are somewhat atypical in many instances. Such animals may react at one time and fail to react at another. When the lesions are removed surgically, gradual loss of sensitivity occurs. The disease is not a serious one, *per se*, although the blemishes produced are distasteful to owners of fine cattle. The most serious feature about them is the fact that they confuse the diagnosis so far as tuberculosis is concerned. Reactions to tuberculin cannot be safely ascribed to the presence of such lesions unless the history of the animal makes the occurrence of genuine tuberculosis in the same animal highly improbable, for the lesions are found in tuberculous as well as in nontuberculous cattle. Until quite recently one could have assumed, because of the absence of references to these lesions in the literature, that the condition did not occur in Europe. This was not true, however. Identical lesions were described in English cattle by Robertson and Hole (10) in 1937, in Danish cattle by Götzsche and Plum (1) in 1938, in Swedish cattle by Krantz (5) in 1938, and in Swiss cattle by Thomann (11) in 1949. As early as 1913 Perard and Ramon (7) described a similar if not identical condition in France.

In 1960 Ressang and Titus (9) reported a case of buffalo leprosy in a Holstein-Friesian cow. The leprosy nodules were located mainly in the lower part of the left hind- and right front-leg. It seems that a disease known as buffalo leprosy is not uncommon in this animal in Indonesia, but cattle ordinarily are not affected. From descriptions of the disease and from the results obtained in transmission experiments by Ressang and Sutarjo (8) it is not entirely clear whether buffalo leprosy is a distinct entity or part of the acid-fast ulcerative lymphangitis complex.

## REFERENCES

1. Götzsche and Plum.  Maanedskr. f. Dyrlaeger, 1938, *50*, 33.
2. Hagan.  Cornell Vet., 1929, *19*, 173.
3. Hastings, Beach, and Weber.  Jour. Am. Vet. Med. Assoc., 1924, *66*, 36.
4. Hedström.  Collected papers from the State Vet. Med. Inst. Stockholm, 1949, p. 180.
5. Krantz.  Skandi. Vet. Tidskr., 1938, *28*, 20.
6. Mitchell.  Jour. Am. Vet. Med. Assoc., 1928, *73*, 493.
7. Perard and Ramon.  Comp. rend. Soc. Biol. (Paris), 1913, *65*, 133.
8. Ressang and Sutarjo.  Commun. Vet., 1961, *5*, 89.
9. Ressang and Titus.  *Ibid.*, 1960, *4*, 47.
10. Robertson and Hole.  Jour. Comp. Path. and Therap., 1937, *50*, 39.
11. Thomann.  Schweiz. Arch. Tierheilk., 1949, *91*, 237.
12. Traum.  Jour. Am. Vet. Med. Assoc., 1916, *49*, 254; 1919, *55*, 639.

## The Tubercle Bacilli of Cold-Blooded Animals

Bataillon, Dubard, and Terre (3) in 1897 isolated an acid-fast organism from fish (carp) that were living in polluted water. Since that time, diseases having some resemblance to tuberculosis of warm-blooded animals and associated with acid-fast organisms have been seen in various cold-blooded animals such as frogs, tadpoles, snakes, turtles, and other species of fish. These organisms are readily cultivated upon media which support growth of true tubercle bacilli. They differ in cultural features but are alike in that they grow rapidly at low temperatures. Several workers have attempted to show a relationship to tubercle bacilli of warm-blooded animals, but it is clear that the two bacilli are quite different. The diseases are seen most often in animals kept in captivity and are the cause of many deaths among animals of this type in zoological parks and aquaria. In many instances the diseases can be reproduced readily by feeding pure cultures (2, 4). Although these organisms resemble closely some of the saprophytic acid-fast organisms commonly found in soil and water, in most instances the tubercle bacilli of cold-blooded animals are true parasites that have a specific affinity for their hosts and are not found commonly in nature except in their hosts and materials contaminated by them (2). Friedman attempted to use a turtle strain for immunizing people to tuberculosis, but the experiments failed. Apparently the tubercle bacilli of cold-blooded animals have little in common with tubercle bacilli of warm-blooded animals other than the fact that both are acid-fast. A good review of the subject of tuberculosis in cold-blooded animals is that of Aronson (1).

## REFERENCES

1. Aronson. Tuberculosis and leprosy. Symposium series, Am. Assoc. Adv. Sci., 1938. Vol. *I.*
2. Baker and Hagan. Jour. Inf. Dis., 1942, *70*, 248.
3. Bataillon, Dubard, and Terre. Comp. rend. Soc. Biol. (Paris), 1897, *10*, Sup. 4, 446.
4. Nonidez and Kahn. Am. Rev. Tuberc., 1937, *36*, 191.

## The Saprophytic Acid-Fast Bacilli

Acid-fast organisms belonging to the mycobacteria are widespread in nature. Nearly all soils harbor them (1), and they are common on vegetation and in the alimentary tracts of herbivorous animals. They have also been found on the mucous membranes and skins of animals. They have been isolated from cases of bovine mastitis (5, 6, 8). Affected animals may or may not react to tuberculin tests. They show granulomatous lesions in the udders and it appears that the condition may result because of a lack of aseptic technic in giving udder infusions of oily therapeutic preparations.

For the most part the organisms seem to be harmless, although abscesses and tubercles may be produced by injecting them into animals. They frequently show a very close resemblance to tubercle bacilli but may be distinguished from them by lack of pathogenicity for animals, rapid manner of growth on culture media, and the fact that they will grow well at room temperature. Most of these organisms will develop luxuriantly on plain glycerol agar, on plain agar, or on solutions of simple mineral salts. They grow on fluid media in the form of pellicles, in most instances, and produce filtrates that resemble tuberculin. Usually these filtrates will not give reactions in animals affected with tuberculosis but will in animals that have been inoculated with the homologous organisms.

The studies of Thomson (7), Gordon (2), and Gordon and Hagan (3) have made it clear that many of the acid-fast organisms that have been isolated from a variety of sources by different persons in the past and have been endowed with different names, depending usually upon the source from which they were obtained, are in reality alike. Thus of a collection of 331 strains, most of which had been isolated by the authors from soil and water but which included about 50 named strains of other authors, the greater part fell into three principal groups. The smegma bacillus of Alvarez and Tavel, *Myco. graminis* and *Myco. stercusis* of Moeller, *Myco. berolinense* of Rabinowitsch, the *nasenschleim* bacillus of Karlinski, several of the so-called leprosy bacilli, and others, with 104 strains isolated from soils, proved to be indistinguishable from each other. Gordon and Smith (4) restudied 124 strains in 1953 and concluded that 62 percent belonged in two species which they designated *Myco. smegmatis* and *Myco. phlei.*

*Myco. fortuitum* is sometimes grouped with these organisms because it is also a rapid grower; however, *Myco. fortuitum* fails to grow at 45 C, whereas *Myco. phlei* and *Myco. smegmatis* will do so. It also possesses a higher order of virulence for mice. Other cultures are regarded at present merely as "saprophytic acid-fast bacilli."

## REFERENCES

1. Frey and Hagan.   Jour. Inf. Dis., 1931, *49,* 497.
2. Gordon.   Jour. Bact., 1937, *34,* 617.
3. Gordon and Hagan.   *Ibid.,* 1938, *36,* 39.
4. Gordon and Smith.   *Ibid.,* 1953, *66,* 41.
5. Richardson.   Vet. Rec., 1970, *86,* 497.
6. Stuart and Harvey.   *Ibid.,* 1951, *63,* 881.
7. Thomson.   Am. Rev. Tuberc., 1932, *26,* 162.
8. Tucker.   Cornell Vet., 1953, *43,* 576.

# XXI | The *Actinomycetaceae*

The actinomycetes are organisms that evidently are somewhat higher in the evolutionary scale than the ordinary bacteria. Usually they grow in the form of a much-branched mycelium. In many forms this mycelium frequently breaks up into fragments that cannot be distinguished from ordinary bacteria. Some have referred to them as the *higher bacteria*. Henrici, in discussing the relationship of these forms to bacteria and molds, mentions three possibilities: (1) that they are bacteria which have evolved into a higher form; (2) that they are molds which have degenerated; (3) that they are forms from which the bacteria have developed by degeneration and the molds by evolution. Some of the actinomycetes are acid-fast and evidently are closely related to the acid-fast bacteria. The family *Actinomycetaceae* is divided into two genera, *Nocardia* and *Actinomyces*.

## THE GENUS *NOCARDIA*

In this genus several species are pathogenic for cattle, dogs, cats, marsupials, and man, causing tuberculosislike diseases or ulcerative lesions. Most are soil saprophytes. In early stages of growth on culture media these microorganisms form a mycelium that is not septate, but eventually the filaments form transverse walls and break up into coccoid cells. Most forms produce aerial hyphae. Members of the genus are nonmotile, aerobic, Gram-positive, and do not form endospores. Their colonies may be rough or smooth, of a soft to a doughlike consistency, or compact and leathery. Many species of the nocardiae form pigments of a blue, violet, red, yellow, orange, or green color, although most of the cultures are colorless. Some are acid-fast, and the small coccoid forms cannot be distinguished with certainty from acid-fast bacilli. This fact should be remembered by those who are dealing with materials that may have been contaminated with soil. Some of these forms have proved pathogenic for experimental animals when cultures were injected, and it is

467

possible that occasional spontaneous animal infections may be caused by such organisms. Some of the acid-fast members of the genus which have been involved in diseases of animals are as follows:

### Nocardia farcinica

SYNONYMS: *Actinomyces farcinicus, Streptothrix farcinica, Streptothrix nocardii, Actinomyces nocardii,* and others

This organism is the causative agent of a disease of cattle first described in France under the name *farcin-de-boeuf* (bovine farcy) (33). The disease is said to be enzootic on the island of Guadeloupe in the French West Indies. It is not known to exist in North America.

**Morphology and Staining Reactions.** Stained films show filaments varying in length and averaging perhaps 0.3 microns in width. Branching is frequently seen. The filaments easily break into fragments, many of which resemble bacilli. These elements are Gram-positive and most of them retain the acid-fast stain (24).

**Cultural Features.** Growth on solid media resembles that of many of the saprophytic actinomycetes which are so common in garden soil. Growth occurs readily on plain agar slants. Small ragged colonies quickly coalesce to form a tough, yellowish-white, dry pellicle, which becomes wrinkled and powdery. The powdery appearance indicates that aerial hyphae are formed. In broth the growth occurs principally as whitish granules, although small islands of growth may appear on the surface. Gelatin is not liquefied and milk is not changed. An abundant, dull pellicle forms on the surface of potato slants. No pigment is formed. Growth is best at 37 C.

**Pathogenicity.** By inoculation this organism is pathogenic for cattle, sheep, and guinea pigs. Musgrave and Clegg (32) produced miliary nodules in monkeys. Other authors say that the monkey is not susceptible to inoculation.

When inoculated intraperitoneally into guinea pigs, the animal usually dies within 10 to 20 days. Autopsy shows general emaciation and numerous tuberclelike nodules scattered over the surface of the peritoneum. When the inoculum is administered intravenously, miliary nodules are formed in the lungs and the animal dies within 1 to 2 weeks, depending upon the size of the dose and the virulence of the strain. Subcutaneous inoculation produces only an abscess.

Cattle and sheep are somewhat more resistant to inoculation than guinea pigs, but death usually occurs after several weeks following intravenous inoculation. The animal becomes very emaciated before death, and the lungs are found to be riddled with myriads of small nodules.

The naturally occurring disease in cattle appears first as a chronic, indurative lymphangitis and lymphadenitis of the subcutaneous tissues, usually of one of the extremities, the lesions eventually breaking through the skin forming sinuses communicating with cold abscesses. The disease is of long duration. Eventually lung involvement generally occurs, the animal becomes emaciated, and death ensues. Cultures are easily obtained from the freshly opened nodules.

**Immunity.** There are no immunizing products. Some affected animals react to tuberculin.

### Nocardia asteroides

SYNONYMS: *Cladothrix asteroides, Streptothrix eppingeri, Actinomyces asteroides*

Eppinger (18) in 1890 isolated an acid-fast actinomycete from a brain abscess of a man who died of a generalized disease which resembled tuberculosis. Besides a purulent meningitis, there were caseated bronchial lymph nodes and miliary lesions of the lungs from which the organism was isolated. In 1921 Henrici and Gardner (24) described another human case, and in 1956 Webster (44) reviewed the literature and reported seven cases of pulmonary nocardiosis. He stated that he had found records of 44 cases with pulmonary involvement.

### Other Pathogenic Nocardiae

Nocardiosis is not an uncommon disease in cattle, dogs, cats, marsupials, and man. It has been reported in tropical fish (13). Numerous isolates have been obtained from these infections, and in some cases the organisms have been given specific names. In others, the generic name alone has been applied. The serologic tests that ordinarily are used in determining strain identity are not applicable, as a rule, to these cultures. In fact, a lack of uniform procedure in characterizing the isolates has made their identification difficult; in many cases the reason for the decision to classify a strain as a variety of a species or to give it species status is not clear. Because *N. farcinica* and *N. asteroides* are widely recognized types, we have considered them separately even though it is believed by some that they are members of the same species, if not identical types. Pier *et al.* (35) have prepared a nocardial antigen from *N. asteroides* and claim that it can be used in allergic, precipitation, and complement-fixation tests to detect present or previous nocardiosis in cattle. Organisms within the genus *Nocardia* are important in producing disease in the following animals:

**Guinea Pigs (Experimental).** Gordon and Hagan (21) in 1936 described several acid-fast actinomycetes which had been isolated directly from the soil and which proved to be pathogenic for guinea pigs, producing in them fatal infections in which the lungs were the principal organs involved. Kurup and Sandhu (27) have assigned the name *N. caviae* to a soil type that was pathogenic for laboratory animals.

**Cattle.** Burnett (11) described two cases in bovine lungs which were caused by the organism now named *Nocardia pulmonalis.*

Bishop and Fenstermacher (5) described an organism that had been isolated from a tuberculosislike process in a cow and decided it was similar to *N. asteroides.*

Munch-Petersen (31) reported a natural case of bovine actinomycotic mastitis. Nodular abscesses were present and the causal organism was similar to, if not identical with, *N. asteroides*. Since then numerous reports (4, 16, 17, 34, 36) have appeared linking *Nocardia* with the bovine mastitis complex. Both *N. asteroides* and *N. farcinica* have been listed as the etiologic agents, and the latter has also been named as a cause of nocardiosis of the testes of bulls.

**Goats.** *N. asteroides* (15) has been found in mastitis in the goat.

**Horses.** Nocardiosis has been diagnosed in equine mandibles where it was associated with bilateral anomalies of the inferior dentition (42).

**Dogs.** Madsen (28) studied an actinomycete that had been isolated from granulomalike nodules on the mediastinum and pleura of a dog. This organism showed a long, slender, branching mycelium in young cultures and rod, oval, and coccoid forms in old cultures. It was weakly acid-fast, grew aerobically, and produced an orange pigment. The organism was listed as *Actinomyces canis* but falls in the genus *Nocardia* under the present system of nomenclature.

Nocardiosis (actinomycosis) has been found on many occasions in dogs (6, 7, 12, 26). Lesions similar to those described by Madsen appear to be most common, and this condition has been diagnosed at Cornell University by Olafson and associates as acid-fast actinomycotic pleuritis. Other forms of nocardiosis occur. Brodey *et al.* (10) have reported a case of chronic subcutaneous infection involving the hind leg of a Pointer, and Moss (30) described an abdominal mass in a Labrador Retriever and an abscess on the neck of a Weimaraner, both of which proved to be granulomas caused by *Nocardia*. Blake (6) has suggested that nocardiosis in the dog often is a complicating factor in some other disease, especially distemper. Rhoades *et al.* (38) have isolated *N. asteroides* from the lungs and brain of a dog that showed multiple, granulomatous lesions of the viscera and central nervous system upon necropsy.

**Cats.** Reports of nocardiosis in cats are not so common as those in dogs, but the disease occurs in cats and a description of two cases with lesions in the submandibular lymph gland, in the pleura, and in the lungs has been given by Akün (2). A review of feline nocardiosis was published by Frost (19). Ajello *et al.* (1) isolated *N. braziliensis* from lacerations on a cat and believed this to be the first authenticated record of an infection of lower animals by this species which is considered to be a human-adapted type.

**Marsupials.** An epizootic caused by *Nocardia* has been reported among kangaroos and wallabies kept in captivity at Brisbane, Australia. It appears that infections in the animals start in the upper respiratory tract and spread rapidly, causing death soon after macroscopic lesions are detected (43).

**Monkeys.** Pulmonary nocardiosis has been observed in monkeys where it mimicked tuberculosis (3).

**Man.** Beginning with the report of Eppinger (18), there have been a number of recorded cases of human nocardiosis. *N. asteroides* appears to be the most

common cause, and although the system usually concerned is the respiratory
45), cerebral involvement is not uncommon (37). Other organs sometimes are
affected, and Cruz and Clancy (14) have reported a case of osteomyelitis with
subsequent embolic abscesses in the heart, brain, kidney, adrenal gland, and
mesenteric lymph nodes. Acid-fast *Nocardia* such as *N. braziliensis* and *N. se-
bivorans* (22) have also been described in human infections. A schema for the
differentiation of *N. asteroides* and *N. braziliensis* was published in 1959 (8)
and expanded in 1961 (20) and in 1963 (9).

A non-acid-fast member of the genus is *Nocardia madurae*. It often is found
in "Madura foot" in man.

**Chemotherapy.** Hager, Migliaccio, and Young (23) reported success in treating human nocardiosis with large doses of penicillin and streptomycin. Sulfonamides are reasonably effective in the treatment of *Nocardia* infections. Reports by Runyon (39) and Strauss *et al.* (41) indicate that sulfadiazine is
effective in animal protection tests, but aureomycin, chloromycetin, and streptomycin give only partial protection. Sapegin and Cormack (40) treated two
cases of canine nocardiosis with hibitane (bis-*p*-chlorophenyldeguanido-
hexane) and reported good clinical recovery. Other reports have indicated
that benzalkonium chloride (29) and the combination of cycloserine and
sulfonamides (25) are effective.

## REFERENCES

1. Ajello, Walker, Dungworth, and Brumfield. Jour. Am. Vet. Med. Assoc., 1961, *138*, 370.
2. Akün. Deut. tierärtzl. Wchnschr., 1952, 59, 202.
3. Al-Doory, Pinkerton, Vice, and Hutchinson. Jour. Am. Vet. Med. Assoc., 1969, *155*, 1179.
4. Awad. Vet. Rec., 1960, 72, 341.
5. Bishop and Fenstermacher. Cornell Vet., 1933, *23*, 287.
6. Blake. Jour. Am. Vet. Med. Assoc., 1954, *125*, 467.
7. Bohl, Jones, Farrell, Chamberlain, Cole, and Ferguson. *Ibid.*, 1953, *122*, 81.
8. Bojalil and Cerbon. Jour. Bact., 1959, 78, 852.
9. Bojalil and Zamora. Proc. Soc. Exp. Biol. and Med., 1963, *113*, 40.
10. Brodey, Cole, and Sauer. Jour. Am. Vet. Med. Assoc., 1955, *127*, 433.
11. Burnett. Rpt. N.Y. State Vet. Coll., 1909–10, p. 167.
12. Christensen and Clifford. Am. Jour. Vet. Res., 1953, *14*, 298.
13. Conroy. Vet. Rec., 1964, *76*, 676.
14. Cruz and Clancy. Am. Jour. Path., 1952, *28*, 607.
15. Dafaala and Gharib. Brit. Vet. Jour., 1958, *114*, 143.
16. Ditchfield, Butas, and Julian. Canad. Jour. Comp. Med. and Vet. Sci., 1959, 23, 93.
17. Eales, Leaver, Swan, and Wellington. Austral. Vet. Jour., 1964, *40*, 321.
18. Eppinger. Beitr. zur path. Anat. (Ziegler's), 1890, 9, 287.
19. Frost. Austral. Vet. Jour., 1959, 35, 22.
20. Georg, Ajello, McDurmont, and Hosty. Am. Rev. Resp. Dis., 1961, *84*, 337.
21. Gordon and Hagan. Jour. Inf. Dis., 1936, 59, 200.

22.   Gorrill and Heptinstall.    Jour. Path. and Bact., 1954, *68*, 387.
23.   Hager, Migliaccio, and Young.    New England Jour. Med., 1949, *241*, 226.
24.   Henrici and Gardner.    Jour. Inf. Dis., 1921, *28*, 232.
25.   Hoeprich, Brandt, and Parker.    Am. Jour. Med. Sci., 1968, *255*, 208.
26.   Johnston.    Jour. Path. and Bact., 1956, *71*, 7.
27.   Kurup and Sandhu.    Jour. Bact., 1965, *90*, 822.
28.   Madsen.    Cornell Vet., 1942, *32*, 383.
29.   Merkal and Thurston.    Am. Jour. Vet. Res., 1968, *29*, 759.
30.   Moss.    Jour. Am. Vet. Med. Assoc., 1956, *128*, 143.
31.   Munch-Petersen.    Austral. Vet. Jour., 1954, *30*, 297.
32.   Musgrave and Clegg.    Phil. Jour. Sci., 1907, *2B*, 477.
33.   Nocard.    Ann. l'Inst. Past., 1888, *2*, 293.
34.   Pier, Gray, and Fossatti.    Am. Jour. Vet. Res., 1958, *19*, 319.
35.   Pier, Thurston, and Larsen.    *Ibid.*, 1968, *29*, 397.
36.   Pier, Willers, and Mejia.    *Ibid.*, 1961, *22*, 698.
37.   Pizzolato, Ziskind, Derman, and Buff.    Am. Jour. Clin. Path., 1961, *36*, 151.
38.   Rhoades, Reynolds, Rahn, and Small.    Jour. Am. Vet. Med. Assoc., 1963, *142*, 278.
39.   Runyon.    Jour. Lab. and Clin. Med., 1951, *37*, 713.
40.   Sapegin and Cormack.    North Am. Vet., 1956, *37*, 385.
41.   Strauss, Kligman, and Pillsbury.    Am. Rev. Tuberc., 1951, *63*, 441.
42.   Tritschler and Romack.    Vet. Med., 1965, *60*, 605.
43.   Tucker and Millar.    Jour. Comp. Path. and Therap., 1953, *63*, 143.
44.   Webster.    Am. Rev. Tuberc., 1956, *73*, 485.
45.   Webster.    Am. Jour. Med. Sci., 1962, *244*, 40.

## THE GENUS *ACTINOMYCES*

Members of this genus produce a true mycelium that fragments into elements of irregular size and may exhibit angular branching. They do not form conidia nor are they acid-fast. They are anaerobic to microaerophilic and are pathogenic for man and animals. Three species currently listed in *Bergey's Manual* are *Act. bovis*, *Act. israeli*, and *Act. baudeti*.

In 1965, Georg *et al.* (9) described a new pathogenic anaerobic actinomycete. It was derived from human clinical material and proved to be antigenically distinct from the recognized types. They named it *Act. eriksoni*. A species called *Act. naeslundi* is generally considered to be a saprophytic component of the normal flora of the human mouth, but it has also been isolated repeatedly from clinical materials associated with disease (5). Two other species now listed in the literature as human types are *Act. odontolyticus* and *Act. viscosus*.

*Act. bovis* grows in soft, smooth colonies that do not adhere to the medium. It does not produce aerial hyphae nor does it cross-agglutinate with strains of *Act. israeli*, while the latter develops colonies that are tough in texture and warted in appearance, produces erect aerial hyphae in an atmosphere of reduced oxygen tension, and agglutinates only in homologous antiserum. Some believe that this rough form is usually responsible for human actinomycosis but is only occasionally found in cattle and that the smooth form (*Act. bovis*) is the cattle type, rarely appearing in man (7, 26). Some success has been achieved in categorizing the antigenic relationships between these organisms by the agar gel diffusion technic of Ouchterlony (15), but much more work is needed.

*Act. baudeti* was regarded as identical with *Act. israeli* until it was shown that it can cause actinomycosis in dogs and cats and that ends of its hyphae found in pus granules absorb basic stains while those of *Act. israeli* stain with acid stains.

Slack and Gerencser (24) have published a serologic grouping of the *Actinomyces* species. They list Group A, *Act. naeslundi;* Group B, *Act. bovis* (two types); Group C, *Act. eriksoni;* Group D, *Act. israeli* (two types); Group E, *Act. odontolyticus* (two types); and Group F, *Act. viscosus* (two types).

Because *Act. israeli, Act. naeslundi, Act. eriksoni, Act. odontolyticus,* and *Act. viscosus* appear to be essentially human types and because there is considerable doubt at present as to the species status of *Act. baudeti,* we will confine our discussion to the types species of the genus, *Act. bovis.*

### Actinomyces bovis

SYNONYMS: *Streptothrix actinomyces, Discomyces bovis, Nocardia bovis, Streptothrix israeli,* and others

This organism is the cause of the common disease of cattle known as *actinomycosis* or *lumpy jaw.* It has been reported in deer, dogs, and a horse. It also affects swine, in which the seat of localization is the mammary gland. Human infections occasionally occur, the manifestations being similar to those in cattle.

It should be pointed out that conditions that resemble actinomycosis clinically, and are often called *actinomycosis,* are due to other organisms, particularly *Actinobacillus lignieresi* and *Staphylococcus aureus.* The true actinomycosis of cattle usually is an affection of the bony structures, particularly the mandible or lower jaw (27). The condition known as *wooden tongue,* which is commonly called *actinomycosis,* really is actinobacillosis in nearly every instance. This is true also of the subcutaneous nodules of the region of the jaw and neck and the nodules which occasionally are found in the liver, lungs, and other internal organs. Magnusson found that actinomycosis of the bovine udder was, in every instance, actinobacillosis, and in the sow, in about a third of his cases, *Staphylococcus* infections. However, pulmonary actinomycosis in swine has been reported by Vawter (28) and *Act. bovis* has been isolated from a bovine lung (2).

In the study of equine poll evil and fistulous withers which appear to be inflammations of the supraatloid and supraspinous bursa, respectively, Roderick, Kimball, McLeod, and Frank (22) regularly have isolated *Actinomyces bovis* and *Brucella abortus. Brucella suis* has also been obtained from these lesions and injection of either *Br. abortus* or *Br. suis* combined with *Act. bovis* into the supraspinous bursa of experimental horses produces a bursitis apparently identical with field cases.

**Morphology and Staining Reactions.** In the "sulfur granules" in the tissues, *Act. bovis* is seen as a tangled mass of filaments around the periphery of which is a considerable mass of acidophilic capsular material. The filaments stain Gram-positively, and also retain the usual basophilic stains. When stains are made of crushed granules, a great diversity of forms, resembling a mixed infection, is seen. They are coccoid, rods of varying size, filaments, branching forms, club-shaped forms, and spiral elements. Actually all of these are forms of the one organism. In cultures it usually appears in the form of diphtheroid bacilli when young; older cultures may show filaments of all kinds. When grown in an atmosphere of carbon dioxide, branching filaments and clubs are frequent.

**Cultural Features.** *Act. bovis* frequently is regarded as an obligate anaerobe. This conception is false. Growth cannot be obtained on the surface of solid media incubated in the air, but it may be obtained when the media are enclosed in a tight vessel in which from 10 to 15 percent carbon dioxide is introduced. When shake cultures are made in solid media, growth does not occur on the surface. The optimum zone, in this case, is about 1 mm below the surface, but scattered colonies usually are found throughout the depths of the medium. Cultures sometimes will develop on the surface if the tubes are hermetically sealed, a procedure which results in an increase in the carbon dioxide content of the imprisoned air.

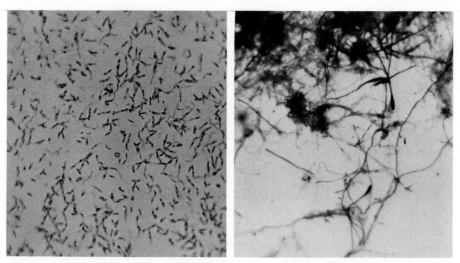

*Fig. 76 (left). Actinomyces bovis,* showing diphtheroid forms in a culture on Loeffler's blood serum incubated for 7 days at 37 C under increased $CO_2$ tension. X 900. (Courtesy L. R. Vawter.)

*Fig. 77 (right). Actinomyces bovis* from a serum-broth culture incubated 6 days at 37 C. Clubs, filaments, and diphtheroid forms are present. X 900. (Courtesy L. R. Vawter.)

*Act. bovis* is a serophilic organism, i.e., little or no growth can be obtained in ordinary media unless animal fluids are present. It does not grow at temperatures very much below those of the animal body.

In stab cultures in serum agar a nodular growth occurs along the lower parts of the stab. There is no growth on the surface or in the upper centimeter of the stab. In shake cultures small, biconvex colonies appear throughout the medium except in the upper layer. Growth on serum agar slants will occur only if the tubes are incubated in a carbon-dioxide-containing atmosphere, or anaerobically.

The growth in serum broth is not abundant. If incubated in the air the medium should be in tall columns, and it should be heated shortly before the serum is added and inoculation is made. The growth is in the form of granules, which collect along the sides of the tube and in the bottom. The fluid is clear except for the granules.

Loeffler's blood serum slants are good for isolation providing they are incubated in a carbon dioxide jar. Growth is evident after 2 or 3 days in the form of fine colonies which may easily be scraped off the medium. After 5 or 6 days' incubation at 37 C the colonies will have reached maximum size, which is about 0.5 mm in diameter. The condensation water at the bottom of the slant usually contains excellent growth in the form of a slimy deposit.

On blood agar plates the colonies are small and nonhemolytic.

Little growth occurs in milk unless serum is added to it. In serum milk

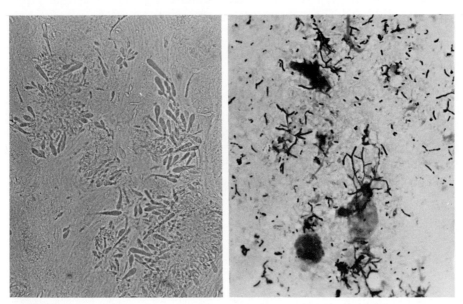

*Fig. 78 (left)*. *Actinomyces bovis,* showing clubs and rosettes in pus of a bone lesion. Unstained. X 360. (Courtesy L. R. Vawter.)

*Fig. 79 (right)*. *Actinomyces bovis,* showing branched filaments and coccoid bodies in actinomycotic pus. X 900. (Courtesy L. R. Vawter.)

there is little change in the appearance of the medium. Sometimes the litmus is bleached in the bottom of the tube.

No growth occurs in gelatin unless serum is added. Serum gelatin is not liquefied.

In serum-containing broth under a vaseline seal, glucose, levulose, maltose, galactose, sucrose, and salicin are slowly fermented without gas formation. By means of agglutination tests Magnusson (19) established three serological types, which he named A, B, and C. Type A was characteristic of cattle, B and C of swine.

**Pathogenicity.** Although *Act. bovis* is nonpathogenic for most laboratory animals, Hazen *et al.* (13) were able to infect male hamsters, 3 to 4 weeks old, by intraperitoneal injection. When these animals were sacrificed 4 to 6 weeks after inoculation, they showed extensive abscess formation throughout the abdominal cavity, in some cases extending through the parietal peritoneum and abdominal wall with resultant sinus. Granules from the pus yielded *Act. bovis* on strained preparations and on culture. (Hazen and Little, 12.)

As a matter of fact, cattle cannot regularly be infected by inoculation with material from lesions or with cultures. Magnusson (19) succeeded in 8 instances in a total of 32 attempts. He succeeded twice in infecting swine: in one instance by injecting culture into the mammary gland, in the other by injecting it into the testicle.

Actinomycotic lesions are characterized by the formation of a soft, granulomatous tissue. After a time this tissue exhibits necrotic areas that break down into abscesses. These abscesses then coalesce to form sinuses or fistulous

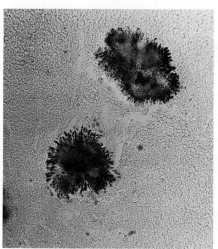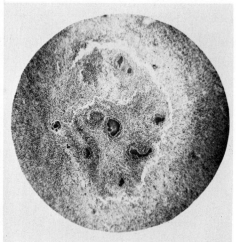

Fig. 80 (left). *Actinomyces bovis*, showing rosettes in pus of a bone lesion. Picrofuchsin stain. X 300 (Courtesy L. R. Vawter.)

Fig. 81 (right). Actinomycotic lesion, showing rosettes embedded in pus in center of the lesion. The greater part of the actinomycotic nodule consists of granulation tissue. X 75.

tracts, and at the same time the connective tissue hardens into dense masses or tumors. A thick, mucoid, tenacious, greenish-yellow, nonodorous pus is characteristic of the disease. The pus contains cheeselike granules varying in size up to 3 or 4 mm in diameter. These are the colonies of the organism and are commonly called *sulfur granules.*

If these granules are examined in the fresh condition, simply by pressing a clean cover glass on them, the ray-fungus appearance can be easily discerned. This is the most rapid way to make a definite diagnosis. The borders of the crushed granules show radiating, swollen, clublike filaments. The clublike

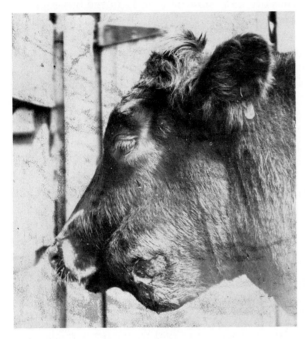

*Fig. 82.* Bovine actinomycosis. This is a case of true actinomycosis, involving the bone of the jaw and caused by *Actinomyces bovis.*

forms are not seen in stained preparations of the pus, as a general rule, but can be observed in histologic sections. Apparently, the swollen filaments are the result of a mantle of capsular material, and this material probably is produced as a result of contact with the tissue fluids.

Sulfur granules are found in the pus of actinobacillosis, and also in those actinomycosislike lesions that are caused by staphylococci. Fresh impression preparations show radiating, clublike forms, not unlike those of true actinomycosis. The sulfur granules in the nonactinomycotic lesions usually are much smaller than those of true actinomycosis, and frequently are so small that they are difficult to find on gross examination. The granules may be differentiated, of course, by making stained preparations, by which means the morphology of the causative organisms can be determined: true actinomycosis shows Gram-positive elements, short rods, filaments, and branching forms; actinobacillosis shows small Gram-negative rods; and staphylococci show their typical morphology. When making such examinations it is well to select the granules from the pus, wash them, and crush them on clean slides. If the slide is made at random from the pus, no organisms at all may be found. The granules can usually be obtained rather easily by placing some of the pus in a tube of broth or salt solution, shaking the tube to dissolve the mucin that holds the pus together, pouring the solution into a flat dish, and searching for the granules, which do not break up.

*Act. bovis* infection occurs more commonly in cattle than in other animals and in the bovine species lesions are seen most frequently in the bones of the face and jaw. That it does occur at times in other tissues is known. Kimball *et al.* (14) have found it in the bovine testis, where it causes orchitis.

In 1953 Ryff (23) described a case of encephalitis in a deer due to *Act. bovis.* In 1952 Burns and Simmons (3) reported a case of actinomycotic infection in a horse. The intermandibular space of this animal was affected. Cases of actinomycosis in the dog have also been recorded. In one case *Act. bovis* was isolated from lung tissue (20). In a second case the right cheek bones of the animal were involved (18), and in a third the infection was localized in the osseous tissue of the mandible (21).

In man orocervical facial actinomycosis is probably the most common form, but anorectal actinomycosis with secondary involvement of the skin and subcutaneous tissues of the perianal, gluteal, and thigh regions has also been reported (10). Although *Act. bovis* may cause actinomycosis in man it is also possible that most cases are caused by other so-called *human types.*

**Sources of Infection.** Formerly it was stated that the organism of actinomycosis was widespread in nature, that it occurred in the soil and on vegetation, and that animal infections were caused by injury of the mucosa of the mouth through which the organism entered. Support for this theory was afforded by the observation that the incidence of this disease was often high when cattle were fed upon very rough forage, especially on barley straw in which sharp awns were found. In fact, it is not uncommon to find fragments of such awns buried deeply in antinomycotic tumors of the jaw.

Because this organism never has been isolated from soil or animal foodstuffs and because it is rather delicate, many have doubted that it could maintain itself outside the animal body. Emmons (6) and Bibby and Knighton (1) have studied actinomycetes from the human mouth, some of which are very closely related to, if not identical with, *Act. bovis.* Grüner (11) found *Actinomyces* granules in material from tonsillectomies and concluded that the organism may be associated in some instances with tonsillar disease.

In the seventh edition of *Bergey's Manual* it is stated that *Act. bovis* frequently is found in and about the mouths of cattle and probably other animals. It formerly was said that the infection of the udder of sows came about from coarse vegetation that injured the low-hanging gland. Magnusson doubts that this is the true explanation and suggests that the infection probably orginates in the mouths of the suckling pigs and reaches the sow's udder through teat injuries made by the sharp teeth of the pigs.

**Immunity.** No attempts have been made to immunize animals against this organism, and there are no records of attempts at diagnosis by serological means.

**Chemotherapy.** This infection is iodine-sensitive. Local lesions are treated with Lugol's solution, and sodium iodide is frequently administered intravenously for internal lesions. A report by Chanton, Hollis, and Hargrove (4) on the treatment of human cases of actinomycosis indicates that penicillin and sulfadiazine therapy is effective. Lane and colleagues (17) used terramycin in treating orocervical actinomycosis, with apparent success. Other reports indicate that aureomycin and penicillin have therapeutic value in treating experimentally infected mice (8) and that the results obtained by treating actinomycosis of the bone in cattle with streptomycin are extremely encouraging (16). Suter (25) studied *in vitro* development of resistance of *Act. bovis* to antibiotics and concluded that none resulted on exposure to erythromycin, carbomycin, and penicillin, while treatment with oxytetracycline, tetracycline, chloramphenicol, and dihydrostreptomycin produced a slow and moderate build-up of resistance.

## REFERENCES

1. Bibby and Knighton.   Jour. Inf. Dis., 1941, *69*, 148.
2. Biever, Robertstad, Van Steenbergh, Scheetz, and Kennedy.   Am. Jour. Vet. Res., 1969, *30*, 1063.
3. Burns and Simmons.   Austral. Vet. Jour. 1952, *28*, 34.
4. Chanton, Hollis, and Hargrove.   South. Med. Jour., 1948, *41*, 1022.
5. Coleman, George, and Rozzell.   Appl. Microbiol., 1969, *18*, 420.
6. Emmons.   Pub. Health Rpts. (U.S.), 1938, *53*, 1967.
7. Erikson.   Med. Res. Council, Spec. Rpt. Ser. 240 (Brit.), 1940.
8. Geister and Meyer.   Jour. Lab. and Clin. Med., 1951, *38*, 101.
9. Georg, Robertstad, Brinkman, and Hicklin.   Jour. Inf. Dis., 1965, *115*, 88.
10. Gordon and DuBose.   Am. Jour. Clin. Path., 1951, *21*, 460.
11. Grüner.   Acta Path. et Microbiol. Scand., 1969, *76*, 239.
12. Hazen and Little.   Jour. Lab. and Clin. Med., 1958, *51*, 968.
13. Hazen, Little, and Resnick.   *Ibid.*, 1952, *40*, 914.
14. Kimball, Twiehaus, and Frank.   Am. Jour. Vet. Res., 1954, *15*, 551.
15. King and Meyer.   Bact. Proc., 1962, p. 68.
16. Kingman and Palen.   Jour. Am. Vet. Med. Assoc., 1951, *118*, 28.
17. Lane, Kutscher, and Chaves.   Jour. Am. Med. Assoc., 1953, *151*, 986.
18. McGaughey, Bateman, and Mackenzie.   Brit. Vet. Jour., 1951, *107*, 428.
19. Magnusson.   Acta Path. et Microbiol. Scand., 1928, *5*, 170.
20. Menges, Larsh, and Habermann.   Jour. Am. Vet. Med. Assoc., 1953, *122*, 73.
21. Migliano and Stopiglia.   *Ibid.*, 1951, *118*, 52.
22. Roderick, Kimball, McLeod, and Frank.   Am. Jour. Vet. Res., 1948, 9, 5.
23. Ryff.   Jour. Am. Vet. Med. Assoc., 1953, *122*, 78.
24. Slack and Gerencser.   Jour. Bact., 1970, *103*, 265.

25. Suter.    Antibiotics and Chemother., 1957, 7, 285.
26. Thompson.    Proc. Staff Meet. Mayo Clinic, 1950, 25, 81.
27. Vawter.    Cornell Vet., 1933, 23, 126.
28. Vawter.    Jour. Am. Vet. Med. Assoc., 1946, 109, 198.

# XXII | The *Dermatophilaceae*

In 1958 Austwick (3) reviewed the histories of *streptothricosis, mycotic dermatitis,* and *strawberry foot rot* and concluded that the causal organisms were congeneric. He proposed that *Dermatophilus,* the earliest generic name, be used for them and recognized three species: *D. congolensis* from streptothricosis in cattle, *D. dermatonomus* from mycotic dermatitis in sheep, and *D. pedis* from strawberry foot rot in sheep. He also suggested that these organisms be assigned to the family *Dermatophilaceae* and placed in the order *Actinomycetales.* In 1964, Gordon (9) studied members of the genus *Dermatophilus* and decided that all isolates can be accommodated in the species *D. congolensis,* with *D. dermatonomous* and *D. pedis* falling into synonymy. This conclusion was supported by serologic studies by Roberts (22) in 1965. Accordingly, we will consider *D. congolensis* to be the cause of the diseases commonly known as *cutaneous streptothricosis, mycotic dermatitis, lumpy wool, strawberry foot rot,* and *cutaneous actinomycosis.*

## THE GENUS *DERMATOPHILUS*

Members of the genus *Dermatophilus* are characterized by the presence of mycelium of narrow, tapering filaments with lateral branching at right angles. Septa are formed in transverse, horizontal, and vertical planes and give rise to parallel rows of coccoid cells that form motile flagellate spores. Both mycelia and spores are Gram-positive. They are aerobic and weakly fermentative.

The organism is pathogenic for cattle, sheep, goats, deer, horses, man, rabbits, and probably cats (18) and experimentally for guinea pigs and mice, causing exudative or pustular dermatitis. Pier *et al.* (20) have described FA and cultural technics available for diagnosis of cutaneous streptothricosis.

481

### *Dermatophilus congolensis*

SYNONYMS:   *Actinomyces congolensis, Streptothrix bovis, Tetragenus congolensis, Dermatophilus dermatonomus, Nocardia dermatonomus, Polysepta dermatonomus, Dermatophilus pedis, Polysepta pedis, Rhizobium pedis*

This organism is the cause of streptothricosis in cattle, horses, sheep, goats, deer, elands, and rabbits. It was first described by Van Saceghem (26), in 1915 in the Belgian Congo. The disease is most common in Africa, but similar cases have been described in Europe, Australia, New Zealand, India, and North and South America (2). It seems to be widespread, although infrequent in occurrence, in the United States and it is found in Canada.

**Cultural Features.** The organism grows well at 37 C. Colonies on solid media are grayish white, becoming yellowish with age, and sometimes viscous and adherent to the medium. They may be smooth, moist, mucoid, and not adherent. *D. congolensis* coagulates milk, usually liquefies gelatin slowly, and may produce a pellicle on liquid media. It ferments glucose and mannitol with acid production. It is variable in its ability to attack dextrin, galactose, levu-

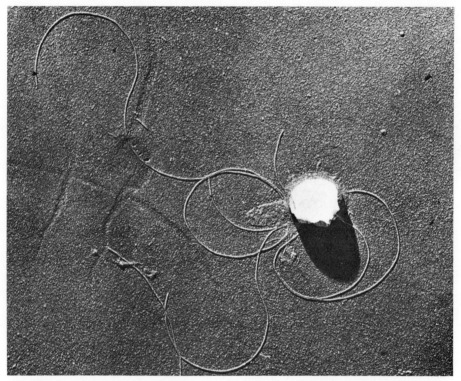

*Fig. 83*. Electron micrograph of *Dermatophilus congolensis* showing flagella. X 28,500. (Courtesy I. Grinyer.)

lose, and sucrose. It does not attack arabinose, dulcitol, lactose, or sorbitol.
**Pathogenicity.** Streptothricosis as it usually is seen in cattle, horses, deer, and
at times in sheep is characterized by small, confluent, raised, and circumscribed crusts composed of epidermal cells and coagulated serous exudate
with embedded hairs appearing on the skin of infected animals. The lesions
may be local or become progressive and sometimes fatal. The disease is essentially an exudative dermatitis followed by extensive scab formation.

Until about 1960 streptothricosis was regarded by the research workers in
North America as an exotic disease. In 1961 it was described in horses by
Bentinck-Smith *et al.* (4) and in a deer and the people who handled the deer
by Dean *et al.* (7). Within a few years the disease was recorded in Texas (5),
Iowa (19), and Kansas (14) cattle. More recently it has been diagnosed in
Mississippi (8), Vermont (13), and in Georgia (13, 24). It has occurred under
natural conditions in rabbits (23) and it has been described in 9-day-old
calves (25).

*For sheep. D. congolensis* is the cause of mycotic dermatitis in sheep. It
was described in 1929 by Bull (6) in Australia. Apparently a similar disease
exists in Africa, where it has been called *lumpy wool.* It has also been reported in India, England, and New Zealand.

The first signs of mycotic dermatitis in sheep are the appearance of small

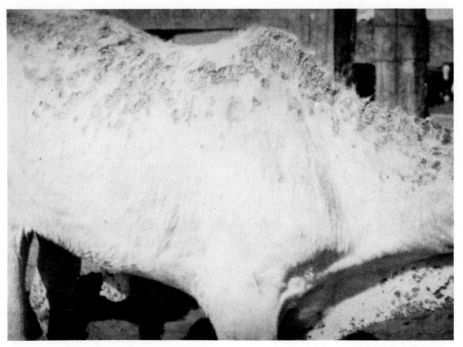

*Fig. 84.* Calf showing streptothricosis. (Courtesy Mario D'Apice, Universidade de São Paulo.)

areas of hyperemia, which persist for 10 to 14 days and are followed by the formation of crusts. Masses of crust material may mat the wool fibers, but usually the crust separates from the skin surface and remains as a zone of hardened exudate or is cast off. Removal of the scab from an active lesion leaves a concave, raw, and moist area. Progressive lesions may result in death and may cause serious losses in lambs.

The organism also causes strawberry foot rot in sheep. It was described by Harriss (10) in 1948 in Scotland, where it has been called *proliferative dermatitis in sheep* and was believed for a time to be caused by a virus (1). Employing the organism derived from sheep Abdussalan and Blakemore (1) were able to infect rabbits and guinea pigs by skin scarification. Papules appeared on the 2nd day after several rabbit passages; originally the incubation period was 5 days. Scabs were soon formed. These dropped off in about 2 weeks leaving smooth, hairless skin. Material from the fourth rabbit passage produced the disease in sheep and goats.

The natural disease in sheep begins with the appearance of dry scabs located on the legs at any point between the coronet and the knee or hock. Papules preceding the scab formation were not observed. It was thought that mechanical injury of the skin probably preceded the formation of lesions. The local lesions show a tendency to spread until sometimes almost the entire skin area of the lower portions of the legs is involved. More often the lesions, after reaching 2 to 4 cm in diameter, heal without further spread. The affected areas become denuded of hair or wool. When the areas are large, the exudate mats the hair and forms a hard, dry casing over the region. This usually can be easily stripped off, leaving a mass of granulation tissue that has the appearance of a strawberry, hence the origin of the common name of the disease. The lesions may remain for long periods but usually they heal within 5 or 6 weeks. The secondary infection rarely invades deeper structures, and usually the animal does not become lame. When lameness occurs, it is because the interdigital space has been invaded. There is little evidence of systemic reaction, although affected animals often do not gain weight as they should. The lesions usually heal without scar formation. They have not been seen on the face, lips, or wooled portions of the body in the natural disease. By inoculation it is possible to produce lesions on the lips, but these do not progress far and they heal rapidly.

After being placed on infected pastures, the animals usually manifest the disease in from 2 to 4 weeks. The longest period between exposure and appearance of symptoms has been 98 days for lambs and 117 days for adult sheep. By inoculation into the scarified skin, typical lesions are produced much earlier.

The mortality is very low but the morbidity is high. Most of the sheep on infected pastures contract the disease.

*For man.* Dean *et al.* (7) described the skin lesions that appeared in individuals who worked with infected deer. Similar lesions have been noted in workers who have come in contact with diseased sheep. Harriss (10) inoculated material that he had obtained from strawberry foot rot of sheep into the skin of the hand of a man. A lesion appeared at the point of inoculation and persisted for 30 days. It itched intensely from the 4th to the 9th day. The dried scab, taken when it was ready to fall off, reproduced the typical disease in sheep.

**Sources of Infection.** The part played by biting insects in producing the disease was established by Richard and Pier (21) when they transmitted *D. congolensis* from infected to normal rabbits by means of stable flies, *Stomoxys calcitrans*, and by house flies, *Musca domestica*. The role of high humidity as a factor in causing streptothricosis has been considered. Macadam (17) claimed that experimental evidence did not support a positive view, but Leriche (15) concluded that transmission of *D. congolensis* can occur by contact between sheep, especially if they are wet, and that therefore the procedures of dipping, showering, or even yarding wet sheep may play an important role in the transmission of dermatophilosis.

**Immunity.** There is conflicting evidence over the development of immunity in these diseases. Apparently immunity is not permanent and not especially solid, even for a short time.

**Chemotherapy.** According to Kammerlocher and Mammo (12) fulvicin administered orally and 1 percent gentian violet in alcohol and 5 percent salicylic acid in alcohol applied topically all proved to be effective during a 30-day treatment period. For successful topical therapy, removal of scabs and exudate from all lesions prior to treatment is essential. Potassium aluminum sulfate (alum) has been used in a dip for sheep with beneficial results (11), copper naphthenate (37.5 percent concentration) has been recommended as a topical medication for horses (13), and a combination of penicillin and streptomycin was credited with producing marked improvement in affected cattle and sheep (24, 16).

## REFERENCES

1. Abdussalan and Blakemore. Jour. Comp. Path. and Therap., 1948, 58, 333.
2. Ainsworth and Austwick. Fungal diseases of animals. Commonwealth Agricultural Bureaux, Bucks, England, 1959, pp. 73–79.
3. Austwick. Vet. Rev. and Annot., 1958, 4, 33.
4. Bentinck-Smith, Fox, and Baker. Cornell Vet., 1961, 51, 334.
5. Bridges and Romane. Jour. Am. Vet. Med. Assoc., 1961, 138, 153.
6. Bull. Austral. Jour. Exp. Biol. and Med. Sci., 1929, 6, 301.
7. Dean, Gordon, Severinghaus, Kroll, and Reilly. N.Y. State Jour. Med., 1961, 61, 583.
8. DiSalvo, Kaplan, McCrory, and Bryan. Vet. Med., 1969, 64, 502.
9. Gordon. Jour. Bact., 1964, 88, 509.
10. Harriss. Jour. Comp. Path. and Therap., 1948, 58, 314.
11. Hart and Tyszkiewicz. Vet. Rec., 1968, 82, 272.
12. Kammerlocher and Mammo. Vet. Med., 1965, 60, 65.

13. Kaplan and Johnston.    Jour. Am. Vet. Med. Assoc., 1966, *149*, 1162.
14. Kelley, Huston, Imes, and Weide.    Vet. Med., 1964, *59*, 175.
15. LeRiche.    Austral. Vet. Jour., 1968, *44*, 64.
16. LeRoux.    Jour. So. African Vet. Med. Assoc., 1968, 39, 87.
17. Macadam.    Vet. Rec., 1961, *73*, 1039.
18. O'Hara and Cordes.    New Zeal. Vet. Jour., 1963, *11*, 151.
19. Pier, Neal, and Cysewski.    Jour. Am. Vet. Med. Assoc., 1963, *142*, 995.
20. Pier, Richard, and Farrell.    Am. Jour. Vet. Res., 1964, *25*, 1014.
21. Richard and Pier.    *Ibid.*, 1966, 27, 419.
22. Roberts.    Nature, 1965, *206*, 1068.
23. Shotts, Jr. and Kistner.    Jour. Am. Vet. Med. Assoc., 1970, *157*, 667.
24. Shotts, Jr., Tyler, and Christy.    *Ibid.*, 1969, *154*, 1450.
25. Thornton and Willoughby.    Canad. Vet. Jour., 1970, *11*, 120.
26. Van Saceghem.    Soc. de Path. Exot. Bul., 1915, *8*, 354.

PART 4

# BACTERIALIKE PATHOGENIC PATHOGENIC ORGANISMS

# XXIII | The Spirochetes

The organisms known as the *spirochetes* are grouped with the bacteria, because of their close resemblance to organisms that undoubtedly are bacteria, the spirilla. It should be recognized, however, that they possess a number of features seen in no other bacteria. Some of the general characteristics of the group are described below.

**Morphology.** The form is spiral. In some species the spirals are tight, in others quite open and variable. Terminal filaments are seen in some types but these do not behave like flagella. Some forms may show an axial filament, a lateral crista or ridge, or transverse striations. When tissue fluids, especially blood, are examined in the dark field for the presence of spirochetes, caution must be exercised in the interpretation of findings inasmuch as mistakes can be very easily made even by experienced workers. Filaments of elastic tissue, fibrin shreds, and other artifacts often resemble spirochetes so closely as to deceive all but the most wary. Such materials even create the illusion of motility.

**Staining Properties.** Most of the spirochetes are difficult to stain. Few of the pathogenic species may be stained with methylene blue. All are Gram-negative. The Giemsa stain is useful, some staining red, others blue. Those that stain blue generally are saprophytes that can be stained with methylene blue. For demonstration in tissues, Levaditi's stain is most useful. This stain contains silver nitrate. After the tissue block has been saturated with the silver compound, it is treated with a reducing agent that removes the silver from the tissues and other bacteria but not from the spirochetes. These are then seen as intensely black organisms. The dark-field method of examination often is used when these organisms are sought, because it is practically impossible to see them unstained in ordinary light due to their extreme tenuousness. India ink, nigrosin, and similar background-filling agents also are useful in making organisms visible in film preparations.

489

**Motility.** The motility of spirochetes is derived from their rotatory motion. In some species it is so rapid as to make it impossible to follow them with the eye. Many spirochetes exhibit various bending movements, which probably have little to do with their movement of translation.

**Resistance.** In general, the resistance of spirochetes is very low. Drying is rapidly fatal. Temperatures of 50 to 60 C generally kill within a short time. Resistance to chemical disinfectants is not great.

**Cultivation.** The spirochetes generally are less easily cultivated than bacteria. Some, especially the *Leptospira,* can be grown without great difficulty, but others require elaborate media and the results are uncertain at best. The majority are strict anaerobes. Even the aerobic forms thrive best when the oxygen tension is lowered. None can be cultivated upon the surface of solid media. Either fluid media must be used, or the inoculum must be incorporated in the depths of solid media. Growth of the pathogenic species practically always requires the presence of serum or other animal fluids.

**Classification.** Two families of spirochetes are recognized. The family *Spirochetaceae* contains the genera *Spirocheta* and *Saprospira,* which include a number of species all of which are free-living and relatively large, and the genus *Cristospira.* Species of the latter genus occur as parasites of various molluscs, principally oysters, mussels, and scallops. The species that are pathogenic for birds and mammals belong to the family *Treponemataceae.*

## THE *TREPONEMATACEAE*

This family contains three genera, *Borrelia, Treponema,* and *Leptospira.* Members of the genus Borrelia are relatively large forms with open, irregular coils, which move by active lashing movements and slow rotation. These forms are readily stained by many of the aniline dyes that stain bacteria. Members of the *Treponema* are smaller, with close, rigid coils, and these do not stain readily with dyes other than the Giemsa stain. The *Leptospira* resemble the *Treponema* in that they have close coils, but these are not rigid, the organism frequently stretching out into a straight filamentous form that relaxes into the coil once more. The *Leptospira* are aerobic but the *Treponema* are strict anaerobes. A further characteristic feature of the *Leptospira* is the almost constant presence of a bend or hook at one or both ends of the organism. Like the *Treponema,* the species of this group are difficult to stain except with Giemsa's stain.

The three genera that contain the species pathogenic for the higher animals (*Borrelia, Treponema,* and *Leptospira*) may be distinguished from the saprophytic groups by the fact that they may be readily dissolved by a 10 percent bile solution. The treponemas may be distinguished from the leptospiras by the fact that they may be dissolved by a 10 percent saponin solution.

Most of the spirochetes known to be pathogenic for animals occur in the genera *Borrelia* and *Leptospira.*

## THE GENUS *BORRELIA*

In this genus are found a number of parasitic forms. They are pathogenic for man, other mammals, and birds. Some are transmitted by the bites of arthropods.

**Morphology and Staining Reactions.** These organisms are loosely spiraled and irregular. They generally taper terminally into fine filaments. They stain easily with ordinary aniline dyes and are Gram-negative. Their refractive indices are approximately the same as those of true bacteria. However, they can be demonstrated best by dark-field illumination, the India ink method, or the Levaditi stain.

**Cultural Features.** Noguchi (13) cultivated a number of species in a medium consisting of a tall column of ascitic fluid that contained a bit of sterile rabbit kidney overlaid with paraffin oil. A few drops of infected blood were used as the inoculum, and the tubes were incubated at body temperature. In such tubes the spirochetes grew rather rapidly for 4 or 5 days, then appeared to disintegrate into granules. The report of Bohls, Irons, and De Shazo (2) indicates that the spirochete of relapsing fever can be cultivated in the developing chick embryo.

### Relapsing Fever Spirochetes (*Borrelia*)

In Europe, India, Africa, and America there occurs a disease of man known as relapsing fever. In the febrile paroxysms of this disease, members of *Borrelia* can be demonstrated in the blood, and these organisms undoubtedly are the cause of the disease. The organisms differ in various localities, although all forms of relapsing fever are clinically identical. Two epidemiological types of the disease are distinguished, the one tick-borne and representing transmission from an animal reservoir of infection to man, and the other louse-borne and spread from man to man (3). The organisms undergo a developmental cycle in these insects; the tick can transmit the infection by biting, but the louse transmits infection by its feces or by being crushed on the skin. The tick-borne disease appears to be the only one that occurs in the United States, and endemic foci of infection exist in Arizona, California, Colorado, Idaho, Kansas, New Mexico, Nevada, Oklahoma, Oregon, and Texas. According to Francis (5), the infection may survive in ticks for as long as 6.5 years and be transmitted to offspring of the third generation. In 1969 an outbreak occurred on Brown mountain near Spokane, Washington in boy scouts and scoutmasters who camped there. *Ornithodoros hermsi* ticks were shown to be infected with spirochetes and it was suggested that chipmunks and pine squirrels were the reservoir for the disease (18).

Mice, rats, and hamsters can be infected by inoculation of relapsing fever spirochetes, but guinea pigs are more resistant. Natural infection of lower animals occurs with some frequency in endemic areas, and it is quite possible that small mammals, especially rodents, constitute a natural reservoir of the tick-borne infection.

Practical laboratory diagnosis is based on mouse inoculation and blood-smear demonstrations of the *Borrelia* organism (4).

### Borrelia theileri

SYNONYMS:    *Treponema theileri, Spirocheta theileri*

This organism was found by Theiler (17) in the blood of South African cattle in 1902. It is a large, loosely twisted spiral, measuring from 20 to 30 microns in length. The organism can be easily demonstrated in the blood during the febrile stage of the infection, but it disappears later. It is actively motile. Artificial cultivation of this organism has not been reported.

The disease apparently is fairly benign. The symptoms resemble those of ana-plasmosis but are less severe. One or more febrile attacks are followed by recovery. Transmission is by the ticks *Margaropus decoloratus* and *Rhipicephalus evertsi.*

The same, or at least a similar, organism has been found associated with febrile attacks in sheep and horses. These diseases are not serious.

### Borrelia anserina

SYNONYM:    *Spirocheta anserina, Spirocheta gallinarum, Borrelia gallin-arum, Spironema gallinarum*

This organism was first described by Sakharoff (16), in Russia, as the cause of "goose septicemia" in 1891. It is probable that it is the same as the cause of "fowl spirochetosis" or "fowl spirillosis," which was recognized in Brazil by Marchoux and Salimbeni in 1903. The disease was found a little later in the Sudan. The spirochete of the chicken disease is regarded as a separate species by some and given the name *Borrelia gallinarum*. A similar disease has been reported in ducks and turkeys. It seems likely that geese, chickens, ducks, and turkeys are affected by the same species. If this is the case, the correct name of the organism, inappropriate as it may seem, is that first applied to the goose infection.

In California, outbreaks of avian spirochetosis have been reported in tur-keys (9) and in Mongolian pheasants. It was readily transmitted from the pheasants to Muscovy ducklings and to chickens (11). The avian spirochete was believed to be the cause of epizootics in Arizona poultry (15). The infec-tion occurs in Australia (7).

The disease is manifested by signs of acute septicemia. The affected birds develop fever, they are depressed, a profuse diarrhea occurs, and they soon die. The mortality rate is very high. Autopsy examination reveals a swollen spleen, a pale and swollen liver, and a serofibrinous exudate in the peri-cardial sac. During the early stages of the febrile reaction the spiral organ-isms can readily be found in the blood. At the time of death they usually are absent, or abnormal or clumped forms may be found.

Al-Hilly (1) claims that the liver of a spirochete-infected chicken yields an antigen that produces positive lines in immunodiffusion agar-gel tests. Gross and Ball (8) have found that the FA technic provides a rapid method of detecting *Borrelia* in blood films. Although the disease is generally believed to be transmitted by ticks such as *Argus persicus* and *A. miniatus* and occasionally by others, the California workers suggested that infected droppings represented the most probable means of transmission in the outbreaks that they studied (9, 11). The fowl mite, *Dermanyssus gallinae* has also been suspected of being a transmitting agent.

**Pathogenicity.** The disease is easily transmitted to a variety of birds, including, besides the ones that suffer from the natural infection, guinea fowl, sparrows, and canaries. Pigeons are fairly resistant, rats and guinea pigs wholly so. The inoculation disease is quite like the naturally occurring type.

**Immunity.** Recovery from the disease leaves the bird refractory to further infection for a considerable period of time. Gabritschewsky (6) found that the fresh serum of recovered geese caused disintegration and destruction of the spirochetes in a short time when incubated at 37 C. This is similar to the action that goes on in the blood of the recovering bird. The same worker found that immune horse serum was effective as a prophylactic agent but was ineffective when administered to birds in which the organism had begun to multiply.

Marchoux and Salimbeni (10) prepared an effective vaccine by heating the fresh blood of affected birds to 55 C for 5 minutes. They also found that the organism loses its virulence when stored in blood for 48 hours, and that such blood may be used as a vaccine. Rao *et al.* (14), Uppal and Rao (19), and Gorrie (7) have developed embryonated egg vaccines that promise durable immunity in vaccinated birds.

**Chemotherapy.** Arsphenamine and its derivatives have been used successfully in treating some of the relapsing fever infections of man. Morcos, Zaki, and Zaki (12) reported that arrhenal, sulfanomides, and penicillin had no curative effect in avian spirochetosis. On the other hand, myosalvarsan, atoxyl, and spirocide were almost specific as curatives and had the further advantage of serving as tonics. Recently, Rao *et al.* (14) reported that penicillin administered as a therapeutic agent at 4,000 units per pound of body weight is fully effective in curing avian spirochetosis at the height of infection.

## REFERENCES

1. Al-Hilly. Am. Jour. Vet. Res., 1969, *30*, 1877.
2. Bohls, Irons, and De Shazo. Proc. Soc. Exp. Biol. and Med., 1940, *45*, 375.
3. Burrows. Textbook of microbiology. 16th ed. W. B. Saunders Co., Philadelphia and London, 1954.
4. Felsenfeld. Bact. Rev., 1965, 29, 46.
5. Francis. Pub. Health Rpts. (U.S.), 1938, 53, 2220.
6. Gabritschewsky. Centrbl. f. Bakt., I Abt., 1898, 23, 365, 439, 635, 721, and 778.

7. Gorrie. Austral. Vet. Jour. 1950, *26*, 308.
8. Gross and Ball. Am. Jour. Vet. Res., 1964, *25*, 1734.
9. Loomis. *Ibid.*, 1953, *14*, 612.
10. Marchoux and Salimbeni. Ann. l'Inst. Past., 1903, *17*, 569.
11. Mathey and Siddle. Jour. Am. Vet. Med. Assoc., 1955, *126*, 123.
12. Morcos, Zaki, and Zaki. *Ibid.*, 1946, *109*, 112.
13. Noguchi. Jour. Exp. Med., 1912, *16*, 620.
14. Rao, Thakral, and Dhanda. Indian Vet. Jour., 1954, *31*, 1.
15. Rokey and Snell. Jour. Am. Vet. Med. Assoc., 1961, *138*, 648.
16. Sakharoff. Ann. l'Inst. Past., 1891, *5*, 564.
17. Theiler. Jour. Comp. Path. and Therap., 1904, *17*, 47.
18. Thompson, Burgdorfer, Russell, and Francis. Jour. Am. Med. Assoc., 1969, *210*, 1045.
19. Uppal and Rao. Indian Vet. Jour., 1966, *43*, 191.

## THE GENUS *TREPONEMA*

These organisms are small and their spirals usually are close and regular. Their ends may be drawn out into extremely fine fibrils. They are difficult to stain and weakly refractive by dark-field illumination. They can be cultivated under anaerobic conditions. They are pathogenic for man and certain animals and generally produce local lesions in the tissues. Within the genus *Treponema* a species, *T. cuniculi*, causes spirochetosis in the rabbit. Other species produce diseases in man. *T. pallidum* is the cause of syphilis, *T. pertenue* the cause of yaws, and *T. carateum* the cause of *mal del pinto* (carate). These species are not naturally infective for animals, but they may be transmitted by injection to the rabbit. The use of penicillin has given dramatic results in the treatment of syphilis (2) and *T. cuniculi* infection (vent disease) of rabbits (1).

### REFERENCES

1. Chapman. North Am. Vet., 1947, *28*, 740.
2. Frobisher. Fundamentals of microbiology. 8th ed. W. B. Saunders Co., Philadelphia and London, 1968.

## THE GENUS *LEPTOSPIRA*

Leptospirae are chiefly saprophytic, aquatic organisms, which are found in river and lake waters, in sewage, and in the sea. Some species are pathogenic for man and animals. Leptospirosis is a not uncommon infection which is widely distributed. The pathogenic types are not known to multiply outside infected animal tissues.

**Morphology and Staining Reactions.** Leptospirae are the smallest of the spirochetes. Individual cells are not more than 0.3 microns in breadth, but vary from 6 to 30 microns in length. Frequently their spirals are so fine and so closely wound that, when observed in the dark field, only the outer curves are seen. They are further characterized by being bent into a hook at one or both ends. Their motion consists of a writhing and flexing movement and a rapid rotation around the long axis. They stain with difficulty except with Giemsa's stain and silver impregnation. They are readily filterable through Berkefeld V and N candles—a means of separating them from bacteria and treponemas.

**Cultural Features.** The leptospirae are readily cultivated. They may be grown on serum diluted with 5 to 10 parts of Ringer or Locke solution. A medium devised by Noguchi which contains a mixture of one part of 2 percent nutrient agar, one part of rabbit serum, and eight parts of physiological salt solution may be used. Semisolid meat infusion agar containing 10 percent serum makes a very good medium (62). Semisynthetic media has also been recommended (24, 38, 77). Incubation at 37 C or slightly below usually produces the best growth. The organisms can be cultivated in embryonated chicken eggs. They will grow in bovine fetal kidney cell tissue cultures (43).

The respiratory mechanism of leptospirae is peculiar in that they require gaseous oxygen, and to this extent are strict aerobes, but in a limited sense they are microaerophilic. In a solid or semisolid media they grow a few mm below the surface, they are cyanide-sensitive, lack catalase, have slight reducing activity, and fail to produce recognizable traces of hydrogen peroxide (21). Apparently they do not ferment sugars. It appears that virulence can be maintained by serial cultivation in animals or embryos but not in artificial media.

**Serotypes.** Although indistinguishable on the basis of morphological, cultural, or biochemical characteristics, pathogenic *Leptospira* can be differentiated by means of their serological properties. Wolff (94) used agglutination-lysis reactions and in his 1954 publication listed 36 serotypes. The serotypes sharing major antigenic components have been placed in serogroups, and within each group complete and incomplete types are recognized, the incomplete types containing part but not all of the antigenic components of the serogroup. By 1960 at least 40 serotypes had been identified in human and animal leptospiroses. In 1967 there were ca. 125 known serotypes divided among 18 serogroups. These groups have been designated Icterohemorrhagiae, Javanica, Celledoni, Canicola, Ballum, Pyrogenes, Cynopteri, Autumnalis, Australis, Pomona, Grippotyphosa, Hebdomadis, Bataviae, Tarassovi, Panama, Shermani, Semaranga, and Andamana.

In general, the leptospiral serotypes are associated with one or more mammalian species. The principal reservoirs are rodents, especially rats, mice, and voles, and domestic animals such as dogs, cattle, and pigs. For many years, rats and dogs were considered to be the primary animal carriers. Although leptospirosis is still prevalent in dogs and infection in rats ranges from 30 to 60 percent, the disease in now a major problem in cattle and swine, and, in some areas, sheep, goats, and horses become infected. There is increasing evidence that there is a wide distribution of leptospires in a variety of wild animals throughout the world.

Besides the rats other rodent carriers are mice and voles, and the wild animal reservoirs include bats, mongooses, shrews, bandicoots, jackals, and hedgehogs. In the United States deer, opossums, raccoons, skunks, foxes, wildcats, beaver, nutria, armadillos, woodchucks, and rabbits have been infected. In these host animals, leptospires will localize in the kidneys and may be found in the lumina of the convoluted tubules. After acute or even inapparent infection, these animals may become carriers and shed the organisms in their urine for long periods. The infected urine of these shedders serves as an important source of infection in man and other animals. In man and the larger mammals the disease varies from mild febrile influenzalike disease to the full blown Weil's disease in man and "canine jaundice" or Stuttgart disease in dogs.

Serotypes such as *L. icterohemorrhagiae, L. canicola, L. grippotyphosa, L. bataviae, L. hebdomadis, L. australis, L. pyrogenes, L. pomona, L. ballum,* and *L. tarassovi* show widespread global distribution. Other serotypes (*L. autumnalis, L. sejroe,* and *L. andamana*) appear to be restricted to particular areas of the world. Primary problems in the United States usually are associated with the more common types, *L. icterohemorrhagiae, L. canicola,* and *L. pomona,* in domestic animals and man (31). Numerous other serotypes have been isolated, and the findings suggest the presence of many more. *L. autumnalis* has been identified in man and in wild animals. *L. ballum* has appeared in mice, opossums, rats, an eastern hog-nosed snake, and man. *L. grippotyphosa* was obtained from wild animals in Florida along with *L. pomona, L. australis,* and *L. autumnalis.* Other serotypes belonging to the Tarassovi serogroup have been isolated from wild animals in southeastern United States and have been designated *L. bakeri* and *L. atlantae.* A new subserotype of the Hebdomadis serogroup was named *L. mimi georgia.* This type has now been derived also from human infection. Serologic evidence suggests the presence of *L. bataviae* infection in man and in cattle. *L. sejroe* occurs in cattle and man and a closely related serotype, *L. hardjo,* has been obtained in Louisiana, Nebraska, and Pennsylvania from animals both with and without signs of disease. A member of the Bataviae serogroup (*L. paidjan*) has been found in Louisiana in nutria (80), and *L. manilae,* a new serotype in the Pyrogenes group, was derived from rats (30).

*L. icterohemorrhagiae* is carried by rats, dogs, and occasionally cattle and swine; *L. canicola* is primarily an infection of dogs but also is seen in swine and cattle; and *L. pomona* is the organism most frequently incriminated as the cause of bovine, equine, and porcine leptospirosis. Although it seems that certain leptospiral serotypes have a primary host, none are completely host adapted. It is not unusual for a so-called *primary host* to become infected with other serotypes. *L. canicola* is found principally in dogs, but has been isolated from cattle, swine, jackals, hedgehogs, and skunks. Serologic evidence suggests that it may infect raccoons. In addition to *L. canicola* dogs have been found to harbor at least nine serotypes, including *L. pomona.*

### Leptospira icterohemorrhagiae

SYNONYM: *Spirocheta icterohemorrhagiae*

This organism is the causative agent of a disease of man known variously as *leptospirosis, leptospiral jaundice,* and *Weil's disease.* Most human infections probably occur through skin contact with fresh rat urine or through consumption of contaminated water and, less often, food. Surveys conducted in various parts of the world indicate that the rat infection is widespread. In a survey of 100 rats obtained in the vicinity of Ithaca, New York, Monlux (67) found 55 that harbored *Leptospira.* The disease ordinarily is sporadic except in situations where men come in intimate contact with rats, e.g., men who work in sewers, in rat-infested mines, and in rat-infested trenches in time of warfare. The disease in rats is chronic, the principal seat of infection being the kidneys.

This organism can easily be transmitted, by inoculation, to dogs and foxes, and natural infections undoubtedly occur (67). The human disease can be contracted from such animals. Although *L. icterohemorrhagiae* can cause infection in dogs, it appears that the majority of infections in this animal are produced by *L. canicola,* which will be described later.

*L. icterohemorrhagiae* infection has been reported in calves (51) and also in pigs (27, 72), but other serotypes, notably *L. pomona,* occur more frequently in these animals.

### Leptospira canicola

A number of European workers had recognized spirochetes in the kidneys of dogs suffering from jaundice and from a hemorrhagic-uremic disease of dogs commonly known as *Stuttgart disease* prior to 1930, and it had been demonstrated that pathologic pictures similar to some of the naturally occurring forms of the disease could be produced by inoculation with the Weil's disease organism. It had been assumed, therefore, that the causative organism was *L. icterohemorrhagiae.* Klarenbeek and Schüffner (54), working in Holland, showed in 1931 that a spirochete which differed serologically from the classical Weil organism was the causative agent of many of the canine cases. This organism later became known as *L. canicola.* It is now known that it differs from the classical type of man and rat in the character of the disease that it produces in the dog and in the fact that it has slight pathogenicity for rats. Present evidence indicates that *L. canicola* is much more prevalent in dogs than *L. icterohemorrhagiae* and that, instead of being a more or less accidental infection, it spreads readily from dog to dog and frequently produces enzootics, especially in large kennels. In many European countries *L. canicola* infections appear to be quite common, and it has become evident that there are many areas in the United States in which the disease is prevalent.

The organism is usually most easily found in the urine (63), in which it should be concentrated by centrifugation. It may also be found in the kidneys and with greater difficulty in other organs. Sometimes it is found only after prolonged search. Occasionally it may be recovered by guinea pig inoculation when it cannot be found in the dog.

**Differentiation between L. canicola and L. icterohemorrhagiae Infections.** Differentiation between these two infections in dogs and man is practically impossible except by the use of serological reactions. Some contrasting characters of the two kinds of infection are given by Walch-Sorgdrager and Schüffner (92) from their considerable experience with both types in Holland. Their principal points of differentiation are summarized below.

1. The disease in dogs. *L. canicola* infection seldom produces icterus, whereas this is a prominent feature of Weil's disease in dogs and in man. (Experience in this country indicates that this feature is not a reliable means of differentiation, because many of the *L. canicola* infections exhibit icterus.)

2. The disease in man. *L. canicola* infection is more benign that Weil's disease, since it seldom results in death. In man icterus is seldom seen in *L. canicola* infection, whereas it is common in Weil's disease. In man *L. canicola* infection is likely to produce severe symptoms of meningitis, whereas these symptoms are not common in Weil's disease.

3. The disease in experimental animals. *L. canicola* infection is not so pathogenic for guinea pigs as is Weil's disease (more than half of injected animals fail to develop clinical disease). The infection sometimes can be established in these animals by several blind passages. In guinea pigs icterus occurs only in a few animals injected with material from dogs when the causative organism is *L. canicola*, whereas 90 percent or more develop icterus when injected with Weil's organism. Guinea pigs injected with *L. canicola*-containing materials, even though they may show no symptoms, usually shed the *Leptospira* in the urine for considerable periods of time. Those injected with Weil's disease organism usually die from an acute infection before they become urinary shedders.

The water rat, which is the reservoir in all parts of the world of *L. icterohemorrhagiae,* and also other varieties of rats are resistant to *L. canicola.* The latter organism usually multiplies for a few days in the tissues and disappears without appearing in the urine, whereas infection with the former practically always results in urine shedders. Furthermore, serological tests of rat populations indicate that the infection carrier is always *L. icterohemorrhagiae* and never *L. canicola.* It is clear, therefore, that *L. canicola* is not a rat-borne infection.

4. Epidemiology. Epidemiological studies indicate that *L. canicola* infection is spread directly from dog to dog. Infected animals usually are urinary shedders. It is probable that the infection is taken in through the mouth and nose when dogs are smelling and licking the urogenital organs of other animals. It is significant that male dogs are infected more than twice as often as females. It is not impossible that the infection is spread through copulation.

5. Serological reactions. These two leptospiras cross-agglutinate only to a

small degree. The greater number of infected dogs agglutinate *L. canicola* to a high titer and *L. icterohemorrhagiae* to a low titer or not at all, whereas naturally infected rats agglutinate Weil's organism and not *L. canicola.*

**Pathogenicity.** Three types of the disease in dogs are recognized: the acute hemorrhagic type, the icteric less acute type, and the uremic type, commonly known as *Stuttgart disease* or *canine typhus. L. icterohemorrhagiae* causes the

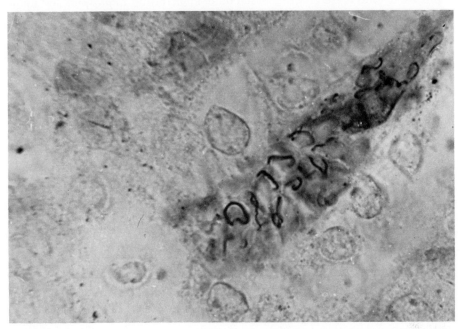

Fig. 85. *Leptospira canicola* in the kidney of an artificially infected guinea pig. Warthin-Starry stain. X 2,300. (Courtesy John T. Bryans and Peter C. Kennedy.)

first and second types but rarely, if ever, the third type. *L. canicola* causes most, if not all, of the third type, some of the second, and a few of the first.

The first type is characterized by high fever, prostration, and early death. Hemorrhages occur throughout the organs, especially in the lungs and alimentary tract. The second type is less acute and is characterized by intense icterus, hemorrhages with blood-stained feces, and pigmented urine. The third type is characterized by uremia because of extensive kidney damage; by a foul odor from the mouth because of ulcerative stomatitis; and by hemorrhagic enteritis, coma, and death in a high percentage of cases.

The clinical picture of the true Weil's disease in man is similar to that exhibited by dogs. Few cases of *L. canicola* infection in man (dubbed *canicola fever* by Meyer) have been reported in the United States. This may be due to the fact that this disease rarely elicits severe icteric or nephritic symptoms such as are seen in Weil's disease. Meyer, Stewart-Anderson, and Eddie (64) have warned veterinarians and dog owners to be careful in the handling of dogs that show symptoms of icterus or of Stuttgart disease, because of the hazard to health.

*L. canicola* has been recovered from swine and cattle but does not appear to be a common cause of infection in these animals.

**Diagnosis.** Although clinical features and autopsy findings may indicate leptospirosis, definitive diagnosis is based on demonstrating *Leptospira* and upon serological findings. The spirochetes may be demonstrated by guinea pig or hamster inoculation, dark-field examination, and cultural means. The FA technic can be used not only to detect leptospires in urine (93) and in tissues (58) but also to identify serotypes (22, 23).

The microscopic agglutination-lysis test is highly sensitive and apparently reliable. It requires dark-field equipment and a knowledge of dark-field technic. A serum sample is titrated against an antigen composed of an actively growing smooth *Leptospira* strain in liquid medium. After several hours' incubation, loopfuls of this mixture of serum and organisms are removed and examined by dark-field illumination. A positive reaction results in either agglutination, lysis, or both. According to Coffin and Stubbs (17), animals suffering from leptospirosis may show serum titers varying from 1:10 to 1:300,000. Antibodies appear in measurable titer 7 to 9 days after the onset of the disease and quickly reach a high level unless the animal succumbs to the infection. A convalescent animal carries this titer for months. More than one agglutination test is necessary to establish the diagnosis because the finding of an increased titer on the second test indicates an active infection, whereas the findings of an equivalent, or a decreased, titer may point to a convalescent case. Furthermore, the frequency of occurrence of agglutinins to leptospiral organisms other than *L. canicola* and *L. icterohemorrhagiae* indicates a need to utilize many test antigens when screening canine serums for leptospiral agglutinins (91).

The macroscopic plate test has been used, but the preparation of a sensitive antigen that will not prove to be autoagglutinable is very difficult. This test can be used in the field but it has no value in the first 5 to 7 days of the illness because antibodies are slow to develop. Too often the animal is dead before agglutinins appear. Furthermore, the concentrated antigen of the macroscopic test fails to detect antibodies as early in the disease as does the microscopic test. Neither test can be relied upon in diagnosing leptospirosis early in the course of the disease. However, the microscopic test is still the standard reference procedure for the serological diagnosis of leptospirosis and classification of leptospires.

A hemolytic test has also been used in the serodiagnosis of leptospirosis (20). Antigen is absorbed on erythocytes which are in turn exposed to complement and the suspect antiserum. The test appears to be even more sensitive than the microscopic agglutination test.

**Immunity.** After recovering from an attack of leptospirosis, both man and animals are thereafter immune. Immune sera have been used in treating Weil's disease in man with fairly good results. Such sera are difficult to produce and can be expected only to ameliorate the symptoms rather than to effect a complete cure. There are no reports of the use of immune sera on dogs.

Vaccination of young dogs with a mixed whole-culture bacterin of *L. icterohemorrhagiae* and *L. canicola* is recommended, but limited experimental evidence suggests that the duration of immunity only persists for a few months.

## Bovine Leptospirosis

A spirochetal jaundice in young calves occurring in the north Caucasus was described by Mikhin and Azinov (65) in 1935. To the causative organism the name *Leptospira icterohemoglobinuriae vitulorum* was given. In 1944 Golikov (37), another Russian, reported a communication from Palestine indicating that a similar, perhaps identical, disease was enzootic there. Later Freund (28) reported that the Palestinian disease was first recognized in 1941 and that more than 500 cases had been diagnosed within the 2 years that followed. The causative organism was named *L. bovis*. It was shown to be serologically different from *L. icterohemorrhagiae* and *L. canicola*. A number of human infections were diagnosed in farmers, veterinarians, butchers, and others who had direct contacts with cattle. Bernkopf (3, 4) and Bernkopf, Olitski, and Stuczynski (7) reported additional cases and the results of experimental infections of cattle in Palestine. Caspar and Reif (15), Padersky (73), Schachtel (81), and Btesh (12) described human cases in Palestine. In 1949 Sutherland, Simmons, and Kenny (90) recorded three outbreaks in calves in Australia.

In the United States bovine leptospirosis has been described by Jungherr (53) in Connecticut, by Marsh (59) in Montana, by Mathews (61) in Texas, by Baker and Little (2) in New Jersey and Pennsylvania, by Sutherland and Morrill (89) in Illinois, and by Reinhard, Tierney, and Roberts (75) in New York. These observations indicated that the disease was widespread in the United States. The causative organism of the American disease was first isolated by Baker and Little, and comparative studies of the American and Palestinian strains were made by Bernkopf and Little (6). These studies revealed that the American and some of the Palestinian organisms were identical with the one first isolated from a dairy farmer in Queensland, Australia, in 1937 by Clayton *et al.* (16) and called *L. pomona*. Extensive evidence of *L. pomona* infection has since been demonstrated in bovine and porcine populations in various sections of the globe, and its infection potential for man in endemic and epidemic proportions has been realized. Apparently this serotype occurs less frequently in dogs, but reports of natural infection are found in the literature (70, 71). It has been observed in the feral cat (26) and it appears that cats may be infected by leptospires, but do not develop overt disease (57).

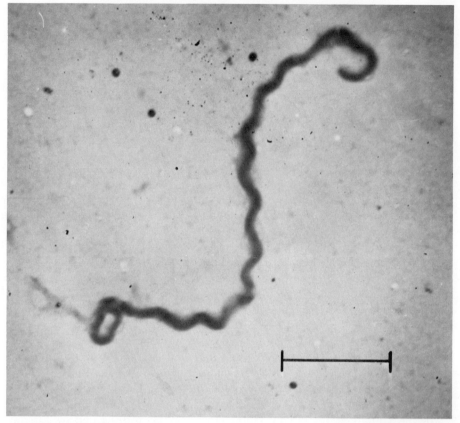

*Fig. 86.* Electron micrograph of bovine *Leptospira*. Scale = 1 micron. X 30,000, approximately. (Courtesy J. A. Baker.)

Although *L. icterohemorrhagiae* and *L. canicola* sometimes occur in cattle, the predominant serotypes in the bovine species appear to be *L. pomona* in the United States and Australia, *L. australis* and *L. hebdomadis* in Japan, and *L. grippotyphosa* in Russia and Israel. Many of the recognized serotypes have been isolated from cattle in widely scattered parts of the world.

**Pathogenicity for Experimental Animals.** The reports on pathogenicity for experimental animals differ in different parts of the world. The Russian strain was found to be virulent for white mice and guinea pigs. The Palestine strains did not produce clinical signs of illness in rabbits, guinea pigs, mice, rats, and hamsters, but induced a temperature rise in guinea pigs about 8 days after inoculation. Bernkopf (5) concluded, however, that the bovine type is infective for chickens. Baker and Little found that the American strains could be transmitted to guinea pigs. These animals developed febrile reactions, and if autopsies were conducted during this period petechial hemorrhages were found in the lungs and whitish areas of focal necrosis in the liver. Those that were not destroyed soon recovered from the febrile attack and appeared normal thereafter. White mice were not affected by inoculation of cultures, but the organism was recovered after serial passage through five animals. Temperature reactions like those of guinea pigs were exhibited by rabbits, but no lesions were found on autopsy. Puppies inoculated with *L. pomona* show no clinical evidence of leptospirosis, but organisms can be found in the blood stream for a short time and the animals become urinary shedders of the spirochete, occasionally remaining carriers for months. These animals develop blood titers, which gradually disappear, but apparently do not produce urinary antibodies.

The cultivation of *Leptospira* in chick embryos has been reported by Morrow *et al.* (68). Gleiser *et al.* (35) showed that the inoculation of *L. canicola*, *L. icterohemorrhagiae, L. sejroe, L. grippotyphosa,* and *L. ballum* into 17-day-old embryonated hens' eggs produced a clinically recognized disease in the newly hatched chicks and that the spirochetes can be readily observed in the circulating blood. They also recommended the use of this chick-embryo technic for the isolation of pathogenic *Leptospira* from blood, urine, or tissue suspensions. Two-day-old chicks uniformly develop leptospiremia, which persists for at least 5 days following intraperitoneal inoculation of leptospirae (48). Roberts and Turner (78) have found the chinchilla to be more susceptible to *L. pomona* than the young guinea pig and have suggested its use in the diagnosis of this infection. Although, the use of 5-fluorouracil, a pyrimidine analogue, and albumin-Tween 80 in serum-containing mediums have raised the frequency of obtaining leptospires on primary culture, it is evident that laboratory animals in isolation procedures cannot be completely supplanted by direct cultural technics.

**The Natural Disease.** Cattle infected with the *Leptospira* usually exhibit an elevated temperature at some time during the course of the disease. Visibly sick animals frequently show icterus and anemia. Pregnant animals may abort. In any outbreak, the number of animals that expel dead fetuses may vary from few to many, but apparently leptospirosis does not result in impaired conception rate or early embryonic death.

Lactating cows may develop mastitis and a drop in milk production. A hemoglobinuria signals the approach of death. During the febrile stage the spirochete frequently is present in the blood. Baker and Little (2) also found the organism in the milk of lactating cows. They concluded that the infection in cattle is generalized, with subsequent localization in the kidney. In this organ the lesions and infectious agent persist for months after the agent has disappeared from the blood and immunity has been established. Stoenner *et al.* (88) have reported neurologic manifestations of leptospirosis in a dairy cow and have claimed survival of the organisms in the cerebrospinal fluid after intensive antibiotic therapy. Sleight *et al.* (85) have produced histologic lesions in the testes of bulls by experimental inoculation of *L. pomona*.

Clinical disease in young calves depends not only on the serotype involved, but also on its origin. It has been shown that strains of the same type coming from different localities vary in pathogenicity (25). Clinical signs in calves may be very mild to severe with acute reactions characterized by high body temperature, anorexia, lethargy, shallow and accelerated respiration, suppressed rumination, diarrhea, and stiffness. There may be mild anemia without hemoglobinuria or jaundice. Focal interstitial nephritis and inflammatory infiltration of the parenchymal cells of the liver may be observed on histologic examination.

**Mode of Transmission.** Because leptospirae are excreted in the urine of affected animals for long periods after recovery from the clinical symptoms, it is quite certain that transmission occurs through this medium. Baker and Little postulate that the splattering of the urine when it falls upon hard surfaces may create infected droplets, which are inhaled by other individuals. Certainly water is a major factor in the circulation of leptospires in enzootic foci. Although the formation and maintenance of water foci are not at all clear it is apparent that contamination with infected urine is important. An attempt by Gillespie and Ryno (34) to incriminate the muskrat was not successful.

The remarkable invasive ability of leptospirae is well known. They readily penetrate the mucous membranes and epidermal surfaces injured or softened by prolonged exposure to water. The nasal, pharyngeal, buccal, and esophageal mucosa, as well as the conjunctival membrane, are probably the most frequent modes of leptospiral infection, although transmission by copulation and artificial insemination involving infected semen has been reported (86).

Rodents have been found to be the most important reservoirs of *Leptospira* serotypes, but other groups of wild mammals, such as the insectivores, carnivores, and ruminants, may play an important role as animal hosts of leptospirosis. Isolation of parasitic leptospires has also been reported from nonmammalian hosts, such as reptiles and birds, but the exact epidemiological role of these hosts has still to be investigated.

**Diagnosis.** Diagnosis is made on the basis of clinical symptoms, the microscopic demonstration of the organism in urine or tissue sections, or the cultivation and identification of the specific organism. The agglutination-lysis test is used as a diagnostic aid. This test does not usually become positive until the 2nd week of the disease. The demonstration of an increasing titer, beginning during the 2nd week of the illness, is regarded as acceptable evidence of the nature of the infection.

Hemagglutination, complement-fixation, and a milk agglutination test, all have been used in the diagnosis of bovine leptospirosis (19, 50, 96). The slide agglutination test, employing four pooled antigens, each comprising three serotypes, is sensitive and broad in genus coverage. These pooled antigens are easy to prepare, simple to use in tests, and are an excellent means of diagnosing leptospiral infections in man and animals (31, 32).

In a study on leptospiral interspecies infections on a single Illinois farm it was shown that *L. grippotyphosa, L. ballum, L. hardjo, L. autumnalis, L. ic-*

*terohemorrhagiae*, and *L. canicola* were present (60). This emphasizes the possibility of multiple infections.

**Immunity.** It appears that an animal which recovers from the infection is immune. In many cases animals in contact with frankly diseased individuals develop immunity or antibody titers without showing any clinical symptoms of the disease.

Apparently the disease can be prevented in cattle by vaccination. Formalinized whole cultures have been used for this purpose as well as suspensions of *Leptospira* that have been grown in embryonated eggs. The latter are inactivated by formalin or by freezing and thawing (97). Another vaccine that has been recommended employs a soluble antigen prepared by acid-heat extraction of living cultures of *L. pomona* (47). According to Gillespie and Kenzy (33), *L. pomona* bacterin induces a high level of immunity which lasts at least 7 to 8 months in calves that are vaccinated at 6 to 8 months of age. By contrast, those vaccinated at 2 months of age usually become infected when exposed 6 to 8 months later.

## Swine Leptospirosis

After 1945 a number of reports came from Switzerland about a disease of man that has been called *swineherds' disease* because it seemed to occur as a result of contact with infected pigs (Gsell, 39, 40; Schmid and Giovanella, 83; Gsell and Weismann, 41; Frey, 29). The same infection has been reported in the Dutch East Indies (18) and also in the United States. This disease is apparently caused by *L. pomona*.

Experimentally, pigs can be infected by subcutaneous or intranasal inoculation or by placing organisms in the eye, but they fail to respond to oral administration. Generally the infected pigs show only mild symptoms of conjunctivitis and some loss of appetite for a short time, or no symptoms at all. They develop a leptospiremia early in the infection, and organisms appear in the urine in the later stages. In such pigs numerous leptospirae are eliminated through the urine over long periods of time, which is in contrast to calves that shed relatively few organisms over a shorter period of time and it is now well known that pigs play a most important part in the epidemiology of the leptospiroses of human beings and animals.

Transmission of the infection by contact exposure occurs readily from infected pigs to susceptible ones and to calves, but not from calves to pigs (13). It is possible that the pig is the primary host of *L. pomona*. Infected pigs agglutinate the spirochete in high dilution.

In the natural disease in swine symptoms vary widely. Many infections may not result in recognizable symptoms, but outbreaks have occurred which were marked by abortion, icterus, and anemia. In baby pigs the main symptoms are jaundice, fever, and inappetence. Icterus and hemoglobinuria are common. Diarrhea, irritability, fever, mild conjunctivitis, tremors of the legs, weakness of the hind limbs, turning of the head from side to side, stiffness of the neck, and convulsions as well as encephalitic symptoms have been described (84).

Diagnosis is made by demonstrating the causal agent or the presence of agglutinins at a sufficiently high titer in the animals examined. The microscopic-agglutination test is the most reliable for diagnosing leptospirosis in swine. The slide agglutination test, although less sensitive, is also useful.

Although *L. pomona* infection appears to be the most common form in swine, *L. canicola, L. icterohemorrhagiae, L. tarassovi,* and possibly other types occur occasionally in this animal.

*L. pomona* bacterins have been used successfully in protecting young swine against leptospirosis (10, 14).

### Equine Leptospirosis

In 1948 Heusser (46) suggested that equine periodic ophthalmia of horses in Switzerland might be caused by infection with leptospirae. He did not succeed in isolating any cultures but based his conclusions on the results of serological tests. Noting that most cases of this disease in Switzerland occurred in areas where swineherds' disease prevailed, he tested 291 affected horses and as many controls. Nine types of leptospirae were used. Positive reactions were obtained with only three—*L. pomona, L. australis,* and *L. grippotyphosa.* The titers varied among these species, but most diseased animals agglutinated one or more of the cultures in dilutions varying from 1:4 to 1:25,-000. The titers of normal horses did not exceed 1:400. Tests made with the aqueous humor of acute cases showed much higher titers than the blood of the same individuals.

On the basis of serological tests Yager *et al.* (95) indicated that *L. pomona* is the cause of recurrent iridocyclitis of horses in the United States, but Bryans (11) in his studies on equine leptospirosis concludes that the disease in horses, as caused by *L. pomona,* does not present pathognomonic symptoms. Because of the mild nature of the disease in horses and the failure to demonstrate a carrier state in experimental animals, it appears that leptospirosis is of little importance to the light horse industry of the United States. However, serological evidence does indicate that a relatively high percentage of horses possess antibodies against leptospirae, and a few naturally occurring cases of *L. pomona* infection have been described with symptoms of fever, anorexia, depression, and icterus (42, 79). Abortion in mares has been reported by Jackson *et al.* (52) to be associated with leptospirosis. Brown *et al.* (8) concluded that satisfactory immunization could be induced in the horse by vaccination.

### Ovine and Caprine Leptospirosis

It appears that leptospirosis occurs in the sheep and in the goat, but only infrequently. *L. pomona* has been isolated from an infected sheep (44) and *L. grippotyphosa* from a goat (49). Experimentally, *L. pomona* produced disease in sheep and goats (55, 69). Clinical signs of the infection appeared to be less severe than in cattle. Pregnant ewes exhibited signs of pyrexia, anorexia, and polypnea. Lambing was normal. The role of these animals in transmitting leptospirosis was considered to be minor.

### Leptospirosis in Other Animals

*L. canicola* infection has been reported in cats and its role in chronic nephritis in this animal discussed (45). Although Lucke and Crowther (57) agree that cats can be infected by several serotypes, they also claim that it is unlikely for leptospiral organisms to cause any recognizable disease, especially nephritis. *Leptospira* are common in rats and in certain areas in field mice. They have been isolated from opossums, raccoons, hedgehogs, foxes, skunks, deer, jackals, beaver, nutria, and various other wild animals, including snakes. It appears that primates, other than man, are not ordinarily infected by leptospirae while existing in their natural state (66).

### Leptospirosis in Man

The epidemiology of leptospirosis in man is not related to age or sex, but to occupation. *L. icterohemorrhagiae* infections are frequently observed in miners and in sewer and abattoir workers. *L. canicola* infections are found predominantly in veterinarians and in breeders and owners of dogs. In Europe *L. grippotyphosa* infection attacks farmers and agricultural and flax workers. *L. pomona* infection occurs in swineherders, creamery workers, cheese makers, and swine slaughterers. *L. australis* infection is found in sugar-cane plantation workers, and *L. bataviae* infection attacks rice-field workers.

Infection of man occurs either directly from urine or tissues of a diseased animal or indirectly through contact with water or soil contaminated by animals; and in the United States the animals most likely to be involved are dogs, rats, cattle, swine, and certain wild animals that may contaminate streams. The portals of entry are most likely to be the mucous membranes of the eyes, nose, and mouth or the broken skin.

Symptoms of leptospirosis in man vary. Although they are frequently severe, the mortality rate is low. The disease is manifested by fever, headache, conjunctivitis, muscle pains, and encephalitic symptoms. There may be muscular tenderness, pharyngeal inflammation, skin rash, and minor hemorrhagic episodes. In some cases meningitis is a conspicuous symptom. Orchitis has been reported. The urine frequently contains albumin, a few erythrocytes, and casts. Jaundice frequently does not occur. Agglutinins and lytic antibodies for *Leptospira* appear in the 2nd week of the disease and reach maximum titers several weeks later. The specific organism has often been isolated from the blood during the febrile period and from the urine later.

Although Weil's disease and canicola fever have been known to exist in the United States for some time, information with regard to the presence of other types is more recent. In 1951 Schaeffer (82) reported a water-borne outbreak of *L. pomona* in Alabama that attacked 50 out of 80 adolescents and young adults. In 1952 Gochenour *et al.* (36) clearly established that the so-called Fort Bragg fever was a leptospiral infection caused by *L. autumnalis*. Since then *L. ballum*, *L. grippotyphosa*, *L. mimi georgia*, and *L. hardjo* have been implicated in human infection.

In Israel where about 30 percent of the cases of leptospirosis appearing annually are canicola fever (74) it seems that jackals are the main reservoir of the spirochete and are responsible for its transmission to pigs and cattle. The source of infection for man is most likely to be swine or rats.

### Chemotherapy in Leptospirosis

Smadel (87) concludes from studies on infected animals that penicillin, streptomycin, aureomycin, and terramycin are effective prophylactic agents but relatively ineffective therapeutic agents. These four antibiotics show appreciable activity against leptospirae in the laboratory but do not produce dramatic results in treating a patient unless given within the first day or two of the disease. On the other hand, Brunner (9) used streptomycin to treat six dogs that had survived experimental infection (five with *L. canicola* and one with *L. icterohemorrhagiae*) and were shedding large numbers of the organisms in the urine. He found the antibiotic to be fully effective in eliminating these organisms. Lococo *et al.* (56) used dihydrostreptomycin and Baker *et al.* (1) employed terramycin in effectively eradicating leptospiruria in swine. Terramycin was used at levels of 500 and 1,000 g per ton of feed. Ringen and Bracken (76) reported no evidence of leptospiruria in cattle treated with high levels of tetracycline. It is possible that the effectiveness of antibiotics varies between species of *Leptospira* and their hosts.

### REFERENCES

1. Baker, Gallian, Price, and White.   Vet. Med., 1957, 52, 103.
2. Baker and Little.   Jour. Exp. Med., 1948, 88, 295.
3. Bernkopf.   Refuah Vet., 1946, 3, 49. (Eng. abstract, Vet. Bul., 1949, 19, 140.)
4. Bernkopf.   Harefuah, 1946, 30, 109. (Eng. abstract, Vet. Bul., 1949, 19, 655.)
5. Bernkopf.   Proc. Soc. Exp. Biol. and Med., 1948, 67, 148.
6. Bernkopf and Little.   *Ibid.*, 69, 503.
7. Bernkopf, Olitski, and Stuczynski.   Jour. Inf. Dis., 1947, 80, 53.
8. Brown, Creamer, and Scheidy.   Vet. Med., 1956, 51, 556.
9. Brunner.   North Am. Vet., 1949, 30, 517.
10. Bryan.   Vet. Med., 1957, 52, 51.
11. Bryans.   Cornell Vet., 1955, 45, 16.
12. Btesh.   Trans. Roy. Soc. Trop. Med., 1947, 41, 419.
13. Burnstein and Baker.   Jour. Inf. Dis., 1954, 94, 53.
14. Burnstein, Bramel, and Jensen.   Vet. Med., 1957, 52, 58.
15. Caspar and Reif.   Harefuah, 1946, 30, 113. (Eng. abstract, Vet. Bul., 1950, 20, 198.)
16. Clayton, Derrick, and Cilento.   Austral. Med. Jour., 1937, 7, 647.

17. Coffin and Stubbs. Jour. Am. Vet. Med. Assoc., 1944, *104*, 152.
18. Collier. Schweiz. med. Wchnschr., 1948, 78, 508.
19. Cox. Proc. Soc. Exp. Biol. and Med., 1955, 90, 610.
20. Cox, Alexander, and Murphy. Jour. Inf. Dis., 1957, *101*, 210.
21. Czekalowski, McLeod, and Rodican. Brit. Jour. Exp. Path., 1953, *34*, 588.
22. Dacres. Am. Jour. Vet. Res., 1961, *22*, 570.
23. *Ibid.*, 1963, *24*, 1321.
24. Ellinghausen and McCullough. *Ibid.*, 1965, *26*, 39.
25. Fennestad. Experimental leptospirosis in calves. Einar Munksgaard, Copenhagen, 1963.
26. Ferris and Andrews. Am. Jour. Vet. Res., 1965, *26*, 373.
27. Field and Sellers. Vet. Rec., 1951, *63*, 78.
28. Freund. Jour. Comp. Path. and Therap., 1947, 57, 62.
29. Frey. Schweiz. med. Wchnschr., 1948, 78, 531.
30. Galton, Aragon, Jacalne, Shotts, and Sulzer. Jour. Inf. Dis., 1963, *112*, 164.
31. Galton, Menges, Shotts, Nahmias, and Heath. Leptospirosis. Epidemiology, clinical manifestations in man and animals, and methods in laboratory diagnosis. USPHS, CDC, Atlanta, Ga., 1962.
32. Galton, Powers, Hale, and Cornell. Am. Jour. Vet. Res., 1958, *19*, 205.
33. Gillespie and Kenzy. Vet. Med., 1958, *53*, 401.
34. Gillespie and Ryno. Am. Jour. Vet. Res., 1963, *24*, 634.
35. Gleiser, Jahnes, and Byrne. Cornell Vet., 1955, *45*, 296.
36. Gochenour, Smadel, Jackson, Evans, and Yager. Pub. Health Rpts. (U.S.), 1952, *67*, 811.
37. Golikov. Veterinariya, 1944, 8–9, 11. (Eng. abstract, Vet. Bul., 1948, *18*, 247.)
38. Greene, Camien, and Dunn. Proc. Soc. Exp. Biol. and Med., 1950, *75*, 208.
39. Gsell. Presse méd., 1945 (Sep), 525.
40. Gsell. Schweiz. med. Wchnschr., 1946, *76*, 237.
41. Gsell and Weismann. *Ibid.*, 1948, 78, 503.
42. Hall and Bryans. Cornell Vet., 1954, *44*, 345.
43. Harrington and Sleight. Am. Jour. Vet. Res., 1966, 27, 249.
44. Hartley. Austral. Vet. Jour., 1952, 28, 169.
45. Hemsley. Vet. Rec., 1956, *68*, 300.
46. Heusser. Schweiz. Arch. f. Tierheilk., 1948, *90*, 287.
47. Hoag and Bell. Am. Jour. Vet. Res., 1955, *16*, 381.
48. Hoag, Gochenour, and Yager. Proc. Soc. Exp. Biol. and Med., 1953, 83, 712.
49. Van der Hoeden. Jour. Comp. Path. and Therap., 1953, *63*, 101.
50. Van der Hoeden. Cornell Vet., 1955, *45*, 190.
51. Ingram, Jack, and Smith. Vet. Rec., 1952, *64*, 865.
52. Jackson, Jones, and Clark. Jour. Am. Vet. Med. Assoc., 1957, *131*, 564.
53. Jungherr. *Ibid.*, 1944, *105*, 276.
54. Klarenbeek and Schüffner. Nederl. Tijdschr. Geneesk., 1933, *42*, 71.
55. Lindqvist, Morse, and Lundberg. Cornell Vet., 1958, *48*, 277.
56. Lococo, Bohl, and Smith. Jour. Am. Vet. Med. Assoc., 1958, *132*, 251.
57. Lucke and Crowther. Vet. Rec., 1965, 77, 647.
58. Maestrone. Canad. Jour. Comp. Med. and Vet. Sci., 1963, 27, 109.
59. Marsh. Jour. Am. Vet. Med. Assoc., 1945, *107*, 119.

60. Martin, Hanson, and Schnurrenberger. Pub. Health Rpts. (U.S.), 1967, *82*, 75.
61. Mathews. Am. Jour. Vet. Res., 1946, *7*, 78.
62. Menges and Galton. *Ibid.*, 1961, *22*, 1085.
63. Menges, Rosenquist, and Galton. Jour. Am. Vet. Med. Assoc., 1960, *137*, 313.
64. Meyer, Stewart-Anderson, and Eddie. *Ibid.*, 1938, *46*, 332.
65. Mikhin and Azinov. Sovyet Vet., 1935, *10*, 23. (Eng. abstract, Vet. Bul., 1937, *7*, 419.)
66. Minette. Am. Jour. Trop. Med. and Hyg., 1966, *15*, 190.
67. Monlux. Cornell Vet., 1939, *29*, 217; 1948, *38*, 57.
68. Morrow, Syverton, Stiles, and Barry. Science, 1938, *88*, 384.
69. Morse and Langham. Am. Jour. Vet. Res., 1958, *19*, 139.
70. Morter, Ray, and Chapel. Jour. Am. Vet. Med. Assoc., 1959, *135*, 570.
71. Murphy, Cardeilhac, Alexander, Evans, and Marchwicki. Am. Jour. Vet. Res., 1958, *19*, 145.
72. Nisbet. Jour. Comp. Path. and Therap., 1951, *61*, 155.
73. Padersky. Harefuah, 1946, *30*, 117. (Eng. abstract, Vet. Bul., 1950, *20*, 198.)
74. Pertzelan and Pruzanski. Am. Jour. Trop. Med. and Hyg., 1963, *12*, 75.
75. Reinhard, Tierney, and Roberts. Cornell Vet., 1950, *40*, 148.
76. Ringen and Bracken. Jour. Am. Vet. Med. Assoc., 1956, *129*, 266.
77. Ringen and Gillespie. Jour. Bact., 1954, *67*, 252.
78. Roberts and Turner. Jour. Am. Vet. Med. Assoc., 1958, *132*, 527.
79. Roberts, York, and Robinson. *Ibid.*, 1952, *121*, 237.
80. Roth, Adams, Sanford, Greer, and Mayeux. Pub. Health Rpts. (U.S.), 1962, *77*, 583.
81. Schachtel. Harefuah, 1948, *34*, 81. (Eng. abstract, Vet. Bull., 1949, *19*, 474.)
82. Schaeffer. Jour. Clin. Invest., 1951, *30*, 670.
83. Schmid and Giovanella. Schweiz. Arch. f. Tierheilk., 1947, *89*, 1.
84. Sippel. North Am. Vet., 1953, *34*, 111.
85. Sleight, Atallah, and Steinbauer. Am. Jour. Vet. Res., 1964, *25*, 1663.
86. Sleight and Williams. Jour. Am. Vet. Med. Assoc., 1961, *138*, 151.
87. Smadel. In: Symposium on the leptospiroses. Army Medical Service Graduate School, Washington, D.C., Med. Sci. Pub. no. *1*, 1953.
88. Stoenner, Hadlow, and Ward. Jour. Am. Vet. Med. Assoc., 1963, *142*, 491.
89. Sutherland and Morrill. *Ibid.*, 1948, *113*, 468.
90. Sutherland, Simmons, and Kenny. Austral. Vet. Jour., 1949, *25*, 197.
91. Thomas and Evans. Jour. Am. Vet. Med. Assoc., 1967, *150*, 33.
92. Walch-Sorgdrager and Schüffner. Centrbl. f. Bakt., I Abt., Orig., 1938, *141*, 97.
93. White, Stoliker, and Galton. Am. Jour. Vet. Res., 1961, *22*, 650.
94. Wolff. The laboratory diagnosis of leptospirosis. C. C Thomas, Springfield, Ill., 1954.
95. Yager, Gochenour, and Wetmore. Jour. Am. Vet. Med. Assoc., 1950, *117*, 207.
96. York. Am. Jour. Vet. Res., 1952, *13*, 117.
97. York and Baker. *Ibid.*, 1953, *14*, 5.

# XXIV | The *Mycoplasmataceae*

In 1898 a group of French workers headed by Nocard (19) succeeded in cultivating a peculiar, very minute organism from the exudates of a destructive cattle disease known as *contagious bovine pleuropneumonia*. The organism is so small that it passes filters as readily as many of the filterable viruses, and for this reason it was long classified as one of the viruses. It now appears that the microbe falls in between the bacteria on one hand and the rickettsiae and filterable virus group of organisms on the other. It is distinguished from the rickettsiae mainly by its extreme pleomorphism and by its ability to grow on culture media in the absence of living cells. According to Dienes (7), the pleuropneumonialike organisms (PPLO) represent stabilized L-phase mutants and are a stage in the life cycle of bacteria.

In 1923 Bridré and Donatien (3) cultivated an organism closely related to the one of pleuropneumonia from the joints of goats that suffered from a disease known as *contagious agalactia*. In 1934 Shoetensack (26) found an organism belonging to this group in dogs suffering from distemper. Dogs frequently carry PPLO in their respiratory and genital tracts, the organisms usually being more prevalent if some pathological condition is present. PPLO have also been found in cats. Van Herick and Eaton (29) reported the finding of PPLO in chick embryos. In 1952 Markham and Wong (15) ascribed etiological significance to PPLO in chronic respiratory disease in chickens and infectious sinusitis of turkeys. Pigeons, parakeets, and ducks are additional avian species from which PPLO have been derived. Saprophytic and parasitic strains have been isolated from the bovine genital tract and from the lungs of calves with shipping fever. They have been found in the genital tract of horses. PPLO have been recovered from infectious atrophic rhinitis of swine, and although their role in this disease has not been determined, Carter (4) has suggested that they are identical with the filterable agents referred to by other workers. Dienes and Madoff (8) found that strains of PPLO isolated

511

from the human urogenital tract were of a different species than those obtained from the buccal cavity. Although there has been some question regarding the importance of PPLO in human disease, it now appears that a highly pathogenic species identified as the transmissible agent of Eaton (*Mycoplasma pneumoniae*) causes most clinical cases of primary atypical pneumonia (5). In 1936 Laidlaw and Elford (14) reported the finding of organisms of this group in filtrates of raw sewage. These were nonpathogenic for experimental animals. PPLO have been found in rats and are very prevalent among mice. In fact, rabbits and hamsters appear to be the only common laboratory animals from which PPLO have not been isolated (17). A major problem for the research worker dealing with tissue cultures has been to prepare and maintain the cells free from contaminating PPLO (1, 20).

The work of the last few years has made it clear that a considerable group of minute bacteria exists of which the bovine pleuropneumonia organism is the type. Borrel and Dujardin-Beaumetz (2) gave the name *Asteroroccus mycoides* to the bovine organism, but the name has been little used. In 1955 Freundt proposed that the PPLO be placed in the class *Schizomycetes*, order *Mycoplasmatales*, family *Mycoplasmataceae*, and given the generic name *Mycoplasma*. In 1967 Edward and Freundt (9) proposed the term *Mollicutes* as the name of the class established for the family, *Mycoplasmataceae*, order, *Mycoplasmatales*. It appears that this nomenclature will be accepted.

The organisms are characterized by the absence of a cell wall. They are highly pleomorphic and reproduce by the breaking up of filaments into coccoid, filterable elementary bodies. They are nonmotile and Gram-negative. They stain poorly with ordinary bacterial stains but fairly well with Giemsa. They grow in agar medium, but pathogenic species require enrichment with serum or ascitic fluid. Both pathogenic and saprophytic species occur, and it appears that much of the confusion in the early literature over the role of the PPLO in producing disease exists because of failure to distinguish between these strains. The designation of the type species is *Mycoplasma mycoides*.

### Mycoplasma mycoides

SYNONYMS: *Asterococcus mycoides, Bovimyces pleuropneumoniae*, organism of bovine pleuropneumonia; abbreviation, CBPP

This organism is the cause of a destructive disease of cattle which occurs in Asia, Africa, and Australia. The disease has been known for more than 200 years. From time to time in the past it has spread over the greater part of Europe. In the early part of the 19th century it became widespread in Europe, and from there it was disseminated to South Africa, Australia, and the United States in exported cattle. According to Moore (16), the disease was imported into the United States in 1843, 1847, and 1859. It was restricted to some of the eastern states until 1883, when it appeared in Ohio. By 1886 it had reached a few herds in Illinois, Kentucky, and Missouri. The spread of this disease led to the establishment in 1884 of the Bureau of Animal Industry of the U.S. Department of Agriculture. In 1887 Congress made available to the Bureau of Animal Industry adequate funds to deal with the disease. During the next 5 years it was hunted down, all affected animals were destroyed, and in September 1892 the Secretary of Agriculture issued a proclamation declaring the country to be free of the disease. It has not occurred in this country since March 1892.

**Morphology and Staining Reactions.** The causative organism of contagious bovine pleuropneumonia (CBPP) is exceedingly pleomorphic and varies widely according to whether it is grown on fluid or solid media, whether the cultures are young or old, and whether one method or another is used for its demonstration. Minute granules and larger bacilliform elements—spirals, ring forms, globules, and budlike forms—are seen. Even amorphous masses containing chromatic bodies are encountered in preparations from solid media. In tissues usually nothing recognizable as organisms can be found. The size varies considerably, but the units capable of reproduction evidently are very small because ultrafiltration studies indicate that they are of the order of 125 to 175 millimicrons in diameter, a size which is comparable to that of many of the filterable viruses. They are not demonstrable in films stained by the usual aniline dyes but are stained by Giemsa and Castañeda's *Rickettsia* stain.

**Cultural Features.** Nocard, Roux, Borrel, Salimbeni, and Dujardin-Beaumetz (19) first succeeded in cultivating this organism by inoculating serum broth with pleural exudate, enclosing the mixture in collodion sacs, and placing the latter in the peritoneal cavity of rabbits. The animals became emaciated and finally died, whereas others treated with similar sacs containing uninoculated media remained well. The broth in the sacs had become slightly clouded, and, when examined with the highest powers of the microscope, minute refractile dots were observed. The organism was cultivated serially in this manner through many generations, remote cultures retaining virulence for cattle. Later it was learned that the organism would grow in broth to which 10 percent serum had been added; hence the collodion sacs were not necessary. Priestley and White (23) have shown that the essential factor in the serum is heat-stable and separable from the coagulable proteins.

Serum broth cultures in which this organism is growing become very faintly clouded. The cloudiness is so faint that it is advisable to incubate uninoculated tubes of the same media for purposes of comparison. Growth occurs under both aerobic and anaerobic conditions, but Turner (28) claims that microaerophilic conditions are most suitable.

In the presence of 2 percent peptone and 10 percent serum in broth, the organism produces acid from a number of carbohydrates: glucose, fructose, mannose, maltose, and dextrin. Sucrose and trehalose are only slightly attacked.

Surface colonies may be obtained on agar containing 30 percent serum or ascitic fluid. Plates or tubes should be sealed to prevent drying. In from 2 to 7 days' incubation at 37 C the characteristic colonies may be seen. These are from 10 to 600 microns in diameter and so transparent that they are very easily overlooked. They may be seen with a hand lens under reflected light or, better, under the 16-mm objective of the compound microscope with oblique illumination. Cultivation is successful on the chorioallantoic membrane of the developing chicken embryo (Tang, Wei, and Edgar, 27).

No growth occurs in plain broth, litmus milk, blood agar, blood broth, and Loeffler's blood serum.

**Resistance.** The organism of pleuropneumonia possesses very little resistance to drying, heat, and chemical action. The virus is kept alive in herds, not because of its persistence on the premises, but because it is harbored and excreted for long periods by apparently recovered animals. However, Hyslop (12) has shown that a lyophilized egg-adapted strain of *M. mycoides* remained viable, infective, and lethal for embryonated eggs after 2.5 years of storage at −20 to −28 C.

**Pathogenicity.** Under natural conditions *M. mycoides* is pathogenic only for cattle. Strains grown in the presence of horse or sheep serum acquire pathogenicity for sheep and goats, and Hyslop (13) has shown that strains can be adapted to rabbits, guinea pigs, hamsters, and mice by intramuscular, intrathoracic, or subcutaneous injection of the organism incorporated in an agar gel. The subcutaneous route is the most satisfactory, and mouse passage has proved valuable for the isolation of *M. mycoides* from contaminated material taken from field outbreaks of bovine pleuropneumonia. Hyslop also states that 50 subcutaneous passages in mice produced adaptation without reducing virulence for cattle, but material from the 30th passage in mice became attenuated in virulence for cattle by 20 subsequent passages in embryonated eggs.

Artificial inoculation of cattle with naturally infected materials or cultures seldom reproduces the pneumonia that is the principal lesion in field cases. Daubney (6) succeeded in producing typical lung lesions by incorporating infective material into small agar plugs, which were injected into the jugular vein. These lodged in the blood vessels of the lung, constituting infective emboli. Exudates and cultures inoculated subcutaneously produce large inflammatory swellings and a toxemia from which the animals may die, but this does not resemble the natural disease, and the inoculation disease is not naturally transmissible. In challenging the immunity induced by vaccines, hypervirulent "lung lymph" obtained from active field cases of CBPP is used (12). This material upon subcutaneous injection into susceptible animals causes death in a high percentage of cases and produces local reactions and immunity in the surviving animals.

**The Natural Disease.** The natural disease spreads slowly and is difficult to eradicate. Walker (30), who has had a great deal of experience with this disease in Nairobi, found that 58 percent of the cattle in a large infected herd had not contracted the infection after a period of 7 months.

The disease may be quite acute, resulting fatally within a week, or it may be chronic. It has a way of becoming arrested by the walling off of infected lung foci, in which case the animal may appear to have recovered, but the sequestration is likely to break down at any time, perhaps weeks or months later, with an extension of the disease, the reappearance of symptoms, and the discharge of virulent material. The movement of such animals into new herds and the reopening of the lesions there spread the disease.

The pleural cavity of acutely infected animals contains a great deal of fluid —as much as 15 or 20 liters. The surface of the lung is injected and covered with a thin deposit of fibrin. The subpleural tissue is thickened and filled with fluid, and the same kind of fluid distends the interlobular septa. When the affected lobes are incised, these fluids run out, coagulating after a few moments' exposure to the air.

The pneumonia begins as nodules or foci, which spread until entire lobes are involved. These areas are hepatized and are bright red, brownish red, or grayish in color depending upon the stage of the process. The surface of the cut section presents a marbled effect, the varicolored lobules being separated from each other by wide bands of infiltrated interlobular tissue. Necrosis occurs in the chronic cases, large portions of lung tissue often being necrotic and sequestered by connective tissue.

**Diagnosis.** Agglutinins, precipitins, and complement-fixing bodies are formed by infected animals and may be used as a means of diagnosis. Antibody formation develops rather slowly, however, and these tests have not proved very successful in detecting early cases. They have been useful, however, in selecting chronically infected animals, which may show few or no clinical symptoms. Newing and Field (18) have described methods of preparing an antigen for a whole-blood, rapid-slide test for diagnosing CBPP. They claim that their test is as satisfactory as the CF test, even in chronic cases. Gel-diffusion-precipitin tests and allergic tests, using extracts of *M. mycoides*, have also been used in the diagnosis of CBPP. Although none of the tests are effective in the very early onset of the disease, Gourlay (10) has reported that later in the acute stage the CF and agar-gel tests detected 100 percent of his CBPP cases, the slide-agglutination test 72, and the allergic test 68. In the late chronic stages none of the tests were entirely satisfactory, the allergic test detecting 74, the CF 72, the slide-agglutination 35, and the agar-gel 21 percent.

**Immunity.** Animals that have recovered from the disease cannot again be infected for a long period of time. Methods of artificial immunization have been used for many years in th badly infected areas. The earlier method consisted in the subcutaneous injection, usually in the tail, of pleural fluid. This method gives protection from the lung disease, but reactions often are severe and some animals even die from the inoculation.

In 1952 and 1953 Sheriff and Piercy (24, 25) isolated and adapted their Tanganyika (TI) strain of CBPP to embryonated hens' eggs. After nine transfers in eggs a lyophilized vaccine was made. It is a living product that retains its viability for years when stored at low temperatures. The vaccine has been tested rather widely and appears to be highly effective in immunizing cattle against CBPP (11, 21). Priestley (22) recommends that 0.5 percent agar be incorporated when reconstituting the vaccine. This acts as an adjuvant and induces rapid and solid immunity.

In the past the disease has been eradicated from many countries by slaughtering all infected herds, and this appears to be the only practicable method now available for dealing with it in areas where most herds are not already infected.

**Chemotherapy.** Sulfonamide drugs and antibiotics have little if any effect on this organism. In fact, these drugs are frequently used to suppress the growth of extraneous bacteria when attempts are made to isolate CBPP organisms.

## REFERENCES

1. Barile and Schimke.   Proc. Soc. Exp. Biol. and Med., 1963, *114*, 676.
2. Borrel and Dujardin-Beaumetz.   Ann. l'Inst. Past., 1910, *24*, 168.
3. Bridré and Donatien.   Comp. rend. Acad. Sci., 1923, *177*, 841.
4. Carter.   Canad. Jour. Comp. Med. and Vet. Sci., 1954, *18*, 246.
5. Chanock *et al.*   Science, 1963, *140*, 662.
6. Daubney.   Jour. Comp. Path. and Therap., 1935, *48*, 83.
7. Dienes.   Jour. Bact., 1945, *50*, 441.
8. Dienes and Madoff.   Proc. Soc. Exp. Biol. and Med., 1953, *82*, 36.
9. Edward and Freundt.   Internatl. Jour. System. Bact., 1967, *17*, 267.
10. Gourlay.   Jour. Comp. Path., 1965, *75*, 97.
11. Gray and Turner.   Jour. Comp. Path. and Therap., 1954, *64*, 116.
12. Hyslop.   Vet. Rec., 1955, *67*, 411.
13. Hyslop.   Jour. Path. and Bact., 1958, *75*, 189.
14. Laidlaw and Elford.   Proc. Roy. Soc. (Brit.), 1936, *120* (B), 292.
15. Markham and Wong.   Poultry Sci., 1952, *31*, 902.
16. Moore.   Pathology and differential diagnosis of the infectious diseases of animals. 4th ed. Macmillan, New York, 1916, p. 412.
17. Morton.   Ann. N.Y. Acad. Sci., 1960, *79* (Art. 10), 369.
18. Newing and Field.   Brit. Vet. Jour., 1953, *109*, 397.
19. Nocard, Roux, Borrel, Salimbeni, and Dujardin-Beaumetz.   Ann. l'Inst. Past., 1898, *12*, 240.
20. Pollock, Kenny, and Syverton.   Proc. Soc. Exp. Biol. and Med., 1960, *105*, 10.
21. Priestley.   Jour. Comp. Path. and Therap., 1955, *65*, 168.
22. Priestley.   Vet. Rec., 1955, *67*, 729.
23. Priestley and White.   *Ibid.*, 1952, *64*, 259.
24. Sheriff and Piercy.   *Ibid.*, 1952, *64*, 615.
25. Sheriff and Piercy.   Proc. 15th Internat. Vet. Cong., Stockholm, 1953, *1*, 333.
26. Shoetensack.   Kitasato Arch. Exp. Med., 1934, *11*, 277.
27. Tang, Wei, and Edgar.   Jour. Path. and Bact., 1936, *42*, 45.
28. Turner.   *Ibid.*, 1935, *41*, 1.
29. Van Herick and Eaton.   Jour. Bact., 1945, *50*, 47.
30. Walker.   A system of bacteriology. Med. Res. Council (Brit.), 1930, vol. *vii*, p. 322.

### Mycoplasma mycoides var. capri

SYNONYMS: *Capromyces pleuropneumoniae, Asterococcus mycoides* var. *capri*

It appears that at least three organisms of the pleuropneumonia group produce disease in goats. One of these, *Mycoplasma mycoides* var. *capri*, causes a disease in this animal that closely resembles pleuropneumonia of cattle. The organism is quite similar to the CBPP type and seems to be a variety of it that has become adapted to goats. In the Near East and Savannah zones of Africa pleuropneumonia of goats is a common disease. It was described in the Sudan as early as 1902 (44). A pathogenic agent similar to *M. mycoides* var. *capri* was isolated from a goat in Connecticut in 1969 (37).

The second organism, *Mycoplasma agalactiae*, causes contagious agalactia (discussed below). It differs serologically, culturally, and biochemically from the pleuropneumonia types (23). The third organism produces a clinical picture different from those seen in pleuropneumonia and contagious agalactia (see below). In this disease the PPLO isolates resemble the pleuropneumonia rather than the contagious agalactia types. An infectious and highly fatal cellulitis, which is endemic in parts of Greece, has been regarded as a hyperacute form of contagious agalactia, but a PPLO isolated from an animal with this disease has been shown to be similar to the pleuropneumonia type.

### Mycoplasma agalactiae

SYNONYMS: *Borrelomyces agalactiae, Anulomyces agalaxiae, Capromyces agalactiae,* organism of contagious agalactia of sheep and goats

The disease caused by this organism is known to occur only in parts of southern Europe and in northern Africa. Agalactia or mastitis in sheep and goats occasionally occurs in the United States, but this disease is related to other causative agents.

The organism undoubtedly belongs to the pleuropneumonia group, but it is distinguishable from the bovine organism on serological grounds, and also on the basis of species pathogenicity (57).

The causative organism was first isolated and studied by Bridré and Donatien (8) in 1923. Its cultural features are not materially different from those of the pleuropneumonia organism of cattle. It can be found in the blood in the early stages of the disease, later in the joints, eye, and mammary secretions.

The name suggests that the disease is localized in the udder and is misleading in this respect. Actually it is a generalized disease that affects males and females alike. The principal lesions are located in the joints, the eyes, and in the mammary glands of females. The disease may be acute but usually is chronic. The involved joints may become ankylosed but usually do not. The mastitis is manifested by the usual symptoms, and milk secretion diminishes and even ceases. Pregnant females often abort. Chronically affected animals become weak and emaciated. There is some evidence that different strains of

*M. agalactiae* may be involved in producing disease in sheep and goats in Asia and Australia as well as in Europe and Africa. Although certain cultures produce the contagious agalactia syndrome others cause edema and nonfatal respiratory disease, accompanied by pleurisy and pneumonia (16, 68).

Most attempts to immunize goats in various ways have proved rather disappointing, but Foggie *et al.* (27) claim that they were able to protect this animal against challenge inoculation by vaccinating with a live culture, attenuated by 40 passes on selective agar. Hyperimmune serum gives only transient protection.

### Other PPLO

The recognized parasitic and pathogenic species are associated with disease in birds, mammals, and man. They have a predilection for the mouth, genitalia, lungs, and joints. A sharp distinction has been drawn between the primary pathogens of cattle, sheep, and goats (PPO); the PPLO that have been isolated from man, dogs, swine, rats, mice, fowls, sewage, and manure; and the L-phase of organisms of bacteria. In morphology and mode of reproduction all three forms belong together. The presence of PPLO that are highly pathogenic for goats, mice, rats, chickens, and turkeys suggests that no useful purpose is achieved by separating the PPO from the PPLO. The status of the L-phase remains controversial.

**Morphology and Cultural Features.** The organisms are small coccobacilli-form bodies with an average mean diameter of 125 to 500 millimicrons (31).

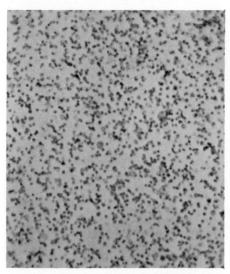 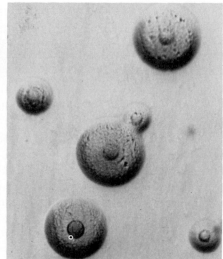

*Fig. 87 (left).* Ring forms of chicken strain of *Mycoplasma gallinarum.* X 1,000. Giemsa's stain. (Courtesy M. S. Hofstad, *Cornell Vet.*)

*Fig. 88 (right).* Colonies of *Mycoplasma gallinarum.* X 140. (Courtesy M. S. Hofstad, *Cornell Vet.*)

They stain readily by Giemsa's stain. They can be propagated in embryonated eggs, they will grow on serum-enriched media (35, 41) and even on synthetic medium (60). On solid media they present small delicate colonies that are just on the border of visibility. Observation with a low-powered lens reveals buttonlike elevations in the centers of these colonies. Some will hemolyze erythrocytes. When grown in cell-free carbohydrate media enriched with 1 to 1.5 percent of a PPLO serum fraction, these organisms vary in ability to split the sugars present. Some commonly ferment glucose, maltose, and sucrose while others exhibit no avidity for these substances.

Although a wide variety of culture media has been used over the years and although it is impossible to predict which ones will be useful in a new situation, Fabricant and Barber recommend (25) the following minimum list, because these media have a wide range of applicability. In each case the broth form of the medium is listed first, the agar-plate form second. It is advisable in media evaluation to use each one both by direct plating and by plating after 3 days of incubation at 37 C in the corresponding broth medium. All plates are examined after 6 days of incubation at 37 C in a candle jar with added moisture. The media are (a) BS and BA (24)—Difco heart infusion broth or agar supplemented with 10 percent swine serum and bacterial inhibitors, (b) II and IIP (26)—the same as BS-BA except that they are supplemented with 10 percent yeast extract (Chanock type), (c) C and CP (13)—Difco PPLO broth or agar supplemented with 20 percent horse serum and 10 percent yeast extract (Chanock type), (d) RYE and RYEP (58)—homemade rabbit infusion supplemented with 10 percent rabbit serum and 10 percent yeast extract (Chanock type), and (e) VFS and VFSP medium (3, 66)—a peptic digest of beef and beef liver—made with pig stomach as the source of pepsin—this medium is never autoclaved but sterilized by filtration.

Because experience has shown that the basal medium, the serum supplement, and the particular yeast supplement used as well as many other factors may stimulate the growth of some *Mycoplasma* or inhibit the growth of others, it is obvious that many other possible varieties of culture media might be useful in different circumstances.

Identification of *Mycoplasma* isolates frequently is complicated because a large proportion of the cultures derived from mucous membranes will contain more than one species of *Mycoplasma*. It is impossible to characterize accurately, identify, or classify such cultures until they are purified. At the present time no simple dependable means exist for culture purification. The presently accepted procedure of cloning (colony picking) three times from terminal dilutions is no guarantee of culture purity. This procedure fails frequently. It should be noted that up to this time no one has successfully initiated growth of a *Mycoplasma* culture from a single organism.

The FA technic has been used both for detecting the presence of PPLO and also for the purpose of identification (14). Complement-fixation and agar gel diffusion tests have shown serologic relationships among human mycoplasmas (65); and Lemcke (42) used complement-fixation tests to distinguish 17 serotypes from 82 cultures derived from man, mammalian cell cultures, laboratory rats and mice, cattle, goats, poultry, embryonated eggs, and sewage. The serotypes of human and lower animal origin were largely host-specific. At this stage in the development of a classification for the mycoplasmas it appears that one of the most useful tools in serotyping isolates is the metabolic-inhibition test (22, 53).

PPLO sometimes contaminate tissue cultures. They tend to develop resistance rather rapidly to antibiotics although showing primary sensitivity to the deoxystreptamines, certain macrolides, and the tetracyclines (52). Some nonionic detergents have proved to be effective in eliminating PPLO from animal-cell cultures (54) and staphylococcal and streptococcal toxins will lyse some *Mycoplasma* strains (5).

**Horses.** Little is known about PPLO infection in the horse. These microorganisms have been isolated from genital tracts in mares that have aborted.
**Cattle.** PPLO have been isolated from milk, from cases of pneumonia and arthritis, from aborted bovine fetuses, from the eyes of calves suffering from keratoconjunctivitis, and from the genital tracts of cows with records of poor breeding efficiency (51). They have been isolated from semen of bulls.

Mastitis associated with *Mycoplasma* was reported by Davidson and Stuart (18) in 1960. In 1962 Hale *et al.* (30) described a severe outbreak in a Connecticut dairy herd. The first isolation was made in New York in 1962 and came from samples of purulent secretions from nine cows in a Lewis County herd. By 1963 *Mycoplasma* had been isolated from a total of 15 herds in New York State (10). It now appears to be present in dairy herds located in widely scattered areas of northern United States and in California. The disease was first described in England.

No acute general febrile symptoms were observed in the *Mycoplasma* infected herds, although all showed elevated temperatures on the 3rd or 4th day following inoculation. Some reached a high of 105.5 F and returned to normal within 24 to 96 hours. These animals showed no general symptoms of depression or inappetence. Leukopenia may appear, however, and the mastitis is characterized by a sharp drop in milk production and extremely swollen udders. The supramammary lymph nodes may be enlarged and firm. The secretion varies in appearance. It may be slightly yellow and on standing deposit a fine sediment on the bottom of the container. In some cases the milk is definitely watery with flakes and a few clots and in others contains large yellow-white caseous chunks or pus. In general, infected cows developed acute mastitis in all quarters.

The disease spreads rapidly in a herd, and it is possible that milking procedures are responsible. Infected cows rarely recover. They may produce reasonably well on the next lactation, but atrophy of glandular tissue and unprofitable production usually result in the sale of the animals. Antibiotics have not proved to be especially effective in curing the disease.

Diagnosis can be made only by culture of the milk and identification of the organism. Kehoe *et al.* (38) demonstrated *Mycoplasma* in the mammary and lymphoid tissues by direct fluorescent antibody procedure.

Stuart *et al.* (62) have indicated that the *Mycoplasma* concerned in an extensive outbreak of mastitis that they studied resembled the organism that has been called *M. bovigenitalium.* Although it appears that *M. bovigenitalium* has been responsible for bovine mastitis in England an organism that has been named *M. bovimastitidis* (*M. agalactiae* var. *bovis*) has been implicated in the United States. The role of the former in reproductive diseases is not yet clear. A third species, *M. laidlawi,* has been isolated from bovine male and female genital tracts, sewage, milk, blood, fetuses, and lymph nodes. Its pathogenic attributes have not been established. In fact the classification of the PPLO strains of bovine origin is not on a firm base. Al-Aubaidi and Fabricant (2) delineated 13 serotypes, exclusive of the so-called *T-strains* and the PPO types. Further study is needed before bovine *Mycoplasma* can be clearly and adequately characterized.

**Swine.** PPLO have been isolated from infectious atrophic rhinitis in swine. Their presence has been reported in polyserositis and other pathologic processes in this animal (40). According to Switzer (64) there are five well-established species of *Mycoplasma* that have been recovered from swine. These are *M. hyorhinis,* a major cause of polyserositis-arthritis; *M. hyosynoviae,* a major cause of arthritis; *M. hyopneumoniae,* the major cause of chronic pneumonia in swine; and *M. granularum* and *M. laidlawi,* both of no known pathologic significance.

In 1963 Roberts *et al.* (56) studied the pathology of *M. hyorhinis* arthritis in swine. They observed acute synovial membrane changes that consisted of mild hyperemia and hypertrophy of the synovial villi associated with a yellowish coloration of the synovial membrane. Histopathologically, these changes were characterized by hypertrophy of the synovial villi, hyperplasia of synovial cells, and lymphocytic infiltration concentrated in nodular foci. Heinze *et al.* (32) encountered acute polyserositis in a herd of swine and isolated PPLO from pleural, peritoneal, and pericardial fluid specimens.

In 1966 Moore *et al.* (47) described a chronic arthritis syndrome in swine caused by an organism that he named *Mycoplasma hyoarthrinosa.* The lesions produced were similar to the early ones that are seen in erysipelas, but no extensive exostosis develops. Histopathologically, there was hypertrophy of the synovial cells at the tip of the villi and an infiltration of lymphocytes and plasma cells. Also in 1966, the same group of workers (48) isolated a *Mycoplasma* from the mucosal surface of the porcine uterus and claimed that the organism was able to induce a metritis-mastitis (postparturient fever) syndrome in sows. This agent was named *Mycoplasma hyogenitalium.* At this time the status of these two cultures is not clear.

In 1967, Switzer (63) indicated that a serious form of arthritis occurring in certain swine herds in Iowa was caused by *M. granularum.* Actually it now appears that the inciting agent is *M. hyosynoviae* and that the status of *M. granularum* is in doubt. The disease evoked by *M. hyosynoviae* differs from the polyserositis-arthritis caused by *M. hyorhinis*.

A very common, chronic respiratory disease of swine long confused with swine influenza was studied in 1952 by Betts and Beveridge (6) in England. It is now known as *enzootic pneumonia of swine* and it is believed that PPLO are the cause (7, 29). The disease has been called *virus pneumonia of swine, infectious pneumonia of pigs,* and *ferkelgrippe.* The etiologic agent (28) bears the name *Mycoplasma hyopneumoniae (suipneumoniae)* and the proper designation for the disease is *mycoplasmal pneumonia of pigs.*

It probably occurs everywhere swine are raised as domestic animals. The disease which is widespread in the British Isles is the same as that which occurs in a very large percentage of all swine herds in the United States. There is little doubt that the diseases described in Australia, Sweden, Finland, Germany, and Kenya are the same.

Pigs usually show signs of illness when 3 to 10 weeks of age. The young animals may suffer from a transient diarrhea and then develop a dry cough. This may last for only a few weeks, or it may persist indefinitely. The affected pigs usually eat well but are unthrifty and do not gain weight as they should. The worst affected may suffer severe stunting of growth and are unprofitable to keep. The less affected may appear to be essentially normal animals after the initial period of coughing.

The incubation period is from 10 days to 2 weeks.

The course of the disease is variable. Actually the animals suffer from the affliction throughout their lives, although in many the signs of the disease may be hardly appreciable.

The mortality from enzootic pneumonia is practically nil. It is the morbidity that makes the disease costly to pig owners.

The lesions of enzootic pneumonia are purplish or grayish pneumonic areas in the apical and cardiac lobes, whereas the remainder of the lungs are usually normal in color and consistency. These lesions have been seen by butchers and pathologists in the lungs of pigs so often and so long that they have been regarded almost as normal. Many have considered the lesions to be atelectatic rather than pneumonic. Bacteria often invade the pneumonic areas, complicating the disease picture. The lymph nodes draining the diseased area are usually enlarged and soft.

The disease is spread by droplets from infected sows to their pigs. It is introduced into herds by the purchase of infected breeding stock.

The diagnosis is easily made from the history of the disease, isolation of the PPLO, and the appearance of the anatomical lesions. The lesions resemble those of swine influenza; but the latter is an acute, rapidly developing disease, whereas enzootic pneumonia develops more slowly and usually causes clinical signs only in very young pigs. CF tests have been used with some success in detecting the presence of enzootic pneumonia in swine herds.

Enzootic pneumonia apparently produces very little immunity. When the disease once becomes established in a herd, it continues indefinitely, the older animals infecting the newborn and any other susceptible pigs that may be introduced into the herd. Several have observed, however, that the disease is more virulent and damaging in herds that have not previously been exposed to it; hence it is surmised that long exposure to it does confer a measure of herd resistance—one that is not great enough, however, to protect the individuals from infection.

No method of effective treatment of the disease is known. Antibiotics show little ability to alter the course of the disease once it is started. It has been claimed that very large doses of the tetracyclines given early will protect exposed pigs and that lincomycin will aid in controlling both mycoplasmal arthritis and pneumonia. Because the breeder animals seldom become free from the disease and serve as sources of infection to those not already infected, it appears that there is little chance of eradicating the disease by measures short of eliminating all stock, cleaning and disinfecting the premises, and starting anew with clean swine. Because purchasing stock that is known to be free of this disease presents a problem, Young and Underdahl (71) advocate obtaining "specific pathogen-free" pigs by removing them from the sow aseptically by Cesarean section, then raising them by hand in rigid isolation from all other swine.

**Sheep and Goats.** In dairy goats PPLO have been reported to cause a highly fatal disease characterized by septicemia and arthritis. Clinically this disease is not typical of contagious agalactia or of caprine pleuropneumonia, and experimentally the PPLO isolate is infective for goats, sheep, and pigs, but not for mice, guinea pigs, and calves (15). PPLO have been isolated from respiratory tracts of sheep.

**Dogs and Cats.** PPLO have been described in respiratory diseases in dogs, and it appears that vaginal samples from this animal often contain these organisms. They were reported to be the cause of a fatal septicemic disease of infant puppies (9), but it now appears that a virus is involved. Barile *et al.* (4) in a study of 249 mycoplasmas isolated from laryngeal and urogenital tissues of dogs concluded that at least four species are commensal inhabitants of dogs. These are *M. spumans, M. canis, M. maculosum,* and *M. edwardi.*

Cats have also yielded numerous mycoplasmas and there are at least three groups with species designations of *M. felis, M. gatae,* and *M. feliminutum* (33).

**Fowl.** In 1935 Nelson (49) found coccobacilliform bodies in association with fowl coryza. He concluded that his "agent" was not a virus and chose the descriptive name of coccobacillus. In 1943 Delaplane and Stuart (19) described chronic respiratory disease (CRD) of chickens and isolated an agent which could be propagated in embryonated chicken eggs. Six years later Hitchner (34) also used this technic to propagate an agent that was present in infectious sinusitis of turkeys (IST). It was soon discovered that these so-called *agents* that were propagated in eggs are constantly found both in sinusitis of turkeys and in CRD of chickens. Although similar agents were first described as rickettsialike, in 1952 Markham and Wong (45) referred to them as PPLO and ascribed to them an etiological role in IST and CRD.

The only avian species listed in the seventh edition of *Bergey's Manual* is *M. gallinarum*. It is a nonpathogen. In 1960 Edward and Kamarek designated the typical pathogen *M. gallisepticum*. In 1969 Fabricant (24) published a tentative reclassification of avian mycoplasmas based on serological and biochemical studies. He delineated serotypes A through S and also two species, of which one has not been established (*M. laidlawi* var. *inocuum*) while another (*M. anatis*) appears to have a valid status. He concluded that *M. gallisepticum* (serotype A), *M. gallinarum* (serotype B), *M. iners* (serotype E-G), *M. anatis*, *M. synoviae* (serotype S), and *M. meleagridis* (serotype H) were valid species. The other previously described (49, 70) serotypes were simplified into three closely related groups C-O, D-P, and I-J-K-N-Q-R. F and L (pigeon types) seem to possess distinct characteristics. Serotype M was discarded because it was identical with B.

*M. gallisepticum infection.* This organism is the primary etiological agent of chronic respiratory disease (CRD) of chickens and turkeys. The disease in turkeys has also been commonly called infectious sinusitis of turkeys (IST).

*In chickens* CRD is typically a disease with a long incubation period (1 to 3 weeks) and a long course. It is accompanied by tracheal râles, nasal discharge, and coughing. Feed consumption is reduced, egg production may be lowered, and the birds lose weight. In chicks the disease often takes the form of a simple coryza. Gross lesions are associated with the presence of mucoid to mucopurulent exudate in the trachea, bronchi, air sacs, and nasal passages. Instances of synovitis involving the synovial membranes of the joints, tendovaginal sheaths, and bursae have been noted. Microscopically, the mucous membranes are thickened, hyperplastic, and infiltrated with mononuclear cells.

*In turkeys* the disease is characterized by swelling of the infraorbital sinuses. These are filled with a thick mucoid exudate. In some cases conjunctivitis and inflammation of the air sacs are observed. The disease runs a chronic course and affected birds lose weight. The death rate usually is not high, but the failure to gain weight may cause considerable economic loss. The lesions are progressive and much more extensive, with severe involvement of the nasal passages, sinuses, lungs, and air sacs. Synovial and joint lesions have also been seen.

*Diagnoses* are made on the basis of history and lesions observed in the affected birds combined with serological confirmation. The rapid serum plate agglutination test, the tube agglutination test, and the hemagglutination-inhibition test have been useful and extensively used tools for mycoplasmal serological studies.

*Egg transmission* of IST and CRD has been demonstrated (11, 36, 67), and it is believed that this method plays a major role, under crowded conditions, in the dissemination of these diseases. It is also transmitted by contact, aerosol, animal vectors, and it has been traced to the use of contaminated live virus vaccines.

*Treatment and control.* Although *M. gallisepticum* is susceptible to many antibiotics *in vitro*, treatments with these substances have had limited usefulness. Antibiotic treatment of hatching eggs has proved to be an efficacious and practical method of producing *Mycoplasma*-free chicks. Through the studies of Chalquest and Fabricant (12) and Levine and Fabricant (43) an egg-dipping procedure has been developed that consists essentially of immersing prewarmed eggs in chilled antibiotic solutions. Under field conditions tylosin has been the most effective antibiotic used in this process. As in chickens, the treatment of turkeys, although often clinically effective, is of limited value because mycoplasmas are not completely eliminated from the birds.

Yoder, Jr. (69) recommends preincubation heat treatment of chicken hatching eggs to inactivate *Mycoplasma*. He suggests the application of an internal egg temperature of 114.5 F during a 12-to-14-hour period to inactivate both *M. gallisepticum* and *M. synoviae*.

M. synoviae *infection*. A transmissible disease of young chickens and turkeys has been known for many years as infectious synovitis (IS). It was first described in chickens by Olson and colleagues (50) in 1954. In the following year it was identified in turkeys by Snoeyenbos and Olesiuk (61). It is now known to occur in many parts of the world. It is a transmissible disease of young chickens and turkeys manifested by joint swellings, lameness, and general unthriftiness. In chickens it is seen mostly in broilers. In turkeys the joint swellings are not as pronounced as in chickens, but lameness and general debility, with failure to grow properly, are the usual signs. In both species the affected joints and tendon sheaths contain a creamy white, viscid, purulent exudate, which sometimes becomes caseous. The hock joints and the bursa on the breast are most commonly affected, but all joints sometimes are involved. The disease does not appear to be highly contagious, the incidence in flocks often being no more than 2 to 10 percent. Rarely it may be much higher, 60 percent or more. The flock mortality usually is less than 10 percent.

*Diagnosis* may be confirmed by isolating the organism or by serum-plate-agglutination test with *M. synoviae* antigen. The organism is unique in its specific DPN (coenzyme I) requirement and demonstration of this characteristic indicates its identity.

*Transmission.* Both egg and contact transmission have been demonstrated.

*Treatment and control.* Feed medicated with chlortetracycline has been useful in preventing the disease, but not in curing affected birds or in eliminating the organism from such birds.

M. meleagridis *infection*. This organism has been found only in turkeys. It was first recognized by Adler *et al.* (1) in 1958. It had been suspected that it caused a decrease in hatchability of turkey poults, then in 1967, Dierks *et al.* (21) demonstrated that it was able to produce airsacculitis in *Mycoplasma*-free poults although the lesions were not as severe as those caused by *M. gallisepticum.*

Transmission of airsacculitis is by means of eggs, the semen-oviduct route, and by the air sac-ovary route (39).

*Other* Mycoplasma *spp.* involved in avian diseases. Apparently isolates of serotypes I, J, K, N, Q, and R have been involved with airsacculitis of turkeys (24).

Mathey *et al.* (46) isolated a PPLO from a mild respiratory disease of pigeons and found that it differed in fermentative ability, antigenicity, and pathogenicity from strains isolated from chickens and turkeys. It now seems evident that avian serotype L occurs in pigeons and is a valid pigeon type.

Roberts (55) isolated a PPLO, which he labeled *M. anatis* from a duck that was suffering from sinusitis. This duck was also carrying an influenza A virus. *M. anatis* is now recognized as a distinct species and although other duck isolates exist they have not been classified.

**Man.** PPLO have been isolated so frequently from the oral cavity and from the male and female urinary tract in the absence of inflammation to suggest that certain strains are a part of the normal flora of the body. It appears that genital strains are transmitted by copulation. That some PPLO are pathogenic for man is indicated by their isolation from children with purpura and from the blood of febrile patients. These organisms have been obtained frequently from a disease known as *Reiter's syndrome,* although their etiologic role has not been established. The disease is characterized by conjunctivitis, nonspecific urethritis, arthritis, and skin lesions (20). Among those species affecting man we find *M. salivarium, M. fermentans, M. pharyngis, M. hominis,* and *M. pneumoniae* (59). The last two appear to be the most important. *M. hominis* plays a role in respiratory- and genital-tract disease. *M. pneumoniae* (Eaton's agent) has been definitely shown to be an important respiratory-tract pathogen. It is the cause of primary atypical pneumonia in man. This disease appeared during World War II in endemic form in army camps and in schools and colleges. The incubation period varied from 5 to 25 days with an average of 13. While many patients were extremely ill, and a few died, very extensive pulmonary infections, with râles and x-ray changes, were found in asymptomatic subjects.

Some progress has been made in vaccinating against *M. pneumoniae* infection with an attenuated culture (17).

The pathogenic human PPLO have been shown to be susceptible to streptomycin, oxytetracycline, and tetracycline.

Mention needs to be made of the so-called *T-strains* (31) of mycoplasmas. They were first isolated in primary agar cultures of exudates obtained from patients with nongonococcal urethritis (NGU). They were originally referred to as "tiny-form colonies of pleuropneumonialike organisms," because colony size at maturity was approximately one fourth the size of the commonly encountered classical (large-colony) human genital *Mycoplasma*, such as *M. hominis*. T-strain organisms in clinical exudates appear as rounded elements 300 to 350 m$\mu$ which assume reddish-purple coloration with Giemsa stain. Although they exist primarily in the genitourinary tract of man they have been isolated from human throats and from a rectal specimen. T-strains have been associated with NGU in human males and they have been isolated from the wives of NGU patients. A "Boston" T-strain was obtained from the chorion, decidua, and amnion of a patient who experienced a spontaneous middle-trimester abortion. Effective and lasting eradication of NGU in the husband in many cases has been accomplished only be simultaneous treatment of both husband and wife and the achievement of negative cultures for T-strains of mycoplasmas in both partners. Present evidence suggests that the female may serve as an *asymptomatic carrier* of T-strain organisms in the genitourinary tract.

In 1967 mycoplasmas having morphologic characteristics of T-strains were isolated from the bovine genitourinary tract. In 1968 similar strains were isolated from pneumonic calf lungs. The role of T-strains in human and lower animal disease awaits further evaluation.

## REFERENCES

1. Adler, Fabricant, Yamamoto, and Berg. Am. Jour. Vet. Res., 1958, *19*, 440.
2. Al-Aubaidi and Fabricant. Cornell Vet., 1971, *61*, 490.
3. Barber and Fabricant. Jour. Bact., 1962, *83*, 1268.
4. Barile, DelGiudice, Carski, Yamashiroya, and Verna. Proc. Soc. Exp. Biol. and Med., 1970, *134*, 146.
5. Bernheimer and Davidson. Science, 1965, *148*, 1229.
6. Betts and Beveridge. Jour. Path. and Bact., 1952, *64*, 247.
7. Betts and Whittlestone. Res. Vet. Sci., 1963, *4*, 471.
8. Bridré, Donatien, and Hilbert. Comp. rend. Acad. Sci., 1923, *177*, 841.
9. Carmichael, Fabricant, and Squire. Proc. Soc. Exp. Biol. and Med., 1964, *117*, 826.
10. Carmichael, Guthrie, Fincher, Field, Johnson, and Linquist. Proc. U.S. Livestock San. Assoc., 1963, *67*, 220.
11. Carnaghan. Jour. Comp. Path. and Therap., 1961, *71*, 279.
12. Chalquest and Fabricant. Avian Dis., 1959, *3*, 257.
13. Chanock, Hayflick, and Barile. Proc. Natl. Acad. Sci. (USA), 1962, *48*, 41.
14. Clark, Bailey, Fowler, and Brown. Jour. Bact., 1963, *85*, 111.
15. Cordy and Adler. Ann. N.Y. Acad. Sci., 1960, *79* (Art. 10), 686.
16. Cottew and Lloyd. Jour. Comp. Path., 1965, *75*, 363.
17. Couch, Cate, and Chanock. Jour. Am. Med. Assoc., 1964, *187*, 442.
18. Davidson and Stuart. Vet. Rec., 1960, *72*, 766.
19. Delaplane and Stuart. Am. Jour. Vet. Res., 1943, *4*, 325.
20. Dienes and Smith. Proc. Soc. Exp. Biol. and Med., 1942, *50*, 99.
21. Dierks, Newman, and Pomeroy. Ann. N.Y. Acad. Sci., 1967, *143*, 170.
22. Edward and Fitzgerald. Jour. Path. and Bact., 1954, *68*, 23.

23.   Edwards.   Vet. Rec., 1953, *65*, 873.
24.   Fabricant.   In: Hayflick. The *Mycoplasmatales* and the L-phase of bacteria. Appleton-Century-Crofts, New York, 1969, pp. 621–641.
25.   Fabricant and Barber.   Proc. 73rd Ann. Mtg. U.S. Anim. Health Assoc., 1969, pp. 573–581.
26.   Fabricant and Freundt.   Ann. N.Y. Acad. Sci., 1967, *143*, 50.
27.   Foggie, Etheridge, Erdağ, and Arisoy.   Jour. Comp. Path., 1970, *80*, 345.
28.   Goodwin, Pomeroy, and Whittlestone.   Jour. Hyg. (London), 1967, *65*, 85.
29.   Goodwin and Whittlestone.   Brit. Jour. Exp. Path., 1963, *44*, 291.
30.   Hale, Helmboldt, Plastridge, and Stula.   Cornell Vet., 1962, *52*, 582.
31.   Hayflick.   The *Mycoplasmatales* and the L-phase of bacteria. Appleton-Century-Crofts, New York, 1969, p. 16.
32.   Heinze, Mortor, and Tiffany.   Jour. Am. Vet. Med. Assoc., 1963, *143*, 267.
33.   Heyward, Sabry, and Dowdle.   Am. Jour. Vet. Res., 1969, *30*, 615.
34.   Hitchner.   Poultry Sci., 1949, *28*, 106.
35.   Hofstad and Doerr.   Cornell Vet., 1956, *46*, 439.
36.   Jerstad.   Vet. Med., 1949, *44*, 272.
37.   Jonas and Barber.   Jour. Inf. Dis., 1969, *119*, 126.
38.   Kehoe, Norcross, Carmichael, and Strandberg.   *Ibid.*, 1967, *117*, 171.
39.   Kumar and Pomeroy.   Am. Jour. Vet. Res., 1969, *30*, 1423.
40.   Lecce.   Ann. N.Y. Acad. Sci., 1960, *79* (Art. 10), 670.
41.   Lecce and Sperling.   Cornell Vet., 1954, *44*, 230.
42.   Lemcke.   Jour. Hyg. (London), 1964, *62*, 199.
43.   Levine and Fabricant.   Avian Dis., 1962, *6*, 72.
44.   Lindley.   Jour. Am. Vet. Med. Assoc., 1967, *151*, 1810.
45.   Markham and Wong.   Poultry Sci., 1952, *31*, 902.
46.   Mathey, Adler, and Siddle.   Am. Jour. Vet. Res., 1956, *17*, 521.
47.   Moore, Redmond, and Livingston, Jr.   *Ibid.*, 1966, *27*, 1649.
48.   Moore, Redmond, and Livingston, Jr.   Vet. Med., 1966, *61*, 883
49.   Nelson.   Science, 1935, *82*, 43.
50.   Olson, Bletner, Shelton, Monroe, and Anderson.   Poultry Sci., 1954, *33*, 1075.
51.   Olson, Seymour, Boothe, and Dozsa.   Ann. N.Y. Acad. Sci., 1960, *79* (Art. 10), 670.
52.   Perlman, Rahman, and Semar.   Appl. Microbiol., 1967, *15*, 82.
53.   Purcell and Chanock.   Med. Clin. North Am., 1967, *51*, 791.
54.   Reynolds and Hetrick.   Appl. Microbiol., 1969, *17*, 405.
55.   Roberts.   Vet. Rec., 1964, *76*, 470.
56.   Roberts, Switzer, and Ramsey.   Am. Jour. Vet. Res., 1963, *24*, 19.
57.   Sabin.   Bact. Rev., 1941, *5*, 1.
58.   Sabry.   Cornell Univ. Thesis, 1968.
59.   Sammons, Gardner, Jr., and Dienst.   Jour. Lab. and Clin. Med., 1969, *73*, 338.
60.   Smith.   Proc. Soc. Exp. Biol. and Med., 1955, *88*, 628.
61.   Snoeyenbos and Olesiuk.   Proc. Northeastern Pullorum Conf., 1955.
62.   Stewart, Davidson, Slavin, Edgson, and Howell.   Vet. Rec., 1963, *75*, 59.
63.   Switzer.   Jour. Am. Vet. Med. Assoc., 1967, *151*, 1656.
64.   Switzer.   Personal communication, 1971.

65. Taylor-Robinson, Somerson, Turner, and Chanock. Jour. Bact., 1963, *85*, 1261.
66. Turner, Campbell, and Dick. Austral. Vet. Jour., 1935, *11*, 63.
67. Van Roekel and Olesiuk. Proc. Am. Vet. Med. Assoc., 1953, p. 289.
68. Watson, Cottew, Erdağ, and Arisoy. Jour. Comp. Path., 1968, *78*, 283.
69. Yoder, Jr. Avian Dis., 1970, *14*, 75.
70. Yoder, Jr., and Hofstad. *Ibid.*, 1964, *8*, 481.
71. Young and Underdahl. Jour. Soc. Farm Mgrs. and Rural Appraisers, 1956, *20*, 63.

PART **5**

# THE PATHOGENIC
# FUNGI

# XXV | The *Eumycetes*

The simplest, least differentiated of known plants belong to the subkingdom *Thallophyta*. These plants have no leaves, stems, seeds, or roots but consist wholly of single cells or chains of such cells forming filaments.

Some of the thallophytes contain chlorophyll and thus are capable of photosynthesis. These are known as *algae*. Others do not have chlorophyll; hence they are not green and are not capable of photosynthesis. These are placed in the phylums *Schizomycophyta* (bacteria), *Myxomycophyta* (slime molds), and *Eumycophyta* (true fungi (1). The bacteria have been considered and the slime molds are of little medical importance.

Among the *Eumycophyta,* sometimes referred to as *Eumycetes,* are forms that are unable to utilize the energy of sunlight, that live a saprophytic or parasitic existence, and generally thrive best in darkness. Here are found molds that are unicellular and others that are multicellular. Some are dimorphic, that is, they may grow as unicellular individuals under some circumstances and as multicellular under others. This occurs among some parasitic fungi, the unicellular stage occurring in tissues and the multicellular in cultures. Most pathogenic species are multicellular. The yeasts, however, are always unicellular.

The multicellular fungi or molds are made up of cells which, placed end to end, form filaments known as *hyphae*. The tangled mass of hyphae forming a single colony is known as the *mycelium*.

In some molds the mycelial filaments are not divided by septa or cross walls but consist of single, multinucleated cells in which the protoplasm streams back and forth as it does in some of the algae. These are said to have a *coenocytic mycelium,* and such species are classified in a group known as the *Phycomycetes*. The greater number of species, however, have *septate myceliums,* and such species belong to the *Basidiomycetes,* the *Asomycetes,* or the *Fungi Imperfecti* (sometimes called *Hyphomycetes* or *Deuteromycetes*).

The *Basidiomycetes* consist largely of the mushrooms, bracket fungi, and other fleshy forms that have no importance in animal infections; hence they will be considered no further here. The *Ascomycetes* are characterized by the possession of membranous sacs called *asci* (sing. *ascus*), which contain spores, generally eight in number, called *ascospores*. Similar to the *Ascomycetes* are the large number of forms that are now relegated to the *Fungi Imperfecti*. Probably the greater part of these forms actually belong to the *Ascomycetes*, but because the sexual or ascospores have not been observed, they are not placed there. The imperfection indicated by the name of the group is probably, in most instances, imperfection in our knowledge rather than imperfection in the fungi themselves. The group is diminished, from time to time, by the discovery of the sexual phases, which permits the transfer of such species to one of the groups previously mentioned.

In all molds except the *Fungi Imperfecti* both sexual and asexual spores are recognized. In most instances the asexual spores are much more readily formed, are more numerous, and are more conspicuous than the sexual types. *Oospores* are sexual spores produced by the fusion of two unlike cells, one of which is regarded as a male element and the other a female. *Zygospores* are sexual spores, occurring among the *Phycomycetes* only, produced by the fusion of two similar sexual cells. *Ascospores* are regarded as sexual spores because the parent cell from which the ascus is formed possesses two nuclei which fuse.

The simplest asexual spore is the *arthrospore,* which is merely a portion of hypha that breaks off and that is capable of reproducing the species. In many species of fungi, spore-bearing hyphae develop and these form spores by a process known as abjointing, i.e., by pinching and breaking off special elements. In some forms special cells appear, generally at the end of the hyphae, which enlarge and balloon into a saclike structure in which the spores are formed. This is known as a *sporangium.* In other forms the spores are formed exogenously at the tip of special hyphae. These are known as *conidia,* and the specialized structure that bears them is called a *conidiophore. Chlamydospore* is a general name used for thick-walled structures of many kinds which are formed in various parts of the thallus and which apparently are resting forms, closely analogous in function to the spores of bacteria.

The next two chapters consider the diseases under two categories, as follows:

1. The *dermatomycoses,* the skin mycoses of the "ringworm" group. These diseases are caused by many different species of fungi, most of which are classified among the *Fungi Imperfecti*. These organisms cause superficial infections of the skin, which are annoying rather than fatal, as a rule.

2. The mycoses of internal organs, consisting of destructive lesions of the mucous membranes, of tumorlike, mycotic granulomas, and of abscesses of the internal organs. Some of these begin as skin infections. These infections generally are chronic in their course and frequently have a high fatality rate.

## REFERENCES

1. Fuller and Tippo.    College botany. rev. ed. Henry Holt and Co., New York, 1954, p. 528.
2. Moss and McQuown.    Atlas of medical mycology. 2d ed. Williams and Wilkins Co., Baltimore, 1960.

# XXVI | The Dermatomycoses of Animals

These infections are common in both man and animals. They are generally known as *ringworm* from the fact that typically they begin in small areas and spread centrifugally, the region of greatest inflammation at the periphery forming an ever-widening circle. If the cases are not treated, new areas usually become infected and finally large areas of the skin may become involved through the coalescence of the primary lesions. Ringworm is also known under the name *tinea*. A certain kind of ringworm is known as *favus*.

The fungi of the ringworm group grow almost wholly on the keratinized layers of the skin, including the hair and other horny structures. They show a preference, in most cases, for the hairy portions of the body; however, some species occur on the glabrous, or hairless, areas. The infections usually involve the hair follicles and the hairs themselves. The latter become brittle and often break off near their bases, or sometimes they split. Commonly they appear dry and lusterless. The skin of the affected areas becomes scaly and harsh, and crusts are formed. Bacterial infection often complicates the picture, pustules being formed in the hair follicles. This condition is known as *sycosis*. The infections differ considerably in appearance, depending in part upon the nature of the infecting species.

Generally speaking, ringworm thrives best in young animals and in older ones that have been devitalized by disease or malnutrition. It is seen more often in stabled animals than in those on pasture, and more often in winter than in summer. Ringworm infection that has become widespread in groups of calves will often clear up spontaneously in the spring several weeks after the animals have been turned out into the sunshine. This may be a result of better nutrition or it may be caused by the direct influence of the light. Ultra-violet light has proved to be useful in treating many forms of ringworm. The infections occur most frequently on the face and neck and around the tail-

536

head, but they may be found on any part of the body. Many types of ringworm are highly contagious, not only for other members of the same species but often also for members of other species. Usually when the infection occurs in an abnormal species, the disease does not spread in the new one but dies out in the initial host. Ringworm of cats, horses, and cattle readily infects people, and most of the other animal types have been known to infect man. These infections are very annoying and sometimes very resistant to treatment.

### Classification and Identification of the Fungi of the Ringworm Group

To most bacteriologists the classification and identification of genera and species in this group are baffling problems. Even the mycologists find it a difficult group and disagree on the classification. According to Conant *et al.* (2), a simplified classification has been made possible by culturing the fungus and selecting certain specific morphologic features as criteria for generic differentiation. By this method only three genera need be considered, *Microsporum, Trichophyton,* and *Epidermophyton.* Thus the genera *Achorion* and *Endodermophyton* have been discarded, and their species have been placed in the genus *Trichophyton.* This genus contains about 11 species; *Microsporum,* about 5 species; and *Epidermophyton,* 1 species.

In diagnosing diseases caused by the dermatophytes, direct microscopic examination should be made of infected hair, skin, or nails. Scrapings from infected areas should be placed in a drop of 10 to 40 percent potassium hydroxide on a slide, a cover glass should be added, and the preparation should be heated over a low flame. This helps to clear the preparation. Kligman *et al.* (5) recommend staining the fungi in skin scrapings with basic fuchsin and claim their method is superior to the KOH technic for demonstrating the organisms. The appearance of the fungus may furnish a clue to the genus to which it belongs, but species identification can be made only after the fungus has been isolated in pure culture. Species of *Microsporum, Trichophyton,* or *Epidermophyton* appear identical in infected skin, and generic or specific identification can be made only by culture. Descriptions of the dermatophytes follow.

*Trichophyton.* Species of this group attack the hair, skin, and nails. Arthrospores may be arranged in parallel rows inside infected hair (*endothrix* type) or arranged in parallel rows outside the hair (*ectothrix* type). In the skin and nails, species of *Trichophyton* appear as segmented, branching mycelial elements, which may or may not break up into arthrospores. Such forms are indistinguishable from those of *Microsporum* and *Epidermophyton.*

The group includes the causative agents of favus, which formerly were placed in a separate genus (*Achorion*). Favus is a type of ringworm characterized by the production of structures called *scutula* which have the general appearance of shields (Latin *scutum*=shield). These are formed because the parasites radiate out from the hair follicles between the Malpighian and the outer cornified layers of the skin, a process that separates the latter from their attachments. The separated layers are thoroughly invaded by the fungus hyphae, which form a felted mass within them. The hairs remain more or less intact, projecting out through the shields. The mycelium can be demonstrated inside the shafts of the plucked hairs, as well as in the substance of the scutula. It tends to break up into fragments of varying lengths, many of which are nearly spherical and thus resemble spores.

*Microsporum.* Members of this genus attack only the hair and skin. The fungus is seen as a mosaic sheath of small spores surrounding the infected hair shaft. In the skin it appears only as segmented, branching mycelial elements and cannot be distinguished from *Trichophyton* and *Epidermophyton.*

*Epidermophyton.* The fungus attacks only the skin and nails, in which it appears as segmented, branching mycelial elements, identical in structure with the forms seen in *Microsporum* infections of the skin and *Trichophyton* infections of the skin or nails.

Specific identification of these dermatophytes can be accomplished only by cultural means. Most of them are rather easily cultivated on artificial media, the principal problem being to separate them from miscellaneous saprophytic fungi, which usually are abundant on animal skins. Even when isolated in pure culture, their specific identification is a task for the expert. It is based upon the gross characteristics of the colonies developing on solid media, to a limited extent upon physiologic characters, and upon microscopic characteristics of the developing hyphae and spores, which often are quite different from those observed in preparations made directly from the skin. The morphology of cultures often varies widely when they are grown for a time on the same kind of medium, and different types of media usually profoundly influence their morphology. The study of such cultures is a very specialized task, which ordinarily will not be fruitful except to one who has had a good basic training in mycology. The scope of this work will not permit further discussion of the subject. Those who desire more information are referred to specific works such as those to which references are given at the end of this chapter.

Before special types of ringworm fungi are discussed, it is of interest to note the fact that certain dermatophytes have the property of fluorescing in ultraviolet light. Not all of them fluoresce and there are other fungi which do; hence the property must be used cautiously as a diagnostic procedure. Often, however, it proves useful in this connection. The patient is examined in the darkroom with a lamp emitting ultraviolet rays from which most of the visible rays have been removed by a Wood's filter. A yellowish-green fluorescence is characteristic of fungi. Plucked hairs and epidermal scales from patients may be examined in the same way, in which case fluorescence of the epidermal material around the root hairs is significant. In making such examinations care must be taken to exclude the possibility of confusing with fungi other fluorescing substances, especially medicaments that may have been used in treatment. Mineral oils and petrolatum, for example, emit a strong bluish-green fluorescence in ultraviolet light.

The brush technic is simple to perform and often is productive (4). Small animals may be brushed with a clean, small brush, giving special attention to areas suggesting infection. Removed hairs are examined by Wood's light to detect any green fluorescence indicative of certain dermatophytes or they may be observed microscopically after treatment with 10 percent KOH.

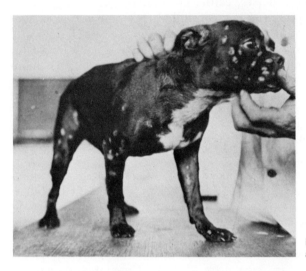

*Fig. 89.* Ringworm infection in a dog. (Courtesy H. J. Milks and H. C. Stephenson.)

An extract of the common dermatophytes has been used in diagnosing ringworm infection. The substance is called *trichophytin,* and by intradermal injection it can be used to detect sensitization to a dermatophyte. It is employed merely as an aid in diagnosis because the results of the test cannot always be interpreted accurately. For instance, penicillin-sensitized individuals may give positive reactions.

Among domestic animals in the United States, ringworm is seen most commonly in cattle, especially in calves. The fungus in this instance belongs to the genus *Trichophyton.* Occasionally serious outbreaks occur in horses, these cases generally being caused by members of the *Trichophyton* group but sometimes by members of the microspora. Ringworm of dogs and cats is common in many localities. Most of these are caused by members of the genus *Microsporum,* but some cases are *Trichophyton* (favus group), which probably are contracted from rodents, especially rats and mice. Chickens and other birds sometimes suffer from favus, which affects their combs principally. Ringworm of sheep has been noted (1), but appears to be of little economic importance in this animal. It has been observed in swine (5), and in the United States it seems to be occurring more frequently in this species since 1964 (3). *Trichophyton* infection has been reported as the cause of a disease called *fur-slipping* in chinchillas (2). It has appeared in New Zealand white rabbits (1). Man is highly susceptible to most species of *Microsporum* and

*Trichophyton* that affect the lower animals. In addition, the genus *Epidermo-phyton* contains a single species, *E. floccosum,* that seems to be a strict human type.

In a survey of domestic, captive, and wild animals Menges and Georg (7) obtained *Microsporum* from dogs, cats, mice, rats, monkeys, and a chinchilla and *Trichophyton* from dogs, horses, cattle, chinchillas, guinea pigs, mice, rats, a kangaroo, and an opossum. They concluded that ringworm is a common disease among animals in the United States. Many cases of ringworm have been described in which the nature of the causative agent is in doubt. Obviously the ringworm infections of animals are in need of much more study.

### Microsporum canis

SYNONYMS:   This species is apparently identical with
*Microsporum lanosum* (of man), *Microsporum felineum* (of cats),
and *Microsporum equinum* (of horses)

Ringworm infection in which this species is the etiological agent is quite common. It has been obtained from dogs, cats, horses, monkeys, chinchillas, and man. The disease spreads readily in kennels and catteries and among household pets which associate with stray animals and pets of other owners in the neighborhood.

The disease appears as small scabby areas on any part of the body but is seen most frequently on the ears, face, neck, and tail. These areas do not appear to cause much irritation, nor do they have any appreciable effect upon the general health of the animal as a rule. The hair is not shed and, in cats especially, if the disease affects the long-haired breeds and occurs on parts that are especially well covered with fur, the lesions may be overlooked until the disease has spread over a considerable part of the body. Such cases are stubborn to treat, and such animals readily infect other cats, dogs, and often

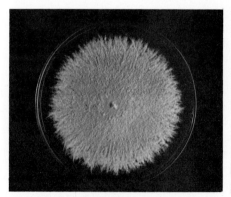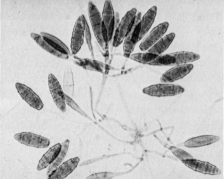

Fig. 90. *Microsporum gypseum.* (*Left*) Cultural appearance on Sabouraud's glucose agar. (*Right*) Macroconidia. X 270. (Courtesy R. W. Menges, *Cornell Vet.*)

human beings with whom they come in contact. Rebell *et al.* (11) have found that kittens react to experimental infection with *M. canis* by producing only a minimal inflammatory response, which reaches a peak in about 28 days and then regresses. They suggest that cats may provide the major reservoir and probably are the natural host of *M. canis*. La Touche (8) expressed the opinion that onchomycosis in cats may be associated with *M. canis*. Guinea pigs may be readily infected experimentally. This species has been obtained from the horse, but apparently it is not so common as the *Trichophyton* type, which will be described later. The lesions are relatively benign. In man the disease may appear on the scalp, or circinate lesions may appear on the relatively hairless parts of the body. There are records of the disease being transmitted from one cat to another through the agency of an intermediate human being.

### Microsporum gypseum

SYNONYM:  *Achorion gypseum*

This organism causes ringworm in dogs, cats, horses, fowl, guinea pigs, rats, mice, wild rodents, monkeys, and tigers (1).

### Microsporum audouini

Rare cases of infection with this species have been observed in dogs, a monkey, a guinea pig, and man. The lesions have been single or scattered, also circular with loss of hair, scaling, and some erythema.

### Microsporum distortum

This species has been reported occasionally in monkeys and man and rarely in the dog.

### Microsporum nanum

Bubash *et al.* (1) recorded the first isolation from swine in the United States in 1964. It occurred in a herd of Yorkshires in Pennsylvania. Lesions begin as small circular areas which gradually enlarge in a circular fashion until they may cover much of the animal's body. Most of them have a somewhat roughened, though not obviously raised, surface that is covered with thin, easily removed, brown crusts. The crusts may cover the area uniformly or they may be more prominent at the periphery, making a band which clearly outlines the infected area. Other lesions have few brown crusts, but have a red cast or a brown speckled appearance. There is no alopecia, pruritus, or general involvement, and lesions may be hidden by dirt and easily overlooked. Since the first report of *M. nanum* infection in swine, it has been found in at least 15 states indicating that porcine ringworm is common and widespread in the United States. It has also been recorded in Australia, Cuba, Canada, Mexico, and Kenya (2, 3).

This organism has been isolated from cases of ringworm in human beings.

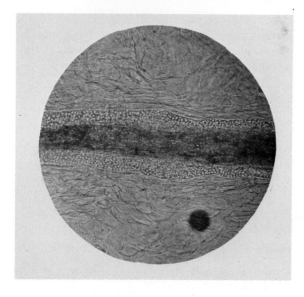

Fig. 91. Trichophyton ver-rucosum. Scrapings from a ring-worm lesion on the skin of a calf, unstained but cleared with caustic potash. The dark band running vertically is a pigment-containing hair in its follicle. Around the shaft of the hair large numbers of fungus spores can be seen. My-celia can be seen in some instances but not in this photograph. X 190.

### Trichophyton verrucosum

SYNONYMS:   *Trichophyton faviforme, Trichophyton ochraceum, Trichophyton album, Trichophyton discoides*

Ringworm of cattle is a very common disease, especially in young animals kept indoors during winter months. The causative agent is easily demon-strated, but the lesions are so characteristic that demonstration of the fungus is unnecessary for diagnosis. Hairs plucked from the margins of the lesions and examined in a strongly alkaline solution, which has a clearing action on the keratinized epithelium, show masses of spherical spores around their bases. These spores are arranged in chains. Filamentous hyphae may also be seen around the hairs, but these are not so easily recognized as the refractile spores.

It has been observed that normal calves placed in quarters where ring-worm-infected animals have previously been kept often will promptly develop the disease. This happens at times when infected animals have been absent from the premises for months. This suggests that fungus survives for long peri-ods, perhaps even from one winter to the next. Muende and Webb (7), in En-gland, succeeded in finding colonies of the calf ringworm fungus growing on semidried fecal material in such a stable. The fungus produced colonies large enough to be macroscopically visible. Blank (1) states that animal dermato-phytes may persist and keep their virulence outside the body on such mate-rial as soil, straw, and wood, especially if mixed with keratinaceous material shed from infected animals.

The lesions are usually found on the face, particularly around the eyes.

They also occur on the neck and occasionally on other parts of the body. Well-developed lesions consist of raised, dry, crusty, grayish-white masses from which a few broken hairs protrude. If the crusty material is pulled loose, bleeding occurs. The disease spreads rapidly among calves kept in a common room, especially if the quarters are dark and damp. It occurs rarely in horses, donkeys, burros, dogs, sheep (4), and man.

This organism does not fluoresce under ultraviolet light.

### Trichophyton equinum

Ringworm of horses occasionally causes a great deal of trouble in large stables and in military units. The disease spreads readily, principally through the use of common grooming tools, harnesses, and blankets. Outbreaks can be controlled only by treatment of the affected animals and by thorough disinfection of all stable equipment.

The disease is seen on parts of the body where harness or blanket straps rub the skin. The face, breast, croup, flanks, and back where the saddle and saddle girth rub are the areas most often involved. The hair on these areas breaks off and much of it comes out leaving semibald patches. The skin becomes progressively thickened and overlaid with flaky crusts. The underlying skin is dry and has a dull luster. Infections often complicate the picture, making the areas moist and reddened. The disease is transmissible to man, although apparently its contagiousness is not so great as that of the type caused by *Microsporum*. These infections seem to cause little inconvenience to the animal. The principal damage is the disfigurement, temporarily, of the animal's coat. If untreated the disease may spread over large areas. One case of infection by this species has been recorded in the dog (4).

### Trichophyton rubrum

SYNONYM:   *Trichophyton purpureum*

Rare cases of dermatomycosis are caused in dogs by *T. rubrum* (9). It has been reported in cows. This organism may also infect man. Although the incidence of infection with this type is low, it is difficult to cure and often persists for long periods regardless of treatment.

### Trichophyton mentagrophytes

SYNONYMS:   *Trichophyton gypseum, Trichophyton granulosum, Trichophyton quinckeanum*

*T. mentagrophytes* commonly infects mice, rats, dogs, cats, rabbits, chinchillas, and guinea pigs. It occasionally is seen in horses, cows, muskrats, opossums, squirrels, and foxes and rarely in swine (3). It has been reported in man. Mice infected with this species have transmitted it to cats, in which the lesions most commonly occur around the paws and on the ears.

### Trichophyton schoenleini

This type occurs occasionally in dogs, cats, mice, and man and appears commonly on the head.

### Trichophyton violaceum

Rare cases of infection have been reported in cows in which it produces lesions similar to those caused by *T. verrucosum*.

### Trichophyton gallinae

SYNONYM:   *Achorion gallinae*

Favus of fowls, particularly of chickens and turkeys, is a disease of considerable importance. It occurs in wild birds, it has been reported in man (1), and one case has been recorded in a dog. It appears as small white patches on the comb (usually of male birds). These enlarge and coalesce, so that finally the comb may be covered with a dull-white, moldy layer several mm thick. The disease usually is self-limiting, healing after several months if untreated. Scutula are not found on the comb lesions, but occasionally the dis-

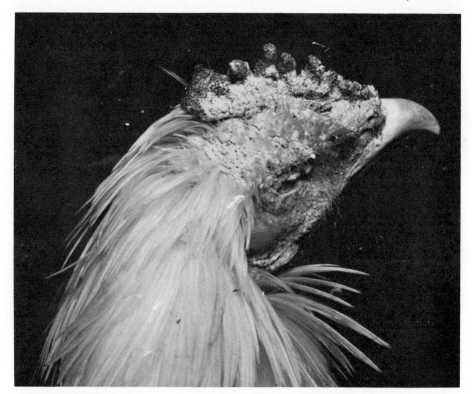

*Fig. 92.* Lesions of favus in a chicken. This condition is caused by *Trichophyton gallinae*.

ease extends into the feathered parts, in which case typical shields are formed. So long as the disease is limited to the comb, there is little effect upon the health of the birds. When the feathered portions are involved, however, the bird becomes emaciated and may die.

## Chemotherapy in Dermatomycoses

*M. canis* has been known to survive on cat hair kept on a laboratory bench at room temperature for 323 to 422 days (7). Certain types of ringworm tend to heal under good environmental conditions without medication, but most of the effort in the control of the dermatophytic infections has centered around the use of chemotherapeutic agents.

Preparations that contain such substances as oils, iodine, sulfur, salicylic acid, and other drugs are used in treating ringworm. Lies (6) recommends spraying cattle with 20 percent sodium caprylate. Hayes (3) used iodochlorohydroxyquinoline as an economical and successful treatment of ringworm in chinchillas. In horses Batte and Miller (1) found that successful healing followed the application of N-trichloromethylthio-tetrahydrophthalimide. Dermatomycosis in man responds to treatment with salts of undecylenic acid, to derivatives of salicyl anilide, and to racemic 2-dehydroemetine (1). Until the discovery of griseofulvin, antibiotics were of little value in curing ringworm. It now appears that oral administration of this antibiotic is highly effective in treating this disease in man (5–7), cats (6), chinchillas (1), Malayan Sun Bears (*Helarctos malayanus*, 1), and cattle (2, 5). The high cost of this antibiotic makes its use on animals practically prohibitive at present.

## REFERENCES

*General References*
1. Ainsworth and Austwick. Fungal diseases of animals. Commonwealth Agricultural Bureaux, Farnham Royal, England, 1959, p. 83.
2. Conant, Martin, Smith, Baker, and Callaway. Manual of clinical mycology. 1st ed. W. B. Saunders Co., Philadelphia and London, 1945.
3. Dodge. Medical mycology. C. V. Mosby, St. Louis, Mo., 1935.
4. Georg. Animal ringworm in public health. USPHS, CDC, Atlanta, Ga., 1960.
5. Kligman, Pillsbury, and Mescon. Jour. Am. Med. Assoc., 1951, *146*, 1563.
6. Lewis and Hopper. An introduction to medical mycology. 3d ed. Year Book Publisher, Chicago, 1948.
7. Menges and Georg. Pub. Health Rpts. (U.S.), 1957, *72*, 503.
8. Moss and McQuown. Atlas of medical mycology. 2d ed. Williams and Wilkins Co., Baltimore, 1960.
9. Plaut and Grütz. In: Kolle, Krause, and Uhlenhuth. Handbuch der pathogen Mikroorganismen. 3d rev. ed. G. Fischer, Jena, 1928, vol. V, p. 204.
10. Sabouraud. Les teignes. Masson et Cie, Paris, 1910.
11. Spinner, Emmonds, and Tsuchiya. Henrici's molds, yeasts and actinomycetes. 2d ed. John Wiley and Sons, New York, 1947.
12. Swartz. Elements of medical mycology. 2d ed. Grune and Stratton, New York, 1949.

*Ringworm in Dogs and Cats*
1.  Botwinick, Peck, and Schwartz.   Pub. Health Rpts. (U.S.), 1943, *58*, 317.
2.  Conant.   Arch. Dermatol. and Syphilol., 1937, *36*, 781.
3.  Davison and Gregory.   Canad. Med. Assoc. Jour., 1933, *29*, 242.
4.  Goldberg.   Jour. Am. Vet. Med. Assoc., 1965, *147*, 845.
5.  Holmes.   Vet. Rec., 1936, *48*, 864.
6.  Kaplan and Ajello.   Jour. Am. Vet. Med. Assoc., 1959, *135*, 253.
7.  Keep.   Austral. Vet. Jour., 1960, *36*, 277.
8.  La Touche.   Vet. Rec., 1955, *67*, 578.
9.  Moss and Dyson.   North Amer. Vet., 1955, *36*, 1031.
10.  Rawson.   Vet. Med., 1936, *31*, 213.
11.  Rebell, Timmons, Lamb, Hicks, Groves, and Coalson.   Amer. Jour. Vet. Res., 1956, *27*, 74.
12.  Young.   Vet. Med., 1936, *31*, 303.

*Ringworm in Horses*
1.  Batte and Miller.   Jour. Am. Vet. Med. Assoc., 1953, *123*, 111.
2.  Curley and Herring.   Vet. Bul., U.S. Army, 1938, *32*, 126.
3.  Lomas.   Vet. Jour., 1939, *95*, 290.

*Ringworm in Cattle*
1.  Blank.   Amer. Jour. Med. Sci., 1955, *229*, 252.
2.  Edgson.   Vet. Rec., 1970, *86*, 58.
3.  Georg.   Trans. N.Y. Acad. Sci., 1956, *18* (II), 639.
4.  Hutyra. Marek, and Manninger.   Pathology and therapeutics of the diseases of domesticated animals. 5th Eng. trans. Alex. Eger, Chicago, 1946, vol. *iii*, p. 595.
5.  Lauder and O'Sullivan.   Vet. Rec., 1958, *70*, 949.
6.  Lies.   Jour. Am. Vet. Med. Assoc., 1949, *115*, 458.
7.  Muende and Webb.   Arch. Dermatol. and Syphilol., 1937, *36*, 987.
8.  Udall.   The practice of veterinary medicine. 6th ed. The author, Ithaca, N.Y., 1954, p. 343.

*Ringworm in Sheep*
1.  Robinson.   Jour. So. African Vet. Med. Assoc., 1952, *23*, 84.

*Ringworm in Pigs*
1.  Bubash, Ginther, and Ajello.   Science, 1964, *143*, 366.
2.  Ginther.   Jour. Am. Vet. Med. Assoc., 1965, *146*, 945.
3.  Ginther and Ajello.   Jour. Am. Vet. Med. Assoc., 1965, *146*, 361.
4.  Ginther, Ajello, Bubash, and Varsavsky.   Vet. Med., 1964, *59*, 1038.
5.  McPherson.   Vet. Rec., 1956, *41*, 710.

*Ringworm in Fowl*
1.  Biester and Schwarte.   Diseases of poultry. 5th ed. Iowa State College Press, Ames. Iowa, 1965.

*Ringworm in Chinchillas*
1. Belloff. Vet. Med., 1967, *62*, 438.
2. Blank, Byrne, Plummer, and Avery. Canad. Jour. Comp. Med. and Vet. Sci., 1953, *17*, 396.
3. Hayes. Jour. Am. Vet. Med. Assoc., 1956, *128*, 193.

*Ringworm in Rabbits*
1. Banks and Clarkson. Jour. Am. Vet. Med. Assoc., 1967, *151*, 926.

*Ringworm in Bears*
1. Groves. Jour. Am. Vet. Med. Assoc., 1969, *155*, 1090.

*Ringworm in Man*
1. Abd-Rabbo and Yusef. Jour. Trop. Med. and Hyg. (London), 1966, *69*, 51.
2. Dalldorf. Fungi and fungous diseases. C. C Thomas, Springfield, Ill., 1962.
3. Dvorak and Otcenasek. Jour. Invest. Dermatol., 1964, *42*, 3.
4. Emmons, Binford, and Utz. Medical mycology. Lea & Febiger, Philadelphia, 1963.
5. Goldman, Schwarz, Preston, Beyer, and Loutzenhiser. Jour. Am. Med. Assoc., 1960, *172*, 532.
6. Halde and Ong. Am. Jour. Trop. Med. and Hyg., 1965, *14*, 1062.
7. McCuistion, Lawlis, and Gonzalez. Jour. Am. Med. Assoc., 1959, *171*, 2174.

# XXVII | The Fungi Causing Mycoses of the Internal Organs of Animals

The dermatophytic fungi are definitely parasitic in habit, existing nowhere in nature, so far as is known, except on the skin of infected animals, on hairs and epidermal scales from such lesions, and to a limited extent on materials in intimate contact with such epithelial debris. On the other hand, the fungi that cause the deep-seated infections generally, if not always, live saprophytically except when chance places them in positions where a parasitic habit is forced upon them. The superficial mycoses are definitely contagious; the deep-seated are not. The agents of the deep-seated infections apparently live in the soil and on vegetation. Some of these diseases occur only rarely and in widely separated localities. They have no definite areas of localization. The causative agents evidently are widespread, the cases of disease depending upon chance infection rather than the distribution of the causative agent. Other fungi of this group are numerous in certain localities and absent in others; hence the diseases are limited to definite areas. The introduction of more-sensitive soil-sampling technics (3) has aided markedly in locating the habitats of the fungi.

The fungi that cause the superficial mycoses are usually associated with disease in young animals. Those which cause the deep-seated infections are found most often in mature and aged animals. Excepting aspergillosis, all of these infections are chronic ones. Henrici (2) believes that animals are highly resistant to infection with such organisms as those concerned in the internal mycoses and that active, progressive disease does not occur until the tissues have become hypersensitized (allergic) through repeated contact. He thinks that repeated minor infections must occur before the conditions become right for the progressive disease to begin. This opinion is based upon considerable

548

experimental evidence, but it cannot be said to have been definitely proved. If this theory is substantiated, an adequate explanation for the relative absence of the diseases in young animals is provided.

The lesions of deep-seated fungus infections usually take the form of tumor-like masses commonly called *infectious granulomas*. These granulomas have necrotic foci in their centers surrounded by heavy walls of fibrotic tissue. Around the margins of the necrotic foci, epithelioid and giant cells may usually be found. The structure, therefore, is similar to that of a tubercle. In the necrotic tissue, instead of tubercle bacilli, one generally can easily demonstrate the hyphae of the fungus, In some cases spores can be found, in others yeastlike cells, depending upon the nature of the fungus present. Frequently stellate bodies made up of fine hyphae radiating from a central mass may be seen. The tips of the radiating filaments often are surrounded by hyaline, acidophilic material, the whole having a distinct resemblance to the colonies of the "ray fungus" of actinomycosis. Henrici believes that these actinomycetoid bodies are produced by the fungus as a result of specific stimulation by the allergic host tissues. That allergic sensitization occurs in fungus infections can easily be demonstrated by making skin tests with extracts of the causative agent.

In the deep-seated mycoses involving the human lungs it sometimes is possible to identify the fungus by examination of the patient's sputum. The technic and procedure of this examination are given in detail by Kurung (5). Pickett *et al.* (6) recommend the use of a simple fluorescent stain in searching for fungi. When stained in sections or films with acridine orange and examined with blue light, fungi fluoresce red, yellow, yellow-green, or green against a dark background.

Fungal immunology has received less attention than that given to viruses and bacteria, but experimentally induced immunity against certain fungi is highly effective suggesting the use of vaccines, especially in selected regions of endemicity (4).

The increasing use of corticosteroids, cytotoxic drugs, and antibiotics in patients whose basic disease process alters their resistance to infection, has resulted in a new spectrum of infectious diseases caused by opportunistic organisms in which saprophytic fungi have played important etiologic roles (1).

## REFERENCES

1. Hart, Russell, Jr., and Remington.  Jour. Inf. Dis., 1969, *120*, 169.
2. Henrici.  Jour. Bact., 1940, *39*, 113.
3. Klite, Kelley, Jr., and Diercks.  Am. Jour. Epidemiol., 1965, *81*, 124.
4. Kong and Levine.  Bact. Rev., 1967, *31*, 35.
5. Kurung.  Am. Rev. Tuberc., 1947, 55, 387.
6. Pickett, Bishop, Chick, and Baker.  Am. Jour. Clin. Path., 1960, *33*, 197.

## PHYCOMYCETES

Members of the family *Mucoraceae* belong to the *Phycomycetes*. Some members are very common in nature, particularly the common bread mold, *Rhizopus nigricans*. A bit of bread, moistened and kept in a Petri dish, will usually furnish a luxuriant growth of this organism within a few days. It is recognized as a maze of loosely felted white mycelium that completely fills the dish. If the lid of the dish is lifted, it will be noted that the hyphae are attached and the disturbance of these attachments results in collapse of the entire structure. Close examination of well-developed cultures reveals black spherical bodies, which are masses of spores encased in sporangia.

*R. nigricans* is not pathogenic, but species quite similar in morphology are encountered in animal infections.

That mucormycosis does occur infrequently in domestic animals has been attested by a number of reports. It appears that these organisms take on pathogenicity when the proper conditions are met. Members of the genus *Mucor* have been isolated from dogs and a heifer (12). In dogs, cases of kidney infection, intestinal infection (mycotic gastritis, 15, 18), and cerebral or cerebellar involvement have been reported. In cattle, the seat of infection is more likely to be the thoracic or mesenteric lymph nodes, although the placentae may also become involved. Systemic mucormycosis has been reported in New Zealand in calves (8), possibly resulting from uterine infection. Abortions have been associated with mycotic infection in sheep (10) and cutaneous mucormycosis (19) has been observed in a gray squirrel (*Sciurus carolinensis*).

Enzootics of mycosis caused by *Absidia lichtheimi* have been reported in mink farms by Momberg-Jörgensen (17). In these cases infection manifests itself by the formation of subcutaneous nodules which perforate the skin and form fistulas. Metastasis to the regional lymph node and the myocardium may occur. Cutaneous (16), subcutaneous (2), pulmonary (1), intestinal (5), and cranial (14) mucormycosis have been encountered in man and in gastric lesions in a rhesus monkey (13).

It has been postulated that the use of antibiotics which suppress the growth of bacteria and thereby permit the invasion of fungi has led to increased frequency of mucormycosis in man and animals. Other species causing infection in animals are discussed below under their specific names.

### Rhizopus equinus

Dodge (9) includes in this species the fungus that Christiansen and Nielsen (7) found in swine and that was regarded by them as a new species, *R. suinus*, also the mucor found by Theobald Smith (20) in bovine fetal membranes. Bendixen and Plum (3), who studied similar, if not identical, infections in Denmark, identified the mucors that they encountered as *Absidia ramosa*. Whether Smith's organism and the one with which Gilman and Birch

(11) worked belong to *Rhizopus equinus* or to *Absidia ramosa*, it is not possible to say. They will be described under the latter name.

*R. equinus*, as its name implies, was found in a horse where it was regarded as the causative agent of a tumor in the region of the withers. Another case, possibly caused by the same species, consisted of a soft, fatlike tissue in the maxillary sinus of a horse. Phycomycosis (mucormycosis) was reported in horses in Texas in 1962 by Bridges *et al.* (4) and the causative agent was identified as *Entomophthora coronata*. In these cases granulomatous lesions occurred on the skin of the nostrils, the nasal mucosa, and the lips of the animals.

### Rhizopus suinus

In 1922 Christiansen (6) described two cases of generalized mucormycosis in swine. One of the cases was attributed to *R. equinus*, the other to *A. ramosa*. In 1929 Christiansen and Nielsen (7) reported a larger series consisting of nine cases, including the two that the senior author had described earlier. The seven additional cases were attributed to *A. ramosa;* therefore the larger series included only the one case caused by *Rhizopus* that had been described originally. In this paper they concluded, however, that the species was not *R. equinus* and they proposed a new name, *R. suinus*.

The affected pig was emaciated. A large vascular tumor was found in the abdominal cavity. This was made up of a conglomerate of small nodules, each surrounded by a connective tissue capsule. The interior of the nodules consisted of dry firm tissue in the center of which there was necrosis. Around the periphery were hemorrhages. In each lung were about 20 nodules similar in structure to those making up the abdominal tumor. A few were also found in the liver. Mycelium was easily demonstrated in the caseous tissue, and the mold was readily cultivated on maltose medium.

### Absidia ramosa

The genus *Absidia* differs from *Rhizopus* only in minor cultural details. This species was originally found in an infection of a human ear, later in head infections of horses. It proved to be the causative agent in eight or nine cases of generalized mucormycosis of swine described by Christiansen and Nielsen (7). It was found by Bendixen and Plum (3) in 9 out of 18 cases of bovine mycotic abortions, being in pure culture in two cases and mixed with *Aspergillus fumigatus* in seven additional cases. The mucor described by Smith and by Gilman and Birch may have belonged to this species.

The swine infections, as described by Christiansen and Nielsen (7), were manifested by the formation of nodules in the wall of the small intestine and in the mesenteric lymph nodes, with occasional nodes elsewhere. The intestinal lesions frequently ulcerated into the lumen of the bowel, forming large ulcers. The histological make-up is similar to that described under the preceding heading. Hyphae were easily demonstrated microscopically, and the mold was readily cultivated.

In the fungus-infected placentas of cattle, the hyphae are readily found in fresh films. The cotyledons are usually necrotic and dry. Sometimes the entire chorion is necrotic, dry, thickened, and leatherlike.

Gilman and Birch (11) and Bendixen and Plum (3) were able to cause placental infections by inoculating pregnant cattle intravenously. Christiansen was able to kill rabbits, guinea pigs, rats, and mice by intravenous and intraperitoneal inoculations. The principal lesions are found in the kidneys, spleen, and liver.

## REFERENCES

1. Baker.   Am. Jour. Path., 1956, 32, 287.
2. Baker, Seabury, and Schneidau.   Lab. Invest., 1962, 11, 1091.
3. Bendixen and Plum.   Acta Path. et Microbiol. Scand., 1929, 6, 252.
4. Bridges, Romane, and Emmons.   Jour. Am. Vet. Med. Assoc., 1962, 140, 673.
5. Calle and Klatsky.   Am. Jour. Clin. Path., 1966, 45, 264.
6. Christiansen.   Comp. rend. Soc. Biol. (Paris), 1922, 86, 461.
7. Christiansen and Nielsen.   Virchow's Arch. Path. Anat. u. Phys., 1929, 273, 829.
8. Cordes, Royal, and Shortridge.   New Zeal. Vet. Jour., 1967, 15, 143.
9. Dodge.   Medical mycology. C. V. Mosby, St. Louis, Mo., 1935, p. 115.
10. Gardner.   New Zeal. Vet. Jour., 1967, 15, 85.
11. Gilman and Birch.   Rpt. N. Y. State Vet. Coll., 1924–25 (1926), p. 127.
12. Gleiser.   Jour. Am. Vet. Med. Assoc., 1953, 123, 441.
13. Hessler, Woodard, Beattie, and Moreland.   Ibid., 1967, 151, 909.
14. Hoagland, Sube, Bishop, and Holding.   Am. Jour. Med. Sci., 1961, 242, 415.
15. Howard.   Vet. Med., 1966, 61, 549.
16. Josefiak, Foushee, and Smith.   Am. Jour. Clin. Path., 1958, 30, 547.
17. Momberg-Jörgensen.   Am. Jour. Vet. Res., 1950, 11, 334.
18. Osborne and Wilson.   Vet. Rec., 1969, 85, 487.
19. Sauer.   Am. Jour. Vet. Res., 1966, 27, 380.
20. Smith.   Jour. Exp. Med., 1920, 31, 115.

## ASCOMYCETES

Most species of *Ascomycetes* are saprophytic, but there are a few fungi within this class that are pathogens. True yeasts belong in the *Ascomycetes* and are generally considered to be nonpathogenic. However, cases of mastitis believed to be caused by yeasts or yeastlike fungi have followed infusion medication in cattle (11, 27). Usually these infections are self-limiting. Of 3,521 specimens from the oral cavity, bronchi, ears, nose, urine, and wounds of man (26) on which simultaneous bacteriological and mycological studies were performed, yeasts were present in 722 (about 21 percent).

Sterile grain on which strains of *Penicillium* and *Aspergillus* were grown has proved to be toxic for chicks. The resulting mycotoxicosis mimics the lesions of the poultry hemorrhagic syndrome (8). Although various strains of *Ascomycetes* produce mycotoxins, the poison known as *aflatoxin* is believed by Wilson *et al.* (29) to be produced only by *Aspergillus flavus* and *Aspergillus parasiticus.* These fungi may grow on many food products including peanuts, cottonseed cake, groundnut meal, country-cured hams, fermented sausages, pecans, flue-cured tobacco, smoked salamis, and fresh meats stored at 20 C. Aflatoxin has been shown to be toxic for cattle, pigs, dogs, chickens, ducks, monkeys, and man. Although the clinical signs differ in the various animal species concerned, in general they include anorexia, dehydration, somnolence, and jaundice. Gross changes may consist of a swollen liver, ascites, and serous atrophy of fat. Microscopically there are fatty changes in the liver, bile-ductule-cell proliferation, hypertrophy of bile ducts, and lymphatic dilation (24). Aflatoxin is also known to produce genetic damage, that is, carcinogenicity, teratogenicity, and mutagenicity (15).

There is a potent mycotoxin that may be produced by the growth of the fungus, *Fusarium tricinctum*, on corn or on tall fescue grass (*Festuca arundinacea*). (Actually the fungus is a member of the *Fungi Imperfecti*, but it is convenient to introduce it here as another fungal toxin.) It affects cattle, causing them to lose weight, to arch their backs, and to develop roughened coats, lameness in the hind legs, and finally gangrene of the tail and feet (13).

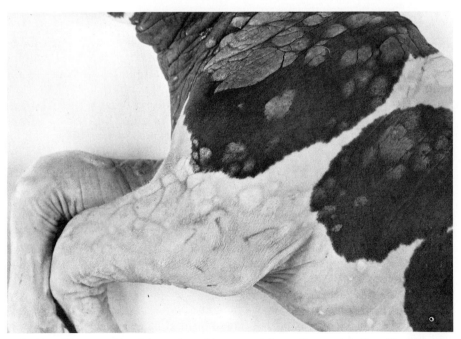

*Fig. 93.* Lesions on skin of fetus aborted because of *Aspergillus* sp. infection. (Courtesy Kenneth McEntee.)

Members of the genus *Aspergillus* also act as pathogens. In man, *Aspergillus* species occasionally cause otomycosis, mycetoma pedis, and onychia and rarely pulmonary infections (18). Spindler and Zimmerman (25) claim that they isolated a mold of the genus *Aspergillus* from swine harboring sarcosporidia and with it transmitted the infection to other domestic animals as well as to pigs (see p. 736 for discussion). In cattle various species have been found to be associated with abortions. Cases of pulmonary and cutaneous aspergillosis have also been reported in this species (6, 17, 19), generalized infection has been recorded in lambs (9), and aspergilli have been associated with abortion in mares (10) and persistent diarrhea in foals (16). Aspergilli have been isolated from frontal sinus infection in the dog (20) and from pulmonary disease in the cat (21).

One of the important animal pathogens among the *Ascomycetes* is *Aspergillus fumigatus*.

### Aspergillus fumigatus

The most characteristic feature of the aspergilli is the structure of the expansions of the tips of certain of the aerial hyphae which bear the spores or conidia. These expansions carry small papillae on which the spores are borne externally. Colonies are woolly, dense, and quite unlike the loose mycelium of the mucors. Most of the aspergilli have pigmented spores, and these give color to the entire colony. *Aspergillus fumigatus* has dark-green spores; hence colonies have a dusty, dark-green color.

*A. fumigatus* is fatal to rabbits and other experimental animals when spores are inoculated intravenously. If the dosage is rather large, the rabbit will die within a few hours, the principal lesions being multiple hemorrhages. If the dose is small, the animal will live longer, and multiple granulomatous lesions will develop, principally in the lungs but also in other organs. Ether extracts from corn on which the organism is grown will produce hyperemia, edema, and subsequent necrosis upon intradermal injection into the rabbit, calf, or horse (3).

This organism was isolated by Bendixen and Plum (2) from the placentae of 15 cows that had aborted. The lesions are identical with those described under *Absidia ramosa;* in fact, in seven of the cases both types of molds were isolated. According to these authors, it was generally possible to distinguish the type present in the fetal tissues by determining the cross walls of the *Aspergillus.* Inoculation of pregnant cows intravenously proved that the organism could localize in the fetal membranes and set up a train of changes that would result in abortion.

Austwick (1) has described seven cases of pulmonary aspergillosis in lambs, one of them subclinical. *A. fumigatus* was recovered from all lung lesions. It has been recovered from amniotic fluid of ewes and from the skin and lungs of fetal sheep (14). Jasmin *et al.* (12) have isolated the organism from pneumonic lesions in captive alligators (*Alligator mississippiensis*). It

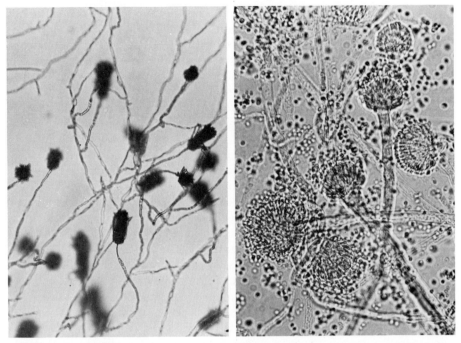

*Fig. 94 (left). Aspergillus fumigatus,* a photograph of the aerial hyphae and the fruiting bodies in a Henrici slide preparation. X 50.

*Fig. 95 (right). Aspergillus fumigatus,* an unstained preparation showing mycelium, fruiting bodies, and free spores. The straight, stiff stalks are aerial hyphae. The bulbous expansions at their free tips contain fingerlike processes (sterigmata) which bear long chains of highly refractile spores of a yellowish-green color. The photograph was made from a bit of culture removed from a solid medium and immersed in a clearing solution. The majority of the spores have broken loose from their attachments. X 500.

has also been found in calves and horses. In man, A. *fumigatus* is an infrequent finding in pulmonary infections where it produces aspergillomas which may develop into lobar pneumonia (22, 31).

For birds this organism is very dangerous, producing a disease known as *aspergillosis.* This infection sometimes occurs in epizootic form, in which case large losses may be sustained. Unlike most of the other fungi that produce deep-seated diseases, this one infects young birds more often than older ones. Hatchery-borne outbreaks have been seen in day-old chicks, although usually the classical disease does not appear before the birds are 5 days of age (5).

The infection is limited to the upper air passages and sometimes the mouth, the lungs, and the air sacs. In these locations the mold has access to air and vegetates readily. Tuberclelike bodies containing giant cells and lymphocytes usually form, and these quickly go on to caseation. The lungs, therefore, may show caseous areas, and the air sac walls may be thickened. Sometimes the air sacs are lined with greenish areas because of the presence of large numbers of spores of the organism. In other cases the air sacs are not uniformly thickened, but many small, whitish bodies of dense composition are present. The mold hyphae in many of these lesions may be recognized by crushing them with a little caustic potash. In the green areas the spores are readily found. In some of the denser lesions it is difficult or impossible to find evidence of the mold except by cultural means.

Encephalitic aspergillosis has been described in very young poults. It appears that the fungus invaded the eggs during incubation and infected the embryos (23).

Culture of the causative organism is very easily accomplished on plain agar, or better upon maltose or wort agar. The organism grows best at about 30 C, although it will grow at body temperature. Fine woolly colonies appear. After a day or so these enlarge, and greenish-yellow specks appear in the aerial hyphae. These are the spores. Later the entire surface is covered with a thick, matted, mycelial growth, yellowish-green in color and dusty.

A. fumigatus apparently is introduced into flocks principally in moldy grain feeds and in moldy litter. The species seems to be widely scattered in nature and can readily multiply in feeds that become wet or are stored in a damp room. The inhalation of spores from such sources seems to be the manner in which outbreaks are produced. The disease is not contagious, but A. fumigatus is an airborne fungus that can penetrate sound and cracked eggs in the incubator (30). One report of systemic infection in 5-week-old chicks that followed caponizing is recorded (4). The disease has been reported in chickens, pigeons, turkeys, ducks, geese, canaries, mynah birds, and many kinds of wild birds. So far as is known all birds are susceptible.

**Chemotherapy.** Experimentally amphotericin B has shown strong antifungal action against A. fumigatus (7) and amidomycin selective activity against yeasts (28).

## REFERENCES

1. Austwick, Gitter, and Watkins.  Vet. Rec., 1960, 72, 19.
2. Bendixen and Plum.   Acta Path. et Microbiol. Scand., 1929, 6, 252.
3. Carll, Forgacs, Herring, and Mahlandt.   Vet. Med., 1955, 50, 210.
4. Chute, Witter, Rountree, and O'Meara.   Jour. Am. Vet. Med. Assoc., 1955, 127, 207.
5. Clark, Jones, Crowl, and Ross.   Ibid., 1954, 124, 116.
6. Davis and Schaefer.   Ibid., 1962, 141, 1339.
7. Evans and Baker.   Antibiotics and Chemother., 1959, 9, 209.
8. Forgacs, Koch, Carll, and White-Stevens.   Am. Jour. Vet. Res., 1958, 19, 744.
9. Gracey and Baxter.   Brit. Vet. Jour., 1961, 117, 11.
10. Hensel, Bisping, and Schimmelpfennig.   Jour. Am. Vet. Med. Assoc., 1961, 139, 883.
11. Hulse.   Vet. Rec., 1952, 64, 210.
12. Jasmin, Carroll, and Baucom.   Am. Jour. Vet. Clin. Path., 1968, 2, 93.

13.  Kosuri, Grove, Yates, Tallent, Ellis, Wolff, and Nichols.    Jour. Am. Vet. Med. Assoc., 1970, *157*, 938.
14.  Leash, Sachs, Abrams, and Limbert.    Lab. Anim. Care, 1968, *18*, 407.
15.  Legator.    Jour. Am. Vet. Med. Assoc., 1969, *155*, 3080.
16.  Lundvall and Romberg.    *Ibid.*, 1960, *137*, 481.
17.  Molello and Busey.    *Ibid.*, 1963, *142*, 632.
18.  Moss and McQuown.    Atlas of medical mycology. Williams and Wilkins Co., Baltimore, 1953.
19.  Nag and Malik.    Canad. Vet. Jour., 1960, *2*, 30.
20.  Otto.    Jour. Am. Vet. Med. Assoc., 1970, *156*, 1903.
21.  Pakes, New, and Benbrook.    *Ibid.*, 1967, *151*, 950.
22.  Parker, Sarosi, Doto, and Tosh.    Am. Rev. Resp. Dis., 1970, *101*, 551.
23.  Raines, Kuzdas, Winkel, and Johnson.    Jour. Am. Vet. Med. Assoc., 1956, *129*, 435.
24.  Sisk, Carlton, and Curtin.    Am. Jour. Vet. Res., 1968, *29*, 1591.
25.  Spindler and Zimmerman.    Jour. Parasitol., 1945, *31* (Sup.), 13.
26.  Stenderup and Pedersen.    Acta Path. et Microbiol. Scand., 1962, *54*, 462.
27.  Tucker.    Cornell Vet., 1954, *44*, 79.
28.  Vining and Taber.    Bact. Proc., 1957, p. 70.
29.  Wilson, Campbell, Hayes, and Hanlin.    Appl. Microbiol., 1968, *16*, 819.
30.  Wright, Anderson, and Epps.    Avian Dis., 1960, *4*, 369.
31.  Young, Vogel, and DeVita.    Jour. Am. Med. Assoc., 1969, *208*, 1156.

### Maduromycosis (Maduromycotic Mycetoma)

These are the mycotic granulomas that may be caused by any one of several fungi of the classes *Ascomycetes* and *Fungi Imperfecti*. It is important to differentiate maduromycosis from norcardiosis, actinomycosis, and botryomycosis and also from such mycotic infections as mucormycosis. Madurmycotic lesions occur not only in the feet of man and animals, but also in the neck, head, and groin (1).

Bridges (1) has stated that most cases of maduromycotic mycetomas seen in the United States have appeared in the southern regions and suggests that the condition is primarily a subtropical or tropical disease. He reported three cases in dogs and one in a horse and identified *Curvularia geniculata* as the etiological agent affecting the feet of one of the dogs. This genus is closely related taxonomically to the *Helminthosporium*, another genus that has been associated with the disease. In 1967 Brodey *et al.* (4) described a case of eumycotic (maduromycotic) mycetoma in a Coonhound. Clinically the dog had intermittent lameness and a progressively enlarged swelling in the right shoulder. *C. geniculata* was determined to be the causative agent. This dog had been used for hunting in Virginia and Pennsylvania. In 1970 two cases of eumycotic mycetoma in dogs were reported (5, 6). In one case the lesion was in the abdominal region and in the other one-half of the spleen and portions of the gastric and duodenal walls were involved. In both cases, *Allescheria boydi*, an ascomycete, was found to be the inciting agent.

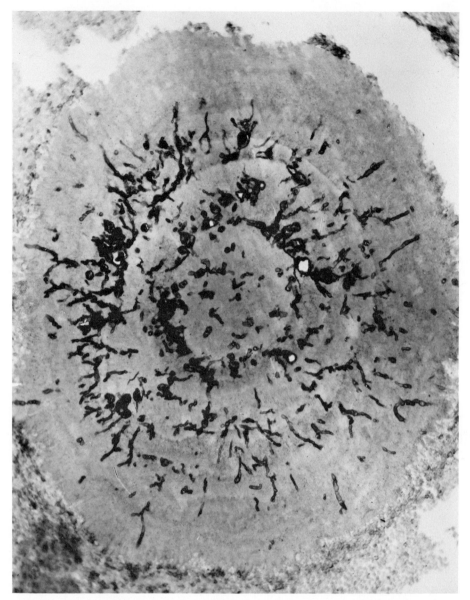

*Fig. 96.* A large laminated acidophilic body from a case of bovine maduromycosis containing many chlamydospores and hyphae. The white holes represent microchlamydospores which extend to both surfaces of the section. Gridley fungus stain. X 200. (Courtesy Charles H. Bridges, *Cornell Vet.*)

It appears that eumycotic mycetomas in man have differed from those in lower animals in that human cases have been worldwide in distribution whereas most of the infections in lower animals have been limited to the United States. The principal cause of the disease in man has been A. *boydi*, a hyaline fungus that forms light-colored granules, while most of the lower animals have developed mycetomas with dark grains as the result of infection with *Curvularia* or *Helminthosporium* (4).

In 1960 Bridges (3) stated that he had diagnosed maduromycotic mycetomas in a cat, a horse, and a dog. *Brachycladium spiciferum* was identified as a causative agent in the cat and the horse. Generally, the clinical signs were manifested by chronic inflammation with formation of nodular granulomatous masses in the foot of the cat, skin of the head and body of the horse, and in a prescapular lymph node of the dog. Pigmented colonies of fungus could be

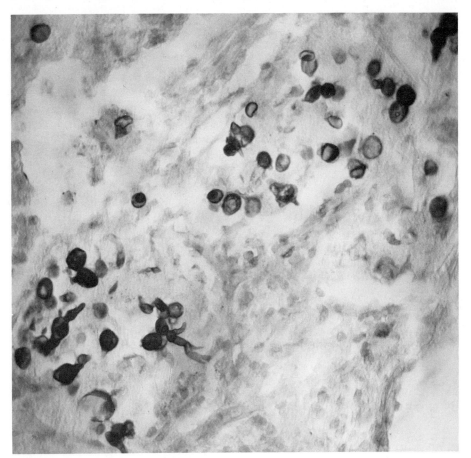

*Fig. 97.* Two fairly discrete collections of chlamydospores with a few hyphae from a bovine maduromycosis lesion. Gridley fungus stain. X 450. (Courtesy Charles H. Bridges, *Cornell Vet.*)

seen as brown to black specks in the lesions from the dog and the horse. Colonies of fungus were easily found in stained smears of pus taken from draining sinuses of the cat's foot. According to Mahaffey and Rossdale (7) *A. boydi* has caused abortion in the horse. They found lesions in the fetal membranes and in the lungs of the fetus.

Bridges (2) in 1960 and Roberts *et al.* (8) in 1963 recorded the finding of maduromycosis (maduromycotic mycetoma) of the bovine nasal mucosa. It appears that nasal granuloma in American cattle was first described in Louisiana in 1933. Since then cases have been seen in Texas and Colorado.

The disease is similar to the so-called *snoring disease* of cattle in India. Growth appears on the turbinate bones causing the animals to sneeze and rub their nostrils on any available object. After several months a thick mucous discharge may block the nasal passages to the point where breathing is difficult. Microscopically there is an eosinophilic granulomatous proliferation of the nasal mucosa and submucosa accompanied by the appearance of deep epithelial crypts, Langhans' giant cells, and thin-walled chlamydospores. In some areas, segmented hyphal elements also can be seen.

A *Helminthosporium* sp. is believed to be the cause of the disease in American cattle.

In man, treatment has consisted of excision of the mycetoma where possible or the application of sulfonamides and penicillin with adequate surgical drainage.

## REFERENCES

1. Bridges.  Am. Jour. Path., 1957, 33, 411.
2. Bridges.  Cornell Vet., 1960, 50, 468.
3. Bridges and Beasley.  Jour. Am. Vet. Med. Assoc., 1960, 137, 192.
4. Brodey, Schryver, Deubler, Kaplan, and Ajello.  Ibid., 1967, 151, 442.
5. Jang and Popp.  Ibid., 1970, 157, 1071.
6. Kurtz, Finco, and Perman.  Ibid., 917.
7. Mahaffey and Rossdale.  Vet. Rec., 1965, 77, 541.
8. Roberts, McDaniel, and Carbrey.  Jour. Am. Vet. Med. Assoc., 1963, 142, 42.

## *FUNGI IMPERFECTI* (DEUTEROMYCETES)

Within this class are many nonpathogenic forms. There are also a few pathogenic types that cause the dangerous mycoses of the internal organs. This class also embraces the dermatophytic fungi discussed in the preceding chapter.

### Chromomycosis (Chromoblastomycosis)

Chromomycosis is a chronic, granulomatous, sometimes ulcerative, cutaneous, mycotic infection which occurs most frequently on the lower extremities, and in man is almost completely confined to these areas and the head. It is worldwide in distribution, believed to be quite common in tropical Africa

(1), often appearing in wood-workers, and not limited as to age, sex, or race.

A small papule appears and spreads peripherally as in an early infection with tinea. Later the organism follows lymphatic drainage and satellite lesions result. These are nodular, firm, verrucous, and purplish-red to gray. Involvement of the lymphatics induces fibrosis and lymphedema. Ulcers, prone to secondary infection with bacteria, occur.

There are a number of fungi that produce this condition, but the types most commonly concerned are classified as *Hormodendrum pedrosoi, Hormodendrum compactum,* and *Phialophora verrucosa.*

Although the disease usually is limited to man, natural infection has been described in a horse and a dog (3).

Small lesions may be eradicated by surgical excision. Amphotericin B has produced good results in therapy. (2).

## REFERENCES

1.  Ive and Clark.   Jour. Trop. Med. and Hyg. (London), 1966, *69*, 184.
2.  Moss and McQuown.   Atlas of medical mycology. 2d ed. Williams & Wilkins Co., Baltimore, 1960, p. 163.
3.  Simpson.   Vet. Med., 1966, *61*, 1207.

### *Coccidioides immitis*

This organism was originally thought to be a protozoon. The form that occurs in the lesions resembles an oocyst of a coccidium, and it is from this resemblance that the generic name was derived.

The fungus is the causative agent of a human disease of considerable importance, especially in the valleys of central and southern California where the disease is endemic. It is not considered to be contagious. Rather, it is generally thought to be contracted from the inhalation of chlamydospores, for it has been observed that the disease is prevalent during the dry dusty season and is rare during the wet season. It has been supposed that the organism lives saprophytically in the soil, but Emmons (13) has recently questioned this belief and has shown that rodents in the infected districts carry the infection. Inasmuch as the organism has been isolated from soil by several workers, there is no question about its existence there, but perhaps it reaches the soil through animal excreta. Most of the early cases of human infection originated in the valley of the San Joaquin River, and the disease became well known as the *San Joaquin Valley disease.* For years only the chronic cases, characterized by the formation of granulomas in the internal organs and especially in the lungs and by a mortality rate in excess of 50 percent, were recognized. In 1938 Dickson (11) showed that the disease occurred in another much more prevalent form. This is the *valley fever* or *desert fever,* an influenzalike disease that had long been known in the valleys of central California without its real nature being suspected. It is now known that large numbers of residents and transient workers in these valleys become infected. Most

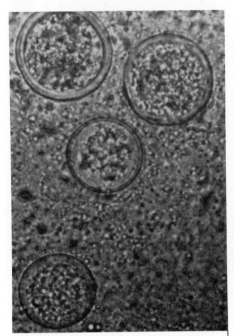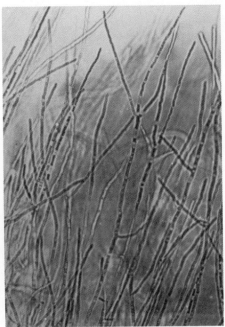

*Fig. 98 (left). Coccidioides immitis,* showing several of the spherules contained in pus expressed from a lesion in a lymph node. X 500. (Courtesy Stiles and Davis, *Jour. Am. Med. Assoc.*)

*Fig. 99 (right). Coccidioides immitis,* a hanging drop preparation from a culture showing mycelium of the organism. X 190. (Courtesy Stiles and Davis, *Jour. Am. Med. Assoc.*)

cases recover in from 3 to 6 weeks. Only a few lapse into the chronic form characterized by granulomatous lesions (*coccidioidal granuloma*).

In 1918 Giltner (15) identified this organism in an infection of a cow that had lived in the San Joaquin Valley. The disease has now been recognized in many cattle, dogs, burros, swine, sheep, horses, a monkey, a gorilla, a chinchilla, a llama, a tapir, and several species of wild rodents (24). Coccidioidomycosis is endemic in California, Arizona, New Mexico, and southwest Texas, but cases may be encountered in almost any area of the United States. It is found in Argentina and Paraguay. Surveys have indicated that it is not present in nationals living in the Middle East (8). An ecological study by Ajello (1) has indicated that *C. immitis* is restricted to desert areas in North, Central, and South America where adaptation to high temperature, low rainfall, and high concentrations of salt enables it to thrive. Outside of the arid regions of the Americas, this fungus seems to be unable to establish itself and survive.

**Morphology and Staining Reactions.** As it occurs in the purulent material and the granulation tissue of lesions, the fungus appears as spherical bodies (spherules or sporangia) that vary greatly in size from 10 to 80 microns in diameter. The wall is double-contoured and highly refractile. The protoplasm is

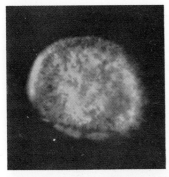 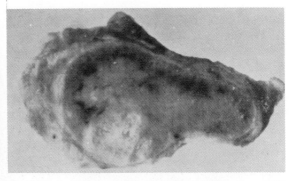

*Fig. 100.* (*Left*) *Coccidioides immitis.* A single colony of the organism growing on a solid medium. Note the cottonlike appearance. X 2. (*Right*) Coccidioidal granuloma. Lesions in a bovine lymph node which strikingly resemble those of tuberculosis. The lesions vary in size. They are caseous in their centers. Note the hemorrhages and the encapsulation. About X 2. (Courtesy Stiles and Davis, *Jour. Am. Med. Assoc.*)

finely granular. In many of the larger spherules a number of endospores may be seen as spherical bodies varying from 2 to 5 microns in diameter. Mycelium is rarely seen in the tissues, although Puckett (31) claims that mycelial growth of *C. immitis* may develop in focalized and stabilized lesions in the human host in the same manner that it develops in cultures. He states that hyphae are more common in cavities (73 percent) than in granulomatous lesions (30 percent).

When tissues are planted on suitable culture media, protoplasmic shoots appear from the spherules. These develop into hyphae, and soon a well-developed mycelium is formed. The hyphae branch extensively and exhibit well-marked septa. In time aerial hyphae appear and a white woolly colony is formed. Microscopically, numerous chlamydospores may be seen and some arthrospores. The spherical structures found in tissues are never present in cultures unless they are incubated under special conditions semianaerobically (3, 20) or in special media (4, 6, 28). It is also claimed that *C. immitis* can be identified readily by the use of specialized media (7). It appears that the yolk sac of the embryonated chicken egg is a good medium for growing the animal phase of *C. immitis* (39).

All forms of this parasite can be stained, but for most purposes fresh material unstained is preferable for study.

**Cultural Features.** *Coccidiodes immitis* will grow on all the common media of the bacteriological laboratory. When cultures on solid media are incubated at 20 C, growth does not appear for 3 or 4 days, but at 37 C it is usually evident within 24 hours. The colonies are circular in outline, or a silvery gray color, and slightly raised. The mycelium penetrates deeply into the medium, so that the colonies cannot be removed except by digging out the medium. After a few days the cultures develop a whitish, moldy appearance because of the development of short aerial hyphae. In some tubes these are abundant and from

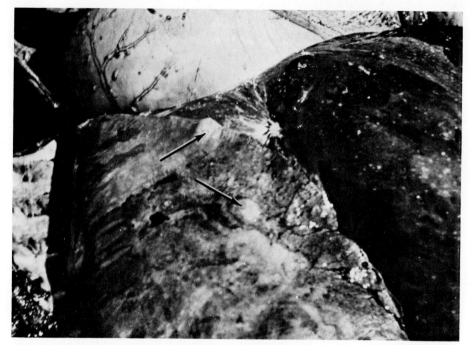

*Fig. 101.* Coccidioidomycosis in a horse. Note raised nodules of coccidioidal granuloma (*arrows*) on surface of the lung. The largest nodule measured 3 cm in diameter. (Courtesy J. A. Rehkemper, *Cornell Vet.*)

2 to 3 mm long; in others they may be scarce and short. In old cultures the medium develops a brownish discoloration but the growth remains white. Gelatin and coagulated bovine serum are slowly liquefied. Milk is gradually digested. Broth cultures produce fluffy masses in the bottoms of the tubes, and some tubes show rather tough pellicles. Sugars are not fermented.

**Pathogenicity.** *For cattle.* Coccidiodomycosis in cattle (2, 9, 15, 38) is a benign disease which ordinarily involves only the lymph nodes of the chest—the posterior mediastinal and the bronchial. In a few cases small granulomatous lesions have been found in the lungs and in the submaxillary, retropharyngeal, and mesenteric lymph nodes. The affected glands are enlarged and contain a yellowish, glutinous pus, similar to that of actinomycosis. The sulfur granules are not present, of course, and microscopic examination readily reveals the spherules. The abscess wall consists of granulation tissue. According to Maddy (22), some degree of calcification is shown by 15 percent of the lesions. Symptoms are not elicited.

With but few exceptions all cases have originated in the inland valleys of California, where the human infection occurs. The diseases in the human and bovine species have no direct relationship to each other because the infection is not transmitted from man to animals or vice versa. Both species contract the disease from the same source, that is, from dust infected with chlamydo-spores. As several cases have been found in cattle that were raised in Colorado and in Arizona, it is evident that the infection is not restricted to California.

*For horses.* In 1958 Zontine (42) reported a case of generalized coccidioido-mycosis in a horse. The main clinical features of the disease were a course of 4 months, severe progressive emaciation, variable temperature, moderate ane-mia, pronounced leukocytosis, edema of the lower parts of the legs, and a pe-culiar attitude of the front feet. At necropsy it was found that the animal had died from recent abdominal hemorrhage resulting from a ruptured liver. Granular abscesses of various sizes were seen scattered throughout the lungs, spleen, and liver. Other cases have been observed in horses and in a pony(10).

*For sheep.* Coccidioidomycosis in a sheep was described in 1931 by Beck *et al.* (2). Since then a number of reports have appeared. The lesions are like those in cattle.

*For swine.* In 1966 Prchal and Crecelius (30) described an infection in pigs raised in the area of Tucson, Arizona. Lesions occurred as granulomas in the bronchial lymph nodes and were found to contain the fungus, *C. immitis.*

*For dogs.* Numerous cases have been described in dogs (14, 16, 29, 32, 37). They have been reported from Arizona, Quebec, Iowa, Kansas, Texas, and California. In general, granulomatous lesions involve the lungs as the primary site, but they are also seen in the pleura, liver, spleen, kidneys, and bones. The picture grossly resembles tuberculosis. In affected animals partial an-orexia, vomition, and distress or collapse after eating are frequent. The dissemi-nated form occurs frequently in this animal and usually produces a hopeless invalid if it does not result in death. It seems that this illness is common in the dog in the Southwest.

*For cats.* Coccidioidomycosis has been diagnosed in two cats in Arizona (34). One animal developed an abscess on the hip, and histologic sections of the subcutaneous tissue, lungs, and thoracic lymph nodes all showed *C. immi-tis.* In the second cat granulomas were found in the liver and kidneys in addi-tion to the sites listed for the first victim.

*For chinchillas.* A case of coccidioidomycosis in a chinchilla has been de-scribed by Jasper (17). The disease was similar to that in the dog.

*For man.* The disease in man may assume one of three forms. Primary pulmonary coccidioidomycosis is seen. This may be subclinical or clinical. The subclinical type occurs with minimal manifestations and is often over-looked. More severe cases show low-grade fever and other symptoms of pul-monary disease. Some patients may develop a hypersensitivity indicated by erythema several weeks later. The coccidioidin skin test becomes positive within about 3 weeks after exposure or within days after symptoms appear. The longer this test remains positive the better the prognosis. A positive CF test is indicative of active or progressive infection.

Rarely the disease is primary in the skin or subcutaneous tissues with or

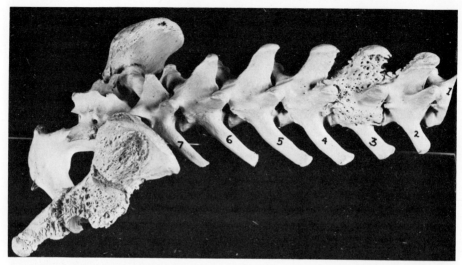

Fig. 102. Lumbar vertebra and pelvis of dog showing coccidioidal lesions. (Courtesy T. J. Hage, *Cornell Vet.*)

without a history of trauma. In these cases lesions appear as painless nodules which break down and ulcerate. Organisms are prssent in the purulent exudate. Healing with scar formation may occur.

The granulomatous type of disease follows extension or dissemination from a primary focus in the lung or in the skin. It is preceded by a rise in CF titer. The skin test may become negative. The symptoms are similar to those of tuberculosis. Any organ or tissue of the body may be involved, although the fungus shows some predilection for bone, skin, and subcutaneous tissue. The dark-skinned races, particularly Negroes and Mexicans, are prone to develop this type.

Between 1957 and 1968, an average of 51 cases per year were reported in Los Angeles County, California (25).

It has been stated that once a child has had the disease and recovered, an immunity has been established and reinfection does not occur. Salkin (35) does not believe that a primary attack confers a lasting immunity. He presents evidence that the disease can resolve and then reappear; that residual nodules and cavities can reactivate; that surgery and debilitating conditions can produce reactivations; and that late disseminations can occur. He also claims that exogenous reinfection can also result from both pulmonary and extrapulmonary routes.

Coccidioidomycosis is a distinct problem in pediatrics in southwestern United States. Maternal infections that occur during the last trimester of pregnancy are a great hazard to the mother and often result in premature birth of the infant (26).

**Artificial Inoculation.** Intravenous inoculation of cultures into guinea pigs, rab-

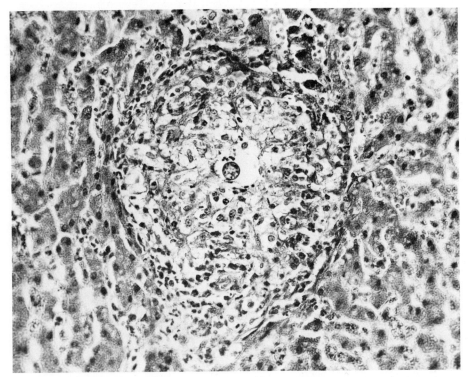

*Fig. 103.* Coccidioidal granuloma in the liver of a dog showing central spherule and surrounding epithelioid cells. (Courtesy T. J. Hage, *Cornell Vet.*)

bits, sheep, calves, and dogs results, ordinarily, in the rapid development of multiple lung lesions and sometimes multiple lesions in other organs. The animals emaciate rapidly and soon die. Swine resist the infection much better than other animals. Lung lesions develop in this species, but the general health of the animals does not seem to be seriously impaired by them.

Subcutaneous inoculations result in the formation of local abscesses, which finally rupture and form ulcers. The larger animals often show no extension of the disease; however, in guinea pigs the disease usually generalizes, giving a picture not unlike that of tuberculosis.

**Mode of Transmission.** The organisms are dust-borne and the endemic areas are arid. The disease is not transmitted from animal to animal. Maddy (23) made a 2-year study of a site in Arizona where a dog had acquired *C. immitis* infection. Soil samples collected from areas not near rodent burrows were negative for this fungus. Some positive results were obtained when soil was taken directly from the burrows. Most of the samples that yielded *C. immitis* were collected during the months of September through December. The fall rains, coming at this time, may have supplied the moisture needed for the growth of the fungus. In 1961 the organism was recovered from an ancient In-

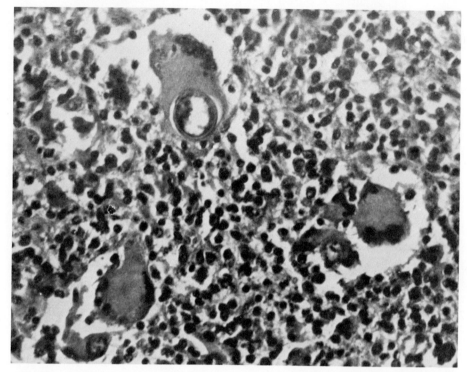

*Fig. 104.* Coccidioidal granuloma section of a bovine lymph node showing granulation tissue and several giant cells, one of which contains a spherule of the causative agent. X 400. (Courtesy Stiles and Davis, *Jour. Am. Med. Assoc.*)

dian camp site in San Diego County, California (40). Although direct transmission is unlikely, bedside interhuman transmission of coccidioidomycosis via growth on fomites has been reported in a hospital epidemic that involved six persons (12). Fifty dogs (33) were exposed in an area where coccidioidomycosis was known to exist and 29 (58 percent) became infected. Most cases developed in the cool months of the year, in contrast to the warm-season pattern of infection reported for man.

**Diagnosis.** Coccidioidin, a product made from filtrates of broth cultures, is used for diagnostic purposes. The CF test also is useful, especially in indicating the progress of the disease. The FA technic applied with absorbed conjugates has been useful in detecting *C. immitis* in clinical materials (18). The agar-gel-diffusion test with soluble spherule antigens is recommended in detecting *C. immitis* antibody in sera from suspect patients (21). Demonstration of the fungus either in the lesions or by cultural means provides a definitive diagnosis.

**Immunity.** Recovered animals appear to be immune to reinfection.

**Chemotherapy.** Moss and McQuown (27) in their discussion of the treatment and prognosis of human coccidioidomycosis recommend a guarded prognosis because no specific treatment has been found to be effective. Apparently the antibiotics commonly used are not active in this disease. Wier *et al.* (41) tried prodigiosin in disseminated infections and from the results obtained concluded that its use seemed warranted. Klapper *et al.* (19) claim that they cured a case of the disseminated form of the disease in man with amphotericin B. Castleberry *et al.* (5) have stated that dogs vaccinated subcutaneously with a formol-killed arthrospore bacterin and treated orally with amphotericin B were able to resist respiratory challenge. It has also been suggested that ethylene oxidehalogenated hydrocarbon be used in fumigating contaminated materials because it is effective in killing both saprophytic and parasitic forms of *C. immitis* (36).

## REFERENCES

1.  Ajello.   Bact. Rev., 1967, *31*, 6.
2.  Beck, Traum, and Harrington.   Jour. Am. Vet. Med. Assoc., 1931, *78*, 490.
3.  Breslau and Kubota.   Jour. Bact., 1964, *87*, 468.
4.  Burke.   Proc. Soc. Exp. Biol. and Med., 1951, *76*, 332.
5.  Castleberry, Converse, Sinski, Lowe, Pakes, and Favero.   Jour. Inf. Dis., 1965, *115*, 41.
6.  Converse.   Proc. Soc. Exp. Biol. and Med., 1955, *90*, 709.
7.  Creitz and Puckett.   Am. Jour. Clin. Path., 1954, *24*, 1318.
8.  Daoud and Schwabe.   Am. Jour. Trop. Med. and Hyg., 1958, 7, 643.
9.  Davis, Stiles, and McGregor.   Jour. Am. Vet. Med. Assoc., 1938, *92*, 562.
10. DeMartini and Riddle.   *Ibid.*, 1969, *155*, 149.
11. Dickson.   Jour. Am. Med. Assoc., 1938, *111*, 1362.
12. Eckmann, Schaefer, and Huppert.   Am. Rev. Resp. Dis., 1964, *89*, 175.
13. Emmons.   Pub. Health Rpts. (U.S.), 1942, 57, 109.
14. Farness.   Jour. Am. Vet. Med. Assoc., 1940, 97, 263.
15. Giltner.   Jour. Agr. Res., 1918, *14*, 533.
16. Hage and Moulton.   Cornell Vet., 1954, *44*, 489.
17. Jasper.   North Am. Vet., 1953, *34*, 570.
18. Kaplan and Clifford.   Am. Rev. Resp. Dis., 1964, *89*, 651.
19. Klapper, Smith, and Conant.   Jour. Am. Med. Assoc., 1958, *167*, 463.
20. Lack.   Proc. Soc. Exp. Biol. and Med., 1938, *38*, 907.
21. Landay, Pash, and Millar.   Jour. Lab. and Clin. Med., 1970, 75, 197.
22. Maddy.   Jour. Am. Vet. Med. Assoc., 1954, *124*, 456.
23. Maddy.   Am. Jour. Vet. Res., 1959, *20*, 642.
24. Maddy.   Vet. Med., 1959, *54*, 233.
25. Matlof, Kamei, and Heidbreder.   Pub. Health Rpts. (U.S.), 1970, 85, 393.
26. Mead.   Jour. Am. Med. Assoc., 1951, *146*, 85.
27. Moss and McQuown.   Atlas of medical mycology. Williams and Wilkins Co., Baltimore, 1960.
28. Northey and Brooks.   Jour. Bact., 1962, *84*, 742.
29. Plummer.   Canad. Jour. Comp. Med. and Vet. Sci., 1941, 5, 146.
30. Prchal and Crecelius.   Jour. Am. Vet. Med. Assoc., 1966, *148*, 1168.
31. Puckett.   Am. Rev. Tuberc., 1954, *70*, 320.

32.   Reed.   Jour. Am. Vet. Med. Assoc., 1956, *128*, 196.
33.   Reed and Converse.   Am. Jour. Vet. Res., 1966, *27*, 1027.
34.   Reed, Hoge, and Trautman.   Jour. Am. Vet. Med. Assoc., 1963, *143*, 953.
35.   Salkin.   Am. Rev. Resp. Dis., 1967, *95*, 603.
36.   Schmidt and Howard.   Pub. Health Rpts. (U.S.), 1968, *83*, 882.
37.   Short, Schleicher, and Rice.   Jour. Am. Vet. Med. Assoc., 1955, *127*, 352.
38.   Stiles, Shahan, and Davis.   *Ibid.*, 1933, *82*, 928.
39.   Vogel, Peace, and Koger.   Am. Jour. Path., 1957, *33*, 1023.
40.   Walch, Pribnow, Wyborney, and Walch.   Am. Rev. Resp. Dis., 1961, *84*, 359.
41.   Wier, Egeberg, Lack, and Leiby.   Am. Jour. Med. Sci., 1952, *224*, 70.
42.   Zontine.   Jour. Am. Vet. Med. Assoc., 1958, *132*, 490.

### Zymonema farciminosum

SYNONYMS:   *Cryptoccus farciminosus, Saccharomyces farciminosus, Endomyces farciminosa, Histoplasma farciminosa, Saccharomyces equi, Blastomyces farciminosa*

*Zymonema farciminosum* (Dodge, 2) is the causative agent of *epizootic lymphangitis* or *pseudofarcy* of horses and mules. A few cases have been reported in cattle, but the latter are not highly susceptible. The infection is endemic in countries bordering the Mediterranean, particularly in Italy and North Africa. It is also found in Central and South Africa, and in parts of Asia and Russia. The disease caused a great deal of trouble during the Boer War, and cases were brought back to England after its conclusion. It also was of much concern during World War I. Some doubtful cases have been reported in the United States. Most of these, possibly all, were cases of sporotrichosis.

The organism was first demonstrated in pus by Rivolta in 1873. It was not successfully cultivated until 1896. The first pure cultures were obtained by Tokishiga (4) in Japan.

**Morphology and Staining Reactions.** In pus the organism appears as a double-contoured oval or ovoid body, measuring 2.5 to 3.5 by 3 to 4 microns. The cells resemble those of yeasts very closely. The cytoplasm is granular, and here and there bits of cytoplasm may be seen extruding from a break in the cell wall, forming buds from which daughter cells are formed. In cultures the organism produces both hyphae and ascospores (Eberbeck, 3).

The fungus cells can be stained, though not very satisfactorily. Structural details are best seen in fresh, unstained preparations. The Gram stain usually is retained.

**Cultural Features.** *Z. farciminosum* is strongly aerobic. It has been successfully cultivated on a variety of media, but growth is slow and uncertain. When incubated under the most favorable cultural conditions now known, growth usually is not evident for 1 to 3 weeks or longer, and of many tubes inoculated similarly a considerable part may fail to exhibit growth. Growth may be obtained on plain agar and broth and on potato, coagulated egg medium, coagulated serum medium, and various other special media. On solid media, growth appears in the form of small grayish-white granules that have a dry appearance and may become leatherlike in structure. In liquid media, growth generally occurs in the form of scanty, granular sediment. Sugar media are not fermented.

**Pathogenicity.** Epizootic lymphangitis of horses is characterized by inflammation of the superficial lymphatic vessels and nodes, principally of the legs, the chest, and the neck. Infection is believed to occur through wounds. In severe cases lesions may be found on any part of the body and even on the mucous membranes.

The lymph channels become enlarged and appear as tortuous cords beneath the skin, connecting the swollen lymph nodes. The nodes soften and rupture, forming craterlike ulcers from which a thick pus exudes. The yeast-like organism can easily be demonstrated in such pus. When mucosal lesions occur, they are most likely to be found in the nasal passages, but there are records of their occurrence on the genitalia and of the transmission of the disease from stallions to mares by copulation.

Bennett (1) described a type of equine pneumonia that was believed to be caused by *Z. farciminosum*. It was of an interstitial type beginning with infiltrations of lymphocytes and then monocytes. Syncytia and giant cells next appeared and in these the *Zymonema* could be seen. The organisms then multiplied profusely, leading to extensive destructive changes and fatality. The condition was not associated with skin manifestations. The organism was not cultivated and therefore was not certainly identified.

The disease is chronic as a rule, though some cases heal spontaneously after a few weeks. The chronic cases usually are incurable. There are no biological agents of value for the diagnosis or control of this disease. Sodium iodide given intravenously has some effect in treating the infection.

**REFERENCES**

1. Bennett.   Jour. Comp. Path. and Therap., 1931, *44*, 85.
2. Dodge.   Medical mycology. C. V. Mosby, St. Louis, Mo., 1935.
3. Eberbeck.   Arch. f. Tierheilk., 1926, *54*, 1.
4. Tokishiga.   Centrbl. f. Bakt., I Abt., 1896, *19*, 105.

### Candidiasis (Moniliasis)

The disease was known for many years as *moniliasis*, but with the changing of the generic name of the fungus from *Monilia* to *Candida*, the designation *candidiasis* has been adopted. This mycotic infection is caused by simple, yeastlike fungi that reproduce by budding, form septate mycelia, and are not known to produce ascospores. The spores are formed by the successive budding of specialized cells at the ends of hyphae, or at nodes in the filaments. Both yeastlike cells and mycelial elements occur in tissues. Colonies on solid media do not form aerial hyphae, and therefore they do not become fuzzy but are fleshy, like colonies of true yeasts.

The etiological agent is called *Candida albicans* and it causes a variety of lesions of the mucous membranes of the skin, and sometimes of internal organs of man. The best known form is the condition called *thrush,* which is an infection of the oral mucosa of human infants, particularly of malnourished ones. It has also been reported in cattle, pigs, colts, dogs, and cats. Apparently it occurs more frequently in birds. Many kinds of *Candida* are observed on normal mucous membranes as *saprophytes;* thus care must be used in attributing pathogenicity to forms found in surface lesions.

### Candida albicans

SYNONYMS: *Odium albicans, Saccharomyces albicans, Monilia albicans*

This is the species that causes thrush in human infants. Members of this genus are also found in animals and in birds.

**Morphology and Cultural Features.** Young cultures consist of oval, budding, yeastlike cells that measure 3.5 by 5.5 microns. *C. albicans* produces chlamydospores when grown on corn meal agar. Other species of *Candida* do not. In lesions the yeastlike cells in process of budding, as well as fragments of mycelium, can be seen.

On Sabouraud's agar, soft creamy colonies that are very convex appear in 24 to 48 hours when incubated at 37 C. In gelatin stabs short villus streaks extend out from the main spike of growth. The medium is not liquefied. Acid and gas are formed from glucose, levulose, maltose, and mannose. A little acid but no gas is formed from sucrose and galactose. Lactose, raffinose, and inulin are not attacked.

Reliable technics for the identification of *C. albicans* have been published (21, 22). Eosin-methylene-blue agar, infused corn meal, and rapid fermentation tests are employed in the procedure.

According to Salvin (19), a soluble endotoxin highly virulent for mice can be prepared from *C. albicans.*

Stallybrass (20) has classified cultures of *C. albicans* into two serologic groups A and B by means of a double diffusion precipitin test. Most of his cultures (75 percent) belonged to group A.

**Pathogenicity.** Some authors refer to *Monilia* infections of the oral mucosa in calves and colts. No additional information about them is available. Presumably they are of little consequence.

Thrushlike lesions of birds—chickens, pigeons, turkeys, pheasants, and grouse—are quite common and often very serious. They involve the mouth, the crop, the proventriculus, and the gizzard. The lesions consist of whitish circular areas or of elongated patches along the crests of folds of the mucosa. The areas may become confluent and finally involve large parts of the linings of these organs. The invaded tissues finally slough off leaving superficial ulcers. Epizootics in very young birds may cause heavy mortality. In older birds the infections occur but recovery is the rule.

A systemic disease of cattle has been reported to be moniliasis (11), and

*Candida* have also been found in bovine mastitis (10). The organism has also been associated with chronic pneumonias, pathologic vaginal discharges, aborted fetuses, specific inflammations of the esophagus, and with associated histologic lesions. In calves following prolonged antibiotic therapy the liver, lungs, brain, kidneys, and forestomachs have become infected. Candidial rumenitis in young calves has been reported in Europe and in Connecticut (5). Thrush has been described in a small pig being reared artificially (12) and in pigs in Wisconsin (2) where the organism appeared to have a predilection for the esophageal region of the gastric mucosa and the lower portion of the esophagus. It has also caused cutaneous candidiasis in swine (18). It has produced cutaneous candidiasis (mycotic dermatoses) in dogs and cats (8, 9).

In man, moniliasis usually involves the mucous membranes of the alimentary or urogenital tracts, but deaths have occurred in which meningitis, pericarditis, endocarditis, or extensive pulmonary lesions were seen. Debilitated infants that succumb to thrush usually show extensive lesions throughout the gastrointestinal tract. *Candida* sepsis has complicated parenteral feeding (1). It has occurred in oral leukoplakias (17).

**Immunity.** According to Comaish *et al.* (4) a clear relation between *Candida* infection and the level of serum agglutinins has been found. Vaccinated mice show a significant degree of resistance to challenge (16). Rabbits respond by producing antibodies of the IgG and IgM classes when injected intravenously with heat-killed *C. albicans* (13).

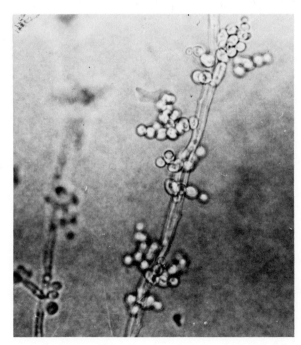

Fig. 105. *Candida* sp., an unstained preparation from a deep colony in agar showing mycelium and the yeastlike spores that arise at the end of filaments and at mycelial nodes. Surface colonies of *Candida* consist largely of yeastlike cells. Mycelium is produced only under conditions of reduced oxygen tension. Both mycelium and yeastlike forms are found in lesions. X 500.

**Chemotherapy.** Therapy in human infections has received much consideration during the past years. It appears that the use of broad-spectrum antibiotics in the medication of infectious diseases of man has enhanced the role of *C. albicans* in producing pharyngitis, glossitis, pruritus ani, pruritus vulvae, vaginitis, and proctitis in the treated individuals (15).

Mountain and Krumenacher (15) recommend the oral use of undecylenic acid whenever oral aureomycin, chloromycetin, or terramycin is administered. Methylparaben and prophylparaben (esters of para-aminobenzoic acid) are also reported to be effective. Brown *et al.* (3) have shown that subcutaneous injection of fungicidin (nystatin) protects mice against a lethal mixture of *C. albicans* and aureomycin. Candicidin is also claimed to be effective in protecting mice infected with *C. albicans* (7).

Present evidence seems to indicate that the expanding use of antibiotics has resulted in an increase of candidial infections in both man and animals and that nystatin is the most effective antibiotic in combating this condition. Amphotericin B and azalomycin F have also been reported to be effective. Haloprogin has been used successfully in treating topical infections (6), candicidin in curing mycotic dermatoses in dogs and cats (9), and formic acid has been sprayed on food, to reduce the severity of lesions in partridge chicks (23).

## REFERENCES

1. Ashcraft and Leape.   Jour. Am. Med. Assoc., 1970, *212*, 454.
2. Baker and Cadman.   Jour. Am. Vet. Med. Assoc., 1963, *142*, 763.
3. Brown, Hazen, and Mason.   Science, 1953, *117*, 609.
4. Comaish, Gibson, and Green.   Jour. Invest. Dermatol., 1963, *40*, 139.
5. Cross, Moorhead, and Jones.   Jour. Am. Vet. Med. Assoc., 1970, *157*, 1325.
6. Harrison, Zwadyk, Jr., Bequette, Hamlow, Tavormina, and Zygmunt.   Appl. Microbiol., 1970, *19*, 746.
7. Kligman and Lewis.   Proc. Soc. Exp. Biol. and Med., 1953, *82*, 399.
8. Kral and Uscavage.   Jour. Am. Vet. Med. Assoc., 1960, *136*, 612.
9. Litwack.   *Ibid.*, 1966, *148*, 23.
10. Loken, Thompson, Hoyt, and Ball.   *Ibid.*, 1959, *134*, 401.
11. McCarty.   Vet. Med., 1956, *51*, 562.
12. McCrea and Osborne.   Jour. Comp. Path. and Therap., 1957, *67*, 342.
13. Matthews and Inman.   Proc. Soc. Exp. Biol. and Med., 1968, *128*, 387.
14. Moss and McQuown.   Atlas of medical mycology. 2d ed. Williams and Wilkins Co., Baltimore, 1960.
15. Mountain and Krumenacher.   Am. Jour. Med. Sci., 1953, *225*, 274.
16. Mourad and Friedman.   Proc. Soc. Exp. Biol. and Med., 1961, *106*, 570.
17. Renstrup.   Acta Path. et Microbiol. Scand., 1970, *78*, 421.
18. Reynolds, Miner, and Smith.   Jour. Am. Vet. Med. Assoc., 1968, *152*, 182.
19. Salvin.   Jour. Immunol., 1952, *69*, 89.
20. Stallybrass.   Jour. Hyg. (London), 1964, *62*, 395.
21. Walker and Huppert.   Am. Jour. Clin. Path., 1959, *31*, 551.
22. Widra.   Jour. Inf. Dis., 1957, *100*, 70.
23. Wood.   Vet. Rec., 1970, 87, 656.

## Oidiomycosis

Closely related to the *Monilia* are the oidia. The latter are simple yeastlike forms consisting of oblong elements that form chains or hyphae. These break up, forming spherical or oblong, sporelike elements. Most of them are saprophytic, the best known being *Oidium lactis*, commonly associated with milk and often found in the mouths of young animals on diets containing milk. Some species have been regarded as pathogenic for man, but recent authors appear to doubt their disease-producing power. Jungherr (2) has found a member of this group associated with the crop and gizzard lesions of birds described above and believes it plays a part in the infection. Pure cultures were shown to be pathogenic for birds. He proposed the name *Oidium pullorum* for the organism.

## REFERENCES

1.  Biester and Schwarte.   Diseases of poultry. 5th ed. Iowa State College Press, Ames. Iowa, 1965.
2.  Jungherr.   Jour. Am. Vet. Med. Assoc., 1934, *84*, 500.

### *Blastomyces dermatitidis*

This organism causes *North American blastomycosis*, a chronic granulomatous and suppurative mycotic infection that occurs occasionally in man and animals. The lesions may be confined to the skin and subcutaneous tissue or the disease may be generalized. The organisms appear as yeastlike bodies in infected tissues, but in cultures they produce a mycelial growth.

*Blastomyces dermatitidis* seems to be confined to the United States, Canada, and Africa, but the reported incidence of blastomycosis in any area is related to interest in the disease. Blastomycosis was recognized in 1912 in dogs by Meyer (14). Since that time the organism has been reported in a number of instances in dogs (15, 16, 18), in a horse (3), in Siamese cats (9), in a sea lion (23), and in man.

**Morphology and Cultivation.** The organism is a spherical, thick-walled, budding, yeastlike fungus in tissue or exudates and in culture at 37 C. In culture at room temperature it develops slowly as a typical, moldlike, filamentous fungus. It grows well on common laboratory media, where it becomes wrinkled, waxy, and yeastlike in appearance. The yeastlike phase is composed of cells (7 to 15 microns) with single buds resembling those found in exudates or tissues. Occasionally pseudohyphae or incomplete hyphae are present.

**Pathogenicity.** The organism causes a chronic granulomatous infection of the skin and internal organs. In dogs it can be characterized as a chronic, debilitating pulmonary condition often accompanied by some degree of lameness. Palpable cutaneous or subcutaneous swellings are frequent. Infection may start as a cutaneous lesion in the form of a papulopustule. In systemic blastomycosis the lungs are most frequently infected and show the most extensive lesions. Most cases reported in animals have been of the systemic type. A case in a dog, studied by Lacroix, Riser, and Karlson (12), showed no cutaneous involvement. Lesions were confined to the lungs, which were dotted with miliary nodules of the type found in infectious granulomas. Saunders (19), however, reported a case of cutaneous blastomycosis in the dog in which it was a primary skin infection, and Foshay and Madden (6) described another case in a dog in which lesions appeared in the subcutaneous tissues, lymph nodes, spleen, liver, kidneys, lungs, and intestines. Ocular involvement has been diagnosed in dogs (21), and also secondary amyloidosis of the kidneys, liver, and spleen (20).

Systemic blastomycosis has been described in Siamese cats (9) and because five out of the six reported cases have occurred in this breed it may indicate a breed susceptibility.

Blastomycotic mastitis has been reported in South African dairy herds (8).

In man the disease may occur as the cutaneous form with the initial lesion appearing on the exposed skin surface following trauma. In these cases healing usually occurs with scar formation of the keloid type.

The systemic infection in man is usually pulmonary in origin but may result from metastasis of a cutaneous lesion. The disease extends mainly by hematogenous routes. A subcutaneous nodule may be the first sign of widespread infection. Any organ or tissue may be involved. Primary laryngeal blastomycosis of man has also been reported (17).

Furcolow *et al.* (7) have indicated that it is an important medical problem in midwestern and southern United States, and have suggested that the disease is endemic throughout most of Kentucky.

**Diagnosis.** Crusts from lesions may be placed in a drop of 10 percent KOH under a cover glass and examined microscopically after the preparation has been gently heated. *B. dermatitidis* appears as a thick-walled, single-budding, yeastlike fungus, 8 to 20 microns in diameter. Cultures can be made on blood agar and Sabouraud's glucose agar. Complement-fixation and FA tests have been used. Because *B. dermatitidis* and *Histoplasma capsulatum* share antigens (10) special caution must be exercised in interpreting these tests.

**Transmission.** Blastomycosis is more prevalent in the middle Atlantic, south central, and Ohio-Mississippi River Valley states. There is no evidence that the disease is contagious or no proof that it is transmitted from man to man or from animals to man. There has been much speculation over the role of soil as a source of infection and in 1961 Denton *et al.* (5) isolated *B. dermatitidis* from a Lexington, Kentucky, soil sample that came from a tobacco-stripping barn that had sheltered a dog that died of blastomycosis 2 years previously. In 1964 it was recovered from 10 of 356 soil samples collected in an endemic area at Augusta, Georgia (4). The organism appears to be a self-sufficient saprophyte, capable of surviving and thriving in nature, but the yeast phase of the organism seems to be the important agent in promoting infection and this phase survives for only a short time in soil (13). Ajello (1) has stated that *B. dermatitidis* presents one of the greatest ecological challenges. As yet, its natural habitat remains unknown. It is difficult to imagine the precise conditions required to permit its existence in such diverse regions as the Americas and Africa.

**Immunity.** Complement-fixing antibodies can be demonstrated in the serum of human patients with extensive or progressive infection, but not in patients with localized cutaneous lesions. A delayed tuberculinlike reaction can be demonstrated in infected individuals by injecting extracts of the organism.

**Chemotherapy.** In an outbreak of North American blastomycosis Smith *et al.* (22) treated nine patients with stilbamidine or 2-hydroxystilbamidine and reported that eight responded rapidly and without toxic manifestations to the therapy. A 7-month-old infant died. Kligman and Lewis (11) protected mice infected with *B. dermatitidis* by administering candicidin. In 1959 Baum and Schwarz (2) reported that North American blastomycosis is an almost-conquered disease due to the effectiveness of amphotericin B and stilbamidine and its derivatives.

## REFERENCES

1. Ajello. Bact. Rev., 1967, *31*, 6.
2. Baum and Schwarz. Am. Jour. Med. Sci., 1959, *238*, 661.
3. Benbrook, Bryant, and Saunders. Jour. Am. Vet. Med. Assoc., 1948, *112*, 475.
4. Denton and DiSalvo. Am. Jour. Trop. Med. and Hyg., 1964, *13*, 716.
5. Denton, McDonough, Ajello, and Ausherman. Science, 1961, *133*, 1126.
6. Foshay and Madden. Am. Jour. Trop. Med., 1942, *22*, 565.
7. Furcolow, Balows, Menges, Pickar, McClellan, and Saliba. Jour. Am. Med. Assoc., 1966, *195*, 529.
8. Giesecke, Nel, and Van Den Heever. Jour. So. African Vet. Med. Assoc., 1968, *39*, 69.
9. Jasmin, Carroll, Baucom, and Beusse. Vet. Med., 1969, *64*, 33.
10. Kaufman and Kaplan. Jour. Bact., 1963, *85*, 986.
11. Kligman and Lewis. Proc. Soc. Exp. Biol. and Med., 1953, *82*, 399.
12. Lacroix, Riser, and Karlson. North Am. Vet., 1947, *28*, 603.
13. McDonough, Prooien, and Lewis. Am. Jour. Epidemiol., 1965, *81*, 86.
14. Meyer. Proc. Path. Soc. Philadelphia, 1912, *15*, 10.
15. Newberne, Neal, and Heath. Jour. Am. Vet. Med. Assoc., 1955, *127*, 220.
16. Ramsey and Carter. *Ibid.*, 1952, *120*, 93.
17. Ranier. Am. Jour. Clin. Path., 1951, *21*, 444.
18. Saunders. Cornell Vet., 1948, *38*, 213.
19. Saunders. North Am. Vet., 1948, *29*, 650.
20. Sherwood, LeMay, and Castellanos. Jour. Am. Vet. Med. Assoc., 1967, *150*, 1377.
21. Simon and Helper. *Ibid.*, 1970, *157*, 922.
22. Smith, Harris, Conant, and Smith. Jour. Am. Med. Assoc., 1955, *158*, 641.
23. Williamson, Lombard, and Getty. Jour. Am. Vet. Med. Assoc., 1959, *135*, 513.

### *Paracoccidioides braziliensis*

SYNONYM:   *Blastomyces braziliensis*

This organism causes *South American blastomycosis* (paracoccidioidal granuloma) of man. It produces a chronic mycotic infection that resembles coccidioidomycosis and blastomycosis of the North American type. The disease may manifest itself in the mucocutaneous form, the lesions occurring around the lips, nose, and buccal mucosa; in the lymphangitic form which starts as a primary lesion in the mouth and spreads to the lymph nodes of the neck; or in the systemic form which involves the digestive tract. Lesions are less common in the lungs than in coccidioidomycosis or North American blastomycosis, but they may occur in any organ or tissue. The tissue lesions resemble those caused by *B. dermatitidis*. Although the disease has been found mostly in Brazil, it has also been reported from other South American countries. Paracoccidioidomycosis has been diagnosed in the United States, but all of the infected individuals have had histories of residing in South or Central America (2). This suggests reactivation as an endogenous reinfection. In one case the disease apparently was acquired in Mexico, a nonendemic area (1). No reports of infection in the lower animals have been seen.

**Morphology and Cultivation.** The mycelial phase resembles that of *B. dermatitidis*. The yeastlike forms which are found in infected exudate and tissues or in cultures grown at 37 C are composed of single cells, which vary in size from 4.5 to 9 microns in diameter and show characteristic multiple-budding forms. The finding of these multiple buds in tissues distinguishes *P. braziliensis* from *B. dermatitidis*.

**Diagnosis.** Serologic tests, such as CF and agar-gel-immunodiffusion, are valuable in making a diagnosis (4).

**Chemotherapy.** Early lesions respond to treatment with the sulfonamides. Iodide therapy also is useful. Fountain and Sutliff (2) treated a case of pulmonary paracoccidioidomycosis and claimed that amphotericin B, even in suboptimal doses, caused a prompt disappearance of the organism from the sputum, and roentgenographic improvement.

### REFERENCES

1. Artiga and Gotelli.   Am. Jour. Trop. Med. and Hyg., 1968, *17*, 576.
2. Fountain and Sutliff.   Am. Rev. Resp. Dis., 1969, *99*, 89.
3. Moss and McQuown.   Atlas of medical mycology. 2d ed. Williams and Wilkins Co., Baltimore, 1960.
4. Restrepo, Robledo, Gutierrez, Sanclemente, Castañeda, and Calle.   Am. Jour. Trop. Med. and Hyg., 1970, *19*, 68.

### *Cryptococcus neoformans*

SYNONYMS:   *Torula histolytica, Cryptococcus hominis*

European blastomycosis is a subacute or chronic mycotic infection of animals and man caused by *Cryptococcus neoformans*. The organism frequently attacks the tissues of the nervous system, but lesions may also be found in the lungs, skin, lymph glands, and other tissues. The disease has been reported from all parts of the world (19). In the United States cryptococcosis (torulosis) has been reported in horses, cattle, sheep, goats, a pig, dogs, cats, foxes, mink, ferrets, koala bears, cheetahs, a civet cat, guinea pigs, monkeys, and man (2, 9, 15, 20).

**Morphology and Cultivation.** *C. neoformans* grows rapidly on Sabouraud's glucose agar. The colony is flat or slightly heaped, shiny, moist, or mucoid, with smooth edges. The color is cream at first, later becoming brown. The organism grows as a yeast at room temperature and at 37 C. It is spherical or ovoid in shape, thick-walled, single or budding, and refractile and measures from 3 to 8 microns in diameter. It develops capsules, but no mycelium. Intravenous infection of chick embryos with *C. neoformans* followed by incubation at 37 C produces almost 100 percent mortality. Incubation at 40 C destroys the organisms (12). Shields and Ajello (21) have developed a selective medium that permits recovery of *C. neoformans* from heavily contaminated materials. It contains creatinine as a nitrogen source, diphenyl ($C_6H_5C_6H_5$) and chloramphenicol as mold and bacterial inhibitors, and *Guizotia abyssinica* seed extract as a specific color marker.

**Pathogenicity.** The pigeon has been used as an experimental animal. Intrace-

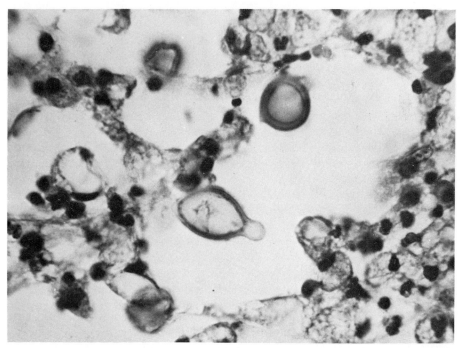

*Fig. 106.* Photomicrograph showing a round cell of *Cryptococcus neoformans* with thick capsule in the upper part of the field. Below is an oval cell in the process of budding. X 900. (Courtesy Jean Holzworth, *Cornell Vet.*)

rebral inoculation induces nervous system disease in pigeons consisting of fine tremors, gait disorders, loss of coordination, and inability to maintain erect posture. Death may occur within 3 to 18 days. Birds that survive for several weeks or more show evidence of meningitis as well as involvement of lung, liver, spleen, kidney, heart blood, and intestine (14). They may continue to harbor the organism for an extended period of time without signs of illness.

In the lower animals involvement of the central nervous system is not uncommon, but other organs and tissues, especially lymph nodes, may be included. The disease sometimes is generalized. Pulmonary and nasal growths, which sometimes give rise to chronic nasal discharges, have also been observed in animals, and localized suppurative lesions have in some instances produced granulation tissue.

In cattle, outbreaks of cryptococcic mastitis with regional lymph node involvement have occurred (2, 10).

Laws and Simmons (13) have reported a case of cryptococcosis in a sheep in which organisms were present in the leptomeninges, brain, mucosa of the nose and maxillary sinuses, and in the lungs. Clinically the sheep presented swollen maxillary sinuses, mucoid nasal discharge, dyspnea, coughing, and anorexia.

In dogs, encephalitis or a chronic respiratory condition may herald the disease. Cases have been accompanied by pulmonary, generalized, and intraocular involvement. The usual pathologic findings reported in dogs are those of a granulomatous destructive process involving nasal mucosa and turbinates, facial sinuses, adjacent osseous structures, and meningitis. Primary pulmonary lesions with secondary meningitis may also occur (16).

Cryptococcosis in cats (7, 9) has also been concerned with lesions in the central nervous system and with granulomas involving the eye, sinuses, and nasal septum.

The disease has been reported in monkeys (8). Although it was not suspected clinically, it was diagnosed on histologic examination by finding typical cryptococcic granulomas in the lungs and deep in the brain parenchyma.

In man, *C. neoformans* may produce a cutaneous form of disease in which healing sometimes occurs spontaneously after several weeks; a pulmonary disease with unilateral or bilateral lesions and a low-grade pneumonia; or a central nervous disease in which symptoms suggestive of a subacute or chronic meningitis, abscess, or brain tumor appear. Meningitis may follow the cutaneous form or it may occur as a primary condition. A case of cryptococcal hepatitis was reported in 1965 (17).

**Diagnosis.** Salvin and Smith (18) have prepared an antigen for the detection of hypersensitivity to *C. neoformans* and claim that it did not cross-react with *Candida albicans* or *Histoplasma capsulatum*. Walter and Jones (24) have stated that contrary to common belief CF, slide-agglutination, and latex-fixation tests are quite reliable in the serodiagnosis of clinical cryptococcosis and that the CF test is most sensitive.

Although a relationship between *pigeon breeders' disease* and *C. neofor-mans* has been suspected Fink *et al.* (6) have indicated that their studies do not support this contention. The antigen that triggers this allergic disease most likely originates with pigeons, but not with the *Cryptococcus*.

**Mode of Transmission.** *C. neoformans* has been isolated from soil (4), which appears to be its natural habitat. Emmons (5) examined pigeon nests and pigeon droppings from 19 premises by mouse inoculation for the presence of pathogenic fungi. *C. neoformans* was isolated from 63 of 111 specimens that came from 16 of these 19 premises. Ajello (1) has indicated that habitats that favor growth of *C. neoformans* occur throughout the world. It flourishes in bird manures, especially that of pigeons. This association may be governed by the presence of creatinine, which is utilizable as a nitrogen source by *C. neoformans* but not by competing microorganisms.

**Chemotherapy.** *In vitro* tests have shown that the thiosemicarbazones, cyclo-heximide (actidione), polymyxin B, ethyl vanillate, prophylparaben, methylpar-aben, and neomycin sulfate are inhibitory for this organism (3, 11, 22). Amphotericin B has been used with varying success. The application of an aqueous solution of hydrated lime and sodium hydroxide has been used to eliminate *C. neoformans* from contaminated pigeon coops (23).

## REFERENCES

1. Ajello.   Bact. Rev., 1967, *31*, 6.
2. Barron.   Jour. Am. Vet. Med. Assoc., 1955, *127*, 125.
3. Eisen, Shapiro, and Fixcher.   Canad. Med. Assoc. Jour., 1955, 72, 33.
4. Emmons.   Jour. Bact., 1951, *62*, 685.
5. Emmons.   Am. Jour. Hyg., 1955, *62*, 227.
6. Fink, Barboriak, and Kaufman.   Jour. Allergy, 1968, *41*, 297.
7. Fischer.   Jour. Am. Vet. Med. Assoc., 1971, *158*, 191.
8. Garner, Ford, and Ross.   *Ibid.*, 1969, *155*, 1163.
9. Holzworth.   Cornell Vet., 1952, *42*, 12.
10. Innes, Seibold, and Arentzen.   Am. Jour. Vet. Res., 1952, *13*, 469.
11. Johnson, Joyner, and Perry.   Antibiotics and Chemother., 1952, *2*, 636.
12. Kligman, Crane, and Norris.   Am. Jour. Med. Sci., 1951, *221*, 273.
13. Laws and Simmons.   Austral. Vet. Jour., 1966, *42*, 321.
14. Littman, Borok, and Dalton.   Am. Jour. Epidemiol., 1965, *82*, 197.
15. Pounden, Amberson, and Jaeger.   Am. Jour. Vet. Res., 1952, *13*, 121.
16. Price and Powers.   Jour. Am. Vet. Med. Assoc., 1967, *150*, 988.
17. Procknow, Benfield, Rippon, Diener, and Archer.   Jour. Am. Med. Assoc., 1965, *191*, 269.
18. Salvin and Smith.   Proc. Soc. Exp. Biol. and Med., 1961, *108*, 498.
19. Saunders.   Cornell Vet., 1948, 38, 213.
20. Seibold, Roberts, and Jordan.   Jour. Am. Vet. Med. Assoc., 1953, *122*, 213.
21. Shields and Ajello.   Science, 1966, *151*, 208.
22. Simon.   Am. Jour. Vet. Res., 1955, *16*, 394.
23. Walter and Coffee.   Am. Jour. Epidemiol., 1968, 87, 173.
24. Walter and Jones.   Am. Rev. Resp. Dis., 1968, 97, 275.

### *Rhinosporidium seeberi*

Rhinosporidiosis is a chronic fungus disease of the nasal and ocular mucous membranes. According to Ashworth (1) and Rao (3), the organism is a slow-growing fungus, although it originally was classed as a protozoon when first described by Seeber. The organisms are found in large cystlike structures, which give rise to nasal polyps in man, cattle, horses, and mules. The human disease has been seen in Argentina and in southern Asiatic countries. It occurs infrequently in man in North America. A case in a horse was described by Zschokke (6) in South Africa. It has been reported in mules in South Africa and in cattle in India (4). The same species probably infects man, cattle, and the *Equidae*. The disease has been infrequently diagnosed in the Western Hemisphere (5). In 1964 it was reported in a mare purchased in South St. Louis (2).

The organism has not been grown successfully on artificial culture media. Diagnosis is made by finding the giant sporangia (20 to 300 microns in diameter) in the polyps, either in tissue sections or in wet mounts. Eradication by means of surgery or by cautery is recommended. Recurrence follows incomplete removal.

### REFERENCES

1. Ashworth.   Trans. Royal Soc. Edinburgh, 1932, *53*, 301.
2. Myers, Simon, and Case.   Jour. Am. Vet. Med. Assoc., 1964, *145*, 345.
3. Rao.   Indian Jour. Vet. Sci., 1938, *8*, 187.
4. Saunders.   Cornell Vet., 1948, *38*, 213.
5. Smith and Frankson.   Southwest. Vet., 1961, *15*, 22.
6. Zschokke.   Schweiz. Arch. f. Tierheilk., 1913, *55*, 641.

### Sporotrichosis

Sporotrichosis is a disease of man, horses, and other species, caused by fungi belonging to the genus *Sporotrichum*. The disease is characterized by chronic granulomatous lesions of the skin, of the skin lymphatics, and occasionally of the internal organs. The superficial lesions have a tendency to ulcerate. Elongated yeastlike bodies occur in the pus, but these frequently can be demonstrated only with difficulty and sometimes not at all. Mycelium is not found in tissues. The condition in horses resembles epizootic lymphangitis. Early in the century epizootic lymphangitis was reported in the United States (11), but Page, Frothingham, and Paige (10) showed that the condition was sporotrichosis rather than zymonemicosis. Sporotrichosis in both man and horses has been reported rather frequently from the states of the upper Mississippi Valley and infrequently from various other parts of this country. It is supposed that the organism is a saprophyte that lives in the soil.

### *Sporotrichum schencki*

SYNONYMS:   *Sporotrichum beurmanni, Sporothrix schencki*

S. *schencki* was first described in the United States in man. It is now known to be widely distributed geographically, affecting both man and animals. It has been observed in horses, donkeys, mules, cattle, a pig, dogs, cats, fowl, camels, rats, and mice. The records of sporotrichosis in animals are far outnumbered by those in man (2).

**Morphology and Staining Reactions.** In pus the organism usually is difficult to demonstrate microscopically. The only forms that can be recognized are cells resembling elongated yeasts, sometimes described as "cigar-shaped." They vary in length from 2 to 10 microns and in breadth from 1 to 3 microns.

In cultures the morphology is best studied in fluids, unstained. The filaments are rather delicate, measuring about 2 microns in diameter. They are septate and branching. Short, irregular lateral branches are numerous. On the ends of the branches clusters of the oval or pear-shaped spores are found. Such spores are also found along the sides of the filaments. The hyphae and spores stain readily with ordinary dyes and with the Gram stain, but the process of staining shrinks the hyphae and dislodges the spores.

**Cultural Features.** Growth occurs on all the ordinary laboratory media, but solid media are more productive than fluid. Acid media are more favorable than those used for the cultivation of bacteria. Maltose favors growth. Good growths are obtained on potato and carrots, and on these media the characteristic brownish-black pigment is best seen.

Small whitish filamentous colonies appear on potato slants on the second day of incubation. These gradually enlarge and darken until finally the color is almost black. The surface is woolly because of the short aerial hyphae. Old cultures develop convoluted surfaces suggestive of the convolutions of the brain.

The growth on sliced carrots is similar to that on potato. On agar the growth is similar to that on potato but the colonies remain a whitish color. They are adherent because of the penetration of the mycelium into the medium. Gelatin is slowly liquified. Most of the growth is near the surface but spikelike growth occurs along stabs. There may be some blackening of the surface growth. Loeffler's blood serum shows a slight depression under the colonies, but general liquefaction does not occur.

In litmus milk there is little growth except on the surface, where white filaments grow around the tube in the form of a ring which becomes black in about 1 week. The milk may coagulate after 3 weeks but the reaction remains alkaline. In fluid media growth occurs principally as a pellicle or a ring, but if undisturbed a few fluffy colonies, which remain permanently white, may form along the sides of the tube or on the bottom. If the pellicle is caused to sink by shaking, a fresh one replaces it.

Poor growth takes place in sugar-free broth and in peptone water. It is much better in glucose and especially in maltose broth. Growth occurs in broth containing chloroform and in broth containing more than 5 percent salt. Acid is formed from glucose but not from lactose, sucrose, maltose, mannitol, dulcitol, adonitol, raffinose, and inulin. Gas is not formed in any medium.

**Pathogenicity.** The disease in horses is characterized by the formation under the skin of spherical nodules of sharp contour. There is no tendency for the nodules to coalesce. Although they may become multiple and spread over areas of the body, in neither the nodular nor ulcerative forms is there any evidence of "cording" of the lymphatics. The skin over the nodules becomes moist, the hair falls out, and crusts form. The pus discharged from the crateriform ulcers is yellowish and rather scanty in amount. The ulcers heal slowly and usually leave hairless cicatrices. Internal lesions have not been reported in horses.

Among the lower animals sporotrichosis appears to be more common in the *Equidae*, but natural infections have occurred in dogs, cats, fowl, the camel, rats, a pig, and possibly cattle. Experimentally, guinea pigs, rats, and rabbits can be infected, but usually only a local abscess is formed.

In 1965 Smith (12) recorded what he believed to be the first reported case of sporotrichosis infection in the joints of a pig.

In man the initial lesion usually begins as a small subcutaneous nodule at the site of trauma. Spreading to the lymph nodes is by way of the lymphatic channels. The lymphatics become thickened, and the lymph nodes become enlarged, then necrotic, and finally ulcerate. Generalized infection may occur through the blood stream with or without a primary cutaneous lesion (3, 5). In 1968, Mahgoub (9) reported a case of pulmonary sporotrichosis in a patient from Khartoum, Africa. The causative agent proved to be *Sporotrichum gougeroti*. Mahgoub has claimed that sporotrichosis is a relatively rare mycotic infection of the skin and subcutaneous tissues, but not an uncommon cause of systemic and pulmonary disease. Cases have occurred in Europe, North and South America, and in Africa. Although the most common cause of sporotrichosis is *S. schencki*, a few cases have been attributed to *S. gougeroti*. The latter is black from the 1st day of growth and does not lose pigment through age or transfers, whereas *S. schencki* is usually white from the 1st day and darkens with age. It occurs in tissues as sclerotic bodies, while *S. schencki* rarely is seen in tissues and occurs as small Gram-positive cigar-shaped bodies or asteroid tissue forms (14).

**Habitat.** There is some evidence of a relationship between *S. schencki* and sphagnum moss. At least, infection has occurred in handlers of this type of moss and the organism grows in moist mixtures of sphagnum and soil (8). Ahearn and Kaplan (1), in an investigation of optimal conditions for cold storage of frankfurters, isolated a fungal agent that they identified as *S. schencki*. Their isolate grew at 5 C in the cold-storage environment.

**Immunity.** Little is known of this aspect of sporotrichosis. The disease is not common enough to warrant special biological treatment. The serum of chronically infected animals will agglutinate spore suspensions, and filtrates of old fluid cultures (*sporotrichin*) will give specific skin reactions. Kaplan and Gonzalez (6) claim that the direct FA technic can be employed as a rapid screening procedure for detecting sporotrichosis.

**Chemotherapy.** The disease yields readily to systemic treatment with iodides. Candicidin has been reported to protect mice infected with S. *schencki* (7). Griseofulvin has been recommended in treating horses (4) and amphotericin B has given favorable results in experiments with mice (13).

## REFERENCES

1.   Ahearn and Kaplan.   Am. Jour. Epidemiol., 1969, *89*, 116.
2.   Ainsworth and Austwick.   Fungal diseases of animals. Commonwealth Agricultural Bureaux, Farnham Royal, England, 1959, p. 26.
3.   Castleton and Rees.   Jour. Am. Med. Assoc., 1952, *148*, 541.
4.   Davis and Worthington.   Jour. Am. Vet. Med. Assoc., 1964, *145*, 692.
5.   Hawks.   Canad. Med. Assoc. Jour., 1955, *72*, 28.
6.   Kaplan and Gonzalez.   Jour. Lab. and Clin. Med., 1963, *62*, 835.
7.   Kligman and Lewis.   Proc. Soc. Exp. Biol. and Med., 1953, *82*, 399.
8.   McDonough, Lewis, and Meister.   Pub. Health Rpts. (U.S.), 1970, *85*, 579.
9.   Mahgoub.   Jour. Trop. Med. and Hyg. (London), 1968, *71*, 313.
10.   Page, Frothingham, and Paige.   Jour. Med. Res., 1910, *18*, 137.
11.   Pearson.   Pa. State Livestock Sanitary Bd. Cir. 8, 1907. See also Mohler. Am. Vet. Rev., 1908–1909, *34*, 198.
12.   Smith.   Vet. Med., 1965, *60*, 164.
13.   Tsubura and Schwarz.   Antibiotics and Chemother., 1960, *10*, 753.
14.   Young and Ulrich.   Arch. Dermat. Syph., 1953, *67*, 44.

### *Histoplasma capsulatum*

Darling (7) first described an intracellular organism in the tissues of natives in the Canal Zone. The organism was thought to be a protozoon. De-Monbreun (8), in 1934, cultured the organism from a human case and proved it to be a filamentous fungus. Spontaneous infections have been reported in dogs, mice, rats, and bats (Ruhe and Cazier, 35 and Tesh and Schneidau, Jr., 47). It has also been found in cats, cattle, a horse, a pig, a woodchuck, a skunk, an opossum, a gray fox, a ferret, and a monkey, but the incidence of the disease in these animals seems to be very low. Sheep, a pig, and fowl have been recorded as histoplasmin-positive. According to Furcolow and Ruhe (16), histoplasmin sensitivity can be demonstrated in cattle, and it is probable that cattle and human beings are infected from the same source, but it appears that cattle are not an important animal reservoir. It is possible that soil that contains certain types of organic matter is the natural habitat of the organism. The disease may be transmitted by infected rodents and dogs, and at least one case of a canine and a human infection in the same household has been reported. In the United States an endemic area of this disease includes Mis-

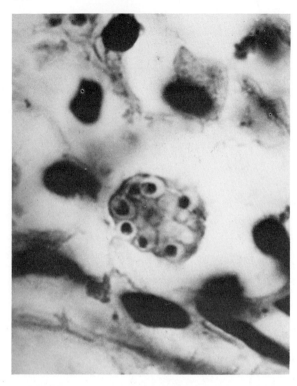

Fig. 107. Histoplasma capsulatum, parasites in macrophage of a dog; natural infection. X 2,700. (Courtesy Oreg. Agr. Exp. Sta., J. W. Osebold.)

souri, Arkansas, Ohio, Tennessee, Indiana, Kansas, and Kentucky. Infection in man has been reported all over the world.

**Morphology and Cultivation.** The organism is a small, oval, yeastlike fungus in tissues and in culture on sealed, blood agar slants or in potato flour-egg medium (24) grown at 37 C. The organisms resemble those seen in the reticuloendothelial cells of tissue. They measure about 1 to 3 microns in diameter. They can be stained by Giemsa's stain. It should be noted that large forms are known to occur in tissue (31). In culture at room temperature, the organism is a typical, moldlike, filamentous fungus. In fact, it is sometimes difficult to distinguish from cultures of *Blastomyces*. In old cultures or under adverse conditions *H. capsulatum* produces the diagnostic chlamydospores. These are round, thick-walled structures that measure from 7 to 15 microns in diameter. Tissue culture has been used to convert *H. capsulatum* to the yeastlike phase (26). Smith and Furcolow (42) studied three technics for isolating *H. capsulatum* from soil and recommend a modified oil flotation method. By employing FA technics, Kaufman and Blumer (22) have demonstrated the existence of five *H. capsulatum* serotypes.

**Pathogenicity.** Histoplasmosis is a mycotic infection primarily involving the reticuloendothelial system of man and animals. It may be acute, subacute, or chronic, localized or disseminated. Primary lesions frequently are located in the respiratory tract, and infection appears to enter by this portal. With dissemination of the infection by the reticuloendothelial cells, splenomegaly, hepatomegaly, leukopenia, anemia, and emaciation may result. Ulcerations of the intestinal tract may occur and produce diarrhea. Nervous symptoms may appear because of invasion of the central nervous system. In lesions the yeast-like cells of the fungus are closely packed in collections of large macrophages. Bone involvement has been noted (28).

Mice, white rats, guinea pigs, hamsters, and dogs can be infected experimentally, but chickens are resistant. Virulence appears to be associated with the yeast phase. Farrell *et al.* (13) found that intratracheal inoculation of the yeast phase into dogs produced infection in all of nine dogs. In gnotobiotic dogs the lesions were limited to the lungs, liver, and lymphopoietic system (15). The same inoculum given to other dogs by stomach tube produced no clinical disease. The mycelial phase given by either of these routes produced no clinical symptoms. Intratracheal inoculation of the yeast phase produced nonfatal infection in horses, cattle, sheep, and swine, whereas intravenous injection resulted in the death of a horse (36).

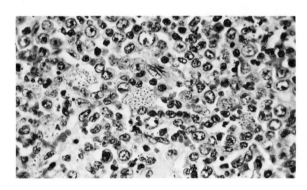

Fig. 108. Hypercellular bone marrow of a horse containing many *Histoplasma*. H and E. X 375. (Courtesy Roger J. Panciera, Cornell Vet.)

The yeast phase, when inoculated intraperitoneally into white mice, may be recovered from the reticuloendothelial tissue as late as 45 weeks after infection. The lungs and heart blood usually are clear within 16 weeks post-inoculation (37).

Naturally infected bats have been located in the United States (Alabama, 2; Arizona, 9; Maryland, 12; Oklahoma, 3; and Texas, 12) and in the Canal Zone (23). The fungus has been isolated from the liver, lungs, spleen, intestines, and feces of this mammal.

A spontaneous outbreak of histoplasmosis has been described in guinea pigs (6). Adult animals showed a chronic disease with progressive emaciation and lameness of the hind legs. The young below 3 months of age died in 2 to 4 weeks presenting ruffled fur, great dorsal curvature, and sometimes closed eyelids and catarrhal conjunctivitis. At necropsy the principal lesions were ulcerative gastritis, hemorrhagic and catarrhal enteritis, and enlarged spleen and mesenteric lymph nodes. Sometimes the liver, lungs, mediastinal lymph nodes, and other organs showed lesions.

In dogs, chronic, debilitating digestive disturbance with enlarged abdomen, hepatomegaly, and ascites are prominent symptoms. Chronic cough and dyspnea are frequent (39). In man, age and sex do not seem to be important factors, although many cases occur in children and infants. The disease in adults differs in several respects from the disease in infants. There is less tendency for widespread visceral involvement in adults. Histoplasmosis of the mouth, nose, and larynx occurs almost exclusively in adults and often as a localized process without dissemination (38).

**Mode of Transmission.** The natural reservoir of the fungus is soil (25), which does not appear to be generally contaminated but which supports concentrations of *H. capsulatum* in particular areas where certain organic matter is found. For instance, the soil of chicken houses and yards located in endemic regions frequently carry high concentrations of this organism (20, 50, 51). Investigations indicate that chickens are not a reservoir of histoplasmosis, and their association with the fungus remains unexplained. There is data suggesting that urban starling-blackbird roosts may harbor *H. capsulatum* and contribute significantly to the prevalence of cutaneous sensitivity to histoplasmin among children residing or attending school near the roosts (48).

*H. capsulatum* has been isolated from the dust in an unused silo and from naturally contaminated air (17, 21).

Emmons (11) reported that dung from bats was the factor responsible for the constant saprophytic infestation of soil in certain premises that he investigated, and Shacklette *et al.* (40) recovered the organism from the liver and spleen of bats. Subsequent investigations concerning the role of bats in the spread of histoplasmosis have shown that they harbor *H. capsulatum*, that their feces contain the organism, and that caves inhabited by bats have been shown to be heavily contaminated with the fungus (41). It seems likely that bats seed the soil with infected feces and that *H. capsulatum* may then be transmitted by air from these foci.

In tap water the yeast phase will change to the mycelial phase and grow (34).

Man has acquired histoplasmosis in the laboratory (32), and feathers from a pillow yielded the fungus in an epidemiologic study of the disease in an infant (4).

The communicability of *H. capsulatum* from dog to dog has been established, and although there is at present no proof of a relationship between the disease in dogs and man, the infected dog must be considered a potentially dangerous source because it can disseminate the organism by saliva, vomitus, feces, and urine (5).

Ajello (1) has concluded that habitats that favor the growth of *H. capsulatum* occur throughout the world and that it has been established that the organism has a predilection for bat and bird habitats, but the basis for this association has yet to be determined.

**Diagnosis.** Fluorescent-labeled antibodies have been used to differentiate *H. capsulatum* from other pathogenic fungi (18). In 1968, Kaufman and Blumer (22) by adsorbing a fluorescent antibody reagent, which they had produced against their most complete *Histoplasma* serotype, obtained a specific FA agent that enabled them to distinguish *H. capsulatum* and *Histoplasma duboisi* from other pathogenic fungi. Differentiation between these two *Histoplasma* species was achieved only by animal inoculation and the demonstration of the large yeast forms of *H. duboisi*.

Peripheral blood, sternal bone marrow, sputum, and biopsies of lymph nodes (14) and mucosal lesions may be examined by FA technics and cultured on blood agar and Sabouraud's glucose agar and incubated at 37 C and room temperature, respectively. Penicillin and streptomycin may be used to prevent the growth of contaminating microorganisms. Colonies of *H. capsulatum* appear in about 1 month.

Mice frequently are used in isolating the organism. As in coccidioidomycosis, extracts of *H. capsulatum* (histoplasmin), when injected in minute amounts into the skin, reveal a state of hypersensitiveness to the infecting organism much like the tuberculin reaction. However, Smith, Saito, Beard, Rosenberger, and Whiting (44) found that histoplasmin cross-reacts with coccidioidin, and a positive test may indicate sensitivity to a fungus other than *H. capsulatum*. Furthermore, a single histoplasmin skin test can stimulate the development of humoral antibodies that can be demonstrated with *H. capsulatum* antigens (29). A hemagglutination test has been described by Norden (33). Complement-fixation tests also are useful, and Sorensen and Evans (45) have described an antigen that appears to be highly specific. Agar-gel tests have been successful.

**Immunity.** Recoveries from localized infections are fairly common, especially in man and cattle. With recovery, the CF test becomes negative, but the skin test remains positive (27). No biological products are available for the control of this disease.

**Control Measures.** In 1949, Smith *et al.* (43) concluded that attempts to eliminate *H. capsulatum* from soil by removal of trees, brush, and leaves and by applying chemical fungicides have failed. Although the investigations of Tosh and coworkers (49), in 1967, agree as to finding no practical and effective procedure for destroying *H. capsulatum* in its natural habitat, they were able to decontaminate soil that contained the fungus by three to four applications of 3 percent formalin.

**Chemotherapy.** *In vitro* studies have shown *H. capsulatum* to be sensitive to ethyl vanillate (19) and fungicidin (nystatin). According to Drauhet *et al.* (10), the treatment with nystatin of fulminating, moderately acute, or chronic disease in hamsters and mice has decreased mortality, inhibited dissemination of the disease in many animals, and sterilized the tissues in selected animals. Also, the administration of sulfonamides, admixed in the diet, proved to be highly effective in the treatment of mice infected with lethal doses of the organism (30). There is evidence that amphotericin B is effective in treating chronic pulmonary histoplasmosis that shows active lesions and positive sputum cultures (46).

## REFERENCES

1. Ajello. Bact. Rev., 1967, *31*, 6.
2. Ajello, Hosty, and Palmer. Am. Jour. Trop. Med. and Hyg., 1967, *16*, 329.
3. Bryles, Cozad, and Robinson. *Ibid.*, 1969, *18*, 399.
4. Campbell, Hill, and Falgout. Science, 1962, *136*, 1050.
5. Cole, Farrell, Chamberlain, Prior, and Saslaw. Jour. Am. Vet. Med. Assoc., 1953, *122*, 471.
6. Correa and Pacheco. Canad. Jour. Comp. Med. and Vet. Sci., 1967, *31*, 203.
7. Darling. Jour. Am. Med. Assoc., 1906, *46*, 1283.
8. DeMonbreun. Am. Jour. Trop. Med., 1934, *14*, 93.
9. DiSalvo, Ajello, Palmer, Jr., and Winkler. Am. Jour. Epidemiol., 1969, *89*, 606.
10. Drauhet, Schwarz, and Bingham. Antibiotic and Chemother., 1956, *6*, 23.
11. Emmons. Pub. Health Rpts. (U.S.), 1958, *73*, 590.
12. Emmons, Klite, Baer, and Hill, Jr. Am. Jour. Epidemiol., 1966, *84*, 103.
13. Farrell, Cole, Prior, and Saslaw. Proc. Soc. Exp. Biol. and Med., 1953, *84*, 51.
14. Fattal, Schwarz, and Straub. Am. Jour. Clin. Path., 1961, *36*, 119.
15. Favero and Farrell. Am. Jour. Vet. Res., 1966, *27*, 60.
16. Furcolow and Ruhe. Am. Jour. Pub. Health, 1949, *39*, 719.
17. Grayston, Loosli, and Alexander. Science, 1951, *114*, 323.
18. Gordon. Jour. Bact., 1959, *77*, 678.
19. Hansen and Beene. Proc. Soc. Exp. Biol. and Med., 1951, *77*, 365.
20. Ibach, Larsh, and Furcolow. Science, 1954, *119*, 71.
21. Ibach, Larsh, and Furcolow. Proc. Soc. Exp. Biol. and Med., 1954, *85*, 72.
22. Kaufman and Blumer. Jour. Bact., 1968, *95*, 1243.
23. Klite and Diercks. Am. Jour. Trop. Med. and Hyg., 1965, *14*, 433.
24. Kurung and Yegian. Am. Jour. Clin. Path., 1954, *24*, 505.
25. Larsh, Hinton, and Cozad. Am. Jour. Hyg., 1956, *63*, 18.
26. Larsh, Hinton, and Silberg. Proc. Soc. Exp. Biol. and Med., 1956, *93*, 612.
27. Loosli, Procknow, Tanzi, Grayston, Combs, and Lowell. Jour. Lab. and Clin. Med., 1954, *43*, 669.
28. Lunn. Jour. Trop. Med. and Hyg. (London), 1960, *63*, 175.
29. McDearman and Young. Am. Jour. Clin. Path., 1960, *34*, 434.
30. Mayer, Eisman, Geftic, Konopka, and Tanzola. Antibiotics and Chemother., 1956, *6*, 215.
31. Moore. Am. Jour. Path., 1955, *31*, 1049.
32. Murray and Howard. Am. Rev. Resp. Dis., 1964, *89*, 631.
33. Norden. Proc. Soc. Exp. Biol. and Med., 1949, *70*, 218.
34. Ritter. Am. Jour. Pub. Health, 1954, *44*, 199.

35.  Ruhe and Cazier.    Jour. Am. Vet. Med. Assoc., 1949, *115*, 47.
36.  Saslaw, Maurice, Cole, and Carlisle.    Proc. Soc. Exp. Biol. and Med., 1960, *105*, 76.
37.  Saslaw and Schaefer.    *Ibid.*, 1956, *91*, 412.
38.  Schulz.    Am. Jour. Clin. Path., 1954, *24*, 11.
39.  Schwabe.    Vet. Med., 1954, *49*, 479.
40.  Shacklette, Diercks, and Gale.    Science, 1962, *135*, 1135.
41.  Shacklette, Hasenclever, and Miranda.    Am. Jour. Epidemiol., 1967, *86*, 246.
42.  Smith and Furcolow.    Jour. Lab. and Clin. Med., 1964, *64*, 342.
43.  Smith, Furcolow, and Tosh.    Am. Jour. Hyg., 1964, *79*, 170.
44.  Smith, Saito, Beard, Rosenberger, and Whiting.    Am. Jour. Pub. Health, 1949, *39*, 722.
45.  Sorensen and Evans.    Proc. Soc. Exp. Biol. and Med., 1954, *87*, 339.
46.  Sutliff (Veterans Administrations—Armed Forces Cooperative Study on Histoplasmosis). Am. Rev. Resp. Dis., 1964, *89*, 641.
47.  Tesh and Schneidau, Jr.    Am. Jour. Epidemiol., 1967, *86*, 545.
48.  Tosh, Doto, Beecher, and Chin.    Am. Rev. Resp. Dis., 1970, *101*, 283.
49.  Tosh, Weeks, Pfeiffer, Hendricks, Greer, and Chin.    Am. Jour. Epidemiol., 1967, *85*, 259.
50.  Zeidberg and Ajello.    Jour. Bact., 1954, *68*, 156.
51.  Zeidberg, Ajello, Dillon, and Runyon.    Am. Jour. Pub. Health, 1952, *42*, 930.

# PART 6

# THE PATHOGENIC PROTOZOA

# XXVIII | The Pathogenic Protozoa

Protozoa are generally regarded as the first, and the lowest, phylum of the animal kingdom. All animals consisting of single cells and capable of carrying on all life processes independently are included. The great English protozoologist Dobell insists, however, that the protozoa are noncellular animals and thus are different from all other members of the animal kingdom, which are cellular. He raises the protozoa to a rank equal to that of all others and calls the others *metazoa*. Although the protozoa are generally regarded as the most primitive of animals, it should be noted that, physiologically, the protozoan cells must be more complex than the cells of the metazoa because they must assume all the necessary functions of life, whereas the cells of multicellular animals have these functions divided among them.

The soil, surface waters, vegetation, and the intestinal tracts of man and animals are teeming with protozoa, which live saprophytic existences. Only a small proportion are parasitic in habit, and a still smaller proportion of all are disease-producing. Nevertheless a number of very important diseases of man and animals are caused by members of the group.

## Structure

All protozoan cells consist essentially of two parts, cytoplasm and nucleus. The nucleus generally is relatively large and easily recognized. It contains a substance (chromatin) that has an affinity for the basic dyes. The cytoplasm stains with acid dyes and consists of a foamy protoplasm in which vacuoles are often seen. In some protozoan forms the nuclear chromatin is stained red and the cytoplasm blue with polychrome stains.

## Locomotion

The ectoplasm gives origin to the structures concerned in motility. In the *Sarcodina* these consist of prolongations of the ectoplasm, called *pseudopodia*,

595

into which the endoplasm flows, producing the form of motility known as *ameboid movement;* in the *Mastigophora,* of long, very delicate, threadlike filaments called *flagella;* and in the *Ciliata,* of fine, needlelike, short filaments that usually cover the entire surface of the cell and are called *cilia.*

## Multiplication

Most protozoa multiply by a process of cell division in which two more-or-less equal individuals are formed. This process is known as *binary fission.* Some forms divide characteristically into two unequal individuals. This form is called *gemmation* or budding. A large group of parasitic protozoa, the *Sporozoa,* reproduce by a process known as *schizogony.* In this method the nucleus divides and the daughter nuclei divide and subdivide until there are a large number of nuclei in one cytoplasmic mass. These nuclei arrange themselves around the periphery of the cell and are pinched off, each with a small amount of cytoplasm, to form a shower of new individuals called *merozoites.* These grow into adults, which may again reproduce by a repetition of the schizogonic process.

## Syngamy

Following the vegetative process of multiplication described as schizogony, many sporozoa form sexually differentiated cells known as *gametes.* The macrogametes are the equivalent of the ovum of higher creatures and the microgametes, of the sperm cell. The fertilization of a macrogamete by a microgamete is a process known as *syngamy.* It results in cells known as *zygotes,* or *oocysts,* which frequently develop resistant capsules and thus are prepared to await more favorable conditions, or a new host, before developing.

In sexual reproduction an alternation of generations, with a life cycle completed within two different hosts, frequently occurs. In the malaria parasites reproduction in man is asexual in type (schizogony), but in the mosquito host it is sexual in type (sporogony).

## Protozoan Cysts

A characteristic of many of the parasitic protozoa in particular, but of many of the saprophytes also, is their ability to form structures that resist drying. These are called *cysts* and are formed by the secretion of substances that harden into rather dense capsules. Cyst walls often are quite clear and refractile. Unlike the spores of bacteria, to which these structures are comparable, at least in function, the protozoan spore is not materially more resistant to high temperatures than the vegetative organism.

## Immunity in Protozoan Diseases

Generally in protozoan diseases the parasite multiplies rapidly for a time, then, if the host continues to survive, gradually diminishes in number until it can no longer be found. In some instances it does not wholly disappear and may give rise to a recrudescence of the disease. This loss of vigor on the part of the parasite is similar to that seen in most bacterial infections and may be due to the same cause, namely, the development of antibodies that are antagonistic to the parasite. Antibodies do develop in protozoan infections, and they may be transmitted passively, often protecting completely an otherwise susceptible host. Agglutinins, precipitins, complement-fixing antibodies, lysins, opsonins, and ablastins have been demonstrated for protozoa. It is probable that developing immunity is not the only factor in causing disappearance of protozoan parasites, for, in many instances, new infections can be superimposed on the old one. Whereas the original infection is fading out, the new one may be vigorous and progressive. This indicates failing vigor in the parasite probably caused by inherent properties that permit only a limited number of generations by one mode of multiplication, after which another mode must intervene. Schizogony, or asexual multiplication, of coccidia of animals and of the malaria parasites of man can go on in the original hosts only for a limited number of generations, after which the parasite assumes the sexual form and further multiplication in the same host does not occur. After a sojourn in another host (as in malaria) or in the soil (as in coccidiosis), the parasite is then ready to institute a new series of generations in another host or in the very host from which it was derived.

In some protozoan diseases, such as human leishmaniasis and East Coast fever of cattle, recovery results in complete and absolute immunity. In most cases, however, the immunity is only a relative matter and the disease may run for years in a single host because of repeated reinfections. Immunity in these instances does not suffice to protect from new infections.

Many attempts have been made to induce active immunity to protozoan infections by vaccinating the animals with attenuated strains, or suspensions of killed cultures. Most of these have met with little success. Vaccination of children against *Leishmania tropica* has been helpful. Usually the only immunity that is successful is that which is produced as a result of suffering from an actual infection. In some instances it has been noted that young animals withstand certain protozoan infections much better than adult animals, and this fact has been put to practical use, as, for example, in Texas fever immunization.

Although it is not within the scope of this book to consider immunity in nematode infestations, tests have demonstrated that pups can be immunized against hookworms by vaccinating them with irradiated infective larvae (3).

## Artificial Cultivation

The pathogenic protozoa fall into two classes: (*a*) those that live in the fluids of the body extracellularly, and (*b*) those that live all or part of their lives intracellularly. Most of the species that live extracellularly have been cultivated in artificial media. The culture media usually are rather simple, but most of them contain blood or blood serum. The species that live intracellularly have been refractory to artificial cultivation, as might be expected. Success has been attained only in tissue cultures in which the host cells are growing, or at least in which the viability of the host cell is preserved for a time.

## Classification

Detailed classification of the protozoa will not be considered. We are concerned only with the disease-producing forms. They fall into four classes: *Sarcodina, Mastigophora, Sporozoa,* and *Ciliata.*

*The Sarcodina* include the organisms that move and ingest food by means of pseudopodia. The only pathogenic species of importance in this group is *Entamoeba histolytica,* the cause of amebic dysentery in man. This protozoon exists in two sizes, normal and dwarf. *Entamoeba hartmanni* (1), a nonpathogenic form, also is found in the minuta form and must be distinguished from the small tetranucleated-cyst form of *E. histolytica* in making a diagnosis. Although amebiasis is usually considered to be a gastrointestinal affliction, accompanied at times by the development of metastatic abscesses in the liver, the possibility that ulceration of the cervix uteri may be amebic in origin must be borne in mind. Cases of amebiasis of the female genital tract have been reported (8). The lesions resembled early carcinoma clinically, and in some instances *E. histolytica* was also found in the intestines.

In nature the incidence of *E. histolytica* infection appears to be low in chimpanzees, but those confined to animal quarters have developed high infection rates to both the small and the large races of the parasite. Deaths have resulted from amebic ulcerative colitis and from amebic abscesses in the livers and lungs of the parasitized animals (10).

Progressive and usually fatal amebic hepatitis can be induced in hamsters by the intrahepatic injection of a strain of *E. histolytica* and its bacterial associates from culture. The amebae appear to be the major etiologic agent (11). This species will develop in young kittens and these animals are frequently used as experimental hosts, but natural infections are unknown. According to Eyles *et al.* (4), dogs may be carriers of *E. histolytica.* They examined 143 dogs from a Tennessee dog pound for intestinal amebae and found the parasite in 12 (8.4 percent). They concluded that cysts of amebae are almost never passed and that trophozoite forms are eliminated in very small numbers in the feces of dogs. On the other hand Jordan (6) believes that subclinical infections may occur in nature and that dogs may spread the disease.

The organism is known to be widely distributed in tropical, subtropical, and temperate regions, although it is more prevalent in warm regions. The incidence of infection depends mainly on the sanitary conditions of the community, because the organism is voided from the host in feces.

Complement-fixation tests may be used as an aid in the diagnosis of amebiasis. The antigen is prepared from *E. histolytica* grown with a single species

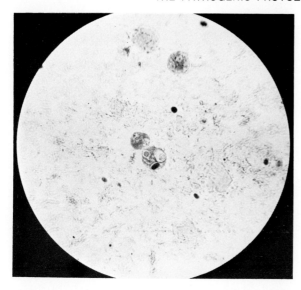

Fig. 109.   Entamoeba histolytica. A fecal specimen from man.
X 700.

of bacteria (5). Skin tests with an extract of *E. histolytica* have also been
employed successfully (9).

Emetine hydrochloride, metronidazole, diiodoquine, chloroquine, and arsenic and iodine compounds are useful in treating amebiasis. It also appears
that many of the antibiotics are amebacides. Among those shown to be effective are penicillin, streptomycin, chloromycetin, aureomycin, terramycin,
neomycin, bacitracin, fumagillin, erythromycin, polymyxin, fradicin, and
prodigiosin. Win 5047, the laboratory designation for N-(2,4-dichloro-
benzyl)-N-(2-hydroxyethyl) dichloroacetamide, is a synthetic nonarsenical
amebacide characterized by high activity and low toxicity (2).

*The Mastigophora* are sometimes called the *Flagellata*. This class includes
all the species that possess flagella during the greater part of their life span.
Flagella are seen temporarily at certain stages of development in some species that are not members of this class. Some members of this group live in
the intestinal and genital tracts and others live in the blood. Trypanosomes,
leishmanias, trichomonads, hexamitae, giardiae, and histomonads are members
of the *Mastigophora*.

*The Sporozoa* include forms that are exclusively parsitic in habit and that
at some stage in their development produce resistant spores enclosing one or
more sporozoites which carry the infection to new hosts. This group includes
the coccidia and many species of blood parasites, the hemosporidia.

*The ciliata* are protozoa that possess cilia in all stages of their development.
Most of them are free-living, nonparasitic forms. Only two genera are of enough
importance to warrant consideration here. They are *Balantidium* and *Tetrahymena*.

## REFERENCES

1. Burrows.   Am. Jour. Hyg., 1957, *65*, 172.
2. Dennis and Berberian.   Antibiotics and Chemother., 1954, *4*, 554.
3. Dow, Jarrett, Jennings, McIntyre, and Mulligan.   Jour. Am. Vet. Med. Assoc., 1959, *135*, 407.
4. Eyles, Jones, Jumper, and Drinnon.   Jour. Parisitol., 1954, *40*, 163.
5. Fulton, Joyner, and Price.   Jour. Trop. Med. and Hyg. (London), 1951, *54*, 27.
6. Jordan.   Vet. Med., 1967, *62*, 61.
7. Kudo.   Protozoology. 5th ed. C. C Thomas, Springfield, Ill., 1966.
8. McClatchie and Sambhi.   Ann. Trop. Med. and Parasitol., 1971, *65*, 207.
9. Maddison, Kagan, and Elsdon-Dew.   Am. Jour. Trop. Med. and Hyg., 1968, *17*, 540.
10. Miller and Bray.   Jour. Parsitol., 1966, *52*, 386.
11. Reinertson and Thompson.   Proc. Soc. Exp. Biol. and Med., 1951, *76*, 518.

# XXIX | The Mastigophora

## THE HISTOMONADS

### *Histomonas meleagridis*

This protozoon is regarded as the causative agent of infectious enterohepatitis or blackhead, a destructive disease of young turkeys. The same disease occurs in chickens, pheasants, quail, and peafowl, but these species are rather resistant and large mortalities are seldom experienced in them. They often are the means of introducing infection into flocks of turkeys.

Originally *Histomonas meleagridis* was thought to be an ameba but later it was found to be a flagellate. Kudo (15) classifies the organism in the family *Mastigamoebidae*. This family includes many free-living and a few parasitic forms. They are simple flagellates that are closely related to the ameba. In certain forms of the genus *Histomonas* one to four extremely fine flagella arise from a blepharoplast, located close to the nucleus.

**Morphology.** The organism is seen embedded in solid tissues as small spherical bodies from 8 to 10 microns in diameter. A few cells are larger. These cells possess a rather small nucleus, usually located excentrically, and a small "extranuclear" body, which was noted quite early (29) but whose function was not known until recently.

When small bits of tissue containing the parasites are placed on a warm slide and crushed in warm fluid, the organisms can be found in abundance. They are quite transparent. Ameboid activity can readily be seen if the slide is kept at a temperature of 42 C, which is the body temperature of the bird, but there is little if the temperature is kept at 37 C. This usually is the only type of motility exhibited by parasites removed from the tissue lesions. If the material is taken from the lumen of the intestine (cecum), the parasites resemble those seen in tissue preparation except that a different type of motility is present. The organisms rotate in a jerky manner, always going anticlockwise;

601

each sudden jerk turns the cell approximately 45 degrees. Tyzzer (24), who first observed this motion, correctly decided that it could be caused only by a kinetic apparatus within the cell. It is a flagellar motion, quite different from the ameboid motion exhibited by the tissue parasites. Tyzzer noted that when warm-stage preparations were left standing for several hours, the original ameboid activity gradually gave way to the pulsating jerky variety. Properly stained preparations indicate that the cells living free in the intestinal lumen have one, sometimes three or four, flagella. These are not seen on the tissue-inhabiting parasites.

The small "extranuclear" body seen by early observers is the blepharo-plast. This is located on the nuclear membrane or near the nucleus. The flagellum or flagella arise from it. These are rudimentary structures which often do not protrude beyond the cell wall.

The parasite of blackhead was first described by Smith (21), who gave it the name *Amoeba meleagridis*, since it resembled an ameba more than any other type of protozoa. Tyzzer (23) showed that it differed from any other protozoon known; hence he created a new genus for it, *Histomonas*.

**Cultural Features.** The first to cultivate the protozoon of blackhead was Drbohlav (7). The media were blood agar slants covered with Locke's solution and coagulated egg medium covered with the same solution. Later he found that slants made of coagulated egg albumen covered with a blood broth containing 1 percent peptone were better than either of the original media. Cultures were obtained from the cecal content and always contained bacteria upon which the *Histomonas* feeds. At times the protozoon also ingested blood cells. He did not succeed in obtaining pure cultures. Tyzzer (26), DeVolt and Davis (4), and Bishop (2) have reported success in cultivating the blackhead organism using methods similar to those used by Drbohlav. DeVolt and Davis found that the addition of a small amount of serum and a little rice starch to the coagulated egg medium gave better growths, but care had to be observed that the bacteria did not overgrow the protozoa. Transfers were made every 48 hours, and incubation was carried on at 42 C. If the bacteria appeared to be overgrowing the parasites, one or more transfers were made on egg medium covered with plain Locke's solution, in which the bacteria do not thrive. Cultures have been maintained by several workers for more than 1 year, and infections have been produced with them by rectal injections. No one has so far succeeded in obtaining cultures free of bacteria. Cultures from the liver lesions usually do not succeed.

In dealing with cultures it is necessary to guard against interpreting other flagellates as *Histomonas*. In practically every normal ceca there are flagellates belonging to the genus *Chilomastix*, and ameba and trichomonads are frequent. All of these will develop in the media described above.

*Histomonas* in cultures has the same appearance as the motile forms found in feces. If examined on a warm stage, the large spherical forms show the pulsating motion and the jerky anticlockwise movement already described. Sluggish ameboid activity may also be observed.

**Pathogenicity.** Turkeys are native American birds, at one time roaming the North American continent from southern Mexico to the northern border of the United States. The domesticated types of today are improved varieties originating in Mexico. Turkeys have been exported to all parts of the world, and blackhead has followed these shipments. This disease has been known in America since domestication of the bird began. In more recent years it has been found in various European countries, South Africa, Brazil, Japan, the Philippine Islands, and Australia. The disease probably exists wherever turkeys are raised.

This disease has been the principal reason for the difficulties encountered in successfully raising this species in flocks. Under flock conditions the disease tends to build up in intensity from year to year, and after a few seasons it becomes economically impraticable to raise these birds without using special methods of husbandry.

The disease is seen most often in young birds, that is, in birds varying in age from 3 weeks to 4 or 5 months. Losses occur in old turkeys but these usually are sporadic. The losses among young turkeys frequently exceed 50 percent, and sometimes all the young birds die. The losses among chickens are almost wholly in those of 5 to 10 weeks of age. Serious losses sometimes occur, but generally the disease disappears spontaneously after a few birds have been lost. An occasional case is seen among adult chickens. In young chickens a combined infection with *H. meleagridis* and *Eimeria tenella* is more likely to be fatal (18).

Affected turkey poults are inactive and refuse their food. They lose weight and walk with a stilted gait. There is diarrhea with light sulfur-colored droppings. They usually show symptoms for a number of days before they die. In chicks the disease runs a short course. The birds are depressed, gather around the brooder stove, and soon die.

The lesions of blackhead occur in the ceca and the liver. Other organs as a rule are normal. Sometimes there is fluid in the body cavity. The lesions have the same appearance in chickens and turkeys. The affected ceca are enlarged and their walls are thickened. Usually a core of grayish-yellow necrotic material mixed with excrement fills their lumen. When this core is removed, the wall of the organ is seen to be necrotic.

The liver lesions are quite characteristic in appearance. They consist of round necrotic areas, varying in diameter from microscopic size to several centimeters. They appear on the liver surface as smooth areas, somewhat firmer than normal liver consistency and somewhat depressed or concave. The color is mottled with green, yellow, and brown intermixed. Often concentric rings occur. Outside these areas, the liver substance is very dark and the entire organ is enlarged.

Allen (1) claims that *Trichomonas gallinarum* sometimes produces cecal and liver lesions that may easily be confused with those of blackhead and also that this trichomonad often is associated with the blackhead organism in the lesions of the liver. She describes three types of liver lesions: (*a*) those caused by pure infections with *Histomonas meleagridis,* already described above, (*b*) those caused by pure infections with *Tr. gallinarum,* which produce yellowish lesions up to 2 cm in diameter but which have less-well-defined borders than those of true blackhead and are raised rather than depressed with respect to the liver surface, and (*c*) those caused by mixed infections with these two organisms, which are large, circular, well-defined lesions, mottled in color and with markedly depressed centers but raised borders. Allen claims that it is possible to distinguish these three types of lesions from one another by gross inspection. When in doubt both organisms are easily identified in preparations made from the lesions. For further consideration of this subject, see *Trichomonas gallinarum* (p. 639).

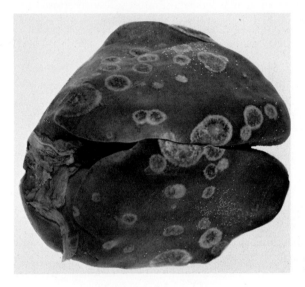

Fig. 110. Lesions of blackhead (histomoniasis) in the liver of a turkey.

Microscopic examination of the cecal wall shows myriads of the characteristic parasites located free in the tissue spaces. They are never found intracellularly except an occasional one that has been phagocytosed and probably is dead. In ordinary sections the parasites usually have shrunk and appear to lie in spaces a little larger than their own diameter. They stain with the acid dyes, and their nuclei are poorly stained and often not visible. The numbers are so great as to account for a considerable part of the thickening of the cecal wall. Necrosis is probably due as much to pressure as to the toxic materials that they may secrete. Parasites may be seen in the necrotic material in the lumen of the organ. These have the same appearance in sections as those embedded in the tissues. When examined in fresh preparations, those forms show flagellate motility, whereas those from the tissues usually show the ameboid type.

The liver lesions are caused by parasites that escape by the blood stream from the cecal lesions. The parasites multiply in the sinusoids of the liver, causing pressure and possibly toxic necrosis of the neighboring liver cells. The lesions attract large numbers of lymphocytes in the early stages. Necrosis occurs and gradually the lesions enlarge. The older lesions consist of myriads of parasites embedded in necrotic tissue. Epithelioid and giant cells usually appear in limited numbers in the older lesions. The necrotic tissue is surrounded by a mild inflammatory zone but there is no capsule formation.

**Mode of Infection.** Experimentally, blackhead is not easily produced by the feeding of tissues or discharges of acutely infected birds. If large amounts of material are given, a few birds will be successfully infected. The disease can be produced much more regularly by injecting infective material per rectum. Very young poults and chicks can be infected fairly regularly in this way. If infected birds are placed among normal birds on clean ground, i.e., ground upon which chickens and turkeys have not previously lived, the disease will not spread (22). If old turkeys or chickens are allowed to run with young turkeys, or if the young turkeys are allowed to run on ground that had previously been used for raising either chickens or turkeys, severe outbreaks can be expected.

These peculiarities were explained by the finding of Graybill and Smith (10) that a common nematode, *Heterakis gallinae*, belonging to the ascarid family and having its habitat in the ceca of turkeys, chickens, and other birds, played an important part in the transmission of this disease. These parasites, living in the lumen of the ceca, ingest the protozoa of blackhead in considerable numbers. The protozoa penetrate the intestinal wall of the worm and reach its body cavity. These stages may readily be followed with the microscope. The succeeding stages have not been followed microscopically but apparently the organism reaches the ovary and in some form exists in the ova of the worm. The evidence for this was furnished by Tyzzer and Fabyan (29), who showed that ova that had been embryonated in 1.5 percent nitric acid, which renders them bacteriologically sterile, were capable of producing blackhead when fed to young turkeys. Tyzzer (25) and others have studiously examined many infected worm eggs without being able to find any morphological evidence of the protozoa. The Japanese investigator Niimi (19) claims to have found minute forms varying from 1 to 1.4 microns in diameter in infected worm eggs; these he believes to be the protozoa. Kendall (14) has also reported the occurrence of parasites in *H. gallinae* which be believed to be *H. meleadgridis*.

The cecal worm is distributed widely and is present in practically every adult chicken, turkey, pheasant, grouse, and other species that is susceptible to blackhead. Apparently also the protozoon of blackhead is widely distributed among adult birds of these species, and therefore most of the ova of the cecal worm carry the parasite of blackhead. To produce blackhead experimentally one has only to feed fairly large doses of the embryonated eggs of the cecal worm, or to place the birds at their most susceptible age on soil that is infected with such ova as a result of having been used previously for poultry range. The feeding of embryonated *Heterakis* ova collected from single adult birds will not always produce blackhead, thus indicating that not all *Heterakis* ova are infective; yet infection seldom fails when ova from several birds are used whether or not there has been clinically recognized blackhead in the flock from which the turkeys originated. Apparently the damage caused by the localization of the young nemotodes in the cecal pouches provides a portal of entry into the cecal wall for the blackhead parasite. It is claimed that grasshoppers can carry infected nemotode ova in a viable form in their intestines for at least 96 hours and initiate infection in poults allowed to feed on them. The feeding of blackhead material without the worm eggs usually fails to infect, presumably because of the lack of the preliminary damage from the larval worms. Lund *et al.* (16) have stated that earthworms from infected premises may act as vectors in the transmission of *Heterakis* and *Histomonas* to turkeys and chickens.

Outside the host, the protozoon of blackhead will maintain viability for only a few hours. It has been well demonstrated, however, that the infective agent of the disease will remain alive in the soil of poultry yards for many months and may survive one or more severe winters. It is obvious that these persistent forms are those which are harbored by the *Heterakis* eggs.

**Experimental Blackhead.** Tyzzer and Fabyan (28) demonstrated that an experimental disease of turkeys, different from the natural form, could be produced by the subcutaneous injection of material containing the *H. meleagridis*. This type of the disease can be propagated indefinitely. It is manifested by the development of a local lesion at the point where the inoculum has been deposited. This can be seen after a few days and then rapidly develops into a granulomatous lesion of considerable size. After several weeks metastasis occurs to the lungs, where several lesions usually develop. From the lung lesions tertiary lesions in many organs develop if the bird lives long enough to permit it. The disease is always fatal. It is characterized by weakness, loss of appetitie, weight loss, and the appearance of sulfur-colored feces—all of which are characteristic of the natural disease—and, in addition, coughing.

McGuire and Morehouse (17) produced fatal cases of blackhead by injecting citrated whole blood withdrawn from veins draining the ceca of diseased donor birds into the wing veins of susceptible turkeys. This procedure produced typical lesions of blackhead in the liver with atypical involvement of lungs, kidneys, heart, spleen, pancreas, and proventriculus, but did not involve the ceca or the lower intestinal tract. It is possible that the liver acts as a filter in usually preventing involvement of other tissues when infection proceeds by natural routes. Peardon and Ware (20) also produced atypical foci of histomoniasis lesions by feeding blackhead-infected tissues to 3-week-old turkey poults. The lesions were found in proventriculi, lungs, kidneys, and hearts, as well as in livers and ceca.

In chickens subcutaneous inoculation results only in the production of a local lesion which rapidly heals. Similar lesions develop in about one-third of inoculated pigeons. Rabbits, guinea pigs, and mice are not susceptible to such inoculations.

DeVolt and Davis (4) produced what they called a *histomonal sinusitis* by placing small bits of infected liver tissue in the facial sinus. Lesions developed causing distortion of the facial bones, metastasis to the lungs, and death. The whole picture is similar to that produced by subcutaneous inoculation.

Experimental infection can be produced by injecting diseased cecal tissue from freshly killed infected turkeys into young poults. According to Farmer *et al.* (9), the infection spreads from the ceca to the liver via the blood stream, and in the latter stages of the disease the spleen may be involved.

Doll and Franker (6) have made the interesting observation that the infectivity of *H. gallinae* or the pathogenicity of *H. meleagridis*, or both, is influenced by the bacterial flora of the host.

**Immunity.** Tyzzer (26, 27) has succeeded in conveying a considerable degree of immunity to young turkeys by inoculating them with a culture strain of *H. meleagridis* that had become avirulent. About 2 weeks after inoculation with the vaccine strain, both turkey poults and chicks showed a high degree of immunity to natural infection with fully virulent strains. The immunity is lost rather early unless the birds are exposed continuously to natural infection. In birds that have lost their immunity, a high percentage of recoveries indicates that all resistance has not been lost. Serum transferred from immune to nonimmune birds does not protect the latter.

**Chemotherapy.** DeVolt and Holst (5) have reported that vioform (5-chloro-7-iodo-8-hydroxyquinoline) and clioform (5-chloro-8-hydroxyquinoline) are effective against this infection. Another drug that has received much attention is enheptin (2-amino-5-nitrothiazole), also known as ANT. According to Jungherr and Winn (13), 0.05 percent of this substance in the feed prevents the disease and 0.1 percent is effective after the appearance of clinical symptoms. However, Grumbles *et al.* (11) have found that the feeding of ANT to turkey hens in a concentration of 0.1 percent for 18 weeks reduces egg production, fertility, and hatchability. At this writing it would appear that enheptin A (2-acetylamino-5-nitrothiazole), dimetridazole (1,2-dimethyl-5-nitroimidazole), and nidrafur (5-nitro-2-furaldehyde acetylhydrazone) all provide effective protection against losses from histomoniasis (12).

**Surgical Prevention.** Durant (8) has shown that blackhead can be prevented by surgical abligation of the ceca. This involves opening the body cavity and ligating the ceca so that no connection exists thereafter with the remainder of the intestinal lumen. Delaplane and Stuart (3) vary Durant's procedure by the use of aluminum clamps, which accomplish the same purpose. The operations are attended with considerable surgical mortality and are time-consuming; hence the methods are not likely to be used as practical procedures. They are, however, of interest as indicating that the walls of the ceca are the only natural points of entry of this infection.

**Practical Control.** Practical control of this disease has been accomplished by large growers through the institution of sanitary measures. The young poults are incubator-hatched and kept in clean surroundings away from adult birds (turkeys and chickens) until they are well grown. Infections are thus prevented by keeping the young birds away from infected feces and cecal worms. Phenothiazine is effective in controlling the latter but will not eradicate the disease.

## REFERENCES

1. Allen. Am. Jour. Vet. Res., 1941, 2, 214.
2. Bishop. Parasitology, 1938, 30, 181.
3. Delaplane and Stuart. Jour. Am. Vet. Med. Assoc., 1933, 83, 238.
4. DeVolt and Davis. Univ. Maryland, Bul. 392, 1936.
5. DeVolt and Holst. Poultry Sci., 1949, 28, 641.
6. Doll and Franker. Jour. Parasitol., 1963, 49, 411.
7. Drbohlav. Jour. Med. Res., 1924, 44, 677.
8. Durant. Vet. Med., 1926, 21, 392.
9. Farmer, Hughes, and Whiting. Jour. Comp. Path. and Therap., 1952, 61, 251.
10. Graybill and Smith. Jour. Exp. Med., 1920, 31, 647.
11. Grumbles, Boney, and Turk. Am. Jour. Vet. Res., 1952, 13, 386.
12. Hall, Flowers, and Grumbles. Avian Dis., 1965, 317, 400.
13. Jungherr and Winn. Poultry Sci., 1950, 29, 462.
14. Kendall. Parasitology, 1959, 49, 169.
15. Kudo. Protozoology. 5th ed. C. C Thomas, Springfield, Ill., 1966.
16. Lund, Wehr, and Ellis. Jour. Parasitol., 1966, 52, 899.
17. McGuire and Morehouse. *Ibid.*, 1958, 44, 292.
18. Ohara and Reid. Avian Dis., 1961, 5, 355.
19. Nimi. Jour. Jap. Soc. Vet. Med., 1937, 16, 183.
20. Peardon and Ware. Avian Dis., 1969, 13, 340.
21. Smith. U.S. Dept. Agr., Bur. Anim. Indus. Bul. 8, 1895.
22. Smith. Jour. Exp. Med., 1917, 25, 405.
23. Tyzzer. Jour. Med. Res., 1919, 40, 1.
24. Tyzzer. Jour. Parasitol., 1920, 6, 124.
25. Tyzzer. Proc. Soc. Exp. Biol. and Med., 1926, 23, 708.
26. Tyzzer. Jour. Parasitol., 1932, 19, 158.
27. Tyzzer. Jour. Comp. Path. and Therap., 1936, 49, 285.
28. Tyzzer and Fabyan. · Jour. Inf. Dis., 1920, 27, 207.
29. Tyzzer and Fabyan. Jour. Exp. Med., 1922, 35, 791.

## THE TRYPANOSOMES

The most important disease-producing members of the *Mastigophora* belong to the family *Trypanosomatidae*. This family contains seven genera. They embrace parasites in vertebrates, invertebrates, and plants. All forms resemble each other in that they possess a nucleus and a single flagellum which arises from a small body, embedded in the cytoplasm and known as the *blepharoplast*. Just posterior to the blepharoplast and very near to it is a deeply staining sturcture known as the *parabasal body*. The composite structure consisting of the blepharoplast and the parabasal body is known as the *kinetoplast*.

During the course of their development in vertebrate and invertebrate hosts members of the family may pass through a number of characteristic stages which are distinguished morphologically. The leishmanial stage comprises an oval body in which the nucleus and kinetoplast are visible but the flagellum is rudimentary or absent, and in no case does it extend outside the cell wall. These cells, therefore, are nonmotile. The leptomonal stage consists of an elongated cell with a nucleus located more or less centrally. The kinetoplast is located near the anterior end of the cell and the flagellum extends well beyond the cell wall, constituting an effective means of locomotion. An undulating membrane is not present in this group. The cell body of the crithidial stage is elongated and similar to that of the previous group, but the kinetoplast is located near but slightly anterior to the nucleus, i.e., near the center of the cell body. The flagellum passes out of the side of the cell into a protoplasmic ridge, known as an *undulating membrane*, of which it constitutes the outer or free margin. At the anterior end of the cell of the flagellum leaves the undulating membrane and extends well forward as a free lash. The trypanosomal stage resembles the crithidial except that the kinetoplast is located well behind the nucleus toward the posterior end of the cell and the flagellum leaves the side of the cell near its posterior end and enters into an undulating membrane which runs nearly the entire length of the cell. At the anterior end of the cell the flagellum leaves the membrane and passes farther forward as a free lash. The free margin of the undulating membrane in both crithidia and trypanosomes is longer than the attached margin; hence it is thrown into folds or ruffles which have an undulating movement when in action.

The family is divided into genera according to the degree of development reached.

1. *Leishmania*. The organisms do not develop beyond the leishmanial stage in vertebrate hosts, but reach the leptomonal stage in invertebrate hosts or in cultures.

2. *Leptomonas*. This genus is confined to invertebrates and does not develop beyond the leptomonal stage.

3. *Phytomonas*. This genus resembles *Leptomonas*, but all species occur in plants and are transmitted by invertebrate intermediate hosts.

4. *Crithidia*. This genus shows leptomonal and crithidial stages during development. It is confined to invertebrates.

5. *Herpetomonas*. This genus develops to the trypanosomal stage but is confined to invertebrates.

6. *Trigomonas*. This genus develops to the trypanosomal stage in plants.

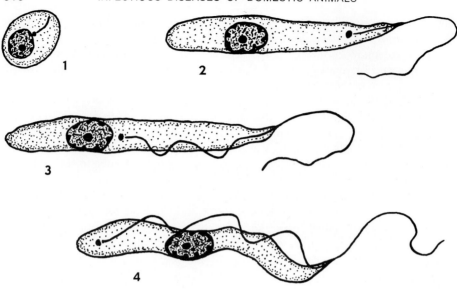

*Fig. 111.* Diagrammatic representation of the *Trypanosomatidae.* (1) *Leishmania.* (2) *Leptomonas.* (3) *Crithidia.* (4) *Trypanosoma.*

7. *Trypanosoma.* This genus develops to the trypanosomal stage in vertebrates.

Only *Leishmania* and *Trypanosoma* have organisms that are parasitic and pathogenic for vertebrates. These are the only genera that will be considered further.

## THE *LEISHMANIA*

Flagellates of the genus *Leishmania* occur in leptomonal and leishmanial forms, and they may be found in both vertebrate and invertebrate hosts. That these organisms are flagellates was first demonstrated by the development of flagellated forms of the leptomonal type in citrate solution to which infected splenic material had been added.

### Leishmania donovani

SYNONYM:   Leishman-Donovan bodies

This parasite is the causative agent of a malarialike disease of man known as kala azar or dumdum fever, which is endemic in India, China, southern Russia, and the countries of Europe that border on the Mediterranean Sea. The disease is found in the northern countries of Africa as well as in Abyssinia, the Sudan, northern Kenya, and Nigeria. It also occurs in South America. The parasite usually is found within large endothelial cells of the capillaries and is concentrated in the spleen, bone marrow, lymph nodes, and liver. Usually very few are found in the blood stream, and diagnosis by means of blood smears, therefore, is very uncertain. For diagnosis, spleen or liver

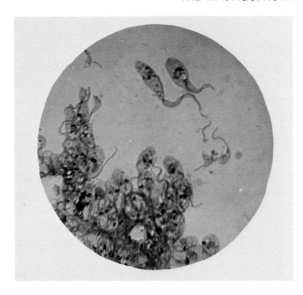

*Fig. 112.* Crithidial form of *Trypanosoma melophagium,* showing stained film of a culture on artificial media. Note that the flagellum originates in a kinetoplast located near but slightly anterior to the nucleus and that an undulating membrane is present.

puncture is frequently done. The endothelial cells of these organs usually contain large numbers of the parasite.

In man another disease, known as *oriental sore* or *Delhi boil,* is caused by a member of the group, *Leishmania tropica.* This is regarded as a separate species although it cannot be distinguished with certainty from *L. Donovani. L. tropica* seems to show a wider range of form and size than the latter. It occurs frequently in regions bordering the Mediterranean Sea, but it is also found in Asia, Australia (9), and Panama (2). The organisms are present in the endothelial cells in and around cutaneous lesions located on hands, feet, legs, face, etc. The lesion and organisms tend to be confined to the primary site of infection.

Another form, *L. braziliensis,* causes the South American naso-oral leishmaniasis. Its morphological characteristics are identical with those of *L. tropica* (9).

Since World War II Packchanian (13) has reported two cases of *L. tropica* infection in United States soldiers who were stationed in Iran, and Levy and Yiengst (10) diagnosed a case of kala azar in a soldier returned from the orient. In the latter case the incubation period was at least 18 months. In 1966 four cases of cutaneous leishmaniasis were encountered in a hospital in Philadelphia (6). One was caused by *L. braziliensis,* acquired in Guatemala, and three were caused by *L. tropica,* probably acquired in Israel.

In Panama it has been shown that both the two-toed sloth (*Cholopeus hoffmanni*) and the three-toed sloth (*Bradypus infuscatus*) are subject to infection with a strain of *Leishmania* that is indistinguishable from the *L. braziliensis* type isolated from man (7).

The transmitting agents of the disease are sandflies, which are dipterous insects belonging to the genus *Phlebotomus* (14). DDT can be used to control leishmaniasis by destroying the sandflies.

**Morphology and Cultural Features.** *L. donovani* usually is ovoid in outline. It measures from 1.5 to 2.5 by 2 to 5 microns. Multiplication is by binary fission, and dividing forms are frequently seen in spleen pulp films. Artificial culture was first obtained by immersing bits of infected spleen pulp in a sodium citrate solution, but continued cultivation by this method is not successful. The best medium for initial as well as continuous cultivation is the well-known NNN medium, now commonly used for the cultivation of most of the pathogenic trypanosomes. This medium consists merely of an agar jelly made up of agar and saline solution to which 10 percent fresh defibrinated rabbit blood is added just before use. The medium is slanted and growth of the flagellates occurs in the water of syneresis. This medium will support vigorous growth of *L. donovani* indefinitely. The medium takes its name from the fact that it was described by Nicolle and is a modification of a medium first used by Novy and McNeal (Nicolle-Novy-McNeal).

**Pathogenicity for Dogs.** Dogs in the kala azar districts, and especially in the Mediterranean region, have frequently been found infected with this parasite (12, 17). Some have suggested, in fact, that the dog is the natural reservoir from which human infections are derived, but there is little support for this idea. In 1968 Bray and Dabbagh (1) examined 132 dogs, 52 rodents, and 2 jackals from the Baghdad area by spleen films and by culture and found that all were negative for leishmaniae. Apparently dogs are exposed to the same sources of infection as man and obtain the infection from them in the same way. There is evidence that rodents, especially certain species of rats, are the vertebrate reservoir (8) and that sandflies of the "*Synphlebotomus*" complex are the chief vectors (16).

The disease in dogs is much like that of man. It may be acute or chronic and the mortality may be great, frequently because of intercurrent infections, sometimes because of the uncomplicated disease. There is great enlargement and hardening of the spleen and liver; there is fever, leukopenia, anemia, and loss of weight and general vitality. In dogs, *Leishmania* are rarely found in the peripheral blood and often they are scarce in the liver. Because the spleen is rather hard to puncture in dogs, bone marrow is often collected by trephining one of the long bones of the legs (5).

What is believed to be the first reported case of visceral leishmaniasis in a dog in the United States appeared in 1955. The dog had been imported from Greece (15). Since then several other cases have been noted in dogs imported into the United States (4, 11). Even though sandflies are found in the areas where the diagnoses were made it does not appear that the disease was transmitted to native dogs.

Duxbury and Sadun (3) have used an indirect FA technic in the serodiagnosis of kala azar in man and claim that it is a reliable test.

**Immunity.** Animals that recover from leishmaniasis are said to be immune thereafter. Vaccination against *L. donovani* infection has not been effective, but vaccination against *L. tropica* infection has proved useful in protecting children from the disease.

**Chemotherapy.** Antimony compounds (e.g., tartar emetic) are used in treating leishmaniasis. They are applied locally or given intravenously and apparently have a marked specific effect on the parasite.

## REFERENCES

1. Bray and Dabbagh.   Jour. Trop. Med. and Hyg. (London), 1968, *71*, 46.
2. Calero and Johnson.   Am. Jour. Trop. Med. and Hyg., 1953, 2, 628.
3. Duxbury and Sadun.   *Ibid.*, 1964, *13*, 525.
4. Gleiser, Thiel, and Cashell.   *Ibid.*, 1957, *6*, 227.
5. Gray.   Bul. Soc. Path. Exot., 1913, *6*, 165.
6. Hambrick, Jr. and Even-Paz.   Jour. Am. Med. Assoc., 1966, *198*, 965.
7. Herrer and Telford, Jr.   Science, 1969, *164*, 1419.
8. Hoogstraal, Van Peenen, Reid, and Dietlein.   Am. Jour. Trop. Med. and Hyg., 1963, *12*, 175.
9. Kudo.   Protozoology. 5th ed. C. C Thomas, Springfield, Ill., 1966.
10. Levy and Yiengst.   Jour. Am. Med. Assoc., 1948, *136*, 81.
11. McConnell, Chaffee, Cashell, and Garner.   Jour. Am. Vet. Med. Assoc., 1970, *156*, 197.
12. Nicolle.   Comp. rend. Acad. Sci., 1908, *146*, 789.
13. Packchanian.   Jour. Am. Med. Assoc., 1945, *129*, 544.
14. Richardson and Kendall.   Veterinary protozoology. 3d. ed. Oliver and Boyd, London, 1963.
15. Thorson, Bailey, Hoerlein, and Seibold.   Am. Jour. Trop. Med. and Hyg., 1955, *4*, 18.
16. Wijers and Minter.   Ann. Trop. Med. and Parasitol., 1962, *56*, 462.
17. Yakimoff and Kohl-Yakimoff.   Arch. l'Inst. Past., Tunis, 1911, *6*, 249.

## THE NONPATHOGENIC TRYPANOSOMES

### *Trypanosoma lewisi*

This species of trypanosome occurs in wild rats the world over and can very easily be transmitted by artificial inoculation to white rats. The rats show very little evidence of the infection, as a rule, but some strains of *Tr. lewisi* appear to possess a certain amount of pathogenicity. There is evidence that cortisone treatment of rats enhances the virulence of the parasite, probably resulting from an impairment of the host immune reaction (2).

**Morphology.** Shortly after inoculation the forms that appear in the blood vary greatly in appearance from *Leishmania*like cells to very broad trypanosomes with long flagella. After the multiplicative stage has passed, the individuals become much more uniform in size and shape. As seen in unstained blood, they are exceedingly active, dashing here and there, knocking the cells about. The parasites are about 25 microns long and have pointed ends and a curved body. The kinetoplast is situated at some distance from the posterior end. The nucleus is a little forward of the center of the body. The undulating membrane is not markedly folded and thus the flagellum is fairly straight. The sharp posterior end and the curved body give this species a characteristic appearance.

During the multiplicative period parasites in various stages of development may be seen in the blood. Division of the kinetoplast first occurs, followed by that of the nucleus. Two flagella are now formed, and the cell splits between them forming two individuals. Before one division is complete others may begin; hence compound structures are sometimes seen.

**Cultural Features.** *Tr. lewisi* is readily cultivated in NNN medium. All the forms of the *Trypanosomatidae* are produced in cultures, the trypanosome form gradually giving way to the simpler ones. The virulence for rats is maintained for a long time.

**Transmission.** Various rat fleas are the transmitting agents. Infection is not conveyed by the bite, because the mouthparts of the fleas are not infected. Transmission apparently occurs through the ingestion, by the rats, of fecal material from the fleas, or from ingestion of whole fleas. The newly diseased flea does not become immediately infective for rats. The parasite undergoes definite cyclical changes in the flea which require about 6 days for completion before the infective stage is again reached.

**Immunity.** The serum of rats that have recovered from infection with *Tr. lewisi* agglutinates and frequently lyses suspensions of the organism. In agglutination the parasites form clumps in which the individuals are attached by their posterior ends. The serum of recovered rats inhibits the development of the parasites in culture.

### Trypanosoma melophagium

This trypanosome occurs in a large percentage of all sheep, in some flocks occurring in 80 percent or more of all animals. It is similar to *Tr. theileri* in form and size and in the fact that it is wholly nonpathogenic. It undergoes its life cycle in the sheep "tick" or ked. Infection of the sheep is not through the bite of the insect, because it is not the head parts but rather the lower parts of the insect's intestine that are infective. Transmission apparently occurs through the rubbing of the excrement of the ked into bite wounds or other abrasions of the skin.

The parasite is found rather sparingly in the blood of the affected sheep but can be demonstrated readily with the cultural method described under *Tr. theileri*. In the ked the parasite develops in the intestinal canal largely in the crithidia form. If all keds are removed from an infected sheep, the parasite rather quickly disappears from the sheep's blood, showing that the reservoir of the infection is really the ked.

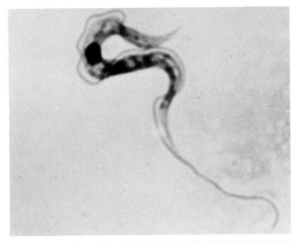

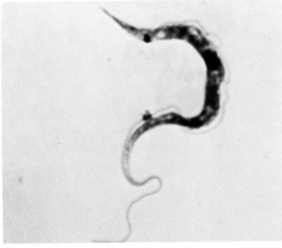

Fig. 113. Trypanosoma theileri from the blood of a cow. X
2,690. (Courtesy G. Dikmans, *Cornell Vet.*)

### *Trypanosoma theileri*

SYNONYMS: *Trypanosoma americanum, Trypanosoma franki,* and others

In 1903 Theiler found a large trypanosome in the blood of an apparently normal cow. Laveran later named it *Tr. theileri* in honor of its discoverer. Many observers in later years have seen such trypanosomes, and many new names have been given to them. All of these may not be identical with Theiler's, but they are similar in morphology and similar in that they are nonpathogenic to their hosts. In 1957 Dikmans *et al.* (3) isolated a trypanosome from the stomach of an aborted bovine fetus and identified it as *Tr. theileri.* In general, the organism continues to be regarded as nonpathogenic, but it has been associated with subnormal milk production, fever and diarrhea, so-called *turning sickness,* abortion, contamination of tissue cultures of bovine origin (4), and with bovine lymphocytosis (2).

**Morphology.** This is a very large trypanosome, some individuals measuring as much as 60 to 70 microns in length. Others are only half as large.

**Transmission.** The parasite evidently is transmitted by several types of bloodsucking flies. Tabanids have definitely been incriminated in a few cases. It is also possible that other biting insects may be involved in the transmission of *Tr. theileri.* Although most species of trypanosomes seem to have a favorite route, none appears to be limited entirely to a single means of transmission. Bats, fleas, ticks, lice, and many species of biting flies, including sandflies, have been implicated in the spread of the various species of trypanosomes from animal to animal.

**Pathogenicity.** Cattle seem not to be affected in any way by the presence of the trypanosome, and no other animals are known to harbor it. The parasite usually is very scarce in the blood, so scarce that it can be found only occasionally on direct microscopic examination. In case the parasite cannot be found, it may often be demonstrated culturally by using a simple technic. One part of the animal's blood is secured aseptically and added to two parts of plain infusion broth. The tube is incubated at 25 C or at room temperature. In about 1 week growth of the trypanosome becomes evident as small whitish colonies that lie on the surface of the mass of sedimented blood cells, contrasting sharply with the dark color of the blood. In these colonies every flagellate type from *Leishmania* to large trypanosomes is seen. In many areas 50 to 75 percent of the cattle may be shown to be harboring *Tr. theileri.*

### Avian Trypanosomes

Trypanosomes occur quite commonly in many species of wild birds. They are rare in the domestic species. Many of these trypanosomes have been given specific names, especially related to the host in which they are found, but these are not of importance in this work.

The morphology varies considerably. Baker (1) has shown that one of the louse flies, *Ornithomyia avicularia,* is a vector, and in some cases mosquitoes have been incriminated. The degree of pathogenicity in most instances is not high, and many of the trypanosomes seem to be practically harmless.

The bird trypanosomes are readily cultivated in NNN medium and even on the surface of blood agar plates. Infections can often be diagnosed by cultural means when the organisms are not readily found microscopically.

## THE PATHOGENIC TRYPANOSOMES

Pathogenic trypanosomes may be divided roughly into four general categories: (1) the brucei group embracing *Tr. brucei, Tr. gambiense,* and *Tr. rhodesiense;* (2) the congolense group consisting of *Tr. congolense* and *Tr. simiae;* (3) the vivax group containing *Tr. vivax* and *Tr. uniforme;* and (4) the evansi group including *Tr. evansi, Tr. equinum,* and *Tr. equiperdum.* The evansi group differs sharply from the others in that the species are never dependent on tsetse flies for transmission. Certain other trypanosomes of Central and South America that are not listed in this grouping are also considered.

### Trypanosoma brucei

This trypanosome was discovered by Bruce in 1895 and is the cause of a destructive disease afflicting domestic animals that are taken into many parts of the African continent, notably Rhodesia, the Sudan, Uganda, Tanganyika, and, in general, nearly all parts of tropical Africa. This disease and certain other African trypanosomal infections of animals are called *nagana.*

**Morphology.** *Tr. brucei* varies considerably in shape and size, even in the same host. There is a short broad form without a flagellum, a long slender form with a long flagellum, and an intermediate form. In some of the broad forms the nucleus is displaced posteriorly, especially when the parasite is growing in rats, mice, and guinea pigs, and this characteristic is of some diagnostic importance. The parasitic cells average 22 microns long, but they vary from 12 to 35 microns.

**Transmission.** *Tr. brucei* is transmitted by various species of tsetse flies (genus *Glossina*), as was shown first by Bruce in 1897. These flies may transmit the disease by contamination, i.e., by carrying the blood parasite directly from one animal to another. A short time after feeding on an infected animal, however, the fly becomes noninfective and remains so for 18 to 20 days. It then again becomes infective and remains so for the remainder of its life. During this time the trypanosome undergoes cyclical changes in the fly, first in the intestine, then in other organs; finally it reaches the salivary glands. Here the crithidia forms await the opportunity to infect a new host at the time the next blood meal is taken by the fly.

**Reservoir Hosts.** In his early investigations in Zululand, Bruce showed that the tsetse flies were infective for dogs that he had taken into the country with him. Because there were no domestic animals in the area, it was obvious that reservoirs of the infection existed in some of the wild animals abundant there. Later studies showed that about 30 percent of the wild animals harbored the parasite in small numbers, apparently without being materially harmed by them.

**Pathogenicity.** Horses, mules, and donkeys are very susceptible to infection. A severe disease also occurs in camels and dogs. Cattle are relatively resistant, but sheep and goats suffer as severely as horses. Pigs appear to be resistant, a chronic infection occurring. The highly susceptible animals usually die from the disease in from 2 weeks to 3 months. Even the more resistant animals eventually succumb to the parasite if untreated. By inoculation *Tr. brucei* is the most virulent of all trypanosomes. It will infect practically all mammals, except certain races of monkeys and man.

Nagana gets its name from a native word that signifies weakness. The disease is manifested by swellings around the neck and legs, fluctuating fever, loss of appetite, and muscular weakness. The affected animals become very anemic. The parasite is found in large numbers in the bone marrow after death, but only a few can be found in the blood stream. The spleen is greatly enlarged and the pericardial sac usually is filled with fluid.

### Trypanosoma gambiense and Trypanosoma rhodesiense

Human trypanosomiasis occurs only in restricted areas of Africa, especially in lowlands close to the water courses in the more tropical parts of the continent. In some of these areas the causative agent is a trypanosome known as *Trypanosoma gambiense*. This parasite is morphologically identical with *Tr. rhodesiense* and with *Tr. brucei*. These organisms differ in their behavior in the vertebrate host. *Tr. gambiense* is transmitted from man to man by means of its insect vector, *Glossina palpalis,* and no important wild animal reservoir has been demonstrated (9). The disease is believed to be confined to forest belts because the parasite is unable to produce a potent infection in the lower animals and because *G. palpalis* is restricted to such areas. Human infections are chronic, leading to final emaciation, weakness, and encephalitis, which gives to the disease its common name, *sleeping sickness.*

In some areas where nagana is prevalent and severe, human cases are practically unknown. In others, however, human infections are frequent and much more acute and fatal than the typical sleeping sickness disease. These cases are caused by *Tr. rhodesiense*. Like *Tr. brucei,* this parasite is transmitted by tsetse flies of the *G. morsitans* group. The strain is maintained in wild animals; man is an accidental host. *Tr. rhodesiense* is far more virulent in man and in animals than *Tr. gambiense*. It is possible that *Tr. rhodesiense* is a strain of *Tr. brucei* that has become specifically adapted to man although *Tr. brucei* is not infective for man. *Tr. rhodesiense* is scattered at present within the savannah fly belts of tropical Africa, but may eventually invade the forest belts because of its ability to infect animals and also to develop in *G. palpalis.*

Sleeping sickness is not unknown in Europeans returning from endemic regions in Africa. Early diagnosis and treatment usually results in a cure (1).

### Trypanosoma congolense

This small trypanosome is the one most commonly associated with the cattle disease known in South Africa as *nagana*. It also affects horses, sheep, goats, camels, and dogs. Most pigs are at least partly resistant. It occurs in many parts of tropical Africa. The parasite averages 14 microns in length, varying from 9 to 18. There is no flagellum; that is, the axoneme or intracellular part of the flagellum is present, arising in the blepharoplast and running along the margin of the undulating membrane, as usual, but it does not extend forward as a free whip or lash as in most forms. The nucleus is located in the middle of the cell.

*Tr. congolense* produces a chronic wasting disease associated with fever and anemia. Transmission is by means of several species of tsetse flies in which a definite life cycle occurs. Wild game animals are the natural reservoir of infection.

### Trypanosoma simiae

This organism resembles some of the longer forms of *Tr. congolense*. It is about 14 to 24 microns in length. It was originally isolated from a monkey. It is highly virulent for pigs, camels, and monkeys. It does not appear to cause disease in horses, cattle, or dogs. It may produce mild infection in sheep and goats. It occurs in Africa and follows the same general distribution as *Tr. congolense*.

### Trypanosoma vivax

This trypanosome is widely distributed throughout the tsetse fly areas of Africa. Wenyon found 76 percent of the humped cattle of the Gold Coast of West Africa to be infected. It occurs most commonly in cattle, sheep, and goats but also affects horses. The disease is similar to, but less virulent than, that caused by *Tr. congolense;* nevertheless the average mortality is high. It produces mild infection in camels. Pigs and dogs are resistant, the dog particularly so. Guinea pigs, rats, and mice are refractory to inoculation. The disease is transmitted by several species of tsetse flies, in which a definite life cycle occurs. Antelopes and other members of the deer family constitute the natural reservoir of infection.

*Tr. vivax* obtained its specific name from the fact that it is an exceedingly active parasite. It measures from 18 to 26 microns in length. The posterior end of the body is broader than the anterior; consequently the greater part of the cytoplasm lies posterior to the nucleus. The undulating membrane is less well developed than in most trypanosomes. The flagellum, as a consequence, is straighter than usual.

*Tr. vivax* was first observed in South America (French Guiana) in 1919 by Leger and Vienne (5). Later it was reported in Venezuela, the islands of Guadeloupe and Martinique, Colombia, Dutch Guiana, and Panama (Johnson, 3). *Glossina* are considered the natural transmitters of *Tr. vivax* but are not indispensable, for the disease has spread on the American continent, where *Glossina* do not occur, probably being carried by bloodsucking insects such as *Stomoxys* and *Tabanus*. There also is evidence that sandflies (genus *Phlebotomus*) transmit certain trypanosomes (6). The pathogenicity is similar to that of the African species.

### Trypanosoma uniforme

This parasite appears to bear a very close relationship to *Tr. vivax*, from which it differs only in its smaller size. Although it is regarded as an African type, in 1970 Woo *et al.* (11) isolated *Tr. theileri* and a smaller type which they considered to be morphologically similar to *Tr. uniforme* from cattle in southern Ontario.

### Trypanosoma evansi

This organism is the cause of a disease that occurs principally in southern Asiatic countries and is known under the name of *surra*. The disease is most virulent for horses but also affects camels, elephants, and dogs. Cattle and the water buffalo (carabao) are susceptible, but the disease in them is very mild and recovery generally occurs. Man is not susceptible.

The disease occurs in India, Burma, Ceylon, South China, Siam, Sumatra, Java, the Philippines, Madagascar, Iran, and Arabia. Infected horses have been imported into Australia and the United States, but vigilance has prevented the disease from getting a foothold. A disease of camels, which apparently is surra of a mild type, occurs throughout Northern and Central Africa. It affects horses as well as dromedaries, the disease being milder in this species than in Asiatic camels.

**Morphology.** The trypanosome of surra is of more uniform morphology than that of the African animal diseases. It averages 25 microns in length. The body is slender, both ends are pointed, and the body usually is bent into the form of a crescent. The nucleus is centrally located and the flagellum is long. The organism is actively motile in blood films.

**Reservoir Hosts.** The water buffalo and other ruminants are the reservoirs of infection in Asia. Camels in other areas are chronic carriers. The greatest losses occur in horses, especially military animals, which are brought into infected areas and quartered near herds of water buffalo.

**Transmission.** Surra is transmitted by a number of bloodsucking flies, principally members of the group of *Tabanidae* or horseflies. There is no evidence of any kind of life cycle, such as occurs in the tsetse flies. Apparently transmission is a purely mechanical process. Flies held in captivity for a few hours after feeding on a surra-infected animal lose their ability to infect other animals. Bloodsucking arthropods other than horseflies have been incriminated experimentally as potential spreaders of surra, but there is little evidence to indicate that any of them have been important natural spreaders.

**Pathogenicity.** The natural disease is almost always fatal for horses, death occurring in from 1 or 2 weeks to as long as 6 months after the date of infection. The affected animals exhibit fever, weakness, wasting, anemia, and edematous swellings. The disease in camels and elephants is similar, but considerably more chronic. Cattle and buffalo are readily infected but the disease does little harm to them. Dogs are highly susceptible and heavy losses have been reported in kennels of hunting dogs. Ticks and fleas have been believed to be the principal transmitting agents among dogs.

Rats and mice are highly susceptible to inoculation and usually die in about 1 week with massive invasion of the blood stream. Guinea pigs and rabbits are more resistant but usually succumb to the disease, without showing great numbers of parasites in their blood, in from 1 to 4 months.

During World War II foreign-bred and raised horses and mules imported into the China-Burma-India Theater proved to be highly susceptible to surra. Although every effort was made to eliminate infected animals before moving them from Burma to China, the disease appeared shortly after their arrival in China (Jennings and Jones, 3).

### Trypanosoma equinum

This parasite is the causative agent of a disease known as *mal de caderas*, which occurs in Brazil, Bolivia, Paraguay, and Argentina in South America. The disease affects horses principally. Mules are less susceptible than horses. Cattle, sheep, and goats have the disease in a very mild form.

**Morphology.** *Trypanosoma equinum* resembles *Tr. evansi* very closely. It is regarded as a variant of the Asiatic species. It has one remarkable feature and that is the fact that it does not have a parabasal body. This is the only species that lacks this structure. The parasite measures about 22 microns in length and shows the general features already described for *Tr. evansi*.

**Transmission.** This trypanosome probably is transmitted by bloodsucking flies of the *Tabanus* and *Stomoxys* groups. Intrauterine transmission has been indicated with several species of trypanosomes (notably *Tr. equinum*) and *Tr. evansi* has been conveyed in the milk to a sucking puppy.

**Reservoir Host.** Although the capybara, a large rodent resembling a guinea pig, held this distinction for many years, most of the evidence points to native cattle as the main reservoir hosts.

**Pathogenicity.** The name, *mal de caderas*, refers to a weakness of the hind quarters and calls attention to one of the prominent symptoms of the disease in the horse. Emaciation, weakness, conjunctivitis, remissions of fever, and edematous swellings are seen. The disease is fatal to horses in from 1 to 4 or 5 months. Rats and mice and other small laboratory animals may be readily infected experimentally.

### Trypanosoma hippicum

This trypanosome is the causative agent of *murrina* or *derrengadera*, a disease affecting horses and mules in the Panama Canal Zone, in the Republic of Panama, and possibly in the Republic of Colombia. The disease is spreading.

**Morphology.** *Trypanosoma hippicum* is indistinguishable from *Tr. evansi* and from *Tr. venezuelense*, which will be described next. Both of these species are considered to be variants of the trypanosome of surra.

**Transmission.** The disease can be transmitted by bloodsucking flies, particularly those of the tabanid family. It is interesting to note, however, that an important means of transmission, perhaps the most important means, is the vampire bat. This creature (*Desmodus rotundus*) is a vicious bloodsucker that preys upon livestock at night by alighting on their backs and puncturing the skin in the region of the withers with its sharp incisors. These bats also prey upon each other. The trypanosome infects these bats, producing a disease fatal to them in from 9 to 27 days. While infected bats are believed to transmit the disease it is possible that a Panamanian species of sandfly, *Phleboto-mus vespertilionis*, may be concerned. This fly is usually associated with bats and has a high infection rate with a trypanosome, but whether or not the sandfly protozoon is the same as the one occurring in bats has not been determined (1, 4).

**Reservoir Hosts.** Cattle and the native burro appear to be important reservoirs of infection.

**Pathogenicity.** The symptoms in horses are characteristic of trypanosome infections in general. There is irregular fever, progressive emaciation, anemia, slight icterus, weakness, and edema of the lower portions of the body. Death usually occurs after several weeks or months. The mortality is very high. Cattle and the native burro contract the disease but in them it is benign.

A large variety of animals can be infected by inoculation, most of them fatally. Cattle, sheep, goats, and swine are susceptible but they recover. Cats, burros, deer, and wild hogs (peccaries) develop chronic infections. Chickens are resistant.

### Trypanosoma venezuelense

This trypanosome occurs in Venezuela, where it causes a disease of horses and dogs resembling surra. The parasite is indistinguishable from those of surra and murrina, and it is doubtful whether it should be regarded as a separate species. Rangel, the discoverer, claims that the parasite occurs naturally in Venezuela in the wild dog, the capybara, and a type of howler monkey.

### Trypanosoma equiperdum

This parasite affects horses and members of the horse family, in which a serious disease known as *dourine* or *maladie du coit* is produced. The disease is transmitted almost exclusively by sexual contact, in which respect it is unique among the trypanosome diseases. Dourine is the only trypanosome disease of importance in the United States. The infection has long been known in Europe. About 1850 it became prevalent in France. It was first recognized in the United States in 1885 by Williams, in DeWitt County, Illinois. It is believed that it was imported from France in 1882 in an infected Percheron stallion. Before it was recognized, the disease had spread from the region in Illinois where it was first recognized to other areas. It later appeared in Nebraska, Iowa, North Dakota, South Dakota, and the western provinces of Canada. Still later it was recognized in New Mexico, Arizona, and southern California. It is presumed that the infection in all these localities had its origin in the early focus in Illinois.

By the use of the complement-fixation test and the destruction of all reacting animals, the disease was brought under control and by 1920 it was believed to have been eradicated. In 1941, however, some infected animals were found in Arizona and southern California. It is believed that the disease had existed in the intervening period in horses owned by Indians living in isolated areas of the southwestern deserts. The infected area is small; hence efforts to stamp out the disease should succeed.

**Morphology.** The trypanosome of dourine resembles that of surra. It varies in length from 25 to 35 microns.

**Transmission.** Dourine is transmitted from stallion to mare and from mare to stallion by contact of the mucous membranes of the genital tract during coitus. It has been proved, too, that the disease can be transmitted by blood-sucking flies (*Tabanidae* and *Stomoxys*), but fly transmission appears to be the exception rather than the rule.

**Reservoir Hosts.** Members of the horse family are the only animals that are known to contract infection naturally. There is no reservoir, therefore, other than naturally infected horses.

**Pathogenicity.** The disease is chronic in nature. In tropical climates it has a tendency to be more acute than in cooler regions. It may continue for months or years, the affected animals alternately improving and relapsing. Finally emaciation and nervous symptoms make the animals worthless, and they are usually destroyed when this stage has been reached.

The symptoms begin with swellings of the genitalia. The prepuce, penis, and testicles of the stallion become swollen and reddened. The vulva and vagina of the mare swell and emit a mucoid discharge. In these discharges the trypanosome generally can be found, and it is through them that the disease is transmitted during coitus. After the acute signs in the genital tracts have subsided, peculiar raised plaques of the skin appear. These are frequently called *dollar* plaques because they have the feeling of a disk, like a silver dollar, under the skin. They vary in size from ones much smaller than a silver dollar to ones several times as large. These appear quickly and disappear within a few hours or after several days to be replaced by others. At this time depigmentation of the mucosa of the genital tract may occur. Symptoms of paralysis gradually develop, an inconstant fever appears, emaciation progresses, and death occurs.

*Tr. equiperdum* often is difficult to demonstrate in cases of dourine. The trypanosome is present in the blood in very small numbers, this probably being the reason why the disease is not more often insect-borne. It may be demonstrated during the acute stages of genital swelling in the mucoid discharge, and it may often be demonstrated by scarifying and squeezing the dollar plaques. The edema fluid frequently will show parasites.

*Tr. equiperdum* is readily inoculable into dogs as a rule, and in diagnostic tests a dog may be given from 100 to 200 ml of blood or other fluids from the suspected horse. Not all strains will infect dogs, however, so a negative test is not conclusive. Rabbits are fairly susceptible—much more so than guinea pigs, rats, and mice. The latter can sometimes be infected, in which case the strain may rapidly become adapted to growing in them. Matsushima, Makita, Ikegemi, and Kano (2) were able to transmit the Manchurian dourine to rab-

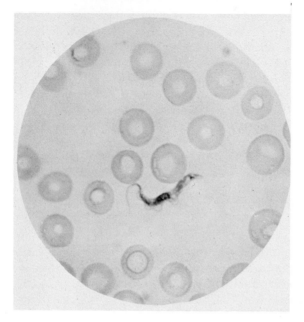

Fig. 114. *Trypanosoma equiperdum*, a stained film of the blood of an artificially infected guinea pig. X 1,200.

bits by intraperitoneal, subscrotal, subpreputial, sublabial, or intravenous injections. Seager (6) was able to transmit *Tr. equiperdum* to week-old duck-lings by injecting them with heavily infected mouse blood. The parasites appeared in the blood stream of infected ducks about 10 days after injection and death occurred in 12 to 14 days.

### Trypanosoma cruzi

This trypanosome causes Chagas' disease or South American trypanoso-miasis, which is mainly a children's disease. It is widely distributed in South America, Central America, and Mexico; and it occurs in Panama (3). It has not been reported in man in the United States, but in the southwestern states natural infection occurs in insects and the wild rodents which they infest (Wood and Wood, 5). Cats, dogs, opossums, monkeys, armadillos, bats, foxes, squirrels, wood rats, etc., are considered as reservoir hosts. It has been re-ported in raccoons in Maryland (4) and in opossums and raccoons in Ala-bama (2).

*Tr. cruzi* is a small curved form, with a central nucleus and a conspicuous blepharoplast located near the sharply pointed nonflagellate end. No multipli-cation takes place in the blood of man, and the predominant phase is a small, rounded nonflagellate stage occurring in cystlike clumps in various tissue cells—heart muscle, macrophages, and endothelium. These forms reproduce in the infected cells by binary fission; some acquire the trypaniform stage and escape into the circulating blood.

Assassin bugs (family *Reduviidae*) transmit the disease. In this family members of the genus *Triatoma* are important. In Lima, Peru, the vector was determined to be *Triatoma infestans* (1), whereas in New Mexico other species of *Triatoma* were found to be carriers of the parasite (6). These bugs obtain the trypanosomes from infected animals in a blood meal. The trypanosomes become intermediate flagellates in the intestinal tract of the vector, multiply, and change to the infective trypaniform flagellates within 2 to 3 weeks after the infecting blood meal is obtained. Then they are shed in the feces of the bug. Man appears to become infected as the result of getting the infected feces into wounds, bites, the mouth, or the eyes.

Irregular fever and edema, particularly of the eyelids, as well as enlargement of lymph nodes, spleen, and liver may be seen in the acute stage of the disease in children. The chronic disease (the usual adult form) is often characterized by myocarditis caused by heart muscle infection. Claims that this organism is concerned with goiter or that extracts of it cause regression of malignant tumors have not been established.

Primates infected with *Tr. cruzi* are known to be imported into the United States from the New World tropics. They have not become established in man to date but laboratory workers should know that *Tr. cruzi* may occur in these animals.

### Trypanosoma ariari

*Tr. ariari* causes trypanosomiasis in man. It was first found in the blood of a man living in the Ariari River valley of Colombia, South America. It has an average length of 31 microns, a nucleus anterior to the equator of the body, and a round, small, and subterminal kinetoplast. Monkeys and dogs are naturally infected with *Tr. ariari*, and an arthropod (*Rhodnius prolixus*) of the family *Reduviidae* has been shown to transmit the trypanosome (1, 2).

### The Diagnosis of Trypanosomiasis of Animals

Diagnosis of trypanosome infections of animals depends upon the recognition of the clinical symptoms and the finding of the parasite in the blood films. Frequently it is impossible, even though thick films have been examined, to find the parasites. This is especially true in dourine. In these cases the complement-fixation test often is useful. Cultural methods are used to demonstrate and identify trypanosomes (12, 13). Many of these species will grow on NNN medium, and others multiply abundantly on the chorioallantoic membrane of the developing chick embryo. *Tr. cruzi* grows readily in mink tissue cells, invading both normal fibroblasts and fibroblasts from Chediak-Higashi mink (8). It has also been grown in the trypanosome form in HeLa cells. The injection of suspected blood into guinea pigs or white rats sometimes is useful. The American opossum is susceptible to infection with *Tr. gambiense* (19). Indirect evidence of the presence of *Tr. cruzi* may be obtained by *xenodiagnosis* (host diagnosis), in which laboratory-reared bugs become infected after feeding on a suspected case. The fluorescent-antibody technic has been used successfully for serodiagnosis of *Tr. cruzi* (2, 18). Gill recommends the use of an indirect hemagglutination test in detecting anti-body for *Tr. evansi* (6). Trager (19) has used a tsetse fly tissue culture to develop trypanosomes to the infective stage.

Dourine has been eradicated from all of Canada and from all of the United States, except for a small area in the southwest, by the use of the complement-fixation test and the elimination of all reacting animals. The test is performed in the usual manner except for the preparation of the antigen. For antigen, a suspension of *Tr. equiperdum* is made from the blood of heavily infected white rats. The rats are inoculated and killed when their blood is teeming with the parasites. The blood is drawn into a citrated saline solution and centrifuged at high speed. The greater number of trypanosomes will be found as a whitish layer on top of the packed red cells, but many will be mixed with the cells. The supernatant serum, which is practically free of parasites, is discarded, and the tube is filled with distilled water, which will hemolyze or lake the erythrocytes. A second centrifuging will give a small amount of sediment, which consists largely of trypanosomes, leukocytes, and cellular debris. This material is washed with saline solution and then suspended in saline solution containing 50 percent glycerol. This constitutes the stock antigen.

Complement fixation with trypanosome antigens is not strictly specific because certain species may cross-react. At present this method is not used in diagnosing African trypanosomiasis. The test has proved very useful, however, in detecting dourine in the United States and in diagnosing Chagas' disease.

### Immunity

Serological treatment of trypanosome infections has been very disappointing. However, it can be shown by serologic tests that antibodies are produced. In *Tr. lewisi* infection of rats, ablastins and trypanolysins appear. These antibodies apparently aid in controlling the disease in these animals. Gill (7) used formolized or freeze-thawed trypanosomes to induce considerable protection in guinea pigs against challenge with homologous strains of *Tr. evansi*.

### Chemotherapy

Some of the compounds most successful in treating trypanosomiasis have been those of arsenic and antimony. Atoxyl, an organic arsenic compound, and potassium-antimony-tartrate (tartar emetic) are two that have been in common use. With both of these drugs, the blood stream may be readily cleared of trypanosomes, but after a few days they usually reappear. Many small doses of arsenic and antimony, given alternately, may bring about a cure, but often the compounds gradually lose their effectiveness because the parasite tends to develop *drug-fastness*. *Bayer 205* (Germanin), a nonmetallic compound with a urea base, was developed by the Germans. In the United States Louise Pearce synthesized *tryparsamide* (monosodium N-phenylglycin-amide-*p*-arsonate). These compounds were more effective in human infections than in those of animals.

Eagle (1) has claimed that early cases of *Tr. gambiense* infection can be cured by treatment with *p*-arsenosophenylbutyric acid. This drug has also been reported to be an active trypanocidal agent for *Tr. equiperdum* and *Tr. rhodesiense,* but it has little effect on *Tr. cruzi* or *Tr. congolense.* According-ing to Mace, Ott, and Cortez (14), it is useful in infections with *Tr. evansi,* but the effective dose for rats and dogs is near the lethal range of the drug. Antimony compounds claimed by Friedheim (4) to be capable of curing *Tr. gambiense* infections when used separately or combined are BSb (*p*-mel-aminylphenylstibonic acid) and MSbB (4-melaminyl-1-[methylolcyclo (ethylenedithiastibina)] benzene). Hornby *et al.* (9) have used phenanthri-dium compound no. 897 as a prophylactic and therapeutic agent for Zebu cat-tle in *Tr. congolense* areas. The phenanthridium derivative, ethidium bro-mide, is reported to be useful in treating both *Tr. congolense* and *Tr. vivax* infection (3, 15). Bayer 7602, another quinoline derivative, is claimed to be effective in treating *Tr. vivax* infection in cattle (Fulton, 5). The use of antry-cide prosalt is recommended in protecting cattle against trypanosomiasis when in transit through tsetse areas (22). This salt is a mixture of antrycide methyl sulfate and antrycide chloride in the proportion of 1 to 5. Antibiotics such as penicillin and streptomycin have proved ineffective in trypanoso-miasis, but Trincao *et al.* (21) report that puromycin is effective. The use of DDT (dichloro-diphenyl-trichlorethane) has had a marked effect in reducing *Trypanosoma* infection in certain areas of Africa by controlling the tsetse flies.

Procedures that aid in preventing trypanosomiasis include prophylactic treatment of susceptible animals; control of the tsetse-fly vector by means of insect repellents, insecticides, and bush clearing; and game control.

## REFERENCES

*General*
1. Eagle. Pub. Health Rpts. (U.S.), 1946, *61*, 1019.
2. Fife and Muschel. Proc. Soc. Exp. Biol. and Med., 1959, *101*, 540.
3. Ford, Wilmshurst, and Karib. Vet. Rec., 1953, *65*, 589.
4. Friedheim. Ann. Trop. Med. and Parsitol., 1953, *47*, 350.
5. Fulton. *Ibid.,* 1943, *37*, 164.
6. Gill. *Ibid.,* 1964, 58, 473.
7. Gill. Jour. Comp. Path., 1965, 75, 233.
8. Hagen. Jour. Parasitol., 1969, 55, 971.
9. Hornby, Evans, and Wilde. Jour. Comp. Path. and Therap., 1943, 53, 269.
10. Kudo. Protozoology. 5th ed. C. C Thomas, Springfield, Ill., 1966.
11. Laveran and Mesnil. Trypanosomes and trypanosomiasis. Masson et Cie., Paris, 1912.

12. Lehmann.   Ann. Trop. Med. and Parasitol., 1964, *58*, 6.
13. *Ibid.*, 9.
14. Mace, Ott, and Cortez.   Bul. U.S. Army Med. Dept., 1949, *9*, 387.
15. Milne and Robson.   Vet. Rec., 1955, *67*, 452.
16. Morgan and Hawkins.   Veterinary protozoology. Rev. ed. Burgess Publishing Co., Minneapolis, 1952.
17. Richardson.   Veterinary protozoology. 3d ed. Oliver and Boyd, London, 1963, pp. 27–71.
18. Sadun, Duxbury, Williams, and Anderson.   Jour. Parasitol., 1963, *49*, 385.
19. Seed and Gam.   *Ibid.*, 1967, *53*, 651.
20. Trager.   Ann. Trop. Med. and Parasitol., 1959, *53*, 473.
21. Trincao, Franco, Nogueira, Pinto, and Mühlpfordt.   Am. Jour. Trop. Med. and Hyg., 1955, *4*, 13.
22. Unsworth and Birkett.   Vet. Rec., 1952, *64*, 351.
23. Wenyon.   Protozoology. Baillière, Tindall, and Cox, London, 1926.

*Trypanosoma lewisi*
1. Laveran and Mesnil.   Ann. l'Inst. Past., 1901, *15*, 673.
2. Sherman and Ruble.   Jour. Parasitol., 1967, *53*, 258.
3. Taliaferro.   Am. Jour. Hyg., 1923, *3*, 204.
4. Taliaferro.   Jour. Exp. Med., 1924, *39*, 171.

*Trypanosoma melophagium*
1. Hoare.   Parasitology, 1923, *15*, 365.

*Trypanosoma theileri*
1. Crawley.   U.S. Dept. Agr., Bur. Anim. Indus. Bul. 145, 1912.
2. Cross, Redman, and Bohl.   Jour. Am. Vet. Med. Assoc., 1968, *153*, 571.
3. Dikmans, Manthei, and Frank.   Cornell Vet., 1957, *47*, 344.
4. Ewing and Carnahan.   Jour. Am. Vet. Med. Assoc., 1967, *150*, 1131.
5. Laveran.   Comp. rend. Acad. Sci., 1902, *134*, 512.
6. Miyajima.   Phil. Jour. Sci., 1907, *2*, 83.

*Trypanosoma avium*
1. Baker.   Parasitology, 1956, *46*, 321.

The African Trypanosomes: *Tr. brucei, Tr. gambiense, Tr. rhodesiense, Tr. congolense, Tr. vivax, Tr. simiae, Tr. uniforme*
1. Duggan and Hutchinson.   Jour. Trop. Med. and Hyg. (London), 1966, *69*, 124.
2. Hutchinson.   Ann. Trop. Med. and Parasitol., 1953, *47*, 156 and 169.
3. Johnson.   Am. Jour. Trop. Med., 1941, *22*, 289.
4. Laveran and Mesnil.   Ann. l'Inst. Past., 1902, *16*, 1.
5. Leger and Vienne.   Bul. Soc. Path. Exot., 1919, *12*, 258.
6. McConnell and Correa.   Jour. Parasitol., 1964, *50*, 523.
7. Plimmer and Bradford.   Veterinarian, 1899, *72*, 648.
8. Theiler.   Schweiz. Arch. f. Tierheilk., 1902, p. 97.
9. Van Den Berghe and Lambrecht.   Am. Jour. Trop. Med. and Hyg., 1963, *12*, 129.
10. Wenyon.   Protozoology. Baillière, Tindall and Cox, London, 1926.

11. Woo, Soltys, and Gillick. Canad. Jour. Comp. Med. and Vet. Sci., 1970, *34*, 142.

*Trypanosoma evansi*
1. Evans. Vet. Jour., 1881, *13*, 1.
2. Holmes. Jour. Comp. Path. and Therap., 1904, *17*, 210.
3. Jennings and Jones. Proc. 4th Int. Cong. Trop. Med. and Malaria, 1948, p. 1331.
4. Mitzmain. Phillipp. Bur. Agr. Bul. 28, 1913.
5. Mohler and Thompson. U.S. Dept. Agr., Bur. Anim. Indus. Circ. 169, 1911.
6. Musgrave and Clegg. Philipp. Bur. Govt. Lab. Bul. 5, 1903.

*Trypanosoma equinum*
1. Migone. Bul. Soc. Path. Exot., 1910, *3*, 524.
2. Voges. Zeitschr. f. Hyg., 1902, *34*, 323.

*Trypanosoma hippicum*
1. Anderson and Ayala. Science, 1968, *161*, 1023.
2. Darling. Jour. Inf. Dis., 1911, *8*, 467.
3. Johnson. Am. Jour. Trop. Med., 1936, *16*, 163.
4. McConnell and Correa. Jour. Parasitol., 1964, *50*, 523.

*Trypanosoma venezuelense*
1. Leger and Tejera. Bul. Soc. Path. Exot., 1920, *13*, 576.
2. Mesnil. *Ibid.*, 1910, *3*, 376.
3. Rangel. Bol. Lab. Hosp. Vargas (Caracas), 1905, *2*, 11.

*Trypanosoma equiperdum*
1. Baldrey. Jour. Comp. Path. and Therap., 1905, *18*, 1.
2. Matsushima, Makita, Ikegemi, and Kano. Jap. Jour. Vet. Sci., 1946, *8*, 41.
3. Mohler. U.S. Dept. Agr. Bul. 142, 1911.
4. Reynolds and Schoening. Jour. Agr. Res., 1918, *14*, 573.
5. Schoening. Jour. Inf. Dis., 1924, *34*, 608.
6. Seager. Science, 1944, *100*, 428.
7. Watson. Jour. Comp. Path. and Therap., 1912, *25*, 39.
8. Watson. Parasitology, 1915, *8*, 156.
9. Williams. Am. Vet. Rev., 1888, *12*, 295.

*Trypanosoma cruzi*
1. Cornejo, Berrocal, and Cubas. Am. Jour. Trop. Med. and Hyg., 1962, *11*, 610.
2. Olsen, Shoemaker, Turner, and Hays. Jour. Parasitol., 1964, *50*, 599.
3. Peralta, Shelokov, and Brody. Am. Jour. Trop. Med. and Hyg., 1965, *14*, 146.
4. Walton, Bauman, Diamond, and Herman. *Ibid.*, 1958, *7*, 603.
5. Wood and Wood. Am. Jour. Trop. Med., 1941, *21*, 335.
6. Wood and Wood. Am. Jour. Trop. Med. and Hyg., 1961, *10*, 155.

*Trypanosoma ariari*
1. Groot. Am. Jour. Trop. Med. and Hyg., 1952, *1*, 585.
2. Groot, Renjifo, and Uribe. Am. Jour. Trop. Med., 1951, *31*, 673.

## THE TRICHOMONADS

The trichomonads are flagellates characterized by the possession of a variable number of flagella, a definite cytostome (an opening into the cytoplasm through which food particles are ingested), and a hyaline rod-shaped supporting structure known as an *axostyle* which arises from the blepharoplasts anteriorly and passes backward through the body to the posterior end from which it usually protrudes. In some species one flagellum is directed backward and there is a well-developed undulating membrane. These organisms frequently are quite pleomorphic and may easily be confused with other types of flagellates. The body usually is more or less pear-shaped. Reproduction is by means of binary fission. Under unfavorable circumstances the organism may assume a spherical form surrounded by mucoid material. This is known as encystment.

Members of this group are rather widely scattered through the animal kingdom as parasites, involving invertebrates as well as vertebrates. Many forms have been found in the intestinal canal of animals. There is disagreement regarding the pathogenicity of some of these. If they are pathogenic, the disease-producing power is low. *Trichomonas hominis* occurs in the intestines of man. Apparently it is relatively harmless. *Trichomonas vaginalis* occurs in the vagina of women, where it causes a vaginitis accompanied by a whitish secretion. The disease is commonly called *leukorrhoea*. Bennett and Franco (4) have described equine intestinal trichomoniasis (EIT) at Trinidad racetracks. Laufenstein-Duffy (22) has indicated that EIT is an infectious disease of horses of all breeds and ages, that it is a functional colitis with partial or complete loss of the normal intestinal flora, and that it is caused by a motile flagellated trichomonad similar to the one found in the intestinal tract of man. The organism has been tentatively named *Trichomonas equi*. Although other species appear to be potential pathogens, the ones of major importance in animal pathology are *Trichomonas fetus* in cattle and *Trichomonas gallinae* and *Trichomonas gallinarium* in birds.

Surveys by Switzer (36) and Shuman *et al.* (34) have demonstrated that a high percentage of pigs affected with atrophic rhinitis harbor trichomonads in their nasal cavities. It has also been shown that such organisms can be isolated from the nasal cavity and from the alimentary tract of nonrhinitic pigs. Spindler *et al.* (35) have set forth presumptive evidence of an etiological relationship between trichomonads and rhinitis of swine, but Fitzgerald *et al.* (9) were unable to show that bacteria-free cultures of trichomonads caused this disease. Fitzgerald *et al.* (11) were able to infect bulls and heifers with trichomonads obtained from the digestive tracts of swine. Abortions occurred in infected pregnant heifers. Studies by Hammond and Leidl (16) indicate that low-level vaginal infections can be produced experimentally in goats and swine by inoculating either *T. fetus* or trichomonads isolated from swine. Intrapreputial infections could not be established in the male animals.

### Trichomonas fetus

SYNONYM:  *Tritrichomonas fetus*

This organism causes early abortions, pyometra, and sterility in cattle. The parasite was recognized early in the 20th century in Europe but its significance was not appreciated until about 1925. The parasite and the condition caused by it in the United States was first described by Emmerson (6) in 1932. It quickly became apparent thereafter that the disease existed in nearly all parts of this country, although the total of all infected herds apparently is not great. It has been reported in South Africa.

**Morphology.** This parasite normally is spindle- or pear-shaped, but there is considerable pleomorphism, some forms appearing almost spherical. It averages about 16 microns in length, the variation being from 10 to 25 microns. The width usually is from one-third to two-fifths of the length.

There are usually three anterior flagella instead of the four that occur in most members of the trichomonad group, and because of this fact Riedmuller

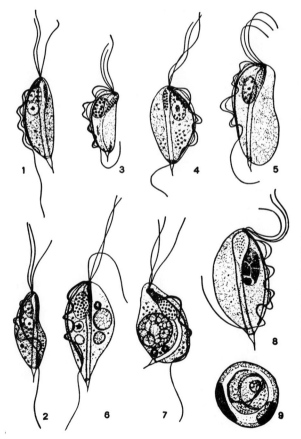

Fig. 115. Morphology of *Trichomonas fetus*. (1-3) Typical individuals. 1 and 3, side views; 2, dorsal view, showing spiral course of undulating membrane. (4, 5) Left-side and right-side views, showing parabasal body; 5 shows cytostome. (6, 7) Individuals showing included food bodies. (8) Individual stained with Giemsa. Note heavy staining of nucleus and axostylar granules. (9) Leukocyte containing an ingested flagellate. Drawings were outlined with the aid of a camera lucida. Magnification about X 2,000. (From plate by Wenrich and Emmerson, courtesy *Jour. Morph.*)

(33) proposed the generic name *Tritrichomonas*. These flagella originate in the blepharoplast located in the extreme anterior part of the body. They extend forward as free lashes, which are approximately as long as the cell body. The posterior flagellum originates in the blepharoplast, runs along the free margin of the undulating membrane, and extends posteriorly as a free flagellum of about the same length as the anterior flagella. The nucleus is large and is located somewhat anterior to the center of the cell. The axostyle extends axially from the blepharoplast to the posterior end of the cell. It is a tubular structure with an expanded portion anteriorly. It projects from the posterior end of the cell as a pointed structure that ends in a slender spine. The mouth or cytostome is not easily seen. It is triangular when open and located at the anterior end of the cell, ventral to the blepharoplast. The cytoplasm of this species is rather dense and only slightly vacuolated. Rounded individuals are seen which superficially resemble cysts, but it is doubtful if true cysts are formed. For a detailed description of this species, see Wenrich and Emmerson (37) and Morisita (30).

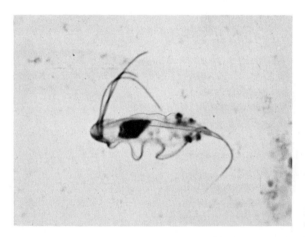

Fig. 116. *Trichomonas fetus.* X 2,000. (Courtesy A. Savage, *Cornell Vet.*)

Well-stained preparations are difficult to obtain. Wet fixation must be employed, otherwise the cells are so shrunken and distorted as to be unrecognizable. In fresh preparations the motility is so great as to make accurate observations difficult. The type of motility exhibited is, however, so characteristic that an experienced observer can recognize the organisms without difficulty. They rotate counterclockwise as they progress forward, jerkily, along an irregular path.

**Cultural Features.** *Trichomonas fetus* is readily cultivated artificially, but there may be difficulty in obtaining pure cultures from exudates in which bacteria are also present. Glaser and Coria (14) made use of a semisolid medium in U-tubes for purposes of isolation. The motile flagellates outdistanced the more slowly moving bacteria and appeared in the opposite arm of the

U-tube before the bacteria. Andres and Lyford (1) used this method successfully. They also succeeded in obtaining pure cultures by inoculating soft
media in Petri dishes and depending upon the flagellates to migrate from the
point of inoculation more rapidly than contaminating forms. Rees (32) claims
to have isolated bacteria-free strains of *T. fetus* by means of microisolation.
Mahmoud (26) was able to isolate the organism by using penicillin to inhibit
the growth of contaminating bacteria.

For obtaining and maintaining pure cultures, coagulated whole egg slants
to which a few ml of defibrinated blood mixed with Ringer's solution have
been added are satisfactory. Loeffler's blood serum slants or liver infusion
agar slants may be substituted for the egg medium. Growth occurs in the fluid
part of the medium. The appearance of the parasite is essentially the same as
that of parasites growing in exudates. Whole blood is not necessary for
growth. Serum may be substituted, or both serum and blood may be eliminated. The organism will grow actively for a short time in serum glucose
broth. Morisita (30) found whole egg slants covered with neutral broth containing 5 percent glucose to be a favorable medium.

The best incubation temperature is from 30 to 37 C. Acid and gas are produced in glucose, lactose, maltose, galactose, mannose, sucrose, raffinose, dextrin, and starch media. Glycerol, adonitol, dulcitol, mannitol, and sorbitol are
not attacked. Cultures on egg-Ringer-blood medium will remain viable for
about 1 month. Those on simpler media often die out in a few days. Jeffries
and Harris (18) were able to maintain *T. fetus* for about 1 year by freezing
suspensions in a liver-infusion broth and storing at $-70$ C with dimethyl sul-
foxide.

Nelson (31) succeeded in propagating *T. fetus* in the allantoic cavity of the
developing chick embryo. Profuse growth was obtained. About 25 percent of
the embryos died within the first 4 days.

**Pathogenicity.** This flagellate is transmitted as a true venereal infection in cattle. The cow is infected at the time of coitus from an infected bull, or vice
versa (5). The disease may rarely be spread in other ways.

The affected cow may show some evidence of vaginitis shortly after infection occurs, but usually this is overlooked. The affliction begins in the vagina
and soon invades the uterus. As a result of this the animal may fail to conceive. If conception occurs, the animal may abort as a result of the infection
within 2 to 4 months. In other instances the fetus dies but is not discharged,
in which case it becomes macerated and lies in a thin, nearly odorless fluid in
which many trichomonads may often be found and from which pure cultures
may be obtained.

Nonpregnant cattle may readily be infected by introduction of the parasite
into the vagina, but in these cases the disease is transitory and the flagellate
can rarely be found after 1 or 2 months. Beattie (3) has described a single
case in an experimental cow where viable organisms were recovered from a
cyst in the right Gärtner duct that was opened after 11 weeks of negative va-

ginal exudate findings had followed a 7-week period of positive tests. Although the disease tends to die out rather quickly in infected cows, it is maintained in herds by infected bulls, in which the disease becomes chronic. In bulls, the organism is found in the prepuce and on the penis. In rare cases the epididymis and vas deferens become involved (Hammond and Bartlett, 15).

According to McNutt, Walsh, and Murray (23), abortions of pregnant guinea pigs and rabbits can be produced experimentally by injection of *T. fetus* into the uterus.

**Diagnosis.** A positive diagnosis depends upon the demonstration of living, motile *T. fetus* in the genital exudate of infected animals or in the tissues or fluids from infected fetuses. Infected bulls may be detected by examining preputial samples. To collect the samples, various pipette, swab, and douche methods are employed (8). Accurate identification of the organism on direct microscopic examination requires technical training. Several egg slant cultures can be inoculated, and some can be incubated at 37 C and others at room temperature. Most free-living protozoan contaminants are unable to withstand the higher incubation temperature but develop abundantly at room temperature. The trichomonads and several of the free-living types will survive and multiply at body temperature. Growth from the cultures incubated at 37 C can be studied and the protozoa identified. See Morgan and Lowell (29) for details. Diagnostic serum agglutination tests have proved to be only moderately satisfactory. The mucus agglutination test, although more useful than the serum test, must be interpreted on a herd basis. It does not detect all the infected animals.

**Immunity.** According to the report of the Chief of the Bureau of Animal Industry for 1939–1940, cows bred to an infected bull may abort on the first pregnancy and a few may abort again on the second pregnancy. Following one or in some cases two abortions, the cow appears to be immune. However, the administration of serum from an immune cow to a susceptible heifer did not prevent infection from developing in the heifer. This may be explained by the findings of Kerr and Robertson (21), who have shown that the introduction of *T. fetus* antigen into the lumen of the uterus results in local production of intrauterine antibody. This antibody can be withdrawn by irrigation. On the other hand, neither free antibody nor sensitization of the uterus is produced by intramuscular injection of antigen, even though antibody is circulating in the blood stream. Actually antibody response to *T. fetus* injection in cattle is quite variable, and studies on the immobilization reaction as a diagnostic test indicate that it is not reliable (27).

**Chemotherapy.** Morgan and Campbell (28) tested 350 compounds for trichomonacidal properties by *in vitro* technic. They grouped the compounds according to their effects, ranging from those that killed in 1 minute to those that had no effect. They did not test these substances for therapeutic action.

It is claimed that intravenous injections of sodium iodide have some curative value in treating infected bulls, but there is no proved specific therapeutic treatment for trichomoniasis in cows. Hess (17) recommends the use of 3 percent hydrogen peroxide to which has been added 1 to 1.5 parts per thousand of a nonionic wetting agent for clearing up infection in the prepuce of the bull. The solution is sprayed into the prepuce through a specially designed spray tube. Bartlett (2) reported curing seven of eight trichomonad-infected bulls by direct application to the genital membranes of a German-developed proprietary compound (*bovoflavin-salbe*). Gabel *et al.* (12) recommend the use of bovoflavin ointment followed by a urethral douche and the feeding of phenothiazine. More recent preparations recommended for the treatment of bulls are p,p′-diguanyl-diazoamino-benzene diaceturate (10) and 1-$\beta$-hydroxyethyl-2-methyl-5-nitroimidazole (13). The former is injected into the prepuce and the latter is given by the intravenous or topical route. It should be noted that *T. fetus* has a tendency to develop drug tolerance and may become unresponsive not only to the specific substance that is employed, but also to related compounds.

In *vitro* tests show that the trichomonads are sensitive to aureomycin, polymyxins A and B, terramycin, and trichomycin, a new antibiotic tested by Magara *et al.* (25). Azalomycin F (24) is claimed to be effective in treating human trichomoniasis in both male and female patients.

**Control.** After the diagnosis of *T. fetus* infection, breeding activity should be suspended for 8 weeks and infected bulls should be eliminated. Recovered cows should then be bred by artificial insemination with semen from clean bulls. The cows with clinical symptoms should not be returned to the herd until they have recovered from the infection. Another method of controlling trichomoniasis in a dairy herd is to withhold service for each cow for three estral periods. No treatment will then be necessary if a clean bull is used.

It has been reported that *T. fetus* can be eliminated from infected semen by storing the latter overnight at 50 C in 20 percent glycerol, by freezing it to −79 C in the presence of 10 percent glycerol (19), or by diluting it 1 to 15 in egg-yolk buffer mixture containing sulfanilamide, streptomycin, and penicillin (7). Joyner and Bennett (20) have restudied this question and confirmed that *T. fetus* failed to survive freezing and thawing in the presence of 10 percent glycerol in egg-yolk citrate diluent, while sperm remained viable. They found that trichomonads were particularly sensitive to the toxic effects of glycerol when suspended in egg-yolk citrate, but survived freezing and thawing when placed in such diluents as egg-yolk phosphate or milk.

The disease is causing some concern in the beef herds of the Rocky Mountain region, because of its nature and rapid spread in areas where it is difficult to apply control measures.

## REFERENCES

1. Andrews and Lyford.  Am. Jour. Hyg., 1940, *31*, 43.
2. Bartlett.  Am. Jour. Vet. Res., 1948, 9, 351.
3. Beattie.  Austral. Vet. Jour., 1955, *31*, 146.

4. Bennett and Franco. Jour. Am. Vet. Med. Assoc., 1969, *154*, 58.
5. Cameron. Rpt. N.Y. State Vet. Coll., 1934–35 (1936), p. 111.
6. Emmerson. Jour. Am. Vet. Med. Assoc., 1932, *81*, 636.
7. Fitzgerald, Hammond, and Miner. Am. Jour. Vet. Res., 1954, *15*, 36.
8. Fitzgerald, Hammond, Miner, and Binns. *Ibid.*, 1952, *13*, 452.
9. Fitzgerald, Hammond, and Shupe. Cornell Vet., 1954, *44*, 302.
10. Fitzgerald, Johnson, and Hammond. Jour. Am. Vet. Med. Assoc., 1963, *143*, 259.
11. Fitzgerald, Johnson, Thorne, and Hammond. Am. Jour. Vet. Res., 1958, *19*, 775.
12. Gabel, Tharp, Thorne, Groves, Koutz and Amstutz. Jour. Am. Vet. Med. Assoc., 1956, *128*, 119.
13. Gasparini, Vaghi, and Tardini. Vet. Rec., 1963, *37*, 940.
14. Glaser and Coria. Am. Jour. Hyg., 1935, *22*, 221.
15. Hammond and Bartlett. Am. Jour. Vet. Res., 1943, *4*, 143.
16. Hammond and Leidl. *Ibid.*, 1957, *18*, 461.
17. Hess. Schweiz. Arch. f. Tierheilk., 1949, *91*, 481.
18. Jeffries and Harris. Parasitology, 1967, *57*, 321.
19. Joyner. Vet. Rec., 1954, *66*, 727.
20. Joyner and Bennett. Jour. Hyg. (London), 1956, *54*, 335.
21. Kerr and Robertson. *Ibid.*, 1953, *51*, 405.
22. Laufenstein-Duffy. Jour. Am. Vet. Med. Assoc., 1969, *155*, 1835.
23. McNutt, Walsh, and Murray. Cornell Vet., 1933, *23*, 160.
24. Magara, Amino, Ito, Takase, Nakamura, Senda, and Kato. Antibiotics and Chemother., 1962, *12*, 554.
25. Magara, Yokouti, Senda, and Amino. *Ibid.*, 1954, *4*, 433.
26. Mahmoud. Vet. Jour., 1945, *101*, 116.
27. Morgan. Jour. Immunol., 1943, *47*, 453.
28. Morgan and Campbell. Am. Jour. Vet. Res., 1946, *7*, 45.
29. Morgan and Lowell. Jour. Am. Vet. Med. Assoc., 1943, *102*, 11.
30. Morisita. Jap. Jour. Exp. Med., 1939, *17*, 1, 7, 27, 43, and 57.
31. Nelson. Proc. Soc. Exp. Biol. and Med., 1938, *39*, 258.
32. Rees. Am. Jour. Hyg., 1937, *26*, 283.
33. Riedmuller. Centrbl. f. Bakt., I Abt., Orig., 1936, *137*, 428.
34. Shuman, Earl, Shalkop, and Durbin. Jour. Am. Vet. Med. Assoc., 1953, *122*, 1.
35. Spindler, Shorb, and Hill. *Ibid.*, 1953, *122*, 151.
36. Switzer. Vet. Med., 1951, *46*, 478.
37. Wenrich and Emmerson. Jour. Morph., 1933, *55*, 193.

## Trichomonas gallinae

SYNONYMS: *Tr. columbae, Tr. diversa, Cercomonas gallinae*

A disease of young pigeons caused by a trichomonad was first described by Rivolta, in Italy, in 1878. This parasite has long been known under the name of *Trichomonas columbae*, but Stabler (8) has called attention to the fact that the name *Cercomonas gallinae*, applied by Rivolta, has priority, so far as the specific name is concerned.

A disease affecting the upper digestive tract of young turkeys and causing serious losses at times has been known for some years to be caused by a trichomonad. Volkmar (12), who suggested the causative connection of the flagellate to the disease process, suggested the name *Trichomonas diversa*, by which it has been generally known. Comparing the organisms from pigeons and turkeys, Stabler (9) could find no significant differences. Furthermore he showed that he could readily infect turkeys with strains derived from pigeons; hence he concluded that the two organisms are identical.

Levine and Brandly (5) encountered a disease of young chickens resembling that of turkeys quite closely. They concluded that the causative agent, a trichomonad, was probably the same as that which occurs in pigeons.

**Morphology.** This organism is usually spherical. Occasionally it is pear-shaped. It measures from 7 to 10 microns in diameter. Active motility is maintained by means of three or four anterior flagella and one posterior, which runs along the free margin of the undulating membrane as far as the posterior end of the cell. In these species the flagellum does not extend beyond the posterior end of the cell as a free lash as it does in most species.

**Cultural Features.** Waller (13) cultivated this organism in Locke's solution to which 5 percent dehydrated Loeffler's blood serum had been added. Evidently most of Waller's cultures contained bacteria. He states that the presence of bacteria is not detrimental to the trichomonads providing the cultures are transferred every 24 hours. Pure cultures were obtained by Cauthen (1), Stabler (9), and others. In Locke-egg-serum medium, and modifications, this flagellate grows readily.

**Pathogenicity.** *For pigeons.* The disease occurs principally in squabs from 3 weeks to several months of age. The most conspicuous lesions are in the liver. This organ is enlarged and congested. The specific lesions consist of necrotic areas of a yellowish color, varying in size from microscopic to 4 or 5 cm in diameter. These areas occur throughout the liver tissue but are readily seen on the surface of the organ. Here they are slightly depressed and smooth. The peritoneum of the body cavity is often eroded and contains a serosanguineous fluid. Lung lesions are seen in some cases. These are somewhat like those in the liver, but softer and darker in color. Both solid lesions and the fluids contain many trichomonads.

This organism occurs commonly in the crop and mouth of older birds, where it appears to do little or no harm. Occasionally ulceration of the crop occurs. Waller believes that the squabs become infected from the adults through the "pigeon milk," a fluid secreted by the glands of the crop, with which the old birds feed their young.

*For turkeys.* This flagellate is believed to be the cause of an unusual type of erosion of the mucosa of the crop, the upper and lower esophagus, and sometimes the back part of the mouth in turkeys. The disease is seen most often in mature birds, but Hawn (2) noted that the young birds (poults) were much more susceptible to inoculation than older birds and suggested that the low incidence of the natural disease in young stock is due to the unusual protection, which is ordinarily given, in not allowing them to associate with older birds and in keeping them off the ground on which birds have previously been raised. This disease was first described by Jungherr (4) in 1927, but he ascribed the disease to the activities of a fungus. The *Trichomonas* associated with the disease was first described by Volkmar (12), who, however, presented little evidence linking the parasite with the disease. Hawn (2) furnished the evidence upon which this protozoon is believed to be the causative agent of the infection.

This disease has been seen in many parts of the United States and probably occurs wherever turkeys are raised. The losses sometimes are very great. The flagellate concerned has been known by the name applied to it by Volkmar, *T. diversa*. It is not entirely certain that the species found in turkeys is the same as that of pigeons, but it seems best, for the time at least, to regard them as identical.

The early lesions in turkeys are found in the crop and upper esophagus. They appear as small, whitish nodules located in the mucous glands and varying in size from 0.5 to 2 mm in diameter. The content is semicaseous and can be expressed by pressure. The lesions may be so numerous that they can quite easily be scraped off the epithelium as a single layer. The characteristic older lesions appear as necrotic areas of grayish color. These become conical, horny growths that project well above the surface of the mucosa and are tipped with thorn-shaped processes from 1 to 3 mm in length. Large areas of the mucous membrane may become necrotic. The lower or thoracic esophagus sometimes becomes totally occluded by masses of such material. The crop usually contains a viscid, colorless mucus with a foul odor. This fluid usually is rich in flagellates.

Hawn succeeded in setting up the characteristic disease in 30 out of 56 turkeys by feeding them with cultures of *T. gallinae* that had been kept in cultures for periods varying from 2 days to 7 months. The cultures were contaminated with bacteria, but those cultures in which the flagellates had died never produced the disease; hence the author felt sure that the pathogenic agent was the trichomonad.

*For chickens.* Levine and Brandly (5) encountered a disease that destroyed a large number of pullets on one farm. Small, multiple lesions and necrotic foci were present in the mucosa of the crops of some of the birds, larger lesions with thickening of the crop well were seen in others, and in still others the crop appeared to be normal. In all, trichomonads indistinguishable from *T. gallinae* (*columbae*) were found. Attempts to transmit the infection to chickens, chicks, turkeys, and pigeons failed except in one case in which a large caseous lesion appeared in the crop of a pigeon 4 weeks after feeding.

*For other birds.* Cauthen found this trichomonad present in a large percentage of ring doves and mourning doves held in captivity on a farm with pigeons, and Stabler (7) found large numbers in the crops of five hawks. Because these prey upon pigeons, he believed the infection to have been contracted from pigeons. Several workers have suggested that this bird may be the normal host of *T. gallinae* and that all infections of other species are derived directly from pigeons. Stabler (10) has shown that strains isolated from doves are less virulent for pigeons but protect exposed pigeons against virulent pigeon-derived strains.

**Chemotherapy.** Jaquette (3) reported that copper sulfate could be used effectively in a concentration of 100 mg per 100 ml of water for nonbreeding pigeons and in a concentration of 35 mg per 100 ml of water for breeding pigeons. Greater concentrations were toxic. Stabler and Melletin (11) recommend the administration of enheptin (2-amino-5-nitrothiazole) in capsules for 7 days. The daily dose varies from 5 to 25 mg depending on the size of the pigeon. McLoughlin (6) freed pigeons of natural *T. gallinae* infection by oral administration of either metronidazole (2-methly-5-nitroimidazole-1-ethanol) or dimetridazole (1,2-dimethyl-5-nitroimidazole) at 50 mg per kg of body weight daily for 5 days.

## REFERENCES

1.  Cauthen.  Am. Jour. Hyg., 1936, *23*, 132.
2.  Hawn.  Jour. Inf. Dis., 1937, *61*, 184.
3.  Jaquette.  Am. Jour. Vet. Res., 1948, 9, 206.
4.  Jungherr.  Jour. Am. Vet. Med. Assoc., 1927, *71*, 636.
5.  Levine and Brandly.  *Ibid.*, 1939, 95, 77.
6.  McLoughlin.  Avian Dis., 1966, *10*, 288.
7.  Stabler.  Jour. Parasitol., 1937, *23*, 554.
8.  *Ibid.*, 1938, *24*, 553.
9.  Stabler.  Jour. Am. Vet. Med. Assoc., 1938, *93*, 33.
10. Stabler.  Jour. Parasitol., 1951, *37*, 473.
11. Stabler and Melletin.  *Ibid.*, 1953, *39*, 637.
12. Volkmar.  *Ibid.*, 1930, *17*, 85.
13. Waller.  Jour. Am. Vet. Med. Assoc., 1934, *84*, 596.

### Trichomonas gallinarum

SYNONYM:  *Pentatrichomonas gallinarum*

This species, according to Allen (2), is associated with a disease resembling blackhead in turkeys and chickens (see *Histomonas meleagridis*). She claims that trichomoniasis occurs as a separate disease, and that it is also often associated with histomoniasis, the two parasites developing in the same lesions. According to her, the liver lesions of trichomoniasis are yellowish and less well defined than those of true blackhead, and furthermore they are raised above the liver surface rather than depressed. The general resemblance of the lesions of trichomoniasis to those of histomoniasis is close enough, however, to cause confusion in diagnosis. In mixed infections, the lesions are similar to those of true blackhead in that they have depressed centers and a mottled appearance, but their margins in these cases are raised and have a netlike appearance. Allen contends that it is possible to distinguish by gross inspection alone between the liver lesions caused by the pure blackhead infection, the pure trichomonad infection, and mixed infections. In addition, it is possible to cultivate the trichomonad rather easily, whereas the histomonad is refractory to cultivation in pure culture. The organisms may also be distinguished morphologically in films from the lesions.

By feeding pure cultures of the trichomonad isolated from liver lesions, Allen produced 10 cases of disease in young poults out of a group of 75. Both cecal and liver lesions were present. The blackhead parsite could not be found in these lesions, but the trichomonad was recognized and recovered in culture. On the other hand, she produced 24 cases of true blackhead by feeding cultures of *Histomonas meleagridis* to 26 poults. In the lesions in these birds the histomonad was present but not the trichomonad.

*T. gallinarum*, according to Allen, is usually found in the ceca of turkeys and only occasionally enters the liver. Chickens carry it in their ceca but only rarely develop liver lesions. In very young poults and chicks, a severe cecal diarrhea sometimes occurs, which she believes to be caused by this trichomonad. Olsen and Allen (3) reported that fever therapy can be used to control trichomoniasis in turkeys. Turkeys were given treatment at intervals of 2 days. They were exposed for 1 to 2 hours to temperatures of 104 to 106 F in a relative humidity of 50 percent.

Allen suggests that the severe losses of chicks in flocks in the northwestern states, described by Weinzirl (5) and attributed by him to a parasite that he called *T. pullorum*, probably were caused by *T. gallinarum*. In 1956 Wichmann and Bankowski (6) reported *T. gallinarum* infection in chukar partridges. Liver and cecal lesions similar to those described by Allen in turkeys were found. The following morphological facts about this parasite are taken from a detailed description by Allen (1).

**Morphology.** The cells usually are nearly spherical; some are pear-shaped. They average 5 by 6.6 microns. There are five anterior flagella and another that runs along the border of the undulating membrane and ends in a free lash. The parabasal body is elongated and located along the base of the undulating membrane. The blepharoplast consists of a small group of granules located at the anterior end of the cell. Below the blepharoplast and nucleus and located on the side of the cell opposite from the nucleus is the cytostome, a small curving opening. The nucleus is round or oval. To obtain the least distorted organisms for morphologic observations osmium-tetroxide fixation is recommended (4).

The parasite has a characteristic type of movement which serves to distinguish it from other trichomonads. It shows rapid jerky motions, which cause the cell to turn from side to side and often to spin around, without, however, making much if any progress from place to place. This is in sharp contrast to *T. gallinae*, which moves so rapidly that it is difficult to follow it under the microscope.

## REFERENCES

1. Allen.   Proc. Helminth. Soc. Wash., 1940, 7, 65.
2. Allen.   Am. Jour. Vet. Res., 1941, 2, 214.
3. Olsen and Allen.   Proc. Soc. Exp. Biol. and Med., 1940, 45, 875.
4. Theodorides and Olson.   Avian Dis., 1965, 9, 232.
5. Weinzirl.   Jour. Bact., 1917, 2, 441.
6. Wichmann and Bankowski.   Cornell Vet., 1956, 46, 367.

# THE HEXAMITAE

The hexamitae constitute a group of flagellates which differ from all others in that the nucleus and other structures are duplicated. This makes them bilaterally symmetrical.

The hexamitae have pear-shaped bodies. Six flagella arise from the anterior end and are directed forward; two arise posteriorly. Dujardin, who first described a free-living protozoon of this type, thought that there were only four anterior and two posterior flagella, six in all, and this was the reason for the name which he coined for the group. The name has been retained although it is known that there are, in reality, a total of eight flagella.

These organisms are found free-living in stagnant water, and others occur in the intestinal tracts of frogs and mice. Members of the genus *Hexamita* and of the genus *Giardia* appear to be the only ones of importance in animal pathology.

### Hexamita meleagridis

This species is thought to be the cause of an enteritis of young turkeys. A similar disease was described by McNeil, Platt, and Hinshaw (6) in quail and chukar partridges and a similar organism found in them. The turkey disease had been recognized as an entity by many workers in various parts of the United States but had been generally regarded as a trichomoniasis. The causal relationship of *Hexamita* to it was recognized by Hinshaw, McNeil, and Kofoid (2) in California in 1938.

**Morphology.** This organism measures about 2.5 by 6 microns but varies considerably in size and shape. The flagella are typical in form and number. There is no undulating membrane and this serves to distinguish it from the trichomonads. The absence of an undulating membrane also is responsible for a different type of motility, active, but lacking the rotating movement of the trichomonads. This species also lacks the axostyle with its posterior projecting "tailpiece," so characteristic of trichomonads.

**Cultural Features.** There have been no reports of the artificial cultivation of this species.

**Pathogenicity.** Hinshaw, McNeil, and Kofoid (2, 3) claim that this organism is the cause of a disease they and other authors previously had regarded as a trichomoniasis. The protozoon affects young turkeys and may be the cause of serious losses. The affected poults are listless, they require more heat than usual, and their droppings are foamy or watery, or both. Greatest losses occur in birds from 3 to 5 weeks of age. The course of the disease in individuals is from 1 to 6 days. The morality varies from 20 to 90 percent. Birds that recover lose a great deal of weight. In the flock the disease usually runs its course in about 3 weeks.

The crop usually is empty, and the intestinal contents are thin and watery and often contain gas bubbles. The ceca frequently appear enlarged, and the wall of the entire intestine is flabby from lack of tone. The specific lesions are in the upper part of the intestine (duodenum and jejunem). Areas of inflammation are located there, and frequently regions of bulbous expansion of the intestinal wall are seen. The other organs show no evidence of disease.

In the upper part of the intestine only *Hexamita* is found, but in the ceca trichomonads and other species of flagellates occur as well and tend to obscure them. The hexamitae have been observed constantly in the bursa of Fabricius. In convalescent cases the parasite disappears from the upper bowel but tends to persist in the lower in association with other flagellates. Adult birds 2 years old have been proved to be carriers.

Inoculation experiments using material from naturally infected birds were carried out by Hinshaw, McNeil, and Kofoid (3). The disease was reproduced regularly when *Hexamita* was present and never when various other flagellates, including the trichomonad which formerly was believed to be the causative agent, were present without *Hexamita*. The authors feel that the failure to recognize the causative agent earlier was due to the fact that most workers had been studying the protozoan fauna of the lower bowel, where the trichomonads are the most numerous and most conspicuous parasites. They evidently feel that the trichomonad is purely parasitic and has nothing to do with the causation of the disease. McNeil and Hinshaw (4, 5) showed that young chicks can easily be infected with *Hexamita meleagridis*. The disease in chicks is relatively harmless, but they remain carriers of the infection for a long time and may be the source of infection for turkeys.

**Chemotherapy.** According to Wilson and Slavin (7), treatment with 2-amino-5-nitrothiazole (enheptin) is partially successful, but di-*n*-butyltin dilaurate (tinostat) appears to be the most promising drug. Almquist and Johnson (1) state that enheptin, aureomycin, penicillin G, and terramycin seem to be beneficial in treating hexamitiasis.

**REFERENCES**

1. Almquist and Johnson.   Proc. Soc. Exp. Biol. and Med., 1951, 76, 522.
2. Hinshaw, McNeil, and Kofoid.   Cornell Vet., 1938, 28, 281.
3. Hinshaw, McNeil, and Kofoid.   Jour. Am. Vet. Med. Assoc., 1938, 93, 160.
4. McNeil and Hinshaw.   Jour. Parasitol., 1941, 27, 185.
5. McNeil and Hinshaw.   Cornell Vet., 1941, 31, 345.
6. McNeil, Platt, and Hinshaw.   Ibid., 1939, 29, 330.
7. Wilson and Slavin.   Vet. Rec., 1955, 67, 236.

## *Giardia lamblia*

SYNONYM: *Giardia duodenalis* race *chinchillae*

Members of the genus *Giardia* are pyriform to ellipsoid. Their anterior ends are broadly rounded and their posterior ends are drawn out. They are bilaterally symmetrical. They inhabit the lumen of the duodenum and other parts of the small intestines and are found in many animals including man. These organisms appear to be host-specific and a number of species have been described, although in some cases very slight morphological variation supports the description. Their ability to cause disease has long been disputed, although they frequently are associated with diarrheal episodes in man and animals.

The parasite designated *Giardia lamblia* by Morgan and Hawkins (7) has been reported to cause enteritis in chinchillas (6, 9). From clinical observations it appears that the organism produces intestinal disturbances in some chinchillas while others seem to have asymptomatic infections. It is probable that severe symptoms and death occur only when heavy *Giardia* populations are present. The soft, discolored, and amorphic droppings of chinchillas heavily infected with giardiasis contain large numbers of the diagnostic cysts. These may be ovoid to nearly spherical in shape, and they average 8 to 12 microns in diameter.

Giardiasis has been described in the horse, but there is some doubt as to its importance (2).

Karapetyan (5) cultivated *G. duodenalis* in media that contained human, horse, or beef serum and inocula of *Saccharomyces cerevisiae*.

According to Hagen (4), atabrine in doses of 3 to 5 mg daily for 9 days or 6 to 9 mg for 4 days has proved effective in treating this disease. In treating giardiasis in man, Rosenberg and Neumann (8) recommend the use of amodiaquin hydrochloride (camoquin hydrochloride). Bassily *et al.* (1) have indicated that metronidazole, at a level of 250 mg twice daily for 10 days, is the drug of choice for treating giardiasis in man, and Cullun (3) has recommended thiabendazole as an economical, safe, and effective treatment for chinchilla.

## REFERENCES

1. Bassily, Farid, Mikhail, Kent, and Lehman, Jr. Jour. Trop. Med. and Hyg. (London), 1970, *15*, 73.
2. Bemrick. Vet. Med., 1968, *63*, 163.
3. Cullum. Canad. Vet. Jour., 1967, 8, 158.
4. Hagen. Calif. Vet., 1950, *3*, 11.
5. Karapetyan. Jour. Parasitol., 1962, *48*, 337.
6. Morgan. Jour. Parasitol., 1949, 35 (Sup.), 82.
7. Morgan and Hawkins. Veterinary protozoology. Rev. ed. Burgess Publishing Co., Minneapolis, 1952, p. 152.
8. Rosenberg and Neumann. Am. Jour. Trop. Med. and Hyg., 1957, *6*, 679.
9. Shelton. Am. Jour. Vet. Res., 1954, *15*, 71 and 75.

# XXX | The Sporozoa

The sporozoa constitute a group of protozoa which live a parasitic existence. Many of them are highly pathogenic to their hosts. All of them are
found, at some stage in their life cycle, intracellularly. The cycle of development is complicated by an *alternation of generation*. A period of repeated
asexual multiplication (*schizogony*) finally terminates in the formation of sexually differentiated cells known as *gametes*. The female gametes are fertilized
(*syngamy*) by the male elements, the product of the union being known as
*zygotes*. This marks the beginning of *sporogony* or spore formation. It is the
function of the spores that develop within these zygotes to carry the infection
into new hosts.

In some instances, as in the coccidia for example, the zygote develops a
protective membrane around itself and is then known as an *oocyst*. The
oocyst escapes from the host into soil. There, in the presence of moisture and
an abundance of oxygen, the zygote multiplies by cell division (sporogony) to
form a number of *sporozoites* within the oocyst. If the "ripened" oocyst is
taken into a suitable host, the walls dissolve liberating the motile sporozoites,
each of which then penetrates an epithelial cell and another period of asexual
reproduction follows.

In other instances, as in the hemosporidia, the alternation of generation involves an *alternation of hosts*. In these cases instead of escaping from the host
into the soil the gametes are taken up by bloodsucking arthropods in which
sporogony occurs. Eventually the sporozoites, the final products of sporogony,
find their way into the salivary apparatus of the arthropod, from whence they
escape into a new host at the time bloodsucking occurs.

The damage to the vertebrate hosts occurs largely during the period of
schizogony, because this is a period of rapid multiplication, each generation
giving rise to greater numbers of new individuals (*merozoites*), each of which
enters and destroys another host cell.

Although the sporozoa are without exception parasitic (1), certain forms are of especial interest to animal pathologists. Those to be considered here can be placed in two orders and in a group of organisms of undetermined status.

The first order, *Coccidia*, contains the commonly recognized genera *Eimeria*, *Tyzzeria*, and *Isospora*, which produce coccidiosis in animals. Another genus, *Hepatozoon*, occurs in the blood of dogs and rats, and it now appears that the infective form of *Toxoplasma gondi* is found as an oocyst (genus *Isospora*) in the feces of the cat (1, 3).

The second order, *Hemosporidia*, contains the following genera: *Plasmodium*, the cause of malaria in man and animals; *Hemoproteus* and *Leucocytozoon*, the cause of malarialike diseases in birds; *Babesia*, the cause of babesiosis (piroplasmosis); *Theileria*, the cause of African coast fever; and *Gonderia*, the cause of gonderiosis.

Among the organisms of doubtful classifications are the *Anaplasmata*, *Globidia*, and *Sarcosporidia*.

### REFERENCES

1. Frenkel, Dubey, and Miller.  Science, 1970, *167*, 893.
2. Kudo.  Protozoology. 5th ed. C. C Thomas, Springfield, Ill., 1966.
3. Sheffield and Melton.  Science, 1970, *167*, 892.

## THE COCCIDIA

Although all animals including man may harbor coccidia, not all are subject to clinical coccidiosis. Most species of coccidia are parasites of the intestinal epithelium. Exceptions most frequently seen are renal coccidiosis in the goose and hepatic coccidiosis in the rabbit. The latter form has also been observed on rare occasions in other animals, especially mink (1).

In many instances coccidia cause extensive destruction of the intestinal epithelium, which results in acute enteritis accompanied by diarrhea. Such cases may result fatally, especially in young animals. The severity of the disease depends in large measure upon the size of the infecting dose and the opportunities for multiple reinfections, because coccidia, unlike bacteria and many other pathogenic organisms, are not able to multiply without limit in the new host but are confined to a definite number of asexual generations, after which they assume the relatively harmless sexual form. If the host survives the acute stages while asexual multiplication of the parasite is occurring, it recovers but retains the infection for long periods and serves as a source of infection for others. If the sanitary conditions are not good, animals usually become reinfected from their own feces, and this serves to keep the infection alive in herds and flocks.

In the process of schizogony the entire growth period is passed within the cytoplasm of host cells. It begins when the host cells are penetrated by sporozoites released from ingested oocysts. The elongated sporozoites are transformed in the host cells to spherical bodies, which grow rapidly at the expense of the cytoplasm. These are known as *trophozoites* or *schizonts*. As they grow, the cell nucleus is crowded aside, and when the schizonts are fully developed, there is little left of the host cell. The cytoplasm of the schizonts undergoes multiple division, forming numbers of smaller elements. The schizont then ruptures, releasing the smaller bodies that are known as *merozoites*. These are motile and immediately seek out other cells, which they penetrate, one merozoite into each host cell, forming a new crop of schizonts.

After a number of generations of merozoites have been formed, the number varying according to peculiarities of the species, a crop of schizonts is formed.

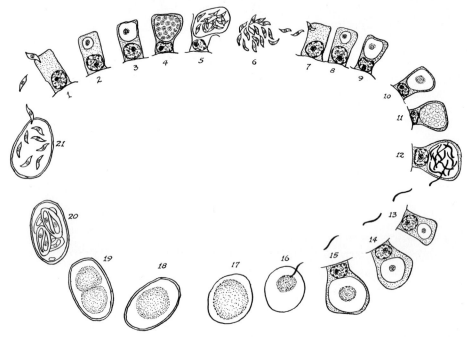

*Fig. 117.* Diagrammatic representation of the life cycle of a coccidium. (1) Sporozoite entering an epithelial cell. (2-4) Schizonts developing in epithelial cells. (5-7) Merozoites released from the schizonts and entering other cells. (8, 9) Second generation of schizonts developing in other epithelial cells. (10-12) Formation of microgametocytes and release of microgametes. (13-15) Formation of a macrogametocyte. (16) Fertilization of a macrogamete by a microgamete. (17, 18) Formation of a zygote or oocyst. (19) Beginning of the process of sporulation of the oocyst, two-cell stage. (20) The fully sporulated oocyst. Four sporocysts are present, each containing two sporozoites, in this instance, thus indicating that the species belongs to the genus *Eimeria*. Members of the genus *Isospora* develop only two sporocysts, each containing four sporozoites. (21) The release of sporozoites from the ripe or sporulated oocyst. Stages 1-18 inclusive occur in a single host. Stage 18 usually is eliminated from the body in the excretions. Stages 19 and 20 usually develop in moist soil. Infection of new hosts or reinfection of the same host occurs through the contamination of food and water with stage 20. Stage 21 occurs in the new host through excystation of the sporozoites through action of the digestive enzymes.

These become transformed into *macro-* and *microgametocytes,* which when mature are usually of about equal size. Each microgametocyte gives rise to a large number of small serpentine elements which are known as *microgametes.* These correspond to the male sperm cells. Released by rupture of the parent cell, these seek out the macrogametes, the female elements, which they fertilize. The fertilized macrogametes then secrete a thick capsule around themselves, forming oocysts. These are discharged into the lumen of the organ and thus escape from the host. The oocysts are more readily identifed than any other stage in the life cycle of coccidia and are commonly sought as a means of diagnosis.

At least three genera of coccidia occur among domestic animals. They can be distinguished from each other by examination of the ripened oocysts. The cytoplasm of the oocyst of *Isospora* divides into two bodies known as *sporoblasts,* each surrounded by a membrane known as a *sporocyst.* In each of these sporocysts four sporozoites are formed. In the *Eimeria* four sporocysts are formed, each containing two sporozoites. In the *Tyzzeria,* sporoblasts are lacking, but eight sporozoites lie free inside a thick oocyst wall. In all three cases, it will be noted, eight sporozoites are formed.

**Host Specificity of the Coccidia.** It was once believed that the coccidia were relatively nonspecific so far as hosts were concerned, that is, infections in one species might readily be transferred to another. It was thought, for example, that rabbits often infected domestic livestock. It is now known that there is a high order of host specificity in this group and that infections seldom are contracted from other species. This is especially true of members of the *Eimeria,* which are responsible for the most serious infections of domesticated animals. Occasionally certain species may be found in closely related species of animals, but this seems to be the exception rather than the rule. The members of the *Isospora* seem to be somewhat less specific than the *Eimeria;* thus we find certain kinds which infect both dogs and cats, and it has been suggested that certain *Isospora* infections in man originate in the dog (6).

**Immunity in Coccidial Infections.** There is definite evidence that animals develop immunity to coccidial infection. Tyzzer showed that young chicks can be readily immunized by infecting them with small doses under conditions in which the birds are unable to reinfect themselves. The mild infections run a definite course and clear up. In some cases the bird may be infected a second, and sometimes several additional times, but eventually it becomes so resistant that additional infections cannot be obtained with the same species. Similar results have been obtained with dogs. It is probable that this is a rule applicable to all coccidia. The idea is at variance with older ideas. It has long been known, for example, that older animals of the species frequently harbored coccidia without showing any symptoms, and that these animals served as sources of serious epizootics among the younger animals living on the premises. It was thought that these animals were chronic carriers; that the disease was not thrown off by such animals but that the parasites were carried in a low stage of activity. This may be true in some cases, but it is quite certain that the carrier state often is a result of constant reinfections, and that when such animals are maintained in such a way as to prevent reinfections they usually eliminate the organism completely.

Studying *Eimeria caviae* of the guinea pig, Henry (3) has shown that these animals not only are immunized by a single contact with the protozoon but that they develop a skin sensitization to proteins derived from the oocysts. She was also able to show evidence of anaphylactic sensitization to these proteins. Clinical coccidiosis is uncommon in man, but human infections are reported from time to time in the United States, usually caused by *Isospora belli* and attributed to exposure to the parasite in a foreign country (7). *Eimeria leuckarti* has been found in horses, but clinical coccidiosis rarely, if ever, occurs in this animal (2). Coccidial parasites have been noted in guinea pigs that were similar to those found in the intestines of mice. These organisms belong in the *Cryptosporidium* (4), another genus of coccidia, which is characterized by the formation of an oocyst which when mature contains four sporozoites but no sporocysts, is found exclusively on the surface of mucous membranes, and has little disease potential among domestic animals.

### REFERENCES

1.  Davis, Chow, and Gorham.   Vet. Med., 1953, *48*, 371.
2.  Dunlap.   Jour. Am. Vet. Med. Assoc., 1970, *156*, 623.
3.  Henry.   Proc. Soc. Exp. Biol. and Med., 1931, *28*, 831.
4.  Jervis, Merrill, and Sprinz.   Am. Jour. Vet. Res., 1966, *27*, 408.
5.  Kudo.   Protozoology. 5th ed. C. C Thomas, Springfield, Ill., 1966.
6.  Routh, McCroan, and Hames.   Am. Jour. Trop. Med. and Hyg., 1955, *4*, 1.
7.  Sanders.   Am. Jour. Clin. Path., 1967, *47*, 347.

### THE COCCIDIA OF DOGS AND CATS

Coccidiosis of dogs appears to be a very common infection. In practically all parts of the world where surveys have been made the incidence has been at least 5 percent and in many places it has been much higher. Lee (9) reports that the incidence in the clinics of the Veterinary Division of Iowa State College over a 10-year period was 13.8 percent. Of 320 dogs examined by Gassner (5) of Colorado State College over a short period of time, 79 percent carried coccidia. All the infections in these studies proved to be *Isospora*, *I. bigemina* being the most frequently encountered. In Gassner's series, for example, *I. bigemina* was found in 74 percent of the dogs, *I. rivolta* in 20 percent, and *I. felis* in 6 percent.

In dogs, the infections with *Isospora* are undoubtedly the most common. A member of *Eimeria*, *E. canis*, is encountered occasionally. Yakimoff and Matschoulsky (16) found that the incidence of this species in Leningrad was about 2.5 percent, whereas *I. rivolta* amounted to 14 percent. *E. canis* has been reported in single cases in Wyoming by Honess (6) and in Nebraska by Skidmore and McGrath (14). These authors think that the species may by more common than reports would indicate. Catcott (3) in 1946 examined 113 dogs at Ohio State University and found that 10.6 percent were infected with coccidia of the genus *Isospora*.

There have been few reports of coccidial infections in cats. Cats are susceptible to experimental infection with all three of the dog species, and natural infections with all three species have been reported. Wenyon (15) states that *I. felis* infections of young kittens are common in London. Lee reports a single natural infection in an Iowa cat.

It appears that the majority of coccidial infections of dogs and cats are light and that there is little evidence of serious damage to the hosts. In some cases, however, diarrhea occurs, with excessive amounts of mucus in the feces, and occasionally there may be a bloody and even fatal dysentery. Evidently the severity of the disease is dependent upon the number of the coccidia present, because Lee has clearly shown that all of the *Isospora* are capable of causing serious damage when large doses are given experimentally.

*Isospora* and *Eimeria* are easily differentiated if some fecal material containing oocysts is kept in a shallow dish diluted with 1 percent potassium bichromate solution ( to prevent putrefaction) for a few days. The presence of four sporocysts in the oocysts, each containing two sporozoites, indicates that the organism belongs to the *Eimeria;* if there are two sporocysts each containing four sporozoites, it belongs to the *Isospora*. The examination can be made with the 4-mm or 16-mm lens of a reasonably good microscope. Differentiation of the species within the genus is more difficult. This is most readily done by noting the characteristics and the measurements of the sporulated oocysts. The measurements of the *Isospora* as reported by Gassner are given in table XXI.

*Table XXI.* MEASUREMENTS OF OOCYSTS AND SPOROCYSTS OF *ISOSPORA* OF DOGS AND CATS

| Isospora | Oocysts | Sporocysts |
|---|---|---|
| | microns | microns |
| felis | 40–42 × 31–32 | 19–22 × 13–15 |
| rivolta | 23–24 × 15–16 | 15–16 × 9.7–11.5 |
| bigemina | | |
| (small variety) | 10–12 × 8–9.6 | 7–8.6 × 8.5–9 |
| (large variety) | 14.8 × 12.5 | 9.5–10.8 × 8–9.4 |

### Isospora bigemina

This coccidium occurs in both dogs and cats, apparently being more common in the former. Lee (9) was able to produce acute infections with a bloody diarrhea in cats with cultures derived from a dog. He also succeeded in infecting a fox with a strain from a dog.

Two types of *I. bigemina* are recognized, one producing a small oocyst and the other a much larger. The small variety is by far the more common. Both ordinarily develop in the subepithelial tissues of the small intestine, but Wenyon and Sheather found one acute case in which the epithelial cells were filled with schizonts and oocysts. It is believed that during acute phases of the infection the epithelial cells are attacked and during the chronic stages the organism remains in the subepithelial tissues. During the chronic stages of the disease the oocysts undergo sporulation in the tissues, frequently rupture there, and release the sporocysts, which are found in the feces instead of the oocysts. Immature oocysts may sometimes be found in the feces along with the free sporocysts but usually they are very scarce. By purging his patients with arecoline hydrochloride, Gassner found that he could force the appearance of oocysts in the feces.

Lee found that when small numbers of sporulated oocysts were fed to dogs, a few oocysts were eliminated on the 6th or 7th day and elimination continued for about one week. No symptoms were observed. When larger doses were given, a profuse, hemorrhagic diarrhea began on the 3rd or 4th day, and oocysts were discharged in abundance on the 6th and 7th days. One dog died of the disease, but the others recovered after a few days although oocyst discharge continued for several weeks. Doses of intermediate size produced a catarrhal diarrhea, the feces often being streaked with blood. Mixed infections of *I. bigemina* with one or both of the other species of *Isospora* occur naturally, and experimentally such infections often are rather severe.

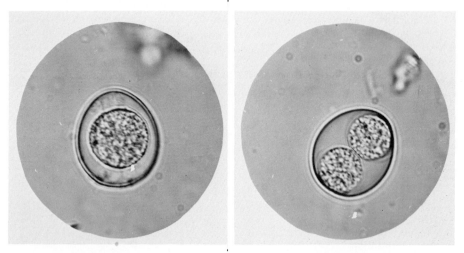

*Fig. 118 (left). Isospora bigemina*, a nonsporulated oocyst of the common coccidium of the dog. Unlike most coccidia, the oocyst of this species often sporulates while in the intestinal canal. X 1,000.

*Fig. 119 (right). Isospora bigemina*, an oocyst in an early sporulating stage. In this instance a dense membrane will form about each of the two cells and each will become a sporoblast containing four sporozoites. This will identify it as a member of the genus *Isospora*. X 1,000.

### Isospora cati

We have followed the nomenclature that has been in general use to date and have designated the *Isospora* infections in dogs and cats as *I. bigemina*, a small type and a large type; *I. rivolta;* and *I. felis*. Frenkel (4) now proposes to restrict *I. bigemina* to dogs and to apply the term *I. cati* to the cat form. *I. felis* will continue to be used to identify the largest *Isospora* of cats and *I. rivolta* the intermediate one.

It is now believed that the small oocyst of *I. cati* is the infective form of *Toxoplasma gondi* (13) and that *I. cati* infects only cats, becoming *Toxoplasma* in other animals. This concept has suggested the abandoning of the genus *Toxoplasma* and the placing of the organism in the genus *Isospora*, but biologic differences from the latter, tissue parasitization, host range, and transmission all favor retaining the conceptual identity of the former, and accordingly toxoplasmosis is discussed under the heading *Toxoplasma* (see p. 714).

### Isospora rivolta

The multiplicative stages of this species occur in both epithelial and subepithelial tissues of the small intestines of dogs and cats. Lee, in his series, found them only in the epithelium near the tips of the villi. The species is regarded as relatively harmless. Coccidia indistinguishable from *I. rivolta* have been found in a number of wild animals and in some cases infections of dogs have been produced with them. This form is frequently found in clinical cases in association with *I. bigemina*.

### Isospora felis

This species is easily distinguished from the others by its very large oocysts. As its name indicates, it is found principally in cats, but dog infections occur. Wenyon states that this species is common in London cats. It has been found less frequently in the United States than the other two species and generally in mixed infections. Pure infections in cats generally are relatively harmless, although diarrhea may be produced. The multiplicative stages are found in the small intestine, being located in the epithelial cells near the tips of the villi. Some are found also in the mucosa of the cecum. Lee reports a pure experimental infection in a dog. Following a rather large dose of sporulated oocysts by mouth, a bloody diarrhea began on the 6th day and continued until the 11th. Oocysts appeared on the 8th day and continued until the 29th day.

### Eimeria canis

This species has been identified on only a few occasions. It was first seen by Wenyon in London. Two isolated cases have been described in the United States, by Skidmore and McGrath (14) in Nebraska and by Honess (6) in Wyoming. The Nebraska dog was said to be unthrifty and suffered from vomiting and diarrhea. Blood was not detected in the stools. Honess sporulated the oocysts from his case and fed them to two experimental dogs. Some of the oocysts were said to have been sporulated when passed. After 3 days all had sporulated. The number fed was not large, and the dogs showed no symptoms at any time. Oocysts appeared in the feces on the 8th day in one case and on the 17th day in the other. The cases were followed for 2 weeks, during which time oocyst shedding continued.

The oocysts were colorless, whereas Wenyon described those of the case with which he worked as being pinkish. They were ellipsoidal and asymmetrical, being more curved on one side than on the other. The sporocysts were elongated. The oocysts averaged 12 by 18 microns in size; the sporocysts 5.8 by 10.4. These measurements are smaller than those given by European workers, but since there was agreement otherwise, Honess regarded his organism as *E. canis*.

### Eimeria felina

*E. felina* was reported in the cat by Nieschulz in 1924. It produces an ellipsoidal oocyst with an average size of 23 by 15 microns (12).

### Eimeria cati

This species was described by Yakimoff in 1933. The oocyst is ovoid and has an average size of 20 by 17 microns (12).

### Eimeria vulpis and Eimeria mustelae

Coccidiosis is a problem at times among foxes and mink raised in captivity. *E. vulpis*, which produces an ovoid oocyst with an average size of 18 by 12 microns, and a micropyle just visible, has been described in foxes. *E. mustelae* occurs in mink. Its oocyst is egg-shaped, 20.5 by 14.5 microns in size, and has no micropyle (12). *E. vison* and *Isospora laidlawi* have also been described in outbreaks of coccidiosis in mink (10).

**Chemotherapy.** Parkin (11) claimed to be successful in treating coccidiosis in dogs by giving 10 ml of 1 percent sodium sulfanilyl sulfanilate per kilogram of body weight as an enema on 3 successive days. Altman (1) recommends the use of aureomycin in treating *I. bigemina* infection. It should be noted that the anticoccidial agent nitrophenide (megasul) is toxic for dogs if fed at the level employed in chicken feeds (7). Knight (8) administered concentrated canine globulins parenterally along with large oral doses of sulfadimethoxine and reported marked success in treating canine coccidiosis. Mepacrine in doses of 0.01 g per kg is effective in cats (2).

### REFERENCES

1.  Altman.  Jour. Am. Vet. Med. Assoc., 1951, *119*, 207.
2.  Brumpt.  Bul. Acad. Vét., 1943, *16*, 66.

3.  Catcott.   Jour. Am. Vet. Med. Assoc., 1946, *108*, 34.
4.  Frenkel.   Jour. Inf. Dis., 1970, *122*, 553.
5.  Gassner.   Jour. Am. Vet. Med. Assoc., 1940, *96*, 225.
6.  Honess.   *Ibid.*, 1936, *88*, 756.
7.  Huang, Marshak, and McCay.   *Ibid.*, 1954, *124*, 212.
8.  Knight.   Vet. Med., 1962, *57*, 52.
9.  Lee.   Jour. Am. Vet. Med. Assoc., 1934, *85*, 760.
10.  McTaggart.   Jour. Parasitol., 1960, *46*, 201.
11.  Parkin.   Jour. So. African Vet. Med. Assoc., 1943, *14*, 73.
12.  Richardson and Kendall.   Veterinary protozoology. 3d ed. Oliver and Boyd, London, 1963, pp. 126–127.
13.  Sheffield and Melton.   Science, 1970, *167*, 892.
14.  Skidmore and McGrath.   Jour. Am. Vet. Med. Assoc., 1932, *82*, 627.
15.  Wenyon.   Protozoology. Baillière, Tindall and Cox, London, 1926.
16.  Yakimoff and Matschoulsky.   Arch. f. Tierheilk., 1936, *70*, 169.

## THE COCCIDIA OF RABBITS

At least six types of coccidia affect the rabbit. Of these, two types are common and destructive. One of these, *Eimeria stiedae*, was the first coccidium known.

### Eimeria stiedae

Young rabbits are especially susceptible to this species, and nearly all deaths from it occur in animals less than 4 months of age. The mortality rate is especially severe in commercially raised rabbits, particularly when they are raised in hutches or confined spaces where opportunities for massive infections are great. Under such conditions heavy losses from this and other coccidial infections can be prevented only by scrupulous cleanliness, frequent changing of bedding, and feeding and watering from containers that cannot readily be soiled with the animal feces. Disinfection in this disease, as in all coccidial infections, can best be accomplished by heat, because chemical disinfectants have little effect upon the oocysts. Moist heat is very effective, but it should be borne in mind that, if it is employed, means of thoroughly drying the hutches and cages should be sought because moisture favors the maintenance of viability of the sporulated oocysts.

*Eimeria stiedae* differs from the other coccidia of the rabbit in that it localizes in the bile ducts of the liver. The liver often becomes greatly enlarged, and white or yellowish lesions that resemble abscesses may be seen on its surface. In acute cases these may not be present. The gross lesions referred to are spherical or elongated and vary in size from minute to 2 cm in diameter. When these lesions are relatively young, they are filled with a thin whitish fluid; when older the content may be thick and caseous; when very old the lesions may be dense and even calcified. The fluid of the fresh lesions consists largely of oocysts, which may be as numerous as leukocytes in pus. In the caseous material they usually may be found but are not numerous, and in the

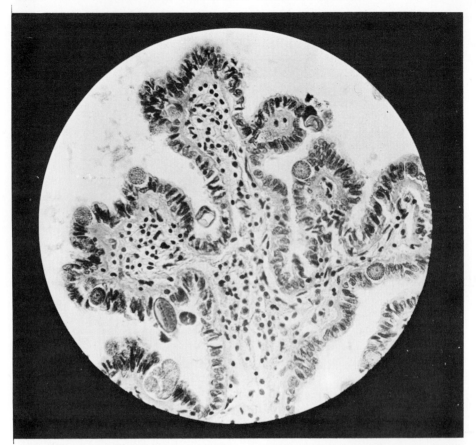

Fig. 120. Hypertrophied bile duct epithelium of a rabbit caused by infection with *Eimeria stiedae*. A number of gametocytes and one oocyst are shown. X 300.

inspissated, calcified material they are usually absent, having degenerated.

Sections of affected livers show that the bile duct epithelium, under the stimulus supplied by the multiplicative stage of the parasite, has proliferated and formed cystic adenomas, the linings of which are filled with every developmental stage of the coccidium. The epithelial growths push out into the liver tissue and become filled with fluid and the products of growth of the parasite, forming the whitish gross lesions already mentioned.

The oocysts escape from the cystic dilations of the bile ducts to the intestine through the gall bladder and the common bile duct, and thus out of the body with the feces. In the presence of an abundance of oxygen and a little moisture they undergo sporulation in about 60 hours under the most favorable conditions. The oocysts are large and have a yellowish color. They average about 35 microns in length by a little more than half this dimension in width. One end is slightly flattened and here there is a thin place in the capsule, the *micropyle*, which the sporozoites penetrate in escaping from the cyst. The cytoplasm of the cell is granular and ordinarily does not occupy more than one-half of the space within the capsule, the remainder being empty. The sporocysts are rather elongated, measuring about 10 by 18 microns.

Horton (3) studied the migration of *E. stiedae* sporozoites between the duodenum and bile ducts of the rabbit. He found sporozoites in the mesenteric lymph nodes, both free and within lymphatic monocytes at between 12 and 84 hours after infecting the animals. He observed no sporozoites in duodenal portal blood. These observations provide morphological evidence compatible with a lymphatic route of migration between duodenum and mesenteric lymph nodes, probably within lymphatic monocytes. After a period in the lymph nodes the sporozoites may leave the monocytes and enter the portal blood, which carries them to the liver, or alternatively they may be carried passively by the monocytes to the liver where they leave these cells to enter the bilary epithelium. When very heavy infections occur, the rabbits die within 3 to 4 weeks. In more chronic infections death may be delayed for 6 weeks or more, or recovery may occur. The affected animals generally become potbellied because of the liver enlargement, and diarrhea usually develops, especially if they are obtaining much succulent feed.

### Eimeria perforans

This species probably is just as common in commercially raised rabbits as the preceding, but the evidence of its existence is not so conspicuous; thus it is not so well known. As a matter of fact, this organism was confused with *E. stiedae* for many years. Infections with this species can be distinguished from those of the liver-infecting variety by a simple fecal examination of the discharged oocysts. Those of *E. perforans* are colorless, i.e., they lack the yellow color of those of *E. stiedae;* furthermore they are much smaller and more nearly spherical. They measure between 24 to 30 by 15 to 20 microns, averaging 15.5 by 25.5 microns. The oocyst walls of this species are slightly thicker than those of *E. stiedae.* Sporulation under favorable conditions occurs in 48 hours or less. After experimental infections, oocysts appear in the feces on the 4th or 5th days, whereas those of *E. stiedae* do not appear in the feces for 6 or 7 days. *E. perforans* can be separated from *E. stiedae* by feeding the mixed culture to a young rabbit and saving the fecal material discharged on the 4th and 5th days, at which time only the oocysts of the first species will be present.

Development occurs in the epithelial cells of the small intestine and, to some extent, of the cecum. The small intestine, especially the duodenum, becomes dilated to several times its normal diameter. The walls of the affected gut are pale and sometimes edematous. Reddened streaks are found on the mucosa. Sometimes almost every epithelial cell in parts of the intestines is infected.

Diarrhea is characteristic of this disease, but if the animal is fed only on dry feed the feces may be soft rather than fluid. The victim becomes potbellied, anemic, dehydrated, and in general presents a miserable aspect. Death usually occurs within 2 weeks of the time when symptoms appear.

### Eimeria magna

This organism originally was regarded as a variety of *E. perforans* but now is believed to be a separate species. Like *E. perforans* it occurs in the epithelial cells of the small intestine, where it reproduces similar changes. The oocyst is much larger than that of *E. perforans* but about the same as that of *E. stiedae*. Like the latter it is of a yellowish or even a brownish color. It measures 28 to 40 by 20 to 26 microns. A broad micropyle is located at the more tapering of the ends. This species is not so widespread or common as *E. perforans*.

### Eimeria irresidua, Eimeria media, and Eimeria neoleporis

These coccidia are also reported to cause infection in rabbits, but they appear not to be so widespread as the species discussed above. Of the coccidia that are found in the intestines of the rabbit, *E. magna* and *E. irresidua* seem to be most pathogenic.

**Chemotherapy.** According to Horton-Smith (4), sulfamethazine incorporated in the feed in a proportion of 1 percent is effective in preventing disease after infection with a dose of *E. stiedae* oocysts that otherwise would be fatal. This preventive treatment is effective in controlling severe hepatic coccidiosis even if postponed up to 10 days after inoculation with sporulated oocysts, but not if delayed to the 15th day. Hagen (2) recommends the use of sulfaquinoxaline in the drinking water to control coccidiosis in domestic rabbits and states that nitrofurazone and furazolidone administered in combination had a detrimental effect on the life cycle of *E. stiedae* by causing the parasite to produce many infertile forms in the bile tracts.

### REFERENCES

1. Becker. Coccidia and coccidiosis of domesticated, game, and laboratory animals and of man. Collegiate Press, Ames, Iowa, 1934.
2. Hagen. Jour. Am. Vet. Med. Assoc., 1961, *138*, 99.
3. Horton. Parasitology, 1967, *57*, 9.
4. Horton-Smith. Vet. Jour., 1947, *103*, 207.
5. Morgan and Hawkins. Veterinary protozoology. Rev. ed. Burgess Publishing Co., Minneapolis, 1952, p. 146.

## THE COCCIDIA OF CHICKENS

Among domesticated livestock coccidial infections do the greatest damage to poultry. Acute infections of young chicks frequently result in mortality rates approaching 100 percent. The more chronic infections of older birds are

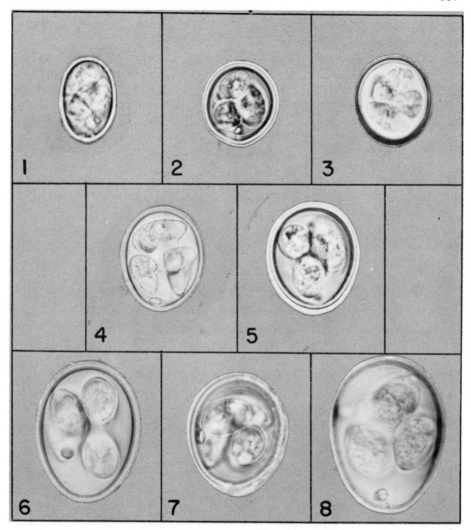

*Fig. 121.* Sporulated oocyst of the coccidia of chickens. All photographs taken at a magnification of X 1,400 to show relative size. (1) *Eimeria acervulina.* (2) *E. mitis.* (3) *E. hagani.* (4) *E. necatrix.* (5) *E. tenella.* (6) *E. brunetti.* (7) *E. praecox.* (8) *E. maxima.*

not often fatal but result in malnutrition, unthriftiness, and decreased production.

Until Tyzzer (33) published his first work on the differentiation of the coccidia of chickens in 1929, it was thought that there was only a single species, and this was known as *Eimeria avium.* Tyzzer called attention to the fact that Railliet and Lucet had differentiated one species adequately in 1891 and had given it the name *E. tenella.* This species was confirmed by Tyzzer, and three additional, *E. acervulina, E. maxima,* and *E. mitis,* were described and

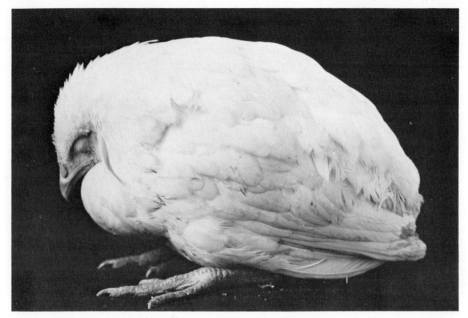

*Fig. 122.* Chicken affected with cecal coccidiosis (*Eimeria tenella*).

named. In the following year, 1930, Johnson (16) differentiated two additional species, *E. necatrix* and *E. praecox*. Levine (19), in 1938, added *E. hagani* and in 1942 *E. brunetti* (21). In 1964 Edgar and Seibold (8) described *E. mivati*. It now appears that there are nine distinct species. Of these, *E. tenella* and *E. necatrix* are highly pathogenic and destructive parasites. *E. brunetti* and *E. maxima* frequently cause acute outbreaks of coccidiosis, and the former is sometimes found in chronic infections. *E. acervulina* and *E. mitis* possess virulence of a medium grade and generally are associated with chronic infections. *E. hagani* and *E. praecox* are nearly harmless. *E. mivati* is not so clearly catalogued, but seems to be similar to *E. brunetti*. All of these species, except possibly *E. hagani*, for which data are not available, are widespread. Several species often occur simultaneously in a single fowl; in fact, this situation generally exists in the infections of older birds.

A study of the incidence of different species of coccidia was made in 1960–62 in England (22). There was a rise in the amount of coccidiosis caused by *E. brunetti* and by *E. maxima* while *E. tenella* showed a decrease. *E. brunetti* and *E. tenella* were more common in birds under 10 weeks of age, whereas *E. acervulina* was most common in chickens over 10 weeks of age.

All of the coccidial infections of birds are self-limiting, that is, birds that survive the original acute attack will recover completely and eliminate all traces of the infection, providing means of reinfection are banished. Chronic coccidiosis of birds, therefore, is a disease kept alive by repeated reinfections

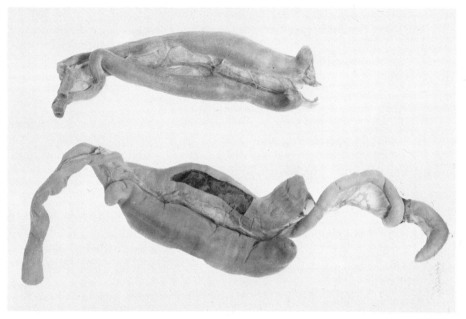

*Fig. 123.* Cecal coccidiosis in a chicken. Normal ceca are shown on top. On the bottom are the diseased. The affected organs are swollen and filled with clotted blood, shown through the incision. The color of the bloody content shows through the thin walls of the organs giving them a dark-red color. (Courtesy E. L. Brunett.)

of the same species, or by repeated infections with different species. Immunity of a rather high order is produced by one or two light infections with some species; with others a number of reinfections are necessary. In all cases apparently enough resistance is established eventually to prevent reinfection or to make it so slight as to be symptomless. Johnson (17) and Tyzzer, Theiler, and Jones (34) have shown that age is not the essential factor in immunity to *E. tenella,* an organism that causes severe infections in young chicks but does not often affect adults. When birds were reared in the laboratory free of all coccidial infection, they were found to be susceptible to *E. tenella* infection when they were more than 2 years old. Infections do not ordinarily occur in old birds reared naturally because almost invariably they come in contact with the organism in repeated small doses earlier in life and are immunized by such contacts. As in other coccidial infections, whether or not symptoms of the disease develop depends upon the size of the infecting doses. Practical control of these diseases requires keeping the environment of the birds sufficiently clean so they will not pick up massive doses of infection at their first exposure. This is accomplished by taking special precautions with the floors of buildings and runs, using feed and water containers that cannot easily be contaminated with droppings of the birds, cleaning and scalding these containers at frequent intervals, keeping the birds on clean range of adequate size so that the infected droppings are scattered widely, and plowing and planting contaminated ranges. The modern practice of using deep litter in poultry houses, the layer of which is built up gradually by additions, does not favor the development of coccidiosis providing the additions are great enough to keep the litter dry, because oocysts do not sporulate in a dry environment. Good poultrymen have found it possible to control coccidiosis in their flocks by the use of these methods.

It is possible to complete the endogenous cycles of *E. tenella*, *E. brunetti*, and *E. mivati* by inoculating their respective sporozoites into chicken embryos. *E. acervulina* and *E. maxima* did not develop under similar conditions, and attempts to infect chicken embryos with *E. stiedae* failed (23).

### Eimeria tenella

This species affects young chickens, most commonly birds from 6 to 12 weeks of age, but they may be as young as 3 weeks and as much as several years old. The affected birds suffer from what is commonly called acute coccidiosis, a disease in which bloody diarrhea is conspicuous and death losses often are large.

*E. tenella* develops only in the ceca or blind pouches, and it is here that the only lesions are found. These consist of gross hemorrhage, the pouches usually being distended with wholly or partly clotted blood. The tissues of the remainder of the body are anemic. The birds actually bleed to death internally in these cases. It was shown by Bradford and Herrick (3) that blood from cecal hemorrhage caused by *E. tenella* produced intravascular coagulation and death in chickens when injected intravenously. Extracts from cecal cores of chickens infected with this protozoon also proved toxic, but extracts from normal ceca did not produce the thromboplastic effect. In 1964 Sharma and Foster (32) prepared bacteriologically sterile extracts from *E. tenella* oocysts and showed them to be lethal upon intravenous injection into rabbits.

The sporozoites liberated from the infecting oocysts enter and develop in the epithelial cells of the ceca. The schizonts that appear, mature, and rupture, each liberating some hundreds of merozoites (first generation). These tend to localize in epithelial cells deep in the glands, where they become another generation of schizonts. The cells that contain these forms are crowded into the subepithelial tissues, where the parasites proceed to grow into huge schizonts, which finally break up into 200 or 300 or more second-generation merozoites. These are much larger than those of the first generation. About the time the schizonts rupture, freeing the merozoites, multiple hemorrhages into the subepithelial tissues occur and the mucosa is undermined and sloughs away, thus releasing the parasites. These invade the remaining epithelial cells and, if the host continues to live, develop into a third generation of schizonts, which is the last, the next generation developing as gametocytes.

The oocysts of *E. tenella* are broadly ovoid, there being little difference between the two ends. They measure 19.5 to 26 by 16.5 to 22.8 microns with an average measurement of 19 by 22.6 microns. The cytoplasm of the oocyst occupies only a fraction of the space within the shell. Sporulation is complete in 48 hours at room temperature. After experimental feeding, oocysts are found in the droppings on the 7th day.

### Eimeria necatrix

Next to the preceding species, this coccidium is the most pathogenic for chickens. The damage that it causes is most likely to occur in old birds, and immediate death losses are not so frequently found, the disease taking a longer course and therefore receiving the name *chronic coccidiosis*.

The developmental phases of this species are quite similar to those of *E. tenella* except that its localization is different. The sporozoites invade the epithelial cells of the small intestine rather than those of the ceca. The schizonts liberate the first generation of merozoites into the lumen of the intestinal glands; these invade cells of the deeper parts of the glands and reach the subepithelial tissues in the same manner as *E. tenella*. The second-generation merozoites escape into the lumen of the bowel with the help of hemorrhages and denudation of the mucous membrane. This occurs on the 4th day of the infection. Instead of invading other nearby cells, the second-generation merozoites allow themselves to be carried with the intestinal content to the lower bowel, whence they enter the ceca. Here another schizogonic generation occurs, and probably several more, but gametes begin to form in the third generation and sporogony thereafter replaces schizogony. Oocysts do not appear in the droppings until rather late in the course of the infection, but oocysts formation continues for a considerable time after it begins.

The oocysts are broadly oval. Some are somewhat egg-shaped, with one end more pointed than the other. They are somewhat smaller than those of *E. tenella*, measuring 11.3 to 18.3 by 13.2 to 22.7 microns, averaging 14.2 by 16.7 microns. Sporulation is completed in 48 hours at room temperature. The shedding of oocysts begins on the 7th day after infection.

Massive infections with this species, especially in younger birds, may result fatally within a week. The usual form is more prolonged. Symptoms begin on the 4th day. The bird stands with dejected attitude, there is roughening of the feathers, and it does not eat. If heavy infections do not destroy the bird by the 7th day, it usually survives, although it may be emaciated and worthless.

The small intestines of birds suffering from this parasite present a characteristic appearance. Showing through the muscular and serous coats, clearly visible on the exterior of the unopened intestines, are many whitish spots which are conspicuous against the dark background made by the bloody content. They are the masses or colonies of the large second-generation schizonts. The wall also generally shows punctate hemorrhages. The intestinal content may be a bloodstained mucus or it may be almost wholly of blood.

Although in nature infection starts in the small intestine, the inoculation of sporozoites of *E. necatrix* into the ceca of coccidia-free chickens results in penetration of the cecal epithelium and the initiation of a life cycle that is similar to the usual one followed in the small intestine. Viable oocysts of *E. necatrix* are produced which can be sporulated and, when given to coccidia-free chickens, produce characteristic infections in the small intestine (15).

### Eimeria brunetti

The oocysts of *E. brunetti* measure 20.7 to 30.3 microns in length and 18.1 to 24.2 microns in width. Of the coccidial oocysts described from chickens, *E. maxima* alone is larger than *E. brunetti*. A fairly constant feature that distinguishes the oocysts of these two species is the presence of a thickening or slight protuberance on the inner surface of the narrow end of the oocyst wall of *E. maxima* at the time the protoplasm has assumed a spherical form prior to division into sporoblasts. The sporulation time of *E. brunetti* is from 24 to 48 hours at 30 C, and oocysts appear in the droppings 5 days after experimental feeding.

In *E. brunetti* infection, oocysts and developing forms are found in the lower half of the small intestine, rectum, cloaca, and ceca and may appear in the anterior part of the small intestine in severe infections. In light infections no lesions appear. In moderately heavy infections a catarrhal enteritis with blood-tinged mucous exudate is found. In severe infections coagulation necrosis and sloughing of the mucosa occur. In some instances the proximal, constricted, tubular entrances to the cecal pouches become dilated and plugged with short, caseous cores (Levine, 21). British scientists have indicated that this protozoon is a widespread cause of avian coccidiosis and that it is similar in pathogenicity to that of *E. tenella* and *E. necatrix*.

### Eimeria mivati

The original isolate of *E. mivati* came from Florida. It is primarily a parasite of the anterior third of the small intestine, but may be found throughout the intestinal tract. Infected areas are slightly swollen, edematous, hemorrhagic, and contain whitish lesions. Severe infections cause growth depression, some mortality, a drop in egg production, and impaired feed conversion in growing and laying chickens. There are four schizogonous asexual and one sexual stages. There is no subepithelial invasion. The oocysts range in size from 10.7 to 20.0 by 10.1 to 15.3 microns, averaging 15.6 by 13.4, and reaching a peak production 5 to 7 days after inoculation. This species is distinguishable from others of the chicken by the region it parasitizes, location of parasite in relation to the nuclei of parasitized epithelial cells, average oocyst size, sporulation time, prepatent period, and antigenic dissimilarity. It appears to be widely distributed throughout the United States, having been identified from 27 states and also in Canada. It has been isolated from fowls in Great Britain, where evidence was presented that heavy experimental infections caused some morbidity and had a marked effect on gain in body weight. Also that the breed or strain of the host influenced the degree of pathogenicity (25).

### Eimeria maxima

This species receives its name from the size of its oocysts, which are larger than those of any of the other chicken species. They measure 21.5 to 42.5 by 16.5 to 29.8 microns, averaging 22.6 by 29.3 microns. They have a yellowish color, and the shells often have a roughened surface. Sporulation is complete in 48 hours at room temperature. Oocysts appear in the droppings on the 6th day after experimental infections.

The schizonts are found in the epithelium of the small intestine, particularly of the middle portion. They are smaller than those of the other species found in the chicken and usually are located above the nuclei of the parasitized cells. Schizogony does not continue beyond the 5th day. The gametocytes develop below the nuclei of the epithelial cells and apparently are more injurious to the host than the schizogonic forms.

The affected portions of the intestine may be somewhat thickened, and the mucosa usually is covered with mucus in which blood flecks are found. There are no extensive hemorrhages such as occur in infections with the four species described above, except in occasional instances when this organism has been observed to cause acute infection.

Heavy doses of pure cultures of this species will produce fatal infections; however, under usual conditions its pathogenicity is not great. It often is associated with other species and in particular with *E. necatrix* in the so-called *chronic* infections of older birds.

### Eimeria acervulina

This species, like *E. hagani*, *E. praecox*, and *E. mitis*, inhabits principally the upper half of the small intestine, although some forms may be found in the lower half and a few in the ceca near their outlets. In the intestine the schizonts tend to concentrate in limited areas, and, because they localize largely in the epithelium of the villi, they form grayish areas that are visible to the naked eye when the bowel has been opened and the contents washed away. The schizonts develop very superficially above the nuclei of the epithelial cells. Dickinson (7) found that the administration of massive doses of oocysts of *E. acervulina* to chickens produced a temporary drop in weight and a complete temporary cessation of egg production. In a short time, however, weights and egg production were almost back to normal. The lesions produced by this species consist of thickening of the intestinal mucosa. A catarrhal exudate may be present, but hemorrhage rarely is observed.

The oocysts are egg-shaped. They sporulate in less than 24 hours, in which respect they differ from the other species found in chickens. They measure 17.7 to 20.2 by 13.7 to 16.3 microns, averaging 14.3 by 19.5 microns. After experimental feeding, oocysts appear in the droppings on the 4th day.

Table XXII.   THE COCCIDIA AFFECTING CHICKENS *

| | E. tenella | E. necatrix | E. brunetti | E. maxima | E. acervulina | E. mitis | E. hagani | E. praecox |
|---|---|---|---|---|---|---|---|---|
| Oocysts | | | | | | | | |
| Average size (microns) | 19×22.6 | 14.2×16.7 | 21.7×26.8 | 22.6×29.3 | 14.3×19.5 | 15.5×16.2 | 17.6×19.1 | 17.1×21.3 |
| Sporulation time | 48 hr | 48 hr | 24 to 48 hr | 48 hr | 21 hr | 48 hr | 48 hr | 48 hr |
| ** Prepatent period | 7 days | 7 days | 5 days | 6 days | 4 days | 5 days | 7 days | 4 days |
| Region of intestine affected | Schizonts and oocysts in the ceca | Schizonts in small intestine; oocysts in ceca | Small intestine, rectum, ceca, and cloaca | Post. half small intestine | Ant. half small intestine | Ant. half small intestine | Ant. half small intestine | Ant. third small intestine |
| Gross lesions | Gross hemorrhage into ceca | Hem. exudate small intestine; petechia and whitish opacities | Hem. streaks in intestinal mucosa; necrotic enteritis in severe cases | Intestinal wall thickened; blood flecks in exudate | Intestinal wall thickened; white streak across mucosa small intestine | Catarrhal exudate in intestine | None | None |
| Degree of severity of the disease | + + + + | + + + + | + + + | + + + | + + | + + | + | + |

* E. mivati is not included in this table, but is described on page 662.
** The prepatent period is the time that elapses between the feeding of the sporulated oocysts and the appearance of a fresh crop of oocysts in the feces.

## Eimeria mitis

This species is occasionally pathogenic. Large and repeated doses of sporulated oocysts produce mild symptoms. It develops in the epithelial cells of the upper part of the small intestine, to a lesser extent in the lower part, and sometimes even in the ceca.

The oocysts are nearly spherical, averaging 15.5 by 16.2 microns in size. The protoplasm practically fills the shell. The sporocysts are elongated, measuring 6 by 10 microns. Sporulation is completed within 48 hours. Oocysts appear in the droppings on the 5th day after experimental feeding.

Schizonts not only develop in the epithelium of the villi but also in the glands. Generally they occur below the nuclei of the host cells but sometimes they are above. Unlike all the other coccidial species of the chicken in which the cycles of development are regular, resulting in the occurrence of certain phases at certain times, all phases of the life cycle can often be found in a single section of intestine infected with *E. mitis*.

## Eimeria hagani

This species was separated from a "culture" of *E. maxima* by Levine, who used a micropipette to pick out the oocysts. The oocysts are broadly oval with both ends of equal breadth. The measurements are 15.8 to 20.9 by 14.3 to 19.5 microns, averaging 17.6 by 19.1 microns. The protoplasm almost completely fills the oocyst shell. Sporulation is complete in 48 hours, the four elongated sporocysts taking up most of the space within the shell. After an infective feeding, oocysts appear in the feces toward the end of the 6th and on the 7th day.

When large numbers of sporulated oocysts are fed to young birds, many hemorrhagic spots about 1 mm in diameter appear in the wall of the duodenum and the first half of the small intestine. The lower end of the small intestine is free from lesions. On the 6th day the mucous membrane appears greatly inflamed. The content of the bowel is thin and watery, and sometimes mucous casts of the lumen of the bowel are present. The birds generally recover.

## Eimeria praecox

This species, like the preceding, is found in the upper third of the small intestine. It is practically nonpathogenic, there being little evidence of change in the intestinal wall except that an excess of mucus appears and mucous plugs often are formed.

The oocysts are ovoidal in form and measure 19.8 to 24.7 by 15.7 to 19.8 microns, averaging 17.0 by 21.3 microns. Sporulation is completed in 48 hours under favorable conditions. The name *E. praecox* was given to this species by Johnson to indicate the precocity which it shows in eliminating oocysts in the droppings on the 4th day after infection. This precocity is shared with *E. acer-*

*vulina.* The schizonts are formed in the epithelium of the sides of the villi and appear below the nuclei of the host cells.

*E. praecox* has been observed in fowl in Great Britain. It was noted that older chickens (6 weeks of age) were more suitable hosts than young ones (1.5 to 3 weeks) for reproduction of the parasite, and that a single exposure conferred a high degree of resistance (24).

### Immunity in Coccidial Infections of Chickens

In 1953 Uricchio (35) showed that 15-day-old chicks could be effectively protected against *E. tenella* infection by feeding them altered oocysts. This was done by giving each chick 100,000 oocysts that had been exposed to −50 C for 5 days. Since then it has been established that complete resistance may be developed to coccidiosis by initiating a regimen of two to three exposures to graded and spaced infections.

Immunity against coccidial infection is species-specific. Now being marketed is a so-called *vaccine* which is composed of a mixture of six species of sporulated oocysts from the chicken. Young chicks running on litter are dosed in the drinking water with a very small number of oocysts. The resulting oocyst discharge in the litter serves to re-expose them with a much larger inoculum. The infection is controlled by a coccidiostat. More time must elapse before an adequate assessment of this product can be made.

### Treatment of the Coccidial Infections of Chickens

At present prophylactic measures appear to afford the best means of controlling coccidiosis in chickens. These may consist of simple sanitary precautions, of sanitary precautions combined with the use of coccidiostatic agents, or a combination of vaccines and coccidiostatic agents. All of these methods are designed to prevent the birds from obtaining massive doses of oocysts.

Some of the chemotherapeutic drugs that have shown varying degrees of effectiveness against coccidiosis are sulfaguanidine (20), sulfamethazine (11), sulfamerazine (12), sulfaquinoxaline (10), nitrophenide (9), amprolium (27), diaveridine (4), nitrofurazone (furacin), pyrimethamine (sulfamezathine), nicarbazin, zoalene, unistat, and glycamide (5, 6, 14, 18, 28). Among the more recently developed anticoccidial agents we find robenzidene (29), methyl benzoquate (31), meticlorpindol (26), and M & B 15,497 (ethyl 6-n-decyloxy-7-ethoxy-4-hydroxyquinoline-3-carboxylate; 13). Combinations of 1, 1'-dimethyl-4,4'-bipyridylium chloride and sulfadimidine (paramez, 30), sulfaquinoxaline and 2-amino-4-dimethylamino-5-(4-chlorophenyl)-6-ethylpyrimidine hydrochloride (1), and sulfaquinoxaline and diaveridine (2) have been highly recommended for treating coccidiosis. None of these has proved to be completely satisfactory. Several facts that help to account for this condition are:

1. The presently known chemotherapeutic drugs are not effective against all species of coccidia that occur in chickens.

2. Some species of coccidia, although sensitive at first, quickly develop drug-resistance.

3. All available medications will break down under heavy exposures of oocysts.

## REFERENCES

1. Ball. Jour. Comp. Path. and Therap., 1964, *74*, 487.
2. Ball and Warren. Vet. Rec., 1965, 77, 1252.
3. Bradford and Herrick. Jour. Parasitol., 1945, *31*, (Sup.), 8.
4. Clarke. Vet. Rec., 1962, *74*, 845.
5. Cuckler and Malanga. Jour. Parasitol., 1955, *41*, 302.
6. Davies and Kendall. Vet. Rec., 1955, *67*, 867.
7. Dickinson. Poultry Sci., 1941, *20*, 413.
8. Edgar and Seibold. Jour. Parasitol., 1964, *50*, 193.
9. Gardiner, Farr, and Wehr. *Ibid.*, 1952, 38, 517.
10. Grumbles, Delaplane, and Higgins. *Ibid.*, 1948, 27, 411.
11. Hawkins and Kline. *Ibid.*, 1945, *24*, 277.
12. Hawkins and Rausch. *Ibid.*, 1946, 25, 184.
13. Hodgson. Brit. Vet. Jour., 1968, *124*, 209.
14. Horton-Smith and Long. *Ibid.*, 1952, *108*, 47.
15. Horton-Smith and Long. Parasitology, 1965, 55, 401.
16. Johnson. Oreg. Agr. Exp. Sta., Director's Biennia Rpt. for 1928–30, 1930.
17. Johnson. Oreg. Agr. Exp. Sta. Bul. 358, 1938.
18. Kendall and Joyner. Vet. Rec., 1956, *68*, 119.
19. Levine. Cornell Vet., 1938, *28*, 263.
20. *Ibid.*, 1941, *31*, 107.
21. *Ibid.*, 1942, *32*, 430.
22. Long. Brit. Vet. Jour., 1964, *120*, 110.
23. Long. Parasitology, 1966, *56*, 575.
24. *Ibid.*, 1967, *57*, 351.
25. Long. Jour. Comp. Path., 1967, 77, 315.
26. Long and Millard. Vet. Rec., 1967, *81*, 11.
27. Morrison. Avian Dis., 1961, 5, 222.
28. Peterson and Hymas. Am. Jour. Vet. Res., 1950, *11*, 278.
29. Reid, Kowalski, Taylor, and Johnson. Avian Dis., 1970, *14*, 788.
30. Ryley. Vet. Rec., 1965, 77, 1498.
31. Ryley. Brit. Vet. Jour., 1967, *123*, 513.
32. Sharma and Foster. Jour. Parasitol., 1964, *25*, 211.
33. Tyzzer. Am. Jour. Hyg., 1929, *10*, 269.
34. Tyzzer, Theiler, and Jones. *Ibid.*, 1932, *15*, 319.
35. Uricchio. Proc. Helminthol. Soc. Wash., 1953, *20*, 77.

## THE COCCIDIA OF BIRDS OTHER THAN CHICKENS

A few years ago it was commonly believed that coccidiosis of domestic birds was spread from flock to flock by wild birds, particularly by sparrows. This belief was disproved by Smith and Smillie (14), who showed that sparrows commonly carried coccidia but that the latter belonged to the genus *Isospora*. The common species of sparrows and other wild birds is now known as *Isospora lacazei*. It is not infective for any of the domesticated birds except some of the cage pets such as canaries and other members of the finch family. That there still is some question with regard to the host specificity of species of *Isospora* for the lower animals has been attested by Levine and Mohan (8) who isolated a form from the feces of beef cattle that was practically indistinguishable from *I. lacazei*. A similar form has been found in sheep (13). They (8) claim that more work is needed to determine whether or not several species are being lumped under this name. Although members of the genus *Eimeria* have been isolated from wild fowl, they likewise appear to be host-specific.

### The Coccidia of Turkeys

Turkeys are occasionally affected with coccidia of the genus *Eimeria*. Under crowded conditions it appears that coccidia sometimes produce serious infections, particularly in turkey poults about 2 weeks old. No characteristic symptoms are evidenced. Infected birds may be listless and may show a lightish-brown diarrhea or abnormally chalky discharges. Turkeys cannot be infected with any of the coccidia of chickens, nor can chickens be infected with species isolated from turkeys. Apparently the coccidia of turkeys are host-specific. Attempts to cultivate coccidia from turkeys in porcine and in bovine tissue culture cells were not successful (2).

*Eimeria meleagridis*, described by Tyzzer (16) in 1927, produces a cecal coccidiosis, and *E. meleagrimitis*, described by the same author (17) in 1929, affects the small intestine. The latter is similar in many respects to *E. mitis* of the chicken but cannot be transmitted to young chickens experimentally; hence it is regarded as a distinct species. Other species of coccidia that have been isolated from turkeys are *E. dispersa*, *E. gallopavonis*, *E. innocua*, and *E. adenoeides* (11, 12).

**Chemotherapy.** Treatment is similar to that in chickens. The addition of sulfa compounds to the mash or drinking water seems to be effective if medication is begun at any time up to 96 hours after infection and if it is continued for 4 days. For controlling mild infections nitrofurazone at a concentration of about 0.01 percent in the feed for a period of 10 days is recommended.

### The Coccidia of Ducks

Coccidiosis of ducks has been described in Europe, but there is little evidence that it is of economic importance.

### *Tyzzeria perniciosa*

Allen (1) isolated a coccidium from the small intestine of the Peking duck and named it *Tyzzeria perniciosa*. The oocysts of this parasite differ from those of *Eimeria* in lacking sporocysts but having eight sporozoites lying free inside a thick wall. Sporulation requires about 24 hours, and oocysts are observed in the feces 6 days after young ducks are infected. The lesions appear to be confined to the small intestine, where they resemble those of *Eimeria necatrix* in chickens. This species was shown experimentally to be highly pathogenic for young ducks.

In 1968 Leibovitz (6) reviewed anatine coccidiosis, and also described a new species which he called *Wenyonella philiplevinei* in honor of Dr. P. Philip Levine. The organism was maintained through 20 consecutive serial passages in White Pekin ducks. It was found to be slightly pathogenic producing low mortality in experimental infections. The prepatent period, from the time of inoculation to the appearance of the oocysts in the feces, was 93 hours. Members of the genus *Wenyonella* are characterized by oocysts that bear four sporocysts, each with four sporozoites, and they have been considered to be of little importance to date.

## The Coccidia of Geese

In geese three species of intestinal coccidia have been described in Europe. These have been named *Eimeria anseris, E. nocens*, and *E. parvula*. Rather severe outbreaks have been ascribed to the first-named. Levine (7) studied fecal samples from 48 Canada geese collected in Illinois. He found *Eimeria magnalabia* in 5 and a member of the genus *Tyzzeria* in 32. Other species that have been isolated from the Canada goose are *E. crassa* and *E. pulchella* (3).

The most important species occurring in geese is *Eimeria truncata*, which produces a severe form of renal coccidiosis. This disease has been known in several European countries for many years. In 1929 McNutt (10) described an outbreak that occurred in northern Iowa. Since then *E. truncata* infection has been reported from Maryland, the District of Columbia, Washington, Illinois, Long Island, and Canada (4, 5, 9). The disease affects goslings from 3 weeks to 3 months of age. When heavy infections occur, the goslings die within 2 or 3 days after the symptoms are first seen. The mortality is often very severe and may be 100 percent. Milder infections occur, however, in which case no symptoms may be observed. Yellowish-white spots are seen under the capsule of the kidney. Sections show large numbers of developmental forms in the epithelial cells of the uriniferous tubules. The oocysts are ovoid in shape and average 16.3 by 23.5 microns in size. A protuberance at the smaller and flattened end is the site of the micropyle. Ducklings raised with the geese were not affected.

## The Coccidia of Pheasants

*Eimeria phasiani* and *E. dispersa* have been reported in pheasants. These species invade the epithelium of the small intestine and may be highly pathogenic. Trigg (15) has shown that *E. phasiani* has three distinct asexual stages prior to the onset of the sexual cycle.

**REFERENCES**

1.   Allen.   Arch. f. Protistenk., 1936, *86*, 262.
2.   Doran and Vetterling.   Proc. Helminthol. Soc. Wash., 1967, *43*, 59.
3.   Farr.   *Ibid.*, 1963, *30*, 155.
4.   Farr and Wehr.   Cornell Vet., 1952, *42*, 185.
5.   Hilbert.   *Ibid.*, 1951, *41*, 54.
6.   Leibovitz.   Avian Dis., 1968, *12*, 670.
7.   Levine.   Cornell Vet., 1952, *42*, 247.
8.   Levine and Mohan.   Jour. Parasitol., 1960, *46*, 733.
9.   McGregor.   Jour. Am. Vet. Med. Assoc., 1952, *121*, 452.
10.   McNutt.   *Ibid.*, 1929, 75, 365.
11.   Moore and Brown.   Cornell Vet., 1951, *41*, 124; 1952, *42*, 395.
12.   Morgan and Hawkins.   Veterinary protozoology. Rev. ed. Burgess Publishing Co., Minneapolis, 1952.
13.   Shah.   Jour. Parasitol., 1963, *49*, 799.
14.   Smith and Smillie.   Jour. Exp. Med., 1917, *25*, 415.
15.   Trigg.   Parasitology, 1967, *57*, 135.
16.   Tyzzer.   Jour. Parasitol., 1927, *13*, 215.
17.   Tyzzer.   Am. Jour. Hyg., 1929, *10*, 269.

## THE COCCIDIA OF CATTLE

For many years cattle were thought to harbor only one species of coccidium. In 1918 Smith and Graybill (24) showed that there were two kinds of oocysts in the feces of calves which they studied in New Jersey, one being very much larger than the other. Yakimoff and Galouzo (27), working in Europe, decided that the one with the smaller oocyst was identical with the form which had long been regarded as the causative agent of bloody dysentery in Switzerland and which had been called *Eimeria zürni*. They proposed the name *E. smithi* for the other. According to Morgan and Hawkins (20), the name *E. bovis* proposed by Zublin in 1908 has priority over the name *E. smithi*, and *E. bovis* will be used in this discussion. They also state that there are 12 valid species of bovine coccidia, but, according to Boughton (4), *E. zürni*, *E. bovis*, and *E. ellipsoidalis* are of greater economic importance than the others. Richardson and Kendall (22) list 19 valid species in their text on *Veterinary protozoology*.

Practically all adult cattle harbor coccidia. The oocysts usually are not numerous in the feces, and methods of concentration must be used to demonstrate them. Marsh (19) noted that *E. bovis* and *E. ellipsoidalis* were found most often in apparently normal cattle, and *E. zürni* when clinical evidence of coccidiosis in the herd existed. He found small numbers of *E. zürni* in healthy cattle, however, and therefore believes that outbreaks of coccidiosis in cattle are not caused by the entrance of new infection into the herd but to the release of dormant infection already there. Baker (1) studied a herd of 63 dairy heifers in New York for a period of 18 months and found four species of coccidia regularly present although no evidence of clinical coccidiosis, except possibly an occasional case of mild diarrhea, appeared. The species most frequently encountered were *E. zürni* and *E. bovis*. In dairy districts where cattle are kept in many small units fairly well isolated from each other, coccidiosis occurs sporadically, that is, isolated cases appear here and there with no physical connection between them. Occasionally sporadic outbreaks involving a considerable number of calves and heifers are seen. The evidence indicates that the parasite is widespread and that clinical disease depends upon conditions which permit massive infections. It is significant that in Switzerland where the disease is frequent and serious during the summer months, the cattle are then on mountain pastures and drinking from shallow pools where conditions for sporulation of oocysts are excellent. In the eastern part of the United States the disease is found throughout the year, but mostly during the warmer months and particularly during the early fall. In Montana, according to Marsh, the disease occurs mostly during the winter, often at times when the temperature is very low. This situation must be caused by the fact that the young animals are concentrated on small areas of ground at that time of year, and thus opportunity for massive infection is better than during the grazing season. Davis *et al.* (12) have indicated that the presence of nematodes in the intestine may have a synergistic effect on the development of coccidia in calves.

Acute coccidiosis of cattle occurs principally among young animals from 2 months to 2 years of age; however, sporadic cases are not infrequent in much older animals. The affected animals lose their appetites and rapidly decline in condition as the disease progresses. Dysentery associated with fetid, watery discharges streaked with blood is characteristic. In many cases the amount of blood discharged is considerable; sometimes the discharge appears to consist largely of blood clots, which, as a rule, are bright red in color, indicating that the hemorrhage originated in the lower bowel and, as a consequence, has not been blackened by the action of the intestinal enzymes. The animals frequently show tenesmus. As a result of the loss of blood, affected animals often show severe anemia and, because of the loss of fluids, severe dehydration of their tissues.

The lesions that are frequently observed in acute field cases of coccidiosis of cattle are located in the cecum, large intestine, and rectum. These organs are greatly thickened and edematous. The mucosa is highly hemorrhagic and thrown into thick folds. In the rectum these folds run longitudinally with large ecchymotic hemorrhages, which tend to appear principally along the crests of the folds. The thickening is so great as to be easily recognized by manual examination. In some cases the tenesmus results in prolapses, the exposed rectal tissue presenting a visual picture of the lesions present. Clots of blood of considerable size are often found, at autopsy, attached to the mucosal surface of the cecum and large intestine. Catarrhal enteritis is frequent in both the small and large intestines. The mortality rate is considerable, probably averaging from 30 to 50 percent in severe outbreaks.

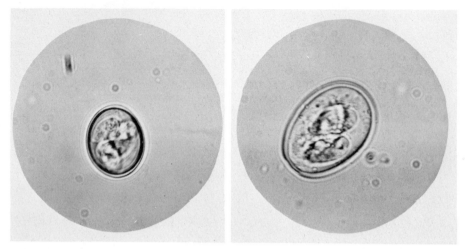

Fig. 124 (left). *Eimeria zürni*, a sporulated oocyst. X 1,000.
Fig. 125 (right). *Eimeria bovis*, a sporulated oocyst. X 1,000.

Boughton (6) in his study of experimental infections has described lesions in the small intestine similar to those seen years ago, but not identified, by Smith (23). In the fatal experimental cases, Boughton observed that the mucosa of the posterior half of the small intestine often was dotted with small, white, cystlike bodies that were macroscopic in size. He believed these bodies to be large asexual stages (schizonts). Hammond *et al.* (14, 15) in their studies on experimental coccidiosis in calves found that a second asexual generation is included in the life cycle of *E. bovis* and occurs in the epithelial cells of the cecum and colon. This would account for the localization of the protozoon first in the small and then in the large intestine. Although the finding has had no practical value to date they also determined that immunization by the use of oocysts of *E. bovis* is possible, the immune reaction being more significant in the large than in the small intestine.

**Chemotherapy.** Frank (13) reports that sulfamerazine is effective in treating young calves in which the coccidia are in the mucosa of the small intestine, cecum, colon, or rectum. In the older animals that are passing pure blood and in which the coccidia usually are located in the rectum, an enema of sulfaquinoxaline is administered. Boughton (6) used sulfaguanidine to treat *E. bovis* infection. Many clinicians prefer to give a 3-to-5-day course of sulfamethazine or sulfamerazine in treating coccidiosis. Nitrofurazone (16) is recommended as a prophylactic agent, and Peardon *et al.* (21) presented evidence that amprolium and lincomycin, administered orally, and sulfamethazine, given intravenously, were strongly coccidiostatic or coccidiocidal. Because cattle suffering from coccidiosis are anemic, blood transfusions are recommended in treating the disease.

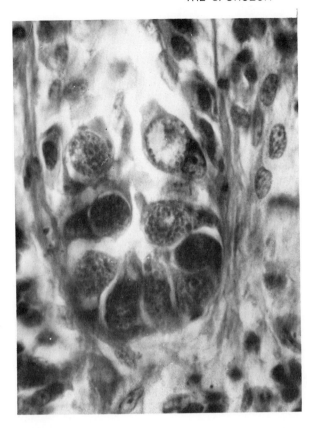

*Fig. 126.* Bovine coccidiosis (*Eimeria zürni*), showing developmental forms in epithelial cells in the base of an intestinal gland. X 690.

### Eimeria zürni

This species is often associated with outbreaks of clinical coccidiosis and is believed to be the most important species affecting cattle. The developmental forms frequently are located in the cecum and lower bowels, but they may also be found in the small intestine. Schizonts are found largely near the base of the glands, and they cause considerable denudation of epithelium, which is the cause, of course, of the extensive hemorrhages. The oocysts are nearly spherical and measure from 14 to 18 microns in diameter, averaging about 16 microns. No micropyle is visible. The color is slightly greenish. Sporulation under favorable conditions takes place in from 48 to 72 hours. The endogenous development of *E. zürni* has been studied in detail by Davis and Bowman (11).

### Eimeria bovis

SYNONYM: *Eimeria smithi*

*E. bovis* is found in clinical cases of coccidiosis, but frequently in association with other coccidia. In some of their cases that were mixed infection of

*E. zürni* and *E. bovis*, Smith and Graybill (24) mention developing forms in the villi of the lower small intestine. Becker (2) quotes Wilson as saying that, in pure infections with *E. bovis*, oocysts were as numerous in the contents of the ileum as in those of the large intestine, and Boughton (5) has demonstrated the presence of *E. bovis* in the small intestines of experimentally infected calves.

The oocysts are much larger than those of *E. zürni* and are egg-shaped. They are quite uniform in size, measuring about 21 by 29 microns. At the smaller end a micropyle is easily visible. The oocyst wall is slightly tinged with brown. The sporulation time, under favorable conditions, varies from 3 to 5 days.

### Eimeria ellipsoidalis

Becker and Frye (3) found the oocysts of this species in the feces of a healthy calf. They were also encountered by Baker (1) in a herd of calves in which clinical disease was absent. The specific name is derived from the shape of the oocysts, which are ellipsoidal, occasionally ovoidal. They measure about 15 by 22 microns, thus being considerably smaller than those of *E. bovis*. The protoplasm of the oocyst practically fills the shell when freshly passed but contracts later into a spherical mass, leaving open spaces at the end. A micropyle can be seen at one end where the shell is slightly thinned. The oocyst is colorless. Its sporulation time is rather long and variable—2 to 10 days according to Baker. Nothing is known of the developmental forms of this species, and nothing of its pathogenicity.

### Eimeria bukidnonensis

This species was described by Tubangui (25) in the Philippine Islands in 1931. Only the oocysts were observed and nothing is known about the developmental forms or its pathogenicity. Subsequently it has been seen by the Russian worker, Yakimoff, and by Baker (1) in New York, whose identification was confirmed by Christensen (7). The oocysts have very thick walls (2 microns), which are dark brown in color and show radial striations. They are distinctly egg-shaped and have a conspicuous micropyle at the smaller end. Baker's measurements indicate that the average size is about 30 by 42 microns. This is somewhat smaller than was reported by Tubangui. The sporulation time is long—from 24 to 27 days according to Baker, but only 5 to 7 according to Christensen and Porter.

### Eimeria cylindrica

Little is known about the incidence of this species. Wilson (26) described its oocysts from Virginia cattle in 1931. The shape is quite elongated, the ratio between breadth and length being greater than it is in any other bovine species. Its average size is 14.4 by 23.7 microns. Sporulation occurs very rapidly, being complete in 48 hours under favorable conditions. Wilson reports artificial infection of one calf. Blood-streaked feces were noted on the 4th day. Oocysts were not eliminated until the 7th day. Nothing is known about its developmental stages.

### Eimeria canadensis

SYNONYM: *Eimeria zurnabadensis*

According to Morgan and Hawkins, this species was named *E. canadensis* by Bruce in 1921. In 1931 it was described from oocysts found in Russian cattle by Yakimoff and called *E. zurnabadensis*. The species also occurs in the zebu and the buffalo. The oocysts vary in shape from nearly cylindrical to ellipsoidal. They are 28 to 37 microns long and 24 to 28 microns wide. Oocysts are brown to pale brown in color and sporulate in about 72 to 96 hours. The micropyle is inconspicuous.

### Eimeria auburnensis

This species was described by Christensen and Porter (9) in 1939. Oocysts were found in a calf at Auburn, Alabama. Later *E. auburnensis* was found in other animals there, and the authors think that the large oocysts mentioned by Smith and Graybill in New Jersey, by Marsh in Montana, and by Wilson and Morley in Virginia were undoubtedly those of this species.

The oocysts are larger than those of any other bovine species except *E. thianethi*, measuring 23.1 by 38.4 microns (average). They are the shape of an elongated egg. The oocyst wall usually is clear, smooth, and moderately thick (1 to 1.5 microns). Sometimes, however, they have rough, mammillated walls. The color is noticeably brownish but they are not so deeply stained as the oocysts of *E. bukidnonensis*. A small micropyle is located on the smaller end. All variations from the heavily mammillated type to the perfectly smooth types are found, but the smooth types greatly outnumber the others. Sporulation is complete in about 48 hours under favorable conditions.

A calf that was free of all coccidia was fed a dose of 8,000 sporulated oocysts. A profuse, watery, greenish diarrheal discharge was noticed from the 9th to the 13th day, accompanied by slight apathy on the part of the host. Oocysts were not found until the 24th day, when large numbers were encountered. The oocyst count rapidly diminished during the next 3 days, but they were discharged in small numbers for several weeks.

Nothing is known about the developmental stages.

### Eimeria subspherica

This type was described by Christensen (8) in 1941. The oocysts are small measuring 9 to 13 microns long by 8 to 12 microns wide. The shape is typically subspherical. Oocysts are colorless to a light yellow and sporulate in approximately 96 to 120 hours. No micropyle is visible.

### Eimeria alabamensis

Christensen (8) described this type in 1941. The oocyst is nearly colorless and measures 13 to 24 microns in length by 11 to 16 in width. The shape is typically pyriform. There is no micropyle. The sporulation time is 96 to 120 hours. According to Davis *et al.* (10), the endogenous stages of *E. alabamensis* are limited to intranuclear sites.

### Eimeria brasiliensis

According to Morgan and Hawkins (20), this type was described by Torres and Ramos in 1939. Oocysts are 34 to 42 by 24 to 29 microns. They are ovoidal, possess a micropyle, and are greenish yellow in color. Sporulation time is about 6 days. Since its discovery in cattle in Brazil it has been found in India, Australia, Nigeria, and the United States (18).

### Eimeria ildefonsoi

This type was also described by Torres and Ramos in 1939 (20). Oocysts are 31 to 54 by 22 to 34 microns. They are ovate, brown, and possess a micropyle. Sporulation occurs between 36 to 72 hours.

### Eimeria wyomingensis

Huizinga and Winger (17) described this type in 1942. Oocysts measure from 37 to 45 by 26 to 30 microns. The shape is typically ovoidal, but occasionally it is slightly pyriform. Oocysts are yellowish to greenish brown in color and possess a conspicuous micropyle. Sporulation time is 120 to 168 hours.

### Other Coccidial Species of Cattle

Richardson and Kendall (22) have listed seven species of coccidia, that are harbored by cattle, in addition to the 12 described above. They are *E. azerbaidschanica*, cylindrical, 45 by $22\,\mu$; *E. böhmi*, ellipsoidal, 34 to 49 by 24 to $33\,\mu$, prominent polar cap; *E. bambayensis*, ellipsoidal, 37 by $22\,\mu$, well defined micropyle 2 to $4\,\mu$ in diameter; *E. khurodensis*, ellipsoidal, 40 to 44 by 28 to $30\,\mu$, thick brown wall with mammillations and a micropyle up to $9\,\mu$ wide; *E. mundaragi*, ellipsoidal, 37 by $27\,\mu$, thin yellow wall with distinct micropyle; *E. pellita*, ovoidal, 40 by $28\,\mu$, thick brown wall with fine projections; and *E. thianethi*, ellipsoidal, 43 by $29\,\mu$, thick yellow wall with transverse striations.

### REFERENCES

1. Baker. Rpt. N.Y. State Vet. Coll. for 1937–38 (1939), p. 160.
2. Becker. Coccidia and coccidiosis of domesticated, game and laboratory animals and of man. Collegiate Press, Ames, Iowa, 1934, p. 65.
3. Becker and Frye. Jour. Parasitol., 1929, *15*, 175.

4. Boughton. Yearbook of Agr., U.S. Dept. Agr. U.S. Govt. Printing Office, 1942, pp. 565–571.
5. Boughton. North Am. Vet., 1942, *23*, 173.
6. Boughton. Am. Jour. Vet. Res., 1945, *4*, 66.
7. Christensen. Proc. Helminthol. Soc. Wash., 1938, 5, 24.
8. Christensen. Jour. Parasitol., 1941, 27, 203.
9. Christensen and Porter. Proc. Helminthol. Soc. Wash., 1939, *6*, 45.
10. Davis, Boughton, and Bowman. Am. Jour. Vet. Res., 1955, *16*, 269.
11. Davis and Bowman. *Ibid.*, 1957, *18*, 569.
12. Davis, Herlich, and Bowman. *Ibid.*, 1960, *21*, 188.
13. Frank. North Am. Vet., 1949, *30*, 238.
14. Hammond, Andersen, and Miner. Jour. Parasitol., 1963, *49*, 415.
15. *Ibid.*, 428.
16. Hammond, Sayin, and Miner. Am. Jour. Vet. Res., 1965, *26*, 83.
17. Huizinga and Winger. Trans. Am. Micro. Soc., 1942, *61*, 131.
18. Marquardt. Am. Jour. Vet. Res., 1959, *20*, 742.
19. Marsh. Jour. Am. Vet. Med. Assoc., 1938, *92*, 184.
20. Morgan and Hawkins. Veterinary protozoology. Rev. ed. Burgess Publishing Co., Minneapolis, 1952.
21. Peardon, Bilkovich, Todd, and Hoyt. Am. Jour. Vet. Res., 1965, *26*, 683.
22. Richardson and Kendall. Veterinary protozoology. 3d ed. Oliver and Boyd, London, 1963, p. 124.
23. Smith. U.S. Dept. Agr., Bur. Anim. Indus. Bul. 3, 1893.
24. Smith and Graybill. Jour. Med. Res., 1918, *28*, 89.
25. Tubangui. Phil. Jour. Sci., 1931, *44*, 253.
26. Wilson. Va. Polytech. Inst. Tech. Bul. 42, 1931.
27. Yakimoff and Galouzo. Arch. f. Protistenk., 1927, *58*, 185.

## THE COCCIDIA OF SHEEP AND GOATS

Coccidiosis of sheep often assumes serious proportions. At least 11 species exist, but the most common species are *Eimeria arloingi, Eimeria parva,* and *Eimeria faurei.* This does not mean that they are the most pathogenic. Also, as in the bovine group, mixed infections with two or more species is the rule rather than the exception. It appears too that most adult sheep harbor coccidia (1, 5) and that the clinical disease develops only when conditions favoring massive invasion exist. As a rule, the clinical disease is seen in lambs, seldom in old animals. In the western states of this country where lambs are raised on the range and brought in to be fattened in the feed lot, the disease is seen most often within the first month they are on feed. This has been noted by Newsom and Cross (10) and by Deem and Thorp (2) in Colorado in a number of successive years, even when sanitary conditions are well maintained. They believe, therefore, that the change of feed has an important influence in favoring the development of the parasites—that this may be more important than the increased opportunity, usually presented in the feed lot, of picking up massive doses of oocysts. It has been noted, for instance, that lambs fed on beet tops are more likely to develop severe clinical cases of coccidiosis than those that are fed alfalfa or other roughage. Newsom and Cross (10) report that the incidence of clinical coccidiosis seen by them in a number of large bands of feeder lambs in the 1929 and 1930 seasons averaged 24 percent, and deaths from the disease, about 2.8 percent. In addition to the actual mortality, however, a considerable number of lambs survived but failed to feed out satisfactorily as a result of the disease. Deem and Thorp (2) noted that as a rule the lambs arriving at the feed lots are already infected. During the first month there is a rapid increase in the oocyst count, which is maintained for 1 to 3 weeks and then declines sharply until very few can be found. Occasionally they have noted secondary rises in the count in the 3rd and 4th month. They attribute this to infection with new species against which the lambs have not developed immunity. They also noted that E. parva usually is responsible for the initial high counts and that E. arloingi later prevails in the same animals. All clinical cases were associated with the E. arloingi infection.

The clinical disease is also seen in lambs at pasture, and even in very young ones that are confined before being turned to pasture. That oocysts survive the winter in soil was demonstrated by Helle (3) in Norway and it appears that lambs become infected by consuming contaminated soil. Such animals suffer from diarrhea and the feces usually are streaked with blood.

An indication of the relative frequency of the various species of coccidia of sheep is given in the study by Christensen (1), who surveyed 100 animals originating in Idaho, Wyoming, and Maryland, with a single animal from New York. Analysis of the types of oocysts indicated that mixed infections predominated. There were only 4 negative animals in the series, 62 showed mixed infections (2 or more species), and 34 showed pure infections (1 species). Oocysts of E. arloingi were found in 28 of the pure infections, those of E. parva in 4, and those of E. granulosa and E. nina-kohl-yakimovae in 1 each. In total incidence E. arloingi occurred 90 times, E. parva 50, E. intricata 14, E. faurei 11, E. pallida 10, E. granulosa 10, and E. nina-kohl-yakimovae 3. In none of these cases was there any evidence of clinical coccidiosis.

It is presumed that all the species that affect sheep will also infect goats, but this presumption may not be correct. E. arloingi occurs in goats, in fact was first described in goats, and in this animal is capable of causing the same type of disease as in sheep. That E. faurei also occurs in both animals has been demonstrated by Lotze (7).

**Chemotherapy.** It is claimed that crude sulfur added to the ration of lambs at a level of 0.5 to 1.5 percent protects them against coccidiosis. Tarlatzis et al. (13) recommend nitrofurazone (furacin) over sulfaguanidine. They employed 10 mg per kg of body weight daily for 7 days. Ross (11) reported the successful treatment of 16 naturally infected lambs with a mixture of amprolium and ethopabate.

### Eimeria arloingi

The developmental stages of this species are found in the small intestine, particularly in the middle portions, although it may involve the greater part from the duodenum to the ileum. The schizonts are found in the epithelial cells, usually above their nuclei. The macrogametocytes tend to collect in patches from 0.5 to 6 mm in diameter, and these show to the naked eye as yellowish-white areas. They are best seen when the bowel is opened but may also be detected from the serous surface. These areas tend to stand up above the level of the mucous membrane and often are very conspicuous. The contents of the bowel are thin, watery, mucoid, brownish, and often streaked with blood.

The oocysts vary considerably in shape and size. Usually they are ellipsoidal, and conspicuous because of a mucoid cap that covers the operculum at one end. They measure 13 to 27 microns in width and 17 to 42 microns in length (average is 18 by 27 microns). The cap apparently is a tough structure, but it is often dislodged and even absent, having been lost. The micropyle, covered by the cap, is rather wide, averaging 5 microns. The smaller oocysts have little color but the larger are yellowish or brownish. Sporulation occurs between 24 and 48 hours under favorable conditions.

### Eimeria parva

Except for *E. arloingi* this seems to be the most prevalent species of coccidium of the sheep. There is little precise information about the pathogenicity of this species but evidently it is low, judging by the reports of the Colorado workers referred to above. The developmental stages in the sheep have not been described. The oocysts are small and only a little longer than broad (subspherical). They measure 10 to 18 microns wide by 12 to 22 microns long (average 14.1 by 16.5 microns). There is no perceptible micropyle. The color is very faintly yellow or yellowish green. A heavy diffraction line along the inner surface of the capsule gives this oocyst a distinctive "double contour." In solutions used for concentrating the oocysts, they frequently collapse if left for long. Sporulation occurs between 24 and 48 hours. These oocysts may be confused most readily with those of *E. pallida*, but they may be distinguished because they are more nearly round and have a double-contoured appearance.

### Eimeria pallida

This species was differentiated from *E. parva* by Christensen (1) in 1938. Only the oocyst is known. This is more elongated than that of *E. parva*. Measurements average 10 by 14.2 microns. The shape is ellipsoidal. A micropyle is not apparent. The wall is thin, transparent, and slightly yellowish green in color. Sporulation is nearly complete in 24 hours under favorable conditions.

### Eimeria faurei

At one time all coccidia of sheep were considered to belong to this species. Although it is among the more common types, it is believed to have little pathogenicity.

The oocysts are distinctly egg-shaped, with a small micropyle located at

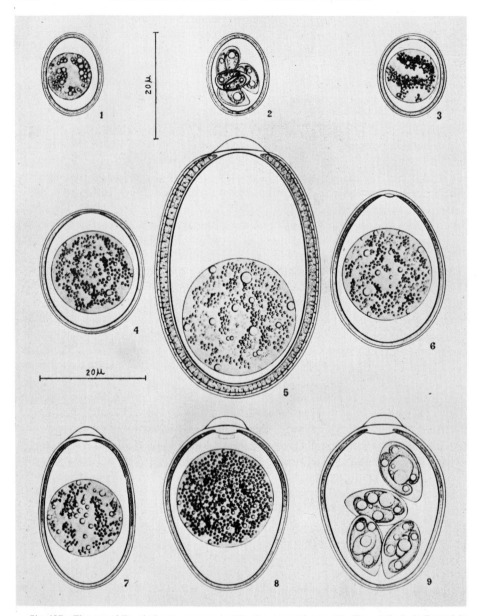

*Fig. 127.* The coccidia of sheep, camera lucida drawings of oocysts. The scale is indicated in the illustration. (1) *Eimeria pallida*, unsporulated. (2) *E. pallida*, sporulated. (3) *E. parva*, unsporulated. (4) *E. nina-kohl-yakimovae*, unsporulated. (5) *E. intricata*, unsporulated. (6) *E. faurei*, unsporulated. (7) *E. arloingi*, unsporulated. (8) *E. granulosa*, unsporulated. (9) *E. granulosa*, sporulated. (From Christensen, courtesy *Jour. Parasitol.*)

the smaller end and without a polar cap. They average 21 microns in width and 28.9 microns in breadth. The wall is clear and discontinuous at the micropylar end. It is of a pale yellowish-brown color. Sporulation occurs between 24 and 48 hours. The shape of this oocyst serves to distinguish it from all others occurring in sheep.

### Eimeria intricata

The oocysts of this species are large, ellipsoidal, dark brown, and opaque. They average 32 by 47 microns in size. The micropyle is seen as a wide gap (averaging 8 microns) in a heavy wall, and it is covered by a prominent, transparent, yellowish-green cap. The wall averages 2.5 microns in thickness and consists of two layers, the inner being twice as thick as the outer, more deeply colored, and more prominently striated. The outer surface of the outer layer is irregularly corrugated. Sporulation occurs in from 72 to 120 hours.

### Eimeria granulosa

This species was described on the basis of the oocysts alone by Christensen (1) in 1930. The oocysts are egg-shaped but differ from most forms in that the micropyle is located on the broad end. This suggests the form of a broad urn. A rather prominent polar cap covers the micropyle. This cap is easily displaced and often lost. The wall is moderately thick, transparent, smooth, and yellowish brown. The oocysts average 20.9 microns in breadth at the widest point and about 29.4 microns in length. The sporulation time is from 72 to 96 hours.

### Eimeria nina-kohl-yakimovae

This species was described on the basis of its oocysts from Russian goats. Christensen (1) found them in three sheep in his series of 100, two animals coming from Idaho, the other from Maryland.

The oocysts resemble those of E. parva but are distinguished, according to Christensen, by their faint, brownish-yellow tint, somewhat larger size, a thin and double-contoured wall at the micropyle end, and a single heavy refraction line marking the inner surface of the wall.

The shape of the oocysts usually is ellipsoidal, but they are rather broader than most ellipsoidal forms. The micropyle is inconspicuous but can be found by careful examination. There is no polar cap. The wall is thin, pale, and almost imperceptibly brownish yellow. The oocysts' average measurement is 18.3 by 23.1 microns. Sporulation is completed in the interval between 24 and 48 hours.

### Eimeria ah-sa-ta

In 1942 Honess (4) described a coccidium from Rocky Mountain bighorn sheep which he named E. ah-sa-ta. It is difficult to differentiate from E. arloingi and may not be a distinct species. The oocysts are about 22.5 by 31.5

microns in size and have a faint pink color. In 1965 Mahrt and Sherrick (8) claimed that *E. ah-sa-ta* was the species of major importance in feeder lambs in east central Illinois.

### Eimeria crandallis

This species has been described from bighorn sheep in Wyoming (4) and has been observed in domestic sheep in Michigan (9). The oocysts measure approximately 19 by 21 microns. They resemble those of *E. arloingi* but are of a somewhat larger size and the oocyst wall presents a double-contoured appearance. The peak of infection with this coccidium in Michigan is supposed to occur at a different time from that of *E. arloingi*.

### Eimeria punctata (Eimeria honessi)

This species was described in 1952 by Landers (6). It is distinguished by its size, the average being 21.17 by 17.68 microns, by the presence of a polar cap which covers a conspicuous micropyle, and by uniform pits that occur in the external surface of the oocyst wall. Sporulation time at room temperature is from 36 to 48 hours.

### Eimeria oreamni

Shah and Levine (12) described *E. oreamni* in 1964. It was found in a Rocky Moutain goat in Montana. The oocysts are elongate ovoid, 26 to 34 by 17 to 20 microns, with a mean of 29 by 9.

### REFERENCES

1. Christensen.   Jour. Parasitol., 1938, *24*, 453.
2. Deem and Thorp.   Jour. Am. Vet. Med. Assoc., 1940, *96*, 733.
3. Helle.   Acta Vet. Scand., 1970, *11*, 545.
4. Honess.   Univ. Wyo. Bul. 249, 1942.
5. Jungherr and Welch.   Jour. Am. Vet. Med. Assoc., 1927, *72*, 317.
6. Landers.   Jour. Parasitol., 1952, *38*, 569.
7. Lotze.   Proc. Helminthol. Soc. Wash., 1953, *20*, 55.
8. Mahrt and Sherrick.   Jour. Am. Vet. Med. Assoc., 1965, *146*, 1415.
9. Morgan and Hawkins.   Veterinary protozoology. Rev. ed. Burgess Publishing Co., Minneapolis, 1952.
10. Newsom and Cross.   Vet. Med., 1931, *26*, 140.
11. Ross.   Vet. Rec., 1968, *83*, 189.
12. Shah and Levine.   Jour. Parasitol., 1964, *50*, 634.
13. Tarlatzis, Panetsos, and Dragonas.   Jour. Am. Vet. Med. Assoc., 1955, *126*, 391.

## THE COCCIDIA OF SWINE

According to Vetterling (8) there are eight valid species of *Eimeria* and one of *Isospora* that occur in swine. Of these the two most pathogenic species appear to be *Eimeria debliecki* and *Eimeria scabra*. Coccidial infection of swine has been reported from Russia, Germany, Holland, France, and the United States (Iowa and California). There is little doubt that coccidia of swine occur wherever swine are raised in considerable numbers.

Many of the earlier authors contended that coccidial infections of swine were benign. Feeding trials by Nöller and Frenz (7) in Germany and by Biester and Murray (2) in the United States disproved this idea, although they did show that the swine strains are probably less pathogenic for their hosts than those of any of the other species. Both groups showed that large doses are capable of producing severe diarrhea and an occasional death among young pigs. Constipation frequently follows the diarrheal period. The pigs that recover from the acute infections frequently show severe emaciation, potbellies, and general unthriftiness, which persists long after all evidences of the coccidia have disappeared. Older swine usually are resistant to infection, probably because they have passed through minor infections early in life and have developed a considerable degree of immunity.

**Chemotherapy.** Sulfa drugs such as sulfaguanidine and sulfamethazine appear to have some value in treating coccidiosis of swine.

### Eimeria debliecki

This appears to be the most common and most pathogenic of the species affecting swine. Vetterling (8) lists it as *Eimeria debliecki* Douwes, 1921 and indicates that it is synonymous with *Eimeria scrofae* Galli-Valerio, 1935 and *Eimeria polita* Prellérdy, 1949. Developmental forms of *E. debliecki* are found in the small intestine, and to a lesser extent, in the cecum and colon. They occur in the epithelial cells. Oocysts are 20 to 30 by 14 to 19 $\mu$ and sporocysts 15 to 20 by 6 to 7 $\mu$. The shape of the oocyst varies from subspherical to ovoid. A micropyle is not present. The protoplasm of the unsegmented oocysts practically fills the shell. At one end of each sporocyst a knoblike protuberance occurs. The sporulation time varies from 7 to 9 days, and oocysts may be recovered from the feces in from 6 to 7 days after feeding sporulated oocysts. When reinfection is prevented, oocyst shedding continues for 10 to 15 days, then ceases. The infection is self-limiting. Second infections can be induced, according to Biester and Schwarte (4), but the animal shows evidence of considerable resistance. Nearly absolute immunity to reinfection can be induced by continued day-to-day feeding of small numbers of oocysts, but this immunity is short-lived because it is possible to set up a new infection with the same species after a lapse of about 3 weeks. Chronic coccidiosis of swine, according to these authors, is a result of continued reinfections.

### Eimeria scabra

This species was described by Henry (5) in California in 1931. Developmental forms occur in the villi of the small intestine. The oocysts are characterized by a thick (1.5 to 2.0 microns) shell with a rough outer surface and a brown color. The size varies from 16 to 25 microns in width by 22.5 to 35.5

microns in length. The shape is ellipsoidal or slightly ovoidal. At one end, the small end of the ovoidal forms, the shell wall is considerably thinner than elsewhere, but a definite micropyle is not present. The nonsegmented oocyst presents a shell nearly filled with the cytoplasm when freshly passed, but later the cytoplasm contracts into a spherical form before dividing. Sporulation is completed in from 9 to 12 days under favorable conditions.

### Eimeria perminuta

This species was described by Henry (5) in California in 1931 and apparently has not been encountered elsewhere. Nothing is known about it except that the oocysts, which resemble those of *E. scabra,* are much smaller. They resemble the oocysts of *E. debliecki* in form and shape, but the latter does not have the roughened surface of this species. The color is yellowish. They measure 9.6 to 12.8 microns in width by 11.2 to 16 microns in length. The sporulation time is about 12 days.

### Eimeria spinosa

This species was discovered and described by Henry (5) in 1931 and has not been reported elsewhere. Only the oocysts are known. These are characterized by small spiny structures that arise in the shell and project about 1 micron beyond its surface. They are spaced about 1 micron apart over the entire surface. The color is brown. The form is ellipsoidal and no micropyle is visible. The measurements vary from 12.8 to 16 microns in breadth by 16 to 22.4 microns in length. The sporulation time is about 12 days.

### Other *Eimeria* Species of Swine

In addition to the four species described above, Vetterling (8) lists the following. *Eimeria suis* Nöller, 1921, previously a synonym of *E. debliecki,* has oocysts 13 to 20 by 11 to 15 $\mu$ and sporocysts 8 to 12 by 4 to 6 $\mu$; *Eimeria neodebliecki* n. sp. with oocysts 17 to 26 by 13 to 20 $\mu$ and sporocysts 12 to 14 by 5 to 7 $\mu$; *Eimeria porci* n. sp. with oocysts 18 to 27 by 13 to 18 $\mu$ and sporocysts 8 to 12 by 6 to 8 $\mu$; and *Eimeria credonis* n. sp. with oocysts 26 to 32 by 20 to 23 $\mu$ and sporocysts 15 to 18 by 7 to 9 $\mu$.

### Isospora suis

In 1934 Biester and Murray (3) published a brief note on their finding of a coccidium belonging to *Isospora* in swine. A few additional details are given by Biester in a note appearing in Becker's (1) book on the coccidia.

The oocysts are thick-walled (1.5 microns), yellowish brown, and subspherical. A micropyle was not seen. In breadth they average about 19.5 microns, in length about 22.5 microns. Sporulation is completed in about 4 days. Oocysts are eliminated in from 6 to 8 days after a single infective feeding, and this continues for about 8 days.

The developmental forms occur in the epithelium of the villi of the small intestine. Diarrhea occurs on the 6th or 7th day after feeding. There is no blood in the diarrheal discharge. Constipation follows the period of diarrhea. The species appears to be host-specific. Dogs, guinea pigs, and rats did not become infected when fed sporulated oocysts, and, conversely, pigs failed to develop infection when fed sporulated oocysts of *Isospora bigemina* from the dog.

### REFERENCES

1. Becker. Coccidia and coccidiosis of domesticated, game, and laboratory animals and of man. Collegiate Press, Ames, Iowa, 1934.
2. Biester and Murray. Jour. Am. Vet. Med. Assoc., 1929, *75*, 705.
3. *Ibid.*, 1934, *84*, 294.
4. Biester and Schwarte. *Ibid.*, 1932, *81*, 358.
5. Henry. Pub. Zool., Univ. Calif., 1931, *36*, 115.
6. Morgan and Hawkins. Veterinary protozoology. Rev. ed. Burgess Publishing Co., Minneapolis, 1952.
7. Nöller and Frenz. Deut. tierärztl. Wchnschr., 1922, *30*, 1.
8. Vetterling. Jour. Parasitol., 1965, *51*, 897.

## THE GENUS *HEPATOZOON*

In the genus *Hepatozoon*, schizogony occurs in the cells of the liver, spleen, and other organs of mice, rats, jackals, and dogs (3); merozoites enter erythrocytes or leukocytes and develop into gametocytes. Sporogony takes place in bloodsucking arthropods (ticks and mites) where the oocysts are developed.

### Hepatozoon canis

In 1925 Rau (2) published an account of *Hepatozoon canis* infection in the dog. It was also seen in the blood of a dog by Chaudhury (1) in Assam, India. The dog presented the symptoms of a subacute disease—increased temperature, impaired appetite, and general emaciation. The infection occurs in Asia and in Africa and it appears that the tick, *Rhipicephalus sanguineus*, is the vector where the protozoon undergoes syngamy and sporogony.

### REFERENCES

1. Chaudhury. Indian Vet. Jour., 1943, *20*, 22.
2. Rau. Vet. Jour., 1925, *81*, 293.
3. Richardson and Kendall. Veterinary protozoology. 3d ed. Oliver and Boyd, London, 1963, pp. 98–99.

## THE HEMOSPORIDIA

The hemosporidia are blood-inhabiting protozoa that are closely related to the coccidia, and may possibly have originated as coccidia. The stages in the life cycles are very much alike as will be seen by comparing them. In both cases infection of the vertebrate host occurs as the result of the invasion of suitable cells by sporozoites coming in from the outside. These sporozoites, developing inside cells of the host, become schizonts, which produce a crop of merozoites. These give rise to a second generation of schizonts. In the case of the coccidia all of this goes on in epithelial cells, usually in the intestinal tract. In the case of the hemosporidia the cells are those of the vascular system. In both cases the schizogonic multiplication finally ceases, an alternation of generation occurs, and gametocytes are formed. At this stage there is divergence. In the group of coccidia, fertilization occurs in the original host, zygotes are formed which are protected by oocysts, and these leave the host to undergo sporulation as free bodies in moist soil or in water. In the process of sporulation sporozoites are formed, which are then ready to infect another host if chance causes them to be ingested. In the group of hemosporidia, the gametocytes are not fertilized in the vertebrate host but must wait until they reach the stomach of a bloodsucking arthropod. The zygotes resulting from fertilization in the stomach of the arthropod, instead of being motionless bodies as in the coccidia, are wormlike organisms (*ookinetes*), which bore their way through the stomach wall to form oocysts in the tissues. The oocysts increase in size and their cytoplasm divides into many small cells, each of which eventually becomes a highly motile sporozoite. These sporozoites migrate to the mouth parts of the arthropod and are ready to infect another vertebrate host at the time of the next blood meal. Since the advent of DDT and related insecticides, it has been possible to control certain protozoan diseases by destroying their insect vectors.

The order *Hemosporidia* contains seven genera that play important roles in producing disease in animals. They are *Plasmodium, Hemoproteus, Leucocytozoon, Babesia, Theileria,* and *Gonderia*. Because the *Toxoplasma* possess characteristics somewhat unique for the classical members of the order *Coccidia* we will continue to discuss them with the hemosporidia, at least until their position is clearly and firmly established.

## THE GENUS *PLASMODIUM*

A single genus, *Plasmodium*, embraces the malarial parasites of man and the lower animals. Schizogony takes place in the erythrocytes and also probably in endothelial cells of man, mammals, birds, and reptiles; sexual reproduction occurs in bloodsucking insects. Although it has generally been believed that the sporozoites, upon entering the blood vessel, penetrate the erythrocytes and begin their development, recent workers have indicated that the early growth takes place in cells of the reticuloendothelial system and that the red cells later are invaded by the forms that have developed in that system (Kudo, 14). The studies of Bray (1) on the tissue phase of malaria parasites in the monkey add further support to this contention. Following a bite by an infected mosquito the sporozoites make their way to the liver of the monkey. Here they penetrate parenchymal cells and begin a process of schizogony which consists of simple growth in size associated with continuous di-

vision of the nuclei. The parasite then ruptures releasing about 5,000 daughter parasites into the blood stream. These enter erythrocytes and initiate the
blood cycle. Asexual reproduction in the blood brings about the clinical
symptoms of malaria. However, a very small minority of the parasites re-enter
liver cells to begin again their 8-to-10-day cycle of development. Sooner or
later the blood cycle will die out because of drugs or natural reasons, but the
cycle in the liver goes on, forming a reservoir from which parasites can again
break out into the blood stream to bring about the so-called *malarial relapse.*
In contrast to the blood cycle, this tissue cycle may take years to burn itself
out. Similar observations on the exoerythrocytic stages of simian malaria have
been made by Held and Contacos (11).

Malaria is a very important disease in man, but it appears to be of little
economic importance in domestic animals. In man, malaria is caused by at
least four species of *Plasmodium* (*P. vivax, P. falciparum, P. malariae,* and *P.
ovaie*). The disease is world wide and is transmitted in nature by anopheline
mosquitoes. Among animals, plasmodial infections occur in monkeys, a number of species of oriental mammals, and in certain reptiles, but they occur
most frequently in birds. In general, the species are rather host-specific but
this does not always apply in the bird malarias, and it has been shown that *P.
cynomolgi* and *P. brazilianum* can be transmitted with relative ease from
monkey to man through the bites of infected mosquitoes, making simian malaria a true zoonosis (8). In fact, it has been adequately demonstrated that a
number of simian malaria species can be transmitted to man and that the so-
called *human species* can be transferred to monkeys, thereby establishing
routes leading from monkey to man, from man to man, and from man back to
monkey (5, 9, 20). Although a number of species of anopheline mosquitoes are
involved in transmitting human and simian malaria, Chin *et al.* (4) have reported that *Anopheles freeborni* is the first recorded vector to transmit all
four species of human malaria.

According to Herman (12), at least 30 North American species of birds harbor malaria parasites. A great many bird-infecting species of plasmodia have
been described, but many of these may not be valid and the known valid species may not number more than a dozen. Herman (12) limits them to eight,
and Manwell (16) to twelve.

A great deal of work has been done on the malarias of birds, partly because
of their intrinsic interest but more especially because they are easily transmitted and handled in the laboratory and have yielded much information that
has led to important advances in our knowledge of human malaria. All but
three of the known avian species are infective for canaries, and because this is
a convenient bird with which to work, it has been commonly used. Acute and
fatal infections, or chronic infections, can be produced experimentally at will.
Besides the malarial parasites that can be readily identified microscopically
in the blood of these birds, a brownish-black pigment known as *melanin* or
*hemozoin,* which results from incomplete destruction of hemoglobin, appears

as granules in the parasitized erythrocytes. In a general way the forms seen resemble those that occur in the blood of human infections.

The malarial infections of birds are transmitted by mosquitoes, but, unlike the human infections, they are usually transmitted by culicine species.

Three species of bird-malaria parasites, *Plasmodium praecox, P. circumflexum,* and *P. cathemerium,* are relatively common in passerine birds in North America. Ordinarily they do not appear to do a great deal of damage to their hosts, but all three are capable, experimentally, of causing fatal infections. Manwell (15) has demonstrated that all three of the species mentioned are capable of developing in chickens, but the developmental level in this abnormal host is so low that parasites could not ordinarily be demonstrated in their blood by microscopic examination but had to be detected by massive inoculations of blood into more susceptible birds. In no cases did infections last more than 10 days. Taliaferro and Taliaferro (19), working with another species (*P. lophurae*), succeeded in producing an acute rise in blood parasites by inoculating chickens with large doses, but the numbers disappeared rapidly and this was followed by a period of latency that lasted as long as 4 months. Avian malaria is discussed in detail by Hewitt (13).

The only species of bird malaria that is of any economic importance in domesticated birds is *P. gallinaceum.* This species does not occur in North America, except in certain laboratories, where it is being studied because its relation to human malaria is closer than that of the common bird types. *P. gallinaceum* was described and named by the French parasitologist Brumpt (2), who obtained it from Ceylon. According to Brumpt (3), this species develops rapidly in all of the yellow fever mosquitoes and other anopheline types but not in the culicine species. It is highly pathogenic for chickens, particularly for young birds. Older birds are more resistant and often become chronic carriers. Geese are also readily infected, but ducks, pigeons, and canaries are refractory.

Hass (10) reported the transmission of sporozoites of *P. gallinaceum* to chick embryos by allowing infected *Aedes aegypti* to feed through the shell membranes of the developing hen's eggs. Because lower animal hosts are not available for the human malarial parasites, the natural species of birds have been used extensively in experimental studies.

**Immunity.** Birds that recover from malarial infection are resistant to reinfection, and, according to Coffin (7), serum from such birds will protect susceptible ones.

**Chemotherapy.** Among the important discoveries are the chemotherapeutic activity of the quinine derivatives such as quinacrine, poludrine, chloroquine, pamoquine, pentaquine, isopentaquine, primaquine, amodiaquine (camozuin), and propoquin. Terramycin (17), sulfamerazine, and pyrimethamine (daraprim) have been reported to be of value in treating malaria. Coatney *et al.* (6) have indicated that a repository preparation of the dihydrotriazine metabolite of chlorguanide (proguanil) known as CI-501 (camolar) has the capacity to exert long-term protection against vivax malaria. The insecticides, DDT, dieldrin, gammexane, and their relatives, have given malariologists a weapon of tremendous value. Whole areas and even countries have been freed from this disease mainly by the use of these drugs (18), but until malaria disappears from the world there are grave risks in losing all that has been accomplished and it will be necessary to maintain vector-borne-disease control service for many years to achieve global eradication of this disease.

## REFERENCES

1. Bray. Jour. Trop. Med. Hyg. (London), 1954, 57, 41.
2. Brumpt. Comp. rend. Acad. Sci., 1935, 200, 783.
3. Brumpt. Ann. Parasitol., 1936, 14, 597.
4. Chin, Contacos, and Buxbaum. Am. Jour. Trop. Med. and Hyg., 1966, 15, 690.
5. Coatney. Ibid., 1968, 17, 147.
6. Coatney, Contacos, and Lunn. Ibid., 1964, 13, 383.
7. Coffin. Jour. Inf. Dis., 1951, 89, 8.
8. Contacos and Coatney. Jour. Parasitol., 1963, 49, 912.
9. Cantacos and Collins. Science, 1968, 161, 56.
10. Hass. Public Health Rpts. (U.S.), 1945, 60, 185.
11. Held and Contacos. Jour. Parasitol., 1967, 53, 910.
12. Herman. Bird-Banding, 1938, 9, 25. (Abs. in Exp. Sta. Rec., 1938, 79, 217.)
13. Hewitt. Bird malaria. Johns Hopkins Press, Baltimore, 1942.
14. Kudo. Protozoology. 5th ed. C. C Thomas, Springfield, Ill., 1966.
15. Manwell. Am. Jour. Trop. Med., 1933, 13, 97.
16. Ibid., 1938, 18, 565.
17. Ruiz-Sanchez, Casillas, Paredes, Velazquez, and Riebeling. Antibiotics and Chemother., 1952, 2, 51.
18. Russell. Am. Jour. Trop. Med. and Hyg., 1952, 1, 111.
19. Taliaferro and Taliaferro. Jour. Inf. Dis., 1940, 66, 153.
20. Young, Porter, Jr., and Johnson. Science, 1966, 153, 1006.

## THE GENUS *HEMOPROTEUS*

Members of the genus *Hemoproteus* occur only in birds. A great many species of wild birds harbor them. The gametocytes are found in the erythrocytes, the fully developed forms being horseshoe-shaped, forming a sort of collar or halter around the nuclei. This suggested the name *Halteridium*, by which these forms are commonly known. Schizogony takes place in the endothelial cells of viscera of the vertebrate hosts, sexual reproduction in blood-sucking insects.

### *Hemoproteus columbae*

This protozoon occurs in pigeons and is found in the Mediterranean region of Europe and Africa, in India, in Hawaii, and in South America. In 1954 Simpson and Swarthout (4) reported that 10 pigeons taken at random in a

Florida city park were found to be parasitized with *Hemoproteus columbae*. No evidence of morbidity was observed in these birds. The transmitting agents are bloodsucking flies, of which several species belong in the genus *Lynchia* (1).

### Hemoproteus lophortyx

This parasite has been found in quail in California. Gametocytes are present in erythrocytes and occasionally in leukocytes. In nature sexual reproduction takes place in the fly, *Lynchia hirsuta* (2).

Members of the genus *Hemoproteus* have also been reported in a turkey poult, in ducks, and in geese in the United States (1, 3).

### REFERENCES

1.  Herman.  Jour. Parasitol., 1951, 37, 280.
2.  Kudo.  Protozoology. 5th ed. C. C Thomas, Springfield, Ill., 1966.
3.  Morgan and Hawkins.  Veterinary protozoology. Rev. ed. Burgess Publishing Co., Minneapolis, 1952.
4.  Simpson and Swarthout.  Vet. Med., 1954, 49, 491.

## THE GENUS *LEUCOCYTOZOON*

Members of this group of hemosporidia are found only in birds. The name was given by earlier workers who believed that the greatly distorted cells seen in the circulating blood which harbored the gametocytes were leukocytes. These cells are devoid of hemoglobin, but it is now believed that they are immature erythrocytes rather than leukocytes. Schizogony occurs in the endothelial cells as well as in the visceral cells of vertebrates, sexual reproduction in the bloodsucking insects.

Leucocytozoa occur in the blood of many species of wild birds. They have been observed also in the domestic duck and turkey, in which they cause serious losses. Reports have also been made of infections of chickens, guinea fowl, and geese, but little is known about such infections. Heavy losses of wild ducks, wild turkeys, and wild grouse have been attributed to members of the group. The transmitting agents, in the cases in which the life cycle has been worked out, have been gnats or black flies of the genus *Simuliidae*.

### Leucocytozoon smithi

In connection with his studies on enterohepatitis (blackhead) in turkeys, Theobald Smith (5) in 1895 mentioned certain structures in the blood which undoubtedly were the gametocytes of this organism; hence the organism has been named in his honor. Laveran and Lucet (2) saw the parasite in France in 1905. It was described again by Volkmar (7) in this country in 1930. Skidmore (4) reported a serious outbreak of the disease in a turkey flock in Nebraska in 1932. Johnson and co-workers (1) in Virginia published a number of papers between 1935 and 1938 on the parasite and the disease, which apparently is rather serious in many parts of southeastern United States. Travis, Goodwin, and Gambrell (6) described the disease in the same area in 1939.

The disease affects young birds, principally those under 12 weeks of age. The mortality rate may be very high. In the flock described by Skidmore, only 40 poults remained at the end of the summer out of an original number of 385. Symptoms in the young may be seen for only a day or two before death intervenes. The sick birds lose their appetites, appear depressed, and have a tendency to lie down. When disturbed they move with difficulty. Often they fall over, gasp a few times, and are dead. Infections of older birds usually are not so severe and many show no symptoms. They may be carriers for several months, and constitute the means by which the infection is propagated from one year to the next. Johnson mentions a common symptom of moist tracheal *râles* which he believes is a part of this disease. Older birds may become severely emaciated and anemic. The liver generally is enlarged and the gall bladder distended. The lungs, liver, and spleen usually are congested. The proventriculus and the first portions of the small intestine are often congested and edematous. The pericardial sac may be filled with fluid.

**Morphology and Staining Properties.** As they occur in the blood, the gametocytes are elongated structures of such size that they are quite conspicuous. Some authors refer to them as "cigar-shaped." According to Newberne (3), the mature gametocytes occur in the peripheral blood and tissue blood spaces. The schizonts are found in the liver. The gametocytes stain rather darkly with Wright's and Giemsa's stains. The cells in which they are located have pointed ends. This form is seen only when the blood films are quickly made, for, shortly after blood is drawn from the bird, the protoplasm of these cells tends to assume a spherical form. Two nuclei are found in most of these forms, one presumably being the nucleus of the parasitized cell. Skidmore does not give measurements, but his photomicrographs indicate that the parasites are from three to four times as long as the greatest diameter of the normal erythrocytes. Johnson and co-workers, also West and Starr (9), point out that differentiation of the microgametocytes from the macrogametocytes is not

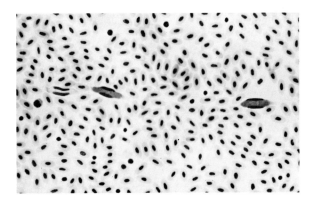

Fig. 128. *Leucocytozoon smithi,* a stained blood film of a turkey showing two macrogametocytes and one microgametocyte. Each body has two nuclei, one being that of the parasite and the other that of the parasitized erythrocyte. X 350. (Courtesy E. P. Johnson.)

difficult, the male cells being much more lightly stained than the female. The latter give the average measurements as 10.5 by 20 microns.

**Transmission.** The disease cannot be transmitted by the inoculation of blood. A few gametocytes may be found in the blood after such inoculations but they tend to disappear, and the bird shows no symptoms of the infection.

In Virginia the natural transmitting agent, according to Johnson and co-workers (1), is *Simulium nigroparvum,* a black fly that breeds abundantly in the small streams of the western part of that state. In Nebraska, Skidmore showed that the transmitting agent was a black fly but one of a different species, *Simulium occidentale.* Both of these flies are active bloodsuckers, and turkeys are attacked vigorously, especially in the region of the head. The small insects act as true hosts, the life cycle in them being very much like that of the other hemosporidia. Zygotes and ookinetes have been identified in the stomach contents of infected flies. Oocysts have not been definitely identified, but sporozoites have been recognized in the salivary glands in from 3 to 5 days after infective feedings. In experimentally infected turkeys gametocytes have been found in the blood on the 9th day. In 1962 Wehr (8) published details on the schizogony, transmission, and control of *L. smithi.*

## REFERENCES

1. Johnson, Underhill, Cox, and Threlkeld.   Am. Jour. Hyg., 1938, *27,* 649.
2. Laveran and Lucet.   Comp. rend. Acad. Sci., 1905, p. 673.
3. Newberne.   Am. Jour. Vet. Res., 1955, *16,* 593.
4. Skidmore.   Centrbl. f. Bakt., I Abt., Orig., 1932, *125,* 329.
5. Smith.   U.S. Dept. Agr., Bur. Anim. Indus. Bul. 8, 1895.
6. Travis, Goodwin, and Gambrell.   Jour. Parasitol., 1939, *25,* 278.
7. Volkmar.   *Ibid.,* 1929, *16,* 24.
8. Wehr.   Avian Dis., 1962, *6,* 195.
9. West and Starr.   Vet. Med., 1940, *35,* 649.

### *Leucocytozoon simondi*

SYNONYM:   *Leucocytozoon anatis*

The probable importance of this species was pointed out in 1915 by Wickware (6), who investigated a serious outbreak of disease in ducks near Ottawa, Canada, which he believed was caused by this parasite. Thinking that the parasite had not been described previously, he proposed the name *Leucocytozoon anatis,* by which it is best known. In 1938, however, Herman (3) called attention to the fact that Mathis and Leger had described what seems to have been the same organism in 1910. This being the case, the name proposed by the latter takes precedence over that of Wickware. Most of the details of the incidence of this species and its life cycle were clarified by O'Roke (4, 5), working in Michigan.

Cook (1) states that the gametocytes of *L. simondi* found in the circulating blood of the duck develop exclusively in the erythrocyte series. Both round and elongate gametocytes appear to be mature.

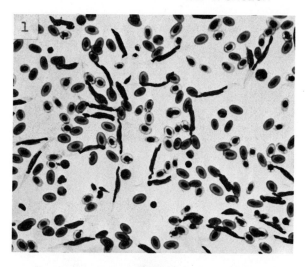

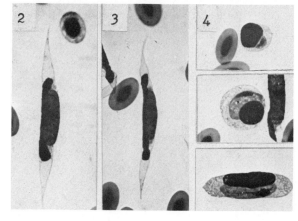

Fig. 129. Leucocytozoon disease in ducks. (1) Stained blood film showing numerous leucocytozoa. X 430. (2) and (3) Macro- and microgametocytes, L. simondi. X 1,000. (4) Early stages of gametocyte development. X 1,000. (Courtesy Savage and Isa, Cornell Vet.)

**Morphology.** The microgametes are spindle-shaped structures oriented parallel to the cell nucleus, which becomes very elongated. The host cells average 46.6 microns in length, the parasite 3.1 to 4.3 by 14.7 to 18.9 microns. The cytoplasm stains a pale blue with Giemsa's stain. The nucleus is centrally located, oval, pale pink in color; it shows no karyosome. The macrogametes occur in the same kind of host cell, but these cells become more elongated, measuring 55.4 microns in length on an average. The spindle-shaped parasite measures 3.2 to 4.4 by 14.5 to 22 microns. The cytoplasm is stained dark blue with Giemsa's stain, and it is granular. The nucleus is spherical, centrally located; it contains a distinct karyosome. No evidence of pigment is seen in either form.

**Pathogenicity.** This parasite attacks both wild and domestic ducks. The mortality rate in young ducks, according to O'Roke, amounts to about 35 percent. Adult birds carry the parasite with no evident effect on their health. The infected ducklings refuse their food and show evidence of stupor. When aroused they often show violent paroxysms. The head is usually carried in a peculiar position and sometimes is waved in a strange fashion. Often there is difficulty in maintaining equilibrium, the wings frequently being called into play in the effort to stand. Wickware mentions a purulent ophthalmitis as a frequent symptom. Death usually occurs within a day to two after symptoms are first observed. The only gross lesion, aside from anemia in the more chronic cases, is a hemorrhagic enteritis.

**Transmission.** At the place where he worked in Michigan, O'Roke found that all ducks not protected from the bites of the black fly, *Simulium venustum*, which was very prevalent, became infected with the protozoon. Those that were kept under screens escaped. Fallis *et al.* (2) have also incriminated *Simulium parnassum* as a vector.

**Life Cycle.** Schizonts are found in the capillaries of the lungs, liver, spleen, and kidneys, but only gametocytes occur in the blood. Following the bite of infected black flies, gametocytes are first found on the 7th day. By the 10th day these have matured. The bird shows symptoms and may die at this time, although it usually dies on the 12th day.

O'Roke was able to follow the entire life cycle in the fly. Gametogenesis and ookinete formation take place in the stomach. The oocysts form in the outer layers of the stomach wall and the sporozoites escape to the salivary glands. O'Roke estimated that the entire cycle in the black fly requires about 5 days, and, because that in the duck requires about 10, the whole life cycle of the parasite can be completed in about 15 days.

## REFERENCES

1.  Cook.   Proc. Helminthol. Soc. Wash., 1954, *21*, 1.
2.  Fallis, Davies, and Vickers.   Canad. Jour. Zool., 1951, *29*, 305.
3.  Herman.   Jour. Parasitol., 1938, *24*, 472.
4.  O'Roke.   *Ibid.*, 1930, *17*, 112.
5.  *Ibid.*, 1931, *18*, 127.
6.  Wickware.   Parasitology, 1915, *8*, 17.

### *Leucocytozoon bonasae*

This parasite was discovered by Clarke (2) in 1934 in ruffed grouse that were dying in large numbers in Algonquin Park, Ontario. The mortality was largely among the young birds, of which about 60 percent had died by midsummer. All dead birds showed this parasite in their blood, and no other cause for the mortality could be found; hence he was inclined to attribute the deaths to it. Because it has long been known that grouse mortality is periodic in the northern countries, the population rising and falling in cycles, the author (3) suggests that this parasite may possibly be the causative agent.

Borg (1), however, made a comprehensive study of *Leucocytozoon* infection in Swedish forest game birds and concluded that it was not possible to trace any connection between the widespread mortality among these birds and the presence of this blood parasite.

## REFERENCES

1.  Borg. On *Leucocytozoon* in Swedish capercaillie, black grouse, and hazel grouse. Berlingsha Bobtryckeriet, Lund, 1953.
2.  Clarke. Science, 1934, *80*, 228.
3.  Clarke. Canad. Jour. Res., 1935, *12*, 646.

### *Leucocytozoon* Species in Chickens

In 1953 Atchley (1) found *L. andrewsi* in the blood of chickens in South Carolina, and in 1963 Pan (3) described and discussed the gametogony of *L. caulleryi* in chickens. While making histopathologic studies of an outbreak of Marek's disease, Chew (2) discovered schizonts (megaloschizonts) of a *Leucocytozoon* not only in the visceral organs but also in the eyes and sciatic nerves of two hens. He concluded that these parasites may cause cataractlike eye lesions and paralysis of the legs in the absence of Marek's disease.

## REFERENCES

1.  Atchley. Jour. Parasitol., 1951, 37, 483.
2.  Chew. Vet. Rec., 1968, *83*, 518.
3.  Pan. Avian Dis., 1963, 7, 361.

## THE GENUS *BABESIA*

These parasites occur in the erythrocytes of mammals. They are pear-shaped and arranged in couples. With Giemsa's stain the cytoplasm stains bluish and the nucleus red. Sexual reproduction occurs in the female tick and is carried through developing ova to young ticks.

### THE BABESIAE OF CATTLE

In 1893 Smith and Kilborne (14) described the blood parasite of the so-called *Texas fever* of cattle and gave it the name *Pyrosoma bigemina*. Because this generic name was found to have been pre-empted for another organism, it was shortly changed to *Piroplasma*, under which it is best known. The group of diseases which later were found to be caused by this and similar organisms are frequently called the *piroplasmoses*. It appears, however, that Babes (1) had seen and described this organism in Romanian cattle in 1888, although he was mistaken as to its nature, and that the generic name *Babesia* had been suggested for it in his honor before Smith and Kilborne applied their name. The name *Babesia* accordingly has priority. The generic designition should be *Babesia* and the disease babesiosis, but the name piroplasmosis will continue to be used.

At least four types of piroplasmoses of cattle are recognized. The diseases are similar, but the parasites are morphologically and immunologically different and the transmitting agents differ. North American students are particularly interested in one of these, *Babesia bigemina*, because it is the only one that occurs in this part of the world.

### Babesia bigemina

SYNONYM:   *Piroplasma bigemina*

This organism was first accurately described by Smith and Kilborne (14) in the United States in 1893. These workers also made the discovery that the infection was transmitted by an arthropod, a discovery of epochal importance because this was the first protozoan disease shown to be so transmitted.

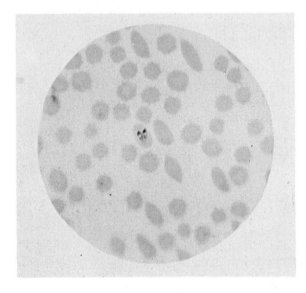

Fig. 130. *Babesia bigemina*, a stained film of blood from a cow suffering from Texas fever. One parasitized erythrocyte is located near the center of the field. This cell contains two parasites. X 1,000.

**Morphology.** *Babesia bigemina* occurs in the erythrocytes as pear-shaped forms, principally, although round and irregular forms are not uncommon. Generally the pear-shaped forms are seen in pairs and this accounts for the specific name. The two individuals of the pair lie side by side with their pointed ends in contact with each other. They are about 4 microns in length and lie crosswise of the erythrocytes. Sometimes only one form appears; in other cases there may be four, arranged in fan-shaped formation. Multiplication is by cell division, two individuals resulting from division of each of the mature forms. The chromatic material is divided equally between the newly formed individuals, taking its place as a distinct granule located near the small end of the pear-shaped cells. Details of the growth process at this stage are rather meager. Apparently the host cells are destroyed because hemoglobinemia is a prominent part of the pathological picture. It is believed that the pear-shaped elements, freed from one cell, proceed to invade others, repeating the process in the second cell. In acute piroplasmosis large numbers of infected cells are seen in blood films. In chronic cases it is difficult and often impossible to demonstrate parasites in blood films, but the infection can be shown to be present by inoculating young susceptible calves with the blood. In Giemsa-stained blood films the cytoplasm of the parasites stains bluish and the chromatic material red. The erythrocytes take a yellowish-pink color, although many of them are low in hemoglobin and stain a pale straw color as a consequence.

**The Transmitting Agents.** In the United States almost the only transmitting agent in the past has been *Boophilus annulatus* (*Margaropus annulatus*), known locally as the *blue tick*, the *Texas fever tick*, the *fever tick*, or the *southern cattle tick*. At one time this agent was prevalent in the southern half of the United States, but the eradication campaign against it, waged since 1906, had practically eliminated it by 1940. A few specimens are occasionally found in country lying along the Mexican border, most of these having come across the border on horses. These specimens are uninfected with the fever parasite. They are known locally as *cold* ticks in contrast to the *hot* ticks which carry the infection. The latter have not been found in the United States since 1939.

In a very limited area of southern Florida the transmitting agent was another species, *B. microplus* (*australis*). This species has a wider host relationship than *B. annulatus*. The campaign for eliminating this species was a difficult one because it was prevalent in the deer and semiwild cattle of the Everglades. By 1940 it was thought that this species had also been eliminated, but in 1948 it was discovered that this was not so. Up to this time (1971) there has been no evidence that the remaining specimens harbor the piroplasms. So far as is known, the United States is entirely free from piroplasmosis at the present time. The island of Puerto Rico and some of the Virgin Islands have also been freed from the disease by the same methods employed in the United States.

In other parts of the world species of *Margaropus or Boophilus*, which some regard as synonymous and others as distinct genera (6), are responsible for transmitting this parasite. In South and Central America and Australia it is *B. microplus*, in South Africa *B. decoloratus,* and in North Africa and the USSR *M. calcaratus*. Members of the genera *Hemaphysalis* and *Rhipicephalus* are important in Europe and also in Africa, transmission taking place through the egg in all species of these ticks. Because babesiosis is spread by ticks, the disease can be eradicated by eliminating them. In the United States, where *B. annulatus* was essentially the sole transmitting agent, systematic dipping of cattle in an arsenical solution poisonous to the ticks produced this effect. In areas where the ticks have a wider host range it is often necessary to dip all of the involved animals.

The life cycle of the protozoon in the tick is unknown. Certain developmental forms in the stomach of the arthropod have been followed, but nothing further is known except that some form of the parasite is carried from the adult female tick through its eggs to the larval form, which, when feeding upon the blood of the bovine animal, introduces the infection into this host.

Callow (3) has indicated that ticks infected with *Babesia bigemina* fail to rid themselves of the parasite while feeding on nonbovine hosts.

**Pathogenicity.** Texas fever ordinarily affects only cattle. Cases in deer have been reported. Other animals harbor the ticks that transmit the disease and may keep the disease alive in a community by propagating the transmitting agent, but they are not affected by the disease, nor do they harbor the protozoon, so far as is known, except possibly for a temporary period when an infected tick is feeding on them.

Calves are much less susceptible to the disease than older animals. Where the disease is prevalent, most calves contract it early, recover from it, and become chronic carriers throughout the remainder of their lives. Such animals frequently are unthrifty and anemic, but they show no acute symptoms and are able to resist severe exposure indefinitely. When disease-free cattle are placed with such animals, acute Texas fever appears only if the transmitting tick is present. These facts explain why Texas fever used to appear among northern cattle that had been shipped into the southern part of the United States and why it appeared in the northern states among native cattle when apparently normal southern cattle were placed among them.

The early history of Texas fever in the United States is rather vague. In the early summer of 1868, however, attention of the people was focused on this disease because of large losses in northern stock following a shipment of Texas cattle sent by Mississippi boat to Cairo, Illinois, and from there by rail to points in Illinois and Indiana. Cattle shipped from these states to other northern points carried the disease with them. Little progress was made in determining the nature of the disease at that time. Salmon, Chief of the Bureau of Animal Industry of the U.S. Department of Agriculture, surveyed the country to determine the areas where the disease was enzootic and defined this area by what came to be known as the *Texas fever line*. This line ran across the country a little north of the 35th parallel of latitude, corresponding roughly with the Mason and Dixon line. Although it was not known at the time, this line marked the northern limit of the distribution of *Boophilus annulatus*. Work on the causation of the disease was begun in the Bureau laboratories under Salmon's direction, the actual work being carried on by Smith, Kilborne, and Curtice, assisted by Moore. Smith (13) published preliminary observations upon the blood protozoon in 1889 and Smith and Kilborne (14) the completed study in 1893. Curtice (4) published his studies on the biology of the Texas fever tick in 1891. Its relationship to Texas fever was clearly exposed in the paper by Smith and Kilborne.

Susceptible cattle placed among the chronically infected will, in the presence of the transmitting tick, develop the first symptoms in not less than 10 days. A few instances are on record in which the disease has been transmitted by surgical operations, such as dehorning, when the instruments had not been sterilized between animals. In these cases the disease should make itself evident in from 8 to 10 days. The onset is marked by a high fever, sometimes reaching 107 F. Hemoglobinuria frequently occurs, although the brownish-red urine may not be noticed during life but is found at autopsy in the urinary bladder. The blood is pale because of severe anemia. The mucous membranes are pale and jaundiced. The animals do not eat, are depressed and weak, and usually die within 10 days, often by the 5th to 8th days. Less severe cases occur, the animals recovering after 10 days. Undoubtedly still milder forms appear in which few or no symptoms are seen.

**Pathological Changes.** Except for the usual changes accompanying severe anemia and icterus, the principal lesions are found in the spleen, liver, and kidneys.

Edematous areas often occur in the subcutaneous tissue of the ventral part of the body and in the fatty tissue around the kidneys. Hemorrhages are frequent in the subcutaneous tissue, on the walls of the heart, and on the mucosa of the urinary bladder. The most conspicuous changes are in the spleen, and these are responsible for the old name for this disease, *splenetic fever*. The organ is much enlarged—from two to four times its normal size. The color is reddish brown; it is often much softer than usual; and the normal structure, the Malpighian bodies and trabeculae, are obscured. The organ is engorged with blood cells and with phagocytic cells filled with blood pigment. A great deal of free blood pigment, in the form of granules, may be seen.

The liver is swollen and pale in color because of fatty degeneration. The surface and cut sections are yellowish and mottled. The bile ducts are engorged and the gall bladder is distended with thick, viscid, dark-colored bile containing flocculi in suspension. The kidneys often are swollen and dark in color. The urine in the bladder frequently, but not always, is tinged with blood pigment.

The changes are those associated with extensive blood-cell destruction. The count of erythrocytes, which normally is about 7 million per mm³, often sinks to less than 1 million at the time of death. Regeneration of blood cells occurs in the disease, as is manifested by the presence of nucleated erythroblasts and other juvenile types in the blood stream. Extreme poikilocytosis, associated with severe anemia, generally occurs.

**Immunity.** A number of methods have been tried for immunizing susceptible cattle that are to be shipped to areas where they will come in contact with piroplasmosis. Small doses of virulent blood will usually accomplish the purpose although the method is, of course, somewhat hazardous in itself. If given to calves from 2 to 6 weeks of age, as was advocated by Francis and Connaway (5) in Texas, the reactions usually are not severe. In older animals they are likely to be severe but nonfatal. Barnett (2) has indicated that bovine blood that contains *B. bigemina* will remain infective for cattle if stored with glycerol (7 percent) at −79 C for up to 720 days. Another method of immunizing young calves, practiced in Texas and elsewhere, was to deliberately liberate one or two infected ticks on the animal before it was turned out on pastures where heavy tick infestations would be picked up. Within 2 weeks the animal will have passed through a mild acute attack, which will protect it thereafter from more severe exposure. Antigens prepared from the blood of cattle heavily infected with a pure infection of either *B. bigemina* or *B. argentina* can be used in complement-fixation tests to detect antibodies against these parasites (8). The indirect fluorescent antibody test has also proved to be useful in detecting *B. bigemina* infection in cattle (12).

**Chemotherapy.** According to Ramanarayanan (9), good results were obtained in India in treating cattle acutely ill with piroplasmosis by injecting acriflavine or euflavine intravenously. Ranali *et al.* (10) eliminated the clinical manifestations of piroplasmosis in cattle by giving 2 mg per kg of body weight of *p,p'*-diguanyl-diazoamino-benzene (ganaseg) intramuscularly in a single dose. This did not clear the blood completely of *Babesia*. Mack (7) reported that the drugs hemosporidin [*N,N'*-di (4-dimethylaminophenyl) urea methyl methosulfate] and thiargen (silver-thiosulfate complex) appeared to be highly effective in treating piroplasmosis in horses, cattle, and sheep. Riek (11) used a diamidine compound (3,3' diamidino carbanilide diisethionate) in treating cattle infected with *B. argentina* and with *B. bigemina*. Acaprin has also proved to be effective.

## REFERENCES

1. Babes.    Virchow's Archiv. Path. Anat. u. Phys., 1889, *115*, 81.
2. Barnett.    Vet. Rec., 1964, *76*, 4.
3. Callow.    Parasitology, 1965, *55*, 375.
4. Curtice.    Jour. Comp. Med. and Vet. Arch., 1891, *12*, 313; 1892, *13*, 1.
5. Francis and Connaway.    Texas Agr. Exp. Sta. Bul. 53, 1899.
6. Gothe.    Onderstepoort Jour. Vet. Res., 1967, *34*, 81.
7. Mack.    Vet. Rev. and Annot., 1957, *3*, 57.
8. Mahoney.    Austral. Vet. Jour. 1962, *38*, 48.
9. Ramanarayanan.    Indian Vet. Jour., 1943, *19*, 205.
10. Ranali, Gonzalez, Rake, and Koerber.    Jour. Am. Vet. Med. Assoc., 1958, *132*, 63.
11. Riek.    Austral. Vet. Jour., 1964, *40*, 261.
12. Ross and Löhr.    Res. Vet. Sci., 1968, 9, 557.
13. Smith.    Med. News, 1889.
14. Smith and Kilborne.    U.S. Dept. Agr., Bur. Anim. Indus. Bul. 1, 1893.

### *Babesia bovis*

SYNONYMS: *Babesiella bovis, Microbabesia bovis, Piroplasma bovis*

The disease caused by this species is essentially like Texas fever. The principal transmitting agent is *Ixodes ricinus;* other ticks occasionally are vectors. Like the piroplasm of Texas fever, *Babesia bovis* passes through the egg of the adult female to the larvae, and these, feeding upon other animals, transmit the disease to them. In morphology this species resembles *Babesia bigem-*

*ina*, but the organisms are much smaller. The largest diameter does not exceed 1.5 microns. They are pyriform and commonly occur in pairs with their pointed ends together. Some of the forms are so small that they appear to consist entirely of chromatic material without cytoplasm.

Stockman and Wragg demonstrated that cattle that survived infection with *B. bovis* were still susceptible to *B. bigemina*. This seems to indicate that these forms are different species; however, there is much confusion with regard to cross immunization among the piroplasms, and some authors hold that immunity tests do not indicate relationships in this group.

Although *B. bovis* inhabits Europe it now appears that it is characteristically found in southern Europe and also in Africa, Asia, and the East Indies, while a smaller type (*Babesia divergens*) occurs in northern Europe, including Britain. Because there is no clear demarcation between these two parasites we are considering them together. They produce similar clinical pictures, causing a disease usually not as severe as that associated with *B. bigemina*, although rapidly fatal cases of fulminating infection are occasionally seen. Both species appear to be transmitted by *Ixodes ricinus* and possibly other ticks. Affected cattle do not respond to treatment with trypan blue, but do react favorably to drugs of the acaprin series, phenamidine, and gonacrine.

### Babesia argentina

This form is regarded to be synonymous with *B. berbera*. The pear-shaped forms measure about 1.5 by 2.0 microns and are commonly found in the center of the erythrocyte.

It is widely scattered throughout the tropics of America, Africa, and Asia and in the subtropics of southern Europe and Australia. It is transmitted by species of *Boophilus*, *Margaropus*, and possibly *Rhipicephalus*.

*B. argentina* produces a severe disease, which often takes the form of cerebral babesiosis. The parasites are comparatively rare in the peripheral blood but may be found fairly easily in films from the gray matter of the cerebral or cerebellar cortex and from the heart or kidney. Parasitized erythrocytes appear to adhere to the endothelium of the capillaries.

Hall (12) has demonstrated immunity in calves to tick-transmitted *B. argentina* infection. It is not effective against *B. bigemina*. In Australia (21), chemoprophylaxis is used to prevent the development of clinical babesiosis caused by *B. argentina*. The procedure consists of administering the quinuronium compound, 5,5'-methylene bis salicylate, in arachis oil in 1-g doses subcutaneously to young calves and then inoculating them with *B. argentina* vaccine.

### Babesia major

This parasite is present in Africa, Israel, South America, and the Balkans. It resembles *B. bigemina* but is smaller. It is morphologically distinct from *B. bovis*, being elongated and subpyriform in shape, greater in size, and located in the center of the red blood cell. *Hemaphysalis* spp. are suspect as transmitting agents.

## THE BABESIAE OF SHEEP AND GOATS

Piroplasmosis in sheep was first noted by Babes in Romania, who found the parasites in the blood of animals suffering from a disease known as *carceag*. He believed the parasite to be the same as the one that he had described in hemoglobinuria of cattle. Later studies have shown that there are at least two types of piroplasmosis in sheep. Cross inoculations do not succeed, however; hence they are regarded as distinct species. There is a relatively large form, to which Wenyon gave the name *Babesia motasi*, which is comparable to *B. bigemina* of cattle. The disease produced often is severe, there being high temperatures, much blood cell destruction, icterus, and hemoglobinuria. This is the carceag of eastern and southeastern Europe. Transmission is by means of *Dermacentor, Hemaphysalis,* and *Rhipicephalus.*

The second type, corresponding to *B. bovis* of cattle, is *Babesia ovis*. The disease produced is much milder than that caused by the preceding species. Fever, jaundice, and anemia are produced but recoveries generally occur. The transmitting agents are species of *Rhipicephalus*.

## THE BABESIAE OF HORSES

Piroplasmosis of horses was recognized in central Europe quite early. In 1910 Nuttall and Strickland described two kinds of parasites of horses, one of which they named *Piroplasma caballi*, the other *Nuttallia equi*.

### Babesia caballi

SYNONYM:    *Piroplasma caballi*

This species resembles *Babesia bigemina* in size and morphology. The disease also is similar to Texas fever, there being high fever, icterus, anemia, and hemoglobinuria. It occurs in southern and southeastern Europe and in the Caucasus region of southern Russia. Darling reported the existence of *B. caballi* in Panama, but it was not until 1961 that the first confirmed case of equine piroplasmosis (babesiosis) from a native horse was disclosed at Miami, Florida (36). There is evidence that the parasite is present in South America, especially in the northern countries. It is transmitted by species of *Dermacentor, Hyalomma,* and *Rhipicephalus*. In Florida the tick concerned was found to be *Dermacentor nitens* (32).

The clinical signs of equine piroplasmosis are icterus of the oral and conjunctival membranes; edema of the limbs; and intermittent temperature rise, with the afternoon recording considerably higher than the morning reading. Hematologically, the horse shows leukopenia, with neutropenia and lymphopenia occurring just prior to the appearance of the organisms in the erythrocytes. The lesions consist of generalized icterus, enlargement of the spleen, and pulmonary edema. The liver shows hematogenous pigment and the spleen is congested (31). Cases of babesiosis in aborted equine fetuses have been reported (27).

Sibinovic *et al.* (35) obtained a soluble antigen from the blood of acutely infected horses and used it in gel-diffusion studies to detect antibody in those animals suspected of having the disease. Frerichs *et al.* (7) have indicated that the CF test is highly specific for detecting infection with *B. caballi*, and Madden and Holbrook (18) have used the indirect fluorescent antibody test.

### Babesia equi

SYNONYM: *Nuttallia equi*

This species is smaller than *B. caballi*. It is pyriform in shape. In the process of division it regularly forms four individuals, these being attached by their pointed ends forming a sort of Maltese cross. Later they break apart, each cell escaping from the parasitized erythrocyte to enter other cells in which the process is repeated. The disease is highly virulent for adult horses and other species of the horse family but is mild in young animals. Inoculation of colts as a means of protection later in life is commonly practiced. The infection has been reported in southern Europe, Africa, southern Asia, and North and South America. The transmitting agents are the same as for *B. caballi*.

**Chemotherapy.** Jansen (15) has indicated that aureomycin will not sterilize infection in the donkey but will delay relapse and allow a true state of premunition to develop. Trypan blue, acaprin, acriflavine, and pentamidine have been used with success against piroplasmosis in the horse.

In Florida, equine babesiosis (piroplasmosis) has been controlled by using a 0.5 percent aqueous solution of toxaphene as a spray and an ear instillation of 1.0 percent solution of lindane in vegetable oil, along with quarantine and the treatment of the babesia-infected horses with amicarbalide isethionate (37).

## THE BABESIAE OF DOGS

Piroplasmosis of dogs occurs in southern Europe, in various parts of Africa, and in Asia. It has been reported in Puerto Rico and in Brazil. It was seen by Clark in Panama in imported hunting dogs. It was recognized in the United States for the first time in 1934. Since then reports of its occurrence in many of the southern states have appeared (1). The two principal species are *Babesia canis* and *B. gibsoni*. Animals susceptible to infection with these parasites are dogs, jackals, wolves, and foxes.

### Babesia canis

SYNONYM: *Piroplasma canis*

The disease caused by this parasite in dogs is essentially like Texas fever in cattle. Young animals are fairly resistant; hence dogs that are raised in an infected environment usually suffer only from the mild, chronic form, which may be practically symptomless, yet the parasites in their blood are exceedingly virulent for animals that have never been in contact with the disease. Imported dogs usually suffer from the acute form of the disease for this reason. In the acute disease there is high fever, progressive anemia, icterus, and hemoglobinuria, and the disease frequently is fatal. The lesions consist of splenic enlargement, fatty degeneration of the liver lobules with distention of its bile ducts, nephritis, and icterus. The cerebral form of babesiosis has been reported in the dog (2, 3) and it is possible that a strain other than *B. canis* may be the cause. Cases have been seen where babesiosis was concurrent with ehrlichiosis. In these instances grave illness accompanied a severe anemia in which it appeared that the destruction of mature erythrocytes was caused by the *Babesia* and the impediment of erythropoiesis by the *Ehrlichia* (6).

The parasites are relatively large. Typical pear-shaped forms occur in pairs as in the cattle disease, but large ameboid forms with large vacuoles are also seen. The cycle of development was studied and described by Nuttall and Graham-Smith (22-25). Often parasitized cells are much more numerous in the capillaries of the internal organs than in the peripheral circulation; in fact it is often difficult to find infected blood cells in the blood of acutely ill patients. In these cases a diagnosis can be made by the inoculation of blood into nonimmune animals. Such animals promptly give a febrile reaction and the other symptoms of piroplasmosis, but in these animals too it may be impossible to find the parasites. Sanders (33) recommends, as a more satisfactory procedure, the inoculation of young, splenectomized dogs, because in these it is usually easy to find parasites in the peripheral blood during the febrile period, 2 or 3 days after inoculation. Popovic and Ristic (28) claim that the gel precipitation test is useful in diagnosing canine babesiosis.

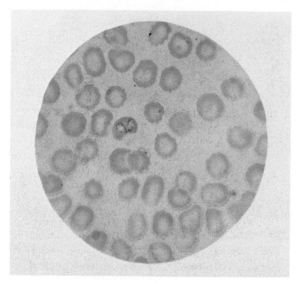

Fig. 131. *Babesia canis*, a stained blood film of a dog suffering from canine babesiosis showing one parasitized erythrocyte near the middle of the field. This cell contains two parasites having the shape of apple seeds and lying characteristically with the pointed ends together. X 1,000. (Courtesy D. A. Sanders.)

Canine piroplasmosis was first recognized in the United States by Eaton (5) in 1934. Since then it has become evident that the disease is not uncommon in Florida, and it is present in Texas, Arizona, and California. Grogan (9) reported it in a dog in Virginia in 1953. It is not unlikely that it occurs in other southern states where the brown dog tick, *Rhipicephalus sanguineus*, the transmitting agent, is found. Inasmuch as this tick is becoming common in the more northerly states, the disease should be watched for in areas where the tick is known to occur (20).

Canine piroplasmosis is naturally transmitted by several different ticks. In Europe the principal vector is *Dermacentor reticulatus*, in India and the United States it is *Rhipicephalus sanguineus*, and in South Africa it is *Hemaphysalis leachi*. The *Hyalomma* are also concerned in transmitting the disease. The parasite passes through the eggs of the ticks to the next generation. Christopher, in India, claims to have followed the developmental cycle in *Rhipicephalus sanguineus* and to have found it to be not unlike that of the plasmodia.

### Babesia gibsoni

This organism occurs in Asia and has been found in Africa. It has been observed in the United States in a dog transported from Malaysia (11). It differs from *B. canis* in being smaller and pleomorphic. Species of *Rhipicelphalus* and *Hemaphysalis* act as transmitting agents, and the disease in dogs is usually less severe than that produced by *B. canis*. The principal signs of infection are anemia, hemoglobinuria, constipation, splenomegalia, and hepatomegalia. Icterus rarely appears.

Experimentally, *B. gibsoni* has been transmitted to jackals, foxes, and dogs (19).

**Chemotherapy.** In treating canine piroplasmosis with novarsenobillon, sulfarsenol, and tryparsamide, Kapur (16) reported that novarsenobillon was the most effective, producing complete recovery in 10 of 11 cases treated. Acaprin [1,3-bis-(6-quinolyl)-urea dimethosulfate], trypan blue, and phenamidine are also reported to be effective in treating piroplasmosis in dogs.

*B. gibsoni* differs from *B. canis* in failing to respond to treatment with trypan blue or acaprin. It is affected by arsenical compounds (29), and a recommended drug is phenamidine isethionate (10).

### THE BABESIAE OF SWINE

Piroplasmosis of swine was apparently first reported from Russia. It has been observed in Italy, Bulgaria, Sardinia, and Africa. *Babesia trautmanni* and *Babesia perroncitoi* are reported to be the causal agents, but the former seems to be the more widely distributed.

*B. trautmanni* resembles *B. bigemina* and *B. canis*. It occurs as an endoglobular parasite of the erythrocytes in the form of round, oval, or pear-shaped bodies varying in size from 2.5 to 4 microns in length and from 1.5 to 2 microns in width. In Italy *Rhipicephalus sanguineus* has been incriminated as the vector (26), and in Africa *Boophilus decoloratus* is believed to be concerned in transmitting the piroplasm (17).

In 1955 Lawrence and Shone (17) reported an outbreak of porcine piroplasmosis in Southern Rhodesia. The disease is characterized by high fever, anemia, hemoglobinuria, and abortion. Diagnosis is made by finding the parasite in Giemsa-stained blood films. Both acaprin and phenamidine are reported to be highly effective in treating piroplasmosis of swine.

## BABESIAE OF OTHER ANIMALS AND MAN

Piroplasms have been described in the domestic cat (B. *felis*) in India, in rodents (*B. rodhaini*) in the Belgian Congo, in the rock hyrax (8) and cape dassie (14) of South Africa, and in the genet cat and a ground squirrel of Kenya (13).

In 1968, a case of babesiosis was diagnosed in man in California (34). This appears to be the second documented case in man in the world, the first occurring in Yugoslavia. Both were observed in splenectomized persons. In the California case *Babesia* antibodies were demonstrated in both CF and tube-latex-agglutination tests and this serologic evidence for diagnosis was supported by the presence of a distinct mature parasite. In 1971, Ristic *et al.* (30) isolated a *Babesia* strain from a woman with clinical babesiosis. The parasite was morphologically similar to *B. rodhaini* and serologically related to *B. canis*.

Chloroquine (34) has been used successfully in treating man and ceporan (4) has been recommended in treating biliary fever (B. *felis*) in cats.

## REFERENCES

1. Alperin and Bevins. Jour. Am. Vet. Med. Assoc., 1963, *143*, 1328.
2. Basson and Pienaar. Jour. So. African Vet. Med. Assoc., 1965, *36*, 333.
3. Botha. *Ibid.*, 1964, *35*, 27.
4. Dorrington and Du Buy. *Ibid.*, 1966, *37*, 93.
5. Eaton. Jour. Parasitol., 1934, *20*, 312.
6. Ewing and Buckner. Am. Jour. Vet. Res., 1965, *26*, 815.
7. Frerichs, Holbrook, and Johnson. *Ibid.*, 1969, *30*, 697.
8. Garnham. Jour. Parasitol., 1951, *37*, 528.
9. Grogan. Jour. Am. Vet. Med. Assoc., 1953, *123*, 234.
10. Groves and Vanniasingham. Vet. Rec., 1970, *86*, 8.
11. Groves and Yap. Jour. Am. Vet. Med. Assoc., 1968, *153*, 689.
12. Hall. Austral. Vet. Jour., 1963, *39*, 386.
13. Heisch. Ann. Trop. Med. and Parasitol., 1952, *46*, 150.
14. Jansen. Onderstepoort Jour. Vet. Res., 1952, *25*, 3.
15. *Ibid.*, 1953, *26*, 175.
16. Kapur. Indian Vet. Jour., 1943, *19*, 199.
17. Lawrence and Shone. Jour. So. African Vet. Med. Assoc., 1955, *26*, 89.
18. Madden and Holbrook. Am. Jour. Vet. Res., 1968, *29*, 117.

19. Maronpot and Guindy. *Ibid.*, 1970, *31*, 797.
20. Merenda. Jour. Am. Vet. Med. Assoc., 1939, *95*, 98.
21. Newton and O'Sullivan. Austral. Vet. Jour., 1969, *45*, 404.
22. Nuttall. Jour. Hyg. (London), 1904, *4*, 219.
23. Nuttall and Graham-Smith. *Ibid.*, 1905, 5, 237.
24. *Ibid.*, 1906, *6*, 586.
25. *Ibid.*, 1907, 7, 232.
26. Pavlov and Paschev. Ann. de Parasitol. Humaine et Comp., 1946, *21*, 235.
27. Plessis and Basson. Jour. So. African Vet. Med. Assoc., 1966, *37*, 267.
28. Popovic and Ristic. Am. Jour. Vet. Res., 1970, *31*, 2201.
29. Richardson and Kendall. Veterinary protozoology. 3d ed. Oliver and Boyd, London, 1963, pp. 145–175.
30. Ristic, Conroy, Siwe, Healy, Smith, and Huxsoll. Am. Jour. Trop. Med. and Hyg., 1971, *20*, 14.
31. Roberts, Morehouse, Gainer, and McDaniel. Jour. Am. Vet. Med. Assoc., 1962, *141*, 1323.
32. Roby, Anthony, Thornton, and Holbrook. Am. Jour. Vet. Res., 1964, *25*, 494.
33. Sanders. Jour. Am. Vet. Med. Assoc., 1937, *90*, 27.
34. Scholtens, Braff, Healy, and Gleason. Am. Jour. Trop. Med. and Hyg., 1968, *17*, 810.
35. Sibinovic, Ristic, Sibinovic, and Phillips. Am. Jour. Vet. Res., 1965, *26*, 147.
36. Strickland and Gerrish. Jour. Am. Vet. Med. Assoc., 1964, *244*, 875.
37. Taylor, Bryant, Anderson, and Willers. *Ibid.*, 1969, *155*, 915.

## THE GENUS *AEGYPTIANELLA*

These organisms are closely related to the *Babesia*, but differ in that the forms in erythrocytes divide several times.

### *Aegyptianella pullorum*

This protozoon is a parasite of geese and chickens. It has been found in South Africa, Indochina, and the Balkans and probably exists in most tropical and subtropical countries.

Three forms of the parasite occur in erythrocytes of fowl. They are (1) initial bodies (oval or round and less than 1 micron in diameter), (2) elements in process of developing (resemble *Babesia*), and (3) large, oval, elliptical or round bodies 2 to 2.5 by 3 to 4 microns in size.

Transmission is through the tick *Argas pericus*, and the disease frequently is associated with fowl spirochetosis. Native fowl rarely suffer an acute disease, but freshly introduced stock may die within a few days with diarrhea, anorexia, a high temperature, and paralysis. Ichthargan given intravenously is a specific against the condition (1).

### REFERENCE

1. Richardson and Kendall. Veterinary protozoology. 3d ed. Oliver and Boyd, London, 1963, pp. 176–8.

## THE GENUS *THEILERIA*

Whether or not Neitz's (6) division of the theileriae into *Theileria parva, Gonderia annulata, Gonderia utans, Gonderia lawrencei,* etc. is valid is not clear at this time. Certainly there are some important differences between *T. parva* and *G. annulata* infections. It has been reported on the one hand that *G. lawrencei* is merely a buffalo-adapted strain of *T. parva* (1) and on the other hand that it differs from *T. parva* in its characteristic interactions with lymphocytes (4). For the present we propose to follow the classification of Neitz and consider these hemosporidia as members of two genera.

According to Neitz (6), *Theileria* multiply by schizogony within cells of the lymphatic system but sometimes develop within cells of the monocytic series.

### *Theileria parva*

SYNONYMS:   *Theileria kochi, Piroplasma kochi, Piroplasma parvum*

This parasite is the cause of East Coast fever of cattle, a disease responsible for severe losses in the countries along the greater part of the eastern coast of Africa. The disease was long confused with babesiosis because both diseases occurred in the same area and the same animals often were infected with both. It is now recognized that chronic carriers of piroplasms often suffer from acute attacks because of the stimulation offered by the *Theileria.* In East Coast fever the anemia, icterus, and jaundice, so characteristic of babesiosis, is absent. In from 10 to 20 days after infection, fever begins and the superficial lymph nodes swell. There is difficulty in respiration, emaciation, and weakness and the passing of dry, tarlike, bloody feces. At the height of the fever as many as 90 percent of the red blood cells contain the characteristic parasites; however, the blood cells are not destroyed by them, as in babesiosis. The disease is ordinarily of short duration and the majority of affected animals die. Milder forms of the disease are known. Animals that recover do not continue to harbor the parasite, for ticks cannot be infected from them. In this respect this disease differs from all the babesioses.

Animals that die of this disease present petechial hemorrhages on the serous membranes and in the subcutaneous tissue. All the lymph nodes are enlarged, but the spleen is essentially normal in size and color. Hemorrhagic and sometimes ulcerative enteritis is seen. The kidneys sometimes show wedge-shaped infarcts.

Most characteristic of this disease are the structures commonly called *Koch's blue bodies* (5). These are the schizonts of the parasite, which may be seen in lymphocytes and possibly within cells of the monocytic series. They sometimes are found free. They are usually demonstrable in the spleen, lymph glands, kidney, liver, and capillaries of the lungs. Koch's blue bodies vary in size from 1 to 15 microns in diameter and are roughly spherical. In films or sections stained with Giemsa's stain they appear as masses of bluish-stained cytoplasm in which numbers of red-staining chromatin dots varying from 1 or

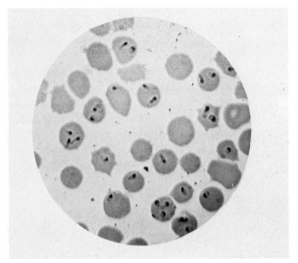

*Fig. 132. Theileria parva,* forms of the parasite found in the circulating erythrocytes during the febrile period of East Coast fever. Unlike the piroplasms, which these bodies resemble, the protozoon of this disease does not ordinarily multiply in the circulating blood, and blood usually is noninfective. When more than one body is found in a red corpuscle, it is believed that a multiple infection has oc-cured. The schizogonic phases of this parasite occur in the tissues in the form of Koch's blue bodies. X 1,000.

2 to 30 or more are seen. When fully mature they break down, releasing min-ute elements, each containing one of the chromatin granules. These either enter other lymphocytes to repeat the multiplicative process, or they pene-trate red blood cells and circulate in the blood. In blood films they are seen as round bodies, 1 to 2 microns in diameter, or they may be ovoid, pear-shaped, or elongated rodlike forms. Most of the erythrocytes contain only one element, but two or even four may be found in a single cell. These forms rep-resent multiple invasions for they do not multiply within the cell. It is possi-ble that the parasites entering the blood stream find only a few lymphocytes to invade and therefore enter the erythrocytes in which they lie dormant until ingested by a suitable tick. Thus it appears that the Koch's blue bodies which sometimes are found in the blood or the forms that invade the red blood cells are both infectious.

*Theileria parva* is transmitted most commonly by the tick, *Rhipicephalus appendiculatus.* Tissues of this tick infected with *T. parva* have induced ex-perimental East Coast fever when fed to cattle (9). Six other *Rhipicephalus* and three *Hyalomma* species have been proved experimentally to be transmit-ters, but the former are less important than *R. appendiculatus* and there is no evidence that the *Hyalomma* transmit the disease in nature. Reichenow (8) states that the ingested parasites pass directly to the salivary glands of the tick, where they lie dormant until the next-stage tick emerges from the molt and begins to feed. Multiplication by binary fission now occurs in the cells of the salivary glands, and the parasites are released into the salivary ducts. This process takes 3 days. It appears that more than 16 days are required for larvae or nymphs to engorge, drop off, molt, and reattach themselves. Accord-ing to Neitz (7) a transovarial transmission does not occur in the vector.

It is of interest that a mildly pathogenic strain of *T. parva* became highly virulent at the 10th passage in cattle (2). Also that preliminary tests in applying agar gel precipitin and intradermal skin tests to the diagnosis of theileriosis revealed common antigens among *T. parva*, pneumogalactan of normal bovine lungs, and *Mycoplasma mycoides* (3).

Aureomycin has some effect on the disease and pamaquin is supposed to cause degeneration of the blood forms of the parasite although it does not appear to affect the clinical picture. Dipping to eradicate the ticks seems to be the most direct form of control.

## REFERENCES

1.  Barnett and Brocklesby.    Brit. Vet. Jour., 1966, *122*, 396.
2.  Brocklesby and Bailey.    *Ibid.*, 1968, *124*, 236.
3.  Gourlay and Brocklesby.    *Ibid.*, 1967, *123*, 533.
4.  Hill and Matson.    Jour. So. African Vet. Med. Assoc., 1970, *41*, 275.
5.  Koch.    Centrbl. f. Bakt., I Abt., 1898, *24*, 200.
6.  Neitz.    Onderstepoort Jour. Vet. Res., 1957, *27*, 278.
7.  Neitz.    Jour. So. African Vet. Med. Assoc., 1964, *35*, 5.
8.  Reichenow.    Arch. f. Protistenk., 1940, *94*, 1.
9.  Wilde, Brown, Hulliger, Gall, and MacLeod.    Brit. Vet. Jour., 1968, *124*, 196.

## THE GENUS *GONDERIA*

According to Neitz (8), members of the genus *Gonderia* multiply by schizogony within cells of the lymphatic system. Schizonts break up into merozoites which either enter lymphocytes to continue the asexual cycle or penetrate red cells which are seen in ordinary blood films. Multiplication also occurs within the erythrocytes.

### Gonderia annulata

SYNONYMS:    *Theileria dispar, Theileria annulata, Theileria sergenti*

*Gonderia annulata* causes a disease quite similar to East Coast fever in its clinical manifestations. It occurs in Egypt, Algeria, Palestine, Iraq, Iran, Transcaucasia, southern Russia, and India. The causal parasite can be differentiated from *Theileria parva* and from the other species of *Gonderia*. It is characterized by the formation of ring-shaped anaplasmatic forms in the red blood cells (3). According to Daubney and Said (2), the Algerian species, which has been known as *Theileria dispar* (*G. dispar*), is the same as *G. annulata*, the cause of gonderiosis in Asia Minor and southern Russia. Accordingly, the name *G. annulata* takes precedence. In enzootic areas the parasite affects chiefly imported cattle but is capable of giving rise to clinical infections in native animals. Mild and acute forms of the disease occur. The erythrocytic stage can be demonstrated in up to 95 percent of the red cells in acute cases. Schizonts are found in the liver, spleen, and lymphatic gland smears and also in fairly large numbers in the peripheral blood. They are seen mostly in lymphocytes, but may develop in cells of the reticuloendothelial

system. In acute cases there is a high temperature (104 to 107 F) with increased pulse rate. There is diarrhea, sometimes nervous symptoms, and
death may occur within a few days. In more chronic cases there may be jaundice. Eye lesions consisting of ulceration and conjunctivitis have been reported
(6). On postmortem examination there are intestinal hemorrhages with ulceration.

Infection leads to the development of a condition of premunity with the
possibility of relapse following stress factors.

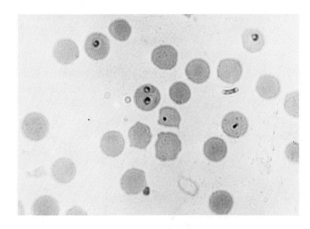

Fig. 133. *Gonderia annulata*,
a stained film from an infected
cow. Note the signet-ring shaped
forms in the erythrocytes. X 900.
(Courtesy Hendrik Versluis.)

Natural and experimental transmission has been demonstrated with six species of *Hyalomma*. Transmission has been effected with nymphs and adults
which were infected in each case by feeding the preceding stage on reacting
or recovered cattle. The infection does not appear to pass through the egg to
the larval stage. Infection can also be transmitted by inoculation of the blood
of a reacting animal in which schizonts are demonstrable.

There is no known drug that is entirely reliable for treating gonderiosis,
and the only effective method of controlling the disease is the destruction of
the tick vectors. As in theileriosis and in all the gonderioses aureomycin administered in repeated doses during the incubation period acts as a schizonti-
cide to prevent the development of the clinical disease, but it is apparent that
this is a form of treatment that cannot be applied in practice.

The species of *Hyalomma* which act as vectors hibernate in buildings and
are more susceptible to control than are the *Rhipicephalus*.

### Gonderia mutans

SYNONYMS: *Piroplasma mutans, Theileria mutans, Babesia mutans*

This parasite was differentiated from other blood protozoa by Theiler in
1906. It occurs in the blood corpuscles of cattle as very small bodies of various shapes. Infections have been recognized in southern Europe, Africa, Asia,
Australia, and Great Britain. It has been seen in a splenectomized calf in the

United States but not in cattle, in which the infection is quite benign. The organisms occur in erythrocytes as rings, rods, commas, or oval forms. Schizogony takes place in the endothelial cells and lymphocytes, particularly in the lymph glands and spleen. The schizonts measure up to 12 microns or more and may be contained in the host cells or free. They are known as *Koch's bodies* or as *blue bodies*.

Theiler succeeded in transmitting this parasite through the agency of *Rhipicephalus evertsi* and *R. appendiculatus*. The parasite was not transmitted through the egg.

### Gonderia lawrencei

SYNONYM:   *Theileria lawrencei*

In 1955 Neitz *et al.* (9) described an enzootic of gonderiosis in cattle following tick infestation in the corridor adjoining the Hluhluwe Game Reserve in Zululand. During 3 weeks of exposure the mortality rate was over 90 percent. Clinical symptoms and pathological changes in the diseased cattle resembled but were not identical with those observed in East Coast fever. Blood and organ smears revealed Koch's bodies relatively smaller than those of *Theileria parva* and the other species of *Gonderia*.

There is considerable speculation at present as to whether or not *G. lawrencei* should be recognized as a host-adapted strain of *Theileria parva*, because it appears to assume the pathogenic characteristics of the latter upon passage through cattle (1), or whether it should rate a separate generic status because it differs hematologically from *T. parva* in its ability to cause a higher degree of terminal peripheral blood lymphocytosis and depression of bone marrow erythropoiesis (4).

The disease has been called *corridor disease, buffalo disease*, and *malignant gonderiosis*. It is a highly fatal peracute, acute, or subacute disease of cattle characterized by pyrexia, anorexia, malaise, lymphadenitis, general weakness, prostration, and pronounced dyspnea before death. Recovered animals develop a durable premunity.

Premune buffalo calves appear to be the reservoirs for the infection of ticks of the species *Rhipicephalus appendiculatus* which act as the transmitting agents.

### Gonderia bovis

This organism causes a malignant form of gonderiosis found to date only in Southern Rhodesia. Whereas corridor disease is a self-limiting disease in the absence of the African buffalo, this infection occurs when buffalo are not present. Cattle, including calves, are highly susceptible to the disease, and the mortality rate may be as high as 90 percent. The transmitting agent is *Rhipicephalus appendiculatus*.

### Gonderia hirci

Malignant ovine and caprine gonderiosis are caused by this organism. The disease has been encountered in Egypt, Algeria, Turkey, Transcaucasia, and Yugoslavia. It occurs in acute, subacute, and chronic forms. The mortality rate is high. It is readily transmissible from sheep to goats or vice versa by means of blood and organ emulsions taken from febrile animals. The vector of *G. hirci* has not been established but *Rhipicephalus bursa* is suspected.

### Gonderia ovis

SYNONYMS: *Theileria recondita, Theileria ovis, Babesia sergenti*

This organism seems to be a rather common parasite of sheep in South Africa. It produces inapparent or mild infection but becomes active on splenectomy. Reaction in infected sheep is manifested by an increased lymphocyte production in the parotid lymphatic glands, a fever, and a relatively mild anemia. Koch's blue bodies are present, but few in number. Transmission by *Rhipicephalus evertsi* has been demonstrated (5). This organism also produces benign caprine gonderiosis.

Protozoon parasites have been reported in deer in the United States (7, 11). They have been designated *Theileria* sp. and *Theileria cervi*, but it seems highly probable that the forms involved belong in the genus *Gonderia* rather than in the genus *Theileria*. There is evidence that *G. mutans* occurs in North America (12) and possibly other species also are present.

In 1948 Neitz and Thomas (10) described a protozoon that was responsible for a disease in the duiker (a species of antelope) of South Africa similar to the rickettsial disease known as heartwater. The protozoon, which they named *Cytauxzoon sylvicaprae*, appears to be closely related to *Gonderia mutans*. Schizogony occurs in the cells of the histiocytes. The mode of transmission is unknown. It is possible that this parasite belongs in the genus *Gonderia*.

### REFERENCES

1. Barnett and Brocklesby.   Brit. Vet. Jour., 1966, *122*, 396.
2. Daubney and Said.   Parasitology, 1951, *41*, 249.
3. Dschunkowsky.   *Ibid.*, 1952, *42*, 70.
4. Hill and Matson.   Jour. So. African Vet. Med. Assoc., 1970, *41*, 275.
5. Jansen and Neitz.   Onderstepoort Jour. Vet. Res., 1956, *27*, 3.
6. Khalifa and Kadhim.   Vet. Rec., 1967, *81*, 76.
7. Kreier, Ristic, and Watrach.   Am. Jour. Vet. Res., 1962, *23*, 657.
8. Neitz.   Onderstepoort Jour. Vet. Res., 1957, *27*, 275.
9. Neitz, Canham, and Kluge.   Jour. So. African Vet. Med. Assoc., 1955, *26*, 79.
10. Neitz and Thomas.   Onderstepoort Jour. Vet. Sci. and Anim. Indus., 1948, *23*, 63.
11. Schaeffler.   Am. Jour. Vet. Res., 1963, *24*, 784.
12. Splitter.   Jour. Am. Vet. Med. Assoc., 1950, *117*, 134.

## THE GENUS *TOXOPLASMA*

The genus *Toxoplasma* was created in 1909 by Nicolle and Manceaux (36) for a parasite that they found in a small mammal, the gondi, which lives around the borders of the Sahara Desert in North Africa. They gave it the name *Toxoplasma gondi*. A little later Splendore (53) described what appears to be the same organism from a Brazilian rabbit under the name *Toxoplasma cuniculi*. Both of these parasites were readily inoculable into pigeons, and Splendore's also infected a dog. Organisms morphologically indistinguishable from *T. gondi* have been found in fowl, mice, rats, guinea pigs, rabbits, other rodents, dogs, cats, mink, swine, sheep, cattle, man, and cold-blooded animals. Transmission experiments have revealed that the parasite is not host-specific; thus Sabin and Olitsky (47) have found that a strain isolated from guinea pigs and another from a human infection could be inoculated successfully into mice, guinea pigs, rabbits, chickens, and rhesus monkeys, producing fatal infections in all cases except in the monkeys. Also, these authors were unable to demonstrate any serological differences between the two strains. These facts suggest that many and possibly all toxoplasmas, irrespective of host, are identical. The organism appears to be ubiquitous and without host specificity.

Until the findings of Sheffield and Melton (51) and Frenkel *et al.* (19) all toxoplasmas were described as minute intracellular parasites that occur in monocytes and endothelial cells of various mammals, birds, and reptiles. They were believed to multiply only by asexual means and the mode of transmission was obscure. In 1970 it was established that cat feces transmitted *Toxoplasma* (19, 51) and that infectivity apparently was associated with the oocysts of *Isospora cati*. This discovery uncovered a sexual cycle for the parasite and provided the missing link in its transmission. Demonstration of the sexual stages permits the classification of *Toxoplasma* as a member of the order *Coccidia*, but unlike other coccidia, which essentially live in the gut epithelium, *Toxoplasma* parasitizes many tissues; also unlike other coccidia that are fairly host-specific, *Toxoplasma* infests a wide variety of animals. For these characteristics and for practical considerations we have retained the genus *Toxoplasma*. It is also possible that cyst-forming parasites such as *Globidium*, *Besnoitia*, *Sarcocystis*, and the protozoon of Dalmeny's disease may possess transmission patterns that are similar to *Toxoplasma*.

### *Toxoplasma gondi*

It is assumed that all forms found subsequently in many kinds of birds and mammals, including man, are members of the same species.

**Morphology.** In the sexual cycle we have the oocyst form of *I. cati* which measures 10 to 14 by 7.5 to 9.6 microns. In fresh preparations the merozoite of the schizogonic stage is somewhat elongated, one or both ends being rather pointed. In stained films it is ovoid or pyriform. In tissue sections it is ovoid or round. It varies in size but averages 2 by 4 microns in width and 4 to 7 microns in length. A solid-staining nucleus is located toward the rounded end of the ovoid forms. In fresh preparations it is motile, but flagella have not been demonstrated.

In tissues the organisms may be found singly or in compact masses in cyst-like structures that contain as many as 50 individuals. They are often abundant in the liver, spleen, bone marrow, lung, brain, kidney, heart muscle, and smooth muscle. *Toxoplasma* multiply by binary fission and schizogony (38) in monocytes, in cells of the reticuloendothelial system, in cells of various viscera, and in cells of the nervous system. In these cells they frequently lie in cystlike vacuoles of the cytoplasm. The individuals are released when the host cell disintegrates. In the peritoneal exudate of infected mice internal budding may take place (20), the parent cell producing two daughter cells, which are in turn released to continue the reproductive cycle.

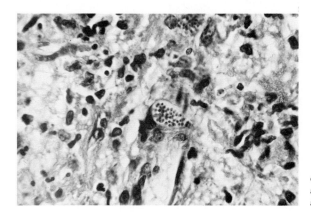

*Fig. 134.* Toxoplasmata in a capillary wall of a lymph node in a cat. X 600. (Courtesy Olafson and Monlux, *Cornell Vet.*)

**Artificial Cultivation.** Sabin and Olitsky (47) succeeded in propagating an organism derived from guinea pigs through six generations without loss of virulence. The medium used consisted of minced chick embryo suspended in Tyrode's solution (Rivers-Li medium). Development was wholly within cells. They did not succeed in obtaining growth in cell-free media. The organism is an obligate intracellular parasite. It can be maintained in embryonated chicken eggs. It will produce plaques in tissue cultures consisting of monolayers of chick embryo fibroblasts (5).

**Pathogenicity.** Cats that have been fed *Toxoplasma*-infected mice develop oocysts and infectivity stimultaneously after 3 to 5 days (17). Experimental animals are readily infected with most strains of *T. gondi* by intraperitoneal, intravenous, or intracranial inoculation. Subcutaneous inoculation is less likely to succeed, and the disease is more chronic when initiated in this way. Sabin and Olitsky succeeded in infecting mice by introducing the inoculum by mouth and nose. The course of the disease depends upon many factors: the dosage, route of inoculation, species of animal, and, particularly, the extent of adaptation of the strain to the species of animal as a result of few or many passages in it. Death usually occurs in from 1 to 3 weeks but may take place as early as the 3rd day; chronic infections may terminate in death after several months, or recoveries may occur.

After intraperitoneal inoculation, a large amount of viscid exudate usually collects in the cavity and often in the pleural and pericardial cavities as well. Many organisms are found in these exudates both free and intracellularly. After subcutaneous inoculation, local inflammation and necrosis appear with or without generalization. Intravenous inoculation causes a generalized disease in the more highly susceptible species. Intracranial injection produces encephalitis, the type depending upon the species of animal used. In the rabbit, the brain usually is not affected unless the inoculum is introduced directly into it. In the mouse, according to Sabin and Olitsky, brain lesions invariably occur no matter how the inoculation is made. The brain lesions of mice inoculated intracerebrally are found near the ventricles and in the midbrain, the organisms apparently spreading by means of the cerebrospinal fluid. When the inoculum is introduced otherwise, the brain is infected by way of the blood stream and lesions are found around the blood vessels. *Toxoplasma* were shown to survive in the brain of a guinea pig for 5 years following intraperitoneal inoculation. The virulence of the strain was unaffected, and only a single passage in mice was needed for its recovery (29).

The rabbit and guinea pig usually show small areas of necrosis in the liver, spleen, adrenals, intestines, and lungs. The parasites are numerous in these areas. The parasites are also found abundantly in the same organs of mice, but, rather oddly, gross lesions are not usually present in mice.

That a toxin is important in producing toxoplasmosis is attested by Woodworth and Weinman (68). They have obtained *toxotoxin* from infected mice and rats and claim that the toxic activity was recovered with certain serum globulin fractions by ammonium sulfate precipitation.

**The Spontaneous Disease.** As our knowledge of toxoplasmosis increases, we find that most of the domestic animals as well as man are subject to infection. Inapparent and clinical forms of the disease occur. Clinically the disease manifests itself by fever in acute cases, respiratory distress, and central nervous disturbances. In pregnant animals premature births and abortions are observed. Retinochoroiditis is not an uncommon finding. Prominent autopsy findings are pneumonia, intestinal ulceration, gray foci and enlargement of the liver, and an increased amount of fluid in the serous cavities.

*In dogs.* The first case described in dogs was that of Mello (34) in Italy in 1910. A dog at the Pasteur Institute of Tunis contracted the infection in 1916, probably from the gondi disease that was being studied there at the time. Another case was reported from Brazil. In 1939 Machattie (31) described two cases seen in Baghdad. In 1942 Olafson and Monlux (37) described the first cases in dogs in the United States. Since then other incidents have been reported in this country.

The affected animals present signs and pathological findings that vary considerably, but all cases have certain things in common. There is gradual emaciation with enlargement of the lymph nodes in all episodes. The abdomen may be tender upon palpation. Dyspnea is common, and a bloody diarrhea sometimes occurs. Nervous symptoms have also been reported in dogs, and pregnant female dogs may abort or undergo premature parturition. That *in utero* transmission exists in the dog was demonstrated by Chamberlain *et al.* (4). They also showed that four lactating females secreted *Toxoplasma* in their milk.

The lesions consist of enlarged lymph nodes, which are often acutely inflamed, the surrounding tissue frequently being edematous and hemorrhagic. Sections of these nodes usually show necrotic areas. Small nodules may occur in the lung tissue, and this organ is often edematous. Nodules and ulceration of the intestinal wall frequently occur. Focal necrotic areas may appear in the liver, spleen, and other organs. The spleen may be moderately enlarged. When extensive involvement of abdominal organs exists, a bloody exudate may be found in the peritoneal cavity.

In the necrotic areas toxoplasmata may often be found in large numbers. Eosinophilic infiltration of these areas is usual. The disease in dogs is usually, if not always, fatal.

*In cats.* In 1942 Olafson and Monlux (37) described a case of toxoplasmosis in a cat in New York. The lesions were not unlike those seen in dogs, and there was a fatal outcome. The pathogenicity of the organism was not proved, the diagnosis being based upon the character of the disease and the demonstration of typical organisms in the lesions. An interesting lesion seen in this animal but not in the three canine cases was a proliferation of epithelial cells in the lung. This adenomalike condition has been reported in human cases. Encephalitic (24), intestinal (30), and generalized cases (32) of toxoplasmosis have been described in cats. Acute feline toxoplasmosis is characterized by anorexia, lethargy, high temperature, dyspnea, and death. There usually is hepatitis, bilirubinuria, leukopenia, mild anemia, lymphadenitis, encephalitis, and retinochoroiditis. Chronic disease shows relapses with anorexia, anemia, central nervous system disorders, myocardial involvement, liver dysfunction, abortion or sterility, and fever. Iritis may be seen in both the acute and chronic forms of the disease, although a positive blood titer is to be expected only in the latter (40). Young kittens may die from pneumonia, encephalitis, and diarrhea. Transplacental infection is a possibility.

*In mink.* Six outbreaks of toxoplasmosis have been recognized in mink on ranches in Ontario. *Toxoplasma* were observed in the brain, liver, intestines, pancreas, and lung sections of affected animals. The mortality ranged up to 100 percent (42).

*In guinea pigs.* A spontaneous outbreak in guinea pigs purchased in Panama City was reported by Rodaniche and DePinzon (44).

Apparently, the organism sometimes produces an encephalitis in wild rodents (52) which mimics rabies and may be mistaken for this disease on clinical diagnosis.

*In sheep.* Toxoplasmosis occurs in sheep (Olafson and Monlux, 37; Wickham and Carne, 64). The animal described by Olafson and Monlux showed nervous symptoms for about 2 weeks and finally became comatose. There was marked dyspnea with some nasal discharge. It was destroyed for autopsy examination.

There were no gross lesions. Examination of the brain revealed a diffuse encephalitis with slight meningitis. The cervical and thoracic regions of the cord showed lesions more severe than those in the brain. These consisted of pronounced monocytic perivascular infiltration, focal areas of cell infiltration, and vacuolization of the white matter. Cystlike structures filled with typical toxoplasmata were present in and around the inflamed areas. Lesions were noted in sections from all levels of the cord. They occurred most frequently in

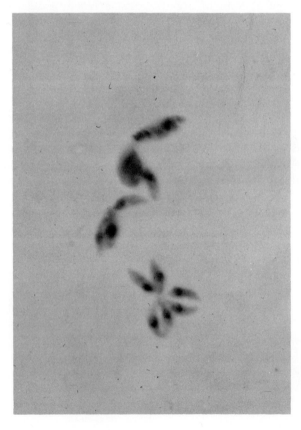

Fig. 135. *Toxoplasma gondi* isolated from a newborn pig. Congenital toxoplasmosis was proved in 3 of 4 pigs at the time of birth. Film showing stages in binary fission; Wright's stain. X 1,700. (Courtesy Clarence R. Cole.)

the white matter about the ventral gray columns. Unfortunately, other tissues of this animal were not examined microscopically, and no inoculation experiments were done because *Toxoplasma* infection was not suspected at the time of the autopsy. It is known that in man the disease is often limited to the nervous system, and sometimes this is true also in rabbits. This incident in a sheep apparently was of such type.

The case described by Wickham and Carne followed the same pattern. Circling disease was suspected but microscopic examination of the brain revealed *Toxoplasma*. It was negative to bacterial culture. The organism has been isolated from ovine fetal membranes (22) and may cause natural outbreaks of abortion in sheep (23, 25, 60). The macroscopic and microscopic pathology of the placenta in ovine abortion caused by *Toxoplasma* has been described by Beverley *et al.(1)*.

*In fowl.* Apparently, toxoplasmosis occurs in fowl but not so frequently as in mammals. Natural infections have been reported in pigeons (16), in chickens (10), in ducks (2), and in wild birds held in captivity (43). In mild infections there may be no predominant lesions. In acute cases foci of necrosis may occur in the liver, spleen, lymph nodes, and lungs. Encephalitis and blindness may be seen. Experimentally, the disease can be established in young chicks (21), and young turkeys are highly susceptible to inoculation (8). The poults develop chronic infections in most cases, and the parasites persist in the organs, especially the brain, for considerable periods of time.

*In swine.* Farrell and co-workers (14) described an outbreak of toxoplasmosis in swine in 1952. The animals were located on a farm in Ohio. Eleven sick pigs representing various ages from 7-day-old piglets to adults over 1 year old

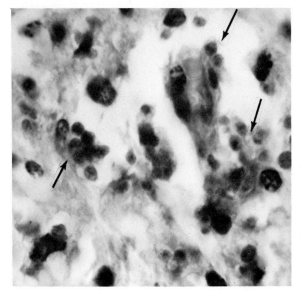

Fig. 136. Active invasion of *Toxoplasma gondi* through a damaged cerebral vessel of a pig. *Arrows* point to organisms in the vascular wall, perivascular space, and adjacent nervous tissue. H and E. X 1,500. (Courtesy Koestner and Cole, *Cornell Vet.*)

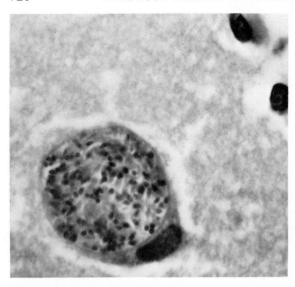

*Fig. 137.* Intracellular *Toxo-plasma gondi* in the cerebral cortex of a pig. The vacuoles indicate the extent of loss of substance. H and E. X 450. (Courtesy Koestner and Cole, *Cornell Vet.*)

were examined. Prominent lesions included pneumonia, lymphadenitis, ulcerative and fibrinonecrotic colitis, and hepatitis. The infection in swine may manifest itself by clinical signs, but it may also be inapparent. Sanger and Cole (49) have isolated *Toxoplasma* from milk, placentas, and newborn pigs of asymptomatic carrier sows. Apparently pigs can be infected by the oral route (65) and the parasite can be isolated from the salivary glands and saliva of pigs with asymptomatic infection (7). The disease has been encountered in piglets where it was believed to be congenital in origin (28).

*In cattle.* Sanger *et al.* (48) demonstrated *Toxoplasma* in three cows, one bull, and two calves originating in four widely separated Ohio herds. Clinical signs observed in spontaneously infected calves were dyspnea, cough, fever, tremors and shaking of the head, extreme weakness, depression, grinding of the teeth, bicycling motions, prostration, and death after a course of 2 to 6 days. In adults, extreme excitability in the early stages was observed more frequently than depression; otherwise, the signs were similar to those seen in calves. They concluded that bovine toxoplasmosis can conceivably be of public health significance because the organism can be demonstrated in the milk as well as in edible portions of infected cows. In addition to milk, feces and sputum may be potential sources of infection for man and animals because *Toxoplasma* may be found in pulmonary and gastrointestinal lesions.

*In wild animals.* In a survey made in Georgia by Walton and Walls (59) *Toxoplasma* were isolated from the opossum, raccoon, gray fox, bobcat, cottontail rabbit, and gray squirrel. They believe that the prevalence of toxoplasmosis in the wild animal population of the United States has been underestimated.

*In man.* Wolfe, Cowan, and Paige (67) described the first human incidents of toxoplasmosis. Their cases occurred in newborn infants and took the form of fatal encephalitis. It is now known that such infections occur *in utero* in apparently healthy mothers (33). Sabin (45) and Pinkerton and Henderson (41) described two cases in children and one in an adult man. All suffered from encephalitis, and the diagnosis was made by finding the organism in the cerebrospinal fluid. One of the children recovered; the other cases proved fatal. Now that toxoplasmosis has been clearly recognized as a human disease, there have been numerous reports of its occurrence in man (26). It may be classified as congenital or acquired and according to the clinical manifestations may be exanthematic, cerebrospinal, ophthalmic, or lymphadenopathic in form.

A nationwide survey for *Toxoplasma* antibodies made in United States military recruits showed a high prevalence of serologic reactions in those from the Appalachian area and a low incidence in those from the Rocky Mountain area (56). In Panama a survey of school children yielded statistically significant differences in prevalence, with the lowest at the highest altitude and the highest near sea level (57).

**Transmission.** There has been much speculation over the mode of transmission of *Toxoplasma*. It is apparent that direct transmission is associated with intimate contact and that spreading occurs readily and quickly. Sabin and Olitsky (47) found it possible to infect mice by feeding them with contaminated material, and they also observed cases traceable to cannibalism in half-starved mice. At the Pasteur Institute in Tunis the disease spread through a large group of rodents (the gondi) kept in captivity. The presence of intestinal ulcers in dogs suggests that the intestinal tract may be the point of entry. Olafson and Monlux (37) reported that the disease spread rather quickly in a litter of puppies one of which had been inoculated intraperitoneally. Eichenwald (9) demonstrated that infected female mice can transmit toxoplasmosis to their offspring through milk. This appears to take place only while the female mouse is undergoing an active, generalized infection. Raw or undercooked eggs from asymptomatic chickens (39) and various arthropods (66) have been suspected transmitting agents.

Weinman and Chandler (62) report that infections are transmitted between swine and rodents when either animal is fed infected tissue from the other, likewise when pigs ingest infected swine offal. They state that the feeding cycles are reminiscent of those in trichinosis. They (63) have postulated that pigs are naturally *Toxoplasma* carriers, deriving the infection by cannibalism or by feeding on infected rodents. Pork cuts may be expected to harbor viable organisms, and people who eat uncooked pork are likely to develop toxoplasmosis because the parasites survive gastric digestion. This could explain the occurrence of toxoplasmosis in carnivorous animals, but not in the herbivorous group.

The observation that oocysts of *I. cati* transmit *Toxoplasma* to herbivores as well as carnivores provides the missing link in the cycle. It appears that these oocysts are excreted only by cats. Because members of this species bury their feces, oocysts are well protected in moist soil. Earthworms distribute them and other vectors such as flies, beetles, and mollusks most likely transmit them. Nematodes, especially *Toxocara cati*, may enter the picture, but are not essential in the transmitting process (18, 50).

**Diagnosis.** Toxoplasmosis may be acquired or congenital. It may be inapparent to acute in its manifestations, and it produces almost the same signs of disease in man as in the lower animals. The most precise way in which to diagnose the infection is to isolate the parasite. For this purpose laboratory-reared mice appear to be the animals of choice. Combined intraperitoneal and intracerebral inoculations should be made.

Serological tests are also of value. One of these is the dye test. Sabin and Feldman (46) demonstrated differences in *Toxoplasma* exposed to normal serum and to immune serum by staining drops of the serum-culture mixtures on a slide with methylene blue. The *Toxoplasma* in the normal serum stained deeply, whereas in the immune serum the cytoplasm of the parasite was completely unstained. This method can be used to detect the presence of antibodies for the *Toxoplasma* antigens. Complement-fixation (CF) tests also are used. Antigens of either egg or mouse peritoneal exudate origin are employed, although the latter antigen is usually preferred (55). The different rates at which the dye test and CF antibodies develop may be used to advantage for diagnostic purposes. Animals that are born with active infections will usually have negative CF tests while their dye test titers will be quite high. Their mothers ordinarily have high titers of both CF and dye test antibodies. If the newborn animals survive, they develop significant amounts of CF antibodies. A combination of a high titer by the dye test and a negative CF result may mean in older animals either that the infection was acquired some time in the past (CF antibodies have already disappeared) or that it is an early infection and that the CF antibodies will increase to significant levels within the next few weeks. Consequently, if we suspect that we are dealing with an active infection, it is mandatory that the CF test be repeated at least 1 month after a negative test was obtained.

Hemagglutination tests have also been used in the diagnosis of toxoplasmosis (13, 27), and by means of fluorescein-labeled antibody the parasites have been identified in tissue sections (3, 58).

Frenkel (15) has described a skin test, using toxoplasmin prepared from species of *Toxoplasma*, to produce the delayed (tuberculin) type of reaction in infected individuals.

**Immunity.** Sabin and Olitsky, working with monkeys, which frequently recover, were able to show that they were immune to reinoculation. They also showed that the serum from recovered monkeys had the power of protecting other monkeys. The tests were performed in the manner customary in virus research, that is, by mixing the organismal suspensions with serum from recovered animals and incubating the mixture for a short time before injecting it into the test animal. For test animals rabbits and mice were used. The test in mice involved the life and death of the animal; in rabbits, however, the mixtures were injected intradermally and immunity was judged by the presence or absence of the local lesions. It was possible to run a number of such tests simultaneously on a single animal. Because the parasites in the mixtures with immune serum seemed not to be changed in any way, they were separated from the immune serum by centrifuging and found to have retained full virulence. In some manner not understood, the serum inhibits infectivity of the organism without directly damaging it, *in vitro*. In studying immunity patterns in guinea pigs following *Toxoplasma* infection or vaccination by killed parasites, Cutchins and Warren (6) found that the convalescent animals were able to resist intracerebral challenge while the vaccinated ones were immune only to intradermal and intraperitoneal challenge.

**Chemotherapy.** According to Weinman and Berne (61), sulfapyridine is strikingly successful in curing acute toxoplasmosis in mice, but even while curing the disease the drug does not sterilize the infection, because some of the cured mice retain virulent organisms and remain carriers. Eyles and Coleman (11) claim that sulfapyrazine shows great activity against mouse toxoplasmosis, but sulfadimetine and sulfisoxazole are ineffective. They (12) also state that the curative effect of pyrimethamine and sulfadiazine administered jointly to infected mice is outstanding. This combination appears to be very effective both *in vitro* and *in vivo*. Steen (54) has reported that aureomycin is effective in treating acute toxoplasmosis in mice, but it suppresses rather than sterilizes the infection. Midtvedt (35) reports that a derivative of sulfamethoxypridazin (bayrena) is the most effective sulfonamide that he has tested.

## REFERENCES

1. Beverley, Watson, and Payne.   Vet. Rec., 1971, 88, 124.
2. Boehringer, Fornari, and Boehringer.   Avian Dis., 1962, 6, 391.
3. Carver and Goldman.   Am. Jour. Clin. Path., 1959, 32, 159.
4. Chamberlain, Docton, and Cole.   Proc. Soc. Exp. Biol. and Med., 1953, 82, 198.
5. Chaparas and Schlesinger.   *Ibid.*, 1959, *102*, 431.
6. Cutchins and Warren.   Am. Jour. Trop. Med. and Hyg., 1956, 5, 197.
7. Dienst and Verma.   *Ibid.*, 1965, *14*, 558.
8. Drobeck, Manwell, Bernstein, and Dillon.   Am. Jour. Hyg., 1953, 58, 329.
9. Eichenwald.   Am. Jour. Dis. Children, 1948, 76, 307.
10. Erichsen and Harboe.   Acta Path. et Microbiol. Scand., 1953, 33, 56.
11. Eyles and Coleman.   Antibiotics and Chemother., 1955, 5, 525.
12. *Ibid.*, 529.
13. Fairchild, Greenwald, and Decker.   Am. Jour. Trop. Med. and Hyg., 1967, *16*, 278.
14. Farrell, Docton, Chamberlain, and Cole.   Am. Jour. Vet. Res., 1952, *13*, 181.
15. Frenkel.   Proc. Soc. Exp. Biol. and Med., 1948, *68*, 634.
16. Frenkel.   Am. Jour. Trop. Med. and Hyg., 1953, 2, 390.

17. Frenkel. Jour. Inf. Dis., 1970, *122*, 553.
18. Frenkel, Dubey, and Miller. Science, 1969, *164*, 432.
19. *Ibid.*, 1970, *167*, 893.
20. Goldman, Carver, and Sulzer. Jour. Parasitol., 1958, *44*, 161.
21. Harboe and Erichsen. Acta Path. et Microbiol. Scand., 1954, *35*, 495.
22. Hartley and Marshall. New Zeal. Vet. Jour., 1958, *5*, 119.
23. Hartley and Moyle. Austral. Vet. Jour., 1968, *44*, 105.
24. Holzworth. Jour. Am. Vet. Med. Assoc., 1954, *124*, 313.
25. Hulland and Tobe. Canad. Vet. Jour., 1961, *2*, 45.
26. Jacobs. Am. Jour Clin. Path., 1956, *26*, 168.
27. Jacobs and Lunde. Science, 1957, *125*, 1035.
28. Jolly. New Zeal. Vet. Jour., 1969, *17*, 87.
29. Lainson. Ann. Trop. Med. and Parasitol., 1959, *53*, 120.
30. Lieberman. North Amer. Vet., 1955, *36*, 43.
31. Machattie. Vet. Jour., 1939, *95*, 70.
32. Meier, Holzworth, and Griffiths. Jour. Am. Vet. Med. Assoc., 1957, *131*, 395.
33. Mellegren, Alm, and Kjessler. Acta Path. et Microbiol. Scand., 1952, *30*, 59.
34. Mello. Bul. Soc. Path. Exot., 1910, *3*, 359.
35. Midtvedt. Acta Path. et Microbiol. Scand., 1964, *61*, 67.
36. Nicolle and Manceaux. Comp. rend. Acad. Sci., 1909, *148*, 269.
37. Olafson and Monlux. Cornell Vet., 1942, *32*, 176.
38. Olisa. Parasitology, 1963, *53*, 643.
39. Pande, Shukla, and Sekariah. Science, 1961, *133*, 648.
40. Petrak and Carpenter. Jour. Am. Vet. Med. Assoc., 1965, *146*, 728.
41. Pinkerton and Henderson. Jour. Am. Med. Assoc., 1941, *116*, 807.
42. Pridham and Belcher. Canad. Jour. Comp. Med. and Vet. Sci., 1958, *22*, 99.
43. Ratcliffe and Worth. Am. Jour. Path., 1951, *27*, 655.
44. Rodaniche and DePinzon. Jour. Parasitol., 1949, *35*, 152.
45. Sabin. Jour. Am. Med. Assoc., 1941, *116*, 801.
46. Sabin and Feldman. Science, 1948, *108*, 660.
47. Sabin and Olitsky. *Ibid.*, 1937, *85*, 336.
48. Sanger, Chamberlain, Chamberlain, Cole, and Farrell. Jour. Am. Vet. Med. Assoc., 1953, *123*, 87.
49. Sanger and Cole. Am. Jour. Vet. Res., 1955, *16*, 536.
50. Sheffield and Melton. Science, 1969, *164*, 431.
51. *Ibid.*, 1970, *167*, 892.
52. Soave and Lennette. Jour. Lab. and Clin. Med., 1959, *53*, 163.
53. Splendore. Rev. Soc. Sci., São Paulo, 1910, *5*, 167.
54. Steen. Acta Path. et Microbiol. Scand., 1950, *27*, 844.
55. Steen and Kass. *Ibid.*, 1951, *28*, 36.
56. Wall, Kagan, and Turner. Am. Jour. Epidemiol., 1967, *85*, 87.
57. Walton, Arjona, and Benchoff. Am. Jour. Trop. Med. and Hyg., 1966, *15*, 492.
58. Walton, Benchoff, and Brooks. *Ibid.*, 1966, *15*, 149.
59. Walton and Walls. *Ibid.*, 1964, *13*, 530.
60. Watson and Beverley. Vet. Rec., 1971, *88*, 120.
61. Weinman and Berne. Jour. Am. Med. Assoc., 1944, *126*, 6.
62. Weinman and Chandler. Proc. Soc. Exp. Biol. and Med., 1954, *87*, 211.
63. Weinman and Chandler. Jour. Am. Med. Assoc., 1956, *161*, 229.

64. Wickham and Carne. Austral. Vet. Jour., 1950, *26*, 1.
65. Wilson, Folkers, Kouwenhoven, and Perie. Vet. Rec., 1967, *81*, 313.
66. Woke, Jacobs, Jones, and Melton. Jour. Parasitol., 1953, *39*, 523.
67. Wolfe, Cowan, and Paige. Am. Jour. Path., 1939, *15*, 657.
68. Woodworth and Weinman. Jour. Inf. Dis., 1960, *107*, 318.

### Encephalitozoon cuniculi

This name was given by Levaditi, Nicolau, and Schoen (1), in 1923, to an organism which several had noted previously in the brains of rabbits suffering from encephalitis. It has also been reported in brain lesions in mice (2) and apparently can be transmitted readily to rabbits, mice, and rats by intracerebral and intraperitoneal inoculation, but not to guinea pigs (3).

The infection is associated with a form of encephalitis, the organism occurring in the brain, kidneys, spleen, and liver of diseased animals. Petri (4) has noted the occurrence of *Encephalitozoon (Nosema) cuniculi* in the cells of transplantable, malignant ascites tumors of the Yoshida rat.

According to Ray and Raghavachari (5), the parasite multiplies by binary fission and a form of schizogony occurs in the ephithelial cells of the urinary tubules. The disease is transmissible by inoculation of urine, and it is thought to be transmitted through urine in nature.

*Toxoplasma* and *Encephalitozoon* closely resemble each other, but, according to Perrin (3), the former are larger and crescentic or fusiform with size ranges of 1.5 to 2.5 by 2.5 to 3.5 microns and the latter are rods with rounded ends. Their size range is 0.8 to 1.2 by 1.5 to 2.5 microns.

### REFERENCES

1. Levaditi, Nicolau, and Schoen. Comp. rend. Acad. Sci., 1923, *177*, 985.
2. Malherbe and Munday. Jour. So. African Vet. Med. Assoc., 1959, *29*, 241.
3. Perrin. Arch. Path., 1943, *36*, 568.
4. Petri. Acta Path. et Microbiol. Scand., 1966, *66*, 13.
5. Ray and Raghavachari. Indian Jour. Vet. Sci., 1941, *11*, 38.

### Dalmeny Disease

Corner *et al.* (1) have described a probably hitherto unrecognized condition in cattle in Canada and have named it Dalmeny disease. The infection occurred in a herd of Holstein cattle and was characterized by high morbidity and mortality in the adult animals. The striking feature was the presence in the vascular endothelium throughout the body of affected animals, of an unidentified, presumable protozoan parasite, morphologically similar to *Toxoplasma gondi*. The parasites were most numerous in animals dying at the acute stage of the disease. Serological tests failed to reveal the cause of this condition and all transmission attempts were unsuccessful.

### REFERENCE

1. Corner, Mitchell, Meads, and Taylor. Canad. Vet. Jour., 1963, *4*, 252.

# XXXI | Pathogenic Protozoa of Undetermined Classification

Several organisms believed to be protozoa but not covered by the established classifications are considered under this heading. When sufficient information about them has been acquired, they will, of course, be placed in their proper relationship to other forms. They are grouped here for convenience only and not because they have features in common.

## THE ANAPLASMATA

In the course of their classical work on piroplasmosis (babesiosis), or Texas fever of cattle, Smith and Kilborne observed and described small coccuslike bodies located near the periphery of many of the red blood cells in animals suffering from the disease. They interpreted these bodies as a stage in the life cycle of the Texas fever parasite. It is clear today that these small bodies were not piroplasms and that Smith and Kilborne were dealing with animals that suffered from two diseases simultaneously, anaplasmosis and piroplasmosis. In 1910 Theiler (35) in South Africa differentiated the two diseases, but because both occurred in the same regions there were many who disagreed with Theiler and continued to look upon the small marginal bodies either as artifacts or as piroplasms. The matter was not fully resolved until recent years when anaplasmosis was found to be prevalent in most of the southern and many of the northern states of the United States, regions that are now free of piroplasmosis (33) or, in some cases, regions that have never been known to have this disease. The parasite is widely distributed throughout the tropics, Africa, the Middle East, some parts of southern Europe, and the Far East.

Considerable uncertainty continues to exist as to the proper place the Anaplasmata should occupy in the schema of parasite classification. In 1934

Neitz, Alexander, and Du Toit (18) described *Eperythrozoon ovis* infection in sheep. In this discussion they compared the organisms found in the genera *Anaplasma, Grahamella, Bartonella,* and *Eperythrozoon* and proposed that all four groups be united into one family *Anaplasmidae.* This proposal has not been accepted, and in the present edition of *Bergey's Manual* the *Bartonella, Hemobartonella, Grahamella,* and *Eperythrozoon* are placed in the family *Bartonellaceae,* and the Anaplasmata have been assigned to the family *Anaplasmataceae;* both families fall in the order *Rickettsiales.* Foote (11; 1954) states that anaplasmosis is caused by a filterable agent that has a single-phase life cycle in the bovine subject. The hemapoietic system of the infected animal is paralyzed by this agent, and the *Anaplasma* body is probably an inclusion body. Lysates of infected blood, prepared and filtered by Ristic (24), were able to produce disease upon injection into susceptible animals. Foote *et al.* (12) also claim that an interference phenomenon exists between anaplasmosis and eperythrozoonosis infections in splenectomized calves and that this interference is reciprocal.

Because the classification of the Anaplasmata is still in doubt, we prefer, for the present, to consider these parasites as protozoa of undetermined classification.

### Anaplasma marginale

This name was given to the organism by Theiler. The word *Anaplasma* means "without plasma" (cytoplasm) and refers to the fact that the parasite seems to consist of nothing but a small bit of chromatic material without any evidence of cytoplasm. The specific name is derived from the fact that these bodies are located, characteristically, near the periphery of the red blood cells and thus appear, in smears, as if on the margin of cells.

**Morphology.** The parasites of anaplasmosis are seen in the red blood corpuscles as minute, deeply staining points usually located near the margin of the cell. If stained with the Giemsa stain, they are deep red in color; with other stains they are apt to be so dark that color in them is not distinguished, but a one-step toluidine blue staining technic has proved to be useful for rapid detection of *Anaplasma* in erythrocytes in the field or laboratory (31). They are spherical in form and ordinarily there is but one organism per cell, although two or more may be seen in some cells. In the early stages of the disease before the temperature rise occurs, few or no parasites can be found. When the febrile period begins, the percentage of infected cells may reach 25 percent or even more than 50 percent. If the animal recovers, the number of cells containing the marginal bodies diminishes rapidly until none can be found microscopically. The blood of recovered animals is infectious for many years and probably for life; hence it is probable that a few bodies are present indefinitely—so few as to make the finding of them impossible.

In 1959 Espana *et al.* (10) employed phase contrast and electron microscopy in studying hemolyzed erythrocytes from cattle infected with *A. margin-*

*ale.* They found ring, match, comet, and dumbbell-like forms in natural and experimental infections. They also stated that the organism is motile, that it is a true parasite, and that it probably belongs in the protozoa.

Bedell and Dimopoullos (1) claim that infectivity of *A. marginale* is destroyed by exposure to 60 C for 50 minutes and by sonic energy treatments for 90 minutes when the blood is maintained at 30 to 35 C (2). Storage of heparinized, glycerolated, and infected *A. marginale* bovine erythrocytes for 4.5 years at −70 C did not alter the infectivity or the virulence of the parasite (34).

**Life History.** The life history of the parasite of anaplasmosis is not completely known. Binary fission is believed to be the usual means of multiplication, but Lotze (17) has described multiple fission with the formation of eight small spherical bodies. Freidhoff and Ristic (14) demonstrated *A. marginale* in the gut contents and in the Malpighian tubes of engorged *Dermacentor andersoni* nymphs by the fluorescent-antibody technic and stated that the anaplasms multiplied in the Malpighian tubes by the process of binary fission.

**The Natural Disease.** Although cattle appear to be the specific host for the Anaplasmata, they have been found in deer (Boynton and Woods, 6). As in piroplasmosis, young animals are quite resistant. Cases in calves under 1 year of age are rare, although in infected territories many calves pass through the infection and become immune carriers. The natural resistance of young calves is removed by splenectomy. The marginal bodies appear in great numbers in such animals; hence they are suitable for diagnostic purposes.

In older animals the disease may be acute or chronic. Those affected with the acute form may die within 2 or 3 days after the appearance of the first symptoms. The disease begins with a high temperature, 105 to 107 F. After a day or two, signs of anemia and icterus appear, and about this time the temperature falls to normal and even subnormal as death approaches. The mucous membranes are pale and yellowish. The yellow color is evident also in the thin-skinned parts of the body. Urination is frequent but the urine is not blood-tinged, as it often is in piroplasmosis. The animal is usually constipated, the feces being dark, often bloodstained, and covered with mucus.

In chronic cases the animals live longer, are weak, become progressively emaciated, and show icterus and anemia. The red blood cell count may fall from a normal of about 7 million to less than 1 million per mm $^3$; the hemoglobin may be less than 10 percent.

The mortality is quite variable. It may be greater than 50 percent, or less than 5 percent. Losses are greatest in hot weather, and in older animals.

In natural infections the period of incubation varies from 20 to 40 days. Experimentally, symptoms may be produced much earlier by inoculation with large doses of acutely infected blood.

The principal lesions are those associated with blood destruction, anemia, and icterus. The spleen is enlarged and the pulp is dark and soft. The blood appears as if diluted with water. A catarrhal enteritis is common. There may be a few petechial hemorrhages on the heart wall and on the mucosa of the urinary bladder. The lymph nodes are swollen and edematous. The liver shows marked icterus with the bile channels engorged and the gall bladder distended with dark green, mucilaginous bile. Kreier *et al.* (16) have indicated that the anemia in *Anaplasma* infected animals is caused by intensive erythrophagocytosis initiated by parasitic damage to red blood cells and to antierythrocytic autoantibody.

The diagnosis is made conclusive, of course, by the finding of the characteristic marginal bodies in the red blood cells. In this connection it is well to warn the examiner to be cautious in his identification, so as not to confuse such structures as basophilic stippling and the "Jolly" bodies, seen in severe anemias, with Anaplasmata. Artifacts resembling these bodies are often seen also. The examinations should be made only on good films which are well stained. Ristic *et al.* (28) have detected A. *marginale* by means of fluorescein-labeled antibody.

In using splenectomized calves to diagnose anaplasmosis, Gates *et al.* (15) noted that blood obtained from cattle whose sera showed a high complement-fixation titer had a much lower degree of infectivity than that of other cattle. It should also be noted that the splenectomized cow is even more susceptible to infection than the splenectomized calf (30).

Boynton and Woods (5) have reported a simple test that seems to have some value in the diagnosis of anaplasmosis. The blood is allowed to clot and a little clear serum is obtained. Two drops are added to 2 ml of distilled water in a tube. The serum of normal animals does not cloud the water; that of animals affected with anaplasmosis causes an immediate clouding and,

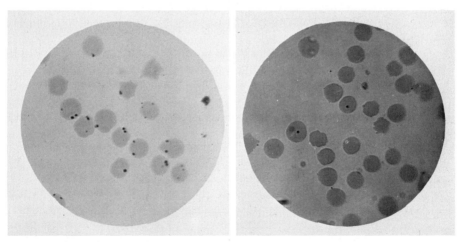

*Fig. 138 (left). Anaplasma marginale,* a stained blood film from a cow suffering from acute anaplasmosis and showing many organisms in its blood. X 700.

*Fig. 139 (right). Anaplasma centrale* in bovine blood. Two typical parasites are seen as sharply staining dots in red blood cells near the center of the illustration. Poikilocytosis and anisocytosis are present as a result of anemia. X 700.

after the tube stands overnight, a white precipitate covers the bottom. Animals affected with acute anaplasmosis and recently recovered carriers give this reaction. The test depends upon the precipitation of euglobulin, which appears to be present in increased amount in this disease. Splenectomized, disease-free calves are suitable for use in locating carrier animals. The complement-fixation test also is used in detecting the disease. According to Price *et al.* (21), it is highly accurate. The antigen is obtained from the blood of infected splenectomized calves (13, 22).

Ristic and co-workers have employed a gel diffusion (26) and a capillary tube agglutination test (25). They claim that the latter test is as accurate as the complement-fixation test and has the advantages over gel diffusion or complement fixation of simplicity, economy, and speed of reaction in detecting anaplasmosis.

**Transmission.** At least 17 species of ticks have been shown to be capable of transmitting anaplasmosis. Most of these probably are mechanical rather than biological carriers, but several are biological carriers (3, 4). Among the latter are *Boophilus* (*Margaropus*) *annulatus, Dermacentor occidentalis,* and *Dermacentor andersoni,* which occur in the United States. In these species the infective agent passes through the egg into the next generation of the species.

The fact that deer are susceptible to anaplasmosis indicates that they may constitute an important resevoir of infection in areas where they occupy the same range land as cattle (8, 19).

Nothing is known about the life cycle of the *Anaplasma* in the invertebrate biological vectors.

In addition, at least seven species of horseflies (*Tabanidae*) have been shown to be mechanical carriers, and certain mosquitoes have also been incriminated. The stable fly (*Stomoxys calcitrans*) and the horn fly (*Hematobia serrata*) apparently seldom, if ever, act as transmitters.

An important means of transmission is through the use of common surgical instruments which have not been thoroughly disinfected after being used on one animal and before being used on another. Reese (23) has shown that anaplasmosis can very easily be carried on a lancet for drawing blood if it is merely wiped after being used on an infected animal. Outbreaks have occurred in herds after dehorning operations, the drawing of blood samples, castrations, and minor operations. In areas where anaplasmosis occurs, veterinarians should be exceedingly cautious in carrying out these mass operations to avoid serious consequences resulting from the spreading of this disease to many animals from a few, or even one, carrier animal. Uterine transmission has also been reported and Davis *et al.* (9) have demonstrated that *Anaplasma* has the ability to infect via the ocular route.

**Immunity.** Animals that recover from anaplasmosis remain carriers for long periods and probably for life. Such animals are resistant to additional infection. Young calves are relatively resistant to the infection. Symptoms are seldom seen in calves less than 1 year of age. Such animals can be inoculated with virulent blood, especially in the winter months when the disease is not so severe naturally as it is in the hot months, and made immune thereafter. Because they become permanent carriers and because the number of vectors is great, such animals are a source of danger to any nonimmune animals with which they may come in contact at any time later in life.

Recent vaccine trials, using a killed antigen, have indicated that the antigen may increase resistance to the *Anaplasma* organism and reduce losses from the disease. Use of the vaccine, however, may complicate control of the disease, because it prevents differentiation of vaccinated and infected cattle by serologic tests (7).

Eradication programs have consisted of continuing testing and stray-dipping of imported cattle, or the selection of uninfected replacement heifers from infected dams by means of the CF test conducted 30 to 60 days after weaning and by placing them in CF-negative groups.

**Chemotherapy.** According to Splitter and Miller (32), anaplasmosis carrier infection can be eradicated by treatment with terramycin (5 mg per pound of animal weight per day in single or divided doses for 12 to 14 days) or by aureomycin (15 mg per pound per day in single doses for 16 days). Pearson *et al.* (20) used intramuscular injections of tetracycline at the rate of 5 mg per pound of body weight daily for 10 consecutive days. Aralen hydrochloride, 5 percent sterile aqueous solution, has been approved for the parenteral treatment of anaplasmosis in cattle, and Roby *et al.* (29) recommend dithiosemicarbazone.

It has been stated that the relapse which ordinarily follows splenectomy in *Anaplasma*-infected calves does not occur in those animals that have been previously treated with cortisone (27).

## REFERENCES

1. Bedell and Dimopoullos.   Am. Jour. Vet. Res., 1962, 23, 618.
2. *Ibid.*, 1963, 24, 278.
3. Boynton.   Cornell Vet., 1928, 18, 28.
4. *Ibid.*, 1929, 19, 387.
5. Boynton and Woods.   Jour. Am. Vet. Med. Assoc., 1935, 87, 59.
6. Boynton and Woods.   Science, 1940, 91, 168.
7. Brock.   Proc. Am. Vet. Med. Assoc., 1963, p. 258.
8. Christensen, Osebold, Harrold, and Rosen.   Jour. Am. Vet. Med. Assoc., 1960, 136, 426.
9. Davis, Dimopoullos, and Roby.   Res. Vet. Sci., 1970, 11, 594.
10. Espana, Espana, and Gonzolez.   Am. Jour. Vet. Res., 1959, 78, 795.
11. Foote.   North Amer. Vet., 1954, 35, 19.
12. Foote, Levy, Torbert, and Oglesby.   Am. Jour. Vet. Res., 1957, 18, 556.
13. Franklin, Heck, and Huff.   *Ibid.*, 1963, 24, 483.
14. Freidhoff and Ristic.   *Ibid.*, 1966, 27, 643.
15. Gates, Madden, Martin, and Roby.   *Ibid.*, 1957, 18, 257.
16. Kreier, Ristic, and Schroeder.   *Ibid.*, 1964, 25, 343.

17. Lotze.   Proc. Heminthol. Soc. Wash., 1946, *13*, 56.
18. Neitz, Alexander, and Du Toit.   Onderstepoort Jour. Vet. Sci. and Anim. Indus., 1934, *3*, 263.
19. Osebold, Christensen, Longhurst, and Rosen.   Cornell Vet., 1959, *49*, 97.
20. Pearson, Brock, and Kliewer.   Jour. Am. Vet. Med. Assoc., 1957, *130*, 290.
21. Price, Brock, and Miller.   Am. Jour. Vet. Res., 1954, *15*, 511.
22. Price, Poelma, and Faber.   *Ibid.*, 1952, *13*, 149.
23. Reese.   North Am. Vet., 1930, *11*, 7.
24. Ristic.   Am. Jour. Vet. Res., 1960, *84*, 890.
25. Ristic.   Jour. Am. Vet. Med. Assoc., 1962, *141*, 588.
26. Ristic and Mann.   Am. Jour. Vet. Res., 1963, *24*, 478.
27. Ristic, White, Green, and Sanders.   *Ibid.*, 1958, *19*, 37.
28. Ristic, White, and Sanders.   *Ibid.*, 1957, *18*, 924.
29. Roby, Amerault, and Spindler.   Res. Vet. Sci., 1968, *9*, 494.
30. Roby, Gates, and Mott.   Am. Jour. Vet. Res., 1961, *22*, 982.
31. Rogers and Wallace.   *Ibid.*, 1966, 27, 1127.
32. Splitter and Miller.   Vet. Med., 1953, *48*, 486.
33. Stiles.   U.S. Dept. Agr. Cir. 154, 1931.
34. Summers and Matsuoka.   Am. Jour. Vet. Res., 1970, *31*, 1517.
35. Theiler.   Transvaal Dept. of Agr., Rpt. Govt. Bact., 1908–09, p. 7.

### Anaplasma ovis

Anaplasmosis of sheep has been described by DeKock and Quinlan (1) in South Africa. In 1955 Splitter *et al.* (5) reported on a flock of sheep in Kansas. They were investigated because of an obscure debilitating condition. Routine blood examination revealed marginal bodies in the erythrocytes identical in appearance with *Anaplasma marginale*, together with extracellular forms characteristic of *Eperythrozoon ovis*. Splenectomized calves inoculated with this sheep blood did not develop evidence of *A. marginale* infection. It seems probable that they were dealing with *A. ovis*.

In 1956 an organism identified as *A. ovis* was recovered from sheep originating in the Rocky Mountain area of the United States (4). The organism produced variable degrees of subclinical anemia in sheep and goats. Cattle could not be infected with the parasite, nor did it produce any detectable immunity in these animals against *A. marginale*. This agrees with the findings of the South African workers, who have shown that cattle are not infected by *A. ovis*.

In 1963 Kreier and Ristic (2) infected two Virginia white-tailed deer (*Dama virginiana*) experimentally with *A. ovis*.

Electron microscopy studies of erythrocytes infected with *A. ovis* have revealed a membrane-enclosed body, usually marginally located and filled with two initial bodies (3).

### REFERENCES

1. DeKock and Quinlan.   11th and 12th Rpt. Dir. Vet. Ed. and Res., Union of So. Africa, 1926, p. 369.

2.  Kreier and Ristic.    Am. Jour. Vet. Res., 1963, *24*, 567.
3.  Jatkar.    *Ibid.*, 1969, *30*, 1891.
4.  Splitter, Anthony, and Twiehaus.    *Ibid.*, 1956, *17*, 487.
5.  Splitter, Twiehaus, and Castro.    Jour. Am. Vet. Med. Assoc., 1955, *127*, 244.

### *Anaplasma centrale*

Theiler (2), in his studies which led to differentiation of the anaplasms from the piroplasms, distinguished two kinds of the former, the marginal bodies, which have already been described and which are the only ones found in anaplasmosis in the United States, and central bodies, which are identical in appearance with the marginal bodies but are located characteristically in the central part of the red blood cells. They have come to be called by the name that heads this paragraph.

Theiler showed that animals which had recovered from an infection with blood containing the central bodies could still be infected with blood containing the marginal bodies. He also noted that the disease caused by *A. centrale* was much milder than the other. In South Africa, according to Schmidt (1), adult cattle coming from Europe are first injected with blood containing *A. centrale* and later with *A. marginale*, the first and milder infection giving some protection against a severe second. In Australia, where premunizing with *A. centrale* is practiced, it has been found that citrated calf blood infected with this parasite retains its effectiveness for 254 days when frozen in 1-ml doses and maintained at $-72$ to $-80$ C (3).

### REFERENCES

1.  Schmidt.    Jour. Am. Vet. Med. Assoc., 1937, *90*, 723.
2.  Theiler.    Zeitschr. f. Infektionskr. Haustiere, 1912, *11*, 193.
3.  Turner.    Austral. Vet. Jour., 1944, *20*, 295.

## THE GLOBIDIA

Closely related to the sarcosporidia, in appearance and probably zoologically as well, is a group of parasites that are found in the mucosa of the alimentary tract and in the subcutaneous tissues of herbivorous animals. These have been given various names but Wenyon groups them together in a single genus, *Globidium*. The relationship of these parasites to the Anaplasmata and the Sarcosporidia, described below, is not clear. Some globidial parasites resemble the schizont forms of coccidia described by Boughton (2) in the small intestines of cattle. It is possible that certain structures seen in the intestines are actually coccidia that have been mistaken for globidia, but it also appears that the skin globidia do not fit this category.

Some authors have indicated that the alimentary tract form should be classed with the coccidia or at least be separated from the skin form. They suggest that the former retain the generic designation of *Globidium* and that the latter be placed in a separate genus, *Besnoitia*.

## Globidiosis of the Intestine

Globidia are common in sheep in England. A form known as *Globidium gilruthi* was found by Triffit (12) in more than nine-tenths of the series that he examined. Marsh and Tunnicliff (5) have described it in Montana sheep, where it is associated with severe diarrhea. Mugera and Bitakaramire (7) have observed globidiosis in goats in Kenya. Infection was indicated by the development of gastroenteritis.

*G. gilruthi* is usually found in the wall of the abomasum, but Marsh and Tunnicliff found it in the intestines. It appears as spherical cysts which vary from 200 to 500 microns in diameter. The cysts consist of a rather thick wall enclosing enormous numbers of spores not unlike those of sarcocysts. They are sickle-shaped and measure 1.5 by 10 microns. The cysts may be seen with the naked eye as minute, opalescent nodules beneath the mucosa. They evidently are formed within cells, for often the cell nucleus can be observed along one border of the cyst. These forms rupture into the lumen of the bowel and often cause hemorrhages. In heavy infections symptoms may be produced, but in most instances the numbers are so few as to cause little damage.

## Cutaneous Globidiosis (Besnoitiosis)

In 1960 Pols (10) reviewed the status of the genus *Besnoitia*. He claims it to be valid and related to the genera *Fibrocystis* and *Toxoplasma*, but distinct from them. The species of veterinary interest cause serious skin disease in horses and cattle in Europe and Africa. Besnoitiosis also occurs in the latter continent in the blue wildebeest, impala, and kudu. There are reports of this condition in Panamanian lizards (11), in Mexican cattle, in rodents in Utah (4), in an opossum in Kentucky (3), and a species has been identified in Alaska in reindeer and caribou. Pols separates the parasite found in the horse (*Besnoitia bennetti*) from the one (*Besnoitia besnoiti*) seen in cattle. The designations *Besnoitia jellisoni, Besnoitia darlingi, Besnoitia panamensis,* and so forth have been applied to the parasites isolated from antelopes, rodents, and lizards. At present there is little evidence to constitute more than one species.

Horses infected with *B. bennetti* may have a history of 7 or 8 months of illness with extreme weakness and dejection, thickened eyelids, swollen legs, loss of hair, scab formation, and general thickening of the skin. The bursting of skin cysts may cause considerable damage. These cysts occur in the matrix of the areolar or adipose tissue of the subcutis or in the intercellular spaces of the more highly differentiated layers.

In cattle *B. besnoiti* produces a disease characterized by involvement of the dermis, subcutaneous tissues and fascia, the connective tissue of the scleral conjunctiva, and the laryngeal mucosa. As the disease progresses the hair falls out and the skin thickens and may crack with exudation of blood.

The parasites are 5 to 9 microns in length by 2 to 5 microns in width. With

Giemsa stain the nucleus is reddish-purple and the cytoplasm blue. Fully developed cysts may reach a diameter of 600 microns in cattle.

According to Pols (8), *B. besnoiti* can be transmitted to cattle and rabbits by the injection of blood collected during the primary stage of the disease. The incubation period for his experiments varied from 6 to 16 days and was followed by a thermal reaction, which persisted for 2 to 5 days. In cattle, the primary stage usually was mild and only one out of five developed skin lesions. Rabbits died within 2 to 5 days after an initial rise in temperature. Trophozoites of *B. besnoiti* were encountered in the monocytes of some of the cattle and in all of the rabbits during the primary stage of the disease. Morphologically these structures resemble those of *Toxoplasma gondi.* Cysts could be demonstrated in the cattle 6 to 28 days after the initial rise in temperature. Pols was unable to transmit *B. besnoiti* to guinea pigs, rats, or mice, but parasites established in the rabbit were transferred successfully to sheep and goats and to a limited extent to guinea pigs. Attempts to transmit from rabbits to the horse or dog were unsuccessful.

In the early stages of besnoitiosis there is a febrile reaction and at this time the parasites appear in the blood. Under field conditions there is a seasonal incidence of infection suggesting an arthropod vector which is active at the time the organism is found in the blood. Attempts to transmit the cutaneous parasites using ground skin tissue have not been successful.

By decreasing the amount of inoculum, Pols (9) was able to protract the course but not the incubation period in the rabbit. Symptoms varied from a febrile reaction only to severe swelling of head and body. In males scrotal swelling appeared first. The besnoitial cysts were formed in the cutis vera, subcutis, and connective tissue of the testis by invasion of histiocytes with trophozoites. Pols infers that simple binary fission is the usual mode of multiplication, but multinucleate aberrant forms occur.

In cattle the mortality is less than 10 percent, but the animals lose condition and their hides become valueless for tanning. Cows may abort and bulls become sterile. At autopsy there is no characteristic change in the internal organs.

Salient findings observed in studying besnoitiosis in wild antelopes and domestic cattle in Africa were (a) an absence of clinical signs of the disease in the antelopes, (b) an almost exclusive confinement of the cysts to the cardiovascular system of the antelope, and (c) a marked incidence of cysts in the subcutaneous lymphatics of the impala, in the peripheral veins of the limbs of cattle and antelopes, in the head of cattle, and in the jugular vein of antelopes (6).

In the febrile stage of the disease diagnosis is made by injecting blood into a rabbit. Later skin biopsies reveal the cysts. At autopsy the cysts may be visible in the mucous membranes of the trachea, in the cutis, and in the subcutis.

According to Bigalke (1) transmission of besnoitiosis may occur through cohabitation, but all evidence points toward the fact that it is self-contained. The only other requirement for transmission to take place is apparently a mechanical vector in the form of a blood-sucking insect.

Pols (10) states that animals that survive either a natural or an artificial infection develop a durable premunity. At present there appears to be no specific cure for besnoitiosis.

## REFERENCES

1. Bigalke. Onderstepoort Jour. Vet. Res., 1968, *35*, 3.
2. Boughton. North Am. Vet., 1942, *23*, 173.
3. Conti-Diaz, Turner, Tweeddale, and Furcolow. Jour. Parasitol., 1970, *56*, 457.
4. Ernst, Chobotar, Oaks, and Hammond. *Ibid.*, 1968, *54*, 545.
5. Marsh and Tunnicliff. Am. Jour. Vet. Res., 1941, *2*, 174.
6. McCully, Basson, Van Niekerk, and Bigalke. Onderstepoort Jour. Vet. Res., 1966, *33*, 245.
7. Mugera and Bitakaramire. Vet. Rec., 1968, *82*, 595.
8. Pols. Jour. So. African Vet. Med. Assoc., 1954, *25*, 37.
9. *Ibid.*, 45.
10. Pols. Onderstepoort Jour. Vet. Res., 1960, *3*, 265.
11. Schneider. Jour. Parasitol., 1965, *51*, 340.
12. Triffit. Protozoology, 1925, *1*, 7.

## THE SARCOSPORIDIA

The parasites included in this group make up a single genus, *Sarcocystis.* As intracellular parasites, they are found in the striated muscular fibers of all the domestic animals, but they are especially common in horses, cattle, sheep, and swine. They are rare in dogs and cats. They occur frequently in wild herbivorous animals and in a number of species of birds. Ducks are more frequently affected than other birds. They have been seen in the heart muscle of the lion (3). A few cases in man have been reported. They are not often seen in young animals. Reiten *et al.* (8) have suggested that there is a relationship between eosinophilic myositis and sarcosporidiosis.

The literature contains the names of many species of *Sarcocystis,* most of them having been named with respect to the animals in which they were found. It has been demonstrated, however, that these organisms are not always host-specific, as Erdmann (5) has shown that mice may be infected by feeding them infected sheep muscle, and Darling (4) infected guinea pigs with an organism found in an opossum. There are some morphological differences between the sarcosporidia of different animals. The sarcocysts found in sheep and the species seen in ducks and mice are macroscopic in size, whereas other mammalian forms are usually microscopic. The spores in the microscopic sarcocysts usually are scattered throughout the cysts, but in the macroscopic cysts of sheep and ducks they are arranged around the periphery, leaving a network of undifferentiated material in the center. However, there are no basic criteria for establishing different species within the group except the host relationship. It is possible that all represent a single species. This question cannot be answered at present.

Spindler (11; 1947) stained sections of *Sarcocystis* sacs and showed that they contained a network of jointed, hyphalike structures. These structures exhibited the staining reactions characteristic of fungi rather than protozoa. So far this work has not been confirmed. Although it is likely that the sarcosporidia will prove to be fungi, their exact classification is undetermined at this time.

### Sarcocystis miescheriana

SYNONYMS: From the discussion above it will be seen that the question of whether all sarcocysts belong to one or to many species cannot be answered at present. If they are regarded as a single species, the name given above has priority. If it is shown that there are many species, this name will be valid only for the parasite of the pig, to which it was applied by Kuhn in 1865. The specific names often used for the forms found in domestic animals are as follows:

Horse—S. *bertrami*          Goat—S. *moulei*
Cow—S. *hirsuta* and S. *cruzi*     Mouse—S. *muris*
Pig—S. *miescheriana*        Rabbit—S. *cuniculi* and S. *leporum*
Sheep—S. *tenella*           Duck—S. *rileyi*

**Morphology.** Sarcosporidia, in whatever host they may be found, have a similar appearance. They are seen in striated-muscles as elongated structures, the long axis of which is parallel to the muscle fibers. In some instances the structures are large enough to be seen with the naked eye, in which case they appear as white streaks. If great numbers are present, the muscles may become grayish white instead of the normal color. These bodies were first seen in muscular tissue by Miescher in 1843 and have become known as *Miescher's tubes*. In most instances the number of these structures is so few and their size so small that they are not detected except in microscopic sections. Sections of muscles of old horses, cattle, and sheep nearly always show a few of these structures.

The sarcocysts develop inside muscle fibers, but as they become larger the fibers containing them disintegrate so the larger forms are embedded in connective tissue. All sizes may be seen from forms about 25 microns to others 4 or 5 cm in length. The elongated structure is surrounded by a definite capsule from which fine trabeculae or septa extend into the interior, dividing it into chambers that are filled with the characteristic banana-shaped spores varying from 3 to 7 microns in length. These spores, in hematoxylin-stained sections, take the blue dye, staining intensely. The trabeculae usually are not easily seen; thus the parasite appears like a sac filled with spores. In cross sections these appear spherical, being many times as large as the normal muscle cells; in longitudinal section they are, of course, elongate.

The spores apparently are formed from a germinal layer around the periphery, and this layer continues to function for long periods of time. Very old sarcocysts not infrequently show nothing but debris and degenerated spores in their interiors, with normal spores around the periphery. A fully developed parasite often contains many thousands of spores, which escape only when the organism ruptures. There is no evidence that this happens during the life of the animal.

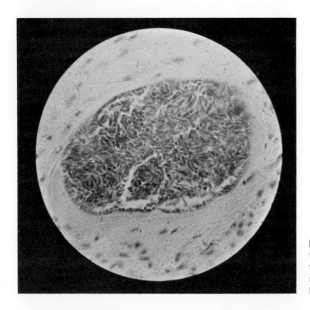

*Fig. 140.* Sarcocyst in the heart muscle of a horse. The photograph is of a stained cross section. The sickle-shaped spores are shown crowding a capsule that is lined with germinal cells. X 1,000.

**Transmission.** Theobald Smith (10) demonstrated in 1901 that mice could be infected by feeding them spores contained in the muscles of other mice. Erdmann (5) infected mice by feeding infected sheep muscle. It seems evident that meat-eating animals can acquire the infection by ingestion, but this does not serve to explain the infections in herbivorous animals. The mode of infection in these animals is unknown. It has been suggested that bloodsucking flies may be responsible. Several observers have found what they believed to be spores in blood films.

Scott (9), who studied the infection in Wyoming sheep, decided that infections occurred only during the summer months. He was not successful in showing that the ingestion of insects, or insect excreta, had anything to do with the infection. Approximately 100 percent of the older sheep became infected on the range, but experimental sheep, kept on a dry lot, watered with deep-well water, and fed only on dry feed, also became infected.

Spindler and Zimmerman (12) removed sarcocysts aseptically from swine muscle and cultured the ruptured sacs on glucose agar. A fungus of the genus *Aspergillus* grew. Young pigs fed conidia from the cultures harbored typical sarcocysts in their muscles upon autopsy, 4 to 6 months after the feeding. Cultures from these cysts yielded the fungus. Later Spindler and Zimmerman (13) showed that pigs, dogs, cats, rats, mice, and chickens, after consuming the flesh of infected swine, are capable of transmitting infective *Sarcocystis* spores to swine. The infective stage is eliminated in the feces and urine of these animals, and pigs become infected by consuming such feces or urine. The animals fed infected swine muscle did not pass infective urine or feces until the 15th day following the feeding. Pigs fed infected flesh did not acquire sarcocysts. The disease in pigs was manifested by vomiting, diarrhea, inappetence, weakness, and temporary posterior paralysis.

**Life Cycle.** Erdmann (6) studied the infection in mice. She found that the cyst walls disintegrated in the intestines releasing the spores which, after assuming an ameboid form, penetrated the intestinal epithelium. Here the trail was lost. It was picked up again only after about 40 days, when the developing sarcocysts in the muscles were found.

**Pathogenicity.** There is evidence that sarcosporidia may cause some injury in swine when heavy infections occur. Deaths of sheep have been attributed to sarcocysts, but the evidence is not convincing. Occasionally sheep and swine that have appeared to be normal during life have so many sarcocysts in the muscular tissue as to lead to the condemnation of the carcass by meat inspectors, principally because of the altered appearance of the meat. However, mice may be killed by large doses of infected material, and this suggests that the same thing may possibly be true occasionally in the larger animals.

Pfeiffer (7) in 1890 made the discovery that extracts of the sarcosporidia of sheep were markedly poisonous for mice, rabbits, and sheep. Small animals may be killed within a few hours by injecting them with aqueous or glycerol extracts of sarcocysts. The dosage required is small. The poisonous property is a toxin to which the name *sarcocystin* has been given. Teichmann and Braun (14) produced an antitoxin with which they succeeded in passively immunizing other animals. The toxin is contained in the spores, and apparently little of it is released from the encapsulated parasite in the naturally infected hosts.

Complement-fixation and dermal sensitivity tests have been used in the diagnosis of sarcosporidiosis. The former employs a frozen and thawed extract of the cysts as antigen and the latter makes use of sarcocystin (1, 2).

## REFERENCES

1. Awad.   Am. Jour. Vet. Res., 1957, *18*, 703.
2. Awad.   *Ibid.*, 1958, *19*, 1010.
3. Bhatavdekar and Purohit.   Indian Vet. Jour., 1963, *40*, 44.
4. Darling.   Jour. Exp. Med., 1910, *12*, 19.
5. Erdmann.   Centrbl. f. Bakt., I Abt., Orig., 1910, 53, 510.
6. Erdmann.   Sitzungsb. Ges. naturf. Freunde, 1910, 8, 377.

7. Pfeiffer.   Die Protozoen als Krankheitserreger. Jena, 1910.
8. Reiten, Jensen, and Griner.   Am. Jour. Vet. Res., 1966, *27*, 903.
9. Scott.   Jour. Parasitol., 1918, *5*, 45.
10. Smith.   Jour. Exp. Med., 1901, *6*, 1; 1905, *13*, 429.
11. Spindler.   Proc. Helminthol. Soc. Wash., 1947, *14*, 28.
12. Spindler and Zimmerman.   Jour. Parasitol., 1945, *31*, (Sup.), 13.
13. Spindler and Zimmerman.   Proc. Helminthol. Soc. Wash., 1946, *13*, 1.
14. Teichmann and Braun.   Arch. f. Protistenk., 1911, *22*, 351.

# XXXII | The Pathogenic Ciliates

Protozoa belonging to the class *Ciliata* are exceedingly numerous in nature. They occur as free-living organisms in stagnant water everywhere, and "cultures" can easily be obtained by placing straw, grass, or almost any kind of vegetable material in ordinary tap water and keeping the dilute infusions at room temperature for a few days. Pathogenic species belonging to this group are not numerous. All of the known pathogens belong in the genera *Balantidium* and *Tetrahymena*. Species belonging to the genus *Balantidium* are intestinal parasites, and members of the genus *Tetrahymena* have been found in the eye lesions of birds (Knight and McDougle, 4). *Balantidium coli* occurs commonly in the intestines of pigs and occasionally in man. A smaller species, *Balantidium suis*, is found in pigs, and this species appears to be specific for swine. Members of this genus have been reported in various types of monkeys, cattle, sheep, and horses. It is not known whether these are separate species or whether they are *B. coli*. It is quite certain that many of the monkey types are *B. coli*, for many cross infections have been secured experimentally (6).

### Balantidium coli

The organism apparently occurs in swine everywhere. In the greater part of the infections no apparent damage is done; however, in animals that are debilitated for other reasons severe lesions result. The same situation exists with respect to the human infections. Most of these have been seen in persons who have had close contact with swine; hence it is believed that human infections are incidental. The organism occurs in the intestines, particularly in the large intestines. Occasionally it is found in the lower end of the small intestines as well.

**Morphology.** *Balantidium coli* is a relatively large protozoon. It is ovoid or pear-shaped, generally measures from 50 to 80 microns in length, and is about two-thirds as broad. Some individuals are considerably larger, measuring as much as 150 microns in length. The surface presents longitudinal ridges which run slightly spirally. In the grooves between these ridges are rows of cilia which vary from 4 to 10 or 12 microns in length. These cilia occur on all parts of the body. In active individuals they are in constant motion.

At the anterior end of the organism there is a slightly oblique depression, the *peristome*, at the bottom of which is an opening, the *cytostome*, which leads into a tubular structure, analogous to an esophagus, which ends blindly in the cytoplasm of the cell. The peristome contracts into a slitlike structure at times and at others relaxes into a broad funnel. Large cilia surround the opening of the cytostome and line a considerable part of the wall of the tube which extends from it into the interior of the organism. At the posterior end of the organism a small opening in the body wall, the *anal aperture*, occurs. The nucleus is a large sausage-shaped structure lying somewhat diagonally across the long axis of the organism. Vacuoles, red blood cells, leukocytes, and other foreign bodies are often seen in various parts of the cytoplasm.

Reproduction is by transverse division. The nucleus divides prior to the division of the cytoplasm, one-half going into each of the new individuals. The cytostome remains in the new individual constituted by the anterior half of the parent cell. The other daughter cell forms a new cytostome.

Round or oval cysts are formed; these are protected by thick walls consisting of two distinct layers. These cysts usually contain but a single individual, but sometimes two individuals appear to fuse (conjugation) within the cyst wall. The rounded parasites may be seen within the cyst, the cilia moving slowly. These cysts are the means by which the species is propagated. They are passed to the ground in the feces and by fecally contaminated food into a new host.

**Pathogenicity.** As has been stated above, *B. coli* occurs in many swine that show no symptoms, and apparently little harm is done by it. Occasionally, however, in stunted, heavily parasitized pigs, especially young pigs, the organism is found in association with an ulcerative colitis and severe bloody diarrhea. Cases of this type have been seen in the United States, and others have been reported from nearly all parts of the world. These cases apparently are not numerous, and it is not clear whether the malnutrition is caused by the *Balantidium* or whether the parasite takes advantage of a host whose resistance has been depressed by other factors. The ulcers are not unlike those seen in amebiasis of man. Sections show the parasite both on the surface and deeply embedded in the intestinal wall around the ulcers. *B. coli* multiplies in the tissues, and it is supposed that the ulcers are formed by the rupture of abscesses formed in the submucosa by organisms that have forced their way into this location by purely mechanical means.

Dewes (2) has reported the occurrence of *B. coli* in calves where lesions of acute ulcerative proctitis were observed. Signs of the illness were the passage of softer than normal feces followed by bright blood and tenesmus. *Balanti-*

*dium* sp. have been seen in sheep, but there was no evidence of pathogenicity (3). They have been reported as the cause of balantidiosis in the capybara (5). The disease in man may be very severe, at times causing fatal dysentery. Lesions similar to those seen in amebic dysentery are found deep in the intestinal wall, commonly within lymphatic vessels. Occasionally they are observed in the regional lymph nodes. Rarely is the terminal ileum affected (1). **Chemotherapy.** Young (7) reported that two out of four human cases of balantidiosis treated with carbarsone (arsenic compound) were cured with one treatment; the other two required a second treatment.

### *Tetrahymena*

Members of this genus are pyriform, small, and of uniform ciliation. They usually are considered to be saprophytic; however, Knight and McDougle (4) found a protozoon of this genus in large numbers in the exudate in eye lesions of birds deficient in vitamin A. It also occurred in the digestive tract. A similar, or identical, form was present in a pond on the premises. The pathogenicity of the protozoon has not been determined.

### REFERENCES

1. Arean and Koppisch.   Am. Jour. Path., 1956, *32*, 1089.
2. Dewes.   New Zeal. Vet. Jour., 1959, 7, 42.
3. Hegner.   Jour. Parasitol., 1924, *11*, 58.
4. Knight and McDougle.   Am. Jour. Vet. Res., 1944, 5, 113.
5. Moulton, Heuschele, and Sheridan.   Cornell Vet., 1961, *51*, 350.
6. Walker.   Phil. Jour. Sci., 1913, 8, 333.
7. Young.   Pub. Health Rpts. (U.S.), 1943, 58, 1272.

# PART 7

# THE MICROTATOBIOTES (RICKETTSIALES AND VIRALES)

# XXXIII | The Rickettsiae

In the seventh edition of *Bergey's Manual* a group of small rod-shaped, co-coid, and often pleomorphic microorganisms that occur intracellularly as elementary bodies, but may occasionally be extracellular, are placed in the order *Rickettsiales*. The rickettsiae appear to be intermediate between the bacteria and the viruses. They are usually nonfilterable and Gram-negative, and can be cultivated outside the host only in living tissues, embryonated chicken eggs, or rarely in media containing body fluids. They are associated with reticuloendothelial, vascular cells, or erythrocytes in vertebrates and also in invertebrates which may act as vectors. They cause diseases in man and animals. Rickettsiae seldom kill invertebrate hosts.

## THE FAMILY *RICKETTSIACEAE*

The rickettsiae comprise a group of small, bacterialike organisms that are commonly found in the tissues of arthropods. In 1909 Ricketts saw and described the one which causes Rocky Mountain spotted fever of man. He demonstrated that the disease was transmitted to man by ticks, principally *Dermacentor andersoni,* and showed that the disease occurs commonly in the tick, the human infections being merely incidental. During Ricketts' studies of typhus in 1910 he contracted the disease and died. Another scientist, Von Prowazek, who was one of the early workers in this field, also died of typhus, and in 1916 Da Rocha-Lima named the causative agent of louse-borne typhus fever *Rickettsia prowazeki.* It is the type species of the group.

**Morphology and Staining Reactions.** Typical rickettsiae resemble small bacteria morphologically. In some instances there is a great deal of pleomorphism; in others they are quite uniform in size and shape. Most of them occur in groups in the cytoplasm of the parasitized cells; sometimes they occur intranuclearly. Nearly all measure less than 0.5 microns in diameter. They stain

747

poorly with ordinary dyes but can be well and characteristically stained by May-Gruenwald-Giemsa, Gimenez, and Macchiavello stains. *Rickettsia tsutsugamushi* cannot be stained by Macchiavello stain and requires a modification of the standard Gimenez staining procedure for success. With Macchiavello and Gimenez stains the rickettsiae stain bright red against a blue (Macchiavello) or greenish (Gimenez) background. By the modified Gimenez staining procedure *R. tsutsugamushi* organisms appear reddish-black against a green background. With Gram's stain they are negative.

**Cultural Features.** Most species of rickettsiae have been cultivated successfully in tissue culture. A few, including *Rickettsia melophagi,* a nonpathogenic form found in the sheep tick, are said to have been cultivated in special lifeless laboratory media, but none of the pathogenic forms has been cultivated in the absence of living cells. They can readily be propagated in chicken embryos and in tissue cultures. Although they may be grown on the chorioallantois of the developing chick embryo, a more successful method of growing rickettsiae has been devised by Cox (13). It consists of cultivation in the yolk sac of a developing hen's egg. It was demonstrated by Rabinowitz, Aschner, and Grossowicz (45), however, that growth of *R. prowazeki* could be obtained by inoculating the yolk sac of dead embryos. In this case 3-day-old embryos were killed by chilling. Upon reincubation at 37 C, living cells could be demonstrated for as long as 16 days and apparently the rickettsiae grew in these cells.

**Resistance.** Rickettsiae are killed by pasteurization at 145 F for 30 minutes. In general, they do not survive more than a few hours apart from the host cells. They may be preserved in infected tissues stored at −20 C or in lyophilized material for several months.

**Pathogenicity.** The rickettsiae appear to be well-established parasites of arthropods (Huff, 32). Some are transmitted transovarially in ticks but do not seem to be pathogenic for them. Certain types are pathogenic for the body louse. They also appear to be reasonably well adapted to animals, especially rodents, which may constitute a reservoir of infection in nature. Many varieties of rickettsiae on intraperitoneal inoculation into male guinea pigs will produce a febrile attack within 7 to 12 days, which may be accompanied by orchitis. The disease in the guinea pig often is not fatal. Other laboratory animals such as dogs, cats, rabbits, rats, and mice are more resistant and may show no febrile or other reaction to injection although the organism may become established and persist for months. According to Price (44), guinea pigs that are infected intraperitoneally with a strain of rickettsiae of low virulence are protected against a simultaneous injection of a highly virulent strain, providing the less virulent strain is given in about 10 to 30 times the concentration of the more virulent one. This is known as the rickettsial-interference phenomenon (RIP). Infection with Q fever, scrub typhus, and epidemic typhus protects guinea pigs against a virulent strain of spotted fever under the same conditions.

The rickettsiae cause a number of diseases in man and are found in some diseases of domestic animals. These infections will be discussed below under the headings "Human Rickettsial Diseases" and "Animal Rickettsial Diseases." **Diagnosis.** The diagnosis of rickettsial diseases is based on recovery of the causative agent from acute phase blood-specimens in a suitable host or on a four-fold or greater increase in agglutinin or complement-fixing antibody titer between acute and convalescent phase serums.

Guinea pig and chicken embryo inoculations usually are employed in isolating rickettsiae. At present the complement-fixation test seems to be the most accurate means of differentiating the various types (Bengston and Topping, 4). Several agglutination and toxin-neutralization systems have been developed for research purposes. Each species has group-distinctive antigens which do not cross-react with antiserums to other groups; however, the rickettsias of the spotted-fever and typhus-fever groups share common antigens which cross-react in the complement-fixation test only with other members of their respective groups.

The most reliable serological results are obtained with ether-extracted antigens prepared from yolk sacs of embryonated chicken eggs containing maximum growth of rickettsias (55). Except for *Rickettsia akari*, members of the spotted-fever group achieve maximum growth in 5-day-old embryos inoculated with a dose calculated to destroy most embryos by the 4th day after inoculation into the yolk sac. Inoculated eggs are incubated at 33.5 C for 48 hours after death of embryos before yolk sacs are harvested. Maximum yields of *R. prowazeki* and *Rickettsia typhi* are achieved in 5-day-old embryos maintained at 36.5 C that were inoculated into the yolk sac with a dose calculated to cause death in 60 to 70 percent of the embryos between the 8th and 9th days after inoculation. Maximum growth of *Coxiella burneti* is obtained when given an inoculum producing 50 percent embryo mortality one day earlier. Yolk sacs are harvested from surviving embryonated eggs and from embryos not dead for more than 6 hours. Infected yolk sacs are stored at $-20$ C to $-70$ C for subsequent antigen preparation.

Ether extraction of infected yolk sacs is used for the preparation of rickettsial antigens. Yolk sacs are emulsified in a Waring blender with sufficient 0.66 M phosphate-buffered saline, pH 5.8, to make a 20 percent suspension. The material is held overnight at 4 C after the addition of formalin adequate to make 0.2 percent concentration. This suspension is mixed with 1.5 volumes of ether in a separatory funnel, shaken several times during the day, and permitted to separate overnight at 4 C. The aqueous phase containing the antigen is removed and residual ether removed by vacuum. Antigenic activity is then assayed by cross-box titration against three specific antiserums with adequate controls to evaluate anticomplementary activity. This activity can be removed sometimes by one or more additional ether extractions.

According to Van der Scheer, Bohnel, and Cox (56), soluble antigens can be prepared from infected yolk sacs by ether extraction, followed by treatment with benzene, and precipitation with sodium sulfate. Complement fixation with this antigen does not always distinguish between European and murine typhus.

In 1915 Weil and Felix found that the serum of patients with typhus fever agglutinated certain strains of *Proteus* bacteria. Apparently these *Proteus* strains possess somatic (O) antigens in common with the rickettsiae. This reaction (Weil-Felix) is not specific, but it has proved useful in serological diagnosis and identification of rickettsial infections.

The identification of *Rickettsia rickettsi* in a film from the gut tissues of the wood tick, *Dermacentor andersoni*, can be established by means of the fluorescent antibody technic. The indirect fluorescent antibody method has been used to demonstrate *R. tsutsugamushi* in smears of the serum from patients with scrub typhus.

The cultivation of live rickettsias in the laboratory, particularly during centrifugation, and also in infected animals is hazardous. Consequently, laboratory and animal personnel should be vaccinated and adequate facilities available for isolating and studying these pathogens.

**Immunity.** Recovery from an attack of rickettsial disease usually confers a solid and lasting immunity. Vaccines against these diseases are now being prepared by injecting the yolk sac of developing chick embryos. The rickettsiae are concentrated by a process of grinding, washing, and centrifugation and then purified by the removal of yolk lipids and tissue debris (Craigie, 14). The infected yolk sac material usually is formalinized before the concentration procedure is started. Craigie claims that the ethyl ether used in the process is bactericidal for rickettsiae.

**Chemotherapy.** Streptomycin, aureomycin, chloromycetin, terramycin, and para-aminobenzoic acid (PABA) have been reported to be highly effective in treating rickettsial diseases (25, 30, 35).

## HUMAN RICKETTSIAL DISEASES

The human rickettsial diseases, with some exceptions, are clinically similar, being characterized by fever, skin rashes or dark blotches resulting from lesions of the blood vessels, and nervous symptoms. They may be divided into five groups (see Table XXIII) on the basis of clinical data, insect vectors, locality, serology, and other factors. Both man and animals are susceptible to diseases of all five groups, and various biting insect vectors may transmit each type.

### Typhus Fever

Typhus is found in central Europe, in South and Central America, Asia, Russia, Africa, and the United States. Mortality may be as low as 5 percent or as high as 70 percent. The blood of patients is infectious, but the organisms have not been seen in the blood.

The European type, the classic form of typhus, is transmitted by the human body louse (*Pediculus vestimenti*). The reservoir of infection is not definitely

Table XXIII. HUMAN RICKETTSIAL DISEASES *

| Disease group | Geographic distribution | Causative organism | Major vectors | Primary natural hosts | Suggested experimental hosts |
|---|---|---|---|---|---|
| I. Spotted fever group | | | | | |
| Spotted fever | North and South America | *Rickettsia rickettsi* | *Dermacentor andersoni* *D. variabilis* *Rhipicephalus sanguineus* *Amblyomma americanum* *A. cajennense* | Many species of feral mammals, chiefly rodents; dogs; birds | Male guinea pigs, *Microtus* sp., and fertile hens' eggs |
| Siberian tick typhus | Siberia | *R. siberica* | *Dermacentor nuttalli* *D. silvarum* *D. marginatus* *D. pictur* *Hemaphysalis concinna* *H. punctata* | Many species of feral mammals, chiefly rodents | Male guinea pigs and fertile hens' eggs |
| Rickettsial pox | Russia North America | *R. akari* | *Allodermanyssus sanguineus* | *Mus* species and *Rattus* species | Mice and fertile hens' eggs |
| North Queensland tick typhus | Australia | *R. australis* | *Ixodes holocyclus* | Small marsupials and rats | Mice and fertile hens' eggs |
| Fievre boutonneuse | Mediterranean area of Africa and Europe | *R. conori* | *Rhipicephalus sanguineus* | Dogs and small feral mammals | Male guinea pigs and fertile hens' eggs |
| South African tick-bite fever | S. Africa | | *R. appendiculatus* | | |
| Indian tick typhus | India | | *Hemaphysalis leachi* | | |
| Kenya tick typhus | Africa | | *Amblyomma hebraeum* | | |

Table XXIII. HUMAN RICKETTSIAL DISEASES * (Continued)

| Disease group | Geographic distribution | Causative organism | Major vectors | Primary natural hosts | Suggested experimental hosts |
|---|---|---|---|---|---|
| II. Typhus fever group | | | | | |
| Epidemic typhus (European type) | World-wide (colder climates) | *R. prowazeki* | *Pediculus humanus* *Amblyomma variegatum* *Hyalomma* spp. | Man (cattle, sheep and goats?) | Male guinea pigs, cotton rats and fertile hens' eggs |
| Murine typhus | World-wide (warmer climates) | *R. typhi* | *Xenopsylla cheopis* | *Rattus norvegicus* | Male guinea pigs and fertile hens' eggs |
| New typhus member | North America | *R. canada* | *Hemaphysalis leporispalustris* | Man and rabbits | Rabbits and fertile hens' eggs |
| III. Scrub typhus | Eastern and southern Asia Islands of southwest Pacific | *R. tsutsuga-mushi* | *Leptotrombidium akamushi* *L. deliensis* | Many species of small feral mammals, chiefly rodents | Mice, cotton rats, and fertile hens' eggs |
| IV. Q fever | World-wide | *Coxiella burneti* | Chiefly airborne, also found in many species of ticks | Cattle, sheep, goats and many species of feral mammals | Guinea pigs, hamsters, and fertile hens' eggs |
| V. Trench fever | Europe North Africa Mexico | *Rochalimaea quintana* | *Pediculus humanus* | Man | Laboratory-reared body lice |

* Table modified slightly from one kindly supplied by Dr. Herbert G. Stoenner, Rocky Mountain Laboratory, Hamilton, Montana.

known. It is not transmitted transovarially in lice, and infected lice usually die within 2 weeks. The disease may be maintained in endemic form by mild infections, or possibly man may act as an asymptomatic carrier. It has spread to the Atlantic seaboard of the United States, where it appears in a mild form sometimes called *Brill's disease* (Zinsser, 58). Brill's disease also occurs in Europe, and Murray *et al.* (39) after studying 26 cases in Yugoslavia, which is a louse-borne typhus zone, concluded that they had obtained further support for Zinsser's hypothesis that man is the interepidemic reservoir of epidemic typhus fever.

Murine typhus, which prevails in the southern United States and in Mexico, is a disease associated with rats (Maxcy, 37). It is transmitted to man by the rat flea (*Xenopsylla cheopis*) and the rat louse (*Polyplax spinulosa*). In an epidemic it may be transmitted from man to man by the human louse.

The European type is called *R. prowazeki*, while the murine type is called *R. typhi*. A third type, *R. canada*, produces a febrile illness in man that resembles Rocky Mountain spotted fever in man (Bozeman *et al.*, 5). The three may be differentiated by the complement-fixation test.

### Rocky Mountain Spotted Fever

Clinically the disease resembles typhus. However, there appear to be at least three forms of the disease: (a) the eastern form, occurring in the eastern United States, less frequently fatal, and transmitted by the dog tick (*Dermacentor variabilis*); (b) a more highly fatal form occurring in the Rocky Mountain area and transmitted by the sheep tick (*Dermacentor andersoni*); (c) a Brazilian form (São Paulo typhus) transmitted by a tick (*Amblyomma cajennese*). The ticks probably maintain the disease among dogs, rabbits, field mice, sheep, etc., by their bites, and in the western form at least transmit the infectious agent to their progeny (Philip, 41). The rickettsiae of spotted fever usually are called *Rickettsia rickettsi*.

Other rickettsial diseases that may be included in the spotted fever group are Marseilles fever, Kenya fever, South African tick-bite fever, rickettsialpox, Bullis fever, North Queensland tick typhus, Indian tick-bite fever, and Russian tick-bite fever.

### Scrub Typhus

SYNONYMS: Mite typhus, Tsutsugamushi disease

This disease, resembling typhus clinically, is found principally in Japan, Malaya, and the islands of the South Pacific. The common transmitting agent (*Trombicula akamushi*) is much like the American "chigger." Rodents serve as a reservoir for the disease (Ahlm and Lipshutz, 1). The causative agent is *R. tsutsugamushi*.

### Trench Fever

SYNONYMS: Wolhynian fever, shin-bone fever, five-day fever

This disease occurred in World War I in the armies in France, Mesopotamia, and Salonika (3). According to Jacobi (33), it appeared in World War II in the German Army in Russia. Usually it produces a high fever of the relapsing type and the most constant symptom is pain in the legs. Natural transmission is through the human body louse, *Pediculus humanus*. The cause is *Rochalimaea quintana*.

### Q Fever

SYNONYM: Nine-mile fever

This is a febrile disease of man resembling influenza. It is an acute and specific rickettsial infection of variable severity and duration. Its clinical course is characterized by sudden onset, severe headache, malaise, and patchy infiltration of the lungs. It is distinguished from most other rickettsial diseases of man by the failure of patients to develop a cutaneous rash.

Q fever was first described as a human disease in 1937 in Queensland, Australia, and its etiologic agent was named *R. burneti* by Australian workers (Derrick, 16, 17; Burnet and Freeman, 6). In 1938 Davis and Cox (15) recovered a *Rickettsia* from infected ticks at Nine-Mile Creek, Montana, which upon subsequent study proved to be *R. burneti*. In *Bergey's Manual* this organism now bears the name *Coxiella burneti*. The disease appears to be quite common, usually masquerading as "flu" or atypical pneumonia, all over the world. A fever in man may also be associated with hepatitis, pericarditis, meningitis, arthritis, orchitis, epididymitis, phlebitis, esophagitis, and arteritis.

*C. burneti* is a bipolar rod, 0.24 by 1$\mu$ (see fig. 141). It occurs intracellularly in the cytoplasm of infected cells and possibly extracellularly in infected ticks. Some observations suggest existence of a smaller filterable stage, but its true nature has not been identified. Strains newly isolated from animals and ticks are characteristically in Phase I which reacts only with antibodies in late convalescent-phase serums. With repeated passage in embryonated chicken eggs the organism converts to Phase II which reacts with antibodies of early convalescent-phase serums.

The prevalence of infection with *C. burneti* among domestic animals is determined by examining serums by the complement-fixation, capillary-tube agglutination, or radioisotope precipitation (RIP) tests. These technics measure different antibodies so complete agreement cannot be expected. Complement-fixing antibodies are associated with 19S macroglobulins while RIP antibodies seem to occur in the 7S gamma globulins. Furthermore, the rate of antibody response to *C. burneti* and the persistence of antibodies varies in different animal species. The RIP test is the most sensitive and will detect antibodies for longer periods after the infection has occurred than do other tests.

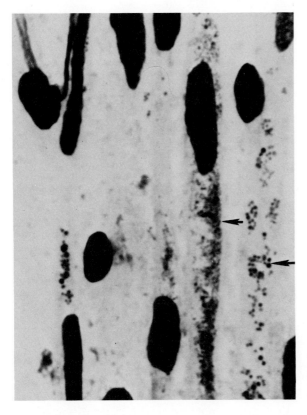

*Fig. 141.* Smear of yolk-sac culture of embryonated hen's egg with *Coxiella burneti.* Macchiavello stain. X 1,150. (Courtesy H. G. Stoenner, Rocky Mountain Laboratory, Hamilton, Mont.)

Infection rates among herds of dairy cattle are most easily determined by testing individual or pooled milk samples by the capillary-tube test.

Q fever is essentially an occupational disease, being limited almost entirely to livestock attendants, farm residents, and laboratory personnel. According to Derrick (18), it is a natural infection of certain wild animals, especially bandicoots in Australia, and is transmitted in nature by ticks. These ticks spread the infection to cattle, which sometimes develop a mild illness. Cattle ticks become infected by feeding on infected cattle. It is then possible that feces deposited on the skins of the animals by the infected ticks may be a source of infection for man. Infection also occurs in such domestic animals as sheep, goats, dogs, cats, and donkeys, as well as in domestic fowl and pigeons. The organisms have been demonstrated in the wool, in birth fluids, in the feces, and in the placental tissues of naturally infected sheep. Apparently *C. burneti* produces only mild or inapparent illness in domestic animals, but they act as reservoirs of the organism. Herd-to-herd transmission among cattle has been demonstrated (47), and dairy farmers and meat packers from areas where there is evidence of Q fever infection in the cattle show serum antibodies against *C. burneti* (34). Infection in a dairy herd may be followed by excretion of rickettsiae in the milk for as long as 32 months (28).

Although the exact mode of transmission of the disease has not been established, epidemiological evidence points to the spread of infection by the inhalation of dust contaminated with infected secreta or excreta of diseased animals or ticks. The fact that outbreaks of Q fever in men who have no contact with livestock sometimes follow dust storms adds weight to this theory. The organism has also been found in cow's milk, where it may survive ordinary pasteurization. It is claimed that a temperature of 145 F for 30 minutes will kill *C. burneti*, whereas 143 F for the same period of time is not sufficient (21). The disease rarely spreads from man to man, although this mode of transmission has been reported. The role of ticks in the spread of Q fever is uncertain, but six strains of ticks common in various parts of the world have been shown to harbor *C. burneti*. Certainly it is not dependent on arthropod transmission in the infectious cycle.

Vaccination appears to have some value in the control of the disease among occupationally exposed individuals and among infected livestock (57). Formalin-inactivated epidemic typhus and Q fever vaccines administered as a mixture have produced an immunity to both organisms in guinea pigs and in man (38).

## ANIMAL RICKETTSIAL DISEASES

Members of the rickettsioses afflicting domestic animals comprise a heterogenous group (Table XXIV) whose members share only a few common characteristics. The morphological and staining characteristics of the eight infectious agents are comparable. Vectors are involved in the transmission of the disease, and intermediate host(s) definitely exist for six of the animal rickettsial diseases. Except for *Colesiota conjunctivae* the disease in the natural host(s) principally involves pathological changes in the blood vascular system. *C. conjunctivae* is limited to the conjunctival sac. Within the limits of our present knowledge each organism is immunologically distinct. Certain of these diseases have been studied extensively in their natural host(s) but their limited host ranges have proved to be a handicap. None of the organisms have been cultivated in the embryonated hen's egg and only *Cowdria ruminantium* and *Ehrlichia phagocytophilia* cause disease or infection in laboratory animals. Difficulties in the preparation of antigens have forestalled the developments of serological tests for diagnosis and research.

There is no evidence that any of the animal rickettsial organisms listed in this section produce disease in man.

### Heartwater Disease

This disease is caused by *Cowdria (Rickettsia) ruminantium*. The organism was first described by Cowdry (12) in 1925, who was working at the time in South Africa. It is the cause of a disease of cattle, sheep, goats, and some wild

*Table XXIV.* ANIMAL RICKETTSIAL DISEASES *

| Disease | Geographic distribution | Causative organism | Major vectors | Cell or tissues affected; natural hosts | Suggested experimental hosts |
|---|---|---|---|---|---|
| Heartwater | East and South Africa | *Cowdria ruminantium* | *Amblyomma hebraeum* and other *Amblyomma* spp. | Sheep, cattle, goats, and some wild ungulates; vascular endothelium | Blue tongue-immune sheep and mice |
| Tick-borne fever; Pasture fever | Great Britain Norway Finland The Netherlands India | *Ehrlichia phagocytophila* | *Ixodes ricinus* | Cattle, sheep, goats, wild ungulates; granulocytes, principally, and monocytes | Cattle, sheep, and goats |
| Benign bovine rickettsiosis | North and South Africa | *Ehrlichia bovis* | *Hyalomma excavatum* and other *Hyalomma* spp. | Cattle; lymphocytes and monocytes | Cattle |
| Benign ovine rickettsiosis | North and South Africa | *Ehrlichia ovina* | *Rhipicephalus bursa* | Sheep; lymphocytes and monocytes | Sheep |
| Canine ehrlichiosis | North and East Africa India Ceylon Aruba USA | *Ehrlichia canis* | *Rhipicephalus sanguineus* | Dogs and jackals; lymphocytes and monocytes | Rabesia-free dogs |
| Equine ehrlichiosis | California | *Ehrlichia* sp. | ? | Horse and burros; granulocytes | Horse |

*Table XXIV.* ANIMAL RICKETTSIAL DISEASES * (Continued)

| Disease | Geographic distribution | Causative organism | Major vectors | Cell or tissues affected: natural hosts | Suggested experimental hosts |
|---|---|---|---|---|---|
| Contagious ophthalmia | Africa Australia New Zealand Europe North and South America | *Colesiota conjunctivae* | Flies | Sheep, cattle, goats, swine and chickens; conjunctival epithelium | Sheep, cattle, goats, swine and chickens |
| Salmon poisoning | Northwest United States | *Neorickettsia helminthoeca* | *Nanophyetus salmincola* | Dogs and wild candidae; reticuloendothelial system, lymph nodes | Dogs |

* Table modified slightly from one kindly supplied by Dr. Herbert G. Stoenner, Rocky Mountain Laboratory, Hamilton, Montana.

ungulates commonly called *heartwater*, because one of the characteristics of the disease is hydropericardium. This disease occurs in East and South Africa. It has long been known in South Africa and is associated with the "bont" tick, *Amblyomma hebraeum*, and other *Amblyomma* species which are the transmitting agents (2).

**Character of the Disease.** Affected ruminants develop a high fever and show gastrointestinal and nervous signs. A high mortality is often reported in cattle, sheep, and goats. The organism infects a variety of feral ungulates without necessarily causing overt disease. Capillaries may be occluded by swollen epithelial cells containing masses of rickettsiae. The disease may assume a peracute form characterized by high fever, sudden collapse, and death or it may be mild or even abortive. In the more common acute form a rise in temperature occurs first followed by depression and loss of appetite although some animals may continue to eat and ruminate. Nervous signs are first manifested by a high-stepping and unsteady gait followed by progressive signs of encephalitis including chewing movements, twitching of eyelids, walking in circles, aggressive and blind charges into objects, and final collapse with attendant convulsions, galloping movements, and twitching of muscles.

Animals that die with the peracute form rarely have gross lesions. Hydropericardium is not always seen in sheep with the acute form and the absence of pericardial fluid in cattle is not uncommon. Mucous membranes are injected. Edema of the lungs is a constant finding. The peritoneal and pleural cavities contain excessive fluid with a variable amount of hemorrhage usually present on the serous membranes of the abdominal viscera and heart. The spleen and lymph nodes, particularly in cattle, are enlarged. The liver is usually enlarged and hemorrhagic and distention of the gall bladder is common. A transparent fluid often infiltrates the mucous membrane of the abomasum. Patches of ramiform injection and diffuse hyperemia of the small intestine, particularly in cattle, produce so-called *zebra markings*.

The principal microscopic changes are leukostatis in all organs and perivascular infiltration in the liver and kidney and occasionally in the adrenal glands.

**Immunity.** Protection is usually afforded against the homologous strain, but this immunity is not complete in all animals. When animals that have recovered from natural or induced disease are challenged with other strains, only partial protection is observed as a rule. These results suggest a multiplicity of immunological strains in nature. Under field conditions animals have continuous exposure to ticks, so repeated infection produces adequate protection. These animals are protected against disease, but not infection, as they may have a rickettsemia sufficient to infect normal bont ticks feeding on them.

Calves up to 3 weeks of age are quite resistant to heartwater disease and can be rendered actively immune by infection with serum from infected animals. This procedure is practiced in certain heavily infected areas of South

Africa where the possible loss of a few young calves, through the use of live vaccine, is preferred to larger losses of older calves from natural infection (Neitz and Alexander, 40).

**Transmission.** Many other kinds of ticks occur in the heartwater districts, but apparently the bont tick and other *Amblyomma* species are the only vectors. Larval ticks retain the infection through the molts to the adult form, but the parasite is not transmitted through the egg to the next generation.

The disease can be transmitted by inoculation with blood taken from sick animals during the early febrile period, but transmission is not always achieved. Subcutaneous inoculation of blood succeeds in not more than 25 percent of the trials, intraperitoneal and intratracheal inoculations are even less certain, and ingestion practically always fails. It is clear that the disease is transmitted naturally solely through the activities of the *Amblyomma* ticks.

**Diagnosis.** Diagnosis is established by demonstration of rickettsiae in tissue smears from suspect cases or reproduction of the disease in sheep. Specimens taken 2 to 4 days after the onset of fever give the best results. After the temperature has returned to normal, blood may not be infectious. Blood should be obtained in sterile containers and inoculated intravenously into test animals as defibrinated blood immediately after withdrawal. If field material cannot be inoculated promptly into sheep, white mice inoculated intraperitoneally will preserve the organism for 90 days and permit later passage into sheep (29). The organism will infect white mice and ferret without signs of illness. The organism is quite labile and only survives in blood for a few hours at room temperature. It is reported to survive for 2 years at −70 C. It is also well to remember that rickettsiae lose their staining properties rapidly in unfixed tissues.

Bluetongue immune sheep should be used for the reproduction of the disease because many cattle and sheep harbor bluetongue virus which may confuse the diagnosis. There is a distinct difference in incubation period since bluetongue virus produces signs in 5 days whereas *C. ruminantium* requires 11 days. To confirm the diagnosis the rickettsial organisms should be demonstrated in endothelial cells of test animals sacrificed 2 to 4 days after onset of illness.

Although *C. ruminantium* cannot be maintained by serial passage in mice, an incubation period in this animal is required for a successful transfer to sheep. Consequently, spleens of infected mice are harvested between 14 and 21 days postinoculation and the suspension injected intravenously into susceptible sheep.

Vascular scrapings and smears from cerebral gray matter (fig. 142) yield equally good results after the preparations are air-dried, fixed with methyl alcohol, and stained with Giemsa. Areas rich in capillaries are sought with low power. Under high power or oil immersion the organisms appear dark blue in the cytoplasm while the nuclei of the endothelial cells are purple. The organ-

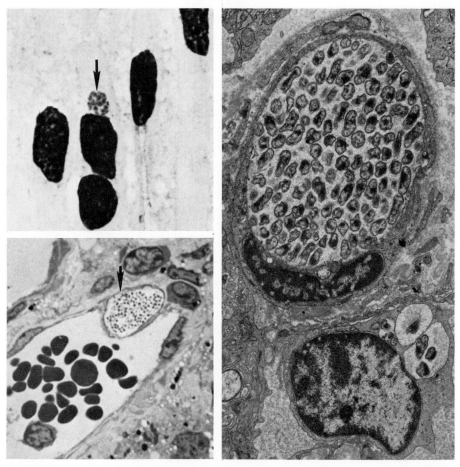

Fig. 142. *Cowdria ruminantium.* In brain smear (*upper left*), stained with Giemsa. X 1,000. In choroid plexus (*lower left*) of sheep, araldite section 0.5 micron thick. X 1,000. A colony of organisms is seen in a distended endothelial cell completely obstructing the lumen of the capillary (*on right*). In adjoining capillary, at the bottom, a monocyte has organisms in a cytoplasmic vacuole. X 7,000. (Courtesy J. D. Smith.)

ism may be coccoid (0.3 μ diameter), bacillary (o.3 μ by 0.5 μ), or diplococcoid (fig. 142).

**Treatment.** Rake, Alexander, and Hamre (46) reported that this disease has proved susceptible to sulfonamide therapy, which suggests a relationship to the psittacosis group of infections, but they believe that the causative agent is neither a *Rickettsia* nor a psittacosis agent but is related to both. Studies by Haig *et al.* (30) indicate that terramycin and aureomycin are quite efficacious as therapeutic agents. Terramycin soluble powder (oxytetracycline) in the water has been used successfully in the treatment of sheep, goats, and cattle.

Control of ticks on sheep by dipping in benezene hexachloride helps in the prevention of the disease (36).

### Tick-Borne Fever

Foggie (26) has described tick-borne fever in sheep and has proposed the name *Ehrlichia* (*Rickettsia*) *phagocytophilia* for the organism. Following an acute attack, the infection may persist up to 2 years in the surviving animal. The organism will infect sheep, cattle, goats, and wild ungulates. The disease has been described in Great Britain, Norway, Finland, The Netherlands, and India.

**Character of the Disease.** This disease is characterized by a sudden rise in temperature with the persistence of an irregular fever for 3 to 5 days in cattle and for 10 days in sheep. Dairy cattle drop in milk production, and may never fully recover. Febrile relapses may occur 2 to 4 weeks after the initial attack. Abortions have occurred in some outbreaks in sheep and cattle that are in the latter stages of gestation. Sometimes clinical disease is complicated by concurrent infection with *Babesia*.

The infecting agents from sheep and cattle are different strains of the same organism. They produce more severe disease in their respective natural hosts. The incubation period varies from 4 to 8 days after exposure to infected ticks and 5 to 12 days after inoculation with infective blood.

**Immunity.** All evidence suggests that strains of *E. phagocytophilia* are immunologically heterogenous. There is little or no apparent cross-immunity between the Scottish and Finnish strains. Experimental cattle and sheep were given successive injections with 11 Finnish strains and some animals reacted to 6 strains. Virulent strains appear more immunogenic than mild strains. Protection appears partial and of short duration, lasting from 3 to 6 months.

In nature, repeated attacks exclusive of relapses are seldom seen. Reinfection from repeated tick bites presumably occurs, confers adequate immunity during the same tick season. The occurrence of tick-borne fever in the same animal during the following tick seasons is not rare.

**Diagnosis.** The ideal time to take blood specimens for demonstration or isolation of *E. phagocytophilia* is during the initial febrile period when large numbers are in the circulation. Some sheep remain carriers for 2 years but most animals rid their tissues of demonstrable organisms within a month. Blood smears may be made directly or later from a citrated blood specimen. The organism usually remains viable for 7 days at 4 C and survives for several months at −70 C.

Either Giemsa or May-Gruenwald-Giemsa are excellent stains for demonstrating the organism in blood smears. The fluorescent antibody method can be used but offers no advantage in ease of technic or in certainty of diagnosis. The organisms have a predilection for granulocytes but monocytes may be infected. At the peak of infection 50 percent or more of the granulocytes may be infected with virulent strains while others may involve 6 percent. At least 100 cells should be examined before a blood smear is called negative.

The pleomorphism of *E. phagocytophilia* is apparent in stained preparations, even in the same cell (fig. 143). The deep-purple-staining coccoid or rod-shaped body usually situated at the periphery of the cell is about 0.5 $\mu$ in diameter. The larger homogeneously staining body more deeply situated in the cell cytoplasm is 1.3 by 2 $\mu$ and often appears to fragment into smaller irregularly shaped bodies. The rounded or oval masses, termed morulae, contain numerous distinct bodies that stain a deeper blue or purple than the surrounding matrix.

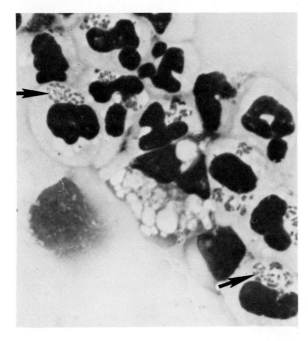

Fig. 143. Ehrlichia phagocytophila in granulocytes of a leukocyte concentrate. May-Grünwald-Giemsa stain. X 1,400. (Courtesy J. Tuomi.)

The intravenous inoculation of infective defibrinated blood into susceptible sheep or cattle constitutes another means of diagnosing the disease. To assure the diagnosis, blood smears from test animals must contain the characteristic organism in the granulocytes.

### Bovine and Ovine Ehrlichiosis

Benign bovine and ovine rickettsiosis is limited geographically to North and South Africa. There is only meager information about the nature of this disease in cattle and in sheep and the immunological relationship between *Ehrlichia bovis* and *Ehrlichia ovina* has not been explored.

**Character of the Disease.** Cattle and sheep show an irregular fever of several weeks' duration. It is rarely a fatal disease in either species. The most significant lesion is excessive pericardial fluid similar to heartwater fever in sheep. Other consistent changes are lymphadenopathy and splenomegaly. Cattle and sheep may remain carriers for 10 months.

**Immunity.** Chronic infections may persist for 10 months in sheep and cattle. Recovered animals develop a solid immunity against challenge with the homologous organism but the duration of immunity is unknown.

**Transmission.** *E. bovis* is transmitted to cattle by ticks of the *Hyalomma* genus whereas *E. ovina* is transmitted to sheep by the tick, *Rhipicephalus bursa*. A 10 percent suspension of spleen, lung, or blood taken during the febrile stage is used to transmit the organism in its natural host. The incubation period in sheep and cattle is approximately 12 days.

**Diagnosis.** The organisms can be readily demonstrated in blood smears from animals in the febrile stage. Tissues from the lungs, liver, and spleen is suitable for *Ehrlichia* demonstration.

These rickettsiae are found in the cytoplasm of the circulating monocytes and monocyticlike cells in the lungs, liver, and spleen. The monocytes in the blood smear usually gather at the edge of the preparation. They frequently assemble in round colonies from 2 to $10\,\mu$ in diameter and also in closely packed granules 0.5 to $1.0\,\mu$ in diameter. With Giemsa they stain similar to *E. phagocytophilia*. Initial bodies, 3 by $6\,\mu$, are described which stain a homogeneous red and later separate into elementary bodies that stain purple with May-Gruenwald-Giemsa stain. A thorough search should be made of smears as the percentage of monocytes with organisms is usually low.

### Canine Ehrlichiosis

This disease has been reported in North and East Africa, India, Ceylon, Aruba, and the United States. *Ehrlichia canis* frequently occurs as a concurrent infection in dogs with *Babesia canis* because both rickettsia are transmitted by the same tick, *Rhipicephalus sanguineus*. Wild dogs, jackals, and coyotes are also susceptible. An excellent review article on canine ehrlichiosis has been written by Ewing (22).

**Character of the Disease.** The onset of the disease is characterized by a high fever and depression. Icterus, vomition, progressive weakness, splenomegaly, and mucopurulent ocular discharge with photophobia are some other signs of illness. A monocytosis occurs and eosinophils almost disappear early in the disease. With disease progression a profound anemia of the normocytic normochromic type develops with depressed values for packed cell volume, hemoglobin, and total erythrocyte counts. The mortality rate among puppies is higher than in older dogs.

At necropsy the gross pathological changes include anemia, hyperactive bone marrow, enlarged spleen, liver, and lymph nodes, and petechiae of the lungs. Less commonly observed changes are hemorrhages and ulcers in the intestinal tract, hydrothorax, and pulmonary edema.

**Immunity.** Animals that recover from an acute attack are immune to reinfection. Persistence of the organism in recovered dogs can be demonstrated by splenectomy with the ensuing appearance of *E. canis* in the circulating monocytes.

**Transmission.** *E. canis* is transmitted to the dog by the tick, *R. sanguineus*, which also transmits *Babesia* to the same host.

Lung, liver, or spleen tissue as a 10 percent suspension or blood taken during the febrile stage of infective dogs produces the disease in susceptible dogs 7 to 21 days after parenteral injection.

Dogs may remain carriers for at least 29 months (23) after an acute attack and constitute a constant reservoir for the infection in nature. Unfortunately carrier dogs may become donors of whole blood used for therapeutic purposes in veterinary hospitals. Buckner (22) has evidence that this has occurred despite efforts to insure that the donor was free of the disease. Puppy inoculation with donor blood is the only known means to detect carriers. Obviously, the same problem exists in other diseases where the organism persists in the blood stream after recovery from signs of illness.

**Diagnosis.** This organism may be recovered from the blood of infected dogs for long periods of time. They are demonstrated most readily 2 or 3 days after the onset of fever until the end of clinical signs. If direct blood smears are negative, smears of the buffy coat of heparinized or citrated blood samples may be positive. During the febrile period *E. canis* may be demonstrated in biopsy material from the lung, liver, or spleen. As there is insufficient data on the survival of the organism, fresh test material should be injected promptly into susceptible dogs.

*E. canis* has the same morphological and staining characteristics as *E. bovis* and *E. ovina*. Because ehrlichiae infections, particularly in the dog, are often complicated by concurrent infections with *Babesia,* a thorough search should also be made for this latter organism in the erythrocytes.

**Treatment.** Certain drugs, such as broad-spectrum antibiotics employed successfully in treating Rocky Mountain spotted fever and salmon-poisoning disease, may alter the course of canine ehrlichiosis (and presumably *E. ovina* and *E. bovis*) but do not prevent the development of the carrier stage.

### Equine Ehrlichiosis

This disease occurs as a distinct entity in horses located in the Sacramento Valley, California, United States. There have been five known naturally occurring cases.

**Character of the Disease.** The information about the nature of this disease has been derived from the five natural cases but principally from the experimental disease produced in horses and burros (27, 54).

The disease is characterized by fever, depression, anorexia, edema of the legs, and ataxia. In experimental cases the incubation period varied from 1 to 9 days with a mean of 2.5 days with fresh blood and of 6.5 days with frozen blood. Hematologic changes are thrombocytopenia, elevated plasma icterus index, decreased cell-packed volume, and marked leukopenia involving first lymphocytes and then granulocytes. Subcutaneous edema of the legs appears first at the metacarpal and metatarsal regions and may ascend to the radius and 6 to 8 inches above the hock.

At necropsy, edema and petechial and ecchymotic hemorrhage occur in the subcutaneous tissues, fascia, and epimysium of the legs distal to the elbow and stifle joints. Carcasses are frequently jaundiced, and orchitis is often seen in mature males. Some horses have excessive fluid in the peritoneal cavity and pericardial sac. Histologically, vasculitis of small arteries and veins involves swelling of endothelial and smooth muscle cells, thromboses, and perivascular infiltrations of monocytes and lymphocytes. The vessels in testes, ovaries, legs, and pampiniform plexus are principally affected.

**Immunity.** Present evidence suggests that one attack confers immunity. Horses recovered from experimental disease withstood challenge with infectious blood given 2.5 to 20 months later. This evaluation was based upon the lack of clinical signs and of organisms in circulating granulocytes.

**Transmission.** No arthropod vector has been incriminated as yet in the transmission of the natural disease, but this is a newly described disease with rather limited opportunity for epidemiological observations.

Infective blood produces the disease in experimental horses. Horses under 2 years of age usually do not show clinical signs other than a fever. Dogs, sheep, and goats develop a mild or inapparent infection after parenteral injection and the organism can be demonstrated in the cytoplasm of the granulocytes.

**Diagnosis.** As with other *Ehrlichia* organisms blood specimens preferably are taken during the febrile period usually 3 to 5 days after its onset. The best smears are made with fresh blood but citrated blood samples in sterile tubes and maintained at 4 C may be used for later examination. Fresh blood is preferred for inoculation into susceptible horses, but defibrinated blood sealed in glass ampoules and stored at −70 C remains infectious but the incubation period is prolonged.

The diagnosis is based upon demonstrating the rickettsiae in the granulocytes contained in blood smears from natural and experimental cases that are stained with Giemsa or Wright-Leishman stains. The inclusion bodies are deep blue to pale blue-gray. They may vary from small darkly stained bodies 200 m$\mu$ in diameter to large granular bodies, 5 $\mu$ in diameter, which represent a cluster of smaller bodies. The percentage of parasitized granulocytes varies with the stage of the disease with mean maximum as 36 percent.

### Contagious Ophthalmia

*Colesiota conjunctivae* produces conjunctivitis in sheep, cattle, goats, swine, and chickens and has been reported on all continents except Asia. Flies apparently play some role in its transmission.

The relationships between these conjunctival agents in livestock have not been well established. The strains are host-specific and not transferrable among livestock. Consequently, some investigators contend that *C. conjunctivae* occurs only in sheep and the rickettsiae which infect the conjunctivae of other livestock should be given another generic name. In this respect Rizvi (49) reported a conjunctivitis in young goats caused by *Rickettsia conjunctivae*. Certain features of its morphological and staining characteristics differed from *C. conjunctivae*.

**Character of the Disease.** The severity of the disease varies from mild cases of purulent conjunctivitis with recovery within a week to severe cases with keratitis, vascularization, and occasionally corneal ulceration. Most severely affected eyes eventually heal without residual blemish.

The disease can be reproduced by instilling conjunctival washings into the eyes of susceptible animals of the same species. The incubation period is 2 to 4 days in the instilled eye and the opposite eye becomes infected 3 to 4 days later.

**Immunity.** In sheep, immunity persists for 3 months but after 8 months approximately 10 percent are again susceptible. The carrier stage persists in some sheep for over 1 year and that fact coupled with the loss of immunity in others may account for the survival of the organism in the flock.

Immunity in animals other than sheep has not been thoroughly studied.

**Diagnosis.** Epithelial scrapings from the inner surface of the conjunctiva are made with a scalpel until a tinge of blood appears. The material is spread on a slide, air-dried, fixed with absolute alcohol and stained. Saline washings from the eyes of sheep during the acute phase of the disease are an excellent source of material for transmission of the disease to experimental animals. The viability of the organism is unknown but it should be considered labile. The organisms will not survive desiccation.

In Giemsa-stained smears several types of inclusions are observed. Many polymorpholeukocytes are observed in smear preparations taken early in the disease. Most of the organisms are found in the cytoplasm and appear as purplish-red small ovoid or short rod-shaped organisms, 0.2 by $0.5\mu$. As recovery ensues, lymphocytes and monocytes replace the leukocytes. At this stage, irregular extracellular organisms, 0.8 by $1.4\mu$, that stain unevenly appear as triangles, imperfect rings, and horse-shoe-shaped clusters.

**Treatment.** In sheep chloromycetin reduces the severity of the disease and also the number of cases developing ulcerative keratitis. Riboflavin in 15-mg daily doses is also effective (36).

### Salmon Poisoning

SYNONYM: Salmon disease

This disease occurs in western Oregon, northwestern California, and southwestern Washington. It is not known to occur elsewhere. It affects several members of the family *Canidae*. Dogs, foxes, and coyotes are known to be susceptible. House cats, mink, raccoons, and swine apparently are resistant. The disease has long been associated with the eating of salmon and trout from streams that flow into the Pacific Ocean in the region described. Although the disease has the appearance of an infection, it was long regarded as a poisoning or intoxication. Several facts about this disease indicated that it was more than a simple intestinal parasitism, and in 1954 Philip *et al.* (41, 42) proposed the name of *Neorickettsia helminthoeca* for the rickettsialike agent that is associated with the fluke infestation and plays an important role in the disease among mammals.

**Character of the Disease.** The first sign in dogs is a slight rise in body temperature. Within 24 hours there is a complete loss of appetite and marked depression, and the temperature rises to 104 to 107 F. The animal appears very dejected and apathetic. After several days the temperature usually decreases. A slight purulent discharge may occur from the eyes during the 4th to 6th day of illness. The eyelids and adjacent tissues become edematous about this time, giving the eyes a sunken appearance. Beginning about the 4th or 5th day persistent vomiting usually occurs. This is accompanied by rapid loss of body weight. The animals become avid for water, but most of it is lost by further vomition. Diarrhea usually begins about the 5th to 7th day. In the beginning the diarrheal discharge frequently is tinged with blood, and later it is heavily impregnated with blood. After a day or two of diarrhea, many animals appear to improve, but usually this is only temporary. Finally the temperature falls to subnormal. At this time the animal is so emaciated and weak that it can hardly stand alone. Most animals die within 6 to 10 days after the appearance of signs, and from 12 to 20 days after eating the infective fish.

Autopsy examinations reveal hemorrhagic inflammation of the intestine as the most characteristic lesion. The inflammatory reaction may be observed throughout the bowel, or it may be limited to certain regions. In many cases the entire bowel is well lined with bloody exudate; in others the content is merely blood-tinged. Ulceration is unusual but is seen in a few cases. The ulcers often are superficial and may vary in size from those barely visible to others 2 to 3 cm in diameter. Flukes and fluke eggs may be found in the intestinal content in large numbers. As many as 200,000 parasites have been recovered from a single dog. Gross changes are found in the lymphocytic tissues. Variable enlargement of the ileocecal, mesenteric, portal, and internal iliac lymph nodes are constant findings. A decrease in the number of mature lymphocytes accompanied by a proliferation of the reticuloendothelial elements in both the cortex and medulla is the predominant and most consistent microscopic finding in the lymph nodes. Similar changes are found in the tonsils, thymus, and lymphoid tissue of the spleen and intestinal tract. Coccobacillary bodies are present in the numerous reticular cells either clustered in morulalike masses or diffusely scattered in the cytoplasm. They are often numerous in the histiocytes of the intestinal villi. Some are seen as free bodies as though released by cell disintegration (10).

Follicles of the spleen rarely contain necrotic foci but often show central hemorrhage. Flukes are found embedded in the villi or duodenal glands of the intestinal tract with no evidence of inflammatory response. Small foci of macrophages and neutrophils, often necrotic, are found frequently in the connective tissue of the lamina propria. Cellularity of the propria also may be increased, principally with plasma cells and neutrophils. Centrolobular lipidosis of the liver is common in foxes, but rare in the dog. In both foxes and dogs a moderate mononuclear infiltration of the liver interlobular connective tissue is seen. Occasionally, a few small hemorrhages beneath the bladder epithelium are observed. An accumulation of mononuclear and neutrophil leukocytes in small areas causes a slight thickening of the alveolar walls of the lungs.

A monocytic leptomeningitis is most intense over the cerebellum. Exudative and proliferative cellular changes in the sheaths of the small and medium-sized vessels in the cerebrum and focal collections of glia of mesenchymal cells (glial nodules) are commonly observed lesions.

Signs of illness usually appear on the 6th or 8th day after eating parasitized fish. In a few cases signs may be observed as early as the 5th day or as late as the 12th day.

Most untreated dogs die of the disease. Simms, Donham, and Shaw (51) observed recovery in only four dogs in a series of 102.

Simms, McCapes, and Muth (52) and Simms and Muth (53) were successful in transmitting the disease to dogs by intraperitoneal injection of blood or of ground, washed flukes from infected dogs and by the injection of metacercariae from parasitized fish, as well as by feeding fluke-infected trout and salmon. The signs produced were the same as those seen in the naturally contracted disease.

**Immunity.** Dogs that recover from salmon poisoning are solidly immune thereafter for long periods and perhaps for life. Simms, McCapes, and Muth (52) found it possible to immunize dogs solidly by the simultaneous injection of virulent blood and hyperimmune serum. Shaw and Howarth (50) showed that strong immunity followed the feeding of parasitized salmon and the curing of the resultant disease with sulfanilamide.

An *Ehrlichia canis*-like organism isolated in Oklahoma, USA, and termed the Oklahoma agent (OA) is pathogenic for dogs but produces fewer deaths than *N. helminthoeca* under experimental conditions (23). Dogs convalescent from infections with either parasite (broad-spectrum antibiotics used late in the disease to permit *N. helminthoeca* infected dogs to recover) had no protection when challenged with the heterologous organism.

**Transmission.** In 1925 Donham (18) reported an association between the disease and an intestinal fluke, the encysted form of which occurred in fish. Chapin (7) studied this fluke and gave it the name *Nanophyetus salmincola*. It is also known as *Troglotrema salmincola*. This fluke is an essential agent in the production of the disease. The encysted form occurs in the musculature of fish of the family *Salmonidae*. When eaten by susceptible carnivores, the adult forms develop in the intestines. Ova escaping from these animals infect a small snail, *Goniobasis plicifera* var. *silicula*, which serves in turn to infect the fish. The limited distribution of this species of snail apparently is the factor which controls the spread of disease.

Donham, Simms, and Miller (19) failed to produce salmon poisoning with ocean-caught salmon in which no encysted flukes could be found. The same species taken in fresh water in the salmon-poisoning area contained metacercariae and produced salmon poisoning when fed to dogs. A survey of the streams of the region showed only one species of snail occurring where fish infection existed. This was the species that was shown to be the intermediate host of the fluke. The parasitized fish included the chinook, silverside, and chum or dog salmon, the brook or speckled trout, the cutthroat or mountain trout, the rainbow trout, and the steelhead trout. Other types of fish occurring in the region were not infected.

Until recently it was assumed that smoke-treated salmon were not dangerous to dogs but Farrell, Dee, and Ott (24) reported signs resembling salmon poisoning in dogs after the ingestion of uncooked, smoke-treated salmon that harbored the organism.

**Diagnosis.** Although signs of illness are rather characteristic, the most certain method of diagnosis is the presence of fluke eggs in the feces of the patient. In most cases the eggs are so numerous that a microscopic examination of the fecal material adhering to the rectal thermometer will result in a diagnosis. These eggs appear in the feces of dogs on the 5th to 7th days after ingestion of infected fish. They are oval in shape, measuring 75 to 80 microns in length and 45 to 55 microns in breadth. There are no embryos in the eggs recovered directly from feces. When stored in cool water, embryonation occurs in from 75 to 90 days.

Microscopic examination reveals intracytoplasmic, rickettsialike, sometimes pleomorphic microorganisms found particularly in the reticuloendothelial cells of lymphoid tissues of infected *Canidae*. Suitable material for this purpose is readily obtained by aspirating cells from the mandibular lymph node with a syringe or by biopsy. Tissue smears require fixation with methyl alcohol prior to staining. Blood contains the organism during the febrile stage but not in a sufficient number for detection by direct microscopic examination. The organisms are about 0.3 of a micron in diameter and Gram-negative; they stain purple with Giemsa, pale bluish with hematoxylin, red or blue with Macchiavello, and dark brown or black with Levaditi. They occur in plaques or loose groups in the cells, often nearly filling the cytoplasm.

The organism can be transmitted in dogs by the inoculation of infective blood or spleen taken during the acute phase of the disease. The rickettsiae are labile but they will survive in fresh frozen tissue stored at −70 C for at least 6 months and will withstand lyophilization. So far they have not been cultivated *in vitro*.

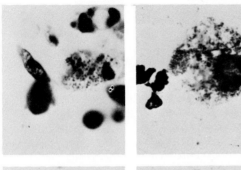

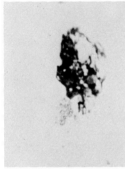 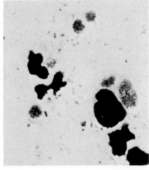

*Fig. 144. Neorickettsia helminthoeca* stained by the Giemsa method in lymph node aspirations. Coccobacillary bodies *(upper left and right)* diffusely scattered in the cytoplasm of reticular cells; bacillary bodies *(lower left)* in a disintegrating macrophage; morulalike clusters *(lower right)* free and in a macrophage. X 800. (Courtesy R. K. Farrell, *Jour. Am. Vet. Med. Assoc.*)

**Chemotherapy.** Coon *et al.* (9) showed that sulfanilamide, administered during the early febrile period of the disease in dogs, brought about rapid recovery from the disease. This was confirmed by Shaw and Howarth (50) and by Cordy and Gorham (11). The latter showed sulfamerazine and sulfamethazine to be effective. They also showed that penicillin and aureomycin were equally effective but streptomycin was ineffective. Philips *et al.* (43) highly recommend the use of either aureomycin or terramycin in treating salmon poisoning.

## REFERENCES

1. Ahlm and Lipschutz. Jour. Am. Med. Assoc., 1944, *124*, 1095.
2. Alexander. 17th Ann. Rpt., Dir. Vet. Services, Union So. Africa, 1931, p. 89.
3. Arkwright, Bacot, and Duncan. Jour. Hyg. (London), 1919–20, *18*, 76.
4. Bengston and Topping. Am. Jour. Pub. Health, 1942, *32*, 48.
5. Bozeman, Elisberg, Humphries, Runcik, and Palmer. Jour. Inf. Dis., 1970, *121*, 367.
6. Burnet and Freeman. Med. Jour. Austral., 1937, *1*, 296.
7. Burrows. Textbook of microbiology. 19th ed. W. B. Saunders Co., Philadelphia and London, 1968.
8. Chapin. North Am. Vet., 1926, 7, 36.
9. Coon, Myers, Phelps, Ruehle, Snodgrass, Shaw, Simms, and Bolin. *Ibid.*, 1938, *19*, 57.
10. Cordy and Gorham. Am. Jour. Path., 1950, *26*, 617.

11.   Cordy and Gorham.   Personal communication.
12.   Cowdry.   Jour. Exp. Med., 1925, *42*, 231 and 253.
13.   Cox.   Science, 1941, *94*, 399.
14.   Craigie.   Canad. Jour. Res., 1945, *23* (Sect. E), 104.
15.   Davis and Cox.   Pub. Health Rpts. (U.S.), 1938, *53*, 2259.
16.   Derrick.   Med. Jour. Austral., 1937, *2*, 281.
17.   *Ibid.*, 1939, *1*, 14.
18.   Derrick.   Jour. Hyg. (London), 1944, *43*, 357.
19.   Donham.   Jour. Am. Vet. Med. Assoc., 1925, *68*, 637.
20.   Donham, Simms, and Miller.   *Ibid.*, 1926, *68*, 701.
21.   Enright, Sadler, and Thomas.   Am. Jour. Pub. Health, 1957, *47*, 695.
22.   Ewing.   Adv. Vet. Sci., 1969, *13*, 331.
23.   Ewing and Philip.   Am. Jour. Vet. Res., 1966, *27*, 67.
24.   Farrell, Dee, and Ott.   Jour. Am. Vet. Med. Assoc., 1968, *152*, 370.
25.   Fellers.   U.S. Armed Forces Med. Jour., 1952, *3*, 665.
26.   Foggie.   Jour. Path. and Bact., 1951, *63*, 1.
27.   Gribble.   Jour. Am. Vet. Med. Assoc., 1969, *155*, 462.
28.   Grist.   Vet. Rec., 1959, *71*, 839.
29.   Haig.   Jour. So. African Vet. Med. Assoc., 1952, *23*, 167.
30.   Haig, Alexander, and Weiss.   *Ibid.*, 1954, *25*, 45.
31.   Horsfall and Tamm.   Viral and rickettsial infections of man. 4th ed. J. B. Lippincott Co., Phila., London, and Montreal, 1965.
32.   Huff.   Quart. Rev. Biol., 1938, *13*, 196.
33.   Jacobi.   Münch. med. Wchnschr., 1942, *89*, 615.
34.   Kitze.   Am. Jour. Hyg., 1957, *65*, 239.
35.   Ley and Smadel.   Antibiotics and Chemother., 1954, *4*, 792.
36.   Marsh.   Adv. Vet. Sci., 1958, *4*, 164.
37.   Maxcy.   Pub. Health Rpts. (U.S.), 1926, *41*, 213.
38.   Morris, Wisseman, Aulidio, Jackson, and Smadel.   Proc. Soc. Expt. Biol. and Med., 1967, *125*, 1216.
39.   Murray, Psorn, Djakovic, Sielski, Broz, Ljupsa, Gaon, Pavlevic, and Snyder.   Am. Jour. Pub. Health, 1951, *41*, 1359.
40.   Neitz and Alexander.   Onderstepoort Jour. Vet. Sci. and Anim. Indus., 1945, *20*, 137.
41.   Philip.   Pub. Health Rpts. (U.S.), 1933, *48*, 266.
42.   Philip, Hadlow, and Hughes.   Exp. Parasitol., 1954, *3*, 336.
43.   Philip, Hughes, Locker, and Hadlow.   Proc. Soc. Exp. Biol. and Med., 1954, *87*, 397.
44.   Price.   *Ibid.*, 1953, *82*, 180.
45.   Rabinowitz, Aschner, and Grossowicz.   *Ibid.*, 1948, *67*, 469.
46.   Rake, Alexander, and Hamre.   Science, 1945, *102*, 424.
47.   Reed and Wentworth.   Jour. Am. Vet. Med. Assoc., 1957, *130*, 458.
48.   Rivers.   Viral and rickettsial infections of man. 2d ed. J. B. Lippincott Co., Phila., London, and Montreal, 1952.
49.   Rizvi.   Jour. Am. Vet. Med. Assoc., 1950, *117*, 409.
50.   Shaw and Howarth.   North Am. Vet., 1939, *20*, 67.
51.   Simms, Donham, and Shaw.   Am. Jour. Hyg., 1931, *13*, 363.
52.   Simms, McCapes, and Muth.   Jour. Am. Vet. Med. Assoc., 1932, *81*, 26.

53. Simms and Muth. Proc. 5th Pacific Sci. Cong., 1933, p. 2949.
54. Stannard, Gribble, and Smith. Vet. Rec., 1969, *84*, 149.
55. Stoenner, Lackman, and Bell. Jour. Inf. Dis., 1962, *110*, 121.
56. Van der Scheer, Bohnel, and Cox. Jour. Immunol., 1947, *56*, 365.
57. Wentworth. Bact. Rev., 1955, *19*, 129.
58. Zinsser. Am. Jour. Hyg., 1934, *20*, 513.

# XXXIV | The Psittacosis-Lymphogranuloma-Trachoma Group (*Chlamydiaceae*)

The name that heads this chapter was suggested by Smadel (46) to designate a number of agents which have in common many characters not possessed by viruses. Jones, Rake, and Stearns (28) regard these agents as belonging to a higher developmental level than viruses. Some authors follow Bergey in using the generic term *Miyagawanella* for them, but most use *Chlamydia* and classify these organisms as bacteria which lack some important mechanisms for production of metabolic energy and thus lead an intracellular existence (39).

Included in this group are the agents of psittacosis, ornithosis, pneumonitis and conjunctivitis, sporadic bovine encephalomyelitis, polyarthritis, placentopathy enteritis and cat-scratch fever. It was first suggested that the agent of salmon poisoning belonged in the family *Chlaymdiaceae;* however, it is now generally regarded as a member of the family *Rickettsiaceae.*

The agents of all these diseases contain a common group antigen. All of them are susceptible to certain chemotherapeutic and antibiotic agents. Most of them are capable of producing pneumonitis in mice and are cultivable in the yolk sac of chick embryos. All of them have elementary bodies—200 to 300 millimicrons in diameter. All of them have the same developmental cycle and contain RNA and DNA in relative amounts of each at different growth stages. They may vary in the specificity of cell-wall antigens, toxins, and species—differentiating biochemical properties.

Bedson and Bland (7) studied the development of the psittacosis agent in the tissues of animals. It was observed that early in the course of infection light-blue or purplish bodies appeared in the macrophages of the spleen and in the epithelial cells of the lungs, intestine, liver, and kidneys. At first these bodies appeared homogeneous, but later they became granular. Eventually they became resolved into masses of distinctly stained elementary bodies, spherical in form. These may be distinctively stained with Giemsa's stain, Macchiavello's stain, or Castaneda's stain for rickettsiae. When these bodies are fully formed, the cells that contain them rupture, discharging showers of infective elementary bodies into the tissue fluids. This developmental cycle is characteristic of all members of this group. Confirmation that the granular material in the plaques consists of psittacoid protein has been supplied by fluorescent antibody studies (17).

The bacteria which cause the psittacoid-lymphogranuloma-trachoma group diseases and which are assigned to the genus, *Chlamydia,* can be separated logically into two species, *C. trachomatis* and *C. psittaci,* according to Page (39). This separation is based on relatively stable morphological and chemical characteristics of the organisms rather than on their presumed natural host(s) or tissue preferences or on the specific serology of their cell-wall antigens. Attempts to classify these bacteria on host specificities or serology has led to great confusion in the past.

Organisms of *C. trachomatis* that are associated with trachoma, inclusion conjunctivitis, or lymphogranuloma venereum of man or mouse pneumonitis have compact intracytoplasmic microcolonies which produce sufficient quantities of glycogen detectable by staining with iodine and which are inhibited by sodium sulfadiazine. In contrast, the members of *C. psittaci* frequently associated with psittacosis, meningopneumonitis, guinea pig conjunctivitis, bovine encephalomyelitis, feline pneumonitis, or caprine pneumonitis have diffuse microcolonies which fail to produce glycogen or to exhibit susceptibility to sodium sulfadiazine. Except for the 6BC parakeet strain which is glycogen-negative, but sulfadiazine sensitive, all strains isolated from many animal species were readily separated into one of the two species, *C. trachomatis* or *C. psittaci.* Until we obtain more concrete information regarding the epidemiology of the *Chlamydia* and develop more specific tests and information as to how they relate to the disease(s) in various hosts, the above scheme as proposed by Page (39), which was reviewed and approved by a majority of the members of the Subcommittee on the *Chlamydiaceae* (Taxonomy Committee, American Society of Microbiology), is logical and acceptable and will be utilized in this textbook. Some of the diseases caused by various strains of *C. psittaci* are given in Table XXV, with principal emphasis on the diseases in domestic animals.

## Psittacosis And Ornithosis

Psittacosis is a disease occurring in birds belonging to the parrot family (*Psittacidae*). Ornithosis is the same disease when it occurs in a variety of nonpsittacine birds. Formerly it was thought that ornithosis, when it affected

*Table XXV.*  CHLAMYDIAL DISEASES

| Disease manifestation | Known geographical distribution | Natural host(s) | Recommended experimental hosts | Epidemiological aspects |
|---|---|---|---|---|
| Psittacosis (Humans) | World-wide | Man, wild and domestic fowls | Embryonated hens' eggs, mice, guinea pigs, wild and domestic birds | Principally transmitted from birds to man, but man-to-man-transmission occurs as aerosol infection. Also associated with cases of lymphogranuloma venereum and abortions in man. |
| Psittacosis Ornithosis (Birds) | World-wide | Wild and domestic fowls | Same | Endemic in psittacine and columbidine birds and probably in water fowl. Carriers exist in all fowl. |
| Placentopathy | | | | |
| Enzootic abortion in ewes | Scotland, England, Hungary, Germany, France, United States | Sheep | Embryonated hens' eggs, guinea pigs, sheep, cattle, pigeons, and sparrows | Endemic in sheep. Arachnids and/or insects may play a role in transmission. Perhaps pigeons, sparrows, and other domestic animals as well. |
| Epizootic abortion in cattle | Spain, Germany, Italy, United States | Cattle | Embryonated hens' eggs, guinea pigs, sheep, and cattle. | Periodically endemic in California and Oregon (USA) cattle. *Arachnida* and/or insects may play a role in transmission as well as sheep, and other domestic animals. |
| Abortions in other domestic animals | United States | Pigs, goats, rabbits, mice | Embryonated hens' eggs, guinea pigs, and respective natural hosts for each *C. psittaci* isolate | Placentopathy not widely observed in these species. Interspecies disease relationships not well known. |
| Sporadic bovine encephalomyelitis | Australia, Canada, Germany, South Africa, United States | Cattle, dogs | Embryonated hens' eggs, guinea pigs, hamsters, cattle, and dogs. | Endemic in U.S.A. cattle. Little known about the infection in dogs. |
| Pneumonitis | | | | |
| Feline | World-wide | Cats, man | Hen's eggs, mice, cats, hamsters, and guinea pigs. | Endemic in the domestic cat. Transmitted by aerosol and infective excretions from cat to cat. |
| Ovine | United States | Sheep | Hen's eggs, mice, guinea pigs, sheep | Probably endemic in sheep raising areas of U.S.A. Sheep-to-sheep transmission |
| Bovine | Czechoslovakia, Italy, Japan, United States | Cattle | Hens' eggs, mice, guinea pig, and cattle | Endemic. Cattle to cattle transmission. |
| Caprine | Japan | Goat | Goat, embryonated hens' eggs, guinea pig. | Endemic |
| Canine | United States | Dog, budgerigars, humans? | Dog, budgerigars, embryonated hens' eggs, guinea pig | Single case only in dog reported |

| Disease manifestation | Known geographical distribution | Natural host(s) | Recommended experimental hosts | Epidemiological aspects |
|---|---|---|---|---|
| Murine | United States | Mice | Mice, embryonated hens' eggs, guinea pig | Endemic in certain mouse colonies |
| Conjunctivitis | | | | |
| Guinea pig | World-wide | Guinea pigs | Guinea pigs, embryonated hens' eggs | Endemic as a conjunctivitis in some colonies. May be transmitted trans-ovarially. |
| Hamster | World-wide | Hamsters | Hamsters, embryonated hens' eggs, guinea pigs | Endemic as conjunctivitis in some hamster colonies |
| Polyarthritis | | | | |
| Ovine | United States (principally intermountain area) | Sheep | Sheep, turkeys, guinea pigs, embryonated hens' eggs. | Endemic in lambs in intermountain area of U.S.A. Transmission from sheep to sheep, intestinal carriers may cause poly-arthritic disease |
| Bovine | United States | Cattle | Cattle, guinea pigs, hens' eggs | Known calf-to-calf transmission. |
| Enteritis | | | | |
| Snowshoe hare and muskrat | Canada, Wisconsin, (U.S.A.) | Snowshoe hares and muskrats | Snowshoe hares, muskrats, embryo-nated hens' eggs | Muskrat may be principal reservoir in nature |
| Bovine | World-wide | Cattle | Cattle, guinea pigs, embryonated hens' eggs, mice. | Endemic in cattle. Many intestinal carriers. |

man, was much milder than psittacosis, but this is not always the case (Meyer and Eddie, 37). The disease contracted from pigeons generally is milder than that contracted from parrots or parakeets, but that contracted from turkeys is fully as severe as any of psittacine origin. The agent causing these diseases generates a toxin which apparently has much to do with the virulence of the strain.

Psittacosis in the United States occurs principally in green Amazon parrots and in shell parakeets. In the tropics it evidently occurs widely in many kinds of parrots and parakeets. Pinkerton and Swank (41) first reported the disease (ornithosis) in the domestic pigeon. Subsequently it has been found in this species in many American cities. Smadel, Wall, and Gregg (47) reported it in New York City, Davis and Ewing (16) in Baltimore, and Zichis, Shaughnessy, and Lemke (51) in Chicago. Meyer and Eddie (36) reported a human case of ornithosis contracted from a flock of chickens, and Wolins (49) a number of cases contracted from domestic ducks. Haagen and Mauer (23) identified the virus in a sea bird, the Fulmar petrel, which is used for food by the inhabitants of the Faroe Islands. During the last several years a new reservoir of or-nithosis infection—the domestic turkey—has come to light.

The disease has attracted wide attention from time to time because of epi-demics in man. During one of these outbreaks which occurred in Paris in

1893, Nocard isolated a bacterium belonging to the *Salmonella* group which he regarded as the causative agent. It was commonly accepted as such until the pandemic that occurred in Europe and the United States in the winter of 1929–1930, during which workers showed that Nocard's organism was not commonly present but that a psittacoid agent regularly could be isolated. The *Salmonella psittacosis* of Nocard is now known to have been *Salmonella typhimurium,* a chance contaminant.

The outbreak in man which occurred in 1929–1930 was traced to green Amazon parrots imported from South America. In 1930 rigid restrictions on the importation of these birds into the United States was instituted to prevent a recurrence of the incident of 1929–1930. In a survey made in 1932 Meyer, Eddie, and Stevens (38) discovered that the disease was well established in southern California in shell parakeets (lovebirds). It was found that more than 1,100 aviaries engaged in breeding and containing more than 100,000 birds existed as a "back-yard industry" in that region, and that nearly one-half of these premises were infected. In 1933 the interstate quarantine regulations were amended to provide for the control of interstate shipment of psittacine birds in order to prevent infected birds being shipped out of the region where the disease was enzootic. Through efforts of health authorities, the incidence of the disease has been greatly reduced in the enzootic region. In addition approximately 98 percent of psittacine birds (245,000 in 1969) are introduced into the U.S. from Public Health Service-approved treatment centers. This program markedly reduces transmission of bird and human psittacosis from imported psittacine birds.

From 1929 to 1942, inclusive, 380 human cases of psittacosis (including ornithosis) were reported to the U.S. Public Health Service (18). Of these, 170 occurred during the epidemic of 1929–1930 and 210 later. Eighty deaths were recorded, of which 33 occurred during the epidemic. The number of cases of psittacosis in man dropped off sharply when restrictions were established by the government on the trade in psittacine birds. These restrictions were lifted in 1953 with the result that the incidence of human infections has again risen (20, 45).

From the public health viewpoint the most serious reservoir of infection in the United States is the domestic turkey. Irons, Sullivan, and Rowen (27) called attention to this in 1951 when they reported 22 human cases with 3 deaths among 78 employees in a small turkey-dressing plant in Texas. Others have since reported outbreaks in Texas, Nebraska, Oregon, California, Michigan, Wisconsin, Minnesota, Ohio, and New Jersey. It is quite obvious that the disease is widespread in turkeys in the United States and undoubtedly exists in many other areas where it has not yet been recognized. Turkey ornithosis has been identified in Canada but, according to the published literature, not in any other parts of the world.

**Character of the Disease.** The virulence of psittacosis and ornithosis agents varies greatly. Many outbreaks in various species have occurred in which the disease was recognized only after human attendants became ill from it, and in others only by the recognition of antibodies for it. On the other hand, some outbreaks have exhibited high mortality rates both among birds and human contacts. In birds the disease generally is manifested by inappetence, great depression, the presence of nasal and eye discharges, and severe diarrhea. Recovered individuals usually continue to eliminate the agent in their discharges for long periods of time.

*In psittacine birds.* Generally speaking, psittacosis presents few or no signs of illness in the older birds. It is the younger birds that are most apt to develop acute and fatal infections, and these are the principal spreaders of the disease. Affected birds refuse feed and are greatly depressed, their feathers become ruffled and soiled with the yellowish-green diarrheal feces, they have mucopurulent nasal discharges, and often their eyes are pasted shut with exudate. Usually they become greatly dehydrated and emaciated before death. Those that recover almost always continue to eliminate the organism in their discharges for long periods of time. It is these birds that keep the disease alive by infecting the younger birds of the flock. Parrots and parakeets that are convalescent carriers remain wholly well, or may at times suffer from transient diarrhea. The carrier state is often discovered only when the pet owners develop psittacosis.

*In pigeons.* Adult birds may be listless, have no appetite, show nasal and eye discharges, and suffer from diarrhea. According to Coles (10), who was the first to describe ornithosis in pigeons, this disease should be suspected in any birds which are affected with conjunctivitis.

Affected squabs are weak and show signs similar to those of adults. Most of these die. Many of the adult birds recover, become convalescent carriers, and serve as sources of infection to fanciers and to those who feed and fondle these birds in city parks and squares.

*In turkeys.* In many outbreaks the virulence of the infection is very low (3), the losses are not serious, and the disease is likely to be undiagnosed. Graber and Pomeroy (22) have shown that strains from such outbreaks may cause human infections. On the other hand, the disease may be serious, with mortality rates of well-developed birds running as high as 25 percent. The signs of the disease often resemble those of fowl cholera or erysipelas. The birds become apathetic, do not eat well, show depression, and develop diarrhea. The diarrheal discharges are fluid, often contain blood, and generally cause matting of the feathers in the region of the vent. Many birds become greatly emaciated.

*In ducks.* Outbreaks in the United States have generally been inapparent. The disease has been recognized either because of human contact cases or by serological or cultural procedures.

*In chickens.* A few cases of ornithosis in chickens have been reported. In these instances the disease has been inapparent.

*In other birds.* Ornithosis has been recognized in geese, gray herons, and pheasants, occurring in an inapparent form. Mention has been made of the occurrence of the disease in the petrels of the Faroe Islands.

The incubation period in parrots varies widely from a few days to several weeks. In pigeons it is from 5 to 9 days. In man it varies from 6 to 15 days, or longer, with an average of about 10 days.

In young birds the course of the disease is short—3 days to about 1 week. In older ones it is chronic, as a rule. Many older birds excrete the agent intermittently over long periods, during this time showing few or no signs.

The mortality varies widely according to species, age, and virulence of the agent. In young psittacine birds it may be as high as 75 to 90 percent. In young pigeons it may be nearly as high. In turkeys it generally is much lower but may be as high as 25 percent. In other species it is generally low and sometimes nil. In man before the advent of antibiotics it varied between 10 and 30 percent, averaging about 20 percent. These cases were of parrot origin. The mortality rate now is much lower because the disease can be effectively treated with antibiotics, if diagnosed sufficiently early.

The lesions vary in different species of birds but the general pattern is the same. In psittacine birds swelling of the spleen is generally observed; in nonpsittacine birds it is frequently absent. In both there is enlargement of the liver and frequently the organ contains necrotic foci. Sometimes it is covered with a layer of fibrin. In all birds inflammation of the air sacs occurs, and this condition varies from mild clouding to the presence of caseous masses of exudate. In many birds fibrinous pericarditis is frequent. In all acute cases there is severe enteritis, often of a bloody character.

In man the disease is principally an atypical, patchy, bronchopneumonia which cannot be clinically differentiated from virus-induced pneumonia of man.

*In experimental animals.* Parrots that have not previously suffered from the disease are readily infected by inoculation parenterally or orally, or by the respiratory route. Java sparrows and reed birds are readily infected by contact and by inoculation. Natural infections in canaries have been recognized. Adult chickens are not readily infected, but young birds can easily be infected by inoculation. White mice are highly susceptible and are commonly employed for diagnostic purposes. Agents of psittacine origin, injected intraperitoneally, results in infection, but that of nonpsittacine origin frequently fails. Ornithosis agents are best inoculated intracerebrally. Guinea pigs, rabbits, and monkeys can be infected by inoculation but in these species the disease often is not fatal.

**Properties of the Agent.** That the disease could be produced by filtrates made from organs of diseased birds was shown, early in 1930, by Krumwiede, McGrath, and Oldenbusch (30) in the United States and by Bedson, Western, and Simpson (8) in England, working independently.

The agent of psittacosis is filterable only through rather coarse filters. Membrane studies indicate that its particulate size is between 200 and 300 millimicrons, a size sufficiently great that the elementary bodies are visible microscopically. The coccoid bodies found in the lesions of parrots, mice, and men are of about this size. There is a general relation between the concentration of these bodies and virulence, and it is known that they are the infectious agents. These bodies were found at about the same time and were described independently in 1930 by Levinthal (32) in Germany, by Coles (10) in England, and by Lillie (33) in the United States. They are generally known as *LCL bodies*, the letters representing the initials of the names of these workers. Lillie at first regarded them as rickettsiae, but now they are considered to be elementary bodies of the psittacoid group. The fluorescent antibody technic has been used in recent years to prove that the LCL bodies contain RNA and DNA. The LCL bodies are Gram-negative, nonmotile organisms that multiply within the cytoplasm by a developmental cycle, unique amongst bacteria. Following penetration of the host cell the elementary bodies increase in size, 900 to 1,000 millimicrons in diameter, to become initial bodies which increase to form clusters or plaques in a matrix. These thin-walled, noninfectious, larger forms multiply by fission and daughter cells change to the smaller infectious elementary bodies, 200 to 300$\mu$, which contain ribosomes and a diffuse nucleus. This process takes place in a vesicle whose wall disintegrates releasing hundreds of elementary bodies into the cytoplasm. Microscopic examination of wet-cell preparations by phase microscopy or of stained preparations by regular light microscopy shows clusters of organisms of various sizes in the cytoplasm of many host cells. The small infectious form, 200 to 300 $\mu$, stains purple with Giemsa's stain, red with Macchiavello's and Gimenez's stains, and blue with Castenada's stain. The large noninfectious form, 900 to 1,000$\mu$, is blue with Giemsa's and Macchiavello's stains, and purple with Castenada's stain. Phase-contrast microscopy avoids time-consuming staining procedures and it also eliminates staining artifacts. By either method it is difficult to distinguish intracellular *Mycoplasma* organisms from chlamydiae so other diagnostic procedures should be included other than smear preparations in order to make a positive diagnosis.

**Cultivation and Resistance of *Chlamydia*.** The elementary bodies of members of this group may be propagated rather easily in a number of ways. Yanamura and Meyer (50) in 1941 reported successful cultivation of the agent in tissue fragments suspended in various fluids, in tissue fragments spread over the surface of serum agar slants, and in the yolk sac of developing chick embryos when the agent was introduced by a technic developed by Cox (12) for the propagation of rickettsiae. It will also develop on the chorioallantoic membrane and in the allantoic cavity of the chick embryo. Because infected cells rupture and discharge their content of elementary bodies, it is possible, in a number of ways, to obtain suspensions comparatively free from extraneous yolk-sac materials. These suspensions can be used for agglutination and complement-fixation tests. (For more information about cultivation see the section on diagnosis.)

The cell walls of chlamydiae contain considerable lipid, which makes them susceptible to lipid solvents and detergents. Consequently, a 1:1,000 dilution of quaternary compound (alkyl-dimethylbenzl-ammonium chloride) is an effective disinfectant for laboratory and hospital use. Phenol, in contrast, is a poor disinfectant. The organisms resist acid and alkali. They are rapidly destroyed by heat but the death time is related to the amount of protective cellular material present.

Various strains produce a cytopathogenic effect in mammalian-cell cultures, but cell cultures are less commonly used than the embryonated hen's egg for research and diagnosis.

**Immunity.** It has been pointed out that after recovery from the active disease birds usually harbor the chlamydiae for long periods of time. During this time they possess a marked resistance to reinfection, as might be expected. The organism tends to remain in mammals also for considerable periods after clinical recovery, and it has been suggested that immunity in this disease is always due to the harboring of latent infection. This has not been proved to be the case.

Unlike most virus diseases, neutralizing antibodies are not always demonstrable in animals immune to chlamydiae and are seldom present in great concentration. Nevertheless, animals that have received chlamydiae intramuscularly without harm are protected against intratracheal inoculations that produce pneumonia in unprepared animals.

Several workers (6, 26) have shown that mice and pigeons could be partially immunized by several injections of inactivated chlamydiae. The protection is not great enough to be useful. Turkeys vaccinated intratracheally, intramuscularly, and subcutaneously with live ornithosis agents of low virulence prepared from yolk-sac and mouse-tissue suspensions stimulated DCF antibody titers. The presence of these titers in the vaccinated turkeys could not be equated to resistance to infection by an ornithosis isolate of high virulence (5). Better immunization can be obtained with virulent organisms administered parenterally, but this has not been used for practical immunization. Whether or not it would be successful in birds has not been demonstrated.

**Transmission.** These diseases apparently are transmitted in both birds and mammals largely by means of infected droplets. Davis, Delaplane, and Watkins (15) and others were unable to find any evidence indicating that virus was ever transmitted through the eggs of birds. A considerable number of laboratory infections have occurred. In many cases these persons actually handled the infected birds and may have contracted the infection otherwise, but there have been a considerable number of persons infected without any direct contacts, and air-borne infection seems the only possible route (see McCoy, 34, and Badger, 2). In turkey-dressing establishments, it was noted that most of the infections occurred in areas where an aerosol was set up by the machinery. Rivers and Schwentker (44) found that monkeys could easily be infected by inhalation but that fully virulent material failed to infect when injected subcutaneously or intramuscularly. A number of volunteers among laboratory workers were immunized by parenteral injection of the fully virulent psittacosis agent without adverse results.

The ornithosis agent has been isolated from several species of poultry ecto-parasites, suggesting that this may also be a vector-borne infection.

**Diagnosis.** The clinical picture may suggest psittacosis or ornithosis but seldom can a positive diagnosis be made without confirmation by laboratory means.

*1. Animal inoculations.* Experienced workers have been quite successful in isolating the agent by inoculating chick embryos into the allantoic cavity or the yolk-sac (25), but the most successful way of recovering the agent is by mouse inoculation (43). Intraperitoneal injection of filtrates of human sputum or of unfiltered sputum, in case organisms are not present which kill the animals prematurely, usually kill these animals in from 5 to 14 days, occasionally as late as 30 days. If any of the mice sicken after the 4th or 5th day, they should be destroyed and examined for the characteristic focal necrosis of the liver. Films are made from the liver tissue, and a search is made for the elementary bodies of psittacosis. If the mice are still living after 30 days, it is well at that time to inject them with the known psittacosis agent to determine whether or not they may have developed immunity from an infection that did not become apparent. A 20 to 40 percent suspension of suspect tissues can be used for transfer in experimental animals.

The method described apparently is efficient for detecting the disease in man or in birds of the parrot family, but the pigeon agent usually does not kill mice or produce the liver lesions. The organism from these birds can usually be recovered, however, by inoculating the mice intracerebrally instead of intraperitoneally. The pigeon agent is more highly virulent for pigeons than that from parrots. The parrot agent will, however, usually produce inapparent infections in pigeons (36).

In using mice and guinea pigs the diagnostician and research worker should be aware that mice and guinea pig colonies may be naturally infected with chlamydiae. The murine pneumonitis strain of *C. trachomatis* has been isolated from the lungs of mice from many colonies. The organisms are demonstrated by repeated passage of homogenized lung suspensions from carrier mice into normal mice by aerosol exposure. Infected mice eventually develop a diffuse pneumonitis and the organisms are readily demonstrated in lung-smear preparations. Guinea pigs may be naturally infected with *C. psittaci* which manifests itself as a conjunctivitis and is readily transmitted by contact.

All strains of chlamydiae can be isolated and propagated in the yolk sac of the embryonated hen's egg. Depending upon the source of inoculum proper treatment must be performed to rid the inoculum of bacteria or *Mycoplasma* which usually grow well in the egg. If bacterial contaminants are suspected the test material should be ground in a phosphate-buffered saline solution (pH 7.2) containing 1 mg per ml each of streptomycin sulfate, vancomycin, and kanamycin. This markedly reduces bacterial contamination without affecting the *Chlamydia* population. Normally, a 10 percent suspension is injected into the yolk sac of 5-to-7-day-old embryonated hens' eggs with death ensuing 5 to 12 days later. The capillaries of infected eggs are not sharply outlined when candled. Infected embryos and yolk-sac membranes are congested and frequently hemorrhagic. Stained smears of yolk-sac membranes show the presence of the chlamydiae organisms (fig. 145). An antigen prepared from an infected yolk sac fixes complement in the presence of a positive chlamydial antiserum in the complement-fixation test. This result constitutes a positive diagnosis of chlamydiae. If no embryos die in first passage three blind passages of yolk-sac material harvested 10 to 14 days after inoculation with no specific embryo deaths are required to conclude that the avian tissue homogenate did not contain *C. psittaci.*

2. *Cell cultures.* Most strains of *C. psittaci* propagate in cultured cells and produce sufficient cell destruction to show plaque formation (41). Intracellular microcolonies (plaques) can be seen 2 to 7 days after inoculation. Presence of chlamydiae can be demonstrated in 2 ways: (a) by the direct fluorescent antibody test (FAT), and (b) by utilization of the tissue-cultured

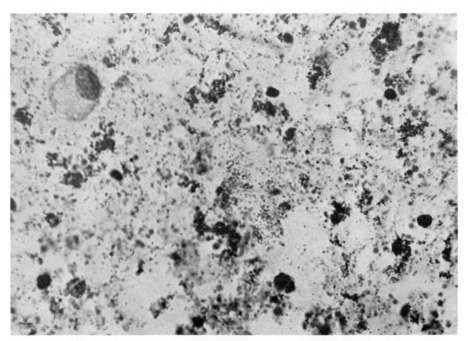

*Fig. 145. Chlamydia psittaci.* A Gimenez-stained impression smear of a yolk-sac preparation infected with a chlamydial strain of mouse pnemonitis. X 1,000. (Courtesy J. Storz.)

preparation as an antigen in the complement-fixation test. The FAT is reputedly more sensitive for their identification in cell cultures, but not in smear preparations from yolk-sac and other animal tissues.

Chlamydial agents multiply in cell cultures derived from various tissues of different hosts. A few such cell cultures are human embryonic skin, muscle, or lung (39), chick embryo (42), and most cells of the McCoy line (48).

3. *Serological tests.* All members of chlamydiae contain a group specific antigen that is a lipopolysacchride. The antigen is resistant to phenol, heat, and various proteinases but inactivated by lecithinase and periodate. Antigens may be prepared in a variety of ways (31) to test for the group-specific antigen in the standard complement-fixation test (CF); in the direct CF (DCF) test that is used principally for detection of CF antibodies in avian sera where normal rooster serum is added as a test component to make the test workable; indirect CF (ICF) test; capillary tube agglutination test; gel-diffusion technics; and hemagglutination test (4). These test procedures can be found in the textbook by Lennette and Schmidt (31).

The cell walls of chlamydiae contain a mosaic of antigens that are distinct from the group-specific antigen. The cell-wall antigens are often shared within a group of strains affecting a certain class of animals (human, mannal, and avian strains) and some antigens cross animal classes. Consequently no precise serological classification of chlamydial strains is possible at present (21).

The complement-fixation test (29) may be used to confirm the presence of the disease in flocks, but it has been shown that carrier birds of all species do not always react to this test and recent infections may not be detected. CF antibodies usually appear in birds and mammals within 7 to 10 days after infection. Some animals with intestinal infection may have no detectable CF antibodies. The height of a titer reflects the antigenic properties and recentness of infection but it may not reflect current infection. Thus, the serologic diagnosis of infection requires demonstration of a 4-fold rise in CF antibody titer using paired sera. If 80 percent or more of individuals in a group have a demonstrable titer and half have titers of 1: 64 or greater this constitutes reasonable proof that the group of animals is currently infected with chlamydiae.

Benedict (9) has used an intradermal test for this detection. It detects fewer chronically infected birds than the complement-fixation test. They become allergic 4 weeks after experimental infection.

4. *Serum neutralization, plaque reduction, and toxin neutralization.* In the neutralization test the embryo is protected from death by the neutralization of the infective particle with the specific antiserum prior to inoculation. In the toxin neutralization test the early death of mice inoculated intravenously with large numbers of organisms is prevented by the injection of specific antitoxin. The mechanism of the plaque reduction is similar to the neutralization test in the hen's egg except cell cultures are used as the indicator system for detecting *Chlamydia* activity.In these three tests high-titered antisera must be used

and results in comparative studies of chlamydiae reflect variation in cell wall antigens responsible for infectivity and provide a means to establish serotypes among some strains of *C. psittaci*.

**Chemotherapy.** Unlike viruses, the psittacosis-lymphogranuloma group show definite susceptibility to the action of some of the sulfonamides and antibiotics. Heilman and Herrell (24) in 1944 showed that large doses of penicillin would save the majority of mice inoculated with the psittacosis agent although most of them developed inapparent infections, which made them resistant to later injections of the same strain. It has been demonstrated by several groups that the same thing is true of the disease in man. Meiklejohn, Wagner, and Beveridge (35) showed that penicillin would inhibit growth of this agent in tissues but it was ineffective in eggs. Early and Morgan (19) found that sulfadiazine in food protected mice from death when the latter were inoculated with the psittacosis agent, but most of the animals became carriers. Streptomycin was not effective. The same workers found that sulfadiazine protected chick embryos from some strains but was ineffective against others.

It is apparent that many of the antibiotics exert an influence on agents of the ornithosis group, but it appears that most are incapable of completely eliminating the chlamydiae from victims of the disease. The most successful are tetracycline compounds (13), chloromycetin, and 5-florouracil. These must be given in rather high concentrations in the feed to accomplish sterilization. Lower doses serve to lower mortality rates but leave many carriers. Davis and Delaplane (14) found that a concentration of chlortetracycline of 200 g per ton in an all-mash ration was required to eliminate the ornithosis agent from a group of 3-week-old poults. Experimentally infected adult turkeys, treated for 2 to 3 weeks with 200 to 400 g per ton of mash, failed to yield organisms.

In view of the initially low rate of psittacosis infection in most wild or uncrowded captive psittacines, group treatment with 0.5 percent chlortetracycline in dry pelleted feed for 45 days was practical, effective, and economically feasible, and might be considered an adequate safeguard against the hazard of psittacosis (1).

Chlortetracycline is used very successfully for treating human infections, providing the diagnosis is made early and the treatment is carried on for a considerable time at a high dosage level. Too small a dosage and too short a treatment time results in relapses.

**The Disease in Man.** Human infections have been discussed in preceding sections. The disease is seldom conveyed from person to person, although it may be unless precautions against droplet infection are taken. Ordinarily the disease in man is derived from the very considerable reservoir that exists in birds, where it often occurs as a latent disease.

## REFERENCES

1. Arnstein, Eddie, and Meyer. Am. Jour. Vet. Res., 1968, 29, 2213.
2. Badger. Pub. Health Rpts. (U.S.), 1930, 45, 1403.

3. Bankowski and Page. Am. Jour. Vet. Res., 1959, *20*, 935.
4. Barron, Jakay-Roness, and Bernkopf. Proc. Soc. Exp. Biol. and Med., 1965, *119*, 377.
5. Bates, Pomeroy, and Reynolds. Avian Dis., 1965, *9*, 220.
6. Bedson. Brit. Jour. Exp. Path., 1938, *19*, 353.
7. Bedson and Bland. *Ibid.*, 1932, *13*, 461; 1934, *15*, 243.
8. Bedson, Western, and Simpson. Lancet, 1930, *1*, 235.
9. Benedict. Am. Jour. Hyg., 1957, *66*, 245.
10. Coles. Lancet, 1930, *1*, 1011.
11. Coles. Onderstepoort Jour. Vet. Sci. and Anim. Indus., 1940, *15*, 141.
12. Cox. Pub. Health Rpts. (U.S.), 1938, *53*, 2241.
13. Cox. In: Beaudette. Psittacosis. Diagnosis, epidemiology, and control. Rutgers Univ. Press, New Brunswick, N.J., 1955, p. 137.
14. Davis and Delaplane. Am. Jour. Vet. Res., 1958, *19*, 169.
15. Davis, Delaplane, and Watkins. *Ibid.*, 1957, *18*, 409.
16. Davis and Ewing. Pub. Health Rpts. (U.S.), 1947, *62*, 1484.
17. Donaldson, Davis, Watkins, and Sulkin. Am. Jour. Vet. Res., 1958, *19*, 950.
18. Dunnahoo and Hampton. Pub. Health Rpts. (U.S.), 1945, *60*, 354.
19. Early and Morgan. Jour. Immunol., 1946, *53*, 151 and 251.
20. Fitz, Meiklejohn, and Baum. Am. Jour. Med. Sci., 1955, *229*, 252.
21. Fraser. Analytical serology of microorganisms. J. Wiley and Sons, N.Y., Vol. 1, 257–330, 1969.
22. Graber and Pomeroy. Am. Jour. Pub. Health, 1958, *48*, 1469.
23. Haagen and Mauer. Centrbl. f. Bakt., I Abt., Orig., 1938, *143*, 81.
24. Heilman and Herrell. Proc. Mayo Clinic, 1944, *19*, 204.
25. Hudson, Bivins, Beaudette, and Tudor. Jour. Am. Vet. Med. Assoc., 1955, *126*, 111.
26. Hughes. Jour. Comp. Path. and Therap., 1947, *57*, 67.
27. Irons, Sullivan, and Rowen. Am. Jour. Pub. Health, 1951, *41*, 931.
28. Jones, Rake, and Stearns. Jour. Inf. Dis., 1945, *76*, 55.
29. Kissling, Schaeffer, Fletcher, Stamm, Bucca, and Sigel. Pub. Health Rpts. (U.S.), 1956, *71*, 719.
30. Krumwiede, McGrath, and Oldenbusch. Science, 1930, *71*, 262.
31. Lennette and Schmidt. Diagnostic procedures for viral and rickettsial diseases. 4th ed., Am. Public Health Assoc., Inc., 1970.
32. Levinthal. Klin. Wchnschr., 1930, *9*, 654.
33. Lillie. Pub. Health Rpts. (U.S.), 1930, *45*, 773.
34. McCoy. *Ibid.*, 843.
35. Meiklejohn, Wagner, and Beveridge. Jour. Immunol., 1946, *54*, 1 and 9.
36. Meyer and Eddie. Proc. Soc. Exp. Biol. and Med., 1932–33, *30*, 484.
37. *Ibid.*, 1953, *83*, 99.
38. Meyer, Eddie, and Stevens. Am. Jour. Pub. Health, 1935, *25*, 571.
39. Page. Internat. Jour. System. Bact., 1968, *18*, 51.
40. Pearson, Duff, Gearinger, and Robbins. Jour. Inf. Dis., 1965, *115*, 49.
41. Pinkerton and Swank. Proc. Soc. Exp. Biol. and Med., 1940, *45*, 704.
42. Piraino. Jour. Bact., 1969, *98*, 475.
43. Rivers and Berry. Jour. Exp. Med., 1935, *61*, 205.
44. Rivers and Schwentker. *Ibid.*, 1934, *60*, 211.
45. Sigel, Cole, and Hunter. Am. Jour. Pub. Health, 1953, *43*, 1418.

46.   Smadel.   Jour. Clin. Invest., 1943, *22*, 57.
47.   Smadel, Wall, and Gregg.   Jour. Exp. Med., 1943, *78*, 189.
48.   Tanami, Pollard, and Starr.   Virology, 1961, *15*, 22.
49.   Wolins.   Am. Jour. Med. Sci., 1948, *216*, 551.
50.   Yanamura and Meyer.   Jour. Inf. Dis., 1941, *68*, 1.
51.   Zichis, Shaughnessy, and Lemke.   Jour. Bact., 1946, *51*, 616.

### Enzootic Abortion of Ewes

SYNONYMS:   Ovine enzootic abortion, ovine virus abortion; abbreviation, EAE.

This disease is caused by *C. psittaci*. It affects pregnant ewes, causing them to abort in late pregnancy. The clinical signs of the disease are indistinguishable from those of ovine vibriosis.

Enzootic abortion of ewes was recognized as an infectious disease by Stamp *et al.* (8) in Scotland in 1950. The disease has since been diagnosed in England, Germany, France, and Hungary. In 1958 a disease which had been under observation for several years in the United States (Montana) was recognized as being caused by an agent of the psittacosis-lymphogranuloma group (14). It was suspected to be the same as the European disease. When comparisons of the agents were made (13), they were found to be identical. This disease is widespread in the United States.

**Character of the Disease.** Abortions occur from midgestation to late pregnancy. Retention of the placenta is frequent, and a vaginal discharge is seen for several days following lambing or abortion. The aborted fetuses may be mummified or quite normal in appearance. The cotyledons are dark red or clay-colored. The ewe is visibly ill and has fever of two or three degrees lasting for periods up to 1 week. The genital organs quickly return to normal and subsequent fertility is not imparied. Experimentally infected sheep react with a febrile response beginning about 3 days after inoculation. Abortions occur at least 56 days following injection or feeding the infectious agent.

The mortality rate in the ewes is virtually nil, although many lambs may be lost. In the ewe, inflammation and necrosis of the placentome is observed. The affected fetus shows hepatopathy, occasionally edema, ascites, vascular congestion, and tracheal petechiae.

**The Disease in Experimental Animals.** Weanling white mice may be killed by intranasal inoculation of yolk sac material. Large doses sometimes kill adult mice when they are administered intracerebrally or intravenously. Some of these mice die as a result of intoxication from the toxin, and within a few hours following inoculation. Others die after a few days as a result of infection. Febrile reactions may be produced in guinea pigs by intraperitoneal injections, but these animals seldom die of the infection. Animals killed during the febrile reaction show enlarged friable livers, containing minute necrotic areas, splenic enlargement, and little else (7).

Guinea pigs are the laboratory animal of choice for the isolation of ovine chlamydiae because these animals are more susceptible than chicken embryos or mice.

Strains of enzootic abortion of ewes (EAE) produce abortions in sheep under natural conditions (10). A strain of enzootic bovine abortion (EBA) also has been incriminated in the production of disease and abortions of sheep (11). The goat EAE agent caused abortion in an experimental ewe and also in two experimental cows (3). The sheep EAE agent causes experimental disease in pigeons and a lethal disease in sparrows under experimental conditions (6). A sheep strain of *C. psittaci* that was isolated from a naturally occurring case of pneumonia caused abortion in experimental ewes but the disease differed from typical EAE infection (11).

The parenteral injection of bovine or ovine chlamydial agents into rams produced seminal vesiculitis with a granulomatous response that was limited mostly to interstitial tissues (2). Excretion of *Chlamydia* in the semen continued until the experimental rams were slaughtered 8 to 22 days after inoculation. During the acute febrile stage the organism was isolated from the blood and somatic organs. Complement-fixing antibodies rose sharply 1 week after inoculation, reaching peak titers of 128 to 512. The leukocytes in semen increased in number during the experiment and the two rams receiving the calf polyarthritis strain of *C. psittaci* had pus in the semen. The frequency of secondary morphologic abnormalities of spermatozoa increased by 20 days after injection.

**Properties of the Agent.** The ovine abortion agent is a typical member of the psittacosis-lymphogranuloma group. It conforms to the general characteristics of the group. Like other members of the group it is sensitive to penicillin and some of the sulfonamides but is unaffected by streptomycin and para-amino-benzoic acid. It is highly sensitive to chloromycetin and the tetracyclines. It forms a toxin which is lethal to mice, but it is believed to play a minor role in the disease of sheep (11).

It has been suggested that the ovine agents of the PLV group isolated from cases of abortion and pneumonia, and from feces, should not be considered to be distinct and separate from one another (1). Later studies by Storz (9) showed that the fecal organism invaded the placenta and the developing fetus just as did the agent causing enzootic abortion of ewes.

**Cultivation.** The agent grows readily and in high concentration in the yolk sacs of embryonated hens' eggs, 5 to 7 days old. The growth of the embryos is retarded and they succumb before hatching. Chlamydiae injected into the allantoic cavity causes death of some embryos.

Strains of EAE multiply only to a limited degree in cell cultures and then only if the multiplicity of infection (ratio of infectious units to host cells) is high. This can be enhanced if suspensions of *Chlamydia* are centrifuged at 1,000 times the force of gravity for 60 minutes and placed directly on a monolayer of host cells growing on the bottom of a flat-bottomed tube.

**Immunity.** The experience of the Scottish workers (4, 5), confirmed in this country, indicates that a single infection solidly immunizes ewes for the normal lifetime of the animal. The presence of complement-fixing antibody resulting from subclinical or clinical infection to the *Chlamydia* group antigen ameliorates the clinical response and may prevent abortion in sheep following inoculation of the epizootic bovine abortion (EBA) agent. The immunity conferred by the antibody is relative because a large challenge dose may cause ewes to abort (12).

**Transmission.** The disease may readily be transmitted to susceptible, pregnant ewes by inoculation. Natural transmission of the disease presumably occurs by ingestion. This explains how the disease spreads in a flock of pregnant ewes. The persistence of the fecal agent may explain how the disease carries over from one lambing season to the next. The susceptibility of pigeons and sparrows to the EAE agent suggests another means of transmission to sheep and a reservoir for it in nature. It has been suggested that arachnids and/or insects may play some role in its transmission. There is no evidence at present that rams are involved. Susceptible sheep, placed on pastures on which the disease occurs one season, seldom will show any evidence of the disease the following season (13).

**Diagnosis.** It is difficult to make a definite clinical diagnosis, because *Chlamydia* abortion and vibriosis exhibit essentially the same signs of illness. Flocks in which vibrios cannot be found should be suspected of harboring the psittacoid agent. The diagnosis can be verified by inoculating stomach contents of aborted fetuses or placental tissues into the yolk sac of embryonated eggs. The complement-fixation test will give evidence of infection with an agent of the group.

The elementary bodies generally can be identified in Giemsa-stained smears of cotyledons of aborting ewes. After some experience this method may be used as a diagnostic procedure.

**Control.** It was found that the disease can be readily controlled by vaccinating all young ewes with a formalinized vaccine made from the infected yolk sacs of embryonated eggs. Commercial vaccine for this purpose is available. The disease has been controlled very successfully in Europe by vaccination of the young ewes prior to first breeding with the adjuvant, yolk-sac vaccine.

**The Disease in Man.** There is no evidence that the EAE agent has produced disease in man but precaution and care should be exercised in handling infectious material from these cases because of the potential health hazard of the *Chlamydia* species to humans.

## REFERENCES

1. Dungworth and Cordy. Jour. Comp. Path. and Therap., 1962, 72, 71.
2. Eugster, Ball, Carroll and Storz. 6th Internatl. Mtg. Dis. Cattle, Philadelphia, Pa., 1971.
3. McCauley and Tieken. Jour. Am. Vet. Med. Assoc., 1968, *152*, 1758.
4. McEwan, Dow, and Anderson. Vet. Rec., 1955, *67*, 393.

5. McEwan and Foggie. *Ibid.*, 1956, *68*, 686.
6. Page. Am. Jour. Vet. Res., 1966, *27*, 397.
7. Parker. Am. Jour. Vet. Res., 1960, *21*, 243.
8. Stamp, McEwan, Watt, and Nisbet. Vet. Rec., 1950, *62*, 251.
9. Storz. Cornell Vet., 1963, *53*, 469.
10. Storz. Jour. Comp. Path., 1966, *76*, 351.
11. Studdert and McKercher. Res. Vet. Sci., 1968, *9*, 48.
12. Studdert and McKercher. *Ibid.*, 1968, *9*, 331.
13. Tunnicliff. Proc. U.S. Livestock San. Assoc., 1958, *62*, 261.
14. Young, Parker, and Firehammer. Jour. Am. Vet. Med. Assoc., 1958, *133*, 374.

## Placentopathy in other Domestic Animals

Placentopathy in the goat, pig, rabbit, and mice caused by *C. psittaci* is not widely observed in the United States. The character of the disease in these species is similar to enzootic abortion in ewes. Comparative studies of the strains of *C. psittaci* that cause placentopathy in domestic animals are lacking.

A well-documented psittacosis abortion epizootic in goats recently appeared in the literature (1). A chlamydial organism was isolated from an aborted goat fetus in an outbreak which caused a 12 percent abortion rate during 1967 in a California flock of 216 milk goats. There was a marked decrease in incidence after penicillin therapy was given to pregnant goats. This isolate of *C. psittaci* produced abortion in two experimental pregnant cows and one experimental pregnant ewe.

### REFERENCE

1. McCauley and Tieken. Jour. Am. Vet. Med. Assoc., 1968, *152*, 1758.

## Sporadic Bovine Encephalomyelitis

SYNONYMS: Buss disease; abbreviation, SBE

This disease affects cattle, particularly those under 3 years of age, and is characterized by encephalitis, fibrinous pleuritis, and peritonitis. It occurs sporadically and is caused by an agent belonging to the psittacosis-lymphogranuloma group. The name Buss was given by McNutt because the first cases were seen on a farm belonging to a man of that name. So far as is known, only cattle are affected. It has been suspected that human infections may occur but the evidence is inconclusive. Dogs apparently are susceptible, but little is known about the disease in this species.

The disease was first recognized and described in Iowa by McNutt (3) in 1940. It has since been diagnosed in Texas, California, South Dakota, Minnesota, and Missouri. In 1956 Schoop and Kauker (5) described a disease in Germany which was caused by a psittacoid agent that may be the same as SBE. In 1961 an outbreak was described in South Africa (6) and in Canada (1). The disease is also present in Australia.

**Character of the Disease.** The disease is manifested by profound depression. Fever occurs early in the course of the disease and is maintained until recovery or death approaches. Inappetence, weakness, emaciation, and prostration are characteristic. A clear mucoid discharge from the nose and eyes frequently occurs. A staggering gait is often seen, and the principal joints may be swollen and tender. Some animals develop a mild diarrhea, and some tend to walk or stagger in circles. Opisthotonos occurs occasionally. The disease appears to spread slowly, and many exposed animals seem to escape infection. This may be more apparent than real. As a rule only a few animals in a herd show illness.

By experimental inoculation the incubation period varies widely from 4 to 27 days. In the naturally transmitted disease it is not known, but apparently it is fairly long. The disease is said to have a course of from 1 to 3 weeks. Enright, Sadler, and Robinson (2) present evidence indicating that there are many mild or inapparent cases. These obviously have a much shorter course. Of the clinically sick animals from 40 to 60 percent die. Many others apparently suffer from the disease without showing detectable signs of illness; hence the mortality rate is really much lower.

The gross lesions are not conspicuous. In many cases the body cavities contain more than the usual amount of fluid, in which strings of fibrin may be found. The brain usually appears normal but shows microscopic evidence of a severe and diffuse meningoencephalitis. The meningitis is most severe at the base of the brain.

**The Disease in Experimental Animals.** The disease is readily produced in young calves by intracerebral or subcutaneous inoculation. Horses, sheep, swine, and mice are not susceptible to inoculation. Guinea pigs, inoculated intraperitoneally, usually die in 4 to 5 days with a fibrinous peritonitis. Hamsters are also susceptible.

**Properties of the Agent.** The causative agent of SBE is a typical member of the psittacosis-lymphogranuloma group. In morphology and growth characteristics in embryonated eggs, and by serology it is difficult to differentiate from other members of *Chlamydia*.

**Cultivation.** The agent reproduces readily in the yolk sac of chick embryos. We have seen no report of its cultivation in tissue cultures.

**Immunity.** No observations on the solidity and duration of immunity in this disease have been reported. It is probable that one experience with this disease would be sufficient to protect the animal thereafter.

**Transmission.** The mode of transmission of this disease is wholly unknown. The disease does not appear to be highly transmissible, but possibly this may be a misconception due to the fact that many mild or imapparent cases occur. Often it appears on a single farm in a vicinity with no other recognized cases near at hand. Frequently only a small number of cases occur in a herd containing many other presumably susceptible animals. Several have shown that the disease may be transmitted to calves through the milk of infected dams (2, 4).

**Diagnosis.** The diagnosis is not easy, because the signs of illness often are vague. Evidence of encephalitis, combined with a stiff awkward gait, and the presence of pleuritis, peritonitis, and sometimes pericarditis are indicative. Isolation of the agent by the inoculation of yolk sacs of embryonated eggs is generally successful, and convincing.

Elementary bodies may be found by appropriate staining procedures in the cytoplasm of mononuclear cells in the exudates in the meninges and from serosal membranes and in microglia of nodules. They are not numerous and often embryonated hens' eggs, guinea pigs, or hamsters are inoculated where the elementary bodies are easier to demonstrate.

**Control.** No means of controlling this disease are known. The apparent sporadicity has not encouraged attempts to develop prophylactic immunization. Because the agent is very sensitive to most of the antibiotics except streptomycin, use of these in treatment is indicated.

**The Disease in Man.** Enright, Sadler, and Robinson (2) reported that 51 of 481 samples of human sera collected from persons who had had contact with cattle in California fixed complement with an antigen made from the McNutt strain of SBE. A number of these persons described clinical syndromes consisting of persisting headache and stiff necks lasting about a week, followed by complete recovery. These data provide circumstantial evidence of infection in man but certainly not conclusive proof.

## REFERENCES

1. Bannister, Boulanger, Gray, Chapman, Avery, and Corner. Canad. Jour. Comp. Med. and Vet. Sci., 1962, *26*, 25.
2. Enright, Sadler, and Robinson. Proc. U.S. Livestock San. Assoc., 1958, *62*, 127.
3. McNutt. Vet. Med., 1940, *35*, 228.
4. McNutt and Waller. Cornell Vet., 1940, *30*, 437.
5. Schoop and Kauker. Deut. tierärztl. Wchnschr., 1956, *23*, 233.
6. Tustin, Mare, and Van Herrden. Jour. So. African Vet. Med. Assoc., 1961, *32*, 117.

### Enzootic Bovine Abortion

SYNONYMS: Foothill abortion; abbreviation, EBA

This disease is caused by selective strains of *C. psittaci* that cause abortion during late gestation in pregnant domestic cows. *C. psittaci* has also been isolated from bulls with the seminal vesiculitis syndrome (8).

The abortion disease was first reported in the United States and occurs principally in California, where it is known as "foothill abortion," and in the adjoining far western states of the United States. A mild form of the disease has been reported from Germany, Italy, and Spain (5). Periodically the abortion disease is endemic in California and Oregon cattle. The seminal vesiculitis syndrome in bulls is known to occur in the same areas as enzootic bovine abortion (EBA).

**Character of the Disease.** The agent usually produces a febrile reaction in susceptible cows of all ages. After a latent period of a few months during which *C. psittaci* propagates in the fetus pregnant animals abort. The disease affects pregnant heifers primarily and the abortion losses are apt to be as high as 60 percent in these animals (3). The delivery of the aborted fetuses are uneventful and the placenta is not retained.

Aborted fetuses in natural and experimental disease are distinctive with similar pathological changes (3). They are usually the size of a full-term fetus and die during delivery or shortly thereafter, but some premature calves may survive the disease.

The seminal vesiculitis syndrome is found in the examination of bulls for breeding soundness and is more common among younger bulls. Ball and his coworkers (1) characterized this condition as a chronic inflammation of the seminal vesicles, accessory sex glands, epididymides, and testicles. Affected bulls have inferior semen quality and some testicles were atrophic. The incidence in a herd may reach 10 percent.

The gross lesions of the abortion disease are limited to the aborted fetus and the fetal membranes (3). The latter are usually thick and edematous. Pale and anemic fetuses usually show petechial hemorrhages of the skin and mucous membranes. Subcutaneous tissues are wet and edematous. Straw-colored peritoneal and pleural fluid is present. A swollen nodular liver caused by chronic passive congestion may sometimes occur. Petechial hemorrhages are often seen in trachea, tongues, thymus, and lymph nodes. Lymphoid tissues are enlarged with associated lymph stasis. Tiny gray foci are irregularly scattered in all tissues that are most difficult to see without proper lighting. Granulomatous lesions may be present in any organ. Histologically, the disease in the fetus is characterized by a diffuse or focal reticuloendothelial hyperplasia which may involve all organs, but the spleen, thymus, and lymph nodes are most apt to be severely affected.

**The Disease in Experimental Animals.** Guinea pigs are the laboratory animal of choice for isolation and study of EBA agents. The embryonated hen's egg and mice are also susceptible. These hosts show the same general signs as described for the EAE (enzootic abortion of ewes) agent.

The injection of pregnant cows with either EBA or EAE agent produces an abortion disease comparable to natural disease. Signs of impending abortion, consisting of a thin, yellowish vaginal discharge, occurred in 6 of 12 heifers that aborted (4). The elementary bodies were frequently demonstrated in stained smears of this vaginal discharge. It was further observed that pathologic changes of extragenital organs occurred only in internal iliac lymph nodes of infected heifers. Because these nodes drain the genital organs the lesions are probably the result of the inflammatory process in the gravid uterus where the EBA agent localizes after a short initial blood infectious stage. Omura *et al.* (7) have induced endometritis by intrauterine inoculation of nonpregnant cows with a *C. psittaci* strain.

A strain of *C. psittaci* isolated from a bull with seminal vesiculitis produced interstitial orchitis and epididymitis, testicular degeneration, and granulomas adherent to the tunica vaginalis propria in inoculated male guinea pigs (8). In contrast, uninoculated male control-guinea pigs failed to show genital lesions.

**Properties of the Agent.** The EBA agent shares the properties of all members of *C. psittaci*. The strain of Storz *et al.* isolated from seminal vesiculitis was indistinguishable from a California EBA strain in the neutralization test (8).

A bull injected intravenously with a strain of *C. psittaci*, which had been recovered from the joint of a calf with polyarthritis, developed a seminal vesiculitis similar to the disease described in rams in the previous section on enzootic abortion in ewes (2). The organism persisted in the semen after recovery from acute disease.

**Cultivation.** The EBA strains of *C. psittaci* have the same cultivation characteristics as the EAE strains.

**Immunity.** All field strains of EBA that have been compared by neutralization tests are immunologically identical. This information helps to explain, in part, the field experience of various investigators and clinicians which indicates that a single exposure to EBA affords protection against this disease for the normal lifetime of the animal. In experimental studies Lincoln *et al.* (4) indicated the presence of CF antibodies and intestinal *Chlamydia* infection, seemingly had no influence on the experimental production of EBA disease in pregnant heifers. Much work needs to be done to elucidate this dilemma. Hopefully, it can be ultimately explained on the basis of two different immunogenic (protective) strains.

The seminal vesiculitis syndrome is observed most frequently in young bulls. After recovery it is possible that they are solidly immune but there is no experimental evidence to support this concept.

**Transmission.** The abortion disease may be readily produced in susceptible pregnant cows. Natural disease may spread by ingestion of infected tissues. Another likely route is venereal transmission (6) because the bull may harbor the organism in the semen. There is some suggestion that *Arachnida* and/or insects may play a role in the transmission of EBA and EAE in a herd.

The persistence of fecal agent results in carriers and may also explain how the disease persists in a herd.

**Diagnosis.** To make a positive diagnosis requires isolation and identification of *C. psittaci*. In making a clinical and pathological diagnosis differentiation from *Brucella abortus* is one principal concern. Granulomatous lesions may be present in any organ of EBA fetuses, and those in the kidney are similar to *Brucella* infection but the bronchopneumonia characteristic of fetal *Brucella* infection is lacking (3). Cultural examinations for *Brucella* and *Vibrio fetus* are indicated in herds troubled with abortions. The cultural smear and serological procedures previously described in this chapter should be utilized for the isolation or identification of *C. psittaci*.

**Control.** No vaccine is currently recommended for the control of this disease.
**The Disease in Man.** There is no evidence that the EBA strains have caused disease in man, but the possibility certainly exists.

## REFERENCES

1. Ball, Griner, and Carroll.   Am. Jour. Vet. Res., 1964, *25,* 291.
2. Eugster, Ball, Carroll and Storz.   6th Internatl. Mtg. Dis. Cattle, Philadelphia, Pa., 1971.
3. Jubb and Kennedy.   Pathology of domestic animals. 2d ed. Academic Press, New York and London, 1970.
4. Lincoln, Rivapien, Reed, Whiteman, and Chow.   Am. Jour. Vet. Res., 1969, *30,* 2105.
5. McKercher.   Jour. Am. Vet. Med. Assoc., 1969, *154,* 1192.
6. McKercher, Wada, Robinson, and Howarth.   Cornell Vet., 1966, *56,* 433.
7. Omuri, Ishü, and Matumoto.   Am. Jour. Vet. Res., 1960, *21,* 564.
8. Storz, Carroll, Ball, and Faulkner.   Am. Jour. Vet. Res., 1968, *29,* 549.

### Feline Pneumonitis

SYNONYMS:   Feline distemper, Feline influenza

This is an infection of the respiratory tract and conjunctiva of domesticated cats caused by *C. psittaci.* In 1944 Baker (1) showed that it was caused by an agent which could be transmitted from cat to cat and, experimentally, from cats to white mice. Later in the same year Hamre and Rake (6) showed that the agent belonged to the psittacosis-lymphogranuloma group. The disease is world-wide in distribution.

**Character of the Disease.** The disease is contagious. Affected animals usually do not die, but they become greatly debilitated and recovery is slow. In the beginning the disease is manifested by fever and inappetence. A mucopurulent discharge appears in the eyes and nose, and the animal coughs and sneezes a great deal. In most cases signs of pneumonia are not detected. The period of incubation varies from 6 to 10 days and the illness usually continues for about 2 weeks after which there is gradual improvement. Much weight is lost during the time when signs are most obvious. It is usually at least a month before the affected animals regain their original body weight. Unless complicated by other factors, the mortality is very slight.

Lesions are confined principally to the upper respiratory tract and the conjunctival membranes. The mucosa of these regions are reddened, swollen, and covered with exudate. Pneumonic lesions may be found when the animal is destroyed during the period of acute signs. These lung lesions disappear promptly as recovery begins. The consolidated portions are of a pinkish-gray color. The bronchial nodes are not noticeably enlarged. Histologic sections of the pneumonic areas show the alveoli to be filled with exudate consisting largely of monocytic and polymorphonuclear leukocytes. Occasional areas of necrosis are found, but in general the epithelium of the air passages is intact.

Elementary bodies are found in the cytoplasm of the monocytic cells. Cello (4) states that significant involvement of the lung is a rare occurrence in the cat.

**The Disease in Experimental Animals.** It is possible to transmit the chlamydiae of this disease to white mice, hamsters, guinea pigs, and rabbits by inoculating them with infective material intranasally while they are under light anesthesia, a technic that has been used successfully in work with the influenza viruses. Using doses 10 to 50 times greater than were needed to infect by the nasal route, Baker (1) was unable to infect mice by parenteral injection. Hamre and Rake (6), however, using much larger doses of yolk sac material, were successful in producing infections by intracerebral and intraperitoneal injection. The disease in adult guinea pigs and in rabbits is manifested by fever and pneumonia, but the animals do not die. Young guinea pigs, hamsters, and mice exhibit the same signs of illness, but the disease usually is fatal, mice dying on the 2nd or 3rd day, hamsters on the 3rd or 4th day, and the young guinea pigs on the 5th to 7th day.

**Properties of the Agent.** The agent of feline pneumonitis usually failed to pass Berkefeld N filters (1). Lung tissue contains bodies similar to those of *C. psittaci*, and large numbers could be produced in the yolk-sac membrane of developing chick embryos by inoculating virus into the sac. In the lungs of mice and hamsters, dense structures or plaques were recognized, which suggested that the agent was undergoing a developmental cycle, now recognized as characteristic of this group of chlamydial agents. Centrifugation at 10,000 rpm for 30 minutes caused sedimentation of large numbers of elementary bodies from suspensions derived from yolk sac membranes. The supernatant fluid lost most of its pathogenicity for mice, but this was regained when these suspensions were shaken and the elementary bodies were resuspended.

Hamre and Rake (6) have shown that the elementary bodies of feline pneumonitis, like those of several other diseases of this group, produce an endotoxin which in large doses ($>10^8$ $ID_{50}$) kills mice within 12 to 24 hours after intravenous injection.

The organism is destroyed when heated at 50 C for 30 minutes and at 60 C for 10 minutes. It is not completely inactivated, but its pathogenicity is reduced, by heating at 45 C for 30 minutes or 50 C for 10 minutes. Lung suspensions in 50 percent glycerol lose most of their disease-producing power in 30 days. Suspensions of yolk-sac material retain their activity for at least a week at room temperature, and for at least a month at 4 C. In the lyophilized state the agent retains its activity for 6 months or longer, but there is a significant loss in titer. Storage at $-70$ C preserves infectivity in most instances.

The group and specific antigens of the feline pneumonitis agent are located in the cell wall. When the cell walls of the feline agent are isolated by treatment of the elementary bodies with deoxycholate and trypsin, the group antigen is found in the deoxycholate extract and the specific antigens remained in the cell wall (7).

The hemagglutination of the feline pneumonitis agent agglutinates mouse erythrocytes only. Differential centrifugation shows that this activity is found in particles distinct from the elementary bodies.

Yerasimides described a strain isolated from a feline case of acute catarrhal conjunctivitis (10). Neutralization tests showed a one-sided relationship because antiserum to Baker's virus did not neutralize Yerasimides' isolate, but equal cross-neutralization occurred with antiserum produced by the Yerasimides isolate. These antiserums were specially prepared for these tests and these data demonstrate a close, but not complete, antigenic relationship.

Cats convalescent from feline pneumonitis infection do not always have demonstrable serum-neutralizing antibodies. Some cats do not have complement-fixing antibodies in their convalescent serum.

**Cultivation.** The agent is readily propagated in the yolk sac of developing chick embryos (1). Using eggs that had been incubated for 5 days, embryonic deaths were found to occur on the 2nd or 3rd day, and large numbers of elementary bodies were present in the cytoplasm of the cells from the yolk-sac membrane. Development of the organism also occurs when infective material is dropped on the chorioallantoic membrane of 10-day embryos. The membranes become thickened but the embryos are not affected by this method of inoculation.

**Immunity.** The degree and duration of immunity to the feline pneumonitis agent in the domestic cat has not been clearly established (2-4). The study of immunity in pathogen-free cats with various strains of the feline pneumonitis agent is needed to clarify the degree and duration of immunity in the domestic cat.

Based upon our meager knowledge of feline pneumonitis immunity in cats and also our general knowledge of immunity to psittacoid agents that produce disease in superficial tissues such as the conjunctiva and upper respiratory tract, it is reasonable to assume that the immunity of cats to the feline pneumonitis agent is partial and transitory. Apparent remissions and exacerbations of the disease in an individual animal may represent recovery and reinfection rather than activation of a latent infection (4). Then, too, some presumed recurrent infections of C. psittaci may be caused by a feline respiratory viral pathogen. We know that carriers of C. psittaci exist as well as viral carriers, such as feline caliciviruses and infectious rhinotracheitis virus, and this obviously leads to considerable confusion in diagnosis. Cello (4) has found that Mycoplasma infection of the conjunctival sac, nasal passages, and sinuses often develops in cats that have had chlamydial infections. This also could lead to the erroneous impression that the original infection had developed into a chronic state or that it had reoccurred unless agent isolation attempts were performed in a complete and precise manner.

**Immunization.** In experimental trials McKercher (8) felt that inactivated elementary body suspensions of the feline pneumonitis agent were relatively ineffective in producing immunity in kittens and in mice so this type of immunizing product has never been produced as an article of commerce.

A modified hen's-egg-propagated vaccine of a feline pneumonitis agent is available for the immunization of domestic cats in the United States. There is a variance of opinion regarding its efficacy and safety. At a recent American Veterinary Medical Association Colloquium on Selected Feline Infectious Diseases a panel of experts with representation from veterinary colleges, from the Veterinary Biologics Division, United States Department of Agriculture, from the veterinary biological industry, and from veterinary practitioners arrived at the following conclusions and recommendations (5). The currently available feline pneumonitis-modified live vaccine of chicken embryo origin stimulates complement-fixing antibodies in the domestic cat. The degree and duration of immunity of protection are unknown. The first vaccination usually is given at weaning time. Until more information is available on duration of immunity yearly vaccination is indicated if exposure is imminent. Care should be exercised in the use of this vaccine because ocular contamination may produce a local inflammation. There is only limited experimental data on the safety of the vaccine in pregnant queens so its use in pregnant cats is not recommended at this time. The panel recognized that a *C. psittaci* of cats is only one of a number of feline pathogens. Consequently, vaccine efficacy in a respiratory outbreak may be questioned at times.

**Transmission.** The natural disease in cats evidently is transmitted by direct

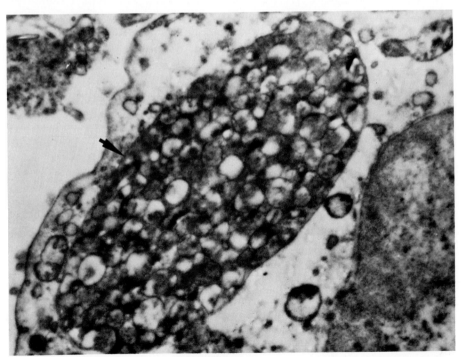

Fig. 146. Chlamydial inclusion in a mononuclear cell from joint of lamb with polyarthritis. X 20,000. (Courtesy of J. Storz.)

contact with infected secretions and by droplet infection. The disease in mice and guinea pigs will not transmit naturally from animal to animal.

**Diagnosis.** The clinical diagnosis is exceedingly difficult because many viruses have been isolated from respiratory cases with signs of illness similar to those described for feline pneumonitis. Only by isolation and identification is it possible to differentiate *C. psittaci* from other respiratory and conjunctival pathogens in the cat such as feline viral rhinotracheitis, feline caliciviruses, and feline reoviruses. Of course, concurrent infections with one or more of these pathogens can and does occur.

According to Cello (4) the large microcolonies (2 to 12 $\mu$ in diameter) with elementary bodies in various stages of development may be seen in Giemsa-stained conjunctival cells from cats infected with feline pneumonitis and represents a reliable and accurate diagnostic feature of infection.

**Control.** This can be best achieved by taking advantage of the feline pneumonitis agents' susceptibility to certain antibiotics. Tetracyclines will free diseased animals of infection, but the problem is to keep them free (4).

**The Disease in Man.** Schachter, Ostler, and Meyer (9) isolated a *Bedsonia* organism from conjunctival scrapings of a man with acute follicular keratoconjunctivitis. The patient owned two cats, one of which had clinical manifestations of feline pneumonitis. *Bedsonia* isolates from the two cats and their owners had the same characteristics as *C. psittaci*. The human isolate produced typical, acute, inclusion-positive conjunctivitis in experimental cats. This suggests that certain strains of feline and human *C. psittaci* with an affinity for the conjunctiva may produce disease in both humans and domestic cats.

**REFERENCES**

1. Baker.   Jour. Exp. Med., 1944, 79, 159.
2. Baker.   Jour. Am. Vet. Med. Assoc., Colloquium (Cornell Univ.), 1971, *158*, *941*.
3. Bittle.   *Ibid.*, 942.
4. Cello.   *Ibid.*, 932.
5. Expert Panel.   *Ibid.*, 835.
6. Hamre and Rake.   Jour. Inf. Dis., 1944, *74*, 206.
7. Jenkin, Ross, and Moulder.   Jour. Immunol., 1961, *86*, 123.
8. McKercher.   Cornell Univ. Thesis, 1949.
9. Schachter, Ostler, and Meyer.   Lancet, May 31, 1969, 1063.
10. Yerasimides.   Jour. Inf. Dis., 1960, *106*, 290.

**Pneumonitis in other Domestic Animals**

In general, the disease in sheep, cattle, goats, dogs, and mice is characterized by a conjunctival and nasal discharge, lethargy, anorexia, labored breathing, signs of pneumonia, and hyperthermia. Diarrhea may occur. The disease is rarely fatal and its severity is largely determined by secondary bacterial infections, but in some instances by other viral or *Mycoplasma* pathogens of the respiratory tract. A lethal pneumonia in animals as in mice can be produced by serial passage in young animals by the intranasal route.

The pulmonary lesions of experimental psittacoid infections are characterized by an intense neutrophilic response whereas viral infections are proliferative (4). Copious mucoid exudates of tracheobronchitis may be present with red, lobular consolidation in the anterior lobes. The histological lesion is an exudative bronchopneumonia of the bronchioles with extension into adjacent alveoli. Demonstration of elementary bodies in smears or in histological sections is difficult. Principal reliance on diagnosis should be placed on their demonstration in smears of yolk sac, of mouse lung, or of guinea pig peritoneal exudate of experimentally inoculated hosts; or on a rising serum titer utilizing paired serum samples.

The strains isolated from pneumonitis of a given animal species can produce experimental pneumonia by intratracheal inoculation in the homologous species. In some instances these strains can produce disease in another body system such as the genital tract of the homologous animal species. Occasionally, a strain that produces a characteristic disease in one species can do likewise in another mammal. One can only conclude that *C. psittaci* organisms contain specific antigen(s) in their structure that has a selective cell-tropism for one or more animal hosts and this dictates the nature of the disease. The carrier state persists in many animals and serves as a source of infection for susceptible animals.

An agent was described by McKercher (5) that causes pneumonia in sheep. A sheep pneumonic strain of *C. psittaci* studied by Studdert and McKercher (10) produces abortion in ewes but the disease differed from typical enzootic abortion of ewes. Dungworth (1) has produced experimental pneumonitis in lambs with an ovine abortion strain while experimental abortions in ewes with an ovine pneumonitis strain was reported by Page (8). Abortion and pneumonia in sheep are caused by similar chlamydial agents although some serotypic differences exist between ovine pneumonic and abortion strains. A pneumonic condition of goats in Japan may be caused by *C. psittaci*. The agent was transmissible to many other domestic animals.

Bovine strains of *C. psittaci* are responsible for pneumonitis in cattle of Czechoslovakia (3) and for pneumoenteritis in cattle of Italy (6) and Japan (7). The disease also has been described in the United States.

Fraser *et al.* (2) have described respiratory signs of illness in a dog that had access to an aviary in which psittacosis occurred. There is strong evidence that the dog as well as three human beings associated with the aviary had a psittacosis disease. *C. psittaci* may also cause nervous manifestations in conjunction with pneumonic signs, or chronic keratitis as a single entity.

Maierhofer and Storz (9) described clinical and serological responses in dogs inoculated parenterally with a chlamydial strain isolated from a case of ovine polyarthritis. The affected dogs had fever, anorexia, signs of depression, pneumonia, incoordination, muscle and joint pain, and diarrhea. The chlamydial agent was isolated from somatic organs, including brain and portions of intestinal tract and also from joints. CF group-specific antibodies were produced with maximum titers 21 to 28 days after inoculation and were still detectable 1 year later. At a local dog pound (Ft. Collins, Colorado) over 50 percent of 119 dogs contained group-specific chlamydial antibodies, with greatest incidence in older male dogs.

## REFERENCES

1. Dungworth. Jour. Comp. Path. and Therap., 1963, 73, 68.
2. Fraser, Norval, Withers, and Gregor. Vet. Rec., 1969, 85, 54.
3. Gmitter. Sborn. Ces. Akad. Ved. Vet. Med., 1960, 5, 475.
4. Jubb and Kennedy. Pathology of domestic animals. 2d ed. Academic Press, New York and London, 1970.
5. McKercher. Science, 1953, 115, 543.
6. Messieri. Atti. Soc. Ital. Sci. Vet., 1959, 8, 702.
7. Omori, Ishii, and Matumoto. Am. Jour. Vet. Res., 1960, 21, 564.
8. Page. Ibid., 1966, 27, 397.
9. Maierhofer and Storz. Ibid., 1969, 30, 1961.
10. Studdert and McKercher. Res. Vet. Sci., 1968, 9, 48.

### Ovine Polyarthritis

Polyarthritis in sheep was first observed in Wisconsin by Mendlowski and Segre in 1957 (1) and further described as an arthritic disease caused by a chlamydial agent (2). The disease was found also by Storz et al. (5) to be widespread in the intermountain area of the United States.

**Character of the Disease.** The main habitat for the polyarthritic agents of sheep may be the intestinal tract. Infections producing polyarthritis are systemic and *Chlamydia* can be isolated from many tissues.

The disease affects lambs up to 6 months of age. The principal feature of the disease is lameness and a few animals become permanently lame. There is also depression, reluctance to move, and a conjunctivitis. Tetanuslike spasms may be occasionally seen. The morbidity is high and the mortality 3 to 7 percent as a rule.

At necropsy, a constant finding is a serous to serofibrinous or fibrinous synovitis. The subcutaneous and adjacent periarticular tissues are edematous with clear fluid with extension around tendon sheaths. Surrounding muscles are hyperemic and edematous with petechial hemorrhages in the fascia. The viscera may show change associated with systemic infection with histologic changes of inflammation of soft tissues, including the central nervous system.

**The Disease in Experimental Animals.** The experimental disease in 5-to-6-month-old lambs is similar to the naturally occurring disease (6).

The sheep polyarthritis agent produced a severe polyarthritis in the leg joints of sheep and in the hock joint of turkeys (3). The sheep polyarthritic agent failed to affect mice inoculated intraperitoneally or pigeons inoculated intracerebrally but caused disease in guinea pigs inoculated intraperitoneally. Both the pigeon ornithosis and sheep polyarthritic agents produced aerosacculitis in intraperitoneally inoculated turkeys. These observations may be important to our understanding of natural interspecies transfer.

**Properties of the Agent.** The isolates of *C. psittaci* from the intestinal tract and affected joints of polyarthritic lambs are antigenically identical but differed from EAE isolates from the same flock or other flocks with EAE (4). All strains of ovine polyarthritis chylamidae seem to be antigenically identical (4).

The organism is readily cultivated in the embryonated hen's egg (2). The guinea pig, turkeys, and lambs readily grow the ovine polyarthritis psittacoid agents (3).

**Immunity.** Convalescent sheep that are injected with ovine polyarthritis strains of *C. psittaci* do not develop polyarthritis although they harbor the organism 21 days after challenge (6).

The natural disease is limited to lambs, so it is a self-limiting disease in this respect. Whether this is an age factor or a very common disease with ensuing protection after recovery is unknown, but it is probably the latter.

**Diagnosis.** Microscopic examination of wet mounts of joint exudates with a phase-contrast microscope often reveal numerous mononuclear cells whose cytoplasm contains elementary bodies. As this is a systemic infection the organism can be isolated from visceral tissues, feces, or from joint exudate in the hen's egg, guinea pig, or turkeys.

The psittacoid organisms are principally responsible for polyarthritis in lambs although *Mycoplasma* have been incriminated.

**Control.** Procedures for control are still being sought.

**The Disease in Man.** Caution must be exercised especially because the turkey can be readily infected with the ovine polyarthritis agent and many human cases are derived from infected turkeys.

### REFERENCES

1. Mendlowski and Segre. Am. Jour. Vet. Res., 1960, *21*, 68.
2. Mendlowski, Kraybill, and Segre. *Ibid.*, 74.
3. Page. *Ibid.*, 1966, *27*, 397.
4. Storz. Jour. Comp. Path., 1966, *76*, 351.
5. Storz, McKercher, Howarth, and Staub. Jour. Am. Vet. Med. Assoc., 1960, *137*, 509.
6. Storz, Shupe, Marriott, and Thornley. Jour. Inf. Dis., 1965, *115*, 9.

### Conjunctivitis

Various colonies of guinea pigs are chronically infected with *C. psittaci* that produce conjunctivitis. The guinea pig organisms also are transmitted transovarially (2).

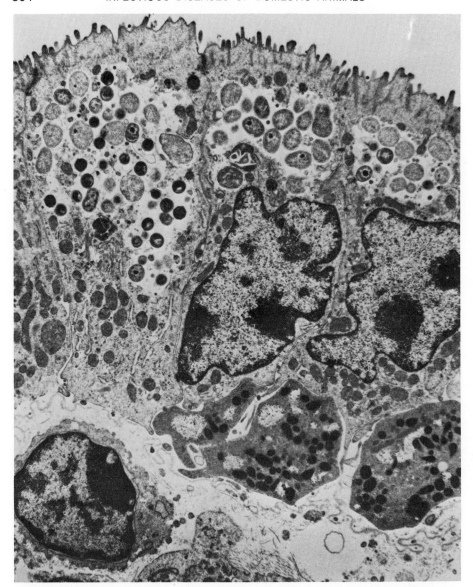

Fig. 147. *Chlamydia*-infected enterocytes of a calf with dense-centered, infectious forms; intermediate and reticulated developmental forms. Microvilli and terminal webb of enterocytes are altered X 15,000. (Courtesy of Doughri, Altera, and Storz.)

C. *psittaci* has been isolated from diseased conjunctiva of hamsters (1). Because guinea pigs and hamsters are used for diagnostic and research studies of C. *psittaci* the worker must be aware of possible latent psittacoid infections in colonies of these species.

Follicular conjunctivitis, sometimes with complicating eye lesions, occurs commonly in sheep. Storz *et al.* (3) have isolated *C. psittaci* from sheep with follicular conjunctivitis in 3 different herds. (fig. 148) The isolates were specifically related to strains of *C. psittaci* causing polyarthritis. Some of the sheep with follicular conjunctivitis also had polyarthritic signs. Parenteral injection of conjunctival *C. psittaci* resulted in follicular conjunctivitis and polyarthritis in lambs.

Conjunctivitis occurs as a disease manifestation of pneumonitis in various domestic animals. These were described earlier in the section under the heading "Pneumonitis."

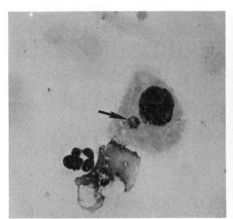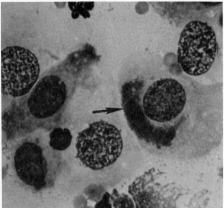

*Fig. 148.* Early (*left*) and mature (*right*) chlamydial inclusions in conjunctival cells of infected sheep. Giemsa stain. X 1,000. (Courtesy J. Storz.)

**REFERENCES**

1. Murray.  Jour. Inf. Dis., 1964, *114*, 1.
2. Storz.  *Ibid.*, 1961, *109*, 129.
3. Storz, Pierson, Marriott, and Chow.  Proc. Soc. Exp. Biol. and Med., 1967, *125*, 857.

**Bovine Polyarthritis**

Polyarthritis in calves has been recognized for years. In this species it is caused by certain bacteria, *Mycoplasma,* and *Chlamydia.* Bovine psittacoid polyarthritis occurs in the United States.

**Character of the Disease.** Chlamydial infection in calves is severe, causing a high mortality. Some affected calves are weak at birth implying intrauterine infection. The infant calves have a fever and develop anorexia, reluctance to move or stand, and swelling of the joints in 2 to 3 days and death ensues 2 to 12 days after appearance of signs of illness. The limb joints are most severely affected with the synovial structures distended with a turbid yellowish fluid and strands of fibrin adhering to the synovium. The surrounding subcutaneous and adjacent periarticular tissues are edematous with an extension around the tendon sheaths. Muscles around the joints are edematous and hyperemic with petechial hemorrhages in the fascia. The visceral organs may show changes attributable to systemic infection.

The natural and experimental disease in calves is similar (1). In the experimental disease of calves, chlamydiae are recovered from the blood within 18 hours after intra-articular inoculation. The *C. psittaci* organisms persist in the blood for 6 days. The organism also is readily isolated from the joint fluids in the embryonated hen's egg by the yolk-sac route.

**Properties of the Agent.** The bovine polyarthritic psittacoid strains are antigenically related to each other and to the ovine polyarthritic psittacoid strains, but apparently are different from epizootic bovine-abortion psittacoid strains (1). There is also a close relationship between one bovine polyarthritis psittacoid strain and one guinea pig psittacoid strain that causes inclusion conjunctivitis and systemic infection.

The guinea pig and embryonated hen's eggs are excellent experimental hosts.

**Immunity.** Little is known about the immunity but one probably expects protection against this systemic disease if the calf recovers from polyarthritic psittacoid infection.

**Diagnosis.** The same diagnostic procedures apply for ovine and bovine psittacoid polyarthritis. In bovine polyarthritis other infectious agents must be sought as well. Certain bacterial organisms such as *Escherichia coli* and streptococci cause polyarthritis in calves and occasionally the former may be present together with *C. psittaci* in the joint exudate. *Mycoplasma* frequently cause polyarthritis in calves but cytopathogenic viruses have not been isolated (2).

**Control.** No effective measures presently exist.

**The Disease in Man.** There are no reports of this agent causing disease in humans but caution should be exercised in handling cases of polyarthritis in calves.

**REFERENCES**

1.  Storz, Shupe, Smart, and Thornley.   Am. Jour. Vet. Res., 1966, 27, 987.
2.  Storz, Smart, Marriott, and Davis.   *Ibid.*, 633.

**Enteritis**

In 1951 York and Baker (4) described an agent isolated from the intestinal tract of calves, which they named *Miyagawanella bovis* and later suggested it may produce enteritis in colostrum-deprived calves. *C. psittaci* is commonly present in the feces of a large proportion of animals in infected herds, and a high percentage of herds in New York State harbor this fecal organism and also have antibodies to this agent. In all likelihood a comparable herd situation exists in other states of the United States and also in other countries of the world. Because there is a close antigenic relationship between many intestinal strains of *C. psittaci* and with many strains that cause EAE, EBA, or ovine and bovine psittacoid polyarthritis, the intestinal-carrier strains may explain, in part, the epidemiology of psittacoid disease in domestic ruminants.

Pneumoenteritis of dairy calves is a very important disease and one of the limiting factor in a successful vealing operation. In all likelihood there is no single pathogenic organism responsible for this disease. Certain respiratory viruses may be responsible and pneumoenteritis reputedly also occurs as a psittacoid disease in cattle of Italy (2) and of Japan (3).

In 1961 a large number of muskrats (*Ondatra zibethicus*) and snowshoe hares (*Lepus americanus*) in Saskatchewan, Canada, died as the result of a chlamydial disease (1). This isolate of *C. psittaci* was highly virulent for the snowshoe hares and moderately virulent for the muskrats.

In snowshoe hares the disease is characterized as an acute, febrile, emaciating, enteric illness. The invariably fatal course is short with terminal signs of opisthotonos, convulsions, and hypoglycemia. The highest titers of *C. psittaci* were found in the liver and spleen where the most marked pathological changes occurred. The organisms were recovered from female rabbit ticks (*Hemaphysalis leporispalustris*) engorging on experimentally infected snowshoe hares.

In the muskrat a febrile illness was observed, and the degree of illness was influenced by the presence of specific antibodies at the time of exposure. In fatal cases a wide-spread focal necrosis of the liver was observed. The organism was readily isolated from the liver. In chronic infections the agent was recovered from the brain and small intestine up to 96 days postinfection. Specific antibodies were found in 11.8 percent of 127 sera of wild muskrats trapped either in Saskatchewan, Canadian Arctic, and Wisconsin. The infection occurs naturally in muskrats in Canada and the United States and this animal serves as one means of maintaining the agent in nature.

## REFERENCES

1. Iversen, Spalatin, Fraser, Hanson, and Berman. Canad. Jour. Comp. Med., 1970, *34*, 80.
2. Messieri. Atti. Soc. Ital. Sci. Vet., 1959, 8, 702.
3. Omori, Ishii, and Matumoto. Am. Jour. Vet. Res., 1960, *21*, 564.
4. York and Baker. Jour. Exp. Med., 1951, *93*, 587.

## Cat-Scratch Disease in Man

SYNONYMS: Cat-scratch fever, Nonbacterial regional lymphadenitis

This is an ulceroglandular disease of man. It does not affect any animals, so far as is known. It is included here because many infections of man appear to be associated with scratches from the household cat. It also occurs when such contact has not occurred. The cat may be a mechanical carrier of the infecting agent, or perhaps the injury by a cat scratch may incite a latent agent of humans such as a herpeslike virus or *Chlamydia psittaci*. Possibly rodents, or other natural prey of the cat, are the original source of the infection.

The disease affects human males and females alike, and all age groups may be involved. Young people appear to be infected more often than older, but this may be because of greater exposure.

In its typical form the disease in man presents an initial skin lesion at the site of the scratch, bite, or abrasions caused by other experiences. Initially this seems to be an ordinary wound infection that occurs within a few days after the infliction of the wound. The local lesion heals slowly, assuming the form of a local ulcer. Two or 3 weeks after the local wound develops the regional lymph glands swell and become painful. Fever and constitutional symptoms usually appear at this time. The nodes may eventually become reduced in size and heal, but in most instances they remain enlarged for a long time. Suppuration occurs, and the nodes have to be lanced, or they will rupture and discharge a thick pus. In rare circumstances, the patient has nervous manifestations characterized by a rapid recovery from encephalitis (8).

Clinical diagnosis of the disease presents some difficulties. Of assistance has been the use of an intradermal test, utilizing aspirated, heat-treated pus as antigen (1). McGovern and his group found that, of 120 persons tested with such an antigen, two out of three reacted when there was a history of an attack of disease sometime in the past. Among 99 persons who had no history of an attack there were 10 reactors. Four of these were members of families in which there had been cases of the disease. A group of the personnel of the hospital were studied. Of the animal house personnel 22 percent gave positive reactions, whereas of the general personnel the percentage was 4.5. It was concluded that there probably were appreciable numbers of undiagnosed, or perhaps inapparent, cases and that the disease probably was much more common than had been supposed.

McGovern *et al.* (5) made a comprehensive study of the disease in patients and animal house attendants. Neither his group nor many others who have worked with this disease were able to isolate any disease-producing agent, but McGovern *et al.* transmitted the infection to human volunteers and monkeys by inoculation with pus from the abscessed nodes. Support for the viral nature of the causative agent was supplied by Dodd and co-workers (2), Manning and Reid (6), and Kalter *et al.* (4). Dodd *et al.* showed that the pus from cases of this disease had the property of agglutinating the red blood cells of rabbits, and that this property was neutralized by the serum of a human case and also by the serum of rabbits prepared by several injections of cat scratch fever pus. The hemagglutinating agent was described in a later paper as a herpeslike virus that lacked cytopathogenicity (9). Kalter, Kim, and Heberling (4) described the presence of numerous herpes-like virus particles in electron microscope photographs of biopsied lymph node material from eight persons with the clinical diagnosis of cat-scratch disease. Attempts to isolate a herpesviruslike agent from this material has not succeeded (3). Manning and Reid conducted studies on patients suffering from this disease, using the complement-fixation test with a psittacosis antigen. Sixty percent of 10 cases with a histologic diagnosis of cat-scratch fever, and 23 percent of 35 persons having positive skin tests fixed complement. No positives were found among 44 persons who were negative to the skin test. These results support previous findings by Mollaret (7) indicating that the causative agent probably belongs to the *Chlamydia* group. Most individuals think in the terms of a single etiology for this disease but it is possible that more than one pathogenic organism may be responsible for the entity that we call *cat-scratch disease*.

## REFERENCES

1. Daniels and MacMurray. Ann. Int. Med., 1952, 37, 697.
2. Dodd, Graber, and Anderson. Proc. Soc. Exp. Biol. and Med., 1959, *102*, 556.
3. Kalter. Personal communication, 1970.
4. Kalter, Kim, and Heberling. Nature, 1969, *224*, 190.
5. McGovern, Kunz, and Blodgett. New Eng. Jour. Med., 1955, *252*, 166.
6. Manning and Reid. Am. Jour. Clin. Path., 1958, *29*, 430.
7. Mollaret. Comp. rend. Soc. Biol. (Paris), 1950, *144*, 1493.
8. Pollen. Neurology, 1968, *18*, 644.
9. Turner, Bigley, Dodd, and Anderson. Jour. Bact., 1960, *80*, 430.

# XXXV | The *Bartonella* Group (*Bartonellaceae*)

Members of this group cause bartonellosis in man and the lower animals. The organisms show a marked preference for intracellular parasitism and both in this respect and in morphology seem to be closely related to the rickettsiae. They are not, however, classed with the rickettsiae but probably fall somewhere between those organisms and the bacteria.

The members of the family *Bartonellaceae* are classifed as small, often pleomorphic, rod-shaped, coccoid, ring-shaped, filamentous, and beaded microorganisms that stain lightly with aniline dyes and are Gram-negative. They stain deeply with Giemsa's stain. They are parasites of the erythrocytes and in some cases are transmitted by insect vectors. Within the erythrocytes they stain solidly, whereas protozoa that parasitize red cells are differentiated, by staining, into a nucleus and cytoplasm.

*Bergey's Manual* lists four genera in the family *Bartonellaceae* as follows:

Genus 1.   *Bartonella*—Parasites of the erythrocytes and of fixed tissues in man.

Genus 2.   *Grahamella*—Parasites of the erythrocytes of lower animals which do not increase on splenectomy and are not eradicated by arsenical compounds. They are nonpathogenic.

Genus 3.   *Hemobartonella*—Parasites of the erythrocytes of lower animals which increase in susceptible animals on splenectomy and are eradicated by arsenical compounds.

Genus 4.   *Eperythrozoon*—Blood parasites, found on the erythrocytes and in the plasma of lower animals. They appear as rings, coccoids, and short rods. Splenectomy activates latent infection.

810

Peters and Wigand (20) question this classification. They agree that *Bartonella bacilliformis* should be classified with the bacteria because of typical characteristics, including small rod-shaped forms; ability to grow on culture media and propagate by binary fission; possession of unipolar flagella, retracted cytoplasm, and bacterialike cell walls; and typical behavior in serological tests. On the other hand, they claim that hemobartonellae and eperythrozoa possess no such criteria. These organisms occur mostly as coccoid and ring-shaped forms. They are nonmotile and do not multiply outside the host's blood. They lack structural details and cell walls like those of bacteria. Furthermore, they are nearly alike in every respect that it is questioned whether or not two generic names are justified for them.

### Bartonella bacilliformis

This organism causes human bartonellosis, which was shown by Carrión, through self-inoculation, to be two stages or manifestations (*Oroya fever* and *verruga peruana*) of a single disease now commonly known as *Carrion's disease*. The first stage (Oroya fever) is characterized by fever and a severe progressive anemia. Although this stage sometimes proves to be fatal it may also be so mild that the patient does not notice it. In a recognized attack of Oroya fever convalescence is accompanied in 2 to 8 weeks by wartlike eruptions (verruga peruana). In the second stage of the disease the case mortality is low and the eruptions persist for several months.

The etiologic agent is a small, pleomorphic bacillus that was observed by Barton in 1905 and named *Bartonella bacilliformis* by Strong, Tyzzer, and Sellards (26). It can be cultivated from the blood in Oroya fever and from the local lesions in verruga peruana. Apparently the microorganism is carried by sandflies, of which *Phlebotomus verrucarum* is the most important species. It should not be confused with sandfly fever (*Phlebotomus* fever), which appears to be a virus disease of man also transmitted by sandflies. Carrion's disease occurs in the Andean Cordillera of Peru, Ecuador, and Colombia (21). This strictly regional occurrence of the disease may be due to limited habitats of the transmitting sandfly.

Experimental animals, with the exception of monkeys, are resistant to infection with *Bart. bacilliformis*.

### Grahamella

These are parasites occurring within the erythrocytes of the lower mammals. Morphologically they bear a resemblance to *Bartonella*, but they are less pleomorphic, more plump, and more suggestive of true bacteria. They are Gram-negative, non-acid-fast, and nonmotile. They can be cultivated on artificial media. Splenectomy has no effect on the source of infection except in rats. They are nonpathogenic and not affected by arsenicals. They cause grahamellosis of rodents.

### Hemobartonella muris (Bartonella muris)

This organism was first described by Mayer (15) in Germany in 1921. It was found in laboratory rats that had been infected with trypanosomes. The organism, like the previous one, is found in and on the surface of the red blood cells. According to Peters and Wigand (20), *H. muris* when stained by Giemsa stain shows mostly coccoid forms in contrast to *Bart. bacilliformis* which shows mostly rod shapes. Electron microscopy studies of *H. muris* do not show structural details, cell walls like those of bacteria, or flagella. Thin sections reveal a spherical or ellipsoidal agent, 350 to 700 m$\mu$ in size (27). It is nonmotile and increases by binary fission, but apparently does not multiply outside the host's blood. It is transmitted by lice and is ubiquitous in geographic distribution. It usually will not cause infection in rats unless the animals are infected with trypanosomiasis, are given certain blood-destroying poisons, or are splenectomized. Of great interest is the fact that rats in many parts of the world, including the United States, carry this organism latently. This can be demonstrated by the fact that removal of the spleen often leads to prompt development of the disease. It appears that the spleen, possibly through a protective activity of its reticuloendothelial system, is able to hold the disease in abeyance. The disease is manifested by a rapidly developing anemia and by the appearance of the organism in the blood. The animals may die or they may recover after a few days. Other animals susceptible to infection with *H. muris* are mice, hamsters, and rabbits.

### Hemobartonella canis (Bartonella canis)

In 1928 Kikuth (10), in Germany, described an organism similar to the other *Hemobartonella* which he believed to be the cause of an infectious anemia of dogs. Workers in other countries have, more recently, seen the same organ-

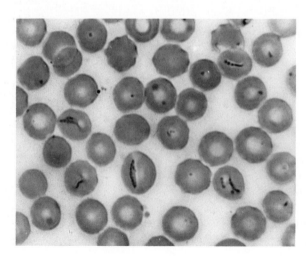

*Fig. 149.* Giemsa stain of blood film from a dog showing *Hemobartonella canis.* X 1,000. (Courtesy M. M. Benjamin and W. V. Lumb, *Jour. Am. Vet. Med. Assoc.*)

ism. None has succeeded in cultivating it, however; hence its relationship to the other *Hemobartonella* has not been proved. The disease appears to be rather mild. Knutti and Hawkins (11), in the United States (1935), encountered the condition in splenectomized, bile-fistula dogs. Spontaneous periods of anemia, associated with excess bile production, were regularly associated, in some dogs, with the appearance of *Hemobartonella*like bodies in the blood. Simple splenectomy would not regularly produce the disease, but the inoculation of dog's blood containing the *Hemobartonella* into such animals was regularly followed by anemia and the appearance of the parasite.

### Hemobartonella felis

Feline infectious anemia was first described by Flint and Moss (7) in 1953. It is an acute, subacute, or chronic infectious disease of cats. When acute, it is characterized by high temperature, a marked hemolytic anemia, anorexia, depression, and rapid loss of weight. Blood smears offer the best diagnostic aid. *H. felis* appears as fine round dots, sometimes as fairly large cocci, and at other times as short rods. Organisms are seldom seen in the plasma, and when they do appear unattached to red cells it is probable that they have just been released by a disintegrating cell. Although the disease was not recognized in the United States until 1953, it appears to be widespread.

### Hemobartonella bovis (Bartonella bovis)

Donatien and Lestoquard (5) reported *Hemobartonella* in the blood of cattle in 1934. Lotze and Yiengst (14) found similar forms in American cattle in 1942. Since they were found in animals infected with anaplasmosis, the American workers were not certain that they did not represent a stage of the life cycle of *Anaplasma marginale*. Later Lotze and Bowman (12) found them in an anaplasma-free calf shortly after it had been splenectomized. It is clear, therefore, that *H. bovis* is not necessarily associated with anaplasmosis. Usually only a very few parasites are found in the blood, but they may become much more numerous during the incubation period following inoculation with anaplasms. There is no evidence, at present, that *H. bovis* is of any economic importance.

*Hemobartonella* are also found in goats (16), but appear to be of little economic importance.

### Hemobartonella tyzzeri

This organism was found by Weinman and Pinkerton (28) in splenectomized guinea pigs from Colombia. The parasite could be transmitted to splenectomized *Hemobartonella*-free guinea pigs by intraperitoneal injection (Groot, 9).

### Eperythrozoon coccoides

This organism was described in 1928 by Schilling and by Dinger (4) a blood parasite of mice. The characteristics of *H. muris* and *E. coccoides* correspond in nearly every respect, there being some trifling differences in morphology. Giemsa stains of both organisms generally show a preponderance of coccoid forms for *H. muris* and a majority of ring-shaped bodies for *E. coccoides*. Like *H. muris* this organism is nonmotile and appears not to multiply outside the host blood. It is ubiquitous in distribution and is transmitted by lice. Rats, hamsters, and rabbits are also subject to infection.

Ott and Stauber (19) observed mice that were infected with malaria and also with *E. coccoides*. In these mice the malarial infection progressed at a low-level, chronic course producing infrequent deaths. When the eperythrozoa were eliminated through treatment with oxophenarsine hydrochloride (arsenoxide), the malarial infection assumed an acute course always ending in death.

### Eperythrozoon suis

In 1950 Splitter and Williamson (25) found an *Eperythrozoon* in swine associated with a clinical entity known as *anaplasmosislike disease* or *icteroanemia*. They saw the organism in three separate outbreaks. Since that time epery-

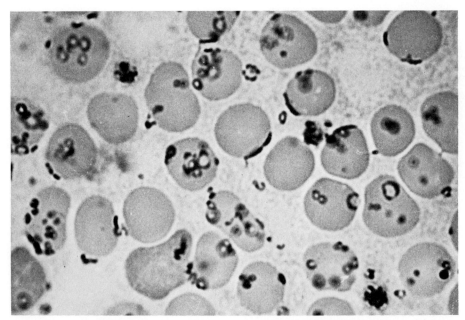

Fig. 150. Eperythrozoon suis in the blood of an infected pig. X 2,500. (Courtesy A. Savage and J. M. Isa, *Cornell Vet.*)

throzoonosis has been found to be rather widespread in the United States (1, 3). The causative agent has been named *E. suis,* and a second species which apparently is a nonpathogenic blood parasite was named *E. parvum.* The latter organism is a common parasite of swine in the Midwest. *E. suis* also shows a high incidence rate in the blood of swine in enzootic areas. The majority of young pigs acquire infection during the summer months and remain immune, latent, clinically unrecognized carriers. The clinical disease depends upon the number of parasites which develop in the blood following infection. In the majority of swine light parasitic attacks take place and cause no visible damage. Pigs heavily infected with *E. suis* show inappetence, lassitude, weakness, anemia, and often icterus. Diagnosis is made by finding small ring-shaped bodies in or on the erythrocytes of diseased pigs. Splitter (24) has found a complement-fixation test useful in diagnosing eperythrozoonosis in swine. He employs an antigen prepared from $CO_2$-precipitated erythrocytes heavily parasitized with *E. suis.*

The exact mode of transmission is not known, but insect vectors such as flies and lice and believed to be concerned. Berrier and Gouge (2) have reported a case of *in utero* transmission.

### Eperythrozoon wenyoni

Neitz (18) reported the presence of this organism in cattle in South Africa, and Lotze and Yiengst (13) observed eperythrozoonosis in the United States in cattle experimentally infected with *Anaplasma marginale.* The economic importance of these organisms is unknown, but they are believed to be important at times in calves. Finerty *et al.* (6) prepared an antigen by ultrasonic disruption of purified suspensions of *E. wenyoni* and claimed that it was specific when used in passive hemagglutination tests for detecting naturally occurring eperythrozoonosis in calves.

### Eperythrozoon ovis

Neitz (17) reports that this organism provokes illness in sheep that are not splenectomized. It is a disease of lambs with considerable mortality and showing postmortem features of anemia, enlarged soft spleen, and an excess of pericardial fluid. Neitz also states that antimony-arsenic compounds are valuable in treating the infection.

In Southern Australia it appears that the majority of anemic conditions of young sheep and the majority of outbreaks of ill-thrift are caused by *E. ovis* infection and that the severity of the disease may depend on complicating factors (23).

### Eperythrozoon felis

In 1959 Seamer and Douglas (22) described a new blood parasite in cats in England and called it *E. felis.* Because the differences between *Hemobarto-*

*nella* and *Eperythrozoon* are very minor, it is possible that they were dealing with feline infectious anemia.

### Chemotherapy

Organic arsenical substances, such as neoarsphenamine and arsenic-antimony compounds, are not effective in bartonellosis, but have a marked influence on hemobartonellosis and eperythrozoonosis. All three diseases are refractory to sulfa compounds. Penicillin, streptomycin, and chloromycetin show a curative effect on bartonellosis. *H. muris* and *E. coccoides* resist penicillin and streptomycin, but are quite sensitive to aureomycin, terramycin, and tetracycline. Chloromycetin has little, if any effect (20). Gledhil *et al.* (8) studied a mouse colony that had a history of long-established infection with *E. coccoides* and claimed that they were able to eliminate the organisms by regular insecticidal treatments designed to reduce infestation with lice and fleas.

### REFERENCES

1. Adams, Lyles, and Cockrell.   Jour. Am. Vet. Med. Assoc., 1959, *135*, 226.
2. Berrier and Gouge.   *Ibid.*, 1954, 98, 124.
3. Biberstein, Barr, Larrow, and Roberts.   Cornell Vet., 1956, *46*, 288.
4. Dinger.   Centrbl. f. Bakt. Abt. I. Orig., 1929, *113*, 503.
5. Donatien and Lestoquard.   Bul. Soc. Path. Exot., 1934, *27*, 652.
6. Finerty, Hidalgo, and Dimopoullos.   Am. Jour. Vet. Res., 1968, *30*, 43.
7. Flint and Moss.   Jour. Am. Vet. Med. Assoc., 1953, *22*, 45.
8. Gledhill, Niven, and Seamer.   Jour. Hyg., (London), 1965, *63*, 73.
9. Groot.   Proc. Soc. Exp. Biol. and Med., 1942, *51*, 279.
10. Kikuth.   Klin. Wchnschr., 1928, 7, 1729.
11. Knutti and Hawkins.   Jour. Exp. Med., 1935, *61*, 115.
12. Lotze and Bowman.   Proc. Helminth. Soc. Washington, 1942, 9, 71.
13. Lotze and Yiengst.   North Am. Vet., 1941, *22*, 345.
14. Lotze and Yiengst.   Am. Jour. Vet. Res., 1942, 8, 312.
15. Mayer.   Arch. Schiffs-u, Trophyg., 1921, *25*, 150.
16. Mukherjee.   Indian Vet. Jour., 1952, *28*, 343.
17. Neitz.   Onderstepoort Jour. Vet. Sci. and Anim. Indus., 1937, 9, 9.
18. *Ibid.*, 1940, *14*, 9.
19. Ott and Stauber.   Science, 1967, *155*, 1546.
20. Peters and Wigand.   Bact. Rev., 1955, *19*, 150.
21. Schultz.   Am. Jour. Trop. Med and Hyg., 1968, *17*, 503.
22. Seamer and Douglas.   Vet. Rec., 1959, *71*, 405.
23. Sheriff, Clapp, and Reid.   Austral. Vet. Jour., 1966, *42*, 169.
24. Splitter.   Jour. Am. Vet. Med. Assoc., 1958, *132*, 47.
25. Splitter and Williamson.   *Ibid.*, 1950, *116*, 360.
26. Strong, Tyzzer, and Sellards.   Jour. Am. Med. Assoc., 1915, *64*, 806.
27. Tanka, Hall, Sheffield, and Moore.   Jour. Bact., 1965, *90*, 1735.
28. Weinman and Pinkerton.   Ann. Trop. Med. and Parasitol., 1938, *32*, 215.

# XXXVI | The Viruses

Quite understandably the early bacteriologists held the belief that all contagious and infectious diseases were caused by bacteria, except for a few which were known to be caused by higher fungi and protozoa. But time showed that bacteria and other known disease-producing agents could not be identified with many diseases. Eventually it was learned that some of these infective fluids retained their ability to produce disease after they had been forced through fine-pored clay filters that retained all ordinary bacteria. This indicated that agents smaller than bacteria were capable of causing infectious diseases. For more than 40 years (1892 to 1935) this was about all that was known of such agents, which became known as filter-passing or filterable viruses. The adjective is not used now because it is known that not all viruses are small enough to be filterable and some well-known bacteria can be made to pass through the so-called *bacteria-proof filters*. The word virus now connotes a series of characteristics among which filter passing is only one probable feature.

The first known virus was that of the tobacco mosaic disease. It was demonstrated by a Russian, Iwanowski (26), in 1892. In 1898 Loeffler and Frosch (28), in Germany, demonstrated that foot-and-mouth disease of cattle was caused by an agent that readily passed bacteria-proof filters and could not be seen with the microscope. It was the first animal virus discovered. In the same year Sanarelli (36) proved that a highly contagious rabbit tumor (myxomatosis) was caused by a virus. In the years that have elapsed since these early discoveries, many viruses and virus diseases have been found or differentiated.

In 1920 D'Herelle (22) described the first of a series of viruses which he named *bacteriophages* because they parasitized bacterial cells, causing them to swell and burst. The ease with which these agents could be studied greatly stimulated the study of viruses, and many of the observations on bacteriophages have been applicable to the viruses which infect plant and animal cells. An even greater stimulus to the study of viruses was given in 1935 by the announcement by Stanley (38) that he had been successful in extracting a crystalline nucleoprotein that had all the properties of the virus from tobacco plants affected with mosaic disease. The virus research field has been very active and productive in recent years because of the introduction of a number of new technics. A new science of *virology* has been formed, manned by individuals who have training in biochemistry, genetics, microbiology, biophysics, statistics, and/or pathology.

## Terms Commonly Used by Virologists

*Virion:* The complete infective virus particle; may be identical to nucleocapsid; more complex virions include the nucleocapsid plus the surrounding envelope.

*Capsid;* The protein shell which encloses the nucleic acid core (genome).

*Nucleocapsid:* The capsid together with the enclosed nucleic acid.

*Structure units:* The basic units of similar structure in the capsid; may be individual polypeptides.

*Capsomeres:* Morphologic units seen on the surfaces of isometric virus particles. They represent clusters of structure units.

*Primary nucleic acid structure:* The sequence of bases in the nucleic acid chain.

*Secondary nucleic acid structure:* The spatial arrangement of the complete nucleic acid chain. For example, is the nucleic acid single- or double-stranded, circular or linear in conformation, or branched or unidirectional?

*Tertiary nucleic acid structure:* Refers to fine spatial detail in the helix such as super-coiling, breakage points, deletions, gaps, catenation, and regions of strand separation.

*Envelope:* The outer coat some viruses acquire as they penetrate or are budded from the nuclear or cytoplasmic membrane. Envelopes always contain altered host-cell membrane components.

*Peplomers:* Morphological units composed of structure units that are embedded in the envelope.

*Complementation:* A general term to describe situations where mixed infections result in enhanced yields of one or both viruses in the mixture.

*Translation:* The mechanism by a particular base sequence in the nucleic acid results in the production of a specific amino acid sequence in a protein.

*Transcription:* The means by which specific information encoded in a nucleic acid chain is transferred to messenger RNA.

*Transcapsidation:* A form of complementation where two viruses "hybridize;" for example, adenovirus capsid is spontaneously transferred to $SV_{40}$ nucleoids (or DNA).

*Helper virus:* Certain viruses are defective and require a closely related "helper" virus to complete their replication.

## THE BIOLOGIC NATURE OF VIRUSES

From the time that viruses were discovered until Stanley initiated a new series of research attacks on their nature, little had been learned. They were known for what they could do, not for what they were. The only criterion for their recognition was their ability to produce recognizable signs of disease in plants or animals and, in some cases, to form certain foreign bodies (inclusion bodies) within parasitized cells. Many speculated about the possibility that a whole host of living beings, too small to be seen with the microscope and many perhaps leading a wholly saprophytic existence, might eventually be found to exist. There were no ways by which such a hypothesis could be proved or disproved. Gradually it became generally accepted that viruses could not be propagated like most bacteria in artificial culture media which was devoid of living cells—that growth and multiplication occurred only in living cells. Whether viruses are living or nonliving entities was a subject of considerable controversy until a decade or so ago. Some virologists still speak of *live* and *killed* viruses. A Dutchman, Beijerinck (9), started the controversy in 1899 with his idea of a *contagium vivum fluidum,* a form of life which, if it existed, would certainly be different from anything known since it would be a noncellular form of life. A still more unorthodox idea appeared—that viruses might be nonliving autocatalytic chemical agents which had the property of instigating abnormal metabolic activities in the cells which they attacked, one of the products of such abnormal activity being more of the instigating substance, which then became available in increased quantity for repeating the process in other cells of the same individual or, if it could escape to another host, of causing in it the same chain of events.

Life in the higher plants and animals generally is easily detectable by a series of well-known criteria. When it comes to determining life in very primitive beings, which probably are at a subcellular level, the usual distinctions fail. Unless new distinctions are made, we must regard viruses as nonliving agents. It is perfectly clear that a strand of nucleic acid, which forms the core of a virus, is a macromolecule with a somewhat simple and definable chemical structure that can perform essential functions of living things in a suitable environment. This macromolecule can replicate itself and also direct the synthesis of proteins. The newly formed nucleic acid and proteins are then assembled to consitute a complete virus particle (17). While the controversy was still ranging in 1945 Burnet (17) suggested that the epidemiologist and public health workers think of viruses as microorganisms. In 1966 Lwoff and Tournier (29) made it clear that viruses differ from other living things including microorganisms by five characters: (a) mature virus particles (virions) have only one type of nucleic acid, either DNA or RNA, whereas microorganisms possess both types; (b) virions are unable to grow or undergo binary fission; (c) virions make use of the ribosomes of their host cell; (d) virions are reproduced solely from their nucleic acid, other agents grow from the integrated sum of their constituents and reproduce by division; and (e) viruses lack genetic information for the synthesis of essential cellular systems such as that responsible for the production of energy with high potential. As our knowledge of viruses increase it is unlikely that Lwoff's concepts will encompass all discoveries; for example, the satellite viruses (27) cannot reproduce from their own nucleic acid and neither the nucleic acid or the virions are infectious. The chlamydiae contain some ribosomes but are partially dependent upon host-cell ribosomes as well. (2)

The contagious living fluid concept is no longer tenable. Although there are many differences among virologists on other points, all now agree that viruses are particulate in nature; that is, they may be filtered out of suspensions with appropriate filters, they may be centrifuged out of suspensions with ultracentrifuges. Many virus particles have been photographed with the electron microscope and their morphology and size accurately determined.

Animal and bacterial viruses contain either RNA or DNA, but not both, while plant viruses have RNA. To release the nucleic acid from its protein outer coat involves lysis of the capsid by a detergent such as sodium dodecyl sulfate and further treatment of the nucleic acid with pronase and phenol. Viruses from various groups, such as the enterovirus, yield infectious RNA by such treatment and members of *Papovaviridae* and bacteriophage have yielded infectious DNA. Infectious RNA and infectious DNA is inactivated by their respective enzymes (ribo- or deoxyribonuclease) whereas the infectivity of intact particles is not affected by such treatment. On the other hand, antiserum produced for intact particles readily neutralizes the virion as the antibodies react with the antigens of the protein coat but fail to inactivate free viral infectious nucleic acid. It is known that purified DNA is not immunogenic, but DNA complexes containing appreciable protein not readily dissociated from DNA are antigenic producing, precipitating, and $C^1$-fixing antibodies in rabbits.

Some viruses are toxic as evidenced by the peracute death of mice within a few hours after parenteral injection of concentrated suspensions of influenza virus. At necropsy these animals show no pathological lesions except marked vascular congestion. In most viral diseases the inflammatory response is characterized by an infiltration of mononuclear cells and lymphocytes whereas polymorphonuclear leukocytes predominate in the lesions of acute bacterial diseases. In many viral diseases pathogenic bacteria play a significant role as secondary invaders in the disease process of ectodermal tissues, so polymorphonuclear leukocytes invade the infected tissues after the mononuclear-type cells.

## CLASSIFICATION AND NOMENCLATURE OF VIRUSES

With the rapid advances in virology during the last decade virologists are producing a reasonable classification and nomenclature of viruses including vertebrate, invertebrate, plant, and bacterial viruses. The responsiblity for

this task lies in the hands of an International Commission for the Nomenclature of Viruses (ICNV), which was established at the IXth International Congress of Microbiology. The Commission approved a number of rules with the
purpose of establishing uniformity and standardized terminology. Many virologists other than the Commission were involved in the task so the final product represents a consensus, but, by no means unanimity.

Many virus groups were proposed for consideration at the International
Congress of Virology in Hungary, 1971. For certain groups family names have
been established, and these end in *idae*. The majority are genera, which end
with the word *virus*, and members of each genus share certain common characteristics. In general an effort has been made to provide for a latinized binomial nomenclature, and existing latinized names are to be retained if possible. Each virus-group description must include a designated type species, its
taxonomic position (genus or family), its main characteristics, a list of viruses
in the group, and a file of probable or possible members belonging in the
group. The description should also include cryptograms for the groups and its
individual viruses. Each cryptogram should contain (1) the type of nucleic
acid/strandedness of nucleic acid, (2) molecular weight of the nucleic acid in
millions/percentage of nucleic acid in virus particle, (3) outline of virus
particle/outline of nucleocapsid, and (4) kinds of host infected/kinds of vector. A proposed classification for viruses should be based upon the features
just cited in the cryptogram and, in addition, (1) the presence or absence of
an envelope; (2) certain measurements for helical viruses such as the diameter
of the nucleocapsid, and for cubical viruses including the triangulation number and the number of capsomeres; (3) the symmetry of the nucleocapsid
(helical, cubical, or binal), and (4) certain characteristic biological and bio-

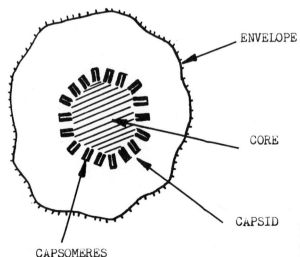

ENVELOPE

CORE

CAPSID

CAPSOMERES

Fig. 151. A diagram of a complete virus particle or virion. The
core is either ribonucleic acid or
deoxyribonucleic acid. (Courtesy
R. W. Horne, *Sci. Am.*)

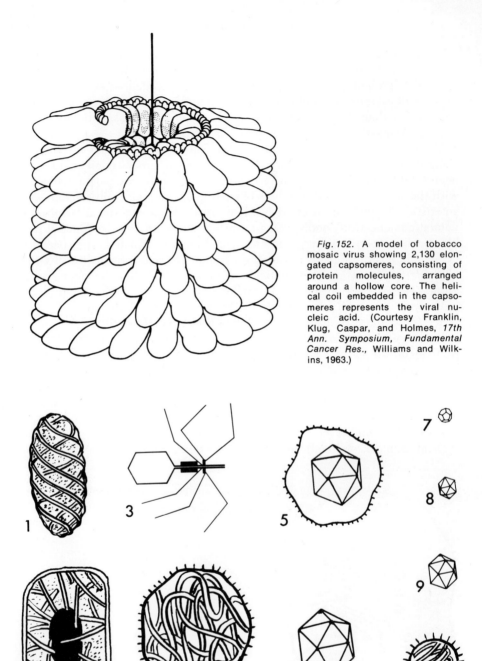

*Fig. 152.* A model of tobacco mosaic virus showing 2,130 elongated capsomeres, consisting of protein molecules, arranged around a hollow core. The helical coil embedded in the capsomeres represents the viral nucleic acid. (Courtesy Franklin, Klug, Caspar, and Holmes, *17th Ann. Symposium, Fundamental Cancer Res.,* Williams and Wilkins, 1963.)

*Fig. 153.* Relative sizes of certain viruses. (1) Contagious ecthyma of sheep. (2) Vaccinia. (3) T-even bacteriophage. (4) Mumps. (5) Herpes. (6) Tipula iridescent (plant virus). (7) Poliomyelitis. (8) Polyoma. (9) Adenovirus. (10) Influenza. (Courtesy R. W. Horne, *Sci. Am.*)

physical features. Ultimately, the classification undoubtedly will include comparisons of the nucleotide sequences of the viral nucleic acids and presently could also include nucleic acid homology (genetic relatedness) and nearest neighbor analyses. Table XXVI depicts the genera proposed (and 2, or possibly 3, families) by the International Commission for Nomenclature of Viruses, and lists the important chemical and physical features of each group.

## Viral Genera

**Parvoviruses.** The members of the genus presently are the only known viruses with single-stranded DNA. The type species is *Parvovirus* n-1. These small DNA viruses, 18 to 24 m$\mu$ in diameter, are divided into subgroups A and B. Subgroup A includes the Kilham rat virus, the X$_{14}$ virus of rats, hamster osteolytic H viruses, minute virus of mice, porcine parvovirus, and infectious feline panleukopenia virus and its closely related mink enteritis virus. Other possible members in subgroup A are avian parvovirus, minute virus of canines, hemorrhagic encephalopathy virus, bovine parvovirus, and densonucleosis virus. The adeno-associated virus 1, 2, 3, and 4 comprise subgroup B. The DNA liberated from adeno-satellites by conventional procedures acts like double-stranded nucleic acid, but the DNA within the virion stains with acridine orange and reacts with formaldehyde as single-stranded. The single-stranded DNA within the satellite particles exist as positive and negative complementary strands in separate particles. Upon extraction of DNA the positive and negative strands unite to form double-stranded DNA helix. The adenovirus satellites are defective and require an adenovirus "helper" to complete its replication. Members of subgroup A are nondefective and replicate without assistance from another virus. Their DNA is single-stranded inside and outside of all particles indicating the strands have a similar polarity. The icosahedral particles probably have 32 capsomeres, 2 to 4 m$\mu$ in diameter, with a buoyant density in cesium chloride of 1.4 per ml and with a molecular weight of 1.5 by 10$^6$ daltons. The nonenveloped particles are acid- and heat-stable and ether-resistant. The guanine-cystine (GC) content is 39 percent.

Viral replication occurs in the nucleus and intranuclear inclusion bodies are formed.

**Polyomaviruses.** The genus is one of two placed in the newly designated family, *Papovoviridae*. The type species is *Polyomavirus* m-1 (murine). Other viruses in the genus are simian vacuolating virus (SV$_{40}$), rabbit-vacuolating virus, and K virus, and possibly the virus associated with leukoencephalopathy in man. The viruses contain double-stranded, cyclic DNA with a GC ratio of 41 to 49 percent. The icosahedral particles, 43 m$\mu$ in diameter and with 5-3-2 symmetry, have a buoyant density in cesium chloride of 1.34 per ml, a molecular weight of 3 by 10$^6$ daltons, and a sedimentation rate of 240 S. The nonenveloped capsid has 72 capsomeres in a skew arrangement. The particles are acid- and heat-stable and ether-resistant.

*Table XXVI.* PROPOSED CLASSIFICATION OF VIRUSES BY INTERNATIONAL COMMISSION FOR NOMENCLATURE OF VIRUSES (ICNV)

| Nucleic acid core and strandedness | Capsid symmetry | Presence of envelope | Acid-lability | Ether-sensitivity | Buoyant density in CsCl₃ g/ml |
|---|---|---|---|---|---|
| Single-stranded DNA | Icosahedral | — | — | — | 1.4 |
| Double-stranded DNA | Icosahedral | — | — | — | 1.34 |
| | Icosahedral | — | — | — | 1.34 |
| | Icosahedral | — | — | —° | 1.34 (RbCl) |
| | Icosahedral | ± | | ±° | |
| | Icosahedral | + | + | + | 1.27–1.29 |
| | Unknown | Complex | + | ±° | 1.1–1.33 |
| Double-stranded RNA | Icosahedral | — | — | — | 1.31–1.38 |
| Single-stranded RNA | Icosahedral | — | ± | — | 1.37–1.38 |
| | | — | + | — | 1.38–1.43 |
| | | — | — | — | 1.34–1.35 |
| | Helical | + | + | + | |
| | Helical | + | + | + | |
| | Helical | + | + | + | 1.2 |
| | Unknown | + | + | + | 1.25 |
| | Unknown | + | + | + | 1.25 |
| | Unknown | + | + | + | |
| RNA-strandedness unknown | Helical | + | + | + | 1.15–1.16 |
| | (probably) unknown | + | ? | + | |

* Diameter, or diameter by length.

* * *Togaviridae* a tentative proposal.

° Some Iridoviruses are ether sensitive; some poxviruses are ether resistant, but all are chloroform sensitive.

The viruses are assembled in the nucleus with the formation of intranuclear inclusion bodies. Some are oncogenic under certain conditions but inapparent infections are the rule in most hosts. Several viruses hemagglutinate by reacting with neuraminidase sensitive receptors.

**Papillomaviruses.** These viruses have many of the characteristics of the polyomavirus group, thus, they also are in the family, *Papovaviridae*, with *papillomavirus* S-1 (Shope papilloma virus) as the type species. Other members of the genus are rabbit oral papilloma, human papilloma, canine papilloma, canine oral papilloma, and bovine papilloma viruses. Probable members include papillomata of horses, monkeys, sheep, goats, and other species. Members of this genus contain double-stranded, cyclic DNA with a GC ratio of 49 percent. The nonenveloped icosahedral particles, 53 mμ in diameter and with 5-3-2

| Capsomere number (C) or diameter of helix (mμ) | Virion* size (mμ) | Molecular weight of nucleic acid in virion (X 10^6 daltons) | Number of genes (approx.) | Virus genus | Virus family name |
|---|---|---|---|---|---|
| probably 32 (C) | 18–24 | 1.5 | 7 | Parvovirus | |
| | | | | | |
| 72 (C) | 43 | 3 | 10 | *Polyomavirus* | *Papovaviridiae* |
| 72 (C) | 53 | 5 | 10 | *Papillomavirus* | *Papovaviridiae* |
| 252 (C) | 70–90 | 20–25 | 50 | *Adenovirus* | |
| 1500 (C) | 130 | 130 | | *Iridovirus* | |
| 162 (C) | 180–250 | 54–92 | 150 | *Herpesvirus* | |
| | 170–250 by 300–325 | 160–240 | 400 | *Poxvirus* | |
| 92 (C) | 75–80 | 15 | 50 | *Reovirus* | |
| | | | | | |
| 32 (C) | 30–40 | 2 | | *Calicivirus* | *Picornaviridae* |
| 32 (C) | 20–30 | 2.4–2.8 | | *Rhinovirus* | *Picornaviridae* |
| 32? (C) | 20–30 | 2.5 | | *Enterovirus* | *Picornaviridae* |
| 9–10 mμ | 90–120 | 2–4 | 10 | *Orthomyxovirus* | |
| 18 mμ | 150–300 | 4–8 | 40 | *Paramyxovirus* | |
| 10–20 mμ | 70 by 175 | 3.5 | 10 | *Rhabdovirus* | |
| | 25–70 | 3 | | *Alphavirus* | *Togaviridae** * |
| | 20–50 | 3 | | *Flavovirus* | *Togaviridae* |
| | 80–120 | 10–13 | 50 | *Leukovirus* | |
| | 70–120 | | | *Coronavirus* | |
| | 50–300 (thin sections) 85–99 (negative stained) | | | *Arenavirus* | |

symmetry, have a molecular weight of 5 by $10^6$ daltons, a buoyant density in cesium chloride of 1.34 g per ml, a sedimentation rate of 280 to 300 S, and 72 capsomeres in a skew arrangement. The virions are ether resistant and heat and acid stable.

The viruses replicate in the nucleus and cause papillomata in many animal hosts. Several viruses hemagglutinate by reacting with neuraminidase-sensitive receptors.

**Adenoviruses.** The genus *Adenovirus* holds a rather large number of viruses represented by the type species, *Adenovirus* h-1 (human). Other members of the genus include human types 2 to 33, seven simian, two canine, three bovine, porcine, murine, avian, and other mammalian adenoviruses from sheep, horse, opossium, and cat. These double-stranded DNA viruses, 70 to 90μ in diameter, have a GC content of 48 to 57 percent. Isometric nonenveloped particles with icosahedral symmetry have 252 capsomeres, 7 m$\mu$ in diameter, arranged in a 5-3-2 axial symmetry. The vertex capsomeres carry a filamentous projection which are antigenically distinct from other capsomeres of the particle. The virions have a molecular weight of 20 to 25 by 10$^6$ daltons, a buoyant density in rubidium chloride of 1.34 g per ml, and a sedimentation rate of 795 S. The particles are ether-resistant and heat- and acid-stable.

The virus replicates in the nucleus where it causes intranuclear inclusion bodies. Some viruses hemagglutinate red blood cells of various species. Some adenoviruses are oncogenic in hamsters. A common antigen shared by all mammalian adenoviruses differs from a corresponding antigen of avian strains.

**Iridoviruses.** The type species of this genus is *Iridovirus* t-1 (tipula iridescent virus). Other members are *Sericesthis* iridescent virus and *Chilo* iridescent virus; probable members are *Aedes* iridescent virus and other iridescent viruses of the mosquito. Possible members include lymphocystis virus of fish, African swine-fever virus, amphibian cytoplasmic viruses, and Gecko virus. The viruses contain approximately 15 percent double-stranded DNA (a single molecule) with a molecular weight of 130 by 10$^6$ daltons and with a guanine-cystine content of 29 to 32 percent. The icosahedral particles, 130 m$\mu$ in diameter, have an icosahedral edge length of approximately 85 m$\mu$ and a sedimentation rate of 2,200 S. The complex particle contains several proteins and the outer icosahedral shell contains approximately 1,500 capsomeres. No lipid is detected in members and probable members, but some possible members in the genus have a lipid envelope.

**Herpesviruses.** The genus *Herpesvirus* holds an exceedingly large number of viruses involved in the production of disease. The type species is *Herpesvirus* h-1 (herpes simplex virus). Other members are herpesvirus simiae (B virus), herpesvirus T (of marmosets), perhaps two herpesviruses of *Cercopithecus*, herpesvirus of patos monkeys, herpesvirus of saimiri, herpesvirus cuniculi (Virus III of rabbits), pseudorabies virus, infectious bovine rhinotracheitis virus, varicella virus, equine rhinopneumonitis and other related equine herpesviruses, malignant catarrah virus of cattle, bovine ulcerative mammalitis (Allerton) virus, feline rhinotracheitis virus, canine herpesvirus, Epstein-Barr virus (associated with infectious mononucleosis and Burkitt lymphoma), Marek's disease virus, avian infectious laryngotracheitis, avian herpesviruses of pigeons, parrots, owls, and cormorants, herpesvirus associated with lymphosarcoma in the African clawed frog, snake herpesvirus, cytomegaloviruses affecting various species including man, porcine inclusion body rhinitis virus, sheep pulmonary adenomatosis (Jasgsiekte) virus and possibly duck plague and mouse thymic viruses.

The herpesviruses contain double-stranded DNA with a molecular weight between 54 to 92 by 10$^6$ daltons and a guanine-cystine content of 57 to 74 percent. The nucleocapsid, 100 to 150 m$\mu$ in diameter, shows cubic and icosahedral symmetry with 162 hollow and elongated capsomeres that usually are hexagonal but some pentagonal in cross section. Lipid membrane surrounding the capsid is 180 to 250 m$\mu$ in diameter. The particles are sensitive to lipid solvents and also are acid-labile. The particle DNA content is approximately 7 percent of its weight and it has a buoyant density in cesium chloride of 1.27 to 1.29 g per ml. The development begins in the nucleus and the particle is completely formed by the addition of protein membranes as the virus passes into the cellular cytoplasm.

Intranuclear inclusion bodies are formed by these viruses. A few contain hemagglutinins. Viruses in this group cause a broad variety of infectious diseases ranging in character from acute catarrhal disease to chronic and even oncogenic disease.

**Poxviruses.** The viruses in the genus *Poxvirus* are divided into subgroups A, B, C, D, E, and F. Subgroup A includes vaccinia, variola, alastrim, rabbitpox, monkeypox, cowpox, and infectious ectromelia viruses, with *Poxvirus* b-1 (vaccinia) as the type species for the genus. Orf, paravaccinia, bovine papular stomatitis, and contagious ecthyma viruses comprise subgroup B, sometimes called the pseudopox viruses. Sheeppox, goatpox, and lumpy-skin disease viruses are in subgroup C. The avian poxviruses are subgroup D, including fowlpox, pigeonpox, canarypox, turkeypox, sparrowpox, starlingpox, and juncopox viruses. The myxoma and fibroma viruses including myxoma, rabbit fibroma, California myxoma, hare fibroma, and squirrel fibroma viruses comprise subgroup E. Subgroup F is a large group including swinepox, horsepox, camelpox, buffalopox, rhinocerospox, molluscum contagiosum, Yaba monkey tumor, Tana, and entomopox viruses. It is interesting to note that no poxvirus has been described in the dog or domestic cat. There are many important animal pathogens in this group that cause fatal diseases and serious economic losses.

The symmetry of the capsid of these largest vertebrate viruses is unknown. The poxviruses contain 5 to 7.5 percent double-stranded DNA with a molecular weight of 160 to 240 by $10^6$ daltons. The guanine-cystine content of the nucleic acid is 35 to 40 percent. Brick-shaped or ovoid complex particles, 170 to 250 by 300 to 324 m$\mu$ have a buoyant density in cesium chloride varying from 1.1 to 1.33 g per ml. The particles have characteristic surface patterns and lateral bodies and some poxviruses have an envelope. Some poxviruses are known to contain RNA polymerase. There is an NP antigen common to all members and members of subgroup A to E also have other antigens in common and can recombine genetically. All poxviruses exhibit nongenetic reactivation and replicate in cytoplasmic foci.

**Reoviruses.** These are the double-stranded RNA viruses. They contain between 10 and 20 percent double-stranded RNA in several pieces with a total molecular weight of 15 by $10^6$ daltons and with a guanine-cystine content of 42 to 44 percent. The particle has an isometric capsid with icosahedral symmetry. It has no envelope as a rule but pseudomembranes, probably of host origin, have been described. Capsid diameter is 75 to 80 m$\mu$ and it has 2 layers. The particle has a buoyant density in cesium chloride of 1.31 to 1.38 g per ml and a sedimentation rate of 630 S. The particle has 92 capsomeres and is resistant to ether. Virus synthesis and maturation occurs in the cytoplasm with the formation of inclusions sometimes containing virus particles in crystalline arrays.

The type species for the genus is *Reovirus* h-1. There are 3 mammalian serotypes common to many species, such as man, dogs, cats, and monkeys, and 5 avian serotypes that are definite members of the genus. Other important animal viral pathogens possibly in the genus include epizootic diarrhea of infant mice, infectious pancreatic necrosis of trout, Colorado tick-fever virus, epizootic hemorrhagic disease of deer, 12 bluetongue disease serotypes, and 9 African horsesickness serotypes. The last two viruses are believed to have a single layered shell (capsid). Reoviruses also are significant pathogens in certain plants and invertebrates.

In mammals, the three mammalian serotypes have been associated with respiratory and enteric disease, but apparently occur most frequently as inapparent infections. In animals, bluetongue and African horsesickness viruses are very important animal pathogens.

**Caliciviruses.** The genus is small and is placed in the family *Picornaviridae*. The type species is *Calicivirus* s-1 (vesicular exanthema type A). The vesicular exanthema virus serotypes are limited to the pig and presently these viruses are not known in nature. Other possible members in this genus are the feline calicivirus (picornavirus) group, which presumably has a large number of serotypes. The feline viruses are principally known to cause respiratory disease.

The caliciviruses contain single-stranded RNA with a molecular weight about 2 by $10^6$ daltons and with a guanine-cystine content about 46 percent. The isometric nonenveloped particles, 30 to 40 m$\mu$ in diameter, with probable icosahedral symmetry have a buoyant density in cesium chloride of 1.37 to 1.38 g per ml and 32 capsomeres. The ether-resistant particles are unstable at pH 3, variably susceptible at pH 5, and stable pH 6 to pH 9.

**Rhinoviruses.** The genus is also a member of the family *Picornaviridae*. The type species is *Rhinovirus* h-1A, one of 90 human rhinovirus serotypes that cause the common cold in humans. The equine and bovine rhinoviruses also cause respiratory disease. The most important animal pathogen in this genus is the foot-and-mouth disease virus.

The particles contain approximately 30 percent RNA with a molecular weight of 2.4 to 2.8 by $10^6$ daltons and a guanine-cystine content of 40 to 52 percent. Isometric nonenveloped particles, probably with icosahedral symmetry and with 32 capsomeres are 20 to 30 m$\mu$ in diameter. The particles have a buoyant density of 1.38 to 1.43 g per ml and a sedimentation rate of 140 to 150 S. Some viruses are stabilized by magnesium chloride. The virions are ether-stable and labile at pH 3. The viruses replicate in the cytoplasm and often achieve maximum growth at 33 to 35 C in cell culture.

**Enteroviruses.** The third member of the family *Picornaviridae* is the genus *Enterovirus*. The type species is *Enterovirus* polio 1. Other human enteroviruses include the other two poliovirus serotypes, Coxsackie A and B viruses, and ECHO viruses. Other members include bovine enteroviruses, porcine enteroviruses, Nodamura virus, EMC (Columbia, SK, Mengo) virus, and murine encephalomyelitis virus. Possible members are acute bee paralysis virus, avian encephalomyelitis virus, and duck hepatitis virus.

The particles contain 20 to 30 percent single-stranded RNA with a molecular weight of 2.5 by $10^6$ daltons and with a guanine-cytosine content between 46 and 54 percent. The nonenveloped isometric particles 20 to 30 m$\mu$ in diameter with icosahedral symmetry and with 32 capsomeres have a buoyant density in cesium chloride of 1.34 to 1.35 g per ml and a sedimentation rate of 150 to 160 S. The particles are stable at pH 3 and in ether. They are naturally occurring protein shells with an approximate sedimentation rate of 80 S. The viruses replicate in the cytoplasm and are principally inhabitants of the intestinal tract.

Many members of this genus are important pathogens, principally those in the human group.

**Orthomyxoviruses.** The genus *Orthomyxovirus* has been known as the myxovirus group. The type species is *Orthomyxovirus* h-A (human influenza A). This well-characterized group includes viruses of types A, B, and C. Type A viruses include human influenza, porcine influenza, equine influenza, and avian influenza. Types B (B/Lee/40) and C (C/Taylor/1233/47) are human-influenza serotypes.

The particles contain 1 percent single-stranded RNA with a molecular weight of 2 to 4 by $10^6$ daltons and with a guanine-cystine content between 40 and 48 percent. Its helical capsid is 9 to 10 m$\mu$, probably in six pieces. The enveloped particle, 90 to 120 m$\mu$ in diameter, is spherical or elongated with characteristic surface projections. The virion possesses neuraminidase and hemagglutinate by virtue of neuraminidase-sensitive receptors. The envelope contains lipid and carbohydrate. The particles are ether-sensitive and acid-labile. The nucleocapsids are formed in the nucleus and maturation occurs by budding. These viruses are sensitive to actinomycin D. Genetic recombination is common and antigenic variation is frequent. Antigenic crossings occur within viral subtypes. There are three distinct antigenic types distinguishable by the specificity of the RNP (ribonucleoprotein) antigen with no cross reaction.

Influenza is one of mans' most important diseases. It causes great concern because pandemics have occurred in the past and its ability to produce variants makes prevention and control difficult.

**Paramyxoviruses.** The viruses in the genus share some of the characteristics of the orthomyxoviruses but major differences exist. The type species for the genus *Paramyxovirus* is *Paramyxovirus* a-1 (Newcastle disease virus). The virions with helical symmetry contain 1 percent single-stranded RNA with a molecular weight of 4 to 8 by $10^6$ daltons and with a guanine-cystine content 48 to 52 percent. The helical capsid is approximately 18 m$\mu$ in diameter and 1.0 micron long. Some particles contain more than 1 nucleocapsid. The spherical-enveloped particles, 150 to 300 m$\mu$ in diameter, contain characteristic projections. Viruses assigned as members hemagglutinate, as do certain other possible members. Some of the viruses possess neuraminidase and all are acid- and ether-labile. Mostly, nucleocapsids develop in the cytoplasm. The viruses are resistant to actinomycin D and antigenically stable with two main serological subgroups. Genetic recombination is not known to occur.

Members of the genus are parainfluenza viruses 1 (human–HA$_2$, murine–Sendai), 2 (human–CA, Simian–SV5, avian), 3 (human–HA$_1$, bovine–SF$_4$) and 4; mumps virus, and other avian parainfluenza viruses including turkey virus (Canada/68) and Yucaipa virus. Possible members include the important triad of measles, canine distemper, and rinderpest viruses; pneumonia virus of mice; and respiratory syncytial virus of humans. Many of the above members are important pathogens of man and/or the lower animals.

**Rhabdoviruses.** Viruses in this genus contain 2 percent single-stranded RNA with a molecular weight of 3.5 by $10^6$ daltons and with a guanine-cystine content of approximately 42 percent. The helical nucleocapsid, 10 to 20 m$\mu$ in diameter, is surrounded by a shell to which is closely applied an envelope with 10 m$\mu$ spikes. The whole particle is bullet-shaped measuring 70 by 175 m$\mu$ and has a buoyant density in cesium chloride of 1.2 g per ml. Infectivity is destroyed by ether and by acid. Some viruses hemagglutinate and antigenic relationships exist between some members. The particles maturate at the cytoplasmic membrane. Most members multiply in arthropods as well as vertebrates.

The type species is *Rhabdovirus* b-1 (vesicular stomatitis virus). Other members are cocal, Hart Park, Kern Canyon, Flanders, and rabies viruses. Most possible members are plant viruses, but also include the hemorrhagic septicemia virus of trout and drosophia virus.

**Alphaviruses.** The genus is tentatively included in the family *Togaviridae* which includes many of the arboviruses. The type species is *Alphavirus sindbis*. The particles contain 4 to 6 percent of single-stranded RNA with a molecular weight of 3 by $10^6$ daltons and with a guanine-cystine content of 51 percent. The spherical-enveloped particles, 25 to 70 m$\mu$ in diameter, of unknown symmetry have a buoyant density in cesium chloride of 1.25 g per ml. The envelope contains lipid that makes the particles sensitive to ether. Hemagglutination is not inhibited by phospholipids and particles are insensitive to trypsin. Replication occurs in the cytoplasm, and maturation results with budding. All members show cross reactions in the hemagglutination test. All members multiply in arthropod vectors and are mosquito-transmitted to vertebrates.

The natural host for most of these viruses is arthropods, and only a few are pathogenic for man and animals. The principal animal pathogens of domestic animals are vesicular stomatitis serotype(s), eastern equine encephalitis, Venezuelan equine encephalitis, and western equine encephalitis viruses.

**Flavoviruses.** The other arboviruses are placed in this newly designated genus with tentative placement in the family *Togaviridae*. These viruses also hemagglutinate like those in the *Alphavirus* genus and all within this genus are serologically related. The virus particles contain 7 to 8 percent single-stranded RNA with a molecular weight of 3 by $10^6$ daltons and with a guanine-cystine content of 49 percent. The spherical-enveloped particles, 20 to 50 m$\mu$ in diameter, of unknown symmetry have a buoyant density in cesium chloride of 1.25 g per ml. The lipid-containing particles are ether-, trypsin-, and acid-labile. Replication occurs in the cytoplasm, and maturation is by budding from the membrane. Not all are proved to multiply in arthropods.

The type species is *Flavovirus febrices* (yellow fever virus). There are 31 other viruses presently recognized as members, some with subtypes. The principal pathogens for humans and/or domestic animals are dengue types (1, 2, 3, and 4), Israel turkey meningoencephalitis virus, Japanese encephalitis virus, louping-ill virus, Murray Valley encephalitis virus, St. Louis encephalitis virus and tick-borne encephalitis viruses.

**Leukoviruses.** This newly designated genus contains subgroups, A, B, C, and D. The type species is *Leukovirus* a-1 (Rous sarcoma virus). The virions contain single-stranded RNA with a molecular weight of 10 to 13 by $10^6$ daltons and with a guanine-cystine content varying from 47 to 57 percent. The enveloped particles, 80 to 120 m$\mu$ in diameter, of unknown symmetry are ether- and heat-sensitive. An RNA dependent, DNA polymerase is present in the virion. Actinomycin D interferes with replication. Most viruses are oncogenic, and some particles are defective and require a "helper" virus of the same subgroup to complete its replication. Hemagglutinins have not been demonstrated for these viruses.

The subgroups were formed because all membranes contain common antigens. Subgroup A contains the avian leukosis viruses and Subgroup B comprises the murine leukemia viruses. Subgroup C contains the feline leukemia and sarcoma viruses while Subgroup D includes the mouse-mammary tumor virus and the nodule-inducing virus.

**Coronaviruses.** The generic name is suggested for a group of viruses that has *Coronovirus* a-1 (avian infectious bronchitis virus) as its type species. The molecular weight and strandedness of these RNA viruses is unknown. The enveloped particles, 70 to 120 m$\mu$ in diameter, have a buoyant density in cesium chloride of 1.15 to 1.16 per ml. The nucleocapsid is probably helical, loosely wound, and probably 7 m$\mu$ in diameter. The virus surface has characteristic pedunculated projections. These ether-susceptible particles replicate in the cytoplasm and are unaffected by DNA inhibitors. Maturation occurs by budding into cytoplasmic vesicles.

Other members besides avian infectious bronchitis virus are mouse hepatitis virus, human respiratory virus, and transmissible gastroenteritis virus of swine.

**Arenaviruses.** These viruses probably contain RNA of unknown strandedness, symmetry, and molecular weight. The virion is round, oval, or pleomorphic with diameters varying from 50 to 300 m$\mu$ in thin electron-microscope sections, and from 85 to 99 m$\mu$ in negatively stained preparations. The envelope consists of unit membrane with regular surface structure and closely spaced projections. The interior of the virion appears unstructured and contains a variable number of electron-dense granules, 20 to 30 m$\mu$ in diameter. Ether-labile virions grow in the cytoplasm and mature by budding from marginal membranes. All strains share a group-specific antigen determined by the immunofluorescence test and in some instances by complement-fixation test.

The type species is *Arenavirus* m-1 (lymphocytic choriomeningitis virus). Other members are Lasso, Juin, Machupo, Amapari, Pichinde, Parana, Latino, Tamiani, Tacaribe, and Portillo viruses—all former members of the arbovirus group.

## VIRAL SIZE AND MORPHOLOGY

**Electron Microscopy.** Electron micrographs are photomicrographs made with an instrument known as an *electron microscope*. This is an instrument of magnification which uses beams of electrons, instead of light rays, and electromagnetic fields instead of lenses of glass or quartz. Because the beams of electrons cannot be seen with the eye, the images are projected on a fluorescent plate, which renders them visible just as x-rays can be visualized on a fluoroscope. The micrographs are the images secured on photographic plates.

With an electron microscope, images with sharp definition can be secured at magnifications as high as 1 : 1,000,000 by enlarging electron photomicrographs. The advantages can be appreciated when it is pointed out that, with the best optical equipment, resolution is difficult to obtain with magnifications greater than 1,200 diameters.

The objects from which electron micrographs are made usually are mounted on very thin collodion films supported on fine metallic screens. Because the density of many of the very small particles is not great, the early micrographs were not clear. This was remedied by the work of Williams (48) who introduced metallic shadowing into the process. This not only provided the needed contrast but also made possible the introduction of a third dimension into the photographs. The prepared films are dried and then introduced into a small chamber, which is evacuated. They are carefully oriented with reference to a focal point where a small particle of the shadowing metal (silver, gold, chromium, etc.) is placed. The metal is then raised in temperature by an electric current until it is vaporized. In the vacuum the vaporized

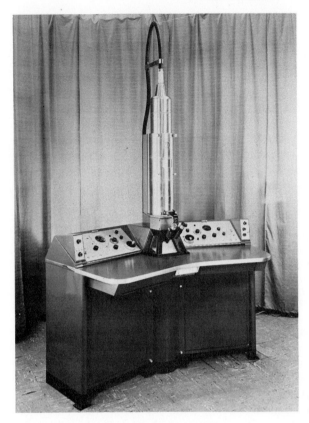

*Fig. 154.* Electron microscope. (Courtesy Radio Corporation of America.)

metal molecules are dispersed in every direction, lodging upon the first surfaces encountered. Because the films on the collodion membranes are deliberately oriented at an angle to the source of the metallic dispersion, the metal film will be deposited on any particles in this film and there will be "shadows" on the side of the particles where the metallic molecules are prevented from reaching the surface by the height of the particles. These shadows give a realistic idea of the third dimension of the particles.

The negative staining technic that employs the use of phosphotungstic is excellent for studying structures of viruses with the electron microscope. The phosphotungstate permeates the virus particle as a cloud and clearly shows the surface structure of viruses by the virtue of negative staining. It also enters the core of particles without nucleic acid that are noninfectious. Thus, it is possible to determine the ratio of infectious particles and noninfectious particles and also to study the development of viral particles at different stages of replication.

Thin sections of infected animal tissues or pellets of centrifuged cells from infected cell cultures have also advanced our knowledge of viral structure.

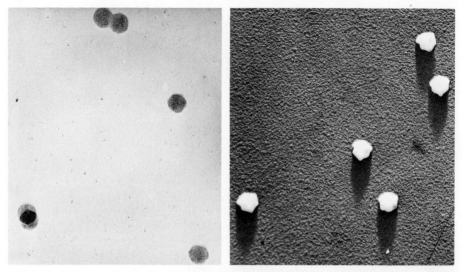

*Fig. 155.* Electron micrographs of air-dried particles of the *Tipula* (crane fly) virus. X 40,000. (*Left*) Unshadowed particles. (*Right*) Metallic shadowed particles. (Courtesy Robley C. Williams and Kenneth M. Smith, *Biochem. Biophys. Acta.*)

Unless special precautions are taken, electron photomicrographs may overestimate the diameter of viruses.

The size of some animal viruses, in comparison with some other microorganisms and protein molecules, is indicated in Table XXVII. It is customary in measuring such small objects to use the millimicron as the unit of measure, this unit being 0.001 of a micron. By such a scale the elementary bodies of chlamydiae measure about 0.3 micron or 300 millimicrons. In the table microns are used as the unit to avoid confusion. Particles with a 2-fold difference in diameter have an 8-fold difference in volume.

*Table XXVII.*  THE APPROXIMATE SIZE OF VIRUS UNITS IN COMPARISON WITH OTHER WELL-KNOWN MOLECULES AND OTHER MICROORGANISMS

| | Microns | | Microns |
|---|---|---|---|
| Staphylococcus aureus | 0.8 to 1.0 | St. Louis encephalitis | 0.025 |
| Psittacosis | 0.3 | Louping ill | 0.015–0.020 |
| Vaccinia | 0.20 | Foot-and-mouth disease | 0.023 |
| Pseudorabies | 0.12 | Poliomyelitis | 0.025 |
| Vesicular stomatitis | 0.176 by 0.069 | Serum globulin | 0.0063 |
| Fowl plague | 0.080 | Serum albumin | 0.0056 |
| Rift Valley fever | 0.030 | Egg albumen | 0.004 |

**Ultrafiltration.** Because it is known that the pore size of silica filters (Pasteur, Berkefeld) is not the sole factor which determines whether or not particles in suspension will be passed, such filters have been discarded as a means of determining the approximate size of virus elements.

To avoid the absorbine properties of silica filters, Bechhold (8) as early as

1907 introduced the use of collodion membranes as filters for virus suspensions. Many years later, Elford (17) and Bauer and Hughes (6) standardized such filters (gradocol membranes) in order that they might be used for determining the approximate size of virus particles. By the use of membranes of differing pore sizes, it was possible to determine the approximate diameter of the elements of many viruses. The size of the limiting APD (average pore diameter), multiplied by 0.64, yields the diameter of the virus particle. Later when other methods of determining particle size were discovered, it was found that the membrane filters had given reasonably accurate results. Early studies for estimation of size by filtration often underestimated the size.

**Ultracentrifugation.** The ordinary laboratory centrifuges, operating at full speed, rarely spin faster than 4,000 revolutions per minute. At this rate most bacteria and larger particles with a specific gravity heavier than the fluids in which they are suspended, gravitate rapidly to the bottoms of the tubes which contain them. Most virus particles, being much more minute, are thrown down at a very much slower rate—so slow, in fact, that it is not practicable to remove most of them from suspensions in this way. More successful are the angle centrifuges in which the tubes are held at an angle while spinning; here sedimenting particles have to travel only a short distance before they come in contact with the fluid-glass interface. For sedimenting the smaller virus particles, ultracentrifuges are needed. These are instruments of several types which can be operated at speeds of 60,000 rpm and more with centrifugal forces up to 198,000 times the force of gravity. One of them is described by Bauer and Pickels (7). These instruments have been used to determine physical characteristics of virus elements, as well as of other minute bodies such as albumin molecules. The approximate size can be calculated from data yielded by the sedimentation constants. The agreement between these calculations and the data derived from filtration studies is very good. It was known before the electron microscope was developed that different viruses varied in size, some being only a little larger than protein molecules and others as large as some of the smaller bacteria.

**Ionizing Radiation.** A beam of charged particles such as high-energy electrons, alpha particles, or deuterons passing through a virus causes a loss in primary ionization. The release of these ions within the virion inactivates particle infectivity, antigenicity, and hemagglutinins.

By ascertaining the number of ionizations per unit volume or area required to inactivate 63 percent of the infectivity of the viral preparation, the average sensitive volume or area per ionization can be determined. This is the point at which there has been an average of one hit per sensitive target, according to the Poisson distribution, so the volume or area per ionization is equivalent to volume or area of the sensitive unit measured. Thus, knowledge of the volume or area permits calculation of the diameter or area of the infective unit in the virus particle. In the same way it is possible to measure the sizes of complement-fixing antigens and hemagglutinins.

Ultraviolet rays and x-rays inactivate viruses. The inactivating dose varies for different viruses.

**Viral Morphology.** The morphology of viruses is determined principally by the use of the electron microscope and x-ray diffraction.

The capsids of animal viruses are arranged in two forms of symmetry, cubic and helical. All cubic symmetry in animal viruses is characteristic of an icosahedron with its 5:3:2 pattern of rotational symmetry. The arrangement of capsomeres to comply with icosahedral symmetry is limited. This limitation in its simplest form can be expressed by the formula $N = 10 (n-1)^2 + 2$, where N represents the number of capsomeres and n signifies the number of capsomeres on one side of each equilateral triangle. The icosahedron has 20 equilateral triangular faces with 12 vertices (see fig. 176 of an adenovirus, in chapter XL), although the face (30 in number) of the *Picornaviridae* members may be a rhomubus thus changing the formula to $N = 30 (N-1)^2 + 2$.

The triangulation number can also be used to group viruses with icosahedral symmetry. The number of capsomeres (morphologic units) is expressed by the formula $M = 10T + 2$. One class has values of 1, 4, 9, 16, and 25; a second class, values of 3 and 12; and a third class, values of 7, 13, 19, and 21.

**Properties of Viral Components**

**Viral Nucleic Acid.** The viral nucleic acid carries the genetic information for the replication of the virus.

The type of nucleic acid can be determined by various means using the intact virus particle or the free nucleic acid. The enzyme digestion tests with free virus nucleic acid constitute a method reliable for determining the nucleic acid type. The type of nucleic acid and its strandedness can be determined by fixing smears of purified virus with an alcohol fixation followed by staining with acridine orange (pH 4.0, dye concentration 0.01 percent). Double-stranded viruses, either RNA or DNA, stain yellow and single-stranded DNA and RNA viruses stain red in the fluorescent microscope. Uranyl acetate is a specific stain for DNA while having no affinity for RNA. This stain is often used in electron microscope preparations for this purpose. Density-gradient centrifugation in cesium salts also is used to differentiate RNA from DNA.

The viral nucleic acids are physically fragile once removed from their capsid protection. This made it difficult to study their structure. It is possible now to examine many nucleic acid molecules in the electron microscope without disrupting them. The molecules are spread in a special inert protein monofilm so their complete contour lengths can be measured with accuracy. In most viruses the nucleic acids are linear, but in some the molecule takes the form of a circle. In the case of the *Papovaviridae* the viruses have a double-stranded circle, often hypercoiled. By using linear densities of approximately 2 by $10^6$ daltons (1 dalton equals the mass of one hydrogen atom) per micrometer for double-stranded forms and one half that amount for single stranded forms the molecular weights of viral genomes can be calculated from direct measurements.

A recent finding of great interest and significance cited the presence of a DNA polymerase in RNA viruses that synthesizes DNA from an RNA template. Thus, it has been demonstrated that an RNA virus can make DNA.

**Viral Protein.** Viral proteins have important functions. These proteins determine the antigenicity of the virus and are very much involved in the immunogenic process. Thus the viral structural proteins are of great interest to individuals concerned in the production of vaccines. In addition, these proteins determine the relatedness of viruses and thus are of importance to the diagnostician. The proteins also protect the viral genome against inactivation by nucleases present in tissues, participate in the adsorption of the virus particle to a susceptible cell, and serve as the structural units providing structural symmetry to the virus. Viral protein as such is not pathogenic.

The structural proteins of only a few viruses have been extensively studied, including those of polio virus. Despite some knowledge of the structural arrangement and chemical composition from polio virus protein, there is little known about the binding of its RNA to the protein. Using polyacrylamide gel electrophoresis, the polypeptides of purified polio virus particles obtained by treatment with detergents were analyzed. Four polypeptides were found to exist in polio virus. Other analyses suggested that these polypeptides exist as precursors of the infectious virus in cells and in some unknown fashion become assembled with the viral RNA to form the virion.

In addition to the structural proteins, other virus specific proteins are formed in an infected cell such as the viral specific enzyme, thymidine kinase, in herpes- and vaccinia-infected cells..

**Viral Lipids.** Lipids are found in those viruses that have an envelope. Those viruses containing essential lipids are ether-sensitive and chloroform-sensitive. It has been observed that certain poxviruses are ether resistant and chloroform-sensitive, but this is the only viral genus showing this distinction among certain of its members.

The study of viral lipids presents real problems because their distinction from contaminating host cell lipids associated with viral particles is difficult. In general the lipids are added to the viral particle as it matures or buds through the cell or nuclear membrane. In the process the host membranes are incorporated into the complete virus particle. The host membrance of the viral-infected cell differs from a noninfected cell. For example, the limiting membrane of myxoviruses contain neuraminidase, an enzyme not found in normal cell membranes. Another RNA virus whose lipid envelopes have been studied with interesting results is the SV5, a simian parainfluenza virus. The lipid content of its envelope is related to the nature of its host substrate. The SV5 virions grown in monkey cells or in baby hamster kidney cells have a lipid composition that is closely similar to the plasma membrane composition of the particular cell in which the virus replicated. In the case of a DNA virus, such as a herpesvirus which is assembled as a nucleocapsid within the nucleus, the nucleocapsid contacts the nuclear membrane whose inner membrane thickens and becomes electron-dense. The nucleocapsid is progressively enveloped by the thickened membrane and finally "buds" off as an enveloped virion in the perinuclear cisterna of the cell. Nucleocapsids can also bud off into nuclear vacuoles which seem to be continuous with the cisterna. The enveloped nucleocapsid is released from the cell by (1) the incorporation of some virions within a cytoplasmic vacuole formed by the outer lamella of the nuclear envelope and sequestration of it from the cytoplasma to the outside of the cell and (2) movement through the cisternae of the endoplasmic reticulum to the cell exterior. In the late stages of infection unenveloped virions appear as breaks in the nuclear membrane occur.

**Hemagglutination.** The hemagglutination phenomenon was described independently in 1941 by Hirst (27) and McClelland and Hare (33) as a property of human influenza virus. A wide variety of animal viruses are capable of agglutinating red blood cells of various animals and under a variety of conditions. The hemagglutination and hemadsorption technics are now widely used in both the diagnostic and experimental laboratory to assay for virus and antibody. This test also serves as a model for host-virus interactions. It is a viral property which is useful in classifying viruses. The same can be said for the hemadsorption test which is a useful manifestation of the hemagglutination phenomenon. This method has been used to demonstrate the presence of some viruses in tissue culture systems. The erythrocytes added to such a culture form red cell clumping at the cell sites of viral activity.

### Certain Physical and Chemical Characteristics of Viruses

**Effects of Heat and Cold.** Most viruses are inactivated by heating at 56 C for 30 minutes although some resist this treatment. Scrapie virus is unusually resistant to heat.

The ideal way to preserve viruses in the laboratory is storage at low temperatures, preferably −60 C or lower. All viral preparations stored under dry ice refrigeration must be tightly stoppered as the liberated $CO_2$ will cause a drop in pH of poorly buffered viral suspensions and inactivate those viruses which are sensitive to acid conditions. Lyophilization is another means by which many viruses can be preserved in the dry state for long periods of time at 4 C. Heat resistant viruses withstand the lyophilization process reasonably well but there usually is some loss in viral titer during lyophilization.

**Inactivation by Vital Dyes.** Vital dyes such as toluidine blue, neutral red, and acridine orange penetrate many viruses to varying degrees. The dyes combine with the viral nucleic acid and when exposed to light inactivation results. These dyes do not penetrate some viruses, such as polio; thus, inactivation does not occur. Others are moderately susceptible such as adeno- and reoviruses while still others such as herpesvirus and vaccinia are readily susceptible. When poliovirus is grown in the presence of a vital dye in the absence of light, dye penetrates the nucleic acid and is then susceptible to photodynamic inactivation. The protein-coat antigen is not affected by this process.

**Effects of pH.** Practically all viruses are stable between pH 5 and pH 9, a notable exception is foot-and-mouth disease virus which is readily inactivated at pH 6.

Electrostatic forces play an important role in hemagglutination reactions. Sometimes a variation of a few tenths of a pH unit may determine a negative or positive reaction.

**Virus Stabilization by Salts.** Many viruses, such as poliovirus, can be stabilized by molar concentrations of salts. The mechanism is unknown. Viruses are preferentially stabilized by certain salts. The *Picornaviridae* family and reoviruses are stabilized by 1 M magnesium chloride. The orthomyxoviruses and paramyxoviruses stabilize in the presence of 1 M magnesium sulfate while 1M sodium sulfate stabilizes herpes simplex virus.

This phenomenon can be utilized to rid certain polio preparations of viral adventitious agents such as SV40, foamy virus, and herpes B virus which are susceptible to heating in 1 M MgCl$_2$ whereas this treatment has no adverse effects on the infectivity of poliovirus.

**Antibiotic Sensitivity.** With one exception, antibiotics and the sulfonamides, which are used so successfully in the treatment of bacteria, have no effects on viruses. The antibiotic rifampin readily inactivates bacterial RNA but not animal RNA polymerase. It also is active against poxviruses, presumably acting against the RNA polymerase of the particle, which is essential to poxvirus replication.

Metabolic analogues or antibiotics that interfere with DNA or RNA synthesis will inhibit viral replication. They also adversely affect RNA and DNA synthesis of the host cell. Consequently they are too toxic for use as viral chemotherapeutic agents.

**Chemical Inactivants.** Several classes of organic compounds are reactive with viruses. Aldehydes and ethylene oxide or imine react with primary valence bonds while others such as urea, phenol, detergents, guanadine, and lipid solvents affect mainly salt linkages or secondary valence bonds. Organic solvents such as ether and chloroform readily inactivate viruses with an envelope (see Table XXVI on classification of viruses).

Phenol and hexylresorcinol are excellent protein denaturants that strip protein from some viruses releasing the infectious nucleic acid, which usually contains sufficient RNase to slowly inactivate the acid.

Formaldehyde, ethylene oxide, acetylethyleneimine, and glycidaldehyde are alkylating agents used for viral inactivation. Formaldehyde has been commonly employed to inactivate viruses for vaccine use. It reacts with amino, guanidyl, and amide groups of the viral protein and with nonhydrogen-bonded amino groups of the purine and pyrimidine bases of the nucleic acid. Ethylene oxide in a humid atmosphere is an effective virocide. Acetylethyleneimine appears to have great promise as an inactivant for foot-and-mouth disease virus vaccine because its kinetic curve for inactivation is essentially first-order, without tailing, and inactivation takes place in 24 to 48 hours without destruction of the viral immunizing properties; any excess can be neutralized with sodium thiosulfate. Organic iodine compounds are relatively ineffective against viruses because small amounts of organic matter rapidly deplete the active iodine.

## Replication of Viruses

Viruses are highly parasitic and require living cells to furnish the energy, the enzymes for metabolic activity, and the low molecular weight precursors for viral protein and nucleic acid. Viruses do contain the essential genetic material for its replication in the host cell. The number of enzymes and structural antigens produced in the cell is a function of the size of the viral genome.

Successful replication studies were first accomplished with the T series of bacteriophages. The bacterial system is relatively easy to prepare and manipulate and the growth cycle is short, being measured in minutes whereas animal viruses take many hours to complete their growth cycle. Lastly, the assay of bacteriophage is accurate and simple.

With the advent of improved methods of *in vitro* cultivation of animal cells, in assay for viral content and for study of biophysical, biochemical, and biological characteristics of viruses, some of the steps of interaction between animal viruses and tissue cells have been elucidated. The principal studies involving the adsorption of viruses to specific receptor sites has been done with the orthomyxoviruses. The receptor sites for these viruses are mucopolysacchrides on the cell surface. Viral adsorption can be prevented by the pretreatment of the host cells with an enzyme (receptor destroying enzyme, RDE) from *Vibrio comma* which destroys the mucopolysacchride receptors involved in the hemagglutination reaction. This test procedure has been extensively used in the study of cell receptor sites. Viruses that contain lipid in their structure are released continuously from the cells. In contrast, viruses without lipid are released in large numbers at the time of cell lysis (burst process) similar to bacteriophage.

The replication of RNA and DNA viruses, in general, is similar but differences do exist. The following two sections cite a replication of a RNA and a DNA virus.

**RNA Viral Replication.** The replication of foot-and-mouth disease virus (FMDV), which contains a single-stranded RNA genome, has been studied in greater detail than any other animal virus, beginning with the process of infection and ending with the release of viral progeny. Moreover, the stage of the cycle dealing with the replication of viral RNA has been accomplished in a cell-free system. The complete growth cycle takes place in the cytoplasm, a known characteristic of all RNA viruses whose replication has been studied in any detail. Further, all steps of the cycle apparently are independent of the cellular DNA genome.

Infection of pig kidney cell cultures by FMDV is a two-step process involving adsorption and penetration. Adsorption of virus requires calcium ions and is temperature-dependent with an activation energy of 6,000 calories per mole. The cells appear to possess between 30 to 100 receptor sites for virus. At low temperatures (2 to 4 C) the virus remains attached without penetration and can be released by certain chemicals. At higher temperatures (37 C) the attached virus penetrates the cell by a first-order reaction with an activation energy of 24,000 calories per mole. The half-time of penetration at 37 C of 30 seconds allows infection of 90 percent of the cells within 3 minutes. Virus attaches itself to dead cells but does not penetrate them. Following engulfment by the cell, fragmentation of the virion into infectious RNA and viral protein subunits occurs within the cytoplasm. Because the host range of the disease is not widened by infection with free FMDV-RNA, this is further proof that cellular engulfment of the virion occurs.

Within 30 minutes after infection, cellular protein synthesis is decreased by 50 percent and followed by bursts of virus-specific protein as a result of translation by viral RNA. The first burst occurs at 60 minutes postinfection. It can be inhibited by guanidine and has a temporal correspondence with the expected synthesis of FMD-specific RNA polymerase. Appreciable amounts of polymerase can be extracted from the cell after 2 hours with a peak activity of 3.5 hours after infection. The VIA (virus infection associated antigen) appears to be enzymatically inactive FMDV-specific RNA polymerase because its antibody inhibits polymerase activity. The VIA-RNA polymerase antigen is formed prior to virions and only when virus replicates in cells indicating that it is translated from noncapsid cistrons of the viral genome.

The nature of the second burst is unknown but the third one coincides with viral maturation. In the interim between the first and third burst of virus-specific protein, single-stranded viral RNA molecules (+ stands) presumably are synthesized from the viral RNA in replicate form. More recently it has been demonstrated that C-type particle RNA tumor viruses contain an enzyme, DNA polymerase, that synthesizes DNA from the viral RNA template thus representing an early event in the replication of RNA tumor viruses and that the newly formed DNA serves as the template for viral RNA synthesis or more likely for a complementary DNA strand. The latter transcribes for viral RNA. It is known that actinomycin D inhibits DNA-dependent RNA synthesis and thus inhibits the multiplication of DNA viruses, and also a few RNA viruses such as Rous sacoma virus and RNA myxoviruses. The exact mechanism for this inhibition of RNA viruses is unclear, but perhaps the answer lies in the above explanation for the C-type particle RNA viruses.

The synthesis of viral capsid proteins apparently occurs at the same time. At a subsequent time the proteins then form procapsids or empty protein shells. In some unknown manner the viral genome is incorporated in the procapsids to form the virion that represents maturation. The FMD viral particles are released when the cell undergoes lysis.

**DNA Viral Replication.** The replication of adenoviruses has been thoroughly studied. Adsorption, penetration, and uncoating of a DNA virus such as an adenovirus is similar to that described for FMDV, an RNA virus. After uncoating, the viral DNA migrates to the nucleus where a viral DNA strand is transcribed into specific messenger RNA that is translated to synthesize virus-specific proteins such as tumor antigen and also to enzymes necessary for the biosynthesis of viral RNA. Host-cell DNA synthesis is initially elevated but becomes suppressed as the cell manufactures viral DNA. Messenger RNA transcribed during the late stage of cellular infection migrates to the cytoplasm where translation into viral capsid protein occurs. The capsid protein is transported to the nucleus where it incorporates the viral DNA to form a mature virus particle. The virions are released after cell lysis.

Infectious viral DNA also has been synthesized *in vitro* by the use of a DNA template molecule from the bacterial virus $\Phi$X-174 which can occur as a single- or double-stranded particle. In the presence of a monomer mixture used for polymerization this covalently closed circular viral DNA template $(+)$ is copied by purified DNA polymerase with the formation of linear $(-)$ strand complementary to the $(+)$ circle that the joining enzyme converts into a covalent duplex circle similar to that which occurs *in vivo*.

### Genetics of Animal Viruses

A tremendous amount of knowledge about genetics has been derived from studies of bacterial viruses. Within the last decade two major advances in the animal virology field have made possible meaningful studies of animal viruses. The first advance was the development of accurate and sensitive plaque assay procedures in cell culture systems permitting quantitation of virus infectivity. Through the study of biophysical, biochemical, and biological characteristics of many animal viruses many stable genetic markers were observed that were amenable to experimental manipulation, easy to recognize, and resulting from single mutations. Some markers that are used include plaque size, pathogenicity, specific viral induced antigens, drug resistance, and inability to grow at a higher temperature. These mutations may occur spontaneously or arise after treatment with a mutagen.

Although no genetic map is available for an animal virus it is known that two different virus particles infecting the same host cell may interact in a variety of ways. In genetic interaction some progeny emerge that are genetically different from either parent. Several types of viral interaction can occur simultaneously under the proper conditions. The true viral genetic reactions are recombination, cross-reactivation, and multiplicity reaction as their progeny are genetically stable and some differ from their parents.

Cross-reactivation takes place between the genome of an infectious particle and the genome of an inactivated virus particle. Certain markers of the inactivated parent are rescued in viable progeny as a result of combination between a portion of the inactivated particle genome with the genome of the active particle. None of the progeny have the same characteristics as the inactivated parent. This phenomenon can be used to produce desirable vaccine strains such as was done with influenza virus.

Recombination occurs when some progeny are produced that carry traits not found together in either parent. It is thought that nucleic acid strands break, resulting in the recombination of a part of the genome from one parent with part of the genome of the second parent. Recombinant progeny are stable and yield like progeny upon replication. Recombination has been demonstrated with polio and influenza viruses.

Multiplicity reactivation involves the combination between the genomes of two inactive particles in the same cell that results in the production of a viable genome that can replicate. None of the progeny produced are identical with either parent. This phenomenon has been demonstrated with vaccinia virus.

Phenotypic mixing has been demonstrated with some of the viruses in the enterovirus group. It involves random incorporation of the genome of one virus such as poliovirus into the capsid of another heterologous virus such as coxsackie virus. A stable genetic change does not occur as the phenotypically mixed parent will produce progeny with a capsid homologous to the genotype because protein synthesis is controlled by the viral genome. In this instance the phenotypically mixed parent would have a coxsackievirus capsid, but its progeny would have a poliovirus capsid.

Genotypic mixing is characterized by a single virus particle that produces progeny of two distinct parental types. This is probably an accidental incorporation of two genomes in a single capsid. This unstable genetic change has been seen in the study of orthomyxoviruses.

Complementation is the interaction between two viruses (one or both may be defective or inactivate), that permits replication of either one or both of them. Neither the phenotype or genotype of the virus changes and the progeny are like the parents. Different types of complementation between viruses is indicated by the following examples: (1) active fibroma virus provides the stimulation for an uncoating enzyme necessary for the genomal release of inactivate myxoma virus, (2) active adenovirus provides the production of the coat protein that is required by defective SV40 (PARA) virus, (3) active adenovirus may provide some essential gene product that induces replication of the defective adeno satellite virus, and (4) viable Rous-associated virus probably supplies genetic material for the replication of defective Rous sarcoma virus particles (25) and murine leukemia virus likewise serves as a "helper" for its defective murine sarcoma virus particles.

**Interference.** In the course of investigational studies it has been noted that simultaneous injection of two viruses into a host may result in interference of one of the two viruses. This phenomenon may occur, wholly or in part, between two viruses of different antigenicity, between two strains of the same virus with differences in virulence, or between inactivated and virulent particles of the same virus. The phenomenon is discussed in detail by Vilches and

Hirst (46) who cite many examples. It is known that monkeys infected with lymphocytic choriomeningitis fail to become paralyzed when given polio virus. Distemperoid (ferret distemper virus) or egg-adapted distemper virus interferes with the multiplication of virulent distemper virus in dogs. Inactivated influenza virus interferes with virulent influenza virus. The protective action in these cases cannot be due to antibodies because ample time had not elapsed for antibody formation. One plausible mechanism is the finding by Isaacs *et al.* in 1957 (29). These investigators described a macromolecular substance which they named interferon. In other instances of interference, interferon is not demonstrated. It is believed that the initial virus may alter either the host-cell surface or its metabolic pathways so the superimposing virus is unable to infect the cells. In either instance the interfering process is generally short-lived as cell susceptibility occurs soon after the disappearance of the interfering virus.

The discovery of interferon and its potential use in the treatment and prevention of viral diseases has created much excitement and considerable study. This viral inhibitor can be produced by cells in animals or in culture after infection with viruses. It appears in appreciable quantities after maximum virus production in the host animal but before circulating antibodies appear, suggesting an important role for interferon in the body defenses against viral infection. The cells of the reticuloendothelial system seem to provide most of the interferon although most cells of the body are believed to contribute to its production.

Interferon is a protein which is heat-labile, acid-stable at pH 2, nondialyzable, trypsin-sensitive, non-neutralizable by virus, and weakly antigenic. It is effective as an antiviral substance on cells from the host species from which it was produced; thus, it is species-specific. It is not viral specific. As a matter of fact interferon can be produced *in vitro* in cultures of cells when stimulated with viruses (particularly double-stranded RNA is produced during replication) or synthetic double-stranded polynucleotides; and also by cells in the intact animal (*in vivo*) with viruses, rickettsiae, bacterial endotoxins, synthetic anionic polymers, or polynucleotides. After stimulation of animals with various interferon inducers different classes of interferon are demonstrable, as evidenced by molecular weight differences. One class with a molecular weight of 8.5 by $10^4$ daltons appears 2 hours after induction whereas one with a molecular weight of 3.4 by $10^4$ daltons appears at 18 hours.

Interferon inhibits viral replication by altering cell metabolism. Its presence in a cell stimulates that cell to produce another protein called the translational inhibitory protein (TIP). This protein attaches itself to the cellular ribosomes and alters those structures so viral RNA is not translated, thus the necessary enzymes and capsid protein for progeny virus are not manufactured. Cellular messenger RNA is not affected so normal cell functions continue.

The use of interferon and interferon-inducers in the prevention and treatment of disease has tremendous potential but many important problems exist that must be recognized and solved prior to general use in man and animals. It has been possible to demonstrate the effectiveness of exogenous interferon, in preventing disease or reducing its severity, if given early enough in the disease. Exogenous interferon is very costly to produce and although interferon-inducers offer the greatest hope in controlling certain virus infections, they often are toxic in therapeutic doses and nontoxic antilogues must be developed that are efficacious and reasonable in cost. The half-life of exogenous interferon is very short and frequent injections are required to maintain effective prophylactic levels.

Enhancement, or dual infection, is the antithesis of interference. The demonstration of dual infection of single cells with viruses producing intranuclear (herpes simplex) and cytoplasmic (vaccinia) inclusions was reported by Syverton and Berry (45). This suggests that interference may not take place between viruses that require different pathways for their replication. Another mechanism may be concerned with the activity of one virus that inhibits the formation of interferon. It is known that parainfluenza virus reduces autoinhibition by Newcastle disease virus, a very potent interferon producer. Often coinfection enhances the production of one of the two viruses involved with the emergence of progeny similar to the parents.

Exaltation of disease may result when dual infection occurs in a host. For example when dogs are given distemper and infectious canine hepatitis viruses simultaneously, a more severe disease results than in dogs given either virus along (22).

## CHEMOTHERAPY OF VIRAL INFECTIONS

The control of disease is based upon health measures, immunization, and treatment. The first two criteria have proved to be successful against many viruses and are responsible for the reduced incidence of serious diseases such as canine distemper, hog cholera, rinderpest, feline panleukopenia, and many other infectious viral diseases of domestic animals. With very few exceptions at present, treatment of viral diseases consists of amelioration of signs rather than reduced replication of the virus.

There are two major deterrents to the effective treatment of viral disease. The first, and perhaps the most important, is the strict parasitic relationship of virus and its host cell. It is quite clear that a virus depends upon the metabolism of the host cell for its replication, and majority of viral inhibitors act against cellular processes. A useful viral inhibitor must prevent completion of the viral growth cycle in the infected cell without causing lethal damage of the uninfected cells. This desirable effect can be achieved by a compound that acts directly on a component of the virus or on a viral product such as a virus-specific enzyme that is essential for successful replication. With the finding of virus-specific enzymes the outlook for viral chemotherapy has brightened considerably. Inhibitors that prevent adsorption or penetration of the cell without damaging it are also being sought. The second problem involves the nature and pathogenesis of viral diseases and the attendant problem of an early and accurate diagnosis. Many viral diseases may be recognized too late for effective treatment with a viral inhibitor. In other instances success depends on the availability of safe and effective viral inhibitors.

Amantadine, a symmetrical amine, inhibits certain members of the orthomyxovirus and paramyxovirus groups, pseudorabies virus (a herpesvirus) and Rous sarcoma virus by blocking the penetration of the virus. It has no effect on adsorption of the virus. When administered prophylactically it is very effective in protecting experimental animals and man against influenza A strains. Therapeutic treatment has little or no effect on the course of the disease.

Many viruses of the *Picornaviridae* family are inhibited *in vitro* (tissue cultures) by guanadine and hydroxybenzylbenzimidazole (HBB). These compounds interfere with the synthesis of viral RNA polymerase, thus, preventing the formation of viral protein and viral RNA. After the RNA polymerase is formed neither drug can prevent viral replication. The inhibitory effect can also be overcome by dilution with fresh tissue culture medium. The therapeutic action of the two drugs with marked structural difference presumably is similar but not identical as some viruses can be inhibited by one drug but not the other. In some instances HBB and guanadine have a synergistic effect. Unfortunately there is no protection by either drug in experimental animal infections. This may be due, wholly or in part, to the rapid production of drug resistant mutants.

Thiosemicarbazones were shown to inhibit the growth of poxviruses. Later isatin B-thiosemicarbozone (methisazone) and its N-methyl derivative were shown to have greater protective capacity in experimental animals. These compounds are also an effective prophylactic for smallpox in man if given within 24 to 48 hours after exposure. The drug is virus-specific without any effect on normal cell metabolism. There is normal synthesis of viral DNA and of the two enzymes (thymidine kinase and DNA polymerase) concerned in DNA synthesis. The synthesis of many, but not all, of the 20 or more soluble viral antigens that are formed during normal viral growth is inhibited, resulting in the formation of immature, noninfectious particles. Mutants resistant to this drug have been isolated.

Actinomycin D (dactinomycin) inhibits the replication of DNA viruses and some RNA viruses such as Rous sarcoma virus and some orthomyxoviruses. The drug inhibits DNA-dependent RNA synthesis by a mechanism that is not clear.

The antibiotic, rifampin, shows a preferential inhibition of bacterial RNA polymerase. Poxviruses carry their own RNA polymerase for synthesizing viral messenger RNA and this antibiotic was very effective against smallpox virus in tissue-culture studies by inhibiting the viral polymerase but not materially affecting cellular polymerase.

Analogues of purine and pyrimidine bases may inhibit both RNA and DNA synthesis. Iododeoxyuridine (IUDR) has been used topically with success in the treatment of corneal lesions caused by herpes simplex, a DNA virus. It cannot be used routinely for systemic infections because it is too toxic. Under heroic circumstances, massive near-lethal doses have been administered in cases of herpesvirus encephalitis with complete recovery ensuing. In tissue-culture studies of *Papovaviridae*-infected or herpesvirus-infected cells, IUDR arrests the synthesis of the virion but not the viral components, because large amounts of viral antigen have been found in the cells. Electron-microscopic examination reveals the presence of immature virus particles in large numbers. Other halogenated deoxyuridines such as 5-fiuoro-$2^1$-deoxyuridine (FUDR), and 5-bromo-$2^1$-deoxyuridine (BUDR), as well as IUDR, inhibit replication of members of the major DNA virus groups by the production of an improperly functioning nucleic acid. Drug-resistant mutants of some viruses have emerged by growth in the presence of IUDR or BUDR.

The activity of a purine or pyrimidine analogue can be enhanced by incorporation of ribose or deoxyribose into its molecule. The action of riboside or deoxyribose can be directed preferentially toward the inhibition of RNA or DNA. It has been found that ribosides of halogenated benzimidazoles are more selective inhibitors of influenza virus replication that the free benzimidazoles or their deoxyribosides.

The size of the halogen atom of the halogenated pyrimidine analogue determines the nature of its viral inhibitory action. The size and shape of 5-bromouracil (BU) is very similar to thymine, and 5-fluorourcil (FU) is similar to uracial. Thus, BU has been shown to inhibit DNA bacteriophage but has no effect on the RNA tobacco mosaic virus. FU inhibits RNA virus, and its action is reversed by the addition of uridine but not by thymidine. In the study of specific viral inhibitors this reversion technic involving the addition of analogous normal metabolic compounds is essential to the proof of drug-specificity, rather than inhibition caused by drug-toxicity.

Certain protein inhibitors have been useful in the study of viral replication. Cycloheximide, p-fluorophenylalanine, and puromycin inhibit synthesis of viral and cell protein. Consequently, they can interrupt the cycle of viral replication at various stages. Because they also inhibit cell-protein synthesis these drugs are not viral chemotherapeutic candidates.

## HOST RESPONSE

Viruses are completely dependent on the living cell for their survival and replication. The alterations caused by viruses in cells are regulated by the cell-virus relationships. Some viruses produce little or no alteration in the biochemical mechanisms of the cell. This represents the ultimate in parasitism, because the virus and cell perform their physiological functions for survival with no adverse structural effects on each other. Others have a severe effect, resulting in pathological changes.

As a result of their marked dependence on cell functions for replication, many newly developed and refined technics and procedures are utilized for the study of the host-virus relationships. With advances in electron-microscope technics this methodology permits the study of many ultrastructural features of cell tissue invaded by virus. Immunofluorescence procedures have enhanced pathogenesis studies, permitting investigators to study the pattern of viral infections in various hosts and in tissue and organ cultures. Improved tissue-culture methods also are used to excellent advantage in assaying virus for pathogenesis studies. Histochemistry and radioautography also are being used for studies of this nature. Both standard and phase microscopy provide the means for correlating the gross lesions of viral disease with the molecular level processes.

**Pathogenesis**

The induction of infection by viruses varies markedly depending upon the viral tropism, cell susceptibility, the means of transmission, and the site of body contact.

As a rule, the initial site of contact occurs in cells that line the superficial tissues of exposed surfaces of various body systems including the reproductive, digestive, and respiratory tracts and also the skin. In some instances, but not in all, initial replication of a virus will occur in these primary sites of contact and adsorption. In some instances viral replication will be limited to these superficial tissues. After a sufficient concentration of virus has been attained its spread involves other cells in neighboring tissues. Prime examples of this type would be parainfluenza in dogs and in cattle, and influenza infection in pigs. This localized process also operates in the case of certain viral skin diseases such as molluscum contagiosum and papilloma. Dissemination of some viruses may extend to other remote areas in the body from initial sites through transport in the lymph and blood streams where replication occurs and pathological lesions are formed. Herpes infection in man and animals constitutes a good example of this type of pathogenesis.

In other instances the virus gains entrance into the body through superficial tissues without viral replication and invades the macrophages, leukocytes, and other cellular elements in the blood stream and is then transported to various tissues throughout the body with adsorption and replication of virus occurring in other fixed, susceptible cells. Canine distemper is an excellent example. In neurotropic canine cases of distemper, virus also penetrates the blood-brain-barrier with virus antigen appearing first in meningeal macrophages, long after viremia occurrs, and then in perivascular cells, ependymal cells, and later in glial and neuronal cells (3).

In the case of arthropod-borne viruses, transmission of the disease is dependent upon insect vectors, which inject the virus through a bite. The virus invades the blood stream and replicates in cells of the endothelial lining of lymph and blood vessels.

A variety of mechanisms operate in the successful adsorption of viruses to cells. Proper receptor sites on cell surfaces are essential to viral adsorption. Certain orthomyxoviruses contain a surface enzyme necessary for union with specific receptors at definite loci on the cell surface. Specific receptor sites also are involved in cell-enterovirus union. Phagocytosis of attached virus by the cell occurs at a time when the viral nucleic acid is released from its protein coat, permitting viral nucleic acid to direct the cellular activity essential to its successful replication (described in section of viral replication in this chapter).

Cells in an animal host at different ages may vary in their susceptibility to viruses producing diverse disease pictures. Infectious bovine rhinotracheitis virus in neonatal calves causes a generalized disease with the most dramatic lesions occurring in the anterior portion of the digestive tract, but with generalized pustular lesions in most body systems. In contrast, lesions in the anterior portion of the digestive tract in older calves or young adults do not occur and lesions are likely to be confined to one body system (5). Less dramatic differences are observed with experimental foot-and-mouth disease in the avian host but prominent heart lesions and the highest virus titers in this organ occur in the 14-day-old chicken embryo whereas lesions and the higher virus titers occur in the gizzard muscle of the 1-day-old chick (18). This demonstrates a remarkable difference in cell susceptibility of the developing avian host to FMDV within a period of 8 days.

The effective transmission of viruses from one host to another is essential in the pathogenesis of any viral disease. This subject is covered in the section on transmission (p. 865).

## Pathology

The various routes of viral transport within the body serve as a means to establish infection in these cells for which each virus has an affinity or tropism. The nature of the infection (and disease) is determined by the degree of parasitism, the number, and type of cells involved in the viral-host relationship, and the nature of viral replication within the cell.

The intracellular processes leading to degeneration and necrosis manifests itself in many different pathological changes in cells. Viral infections are usually characterized by vacuolation, ballooning degeneration, syncytium formations, hypertrophy, and hyperplasia. Nucleolar displacement, margination of nuclear chromatin, and the production of cytoplasmic or intranuclear inclusions are changes at the cellular level. The degree, nature, and type of cellular involvement determines the severity and nature of the disease. In some instances no clinical signs or lesions are associated with the infection, while in others severe disease with resulting death ensues. In most viral infections the initial stages of the pathogenesis are clinically inapparent and in some diseases signs of illness do not occur until late in acute stages of the disease, often when antibodies are first demonstrable.

**Inclusion Bodies.** In many virus diseases round or oval bodies may be found in the cytoplasm or within the nuclei of affected cells. These have long been known to pathologists as *inclusion bodies*. They are indicative of the presence of virus in the cell. Some are so characteristic in appearance and staining qualities that they are of diagnostic importance. They are not used so often as formerly for diagnosis because better methods are available in most cases. The Negri body, found in certain nerve cells of animals suffering from rabies, is an inclusion body still commonly sought as a means of quick diagnosis of that disease.

Inclusion bodies have not been detected in some virus diseases, and in others their presence is not constant. The majority of inclusion bodies stain with acid dyes. A few are basophilic, and others are basophilic and Feulgen positive in their early stages and acidophilic later. The inclusion bodies of trachoma of man, of psittacosis in man and animals, and of some related diseases of the psittacoid lymphogranuloma group are quite different from those of virus infections. They have been described under psittacosis.

The eosinophilic cytoplasmic inclusions vary in size in different diseases, and in variant cases of the same disease, up to 20 or more microns in diameter. There may be only one, or several, bodies within a single cell. Some of these may be large and others much smaller. Some appear to be quite hyaline but most are granular, and some contain distinctly stained "inside" bodies.

Two types of intranuclear inclusions may be distinguished. Cowdry (14) refers to them as A- and B-types. The *Type A inclusions* are found in nuclei in which there is evidence of severe disruption of the chromatic structure. The chromatin fragments are crowded around the nuclear membrane (margination). The inclusion body, or bodies, usually lie near the center of the nucleus and appear as amorphous or granular, generally acid-staining material. The affected tissue often shows cells with bodies in different stages of development; that is, fully developed bodies may be seen in some cells and much smaller ones in neighboring cells. The *Type B inclusions* may vary in size but they are better circumscribed, there is no margination of chromatin, and the nucleus presents a less disorganized appearance than in the other type. Type A bodies are found in such diseases as canine hepatitis, canine distemper, infectious enteritis, and pseudorabies. A good example of the Type B inclusion is the Joest body found in Borna disease.

Some of the earlier workers regarded inclusion bodies as the infective agent; some regarded them as protozoa; others thought them to be aggregates of minute parasites embedded in capsular or other hyaline material. When filtration experiments demonstrated that the viruses of many diseases obviously were much smaller than the inclusion bodies seen in those diseases, there was a tendency to regard them as specific degeneration products of the cell substance. More recently, however, evidence has accumulated that some of the bodies contain aggregates of virus elementary bodies.

Borrel (11) studied the inclusions, known as *Bollinger bodies*, found in pox of fowls. These are rather large structures that occur in the cytoplasm of diseased epithelial cells. Microscopically, minute spherical corpuscles were detected within the larger body, which, when crushed, released smaller bodies. These are now known as *Borrel bodies*. Borrel bodies may be separated from affected tissues by crushing, by tryptic digestion, and by differential centrifugation. After many washings these bodies are capable of inducing fowlpox; that is, they contain virus. Borrel bodies may be specifically agglutinated by the serum of animals that have recovered from the disease or have been immunized against it. They are regarded as the virus particles, or *elementary bodies*. A similar condition can be demonstrated in several other virus diseases.

It has now been established that the intranuclear inclusion bodies may contain virus. It has not been proved that all inclusion bodies are virus carriers. It is possible, of course, that some are specific degenerative structures and others are essentially virus aggregates.

**Inflammatory Response.** The inflammation that accompanies viral infections is usually secondary to the primary cellular alterations. There is little to distinguish viral infections based upon the character of the inflammatory response. Edema is often observed as an early and persistent feature but the reason for its occurrence is unknown. The early cellular response to most viral infections is mononuclear and lymphocytic.

Polymorphonuclear leukocytes are commonly found in bacterial infections, but the initial and in many instances the whole reaction to viruses depends upon mononuclear cells, including macrophages, lymphocytes, and plasma cells. Inflammation is found in most viral diseases. In louping ill, Purkinje cells undergo complete necrosis before any infiltration is observed. In rabies, neuronal cells are completely destroyed and yet there is often no inflammatory response.

When secondary bacterial infection does occur in viral diseases, infiltration of polymorphonuclear leukocytes is presumably a response to cell necrosis and degeneration. The leukocytes predominate in the lesions of infectious bovine rhinotracheitis infection where massive necrosis is observed. Perivascular infiltration with lymphocytes is especially characteristic of various types of viral encephalitis such as the equine encephalomyelides. The lymphocytic pleocytosis in the cerebrospinal fluid usually distinguishes aseptic meningitis from purulent meningitis.

Secondary bacterial infection often complicates viral diseases. This is especially true in viral respiratory and skin diseases, particularly the former. Many potential bacterial pathogens reside on the skin and in the respiratory tract. The initial damage to the superficial cells of these organs by the virus provides the necessary conditions for the rapid invasion and multiplication of the bacterial pathogens, whose influence changes the nature and character of the disease to an acute pyogenic inflammatory infection that is often responsible for the high morbidity and mortality rates encountered in many viral epidemics. This sequence of events is characteristic for most viral respiratory diseases of domestic animals.

Virus infections of cells cause chromosome damage with derangement of the karyotype. Most changes are random in nature. Most frequently breakage, fragmentation, and rearrangement of the chromosomes occur. Abnormal chromosomes and changes in their number also are observed. Cell cultures infected with or transformed to malignancy by certain adenoviruses, as infectious canine hepatitis virus, exhibit such changes as well as random chromosomal abnormalities in addition to fragmentation. Certain viruses, as herpes simplex virus in the Chinese hamster cell, cause chromosome breaks that are not random in distribution. Replication of the virus is necessary for induction of the chromosome aberrations. As yet, chromosome alterations cannot assist in the identification of virus-infected or virus-transformed cells.

**Constitutional Effects.** Each viral infection is recognized by a number of nonspecific constitutional disturbances including fever, myalgias, anorexia, malaise, and headaches. These signs are attributed to a number of factors such as absorption of degradation products from injured cells, viral toxicity, vascular abnormalities producing circulatory disturbances, viremia dose, and other less specific factors. Usually the mechanism that leads to the production of signs of disease, and certainly death, in viral diseases is unknown. Vascular shock, viral toxicity, functional failure of one or more vital organs are believed to account for death.

### Immunopathic Viral Diseases

Certain viruses cause chronic diseases. The presently accepted hypothesis holds that the immunologic response of the host to persisting viruses in these diseases causes the formation of circulating virus-antibody complexes which results in cellular alterations with the production of disease. This mechanism apparently exists in lymphocytic choriomeningitis in mice. If adults are rendered immunologically incompetent by immunosuppressive drugs, x-irradiation, or antiserum produced against the lymphoid elements of the mouse no illness is produced after inoculation with the virus. The virus replicates and persists until immunocompetence is re-established, at which time the mouse becomes ill. Infection of newborn mice before they become immunocompetent results in a lifetime viral infection without illness. Age plays a definite role in the persistence of certain viruses. This may be related to the development of immunocompetence. Other notable examples that may have a similar basic mechanism include Aleutian disease of mink and equine infectious anemia. These are characterized by persisting virus and by pathologic alterations of blood vessels and kidneys not unlike those seen in certain connective-tissue disorders of man. It should be made clear that no proof exists that these are immunopathic diseases.

## Latent Virus Infections

A few decades ago only a limited number of viruses were believed to persist in the host. Now the vast majority of viruses are known to persist, and this has been determined through new and refined technics for the detection of incomplete and complete virus. In some viral diseases the agent is transmitted vertically from mother to progeny and horizontal transmission is not necessary—an ideal situation for the perpetuation of the parasite.

Many viral diseases occur as inapparent (or silent) infections in the human or animal populations. Such infections are important in the epidemiology and immunity of a given population. In many instances these inapparent viral infections end with the elimination of the parasite from the host. In others, especially in subclinical infections, this does not occur but results in the phenomenon known as latent infection. With some diseases such as lymphocytic choriomeningitis in mice and Rous sarcoma infection in chickens, the virus persists but antibody does not develop and the animal remains a virus carrier for an indefinite period. In other diseases caused by herpesviruses, adenoviruses, and varicella-zoster virus, virus persists after the initial infection despite the production of antibody. The basic nature of latent infection with these viruses is poorly understood *in vivo*. For example, herpesvirus is presumed to survive within certain cells of the buccal mucous membranes, lymph nodes, or local sensory ganglia. It is not known if the virus persists as a complete virion or as "occult" virus; or if latent infection is established in all individuals after a primary experience with the virus. It is known that reactivation follows stimulation by a physical, nutritional, or endocrine altercation or during a fever or cold. An interesting observation has been made in a tissue culture system which may explain the pathogenesis of the reactivated latent disease (24). Certain variants of herpesvirus induce the formation of syncytia by which adjacent cells can be invaded by virus through interconnecting cytoplasmic channel ways. By this route virus avoids contact with antibody.

Occult (or masked) virus may account for the long duration of immunity attributed to such diseases as canine distemper, but presently there is no adequate way to detect this type of virus. In the case of certain tumor viruses such as Shope papilloma virus, the course of the infection is long and eventually the virus becomes occult. The phenomenon of masked virus occurs with other DNA viruses such as polyoma, SV40, and human adenovirus 12 and 18. With polyoma, the antigenic components for the virus become undetectable and there is no evidence of virus or viral genome in the transformed cells. It has been postulated that SV40 induced transformed cells carry the viral genome in an noninfectious state and on rare occasions a parasitized cell produces infectious virus. On the other hand, certain RNA tumor viruses such as Rous virus and murine leukemia viruses persist in transformed cells and defective Rous virus can produce transformed cells in culture. For example, growth of cells in culture may occur for many generations despite replication of a virus. Usually, only a small proportion of the cells is infected with virus. This may be likened to slow virus infections in a natural host that are characterized by a prolonged incubation period lasting months or years during which time the virus replicates with progressive destruction of tissue as occurs in diseases like scrapie, visna, maedi, Aleutian disease, and equine infectious anemia. In some viral cell-culture systems the cell continues to survive despite viral replication in that cell, thus, resembling a moderate virus infection. In these virus-carrier cultures the virus seems to be under some control, perhaps, interferon is responsible in some instances. By various means, the virus can be released in these cultures by cell crowding, lowering the temperature, or medium exhaustion. Although cell cultures have helped to increase our knowledge of viral latency the results must be viewed with caution as they may apply to the natural host where defense mechanisms are in operation that are lacking in an *in vitro* system.

## Natural and Acquired Resistance in Virus Diseases

**Natural Resistance.** It is quite clear now that mechanisms for resistance to viral infections involves more than the production of circulating antibodies. This became apparent as a result of viral and bacterial resistance studies with hypogammaglobulinemia patients, absence of an antibody response in certain congenital viral infections, and the role of antibodies in the protection of animals against the production of tumors by oncogenic viruses.

Innate susceptibility or resistance are terms commonly used in discussing so-called *natural resistance* (or susceptibility) of a given species to a particular viral infection. This may also apply to the marked variation in resistance of individuals to a given virus within a species. The mechanisms involved in innate resistance are poorly understood but they may operate at the level of the cell or organism (host). The route of viral entry also is a factor.

At the cellular level, adsorption of the virus to the cell receptors is the first and perhaps most important factor in cellular resistance or susceptibility. In some instances, such as poliovirus, other human enteroviruses, and phage-resistant strains of *Escherichia coli,* cellular insusceptibility is caused by the failure of adsorption and not the ability of the nucleic acid to replicate in cells. Actually little is known about intracellular factors affecting the susceptibility of cells to viral infection but such things as pH, temperature, interferon, and genetics can play a role.

Two known forces operating at the organism level that are generally recognized include the blood-brain barrier and the role of the reticuloendothelial system. These were considered in the section on pathology.

At present, the only effective experimental approach to the study of the mechanisms of innate resistance to virus infections can be made in "inbred" mouse colonies or perhaps in chicken flocks. These animal lines may differ markedly in their resistance to certain viral diseases. The mechanism of resistance in these "inbred" lines to various viruses may differ. Susceptibility by mouse lines to St. Louis encephalitis and louping-ill viruses was correlated with the level of viral multiplication in the mouse brain. The Princeton Rockefeller Institute mice are highly resistant to 17D strain of yellow fever virus and this observation (35) extended to the other group B arboviruses but not the group A arboviruses. In the intact animal it is sometimes possible to produce resistance by transfer of macrophages from resistant to susceptible animals. Macrophages also play the same role in infectious hepatitis of mice. Unfortunately, this does not seem to be the case with mousepox where macrophages apparently had no influence on the susceptibility of mice to this disease. It is well to note that selective breeding to one viral disease does not insure resistance to others.

Natural selection in a population plays an important role in the history (ecology) of a viral disease. Most diseases as we know them represent such a situation where adjustment of the host and virus occur over a long period of time. An excellent opportunity for the study of innate resistance occurred in Australia two decades ago when virulent myxoma virus was introduced into a previously unexposed, highly susceptible wild rabbit population. Initially the case-mortality rate was 90 percent but within 7 years fell to 25 percent under standardized conditions.

Other environmental factors known to operate in disease resistance include age, ambient temperature, and poorly developed thermal regulating mechanism of most species at time of birth. Neonatal animals are often highly susceptible to viruses during the first weeks of life. Consequently, neonatal animals are often used for study of viruses. Certainly, dogs are more susceptible to canine distemper and canine herpesvirus during the first 1 to 2 weeks of life. Fortunately, maternal antibodies are conferred to the progeny counteracting this highly susceptible period. Temperature also may have an effect on the viral multiplication, antibody response, and interferon production of the organism. The aged often are more susceptible to virus infections—for reasons unknown.

**Acquired Resistance.** Acquired resistance (or immunity) is obtained by contact with the antigens of infectious agents and specific antibodies to these substances play an important role in the resistance of the host organism. As stated in an earlier section there are two main segments in the immune response, namely (1) the production and effects of humoral antibodies, and (2) the delayed type of sensitivity, principally mediated by specifically altered cells.

Immunity in a considerable proportion of all virus diseases is absolute and relatively long-lasting. This is quite different from that which is found in bacterial diseases, because these are only relative and usually short-lived. Such solid and lasting immunities do not occur in all virus diseases; in fact in

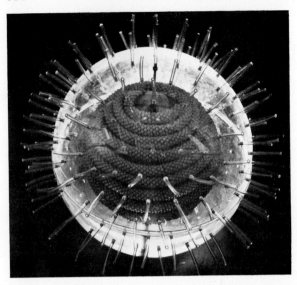

*Fig. 156.* This model shows a possible arrangement of components in myxoviruses. (Courtesy R. W. Horne and P. Wildy, *Virology.*)

many, especially those which affect superficial structures such as herpes infections and foot-and-mouth disease, it is solid but not long lasting.

The prolonged solid immunity found in many virus diseases cannot be explained with certainty. When antigens come in contact with tissues, antibodies are produced, and these usually may be recognized by a variety of established methods. If the antigen is contained in a parasitic or pathogenic organism that multiplies and retains its position in the body for a considerable period of time, antibodies will be stimulated as long as the stimulus remains. If it is a nonviable antigen that is quickly eliminated from the body, antibody formation quickly ceases and the blood titer is soon lost. The same thing ordinarily happens when an animal recovers from an infection. How then can continued virus-neutralizing power be maintained, as it is in many virus diseases, long after all evidence of the disease has disappeared?

No definite answer can be given to this question at present. The fact that viruses develop only intracellularly whereas bacteria usually develop in the body fluids may be responsible for the difference. In these cases viruses may find it possible to continue to exist in certain cells of the recovered host as latent or occult virus in spite of the fact that the body fluids contain virus-neutralizing antibodies. Such an individual may have little or no ability to infect others because the neutralizing antibodies bathing the infected cells would prevent the escape of virus into any of the secretions or excretions of the body under most circumstances, but might not prevent the passage of virus through intercellular bridges to other susceptible cells of the same individual. In virus diseases it is at least theoretically possible that many individuals will continue to harbor the virus as long as they live. Such individuals would be expected to show continuous production of antibodies especially if the virus persisted in cells involved in antibody production and maintain a solid immunity to reinfection. This theory is supported by Poppensiek and Baker (33) who showed that virus in the urine and immunity persisted in dogs that recovered from infectious canine hepatitis.

Rivers, Haagen, and Muckenfuss (34) inoculated rabbit cornea with vaccinia virus and then maintained the viability of the corneal cells by submerging them in antivaccinal plasma. They found that corneal lesions developed in spite of the virus-neutralizing antibodies in the plasma. When the vaccinia virus was first mixed with the plasma before the addition of the corneal tissue, the tissue did not become infected. These experiments prove that viruses may develop in cells that are bathed with antiviral substances. Such experiments serve to explain the frequent clinical experiences indicating that viral antisera may be useful as preventive agents but are useless in treating already existing disease.

Another interesting possibility was pointed up by the findings of van Bekkum and colleagues (10) with animals that have recovered from foot-and-mouth disease. This is a disease in which immunity is relatively short-lived and in which it has always been believed that virus disappears rather quickly after recovery. The Dutch workers discovered that FMD virus could be recovered from the saliva of a considerable portion of recovered cattle for several months after all evidence of the disease had disappeared even though these animals did not transmit the disease to susceptible cattle which were kept in close contact with them. Convalescing animals apparently continued to produce a small amount of virus for a long period, the amount being too small to cause infection by ordinary contacts.

**Passive Immunity.** Specific hyperimmune sera are useful against a number of animal virus diseases. When these sera are administered before infection occurs, or perhaps very early in the course of the infection before the virus has been widely disseminated, they are fairly effective. The protection given by such sera usually is complete and solid, but it is of short duration. It is not safe to depend upon passive immunity lasting for more than 1 to 2 weeks. Additional doses can be given to prolong this period. Antiserum is often used to protect susceptible animals during critical periods. If the passively immunized animal comes in contact with virus during the period of protection, active immunization often occurs.

In general, it is useless to administer antisera to animals that exhibit well-marked signs of virus infections. The virus, in these cases, has already reached the susceptible cells, where it is beyond the reach of the antibodies.

Hyperimmune antisera are used effectively in combating cholera of swine and infectious enteritis of cats. It may be used in many more virus diseases, but in some either it is impracticable, ineffective, or better methods of protection are known.

In *maternal immunity* the temporary immunity is conferred by the mother to her progeny. This is very important in many virus diseases, as neonatal infections are often fatal. Certainly this is true for many human and animal viruses. In general, there is a quantitative relationship between the serum titer of the dam at birth and the duration of the passive protection for the progeny. For example, the duration of maternal protection for puppies against distemper and infectious canine hepatitis viruses, in general, persists from 4 to 15 weeks. Obviously, dams with the highest serum antibody titers confer protection to their progeny for the longest period of time. Most domestic animals receive the major portion of their maternal antibody through the colostrum, thus it is important for them to nurse well in the first 24 to 48 hours of life. For more information about maternal immunity, see the section on canine distemper.

**Active Immunization.** The methods of actively immunizing against virus infections fall into four categories: (*a*) the use of fully virulent virus alone, (*b*) the use of virulent virus and antiserum, simultaneously, (*c*) the use of vaccines made from attenuated virus, and (*d*) the use of inactivated virus.

*Fully virulent virus.* When fully virulent virus is used, it is usually administered by an abnormal route. This is a relatively dangerous method because the virulent material does not always behave in a predictable manner, and at best it is undesirable to spread virulent material to premises where it did not formerly exist. When it is used, *all susceptible stock* on the same premises should be treated; otherwise there is danger of producing an epizootic among the unprotected animals. This method is seldom used on man, but it is employed for the control of a number of animal diseases including contagious ecthyma of sheep and infectious laryngotracheitis and infectious bronchitis of chickens.

*Virus and antiserum simultaneously.* The best-known example of the use of virus and antiserum simultaneously is in hog cholera. In this method of immunization, the antiserum is depended upon to lessen the virus effect so the animal suffers only a mild virus reaction.

*Attenuated virus.* Attenuated viruses for immunization purposes are generally made by adapting them to hosts other than the one on which the vaccine is to be used. In many cases this increases the virulence for the new host but reduces it for others. The first virus vaccine, the rabies vaccine of Pasteur (31), was of this type. This was produced by passing virulent virus through a series of rabbits. Finally when the virus had developed great virulence for the rabbit, it was found that it had lost most of its pathogenicity for other animals and man. This attenuated virus thus could be used to stimulate antibodies that would protect against the more virulent strains. Other examples of such attenuated virus vaccines are the ferret-adapted virus vaccine for canine distemper, the mouse-brain vaccines for yellow fever of man and the horsesickness of Africa, and the vaccines for rinderpest, distemper, and rabies made by cultivating the viruses in fertile hens' eggs. When viruses have been adapted to rabbits, the natural hosts being other species, the virus is said to have been *lapinized.* When a foreign virus is adapted to birds or eggs, it is said to have been *avianized.*

The propagation of viruses in cell cultures from tissues of the same or alien hosts usually results in their attenuation for the natural host. These attenuated virus vaccines now are used to protect individuals against many diseases, and they are rapidly replacing attenuated virus vaccines produced *in vivo*. Tissue-cultured vaccines are usually simpler and cheaper to produce and also easier to assay for viral content because most viruses cause a cytopathogenic effect in cell cultures. They are only approved after the product is determined to be safe and efficacious.

The major concern in the production of attenuated virus vaccines *in vivo* and *in vitro* is the problem of latent viruses and *Mycoplasma* contamination. The latter seems to be easier to detect but it is quite difficult to control. Latent viruses in both systems confront our medical professions with major problems. There is a slow but gradual shift from primary or secondary cell cultures to the use of diploid- or stable-line cell cultures for the production of veterinary and human viral vaccines. These lines are carefully monitored for all known viruses, particularly to the respective hosts from which the cell cultures were derived, and also for *Mycoplasma*. In addition, critical cytological studies including karyography and oncogenic capabilities are made before approval is given for the production of viral vaccines in these cell lines.

The duration of the immunity conferred by vaccines containing active virus depends upon the peculiarities of the virus itself. When the natural disease confers a solid and permanent immunity, attenuated virues vaccines generally will do the same.

*Inactivated virus.* The word "inactivation" is used in viral terminology to avoid the use of the word "killed," which is commonly used in bacteriology. The implications with respect to life are thus avoided.

There are those who do not believe that fully inactivated virus vaccines can induce useful immunity in animals. These have felt, and more recent knowledge of the nature of viruses lends plausibility to their beliefs, that the so-called *inactivated viruses* generally contain some active elements. It is possible that inactivation may prove to be a reversible phenomenon, that inactivated agents may be reactivated in some degree by contact with susceptible cells. It has been conclusively demonstrated many times that so-called inactivated viruses really have contained a very small fraction of active virus, a portion which has much greater resistance to the attenuating agent than most of the virus volume (4, 16).

Replication of foot-and-mouth disease virus produces an enzyme (VIA) detectable in the agar-gel diffusion test (13). Sera from animals given inactivated FMD virus fail to show this enzyme antibody. It is possible that this phenomenon may be used to test other inactivated virus vaccines for infectious virions.

Today most virologists accept the concept that it is possible to induce serviceable immunity with wholly inactivated viruses. To be effective such vaccines must contain relatively large amounts of virus protein, because there can be no increase of protein in the body such as occurs when active virus is used. It is often difficult to produce vaccines with sufficient protein to provide satisfactory antigenic stimulus, and it is believed that this has been the reason for many failures. Moreover, inactivated virus cannot supply continuing stimulation; hence the induced immunity may be initially solid but cannot last. The inactivated virus vaccines for eastern and western equine encephalomyelitis and for feline panleukopenia are excellent biologics.

Viruses may be inactivated with heat, chemicals, ultraviolet rays, ultrasonic vibration, and other processes which commonly destroy life in higher forms. Care must be exercised to be certain that complete inactivation results (16).

### Cross Immunity in Viral Infections

It has been pointed out that antigenicity is a property of the protein fraction of the virus moiety, the innocuous portion which serves to protect the nucleic acid or infectious fraction.

As known for a long time with bacteria, there are antigenic relationships and similarities among viruses. These do not necessarily mean that common pathogenic factors exist, or that the agents are biologically related. The literature contains a number of examples. One of the most intriguing of these is the relationship that exists between measles in man, distemper in dogs, and rinderpest in cattle (1, 32). The protection conferred by measles virus in dogs against virulent distemper virus is based upon the anamnestic response (20). The protection conferred by bovine virus diarrhea virus in pigs against virulent hog cholera virus is based upon a similar phenomenon (37).

### Viral Resistance

In general, viruses seem to possess about the same degree of resistance to heat, drying, and many chemical agents as the vegetative forms of most bacteria. Moist heat at 55 to 60 C for 30 minutes serves all practical purposes of disinfection; yet it has been shown that a very small residuum of active FMD virus remains after exposure at these temperatures for several times as long. This same situation exists for some other viruses. Drying is destructive to most viruses; yet there are some that survive very long periods of ordinary drying. Freeze drying, or lyophilization, is one of the best methods of preserving viruses for long periods of time. Another method is the storage of viruses at −60 C or lower.

To chemical disinfectants, viruses behave in general about like vegetative forms of bacteria, but there are important differences. Most viruses are wholly unaffected by concentrations of most antibiotics that will inhibit and destroy bacteria. In most tissue culture work it is standard practice to incorporate such substances as penicillin, streptomycin, or mycostatin in the culture media to restrain the growth of bacteria and molds and allow unrestricted growth of viruses.

Viruses, it should be remembered, are usually present in necrotic tissue fragments and mixed with coagulable proteins that may serve as effective protective coatings, delaying access of chemicals to the active agents. Because strongly alkaline solutions are effective tissue solvents, it has been believed that they were particularly effective agents in chemical disinfection. Two percent lye solution has been used for many years in disinfection following outbreaks of FMD, apparently with complete success. Recently it has been found that this solution is not very effective in laboratory experiments with this virus, and with the virus of vesicular stomatitis. It is probable that the virtue of the lye has resided not so much in its virucidal properties as in its solvent and detergent properties, because these have resulted in exposing the virus particles, diluting them, and removing them from the environment.

Most viruses are well preserved in strong solutions of glycerol (50 to 100 percent). Such concentrations cause dehydration of the cells containing virus and tend to prevent their autolysis.

## REFERENCES

1. Adams and Imagawa. Proc. Soc. Exp. Biol. and Med.; 1957, 96, 240.
2. Anderson, Hopps, Barile, Bernheim. Jour. Bact.; 1965, 60, 1387.
3. Appel, M. J. G. Am. Jour. Vet. Res.; 1969, 30, 1167.
4. Bachrach, Breese, Callis, Hess, and Patty. Proc. Soc. Exp. Biol. and Med., 1957; 95, 147.
5. Baker, McEntee, and Gillespie. Cornell Vet., 1960, 50, 156.
6. Bauer and Hughes. Jour. Gen. Physiol., 1934–35, 18, 143.
7. Bauer and Pickels. Jour. Exp. Med., 1936, 64, 503.
8. Bechhold. Zeitschr. phys. Chem., 1907, 60, 257.
9. Beijerinck. Centrbl. f. Bakt.; II; Abt., 1899, 5, 27.
10. Van Bekkum, Frenkel, Fredericks, and Frenkel. Tijdschr. v. Diergeneesk., 1959, 84, 1159.
11. Borrel. Comp. rend Soc. Biol. (Paris), 1904, 57, 642.
12. Brenner and Horne. Biochem. et Biophys. Acta, 1959, 34, 103.
13. Cowan and Graves. Virology, 1966, 30, 528.
14. Cowdry. Arch. Path., 1934, 18, 527.
15. Eklund, Bell, and Hadlow. Am. Jour. Hyg., 1956, 64, 85.
16. Elford. Jour. Path. and Bact., 1931, 34, 505.
17. Fenner. The biology of animal viruses. Vol. I, Academic Press, New York, 1968, p. 2.
18. Gillespie. Cornell Vet., 1955, 45, 170.
19. Gillespie, Robinson, and Baker. Proc. Soc. Exp. Biol. and Med., 1952, 81, 461.
20. Gillespie and Karzon. Ibid., 1961, 105, 547.
21. Hanafusa, Hanafusa, and Rubin. Proc. Natl. Acad. Sci. (U.S.), 1963, 49, 572.

22. D'Herelle. The bacteriophage: Its role in immunity. Eng. trans., Williams and Wilkins Co., Baltimore, 1922.
23. Hirst. Science, 1941, *94*, 22.
24. Hoggan, Roizman, and Roane. Am. Jour. Hyg., 1961, *173*, 114.
25. Isaacs and Lindenmann. Proc. Roy. Soc., 1957, *147*, 258.
26. Iwanowski. Bul. Acad. Imp. Science, St. Petersburg, 3rd ser., 1892–94, *35*, 67.
27. Kannanis. Jour. Gen. Microbiol, 1962, 27, 477.
28. Loeffler and Frosch. Centrbl. f. Bakt., I, Abt., 1898, *23*, 371.
29. Lwoff and Tournier. Ann. Rev. Microbiol., 1966, 20, 45.
30. McClelland and Hare. Canad. Pub. Health Jour., 1941, *32*, 530.
31. Pasteur. Comp. rend. Acad. Sci., 1885, *101*, 765.
32. Polding, Simpson, and Scott. Vet. Rec., 1959, *71*, 643.
33. Poppensiek and Baker. Proc. Soc. Exp. Biol. and Med., 1951, 77, 279.
34. Rivers, Haagen, and Muckenfuss. Jour. Exp. Med., 1929, *50*, 673.
35. Sabin. Proc. Natl. Acad. Sci., 1952, 38, 540.
36. Sanarelli. Centrbl. f. Bakt., I, Abt., 1898, *23*, 865.
37. Sheffy, Coggins, and Baker. Proc. Soc. Exp. Biol. and Med., 1962, *109*, 349.
38. Stanley. Science, 1935, *81*, 644.
39. Syverton and Berry. Jour. Exp. Med., 1947, *86*, 145.
40. Vilches and Hirst. Jour. Immunol., 1947, *57*, 125.
41. Webster. Jour. Exp. Med., 1937, *65*, 261.
42. Williams and Wyckoff. Science, 1945, *101*, 594.

# XXXVII | Epidemiology of Viral Infections

The epidemiology of viral diseases is an exceedingly fascinating area of microbiology because of the unique biochemical, biophysical, and biological characteristics of viruses. With their highly parasitic nature and small size, certain problems arise which make the viruses more difficult to recognize in nature than other microorganisms. With the advent of modern tissue-culture technics, as well as improved methods of purification, concentration, and visualization, the detection of viruses in our environment is more easily accomplished now than one or two decades ago. Our increased knowledge of the host spectrum of viruses has also aided in their detection as we still rely heavily upon the effects that viruses produce in various animal species for their recognition. Thus, our knowledge of the epidemiology and ecology of viral diseases has grown at a rate commensurate with our technological advancements in animal virology. Consequently, it becomes obvious that a meaningful program in viral epidemiology requires competent laboratory support utilizing various viral isolation and serological procedures.

According to Shope (9) periodicity and seasonal prevalence are two characteristic features of most viral diseases, but these are incompletely understood. The terms "distemper years," "hog cholera years," "foot-and-mouth disease years," and so on, are expressions used for our recognition of the periodicity of viral diseases. These years of significant disease caused by various animal viruses are explained on the basis of increased virulence or invasiveness of the virus or on the fluctuating ratio of immune and susceptible animals in a population. Thus, the virus and the host both play a major role in the periodicity of disease. Certain viral diseases do have a seasonal prevalence, such as canine distemper, which occurs more frequently in the Fall and Winter. Where arthropod vectors are involved in disease transmission, such as the arboviruses, the disease occurs during the summer season in temperate zones.

863

For many years epidemiologists limited their studies of an outbreak from the time it appeared as a disease in a single host species until it disappeared from that population; with each experience treated as an episode. More recently, epidemiologists have broadened their interests by concerning themselves with the ecology and natural history of viral disease(s) seeking more information about the location and survival of the virus during the interepidemic phase. The epidemiology of animal viral diseases, generally speaking, is less complex and less difficult to study than human viral diseases. Farm and pet animals usually are confined to limited areas of travel and contact with large numbers of animals from outside sources is the exception rather than the rule. Our greatest disease problems in veterinary medicine are usually associated with the movement of animals from one location to another where assembly of animals from many sources occurs. Even wild animals, except certain species of birds and bats, tend to reside within a limited geographic area; thus exposure to various disease agents is restricted. This situation does produce a more susceptible population which leads to more explosive outbreaks when an agent is introduced into a virgin population. For example, rather severe outbreaks of canine distemper with a high morbidity and mortality rate in dogs of all ages has been reported in isolated arctic communities. Obviously, it is simpler to study the natural history of disease under these circumstances than a population in various stages of immunity; thus, animal models are often applied to enhance one's knowledge of the epidemiology of certain human viral diseases. There are many notable examples, but the earliest and perhaps in many ways the most important was the finding, by Smith and Kilbourne (11), of the arthropod transmission of Texas fever in cattle. Of course, many viruses produce infection and disease in animals and man under natural conditions, and these particular infections are of great interest to human and veterinary medicine.

**Persistence of Virus in Nature**

In an account of viral persistence in nature two major factors are taken into consideration: (1) the biophysical and biochemical characteristics of a virus that permit it to retain its infectious nature in the enviroment outside of its natural host(s); and (2) its biological characteristics that facilitate persistence in one or more hosts for varying periods of time. If failure occurs on both counts the virus passes into oblivion.

Most viruses cannot withstand severe environmental conditions. The majority are destroyed in a strong alkali or acid solution, or even in strong salt solutions. In the presence of fat solvents, viruses with a lipid coat are quickly inactivated. High temperatures for relatively short periods of time destroy viral infectivity. Certain viruses are quickly inactivated in direct sunlight. On the other hand many viruses in well-buffered media or in tissue are maintained for long periods of time at exceedingly low temperatures ($-60$ C and lower) and also in a dried state at regular refrigeration temperature for a long time. In a study of viral ecology it is well to know the biophysical and biochemical characteristics in an assessment of their ability to survive in an environment outside of the body of their natural host(s). It soon becomes apparent that the chances for viral survival outside of the host (s) in most instances are rather meager.

The successful spread and the perpetration of virus in the host are the principal mechanisms by which a viral species is maintained in nature. There exist several known epidemiological models which explain the successful spread and maintenance of certain viral diseases. These models will be considered in some depth in subsequent sections of this chapter.

According to Shope (9) the epidemiology of clinically apparent viral illnesses may be classified as intermittent and nonintermittent. The intermittent diseases have no good evidence for the existence of a continuous chain of animal-to-animal infection either by contact or by a vector or intermediate host. The nonintermittent viral diseases apparently are maintained by contact infections either as clinical or subclinical infections. In addition, indigenous viral infections occur in nature and serve as a source of disease in more susceptible hosts. As our knowledge of animal viral diseases has improved, it has become apparent that viruses can readily exist in the host as persisting or occult virus, or even as a virogene, representing a potential source of virus in nature, not necessarily requiring a broad host spectrum to enhance its perpetuity.

### Direct Species-to-Species Transmission

The infections transferred by direct contact from an animal of one species to another animal of the same species are usually spread by salivary contamination, aerosal, or fecal contamination. The examples of this type of situation in the animal kingdom are extremely common—perhaps the most notable examples are vesicular exanthema, transmissible gastroenteritis, hog cholera in swine, virus diarrhea—mucosal disease (VD-MD) of cattle, avian bronchitis of chickens, and murine hepatitis. We know little about these diseases in our wildlife but, in reality, some viruses, such as VD-MD in deer, likely appear in very closely related species and not limited to a single animal species. Subclinical infections often play an important role in maintaining the chain of infection.

Most of the diseases in this epidemiological group have a long-lasting immunity. Earlier, it was believed that these viruses did not persist but it is known now that some of them do remain under certain conditions serving as probable links in any subsequent chain of infection.

### Virus Transmission by Virus Carriers

A large number of animal virus infections now can be placed in this category. After initial infection of an individual the virus persists in a superficial tissue of the body that readily permits elimination of the agent in various body excretions. This includes viruses in various genera such as adenovirus, herpesvirus, picornavirus, and poxvirus to mention a few. The virus carriers are a source of potential infection to all susceptible species.

Some of the diseases in this group such as herpes simplex of man are characterized by clinical relapses that usually occur after some stress such as another infection. The coexistence of immunity and infection are in delicate balance in these persisting viral infections. In an interesting experiment Good and Campbell (3) precipitated latent herpes simplex encephalitis in rabbits by anaphylactic shock, a severe form of stress.

### Arthropod-Borne Virus Transmission

Four principal cycles are involved in the transmission of the arboviruses: (1) arthropod to man with urban yellow fever as an example; (2) arthropod-lower vertebrate cycle with tangential infection of man, examples are jungle yellow fever and equine encephalomyelitis; (3) and arthropod cycle with occasional infection of lower vertebrates and man, an example is Colorado tick fever; and (4) lower vertebrate-arthropod with African horsesickness as a prime example—other probable ones are turkey meningoencephalitis and bluetongue in sheep and cattle although essential insect transmission has not been completely proved.

In the arthropod-arthropod transmission the virus may be transmitted from the adult arthropod to its offspring by transovarian passage not involving a vertebrate host in its successful transmission. Often the virus produces little or no disease in the arthropod host and the agent persists in an infective form in the insect host which serves for its complete life-span as the reservoir for the infection. In contrast, the arboviruses produce a severe disease of short duration in most vertebrate hosts. The disease terminates quickly in survival or death. Survival results in the formation of an excellent immunity that persists for a long period of time. In some arbovirus infections the presence of the virus in the vertebrate is temporary and short and it therefore plays a minor role in perpetrating the agent in nature.

### Transmission of Viral Diseases by Accidental Bite Injection

There are two well-known viral diseases transmitted by a bite. Rabies is a disease of considerable historical importance. This virus has a broad host spectrum and the main means of transmission occurs as the result of a bite by an infected carnivorous animal or by an infected bat. Its epidemiology will be discussed at length in the section on rabies. Another disease is monkey B-virus infection in man, caused by a bite from an infected monkey that shows no evidence of illness. The clinically apparent disease occurs as encephalitis, and is often fatal.

Certain diseases can readily be produced by the accidental infection of a viral contaminant or by blood transfusion from viral carriers to susceptible individuals. These diseases are obviously produced by man, and some simple procedures can correct some of these situations through the observation of sterile technics in the vaccination of animals and by strict control in the production and testing of biologics. When fresh animal tissues (including blood) are used in therapy certain hazards such as the occurrence of persisting microbes must be weighed in their usage. Certain blood protozoan agents and equine infectious anemia virus are readily transmitted by these means.

### Indigenous Viral Infections

Some notable examples include lymphocytic choriomeningitis in mice, viral encephalitides in birds and rodents, bovine malignant fever, and East African swine fever. In these situations healthy carriers exist in a given species that have never shown disease and yet serve as the means of perpetuating and transmitting the viruses that they may carry. Indigenous viral infections have three main features, namely, (1) inapparent infection, (2) persisting virus, and (3) infection at an early age.

Immunological tolerance may be an important characteristic of lymphocytic choriomeningitis, an indigenous infection in mice. In this infection, mice are infected *in utero* and as sucklings from their clinically well mothers. Through the excreta of the latently infected mouse, humans may contract clinical disease. Indigenous viral encephalitis infections in birds and in rodents may play important roles in the epidemiology of these important viruses in which frank disease develops in other hosts, such as the horse and man through the medium of the arthropod that has contact with indigenous viral hosts.

In bovine malignant cattarrhal fever, cattle are the disease (indicator) host of a virus carried as a silent infection in the wildebeests and possibly by sheep. African swine-fever virus is an indigenous viral infection in the wart hog. In contrast, it is a highly acute and fatal disease in domestic swine.

### Parasite Reservoir Hosts for Viral Diseases

There are three animal diseases in whose epidemiology a worm may play a role. Swine influenza and hog cholera are virus diseases of swine and salmon-poisoning of dogs is caused by a rickettsial agent. There are no known human viral or rickettsial agent counterparts.

The causative agent of salmon-poisoning in dogs is carried by the trematode, *Troglotrema salmincola*. The complete life cycle of this fatal disease of dogs has been established by Simons, McCapes, and Muth (10) and Cordy and Gorham (2). The details of the cycle are given in the chapter on rickettsiae.

Shope's studies with influenza and hog cholera viruses incriminated the swine lungworm and its intermediate host, the common earthworm (9). The transmission of these viruses is complicated by the occult (masked) form that the virus assumes in lungworm intermediate host, and once within the swine the virus must be provoked to the infective state by a stress induced in the infected swine. In nature stress is associated with the onset of cold and wet weather.

### The Case for the Virogene and the Oncogene

Lysogeny (prophage) is a state in bacteriophage replication known for a long period of time. Bacteria in the prophage stage may lose the prophage for reasons presently unknown, retain that state, or develop from prophage to vegetative form with phage maturation and eventual lysis. It is believed that there is a comparable prophage stage for animal viruses which has been called by Luria (7) "parasitism at the genetic level." Shope (9) has called it "masked" virus while the terms "occult" or "virogene" have also been suggested. This viral stage is most difficult to prove, especially when it cannot be reactivated into an infective form. There are a number of viruses capable of causing tumors in animals in which the agent presumably becomes integrated into the genetic apparatus of the parasitized cell. Although the virus may lose its infectivity under these circumstances it retains the capacity to elicit the formation of specific antiviral antibodies. The first notable example of this phenomenon involved the Shope papilloma rabbit virus. In cottontail rabbits that are naturally infected with this virus, active virus could usually be demonstrated in the papillomas. In contrast, no infective virus could be demonstrated in the papillomas induced by the cottontail virus in domestic rabbits. Viral antigen was demonstrated in these noninfective domestic rabbit papillomas (8) and also in the carcinomas arising from them (6). This noninfectious antigenic virus was called "masked virus" by Shope. Other oncogenic DNA viruses such as the polyoma and certain adenoviruses behave in a similar manner. Infective virus often is not demonstrable in polyoma-induced tumors in hamsters (4). Similarly Huebner et al. (5) failed to isolate infective virus from tumors in hamsters induced by adenovirus types 12 and 18 or in rats by adenovirus 12 although antigens that produce antibodies capable of reacting with type-specific viral antigens of a given serotype were demonstrated in the tumor mass. The studies of Black et al. (1) with simian virus ($SV_{40}$), hamster tumors, or with cells transformed in culture gave similar results, causing the investigators to conclude that the noninfective antigen is synthesized by information from the $SV_{40}$ viral genome integrated in the tumor and in vitro-transformed cells. Thus, we have four examples of DNA oncogenic viruses that are usually free of infective virus in the tumor tissue but contain viral antigen(s).

### The Epidemiology of Tumor Viruses

There are a number of viral-induced tumors in mammals and birds. Many of these tumors are similar in structure to certain tumors in man. Although no virus has been proved to cause a tumor in man, certain human tumors may eventually be found to be viral-induced.

In general, our limited knowledge of viral-induced tumors suggests that these diseases usually are vertically transmitted, thus, limiting the means by which they may ultimately be controlled from an epidemiological standpoint. The principal method would appear to be the use of drug therapy aimed at the replication of specific viral enzymes.

The Bittner mouse virus that causes mammary carcinoma is an interesting epidemiological model. Virus is present in the milk and other tissues of certain strains of mice. The virus is transmitted to the offspring through the milk at nursing. The agent may remain dormant for the lifetime of the infected mouse without manifesting itself as a disease, but may readily be transmitted to its offspring. In most instances, the infected adults develop mammary carcinoma at a certain stage of hormonal function and subsequently die.

Certain tumor viruses such as the murine leukemia, avian leukemia, and feline leukemia viruses are transmitted directly (vertically) from the dam to the progeny *in utero*. Much must be done to determine the precise pathogenesis. There has been speculation that the virus is transferred in the germ cell of the female and perhaps even in the male germ cell. These viruses may persist within the cells for the lifetime of an individual without disease manifestation. Why some individuals harboring the agent develop leukemia and/or sarcomas and others do not is unknown. This close association of the virus with the genetic apparatus of the cell and its ability to persist for long periods of time assures the viral parasite of perpetuation as long as its natural hosts do not become extinct.

Certain superficial surface tumors such as rabbit fibroma and papillomas of rabbits and some domestic animals can be transmitted surgically and presumably by certain insects as well. For example, there is definite field evidence that the rabbit fibroma is transmitted in nature by a flying biting insect (9). The rabbit papilloma also appears to be insect transmitted in cottontail rabbits.

The epidemiological study of animal tumors has been rather limited. There is considerable interest now in these diseases, particularly those for which good viral assay and serological methods exist. Until the etiology of human tumors is determined, the measure of success in epidemiology in this area will be rather limited. Consequently most of our basic knowledge of tumor epidemiology will be developed with animal tumor models.

## The Epidemiology of Chronic and Degenerative Diseases

This includes a group of diseases caused by agents called slow viruses. The incubation period of the disease manifestation is as a rule extremely long in the natural host, and virus can be isolated from the tissues of these infected animals for long periods of time. There is strong evidence that some of these diseases are autoimmune conditions with lesions resulting from the combined action of antigen, antibody, and complement.

Little is known about the transmission of these diseases. Is vertical or horizontal transmission the main mechanism for its spread from one individual to another? Are vectors required for their transmission? Do they have a narrow or broad host spectrum? How long do these disease agents persist in the host? These are some of the questions still unanswered about the nature of these diseases which are essential to an understanding of their ecology.

### Eradication of Viral Diseases

In veterinary medicine slaughter has been the principal method utilized to eradicate certain viral diseases. Foot-and-mouth disease is the prime example and success has been achieved in certain countries where the infection was limited to a single country bordered by others free of the disease or by navigable waters. It is quite remarkable that this success has been achieved in many instances by slaughtering the afflicted ruminant species and pigs in infected herds with no particular effort pursued in the direction of other domesticated animals or wildlife species that are susceptible to some degree to FMD virus. In Great Britain, where the disease has occurred frequently within the last two decades, the reinfection of the population usually has been traced to the introduction of the virus in an animal product from a country where the disease is epizootic. Yet the virus does persist in recovered animals, in animals given attenuated virus vaccine, or in animals vaccinated with inactivated virus vaccine and subsequently exposed to infective virus. Consequently the slaughter method seems the only reasonable approach to eradication with this virus disease. Where latency and vertical transmission are features of a viral disease, the slaughter method is probably the only means by which it can be eradicated.

Hog cholera has been eradicated from Canada by the slaughter method. A concerted effort now is in progress to achieve this goal in the USA. This disease only affects domestic and wild pigs with no positive proof that the virus affects other hosts naturally so it seems reasonable on the basis of the Canadian experience to expect that the USA program also will be successful. There already is some evidence that this will be the case despite the complex pig-industry system, which involves frequent and rapid movement of hogs over long distances. The latency of the virus presents a problem that is overcome by the slaughter technic. Inactivated virus vaccine is not a very good biologic and has never completely controlled the disease. Attenuated virus vaccine helped to control the disease, but led to latency and chronicity in certain animals, so this procedure was terminated as a method of eradication. Consequently, vaccination was helpful in preventing and controlling the disease, but not in its eradication.

In certain arbovirus diseases, insects are true biological vectors and are essential to disease perpetuation in man and animals. If these vectors are removed from the environment where susceptible animals or humans reside, the disease is eliminated. Of course the eradication of insects also poses a formidable task that it is not usually feasible or practical to execute.

The eradication of viral disease from a country by vaccination has not been too successful. The notable exception is rinderpest of cattle. Inactivated virus vaccines generally provide insufficient immunity to prevent the replication of virus in a vaccinated animal even though disease may not occur. Attenuated virus vaccines provide greater immunity and usually prevent the residence of virulent (street) virus in the animal, but often the attenuated virus may be transmitted to susceptible animals. After repeated transfer of attenuated vaccine virus in nature it may revert to virulence with the production of acute or chronic disease depending upon its nature. With properly attenuated rinderpest vaccines the virus does not produce disease nor transmit to susceptible hosts and constitutes a blind-ended infection in the host. This is an ideal vaccine, which leads to eradication when a large percentage of the population are vaccinated in a unified, country-wide campaign. Theoretically, this should be possible to accomplish with canine distemper in dogs because excellent biologics that do not spread the disease are available. It would require a well-organized nationwide campaign to eliminate a virulent agent that spreads as readily in a susceptible population as does the distemper virus. This may not be a desirable situation unless very strict quarantine and vaccination procedures were enforced. At best it would be difficult to control in pets while international travel is so common and there is a close companionship between man and dog.

## REFERENCES

1. Black, Rowe, Turner, and Huebner.    Proc. Natl. Acad. Sci., 1963, *50*, 1148.
2. Cordy and Gorham.    Am. Jour. Path., 1950, *26*, 617.
3. Good and Campbell.    Proc. Soc. Exp. Biol. and Med., 1948, *68*, 82.
4. Habel and Atanasiu.    *Ibid.*, 1959, *102*, 99.
5. Huebner, Rowe, Turner, and Lane.    Proc. Natl. Acad. Sci., 1963, *50*, 379.
6. Kidd, Beard, and Rous.    Jour. Exp. Med., 1936, *64*, 76.
7. Luria.    Science, 1950, *111*, 507.
8. Shope.    Jour. Exp. Med., 1937, *65*, 219.
9. Shope.    Viral and rickettsial infections of man. 4th ed. J. P. Lippincott, Philadelphia, 1965, pp. 385–404.
10. Simms, McCapes, and Muth.    Jour. Am. Vet. Med. Assoc., 1932, *81*, 26.
11. Smith and Kilbourne.    Investigation into the nature, causation, and prevention of Texas or southern cattle fever. Bul. 1, B.A.I., U.S. Dept. Agri., Gov't Printing Office, Washington, D.C., 1893.

# XXXVIII | Laboratory Diagnosis of Viral Infections

Ideally, disease is diagnosed at the clinical level, utilizing anamnesis, physical examination, and the signs of illness of a single patient or herd for this purpose. The veterinarian, especially the small animal practitioner, often resorts to fluoroscopic x-ray, surgical, and other specialized procedures to facilitate a proper diagnosis. Most cases can be adequately diagnosed in this manner. With the availability of more specialized equipment and increased knowledge, more veterinary practitioners are requiring laboratory examinations involving such disciplines as pathology, microbiology, physiology, and biochemistry. Many laboratory procedures today are simple, rapid, accurate, and inexpensive to conduct, and constitute ideal diagnostic tests. A small laboratory for such tests is maintained and operated in conjunction with many veterinary practices. An occasional case demands more sophisticated equipment and a specialized approach to diagnosis that requires the services of a state or university veterinary diagnostic laboratory. Biological specimens for this purpose must be properly prepared, stored, and sent to the laboratory. These latter points cannot be over-emphasized because a poor specimen often receives (and deserves) a poor answer.

Many viral diseases have rather characteristic features that permit identification at the clinical and pathological level. In other instances it may be deemed essential to establish a diagnosis either by isolation of the virus or by serological methods. Isolation of the virus often entails technics that require a few days or weeks for identification. Most serological tests require the use of paired sera taken 2 to 3 weeks apart for a proper diagnosis of viral disease. It is apparent that most viral diagnostic test results become available after the patient has recovered or passed away. A notable exception is immunofluorescence (fluorescent antibody) testing, which is being rapidly devel-

872

oped for the diagnosis of many viral diseases. Some viral diseases, notably rabies, presently are diagnosed by this method.

## Isolation of Viruses from Infected Animals

The effort and cost involved in a viral etiological diagnosis requires careful selection of case material as well as the proper collection and handling of the right type of specimen. As a rule, a virus isolation is desirable for the following reasons: (1) to identify a virus concerned in a herd health program; (2) to point out a public health problem that may be involved, such as rabies; (3) to establish the viral etiology of a disease not previously encountered in a practice; (4) to determine the immunological type of a given virus when epidemics such as foot-and-mouth disease occur; and (5) to pin point the exact agent when serological-test-methods fail because it shares common antigens with other viruses.

The isolation of a virus from a diseased animal does not necessarily mean that the isolate is the cause of the diseased state. Many viruses, including pathogens, persist in animals for long periods of time and their presence would tend to confuse the diagnosis. Some of these viruses, such as bovine enteroviruses, will be of the orphan type in that they are not proved pathogens. A knowledge of clinical and epidemiological patterns for the various viruses is useful in assessing the significance of a viral isolate from a diseased animal. On occasion more than one virus is isolated from a patient. This can be a difficult problem if both isolates are known pathogens. In a given patient at a particular time, one virus may be causing an inapparent infection while the other is responsible for the observed clinical signs of illness. A knowledge of the clinical signs produced by each virus is important as this may help to establish the primary disease agent in that situation. If both viruses produce comparable signs the etiological diagnosis becomes academic unless it is known that the patient may have had previous experience with one or both agents. It may then be possible to evaluate the facts and decide upon the real culprit in a given situation. It also becomes apparent that the right diagnosis would be missed if antibody (serological) studies were only made for the virus causing the inapparent infection.

There are a number of excellent textbooks, papers, and monographs devoted to the laboratory diagnosis of viral diseases. Perhaps the most desirable single source, which gives an excellent, authoritative, and up-to-date coverage, is the multiauthored book edited by Lennette and Schmidt (3). The book by Kwapinski (2) also is an excellent reference source for methods of serological diagnosis.

## Collection of Clinical Material for Viral Diagnosis

The ideal time to collect biological material for viral isolation is during the acute stage of illness prior to the formation of antibodies.

Various materials such as blood, nasal swabs, nasopharyngeal swabs, feces, urine, pus, vesicular fluid, skin lesions, spinal fluid, and biopsy material as well as tissues obtained at autopsy are used for the isolation of viruses. The biological specimens required for each specific disease can be obtained by referring to the description of the disease in this textbook, particularly the section of each disease dealing with diagnosis.

Some general rules can be stated which apply to the proper selection of tissues for viral isolation. Respiratory illnesses in their acute stage usually are associated with the excretion of virus in the nasal or pharyngeal secretions. Virus can be demonstrated in the fluid of vesicular lesions or in the scabs from pox lesions. Many generalized catarrhal diseases have a viremic state, and the virus can be readily isolated from the blood; virtually all body excretions contain virus during the acute stage of illness. Diseases referable to the central nervous system often present a problem, but it is reasonable to attempt isolation from the blood and also from the brain of animals that succumb to the disease. It is most important to obtain tissue specimens from deceased animals immediately after death—in some instances an owner may agree to sacrifice a moribund animal, which further enhances viral isolation. Often a blood sample is taken from an animal for serologic tests at the same time. It is important that the serum be harvested from the whole blood prior to freezing because lysis of red blood cells often renders a sample useless for certain serologic tests.

The biophysical and biochemical properties of viruses vary markedly. Many viruses are heat-sensitive and acid-sensitive, and great care must be exercised in handling such materials. In particular, fresh tissues must be used and then frozen to $-60$ to $-70$ C immediately after harvesting. Furthermore, a minimum of time is desirable in attempted isolations with these tissues in cell cultures or test animals. If there is no alternative, the tissue specimens may be placed in a deep freeze maintained at $-20$ C until dry ice is obtained for storage and shipment to the laboratory. A wide-mouthed thermos jug or a styrofoam-insulated carton, filled with dry ice after the specimens are inserted, is used for this purpose. If dry ice is not available, 50 percent glycerol can be used recognizing that certain viruses remain viable longer than others in this solution. Small pieces of tissue, fecal material, or mucus are placed in a vial and the vial is completely filled with 50 percent glycerol and stored at 6 C.

Most laboratories do not operate over a weekend so it is wise to ship the biological material during the early part of the week unless other arrangements are made.

Naturally, the tissue specimens should be taken with sterile instruments in a sterile manner. If an individual is concerned with the viral distribution in the tissues, separate sterile instruments must be used for procuring each tissue. Tight, sterile screw-cap vials often are used for storage of suspect tissues and fluids. If the fluid specimens are stored in dry ice, the vials should be air-tight as the gaseous phase of dry ice is $CO_2$, which changes the pH of fluids—resulting in inactivation of acid pH-labile viruses. When vials are not air-tight they can be placed in a sealed, air-tight plastic bag, which accomplishes the same purpose.

## Isolation of Virus

Susceptible animals, cell cultures, and embryonated hens' eggs are used for viral isolation. Fluid specimens that are bacteria-free can be inoculated directly or after dilution with a buffered solution (pH 7.2 to 7.6).

Solid tissues are prepared as 10 to 20 percent suspensions using a buffered solution (pH 7.2 to 7.6) as diluent. This suspension is given a light centrifugation to remove the coarse particles which tend to plug the inoculating equipment and often are toxic to cells in the test system. The supernatant fluid is used as the inoculum after centrifugation at 2,000 rpm for 10 minutes.

Certain test inocula such as feces, oral and nasal swabs, insects, and some infected tissues contain bacteria and these should be eliminated prior to inoculation. Various procedures are used for this purpose, but for various reasons they do not always succeed. Ether is bactericidal but may not be harmful to the virus under consideration. In such instances 10 to 15 percent ether can be added to the test suspension. Antibiotics are used and a mixture of penicillin (1,000 units per ml) and streptomycin (100 mg per ml) is most commonly employed. The dye proflavine is often used to photodynamically inactivate microbes in stool and throat specimens as it has little or no effect on enteroviruses or rhinoviruses. The specimen is treated with $10^{-4}$ M proflavine for 1 hour at pH 9 at 37 C after which the dye is removed by cation resins. The photosensitized bacterial and fungal contaminants are inactivated by exposure to white light. Microbes also can be removed by mechanical means such as ultrafiltration and differential centrifugation. Earthenware, porcelain, and asbestos filters are used for this purpose, but viral concentration is reduced by adsorption to these materials. Differential centrifugation is a convenient and excellent method to remove many bacteria from a heavily contaminated specimen of the smaller viruses. For viruses smaller than 100 m$\mu$ in size a run in the centrifuge at 18,000 rpm for 20 minutes in a 6-inch rotor will sediment the bacteria but not the virus. With specimens containing a minimal amount of virus, centrifugation at 40,000 rpm for 60 minutes in a 6-inch rotor will concentrate most viruses in a small gelatinous pellet at the bottom of the tubes. The supernatant of such runs contains less than 1 percent of the original virus. The pellet is then resuspended in a small volume of buffered solution.

## Isolation of Viruses in Embryonated Hens' Eggs

Marked progress made in the field of virology during the past 25 years has been due, in part, to the utilization of the chicken embryo as a medium for the propagation of viral agents. Most viruses under natural conditions are relatively host-specific. Moreover, they show a marked predilection for groups of highly specialized tissue cells of the host, for example, those comprising nerve tissue, epithelial tissue, etc. Although growing readily in these tissues, they fail to grow in all or most others of the body. This tissue affinity, which is one of the unique properties of viruses, is known as "tropism." While a number of viruses show marked host-specificity or tissue tropism, the great majority can be adapted by various procedures to foreign hosts. Inasmuch as the cells and the extraembryonic membranes of the developing chicken embryo, like most embryonic tissues, lack a high degree of specialization, these provide a general substrate containing some constituents conducive to the growth of all or most viruses. By virtue of the ability to alter their tropism and to adapt to new host species, many viruses become fully capable of growing in chicken embryo tissues wherein they frequently attain a much higher concentration than in the tissues of the natural host species.

A general knowledge of the development, structure, and physiology of the chicken embryo is essential in order for the student to understand fully the technics involved in the cultivation of viruses in this experimental host. The extraembryonic membranes of the chicken embryo arise from three germinal layers, namely; the entoderm, the mesoderm, and the ectoderm. The dorsal somatopleure, which consists of a sheet of tissue cells, is composed of ectoderm on one side and mesoderm on the other, while the ventral splanchnopleure consists of mesoderm and entoderm. By a process of folding, the somatopleure gives rise to both the chorion and the amnion while the allantoic- and yolk-sac membrances develop from the splanchnopleure. The amnion arises from the head and caudal regions of the embryo, the membrane being reflected back to form the serosa or chorion. The amniotic membranes grow rapidly and fuse dorsal to the embryo by the 5th day to form the amniotic sac. Meanwhile the chorion continues to grow and by the 10th day has almost completely enveloped the whole of the egg contents and is in contact with the inner shell membrane. The allantois makes its appearance on the 3rd day as a diverticulum from the ventral wall of the hind gut. By the 10th day it has fused with the chorion to form the allantoic cavity which separates the chorion from the amnion. The fused chorionic and allantoic membranes are referred to also as the chorioallantoic membrane or the chorioallantois. The yolk sac, which arises from the splanchnopleure, envelops the yolk material. The gross and microscopic structure of the yolk-sac membrane closely resembles that of the intestinal mucosa, of which it is essentially an extension.

Inasmuch as the allantoic sac represents a diverticulum of the gut, it serves as the excretory receptacle for the embryo. The sac contains a variety of solids in solution, the solution becoming turbid after the 12th day, owing to the presence of urates. The chorioallantois is primarily the respiratory organ of the embryo and hence is richly supplied with blood vessels. The amniotic fluid, which contains much of the albumen in the egg, appears to serve as a source of protein, which is ingested during the swallowing movements the embryo is observed to make from the 9th day onward. The function of the yolk-sac membranes is to transport nutrients from the yolk sac to the embryo.

## Inoculation Procedures

The methods described below for the inoculation of the chicken embryo do not comprise a complete list but represent rather those that are practiced most commonly. Likewise, while there are a number of technics for inoculating by each of the routes listed, the one most widely used is described herein (fig. 157).

**Yolk Sac.** The large elementary-body viruses and the rickettsiae grow readily in the yolk-sac membranes. Although many of the smaller viruses also are inoculated by the yolk-sac route, they invade the embryo proper and multiply in the body tissues of the embryo rather than in the yolk-sac tissues.

1. *Candling and drilling.* Fertile eggs that have been incubated for 5 to 7 days are suitable because the yolk sac is relatively large at this time. The eggs are candled and the boundary of the air sac pencilled in. The shell over the air space, which is referred to as the shell cap, is disinfected by an application of iodine to one small area. When the iodine is dried a hole is made through the shell over the center of the natural air space by means of a drill.

2. *Inoculation and incubation.* By means of a syringe fitted with a 1-inch 23-gauge needle, the inoculum is deposited in the yolk sac by passing the needle through the hole in the shell cap and directing it downward to its full

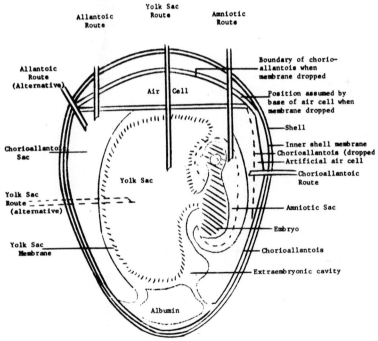

*Fig. 157.* Various routes of inoculation into embryonating hens' eggs for the propagation of viruses.

length, parallel to the long axis of the egg. From 0.2 to 0.5 ml is usually inoculated. The hole in the shell is then sealed with hot vaspar (paraffin-vaseline mixture) and the eggs are incubated at 37 C.

3. *Harvesting procedure.* The egg is placed in a container that maintains it in the upright position during the harvesting procedure. The shell is cracked with sterile forceps and the cap lifted off. The exposed membranes are torn away and the yolk-sac contents may be removed with a special sterile 10-ml pipette with the tip removed. If the yolk-sac membranes are to be harvested, the contents of the egg are quickly emptied into a sterile petri dish. The yolk sac is usually ruptured in the process. The yolk-sac membranes, which are easily recognized by their deep yellow color, are detached from the embryo, separated from the chorioallantois with sterile forceps, and quickly transferred to a sterile petri dish. When the embryo is to be harvested, it is withdrawn by hooking the curved end of a dental probe around the neck. It is then separated from the adherent membranes with sterile scissors and transferred to a sterile petri dish.

**Allantoic Cavity.** The influenza and the Newcastle disease viruses, and most other viral agents that cause respiratory infections, grow readily in the entodermal cells of the allantoic sac wall and are liberated into the allantoic fluid. The encephalomyelitis viruses and the mumps virus also multiply readily when inoculated by this route.

1. *Candling and drilling.* Embryonating eggs that have received a preliminary incubation of from 8 to 11 days are candled and the boundary of the air space pencilled in. The eggs are held in the upright position with the air sac uppermost. A point is selected several millimeters above the floor of the air space on the side of the egg where the chorioallantois is well developed but free of large vessels. Iodine is applied to the area around the site. A hole is then drilled or punched through the shell.

2. *Inoculation and incubation.* A 0.5-inch 24-gauge needle, fitted to a small syringe containing the inoculum, is inserted into the allantoic cavity by passing it through the hole in the shell parallel to the long axis of the egg or at an angle directed towards the apical extremity. From 0.2 to 0.5 ml of inoculum is injected into each egg. The hole in the shell is then sealed with hot vaspar and the eggs are incubated at 37 C.

3. *Harvesting of allantoic fluid.* In order to avoid hemorrhage into the allantoic fluid while harvesting, the eggs are chilled by holding in the refrigerator from 4 to 6 hours prior to the harvesting procedure. They are held in an upright position and the shell over the air sac is removed with sterile forceps. The floor of the air space is exposed. The floor consists of the inner shell membrane overlaying the chorioallantois. With a pair of small sterile curved forceps these membranes are torn away. In order to facilitate the harvesting of the allantoic fluid, the embryo is displaced to one side by placing the forceps against the embryo with the tips toward the shell wall. The allantoic fluid then can readily be aspirated with a 5- or 10-ml sterile pipette.

**The Chorioallantoic Membrane.** Nine-to-eleven-day-old embryonating eggs are candled and an area about 1 centimeter square is outlined with a pencil on the shell over the most vascular underlying portion. The surrounding shell is treated by applying 5 percent phenol, which is permitted to dry. Iodine is not used to sterilize the shell because the alcoholic solution is absorbed through the shell and causes lesions on the chorioallantois which could be mistakenly attributed to the virus. With a drill, the shell is cut along the pencilled lines, great care being exercised to avoid cutting the inner shell membrane. A hole is then drilled or punched through the shell and inner shell membranes into the natural air space, as for yolk-sac inoculation. The egg is now placed on its side in a holder with the drilled side uppermost. With a pair of sharp pointed forceps or a dental probe the excised piece of shell is gently removed, exposing the white inner shell membrane, to the underside of which is attached the chorioallantois. A small drop of sterile saline is placed on the center of this area to soften the membrane. The bevelled surface of a 27-gauge, 0.25-inch needle (depending on the preference of the operator) fitted to a 1-ml syringe is applied at a 45-degree angle to this area with gentle downward pressure and, by traction, a slit is made in the membrane. Care must be exercised in order to avoid damage to the underlying chorioallantois. Because the fibers of the inner shell membrane run obliquely, the syringe should be held at a 45-degree angle to the long axis of the egg so that the pressure exerted will tend to separate rather than to tear the fibers. Suction is then applied with a rubber bulb to the hole in the natural air space. If preferred, a drop of sterile saline may be dropped on the slit before suction is applied. The saline, as it is drawn in, aids in separating the chorioallantois from the inner shell membrane. The former then drops as part of the egg contents is displaced into the space occupied originally by the natural air space. This is indicated by a clearing of the inner shell membrane as the chorioallantois separates from it.

1. *Inoculation and incubation.* By carefully passing the needle through the inner shell membrane from 0.1 to 0.2 ml of inoculum is dropped on the chorioallantois with a 1-ml syringe fitted with a 22- or 23-gauge needle. In very critical studies the egg should be candled during this procedure to insure that the inoculum is deposited on, rather than through, the membrane. After inoculation the egg is gently rocked in order to spread the inoculum uniformly over the surface of the chorioallantois. The opening in the shell is covered with a small square of scotch tape and the inoculated eggs are incubated with the shell window uppermost.

An alternative method for inoculating by this route, which eliminates much of the tedium connected with window cutting, is carried out as follows: At a selected point a hole is drilled through the sterilized shell to the inner shell membrane. Using a 19-gauge needle with the bevel held downward, the inner shell membrane is carefully separated from the shell around the margin of the hole by exerting a slight downward pressure on the needle. The egg is then placed on a candler and suction applied to the hole that has previously been made into the air space. The dropping of the chorioallantois can then be readily observed.

2. *Harvesting of the membrane tissues.* The egg is placed in the horizontal position with the window uppermost. Iodine is applied to the area around the window with a cotton swab and the tape then peeled off. The surrounding shell is broken away with sterile forceps and the chorioallantois exposed. The membrane is grasped with forceps, detached with scissors, and quickly transferred to a sterile petri dish.

Inasmuch as the chorioallantois of eggs that have been incubated for 9 or 10 days adhere firmly to the inner shell membrane, a common practice is to drop these membranes at 7 or 8 days and to hold the eggs in the incubator until they are ready to be inoculated. They are candled during the inoculation procedure in order to insure that the chorioallantois has not risen in the meantime, and that the inoculum is deposited on the membrane rather than in the allantoic sac. The hole in the shell is then sealed with vaspar or scotch tape. Incubation and harvesting is the same as described for the first method.

**Amniotic.** This method is used principally for the isolation of the influenza virus from throat washings. The embryo during the course of its development swallows the amniotic fluid, thereby bringing the inoculated virus which it contains into contact with the tissues of the respiratory and intestinal tracts where multiplication presumably occurs. The amniotic route of inoculation is used also for the isolation of the encephalomyelitis viruses.

1. *Candling and drilling.* Embryos from 7 to 15 days of age are used. The position of the embryo is determined by candling, and then a point is marked on the shell over the air space on the side of the egg in which the embryo is situated. The site is prepared in the usual manner and a hole is drilled or punched as for yolk-sac inoculation.

2. *Inoculation and incubation.* A 1-ml syringe fitted with a 0.75-inch 24-gauge needle is used for the inoculation. The egg is placed horizontally on the candler, the needle is introduced and gently stabbed in the direction of the embryo. Penetration of the amniotic sac is indicated by a sudden movement of the embryo. The needle is then withdrawn slightly and from 0.1 to 0.2 ml of the inoculum injected. The hole in the shell is sealed with vaspar and the eggs are incubated in the vertical position.

3. *Collection of amniotic fluid.* The shell is removed as for the allantoic and yolk-sac routes of inoculation. A few drops of saline are placed on the floor of the air space to render the membrane transparent. Using the eyes of the embryo as a reference point, the amniotic fluid is aspirated by means of a syringe fitted with a short 23-gauge needle.

**Miscellaneous.**   1. *Intravenous.* This method of inoculating chicken embryos is not practiced to any extent. In carrying it out, 12-to-14-day-old chicken embryos are used. A large vein is located by candling and marked. A rectangular piece of shell directly over the vein is removed in the manner already described and a droplet of sterile mineral oil is placed on the inner shell membrane so as to render it transparent. A 27-gauge needle fitted to a small syringe is introduced through the membrane into the vein in the direction of blood flow. From 0.1 to 0.5 ml of inoculum is then injected. Incubation and harvesting of the embryo is carried out as already described.

2. *Intracerebral.* This method was occasionally used for the cultivation of the rabies virus.

## Isolation of Viruses in Tissue Culture

Recent advances in the methods of cell culture has provided the virologist with highly valuable tools for isolation and propagation of viruses. Certain knowledge of the technics of cell cultivation and maintenance is, therefore, a prerequisite to the study of viruses. Tissue cultures are the most widely used methods for isolation of viruses from clinical material. Viruses that replicate in cell cultures can be recognized in various ways, such as: cytopathic effects, viral interference, hemadsorption and hemagglutination, fluorescent antigen, and complement-fixing antigen.

The usage of the following terms has been recommended by the Committee on Terminology of the Tissue Culture Association. Dependent on whether cells, tissues, or organs are to be maintained or grown, two methodological approaches, cell culture, and tissue or organ culture, have been developed in the field of tissue culture. The cell culture denotes the growing of cells *in vitro* including the culture of single cells. In these, the cells are no longer organized into tissues. In tissue or organ cultures, tissues, or whole or parts of an organ are grown or maintained *in vitro* in a way that may allow differentiation and preservation of the architecture and/or function. A single layer of cells growing on a surface is called a monolayer. Suspension culture denotes a type of culture in which cells multiply while suspended in medium. A primary culture may be regarded as such until it is subcultured for the first time. It then becomes a cell line. A cell line may be said to have become established when it demonstrates the potential to be subcultured indefinitely *in vitro*. Diploid cell line denotes a cell line in which, arbitrarily, at least 75 percent of the cells have the same karyotype as the normal cells of the species from which the cells were originally obtained. A diploid chromosome number is not necessarily equivalent to the diploid karyotype, because there are situations in which a cell may lose one type of chromosome and acquire another type. Thus the karyotype of the cell has changed, but the diploid number of chromosomes remains the same. Such cells should be referred to as pseudodiploid.

Primary cultures are prepared from a variety of tissues of human and animal origin and are routinely employed in the cultivation of a large number of viruses. Primary cultures are preferred in many instances for their increased susceptibility to viruses. On the other hand, lack of uniformity in susceptibility in different batches of cells and the possible presence of occult viruses are some of the inherent dangers involved in their use. Certain viruses such as some human coronaviruses will replicate only in organ cultures.

Only under special circumstances can cell lines be grown continuously without changes in karyotype. Usually the conditions of culture select out variants in the cell population. These may differ radically from the predominant cell type in a primary culture. Most established cell lines used today are of this selected type although increasing use is made of diploid or pseudodiploid cell lines. By preserving large batches of these cells in the frozen state it is possible to work with cells of constant characteristics. In addition, cell lines offer advantages for their availability and rapid growth. At the same time, more attention is required to maintain them free of contaminants.

Viruses do not propagate outside living, actively metabolizing cells. For this reason it is necessary to consider the cell, its nutritional requirements, and its susceptibility to viruses, as well as the virus itself, when working with tissue-culture systems. While the body of the natural or experimental animal host species provides the necessary conditions for virus multiplication, it becomes necessary to manipulate the tissue-culture system in such a way that optimal virus-growth conditions are satisfied in the test tube. This has been accomplished to a considerable degree by providing the cells with media designed to assure satisfactory growth and maintenance. The conditions necessary for virus multiplication are intimately associated with and dependent on the maintenance of viable cells and to this end a formidable formulary of media has been devised to suit the requirements for growth of various cell types. In general, all media contain the following general substances in varying combinations and amounts: (1) Balanced salt solutions—Earles, Hanks, and Tyrode solution—to mention only a few media; (2) "Fortification substances"—lactalbumin hydrolysate, embryo extracts, amniotic fluid, vitamins, hormones, amino acids, minerals, and yeast extract; (3) Serum—human, horse, dog, calf, rabbit, sheep, and other species free of inhibitors and antibodies to the virus under study; and (4) Antibiotics—penicillin, streptomycin, mycostatin, tetracyclines, and many others used in dosage levels not toxic to cells.

Cell-culture work was plagued with contamination by unwanted bacteria and molds until the introduction of antibiotics, which allowed a much wider group of workers to do satisfactory tissue culture in mass quantity. Contamination is still, however, one of the major hazards; for this reason strict asceptic technic is necessary.

The many technics of tissue culture applied to virus cultivation are modifications of 5 basic methods:

1. *The suspended-cell method.* An old and still employed method now in more common usage for the production of virus for foot-and-mouth disease.

2. *Plasma-clot method.* Tissue fragments (explants) are made to adhere to the wall of a glass slide or test tube with the aid of clotted plasma, often chicken plasma. A film of plasma is layered onto a glass surface and induced to clot by the addition of embryo extract. Into this matrix are placed tissue fragments which adhere and proliferate. By this method one can observe the cellular proliferation and measure growth of the explants. Growth of viruses

in such cultures can be determined by several methods: (1) sampling the virus in the liquid or cellular phase of the culture and inoculating susceptible laboratory hosts which are known to become infected; (2) note the effect on cellular metabolism (i.e. inhibition of certain metabolic pathways); (3) observe cell-death (necrosis); (4) test for presence of hemagglutinins; and (5) electron microscopy of cells and purified fluids.

3. *Monolayer cell cultures.* Stationary-tube cultures are by far the most widely used in virology. These cultures are prepared from trypsin-dispersed tissues and consist of small clumps of cells and single cells derived from the particular source suited for use; kidney, testicle, skin, tumors, and other tissues. Tissues to be used are finely minced with scissors, washed with saline to remove blood cells and tissue debris, and placed in a trypsin solution that is kept constantly stirred with a magnetic stirring device. When the cells are dispersed (the time depending upon the temperature of trypsinization and the type of tissue being prepared) they are lightly centrifuged, washed with media two or three times to remove the trypsin, filtered through several layers of cheesecloth, diluted to contain sufficient cells per ml to insure good growth (the amount of cells depends upon the type), and inoculated into test tubes. The cell suspensions prepared from kidney fragments produce luxuriant monolayer cultures on any clean glass surface, petri dish or test tube, or bottle held in a stationary position. Tube cultures prepared in this way are used for virus isolations, titrations, neutralization tests, and studying the growth of viruses in cells.

4. *Direct cultures.* The procedure is the same as described for monolayer cell cultures. In this situation, tissues are taken at autopsy or by biopsy from the diseased animal for the production of monolayer cell cultures to enhance the opportunity for viral isolation where little virus is likely to be present or virus may be rendered inactive by antibodies present in the tissues. As little trypsin as possible should be used because some viruses are inactivated by trypsin.

5. *Organ cultures.* These cultures, used for the inoculation of suspect viral material or organ cultures, can be made directly from diseased tissues as indicated in the previous section. Organ cultures contain the differentiated tissues characteristic of a given organ. In some cases a virus—such as certain human coronaviruses—requires a specialized cell essential for its replication that is not present in a monolayer cell culture from the same organ. Organ cultures are used principally in research studies, for the technic is time-consuming and tedious in its present technology. Most viral studies in organ cultures involve the use of respiratory viruses in organ cultures derived from respiratory embryonic tissues with emphasis on viral propagation and its cytomorphological effects in the *in vitro* differentiated tissues. Investigators interested in the pathogenesis and immunity of viral diseases will continue to apply this method in future studies.

The most characteristic change in virus-infected cultures is a degenerative or necrotic change in the cellular elements of the culture (fig. 158). These cytopathic changes (cytopathic effect or CPE) are microscopically visible with a light microscope, and first involve individual cells and then spread to all susceptible cells in a culture. The effect of the virus on the cells depends upon the type of virus and cell. With certain viruses such as IBR, ICH, human adenoviruses, poliovirus, vesicular stomatitis virus, and foot-and-mouth-disease virus, the cells become granular, round up into clumps of degenerated cells, and finally drop from the glass surface, leaving islands of clear spaces. Eventually all the cells of a culture may become infected. In some infections the cells tend to clump together in aggregates to form "giant cells," which are syncytial formations of multinucleate cells. These are characteristic of distemper, mumps, measles virus, parainfluenza viruses, and syncytium-forming viruses of monkeys, humans, cattle, and cats. In such infected cultures there is a liberation of virus into the fluids bathing the cells, although with certain viruses the concentration of virus at any time in the growth cycle may be higher within the cell (cell-associated virus) than in the tissue culture fluid. Certain tumor viruses cause a loss-of-contact inhibition and the cells tend to pile upon each other forming a plaque. The characteristic cytopathic effect produced by some viruses along with their clinical history permits a

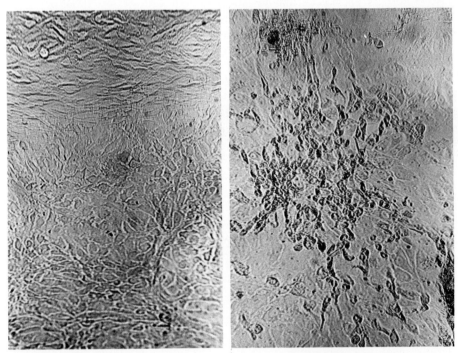

*Fig. 158.* (*Left*) Uninoculated feline kidney cell culture. (*Right*) Cytopathic changes (CPE) induced by a virus in feline kidney cell culture. (Courtesy F. Scott, C. Csiza, and J. Gillespie, *Am. Jour. Vet. Res.*)

rapid presumptive diagnosis. Because some viruses replicate without producing a cytopathic effect other means are used for their identification in cell cultures.

Such viruses as feline infectious panleukopenia virus produce intranuclear inclusion bodies, which can be readily observed after May-Gruenwald staining, without a significant destruction of the cell layer, so staining procedures of cover-slip cell cultures offer a better means for diagnosis (fig. 159). The diagnostician can use immunofluorescent staining with a specific conjugate (fig. 160) or a vital stain such as May-Gruenwald for identification. In instances

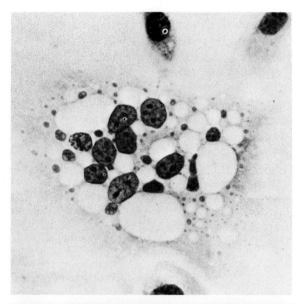

Fig. 159. Cytopathic effects by a bovine syncytium-forming virus characterized by syncytium formation with marked vacuolation and numerous cytoplasmic inclusion bodies clearly demonstrated by staining a cover-slip preparation(s) with May-Grünwald-Giemsa stain. X 1,200. (Courtesy F. Scott.)

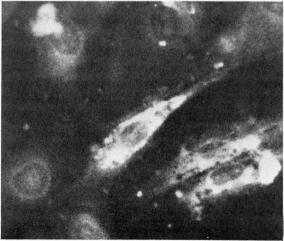

Fig. 160.    Immunofluorescence test (FAT). Specific cytoplasmic fluorescence (white area) in a cell culture infected with mucosal disease-virus diarrhea virus stained with MD-VD antiglobulin conjugate. (Courtesy R. Schultz.)

where a virus such as a noncytopathic strain of virus diarrhea-mucosal disease virus produces absolutely no cell alterations, a fluorescent antibody conjugate or the viral interference test with a cytopathic strain of virus diarrhea-mucosal disease virus can be used to assist in identification. In the interference test the noncytopathic strain interferes with a precalculated amount of cytopathic virus (usually 100 $TCID_{50}$ per 0.1 ml) and prevents the production of a cytopathic effect, often manifested as a plaque (fig. 161).

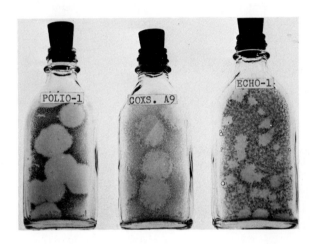

Fig. 161. Rhesus bottle cultures of poliovirus type 1 (Mahoney), Coxsackie virus A-9 (Grigg), and ECHO virus type 1 (Farouk) showing characteristic plaque morphology. (Courtesy Joseph L. Melnick, *Prog. Med. Virol.*)

Some viruses, such as members of the *Orthomyxovirus* and *Paramyxovirus* genera, cause hemagglutination and/or hemadsorption. The hemadsorption phenomenon can be utilized for viral detection by adding 0.15 ml of a 0.25 percent suspension of red blood cells directly to washed tube cell cultures and incubating at 37 C for 48 to 72 hours. In cultures containing virus the red blood cells are adsorbed to the infected cell sheets (fig. 162).

Production of virus in large quantities, as required for production of vaccines or complement-fixing antigens, is possible then using sheets of cells grown in bottles. By using protein-free media (such as Parker-Morgan media 199) virus can be harvested in large quantities by withdrawing the fluid at a time when the maximum yield is expected. Once the immunizing dose is established the fluid can be harvested and either inactivated with formalin or phenol to produce a killed vaccine or, if the agent has been adequately attenuated, diluted properly to contain sufficient virus to immunize.

### Isolation of Viruses in Animals

The selection of a susceptible host for the isolation of a virus is essential to a diagnosis by this means. In certain instances age is important; suckling animals are more likely to develop recognizable infection than older animals. It is not a wise idea to use an animal more than once for viral isolation as subclinical infections do occur, and this would cause a false negative result. In

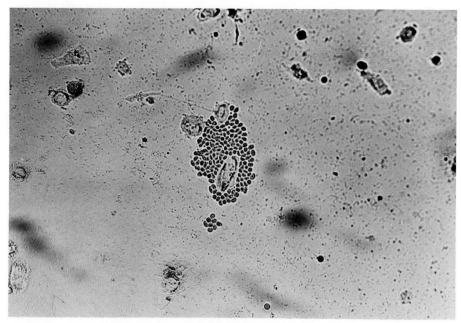

*Fig. 162.* Mumps virus causing hemadsorption (clumping) of chicken red blood cells in a cell culture of Vero cells. X 300. (Courtesy R. Schultz and F. Scott.)

studying a new viral agent the best chance for its successful propagation is in the natural host. In veterinary medicine we have this distinct advantage for the isolation of a virus in an animal. Often the natural host is a large animal, a fact that reduces its usefulness in achieving quick and easy solutions. The researcher then studies the effects of the virus in many other hosts, particularly in caged laboratory animals such as mice, hamsters, guinea pigs, rats, cats, and rabbits. In some instances adaptation to an unnatural host requires the use of a special virus strain, or by alteration of viral transfers between natural host and unnatural host it is possible to select viral particles which can be maintained in serial passage in the new host. The laboratory animal of choice for the various viruses, if one is available, is given under each virus infection discussed in this book. The route of inoculation of the virus in a laboratory host is critical with certain viruses. In unknown situations the most successful route is directly into the body system, where the virus produces lesions in the natural host; for example, suspect brain material from encephalitic cases would be inoculated intracerebrally into suckling and older mice.

The source of animals is exceedingly important as latent viruses occur in many animal colonies. To counteract this problem in part, animal colonies have been established by using caesarian-derived animals as the breeding stock. It is important to maintain these colonies as pathogen-free stocks by the use of isolation procedures. In some instances germ-free colonies are established for selected types of biological research problems. The caesarian-derived animal gives reasonable assurance that it is not harboring a viral agent which is transmitted horizontally. In the case of vertically transmitted viruses, such as the RNA (type C) oncogenic viruses, this procedure does not eliminate the viral agent. Consequently, there is little chance of establishing a colony which is free of all viruses or their viral genomes. Of course the problem of latent viruses also applies to the chick embryo and tissue culture as well. *Mycoplasma* and other microbes constitute a similar problem for all three systems often used for virus isolations. At best one can only hope to achieve a colony which is well defined and can be monitored for diseases for which adequate and specific tests exist for their identification.

With the introduction of the chick embryo technic, and particularly tissue culture technics, animal inoculations are seldom used for diagnosis of viral infections. They are still essential for viral research studies so the student should have some knowledge of their use and the problems associated with their use.

**Intracerebral Inoculation.** The intracerebral route of inoculation in mice is used for the isolation of neurotropic viruses. Either suckling mice or recently weaned mice (3 to 4 weeks old) are used for this purpose. On occasion, guinea pigs and rabbits are used. The inoculum should be virtually free of bacteria because the brain has little resistance to bacterial agents. Mice are lightly anesthetized with anesthetic ether before inoculation of 0.03 ml of test inoculum with a sharp needle, 27-gauge, 0.25-inch long and syringe, above the orbital ridge directly into the brain. Similarly, control mice are given a comparable amount of buffered physiological salt solution in a test to activate a latent brain virus such as lymphocytic choriomeningitis virus if it should exist in the test mice.

After inoculation all mice should be observed daily for signs of illness for approximately 30 days. Any mice that die during this period should be autopsied utilizing sterile technics in an attempt to isolate microbes from the brain and heart blood. Negative cultures rule out contamination with bacteria, fungi, and *Mycoplasma,* assuming the proper type of media were used to isolate these agents. Brain tissue should also be retained for additional viral tests if required to establish the diagnosis. Careful observation is made for macroscopic lesions followed by the study of stained sections of various tissues, particularly the brain, for the microscopic lesions. In viral encephalitides macroscopic brain lesions usually are lacking but microscopic lesions are quite pronounced. If the control mice given sterile buffered PSS develop nervous manifestations the test is declared void and another source of test mice sought if the infection is viral in nature. If all mice appear healthy at 30 days they are sacrificed and examined carefully for lesions.

**Intranasal Inoculation.** As a rule the mouse is the animal of choice for the isolation of pneumotropic viruses. Occasionally ferrets are used but they are generally avoided if possible, because the ferret is a difficult animal to handle.

The mice are anesthetized in a covered jar containing cotton soaked with ether and 0.05 ml of test material applied to the nares with a fine pipette. If properly anesthetized the mice will inhale the fluid preparation with no difficulty; otherwise it will discharge the fluid. Conversely, too much anesthesia or fluid inoculum causes death of the mouse.

Most respiratory diseases have a short incubation period so a 14-day observation period for signs of illness is usually adequate time. Mice that die are examined carefully at autopsy for lesions, especially of the respiratory tract. If the test mice show signs of respiratory illness, some are sacrificed. Some lungs are harvested for future virus studies. Others are used for macroscopic and microscopic study of the lesions. Surviving mice are examined at autopsy at the end of the observation period. Although virus may have replicated in the mouse lung no pneumonic lesions are produced in first passage. Depending upon the virus, it may be possible to detect it by various means such as the hemagglutination phenomenon. Subsequent passages of infective mouse lungs in mice may select a viral population which does cause pneumonia. The number of mouse transfers required will vary with the virus and also with the strain of virus.

**Intraperitoneal Inoculation.** This route of inoculation is commonly used for isolation of agents in guinea pigs, particularly, the psittacoid and rickettsial organisms. Mice are also used but less frequently. The peritoneal cavity of the guinea pig is particularly effective in the destruction of most nonpathogenic bacterial organisms present in feces of various domestic animals; consequently, it serves as an effective filter to eliminate most bacteria from fecal specimens not treated with antibiotics and being tested for psittacoid and rickettsial agents.

The guinea pigs are inoculated directly into the peritoneal cavity with a sharp needle, 24-to-25-guage and 0.5-inch long, and syringe with 0.5 ml of the lightly centrifuged test suspension. Daily temperatures and observations are made of the guinea pigs maintained in a temperature controlled environment. The guinea pig's thermal-regulating mechanism is sensitive to a marked rise in room temperature and its normal temperature range is exceeded at 38 to 39.5 C. This becomes especially important when a rise in temperature may be the only indication of infection. If the guinea pigs sicken, the appropriate tests from spleen, blood, and peritoneal cavity are made for possible bacterial contamination. Tissues also are selected for further study of the pathogenic agent, usually the spleen. Quite often guinea pigs recover from active infection, which is a distinct advantage for serological studies.

### Serological Diagnosis of Viral Diseases

The immunological response of an animal to natural or planned viral infection can be detected and measured by a large number of serological procedures. There are two indispensable elements in any serological test: the antigen and the antibody. The viral antigen(s) may be detected, identified, and quantified by testing it against a number of specific antibody preparations. Conversely, the antibody in the serum of a recovered or vaccinated animal can be identified and quantitated by testing against a number of prepared viral antigens.

At present the greatest number of diagnostic tests performed in a microbiological laboratory are serological tests. The most widely used tests are the serum-neutralization, complement-fixation, and hemagglutination-inhibition. Other methods include the hemadsorption, hemadsorption-inhibition, precipitation, agglutination, immunodiffusion, and flocculation tests. The procedure with the greatest potential as a quick and accurate diagnostic test for viral diseases is the fluorescent antibody technic (FAT) involving immunofluorescence. Kwapinsky (2) and Lennette and Schmidt (3) cover all these tests in detail.

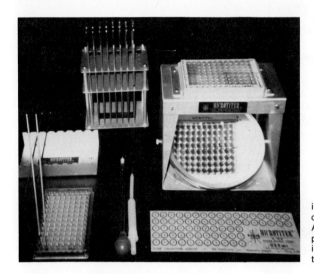

*Fig. 163.* A photograph depicting most of the equipment (produced by Cooke Engineering Co., Alexandria, Va.) essential for the performance of viral and serological microtiter plate tests. (Courtesy R. Schultz and D. Holmes.)

In 1955 Takatsy (5) described the use of spiral loops in serological and virological micromethods and Sever (4) utilized the microtechnic for viral serological investigations in the United States. With the availability of accurately calibrated equipment for measuring small volumes from a commercial source,* microserological technics have been developed for the diagnosis of viral diseases in the United States and elsewhere. At present microtests for the hemagglutination-inhibition, complement-fixation, gel-diffusion, and neutralization tests are in common usage (1) in viral serological diagnosis and they give comparable results to the macromethods. The microtests are preferred because they contribute to an economy in time, space, and reagents.

With most serological methods antibody titers are expressed as the recipro-

* Cooke Engineering Company, Medical Research Division, Alexandria, Virginia, 22314, U.S.A.

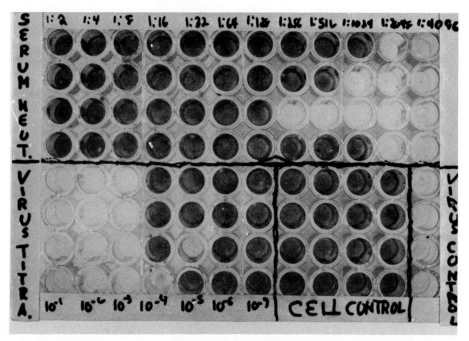

*Fig. 164.* Test results of a microtiter serum neutralization test with an accompanying virus titration using a feline herpesvirus antigen-antibody system. In the SN test 100 $TCID_{50}$ of virus was used against varying 2-fold dilutions of serum. After appropriate incubation at 37 C the nutrient fluid is discarded and cell layers in the plate are rinsed with saline, fixed with methanol, and stained with Giemsa. The stained wells (dark) indicate lack of viral cytopathic effect; the clear wells lack cells as a result of viral cytopathic activity. (Courtesy D. Holmes and R. Schultz.)

cal of the highest serum dilution causing a positive observable antigen-antibody reaction. In such tests as the neutralization test, which is based upon the inhibition of viral replication by specific antibody the level (titer) can be expressed as the neutralization index (alpha test procedure) or as the highest dilution which protests 50 percent of the test host against a precalculated virus dosage (beta test procedure). The 50 percent end points for the beta test procedure can be calculated by the methods of Reed and Muench and Spearman-Karber (3).

To perform satisfactory serological tests blood samples should be collected in sterile sealed units. The recommended unit is the B-D Vacutainer ° (without additive). The specimens should be allowed to clot at room temperature for a few hours before overnight refrigeration. The following day the serum is decanted from the clot into a sterile centrifuge tube. Centrifuge the sample at 2,500 rpm for 20 to 30 minutes and remove the serum into a sterile vial without disturbing the red cells. The nonhemolyzed serum sample can be frozen

° Becton-Dickinson Company, Rutherford, New Jersey, U.S.A.

at $-10$ to $-20$ C and shipped immediately, under refrigeration, or sent later with a second sample drawn from the same animal. Under no circumstances should the blood sample be frozen before the serum is harvested from the collected specimen. Proper labeling of each sample identified with a given animal and with proper date is essential to a correct diagnosis.

## REFERENCES

1.    Casey.   Health Lab. Sci., 1970, 7, 233.
2.    Kwapinksy.   Methods of serological research. John Wiley & Sons, Inc., New York, 1965.
3.    Lennette and Schmidt.   Diagnostic procedures for viral and rickettsial infections, 4th ed. Am. Pub. Health Assoc., Inc., New York, 1969.
4.    Sever.   Jour. Immunol., 1960, 88, 320.
5.    Takatsy.   Acta Microbiol. Acad. Sci., 1955, 3, 1955.

## The Diagnosis of Viral Respiratory Diseases of Domestic Animals

The differential diagnosis of infectious diseases of domestic animals offers the student and veterinary practitioner one of his greatest challenges yet also contributes to his frustrations. This is especially true of the respiratory diseases, principally those of viral origin. Their disease manifestations are so similar that differential diagnosis is possible only through laboratory procedures ranging from simple cytologic examination to the isolation of the agent(s). Some viral respiratory diseases are further complicated by secondary infections with opportunist bacterial pathogens or even another virus. A clinical diagnosis can be no more than a calculated guess as the problem in domestic animals is similar in complexity to the "common cold" in humans.

To assist the practitioner in the proper selection of biological materials for diagnosis of respiratory infections, tables depicting the major characteristics of the principal respiratory viral infections of domesticated animals are given below. In the preparation of tables XXVIII (1) and XXIX (2) some of the information was extracted from information developed by the respective panels of the American Veterinary Medical Association Symposia. The practitioners on these panels felt that this type of table would be quite useful to the student and veterinarian in their understanding of respiratory complexes and as an aid in arriving at a differential diagnosis.

**REFERENCES**

1. American Veterinary Medical Association. Panel, Bovine Respiratory Disease Supplement. Jour. Am. Vet. Med. Assoc., 1968, *152*, 713.
2. *Ibid*. Panel, Feline Infect. Diseases Report. Jour. Am. Vet. Med. Assoc., 1971, *158*, 835.

Table XXVIII. CHARACTERISTICS OF CHLAMYDIAL*

| | Infectious bovine rhinotracheitis (IBR) (respiratory form only) | Parainfluenza 3 Infection (PI-3) ‡ | Bovine rhinovirus (BRH) |
|---|---|---|---|
| Agent | Infectious bovine rhinotracheitis virus, a bovine herpesvirus | Bovine parainfluenza 3 virus | Bovine rhinovirus |
| Known geographic distribution | World-wide | World-wide | Germany, US, England |
| Incubation, natural infection | 4 to 6 days | 5 to 10 days | 2 to 4 days |
| Age | Any, usually in young stock | Any | Any |
| Signs | Respiratory form only—Varies markedly in severity as a herd infection. Characterized by high fever, depression, inappetence, and copious mucopurulent exudate initially followed by nasal ulcers, necrosis of muzzle and nostril wings, dyspnea, mouth breathing, conjunctivitis, coughing, and sometimes bloody feces. WBC mostly normal | Seldom occurs in calves. In adult cattle respiratory signs encompass those associated with a fibrinous pneumonia such as coughing, difficult breathing, extended neck, foamy saliva | Serous nasal discharge, temperature, coughing, depression, dyspnea |
| Course of disease | In respiratory form some cattle may die acutely, but most of them run a disease course for a few days | 4 to 7 days, occasionally longer | Approximately 1 week |
| Morbidity | In US varies from 10 to 35 percent in cattle population | High in infected herds | Probably high |
| Mortality | Varies but in western feedlots the average mortality is 10 percent | Varies markedly, but can be moderate in cattle shipped during cold weather | Little or none |
| Pathologic findings | Highly inflamed mucous membranes of upper respiratory tract with shallow erosions with a glary, fetid mucopurulent exudate. These lesions may be found in the pharynx, larynx, trachea, and larger bronchi. Sometimes patchy purulent pneumonia. Ulceration and inflammation of the abomasal mucosa is found, and catarrhal enteritis may occur | Lesions confined principally to respiratory tract. White fibrinous mass on lung surface. Lungs may be solid and heavy, filling the thoracic cavity. Cut sections show deep red and grayish lobules separated by interlobular tissue, greatly thickened by infiltration of coagulated exudate on serous surface | Principal lesions occur in nasal passages. A pneumonia in calves can occur after experimental intratracheal inoculation |
| Inclusions | Intranuclear inclusion bodies occur in epithelial cells of respiratory tract | Intracytoplasmic inclusion bodies in nasal and bronchial epithelial and alveolar macrophages that show marked fluorescence with specific antibody conjugate | None reported in cattle or in cell culture |
| Other natural hosts | None known; goats can be experimentally infected | PI-3 virus has been isolated from man, water buffalo, horses, and monkeys | None reported |

| Bovine adenovirus (BA) | Bovine viral diarrhea-mucosal disease (BVD-MD) | Malignant catarrhal fever (MCF) | Bovine reoviruses (BRE) |
|---|---|---|---|
| Three recognized serotypes, may be 5 additional ones | BVD-MD virus | Probably a bovine herpesvirus | Bovine reovirus—3 serotypes known |
| US, England, Hungary, Japan | World-wide | Africa, most countries of South and Central Africa, North America | Probably world-wide |
| Several days | 6 to 9 days | Unknown. Exp. infection in cattle 10 to 44 days | Few days |
| Usually in calves | Any | Any | Any |
| Signs associated with a pneumoenteritis | In clinical cases, diphasic temperature reaction, usually a dry, harsh, nonproductive cough, and a watery conjunctivitis, no dyspnea, excessive salivation with erosions in oral cavity, mucoid and sometimes blood-tinged diarrhea, and bluish discoloration of muzzle. Abortions. Leukopenia often followed by leukocytosis | Initially, a fever lasting 1 to 2 days coinciding with inappetence and depression. Then inflammation of nasal passages, oral cavity, and eyes occurs. Difficult breathing follows and fibrinopurulent pneumonia may occur. Nervous signs develop early in most cases with either stupor or excitement | Usually inapparent infection. Presently recognized as a mild respiratory infection |
| Weeks in some instances | Usually subclinical, few days as a rule, occasionally chronic, persisting for months | Varies markedly. Sometimes death in 24 hours; usually 5 to 14 days | Unknown |
| High in infected herds | Moderate to high | Low; usually only 1 to 2 cattle in herd will show signs | Believed high |
| Low to moderate in infected herds | Low to high | Extremely high | Little or none |
| Varying degrees of pneumonia with proliferative bronchiolitis with necrosis and bronchiolar occlusion causing alveolar collapse. Lesions may persist for weeks | The lesions are not confined to the respiratory tract; in fact the principal lesions are found in the oral cavity, digestive tract, and lymphatic system | Dark, swollen glassy membranes of turbinates and nasal sinuses covered with fibrin shreds and purulent excretion with shallow ulcers under this mass. Similar lesions seen in larynx, trachea, bronchi, and sometimes bronchopneumonia. Swollen head lymph nodes. Inflammation and erosion of abomasum and small intestine sometimes occurs. Meninges congested and hemorrhagic. Nonpurulent encephalitis | Interstitial pneumonia and lymphadenitis of regional nodes |
| Intranuclear inclusion bodies in bronchiolar epithelium, septal cells, and bronchial lymph nodes | None | Inconclusive. Some investigators report nerve-cell intranuclear inclusion bodies; others cytoplasmic inclusion bodies in epithelial cells | Unknown but should be present in bronchiolar epithelium |
| Not determined | Perhaps sheep, goats, and also white-tailed and mule deer | Possibly sheep and African wildebeests | May infect man and other animals; not known for certainty |

*Table XXVIII*   CHARACTERISTICS OF CHLAMYDIAL*

| | Infectious bovine rhinotracheitis (IBR) (respiratory form only) | Parainfluenza 3 infection (PI-3) ‡ | Bovine rhinovirus (BRH) |
|---|---|---|---|
| Propagation | Tissue culture; cytopathic effects in kidney cells from cattle, pig, dog, sheep, goat, and horse | Replicates in many types of cell cultures from many species, causing CPE and hemadsorption. Causes syncytia and cytoplasmic and intranuclear inclusion bodies | CPE produced in bovine kidney cell cultures at 33 C |
| Carrier state | Virus may persist for weeks | Known to persist in lungs for at least 18 days | Unknown |
| Diagnosis | Sometimes possible on basis of history and character of the disease. Viral isolation from exudate of nasal passage in tissue culture. SN, FA, CF, gel-diffusion tests | Virus readily isolated from nasal exudate in cell culture. HI, HA-I, FA, and SN tests | Difficult clinically. Virus isolation in cell culture. SN test |
| Immunity | Long-term serviceable immunity | Maternal immunity apparently confers protection. The degree and duration of active immunity is yet to be determined with certainty | Status vague, immunity may be incomplete |
| Prophylaxis | Inactivated and attenuated virus vaccines | Inactivated vaccines, one incorporating PI-3 virus and *Pasteurella* organism, appear to be effective in controlling field disease | No vaccine available |
| Treatment | Antibiotic therapy and supportive measures | Antibiotic therapy is useful, as bacteria play an important role in the pathogenesis of the disease. Warm and dry quarters and supportive measures are important | Antibiotic therapy may be useful; supportive treatment |

* Chlamydial respiratory disease in cattle is similar to that described for sheep and goats in table XXXIII, and it is sometimes called pneumoenteritis in calves.

† See table XXXIII for description of Rift Valley fever in sheep and cattle; the disease is less severe in cattle.

‡ *Pasteurella* organisms are usually involved in this disease.

| Bovine adenovirus (BA) | Bovine viral diarrhea-mucosal disease (BVD-MD) | Malignant catarrhal fever (MCF) | Bovine reoviruses (BRE) |
|---|---|---|---|
| Tissue culture; calf kidney and testes | Tissue culture; cell cultures derived from bovine tissues. Some strains produce CPE, others do not | Tissue culture; thyroid or adrenal gland cultures | Tissue culture—produces CPE in bovine kidney, pig kidney, and monkey kidney |
| 21 days known but probably longer | Possibly, but little known | Unknown | At least 1 month |
| Isolation in calf testes cell cultures from exudate of nasal passages or from feces; SN, HI, and agar gel tests | Clinical signs, but more specifically upon lesions in severe cases; may be confused with rinderpest, malignant catarrhal fever, and certain respiratory diseases. Isolation of virus from blood or excretions and selected tissues in cell culture. Noncytopathic strains are identified in culture by exaltation or interference tests. SN and agar gel tests | Clinical diagnosis is possible when sporadic cases with nervous and eye manifestations occur in a herd | Virus is isolated from nasal passages and conjunctiva in tissue culture. SN, HI tests |
| Duration of immunity presently unknown | Complete and long lasting immunity | Uncertain | No evidence of maternal immunity. Degree and duration of active immunity unknown |
| None | Attenuated virus vaccine available; do not use in pregnant cows | None. Keep sheep away from cattle | None at present |
| Antibiotics to assist in control of bacterial invaders; supportive measures | Supportive measures | None | Antibiotics may be useful in controlling secondary bacterial infections such as *Pasteurella* organisms |

Table XXIX. CHARACTERISTICS OF CHLAMYDIAL AND VIRAL RESPIRATORY INFECTIONS OF CATS

| | Rhinotracheitis (FVR) | Calicivirus infection (FPI) | Reovirus infection (FRI) | Pneumonitis (FPN) |
|---|---|---|---|---|
| Agent | Herpesvirus | Caliciviruses of numerous serotypes (picornavirus) | Reovirus serotypes 1 and 3 | *Chlamydia psittaci* (*Miyagawanella felis; Bedsonia felis*) |
| Known geographic distribution | US, Europe, New Zealand | US, Europe, Australia, New Zealand, Japan | US | US, Europe |
| Incubation, natural infection | Several days | Usually 1 to 3 days shorter than for FVR | 4 to 19 days | 6 to 10 days |
| Age | Any | Any | Any | Any |
| Signs | Sneezing and coughing, sometimes paroxysmal; salivation, ocular and nasal exudation, oral breathing, fever, inappetence, weight loss; pregnant females occasionally abort; some fatal generalized infection in newborn kittens; sinusitis, ulcerative keratitis, panophthalmitis in chronic infections. Leukocytosis when accompanied by bacterial infection | Asymptomatic to severe, depending on virus strain. Conjunctivitis, ocular discharge often unilateral, rhinitis, sneezing, depression, inappetence, dyspnea, râles, other abnormal lung sounds, and pneumonia; fever, often diphasic; ulcers on tongue and hard palate, preceded by salivation; mortality in newborn cats. Early transient lymphopenia in some cases. May initiate urolithiasis | Generally mild, with lacrimation, photophobia, serous conjunctivitis, gingivitis, and depression; nasal discharge and fever rarely. WBC mostly normal; no leukopenia | Sneezing, drooling, lacrimation, ocular and nasal discharge, occasional cough, fever, and inappetence. A related strain thought to cause unilateral purulent conjunctivitis often affects other eye in 5 to 7 days. May be enzootic in catteries. May infect newborn or newly introduced cats. Occasional sneezing and nasal discharge; fever uncommon. Leukocytosis inconsistently |
| Course of disease | Usually 2 to 4 weeks | Average of 7 to 10 days | 1 to 26 days | A few days to several weeks |
| Morbidity | High | High | About 50% among contact controls | Variable |
| Mortality | Low in adults | Variable; up to 30% in experimental infections | Low | Low in adults |

|  | | | |
|---|---|---|---|
| Pathologic findings | Necrotizing conjunctivitis, rhinitis, and tracheitis associated with intranuclear inclusions; sinusitis, resorption of turbinates in chronic infections; in some cases, patchy or general consolidation in anterior lung lobes characterized by necrotizing bronchiolitis and proliferation of alveolar septal cells; secondary bacterial or mycotic infections may occur* | Conjunctivitis, rhinitis, ulcers of the tongue and palate, patchy broncho-pneumonia. Alternately banding of spleen associated with calicivirus infection in some cats | Conjunctivitis | Conjunctivitis, rhinitis, laryngitis, pharyngitis, patchy pneumonic consolidation in anterior lung lobes |
| Inclusions | Intranuclear inclusions in respiratory epithelial cells, nictitating membrane, tongue, and tonsils | None | Paranuclear cytoplasmic inclusions | Intracytoplasmic elementary bodies in respiratory and conjunctival epithelial cells |
| Other natural hosts | None known | None known | Reovirus 1 and 3 isolated from many mammals | Mouse, hamster, guinea pig, rabbit |
| Propagation | Tissue culture; cells of feline origin | Tissue culture; cells of feline origin | Tissue culture, feline and bovine kidney cells | Chicken embryo or cell culture |
| Carrier state | Yes | Yes | Not determined | Yes |
| Diagnosis | Demonstration of intranuclear inclusions early in course of infection, tissue culture isolation, SN, HA, HI, FA tests | Tissue culture isolation, SN, FA tests | Tissue culture isolation, SN, HA tests | Demonstration of elementary bodies in Giemsa-stained material, animal inoculation, CF test |
| Immunity | Weak, transient | Many serotypes; homologous protection likely | Not determined, but likely | Weak, transient |
| Prophylaxis | None | None | None | Vaccine is available |
| Treatment | Antibiotics indicated for secondary invaders, supportive measures | Antibiotics indicated for secondary invaders, supportive measures | Symptomatic | Tetracyclines systemically and in ophthalmic ointment; supportive measures occasionally needed |

* Experimental intravenous inoculation results in necrosis in growth regions of all bones, focal necrosis in adrenal glands and liver, and, in pregnant females, placental necrosis, fetal death, and abortion.

*Table XXX.* CHARACTERISTICS OF VIRAL

| | Equine herpesvirus infection (EHI) | Equine influenza (EI) |
|---|---|---|
| Agent | Equine herpesvirus 1; new equine cytomegaloviruses now under investigation | Equine influenza virus. Two types designated A/Equi-1/Praha/56 and A/Equi-2/Miami/63 |
| Known geographic distribution | US, Europe | World-wide |
| Incubation, natural infection | *Weanling disease*—a few days *Abortion disease*—3 to 4 weeks | 1 to 3 days |
| Age | Any | Any |
| Signs | *Weanling disease*—mild febrile reaction accompanied by rhinitis or nasal catarrh; usually in fall of year. *Abortion disease*—infection in mares causes abortion (usually between 6 to 10 months of pregnancy) with no other signs. Rare cases of nervous disease. Sometimes a leukopenia in weanlings | Coughing is most common sign of illness. High temperature, inappetence, mental depression, photophobia, lacrimation, cloudy cornea, nasal catarrh, swollen lymph nodes of head. If pneumonia develops horse usually dies from bacterial infection |
| Course of disease | Foals usually recover in 8 to 10 days | 1 to 3 weeks, sometimes longer |
| Morbidity | Very high in foals of infected herds; varies from 10 to 90 percent on stud farms | Highly contagious with high morbidity |
| Mortality | No mortality in weanlings. Only rarely in mares, but loss of foals through abortions may be high | Usually does not exceed 5 percent |
| Pathologic findings | *Weanlings*—Reddening of mucous membranes of upper air passages with a collective mucopurulent exudate *Aborting mares*—No lesions *Aborted feti*—Multiple focal liver necrosis, petechial hemorrhages in heart muscle and in capsules of spleen and liver; lung edema | Principal lesions in fatal cases are extensive edema of lungs or a bronchopneumonia with pleurisy; hydrothorax; gelatinous infiltrations around larynx and in the legs; swollen lymph nodes |
| Inclusions | Intranuclear inclusion bodies are found in hepatic cells, and also in epithelial cells and endothelial cells of various organs | None |
| Other natural hosts | None known | Only members of equine family |

# RESPIRATORY INFECTIONS OF HORSES

| Equine rhinovirus infection (ERI) | Equine parainfluenza infection (EPI) | African horsesickness (AHS) |
|---|---|---|
| Equine rhinovirus; all present isolates except one are serologically related | Parainfluenza 3 virus. Limited information about virus and the disease | Equine reovirus. Nine distinct immunological types |
| North America, South America, Africa | US and Canada | Africa, Middle East, parts of Asia |
| 3 to 7 days | Few days | Probably 7 to 9 days |
| Any, mostly young animals | Any | Any |
| Fever, anorexia, serous, followed by mucopurulent nasal discharge, cough | Usually occurs in young horses. Mucopurulent discharge and other signs referable to respiratory tract, fever | Acute form characterized by respiratory signs with death resulting from severe edema in the lungs. There is fever, labored breathing, coughing, severe dyspnea, and copious foamy nasal discharge. Chronic cases also include heart distress coupled with edema of head and neck tissues |
| About 1 week | 4 to 7 days, sometimes longer | 3 to 5 days average; may be longer |
| Infected stables—high morbidity | Moderate to high in limited surveys | Usually high; spreads very rapidly |
| Low | Low | 25 to 95 percent |
| Marked pharyngitis, lymphadenitis, abscesses in submaxillary lymph nodes | Insufficient information | Depends upon severity of case. *In acute type* thoracic cavity contains liters of fluid and lungs are distended. A yellowish fluid separates interlobular tissue from alveolar portions. The lung surfaces are wet and fluid runs from cut surface. Pericardial sac may have excess fluid and subendocardial hemorrhages usually are present. Some fluid is present in abdominal cavity, the liver is swollen and intestines reddened. *In chronic form,* edema of head and neck; hydropericardium and hydropic degeneration of myocardium. Lungs and thoracic cavity have moderate edema |
| None | Unknown | Unknown—should be present in bronchiolar epithelium |
| None known | Unknown | Zebras, dogs, angora goats, mules, donkeys |

*Table XXX.* CHARACTERISTICS OF VIRAL

|  | Equine herpesvirus infection (EHI) | Equine influenza (EI) |
|---|---|---|
| Propagation | It has been adapted to hens' eggs. Replicates and produces CPE in cell cultures of fetal horse kidney, lamb kidney, and rabbit kidney | Embryonated hen's egg is best. Tissue cultures of monkey kidney more susceptible than bovine, equine, or human kidney cells |
| Carrier state | Not studied | Suggested that some horses remain carriers for months |
| Diagnosis | Clinical diagnosis of respiratory disease is difficult; aborting disease less complicated. Intranuclear inclusion bodies help establish diagnosis. Virus can be isolated from affected tissues in cell culture. SN, CF, precipitation tests | Usually can be diagnosed in an outbreak on basis of history, clinical signs and lesions. Virus isolation from nasal exudate in hens' eggs or tissue culture. SN and HI tests |
| Immunity | Probably transitory immunity, lasting few years | Solid immunity to natural disease for 1 year |
| Prophylaxis | In US, planned infection on trouble farms with a hamster adapted live-virus vaccine. Mares kept in small, isolated groups minimizes spread | Two types of inactivated vaccine available. Yearly vaccination required |
| Treatment | None | Antibiotic therapy indicated to control bacterial infection. Supportive measures |

| Equine rhinovirus infection (ERI) | Equine parainfluenza infection (EPI) | African horsesickness (AHS) |
|---|---|---|
| Rabbits, guinea pigs, monkeys and man susceptible to intranasal instillation. Tissue culture: cells of many animal species | Tissue culture | Tissue culture: cell cultures derived from baby hamster, bovine kidney and others with production of CPE and cytoplasmic inclusion bodies; suckling mice |
| At least 1 month | Unknown | *Culicoides* (midges) are probable vectors. Direct transmission does not occur |
| Isolation of virus in cell culture from nasal excretions. SN test | Isolation of virus in cell culture. SN, HA-I, HA, HI, CF tests | May be confused with other diseases, especially when first occurring in virgin territory. Laboratory diagnosis required by virus isolation from infective blood or tissues inoculated intracerebrally into suckling mice. SN, CF, agar gel, FA, HI tests, HI used for viral serotyping |
| Limited knowledge. Evidence of maternal immunity and active immunity protection | Unknown | Apparent excellent immunity to homotypic serotype |
| No vaccine available although one is needed | No vaccine available | Multiple mouse-brain virus vaccine available. Given annually. Stable nonvaccinated horses at night |
| Antibiotic therapy to help control bacterial invaders | Antibiotic therapy may be useful. Supportive measures and good nursing in warm, dry quarters | No treatment is effective |

*Table XXXI.* CHARACTERISTICS OF CHLAMYDIAL*

| | Canine distemper (CD) | Infectious canine hepatitis (ICH) |
|---|---|---|
| Agent | Canine distemper virus | Canine adenoviruses 1 & 2; canine 2 causes its major effects in the respiratory tract |
| Known geographic distribution | World-wide | World-wide |
| Incubation, natural infection | 4 to 6 days | 5 to 9 days |
| Age | Any | Any |
| Signs | Some infections are inapparent; principal signs in others may be respiratory, enteric, or nervous or a combination of them. Respiratory signs include watery discharge from eyes and nose, which may become mucoid in 24 hours; diphasic temperature, and pneumonia may develop as a result of bacterial infection. Leukopenia followed sometimes by leukocytosis | *Classic hepatic form* characterized by fever, intense thirst, sometimes edema of extremities, diarrhea, vomiting, intense pain, serous nasal discharge. *Respiratory form* characterized by 1 to 3 day fever, harsh & dry hacking cough, serous nasal discharge sometimes becoming purulent, muscular trembling, depression, dyspnea. In hepatic form there is a leukopenia, but in respiratory form total WBC are variable |
| Course of disease | Usually 2 to 3 weeks; may last longer in few cases | *Hepatic form*—5 to 10 days *Respiratory form*—5 to 28 days |
| Morbidity | High | High |
| Mortality | Varies markedly in outbreaks, usually related to brain involvement. Probably averages 20 percent in clinical cases | 10 to 25 percent overall; especially high in puppies |
| Pathologic findings | Viremic disease with affinity for epithelial cells thus capable of producing a wide variety of lesions. There is a viral-induced giant cell pneumonia which may be complicated by bacterial infection causing a purulent bronchopneumonia. There may be enteritis, encephalitis, vesicular & pustular skin lesions, atrophied & gelatinous thymus gland, eye lesions, urinary & reproductive system lesions | *Hepatic form*—characterized by edema and hemorrhage. Fibrinous peritonitis with blood tinged fluid in cavity; hydrothorax; marked thickening of gall bladder; swollen liver; lung edema; uveitis. *Respiratory form*—moderate to severe pneumonic changes. Proliferative, adenomatous changes are seen in lungs of dogs with infection for 10 days |
| Inclusions | Cytoplasmic and/or intranuclear inclusion bodies in many epithelial cells; particularly seen in bronchi, bladder, renal pelvis, and glial cells | *Hepatic form*—intranuclear inclusion bodies in hepatic & endothelial cells. *Respiratory form*—intranuclear inclusion bodies in bronchial epithelium, alveolar septal cells, and turbinate epithelium |
| Other natural hosts | Principally members of canine family | Foxes (often show nervous disease), wolves, coyotes, bears, raccoon? |

| Canine parainfluenza (SV-5) | Canine reovirus infection (CRI) | Canine herpesvirus (CH) |
|---|---|---|
| Parainfluenza II virus (SV-5) | Canine reovirus 1 | Canine herpesvirus |
| US | US | US, Great Britain, and Europe |
| 2 to 3 days | Uncertain | 3 to 8 days in puppies |
| Any | Any | Any |
| Sudden onset, copious nasal discharge, fever, and coughing. If *B. bronchiseptica* and *Mycoplasma* are involved, a dry cough persists for weeks | Experimental dogs from conventional sources showed elevated temperature and respiratory signs and pneumonia. Sometimes causes enteritis. Germ-free dogs became infected without signs | *Puppies*—labored breathing, abdominal pain, yellowish-green stool, anorexia, and acute death. *Older dogs*—vaginitis and mild rhinitis |
| 1 to 7 days; weeks in cases with complications | Not well-studied | In 1 to 2 week old puppies one to two days; older dogs—unknown |
| Low to moderate | Low to moderate | Low to moderate |
| Low | Low | High in 1 to 2 week old puppies; negligible in older dogs |
| Usually no gross lesions except petechial hemorrhages in respiratory tract. Microscopic catarrhal changes are present in lower and upper respiratory tract & also in regional lymph nodes | Pneumonia and enteritis | *Puppies*—disseminated focal necrosis and hemorrhages found in virtually all internal organs, especially kidney. Lungs are diffusely pneumonic. Meningoencephalitic lesions frequently seen but without nervous signs |
| Unknown | Unknown | Intranuclear inclusion bodies in cells in areas of necrosis are found |
| Monkeys, man, dogs, perhaps others | Unknown, may infect man & other animals | Not known |

*Table XXXI.* CHARACTERISTICS OF CHLAMYDIAL*

|  | Canine distemper (CD) | Infectious canine hepatitis (ICH) |
|---|---|---|
| Propagation | Tissue culture—primary and cell lines from various tissues support the replication & show CPE. Embryonated hens' eggs with adapted strains. Suckling mice, suckling hamsters, ferrets & many other species are susceptible | Tissue culture; canine, ferret, and swine-kidney monolayer cultures |
| Carrier state | Footpads—4 to 6 weeks. Brain—at least 49 days in some nervous cases of dogs | Urine—39 weeks<br>Kidney—unknown<br>Tonsils—unknown |
| Diagnosis | Demonstration of inclusion bodies constitutes a presumptive diagnosis. Isolation of virus constitutes a positive diagnosis—this can be done in dog macrophage cultures. FA and SN tests are excellent methods | Demonstration of intranuclear inclusion bodies. Isolation of virus from pathological lesions in tissue culture; SN, FA, and CF tests |
| Immunity | Long-term durable immunity to natural disease. Maternal protection may persist for 15 weeks | Solid and long-lasting, perhaps life |
| Prophylaxis | Excellent vaccines are available; for maximum protection yearly vaccination is advised | Inactivated and attenuated virus vaccines |
| Treatment | Antibiotic therapy recommended for control of bacterial disease; supportive measures | Antibiotics indicated for bacterial invaders, especially respiratory form; supportive measures |

* The disease in dogs is similar to that described for sheep and goats in Table XXXIII, except dogs have muscle and joint involvement in addition to respiratory signs.

| Canine parainfluenza (SV-5) | Canine reovirus infection (CRI) | Canine herpesvirus (CH) |
|---|---|---|
| Replicates with CPE and cytoplasmic inclusion bodies in kidney cultures of dog, African green monkey, rhesus monkey, and human embryos. Replicates in amniotic cavity of hens' eggs without death | Produces CPE in dog kidney cell culture | Tissue culture; dog kidney cells |
| Unknown | Spleen—3.5 weeks | Turbinates—3 weeks<br>Kidney—unknown<br>Nasal—3 weeks |
| Clinically difficult. Virus isolation with respiratory exudates in cell cultures; HA, HA-I, HI, SN, FA tests | Isolation of virus from nasal exudate or feces in cell culture | Focal renal hemorrhages not seen in CD and ICH. Intranuclear bodies must be differentiated from ICH intranuclear inclusions. Virus can be isolated from many tissues of dead puppies in dog kidney cell cultures. SN, CF tests |
| Dogs infected naturally or by intranasal route are completely protected. Duration of immunity not known. Level of maternal immunity is low so it has little significance in natural protection | Unknown | Duration of immunity unknown, but puppies from immune mothers are temporarily resistant |
| No vaccine available although there is a need for one | None | No vaccine available |
| Antibiotic therapy is indicated to control secondary invaders; supportive measures and good nursing | Antibiotics may be indicated; supportive measures | Supportive measures and especially warm environment for puppies |

Table XXXII. CHARACTERISTICS OF VIRAL RESPIRATORY INFECTIONS OF SWINE

| | Swine influenza (SI) | Porcine inclusion body rhinitis (PIBR) | Pseudorabies (PR) |
|---|---|---|---|
| Agent | Swine influenza virus—single serotype | Type B herpesvirus of pigs | Pseudorabies virus, a herpesvirus |
| Known geographic distribution | World-wide | World-wide | World-wide |
| Incubation, natural infection | 1 to 3 days | 5 to 10 days | 4 to 7 days, occasionally longer |
| Age | Any | Any | Any |
| Signs | Whole herds seem ill at once. Disease begins with fever, extreme weakness, prostration. Swine exhibit muscular stiffness and pain. Some show lung edema and broncho-pneumonia and usually die. Coughing also is observed | Severe disease in piglets as acute infection. In pigs over 2 weeks a subacute disease. Signs include sneezing, nasal exudate, inappetence, rapid loss of weight, paralysis, and death in 5 days. Subacute infections limited to respiratory tract. Severe anemia | Pruritis does not occur. Signs in sows usually are mild. Characterized by fever, depression, vomition, respiratory signs, and abortions. In suckling and recently weaned pigs the above signs are more severe |
| Course of disease | 2 to 6 days | Several days | 4 to 8 days |
| Morbidity | High | 1-to-2-week-old piglets—probably high. Older pigs—low | May be high |
| Mortality | Usually less than 4 percent, but may go to 10 percent | 1-to-2-week-old piglets—high. Older pigs—low | Young pigs—high Older pigs—very low |

| | | | |
|---|---|---|---|
| Pathologic findings | Principal lesions are in the lungs. Thick, mucilaginous exudate in the bronchioles and bronchi cause a atelectasis while remainder is usually pale because of interstitial emphysema. In some cases pneumonia develops and involves the areas in which atelectasis first occurred. Regional nodes are swollen and wet. Spleen is enlarged and there is hyperemia of stomach mucosa | Mucopurulent rhinitis, sinusitis, and sometimes turbinate atrophy, petechial hemorrhages in kidneys and myocardium | The gross lesions are not extensive; in fatal cases cellular infiltrations and necrosis occur in various parts of nervous system as seen in microscopic sections. Animals may die before virus reaches and causes lesions in anterior part of cord and brain |
| Inclusions | None | Intranuclear inclusion bodies in enlarged cells of many organs, including brain and particularly tubuloalveolar glands of nasal mucosa | Intranuclear inclusion bodies are not found in swine |
| Other natural hosts | Man? | None known | Cattle, cats, dogs, sheep, rats; horses? |
| Propagation | Intra-amniotic and intra-allantoic inoculation of 10-to-12-day-old embryonated hens' eggs. Various tissue cultures useful for cultivation and assay | Primary porcine lung-cell cultures—produces CPE and intranuclear inclusion bodies | Chick embryos. Tissue culture; chick, rabbit, guinea pig, dog, and monkey tissues |
| Carrier state | Complex viral etiology involving earthworms, lung worms, and pigs not completely understood or accepted by all investigators | Unknown | Animals which exhibit no visible signs can transmit the virus |
| Diagnosis | Embryonated hens' eggs with respiratory exudates. SN, FA, HI, CF, HA-I tests | Herd history, signs, and lesions allow good field diagnosis. Virus from lesions can be isolated in cell culture | More difficult in swine than other animals unless nervous signs occur. Virus can be isolated from lesions by inoculating into brain of rabbits; SN test |

*Table XXXII.* CHARACTERISTICS OF VIRAL RESPIRATORY INFECTIONS
OF SWINE (*Continued*)

| | Swine influenza (SI) | Porcine inclusion body rhinitis (PIBR) | Pseudorabies (PR) |
|---|---|---|---|
| Immunity | Believed to be immune after disease but not all investigators agree. Maternal immunity lasts for as long as 13-to-18 weeks | Piglets derive maternal protection from immune dams | Long-lasting, perhaps life |
| Prophylaxis | No vaccine available now; previous ones not effective | None | No vaccine available. Keep swine separated from cattle. Rat control |
| Treatment | Antibiotic therapy. Dry, warm quarters beneficial | None | None |

*Table XXXIII.*  CHARACTERISTICS OF CHLAMYDIAL AND VIRAL RESPIRATORY INFECTIONS OF SHEEP AND GOATS

| | Adenomatosis (sheep) | Psittacosis (sheep and goats) | Parainfluenza virus infection (PIV) (sheep) | Rift Valley (RVF) fever (sheep) |
|---|---|---|---|---|
| Agent | Herpesvirus | *Chlamydia psittaci* | Parainfluenza virus 3. Closely related to bovine and human PI-3 viruses, but not identical | Rift Valley fever virus, an arbovirus |
| Known geographic distribution | Europe, Peru, Iceland, South Africa, India, Israel, US | Probably world-wide | US, Australia | Africa only |
| Incubation, natural infection | Very long | Usually 6 to 10 days | Unknown | 1 to 3 days |
| Age | Any | Any | Any | Any |
| Signs | Signs are seen only in sheep over 4 years of age. As air spaces in lungs become obliterated the animals become dyspneic and emaciated | Conjunctival and nasal discharge, lethargy, labored breathing, pneumonia, and hyperthermia. Sometimes diarrhea | Signs referrable to respiratory tract with production of pneumonia | Fever, prostration, rapid course; some vomiting, also show purulent nasal discharge and bloody stools. Ewes abort sometimes without other signs. Severe leukopenia |
| Course of disease | When sheep become dyspneic they die in a few days to several weeks from anoxia | Varies, but generally 2 weeks | Usually 1 week; longer in some cases | 2 weeks |
| Morbidity | Low | High in affected flocks | Common and widespread in US | High |
| Mortality | High | Rarely fatal and its severity determined by secondary bacterial, viral, or *Mycoplasma* infections | Low | *Lambs*—high, often 95 to 100 percent; *Ewes*—probably less than 20 percent; *Cattle*—less than 10 percent |

|  | Adenomatosis (sheep) | Psittacosis (sheep and goats) | Parainfluenza virus infection (PIV) (sheep) | Rift Valley (RVF) fever (sheep) |
|---|---|---|---|---|
| Pathologic findings | Proliferation of cells in lung-supporting tissues with gradual filling of alveoli causing lung consolidation. Recognized as primary lung carcinoma which may metastasize | Intense neutrophilic response; copious mucoid exudates may be found with red lobular consolidation in anterior lobes of lungs. Histologically, it is a typical exudative bronchopneumonia of bronchioles with extension into alveoli | A fibrinous type of pneumonia | Most characteristic lesion is focal necrosis of the liver. Other lesions are principally hemorrhages in lymph nodes, gastric and intestinal mucosa, endocardium, and epicardium |
| Inclusions | Unknown | Elementary bodies are found in cytoplasm of infected cells | Unknown | Intranuclear inclusion bodies in liver |
| Other natural hosts | None known | Not thoroughly studied. Some strains of *C. psittaci* may cause similar disease in other mammals | Unknown | Cattle and humans |
| Propagation | Unknown except sheep | *C. psittaci* grows well in yolk sac of embryonated egg. Also in certain tissue cultures. Mice and guinea pigs are best laboratory animals for propagation | Sheep kidney cell cultures | Cell cultures of chick, rat, mouse, human, lamb, and hamster. Replicates in embryonated hens' eggs. In white mice |
| Carrier State | Unknown | Carriers do exist | Unknown | Unknown |
| Diagnosis | Typical lesions at autopsy | Demonstration of elementary bodies are difficult in smears or histological sections of lesions. Principal means is by isolation of exudates in hen's egg, in mouse lung, or guinea pig peritoneal cavity. CF, SN, and other serological tests | Isolation of virus from respiratory exudates in cell culture. SN, HA, HA-I, HI tests | Clinical signs and history highly suggestive. Massive liver focal necrosis characteristic. Inoculation of white mice causes prompt fatal infection with liver tissue and other infective tissues. CF, agar gel, HI tests |

| | | | | |
|---|---|---|---|---|
| Immunity | Affected animals do not recover | Immune status is unclear | Maternal immune protection exists. Little known about active immunity | Long-term, durable immunity in animals and humans that recover |
| Prophylaxis | Remove affected sheep from flock | No vaccines are available | No vaccine available | Live-virus vaccines are available but not safe in young lambs or pregnant cattle and ewes. Inactivated vaccines also available. Move animals into mountains away from mosquito vectors if possible |
| Treatment | None | Chemotherapy is useful— various antibiotics are effective | Antibiotic therapy, but it may not be feasible or practical | No effective treatment |

Table XXXIV.   CHARACTERISTICS OF RESPIRATORY

| | Newcastle disease (ND) | Avian infectious bronchitis (AIB) |
|---|---|---|
| Agent | Paramyxovirus a-1 | Coronavirus a-1 |
| Known geographic distribution | World-wide | North America, Japan, England, Europe |
| Incubation, natural infection | 4 to 14 days | 2 to 4 days |
| Age | Any | Any |
| Signs | Outbreaks vary in intensity—older birds may have inapparent infection but chicks usually show marked respiratory distress and nervous manifestations appear in a varying percentage a few days later. When nervous signs occur the death rate is high. In laying birds respiratory signs occur accompanied by a complete cessation in egg production | Severity of respiratory signs is age-dependent, with chicks showing greatest effects, including listlessness, depression, rales, gasping. In laying flocks egg production drops dramatically and full production is not usually achieved until next laying period |
| Course of disease | 6 to 8 days with respiratory disease; with CNS involvement usually longer | 6 to 18 days |
| Morbidity | High | High |
| Mortality | Low to high depending on incidence of birds with nervous manifestations | Chicks—25 to 90 percent. Older birds—none to low |
| Pathologic findings | Gross lesions not particularly striking. Fluid or mucus in the trachea, cloudy air-sac membranes. Spleen may be enlarged. Typical viral encephalitic lesions in birds with nervous signs | Mucoid or caseous plugs overlying a highly inflamed bronchi and sometimes in nasal passages. Chicks that die usually have fibrinopurulent exudate in lower trachea and larger bronchi |
| Inclusions | None seen | None |
| Other natural hosts | Turkeys, pheasants, ducks, geese, and many other species are naturally infected | None |
| Propagation | Readily propagated in embryonated hens' eggs and produces a CPE and also replicates in cell cultures of chick origin. Cytoplasmic and intranuclear inclusions occur in cell cultures | Causes dwarfing and curling of chick embryos. Cytopathic effect in chicken embryo kidney cultures |
| Carrier state | Perhaps as long as 1 month | At least 49 days |

# VIRAL INFECTIONS OF CHICKENS

| Laryngotracheitis (LT) | Fowlpox (FP) | Fowl plague (FP) |
|---|---|---|
| Laryngotracheitis virus, an avian herpesvirus | Fowlpox virus | Avian influenza virus |
| World-wide | World-wide | US, Canada, Europe, South America |
| 2 days | Several days | 3 to 5 days |
| Any | Any | Any |
| Highly contagious. Respiratory signs include mouth breathing, gurgling and rattling sounds, nasal exudate in some birds | As a rule, the pox lesions are confined to head; occasionally they are limited to oral cavity and trachea causing a respiratorylike disease | Mucoid nasal discharge, fever, edema of head and neck, lethargy, bluish-black discoloration of combs and wattles; rapid deaths |
| 5 to 6 days in individual. 3 to 4 weeks as a flock | Most birds recover in 3 to 4 weeks | 1 to 3 days |
| Approaches 100 percent in susceptible flocks | High in affected flocks | High |
| Depends upon time of year and stage of production. Young birds in warm weather have low mortality. In heavy layers during winter months may be 70 percent | Low to moderate | As a rule, high in chickens |
| Lesions confined to larynx, trachea, and bronchi and characterized by a reddened petechiated, slimy exudate containing blood. Sometimes exudate is caseous forming a plug which occludes trachea causing suffocation and death | In respiratory form, the infraorbital sinus is involved and greatly distended as a result of a yellowish or brownish caseous exudate. In mouth and trachea there are whitish canker-like lesions that tend to ulcerate | Usually not numerous. Petechial hemorrhages in heart, gizzard, proventriculus and body cavity serosa. Principal organs may show cloudy swelling and petechial hemorrhages. By microscopic examination, there is a diffuse encephalitis |
| Intranuclear inclusion bodies in epithelial cells of tracheal lesions | Cytoplasmic inclusions in swollen epithelial cells are termed Bollinger bodies | None |
| Occasionally pheasants | Turkeys, pheasants, canaries, and some wild birds | Turkeys (main host in US and Canada), pheasants, and certain wild birds |
| Chicken embryos | Chorioallantoic membrane of hens' embryonated eggs. Tissue-culture cells derived from chick embryo tissues | Embryonated hens eggs and in certain tissue cultures |
| Yes, for months after infection and serve as source for future infections | Some recovered birds are carriers | Unknown |

*Table XXXIV.* CHARACTERISTICS OF RESPIRATORY

| | Newcastle disease (ND) | Avian infectious bronchitis (AIB) |
|---|---|---|
| Diagnosis | Chicks with respiratory and nervous signs suggest the disease is Newcastle disease; in this instance it must be distinguished from fowl plague. Virus isolation from nasal exudate or tissues with lesions. Can be isolated in hens' eggs. SN, HI tests useful in diagnosis | Difficult to distinguish from Newcastle unless nervous signs are observed, then it can be diagnosed as Newcastle. In older birds must be distinguished from other respiratory infections requiring cultural tests for virus & bacteria. SN, FA, agar gel tests |
| Immunity | Immunity persists for years | Immune for at least 8 months after infection |
| Prophylaxis | Vaccines are available. Caution should be exercised in their use in laying flocks | Complicated by multiple serotypes although attenuated virus vaccines are available and apparently useful |
| Treatment | Replacement of laying flock at appropriate time may be required to prevent infection of susceptible young stock | Often flocks are disposed of after disease if vaccination is not feasible or desirable |

| Laryngotracheitis (LT) | Fowlpox (FP) | Fowl plague (FP) |
|---|---|---|
| As flock becomes diseased, diagnosis can be made by signs and lesions. Inoculation of 2 susceptible and 2 resistant birds with trachea exudate provides positive diagnosis | Typical skin pox lesions—or by demonstration of Bollinger bodies in wet preparations. Virus isolation in hens' eggs or tissue culture. SN, HI, CF, agar gel tests | Exceedingly high mortality accompanied by peracute deaths highly suggestive. Confirmation by viral isolation and serology. HI test best |
| Long-term and complete | Permanent | Solidly immune for several months at least |
| Conjunctivally administered vaccine strain 146 provides durable immunity after production of conjunctivitis without permanent damage but carriers may exist | Pigeonpox and fowlpox vaccines available; latter should not be used in laying flock | No vaccine available in US |
| Flock disposal may be indicated | In some instances flock disposal may be desirable | Flock disposal may be indicated |

# XXXIX | The Animal Poxviruses

The assignment of viruses to the genus *Poxvirus* depends primarily on morphology, as they have a very characteristic appearance. Five subgroups are recognized and, in addition, there are several poxviruses which have not been assigned to any of these groups. Subgroup A (vaccinia) includes vaccinia, variola (smallpox), cowpox, rabbitpox, mousepox (ectromelia), and monkeypox viruses. Subgroup B (sometimes called pseudopox or paravaccinia) contains contagious ecthyma (contagious pustular dermatitis), milker's nodule (pseudocowpox), contagious exanthema, and bovine papular stomatitis viruses. Lumpy skin disease, goatpox, and sheeppox viruses comprise Subgroup C. The avian poxviruses also referred to as the true poxviruses are in Subgroup D and include fowlpox, pigeonpox, canarypox, turkeypox, starlingpox, and juncopox viruses. Subgroup E is the myxomafibroma group and consists of myxoma, rabbit fibroma, California myxoma, hare fibroma, squirrel fibroma viruses. Subgroup F contains other poxviruses not included in the other subgroups such as swinepox, horsepox, camelpox, buffalopox, rhinocerospox, molluscum contagiosum, Tana virus, entomopox viruses and also the interesting Yaba-monkey tumor virus. The serological comparison of groups of poxviruses has presented difficulties because some poxviruses cannot be neutralized by specific immune sera. Further studies are needed to decide whether the present subgroup B viruses (pseudopoxviruses) rightfully belong in the genus *Poxvirus.*

The true poxviruses and pseudopoxviruses are readily distinguished by morphology. The true poxviruses are slightly larger and less ovoid than the pseudopoxvirus. There is a pronounced difference in the arrangement of the threadlike structures with the true poxviruses displaying an irregular whorled (mulberrylike) appearance. In contrast, these threadlike structures are wound around the virion creating a highly regular criss-cross pattern characteristic of pseudopoxviruses.

918

The serological relationships of poxviruses are determined by the use of infected cell extracts (6). In these preparations up to 20 antigens are capable of forming precipitin lines with antiviral serum for the vaccinia group (1, 8) and for the myxoma-fibroma group (3). One of these antigens is probably responsible for production of neutralizing antibody (2). Viruses of the vaccinia group differ by no more than one antigenic component according to the gel-diffusion test (9) and the same is true for the myxoma-fibroma-group (3). It is generally assumed that these antigens are structural protein components, but this has not been proved. Viruses of the myxoma-fibroma group are not neutralized by vaccinia antiserum and none of the major antigens are shared by these two groups. The avianpox viruses are not related to other true poxvirus groups. Many poxviruses form a hemagglutinin. Alkaline digestion of all poxviruses yields a fraction called the NP antigen which is shared by all poxviruses. The NP antigen is useful in the classification of poxviruses.

Serological relationships among paraviruses have been less well characterized. It is known that contagious ecthyma and goatpox (4), and bovine lumpy skin disease and sheeppox viruses (7) are antigenically related.

The type species for the genus is *Poxvirus* b-1 (vaccinia). The poxviruses contain 5 to 7.5 percent double-stranded DNA with a molecular weight of 160 by $10^6$. The brick-shaped or ovoid complex particles are 170 to 250 by 300 to 325 m$\mu$. The buoyant density in cesium chloride is 1.1 to 1.33 g per ml and the sedimentation coefficient is 5,000 S. The viruses probably contain enzymes such as RNA polymerase. Some poxviruses are ether-resistant. Members of subgroups A to E can recombine genetically. All members exhibit nongenetic reactivation. Replication takes place in the cytoplasm of cells, principally in epithelial types. Except for contagious ecthyma the parasitized cells contain cytoplasmic inclusion bodies which harbor the virus particles sometimes termed "elementary bodies."

Diseases characterized by the formation of pustules on the skin, with or without general manifestations of illness, occur in all species of domestic animals except dogs and cats. These are the animal poxes. In man, the disease is called *variola*, or *smallpox*. It is believed by some that all of our pox diseases came originally from one or more basic strains, which in the course of time have changed as they became adapted to different hosts. The disease in birds differs from that in mammals in several respects but principally in that the lesions are proliferative and tumorlike rather than pustular. It is seldom possible to establish an infection in a mammal with a bird pox, or vice versa. There are many types of bird poxes but these are related immunologically, and many of them can readily be adapted to new bird-species hosts. The true pox diseases of mammals show immunological relationships, and in many instances they may be adapted to new mammalian hosts.

Man may be successfully infected with cowpox virus, and cattle can be infected with smallpox. Immunologically these two viruses are very closely related to each other and also to that of horsepox. The pox diseases are quite rare today in mammals, especially in western Europe and North America, but this has not always been the case. The pox diseases of man, sheep, and fowl are severe and destructive. The others generally are of rather trivial importance when not complicated with other diseases.

Pox in fowls, turkeys, pheasants, pigeons, canaries, and many wild birds is seen from time to time in the United States. Immunization of domestic fowls has reduced the incidence and importance of this disease.

Excellent review articles have been written by Joklik (4, 5).

## REFERENCES

1. Appleyard, Westwood, and Zwartouw. Virology, 1962, 18, 159.
2. Appleyard, Zwartous, and Westwood. Brit. Jour. Exp. Path., 1964, 45, 150.
3. Fenner. Austral. Jour. Exp. Biol. and Med. Sci., 1965, 43, 143.
4. Fenner and Burnet. Virology, 1957, 4, 305.
5. Joklik. Bact. Proc., 1966, 30, 33.
6. Joklik. Ann. Rev. Microbiol., 1968, 22, 1514.
7. Plowright and Ferris. Virology, 1959, 7, 357.
8. Rodriguez-Burgos, Chordi, Diaz, and Tormo. Ibid., 1966, 30, 569.
9. Rondle and Dumbell. Jour. Hyg., 1962, 60, 41.

### Fowlpox

SYNONYMS: Chickenpox, sorehead, contagious epithelioma

Fowlpox attacks chickens primarily. Occasionally outbreaks in turkeys are observed. It occurs in pheasants, other wild birds, and canaries. The virus differs somewhat in pathogenicity in different species, usually being of greater disease-producing power for the species from which it was recovered than for other kinds of birds. Pigeonpox virus, for example, is only slightly pathogenic for chickens, but it immunizes chickens against fowlpox and constitutes a good vaccine for this purpose. A virus that Brunett (4) isolated from a turkey proved to be identical in every way to that of chickens, but one isolated by Brandly and Dunlap (3) was not typical. Virus recovered from infected pheasants usually is typical of that of fowlpox, but Dobson (5) found a strain in one serious outbreak which resembled that of pigeonpox rather than fowlpox. It seems obvious that all bird pox viruses are closely related but are host-modified. That these modifications become considerable, however, is indicated by the fact that pigeonpox virus does not naturally pass from pigeons to chickens, and that fowlpox virus is transmitted to pigeons by inoculation only with difficulty.

**Character of the Disease.** Pox in chickens is manifested by characteristic lesions on the head. They appear on the comb and wattles and around the corners of the mouth, the nostrils, and the eyes. In some cases the lesions spread into the mouth and even into the trachea, causing whitish lesions that ulcerate forming what is commonly called *cankers*. This form of pox was considered to be a separate disease and was known under the name of *avian*

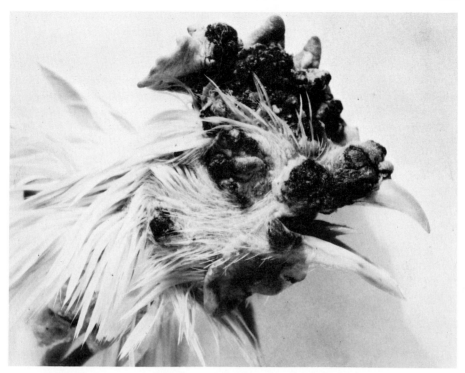

*Fig. 165.* Fowlpox, showing characteristic dry scabs on the comb and around the eye, nostrils, and corner of the mouth.

*diphtheria* for many years. In such infections the infraorbital sinus is frequently involved, becomes greatly distended, and thus distorts the facial features. The content is a yellowish or brownish caseous mass.

The skin lesions consist first of small pustules, which soon dry and become transformed into warty epithelial crusts. These may become quite thick. The affected birds become very ill, refuse to eat, become emaciated, stop laying, and many of them die. The lesions are confined to the featherless part of the head, as a rule, but occasionally pox lesions are found around the vent, and even on the feet. If the infection remains on the skin and does not involve the mucous membranes of the head, the effect on the bird is much less severe and recoveries are more common. In favorable cases the course of the disease is 3 or 4 weeks; in the presence of complications it may be much longer.

**Properties of the Virus.** In 1902 Marx and Sticker (10) proved that fowlpox was caused by a virus. The Borrel bodies (or elementary bodies) have an estimated diameter of 332 by 284 m$\mu$. The elementary bodies have a pepsin-resistant core (12). They are located in the Bollinger body, a cytoplasmic inclusion body which consists of a matrix. This matrix is dissolved by sodium lauryl sulfate but quite resistant to enzymes. It gives a positive Feulgen reaction after previous extraction of lipoids. The developing elementary bodies initially are poorly defined but later acquire the characteristic poxvirus appearance of a dumbbell-like structure within an outer membrane.

Fowlpox virus is resistant to drying. In the dried crusts removed from epithelial lesions, the virulence remains unimpaired for many months providing the drying has been well done. In soil subject to the usual conditions, the viability of the virus is not longer than several weeks as a rule. The disease tends to recur, year after year, on the same premises. It is now known how the virus is preserved in the intervening periods. It is readily destroyed by alkalies and by most disinfectants. It is preserved for long periods by 50 per-

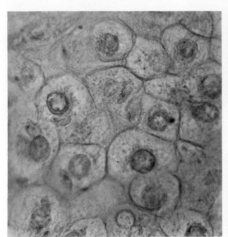 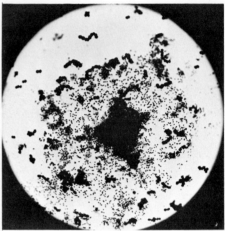

Fig. 166. (Left) Fowlpox. Swollen epithelial cells in an early lesion show the Bollinger bodies. The inclusion bodies are spherical and prominent in the stained section. In several of the cells the nuclei may be seen crowded against the cell wall. X 350. (Right) The Borrel or "elementary" bodies of fowlpox. These minute spherical bodies were obtained free of tissue debris by tryptic digestion of the Bollinger bodies contained in virus-infected cells. The bodies here are stained after admixture with a Streptococcus to indicate comparative size. (Courtesy E. W. Goodpasture, Am. Jour. Path.)

cent glycerol. It is resistant to ether but is chloroform sensitive. It is activated by heating for 30 minutes at 50 C, or 8 minutes at 60 C.

Neutralization tests can be performed involving the use of "pock" counting on chorioallantoic membranes. Precipitating antibodies can be revealed by gel diffusion and complement-fixing antibodies by the complement-fixation test. The hemagglutination test can be used to measure virus and detect HI antibody.

**Cultivation.** Goodpasture, Woodruff, and Buddingh (7) cultivated the virus of fowlpox on the chorioallantoic membrane of the developing chick embryo in 1931. Brandly (2) and others have confirmed these findings, and such cultures are now being used for vaccine production.

Fowlpox and pigeonpox viruses produce a cytopathogenic effect (CPE) in

chick embryo tissue cultures. According to Bang *et al.* (1) growth in chick fibroblasts was not accompanied by CPE or inclusion formation.

**Immunity.** Birds that have recovered from fowlpox are solidly immune thereafter. In flocks in which the disease has occurred for some years, the disease is
seen only in the young birds. In previously uninfected flocks, birds of all ages
develop the disease.

Practical immunization of poultry flocks is carried out in all regions where
pox is prevalent. Two methods are in use. One consists in the use of virulent
fowlpox virus; the other, of pigeonpox virus. Both methods give satisfactory
results.

The fowlpox vaccine may be made in two ways: (*a*) from the epithelial
growths that appear on the combs of cockerels after scarification and inoculation with virulent material, or (*b*) from the epithelial lesions produced on the
chorioallantoic membrane of developing chick embryos following inoculation
with bacteria-free virus. Only the latter of these two vaccines is permitted in
interstate commerce in the United States because of regulations of the U.S.
Department of Agriculture. These are based upon the fact that there is some
danger of transmitting other diseases in pox vaccine made from live birds,
whereas this danger is almost eliminated by viral cultivation in eggs. In both
cases the vaccine is made by drying the affected tissues, grinding them into a
fine powder, and distributing the powder in sealed ampoules. It is mixed with
sterile distilled water or other diluent just before it is used.

The pigeonpox vaccine is prepared by plucking feathers from the breast of
a susceptible pigeon and rubbing pigeonpox virus into the denuded area.
When the inflammation has subsided and the area is covered with crusts,
these are removed after the bird is destroyed and the entire piece of infected
skin removed and dried. This material is made into a coarse powder by
grinding; it is used as described above. Egg-propagated pigeonpox vaccine is
also available for use on chickens.

There are two accepted ways of applying the vaccines, the "feather follicle"
method and the "stick" method. The method used depends upon the preference of the operator.

In the follicle method of vaccinating, six or eight feathers are plucked, preferably from the outside of the leg about the middle of the tibial region. The
virus suspension is then applied to the exposed follicles with a small, stiff
brush. The "stick" method, suggested by Johnson (8), is performed with a
small, sharp-pointed scalpel, which is wrapped with adhesive tape leaving
only about one-eighth inch of the tip exposed. This instrument is used to
make several pricks in the skin, the blade having been dipped in the vaccine
suspension just prior to use. Some operators have made use of the under surface of one of the wings in vaccinating in this way; others use an area on the
outside of the leg. The latter is preferable because the bird is less likely to
contaminate its head from surface virus in this case. With either method a
"take" is meanifested by swelling of the feather follicles and the appearance

of cheesy material and finally scabs, which generally fall off within 3 or 4 weeks leaving a fully healed lesion.

**Transmission.** Fowlpox is believed to be transmitted principally by direct inoculation from bird to bird through fighting wounds and by the birds' picking at one another. The disease may also be spread by the bites of mosquitoes (Kligler, Muckenfuss, and Rivers, 9; Matheson, Brunett, and Brody, 11) and possibly by other arthropods. Arthropod transmission is certainly not as important as direct contact in the spread of this disease within flocks, but it may be the usual way by which the infection is spread from one flock to another. Doyle and Minett (6) placed susceptible birds in cages that had just been occupied by infected birds. Transmission did not occur except when the skin or mucous membranes of the susceptible birds had been scarified. Infection seems to depend, therefore, upon breaks in the continuity of the skin.

**Control.** When pigeonpox virus is used, the constitutional effect upon the birds is minimal. For this reason this material is recommended when birds are not in first-class physical condition or when birds are in full production. The immunity conferred is not so complete and so lasting as that conferred by the fowlpox virus. In field use it, nevertheless, appears to give excellent satisfaction.

Fowlpox vaccine gives satisfactory results when used properly and at the right time. The birds should be in good physical condition and about 2 months before coming into production. The resulting immunity is solid and lifelong. The birds usually suffer a physical reaction from it. They become anorectic and, when in production, stop laying for a considerable time. It should be kept in mind that fowlpox vaccine is fully virulent material. It should not be spilled, it should be kept away from the head region of the birds as they are handled, and utensils, empty bottles, and other contaminated objects should be destroyed or sterilized immediately after use.

**The Disease in Man.** Fowlpox does not affect man. The disease in man commonly known as *chickenpox* or *varicella* is not identical with this disease nor is it contracted from chickens or other fowls.

## REFERENCES

1. Bang, Levy, and Gey.   Jour. Immunol., 1951, *66*, 329.
2. Brandly.   Jour. Am. Vet. Med. Assoc., 1936, *88*, 587; 1937, *90*, 479.
3. Brandly and Dunlap.   Poultry Sci., 1938, *17*, 511.
4. Brunett.   Rpt. N.Y. State Vet. Coll., 1932–33 (1934), p. 69.
5. Dobson.   Jour. Comp. Path. and Therap., 1937, *50*, 401.
6. Doyle and Minett.   *Ibid.*, 1927, *40*, 401.
7. Goodpasture, Woodruff, and Buddingh.   Science, 1931, *74*, 371; Am. Jour. Path., 1932, 8, 271.
8. Johnson.   Jour. Am. Vet. Med. Assoc., 1929, 75, 629.
9. Kligler, Muckenfuss, and Rivers.   Jour. Exp. Med., 1929, *49*, 649.
10. Marx and Sticker.   Deut. med. Wchnschr., 1902, *28*, 893.
11. Matheson, Brunett, and Brody.   Poultry Sci., 1930, *10*, 211.
12. Woodruff and Goodpasture.   *Ibid.*, 1929, 5, 1; 1930, 6, 713.

## Pigeonpox

Pigeonpox frequently causes considerable trouble in squab-raising plants. The squabs may become infected while still in the nest, but more often the disease appears in well-developed birds. Cankers are found in the mouth, and the corners of the mouth are covered with crusts. The eyelids may also become affected and the birds be blinded. The legs and toes are sometimes involved. The death rate may be high. Pigeons may be protected against the disease by vaccination with pigeonpox vaccine, used in the same way as for chickens.

## Vaccinia

SYNONYMS:  *Vaccinia variolae, Poxvirus officinalis*

In the first half of the 19th century and earlier, evidence indicates that true cowpox prevailed rather frequently in both Europe and America, and that these outbreaks were often related directly to epidemics of smallpox in man (Reece, 5). This evidence suggests that smallpox infection was not infrequently transmitted from milkers to the cattle that they milked, and that this disease was then known as *cowpox*. There is evidence, too, that horsepox was often transmitted to cattle by the infected hands of milkers, the disease being indistinguishable from that which sometimes came from human beings and sometimes from other cattle. Although smallpox, cowpox, and horsepox are regarded as separate and distinct diseases, it is rather clear that they are related, and differences in the viruses may result from adaptation to different hosts. These relationships were first recognized by Jenner (3), who utilized the knowledge to immunize man against the deadly smallpox by vaccinating children and susceptible adults with vaccinia or cowpox virus. Some people differentiate between cowpox and vaccinia virus, believing that the latter is really a smallpox virus which has been modified by passage through cattle whereas the former is a true cattle virus (Downie, 2). The difference does not seem to be very important.

Vaccinia in cattle is a rare disease in the United States now. Indeed, there is no evidence that it exists at all today, except occasionally as an accident caused by contact between cattle and persons who have been recently vaccinated against smallpox with vaccinia virus. A disease commonly called *cowpox* occurs frequently in cattle in the United States and other countries. It is more frequent in dairy cattle. The available evidence indicates that this condition is caused either by cowpox or pseudocowpox virus, separate and distinct agents from vaccinia.

A number of cases were described formerly in the U.S.A. in which cattle were infected by recently vaccinated persons (Boerner, 1; Sayer and Amos, 6). The cattle become infected from virus on the hands of the milkers. The disease often spreads to many cows in the milking herd and from these cows to other people. In some cases nearly every unvaccinated person on the farm who had contact with the cows, or who used the raw milk from them, became

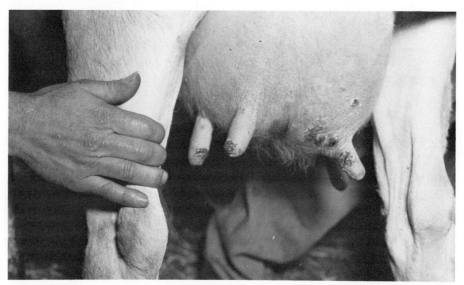

*Fig. 167.* Cowpox, showing well-advanced lesion on the teats and udder. (Courtesy Robert Graham.)

infected. These individuals developed typical vaccinia lesions on their hands, arms, faces, and other parts of their bodies. It is obvious that recently vaccinated persons should not be permitted to milk, or have other close contact with dairy cattle.

**Character of the Disease.** The lesions of vaccinia occur on the teats and udder. They appear as small papules which gradually change to pustules. A reddened areola appears around each lesion. The pustule has a tendency to develop a small pit, or umbilication. The lesions may be numerous but generally they appear in rather small numbers, most of them being on the teats. The friction of the milking process generally causes the lesions to break, forming raw areas that are very tender. When the lesions are not broken in this way, the pustules dry up and become covered with dry scabs, which fall off in about 10 days leaving an unscarred surface. The healing process is greatly delayed by the friction of milking, and bacterial invasion of the udder often results in mastitis.

**The Disease in Experimental Animals.** The vaccinia virus can be transmitted experimentally to the skin of many mammals. It can readily be transmitted to the cornea of the rabbit's eye. Paschen (4) believes that the cornea test (Paul's test) is a reliable indicator of the presence of vaccinia or variola virus. This test is performed by placing a suspension of the suspected material on the cornea of a rabbit, introducing it very carefully to avoid mechanical irritation. After 36 to 48 hours the animal is destroyed, and the enucleated eye is placed for a few minutes in a sublimate-alcohol mixture. The presence of pox virus is indicated by grossly apparent, opaque lesions, circular in outline, which were not apparent before they were acted upon by the fixative solution.

Guinea pigs and mice also react to inoculation with vaccinia. Big doses given intravenously to suckling mice will kill them without the multiplication of virus.

**Properties of the Virus.** The mature *elementary bodies* known as *Paschen bodies* vary in size from 240 to 380 by 170 to 270 m$\mu$. The outer membrane is 9 to 12 m$\mu$ thick and the virus contains an inner central nucleoid with a smaller body beside it. The nucleoid is probably nucleoprotein. Negative staining subunits exist on the surface of the particle but within the outer membrane. The Paschen bodies probably develop within the cytoplasm causing the formation of large *Guarnieri bodies*. They can be readily seen with light microscope.

The virus contains biotin and flavin besides carbon, phosphorous, nitrogen, copper, lipids, carbohydrates, and thymonucleic acid.

This agent is quite stable and resistant. Suspensions of the virus are inactivated in 10 minutes at 60 C, but dried virus withstands 100 C for 10 minutes. It is quite stable between pH 5 and 9. The virus is resistant to ether in the cold but is inactivated by chloroform. Oxidizing agents such as potassium permanganate or ethyl oxide readily inactivate the particle.

The hemagglutinin is separable from the virus particle, resists boiling, and agglutinates the red cells of some fowls.

The nucleoprotein antigen (NP) is involved in the complement-fixation and precipitation reactions. Neutralizing antibody is demonstrated by the use of tissue culture, embryonated hens' eggs, or rabbit skin reaction.

Interference has been reported between vaccinia and fowlpox, foot-and-mouth disease, and influenza. Interferon has been demonstrated in the latter instance.

**Cultivation.** Vaccinia grows in primary cultures of chick embryo, rabbit kidney, rabbit testis, bovine embryo skin, and also in continuous cell lines such as HeLa and L. Cell destruction occurs early and includes the formation of giant cells. Plaques are formed in agar overlay systems.

In the embryonated hens' eggs, 7 to 13 days old, the virus grows well on the chorioallantoic membrane producing pocks, the formation of which may be used to titrate the virus. Embryo mortality varies from low to 100 percent depending upon the strain and test conditions. Less sensitive routes of inoculation are the allantoic cavity and the yolk sac.

**Immunity.** After recovery from vaccinia, cattle are immune for a considerable time and perhaps for life. Second attacks have been reported but these may have been infections of the pseudopox disease. Experimentally, solid resistance is conveyed by one exposure.

**Transmission.** Vaccinia is clearly transmitted largely in the milking process on the hands of the milker. There is little evidence of any other mode of transmission.

**Diagnosis.** Except for differential diagnosis between vaccinia and the pseudopox diseases, the diagnosis can readily be made from the appearance of the lesions. Neither of these diseases is particularly serious, and in most instances differentiation is more or less academic. This matter will be discussed further under pseudopox (p. 929).

**Control.** Infections of herds with vaccinia virus through exposure to recently vaccinated milkers should be avoided. When the disease appears in a milking herd, affected animals should be segregated from the others as far as practicable. They should be milked last, and the milkers should scrub their hands thoroughly with soap and water after milking them and before handling others.

The use of 5-iodo-2-deoxyuridine for the treatment of vaccinal keratitis is attended with some success.

**The Disease in Man.** The presence of poxlike lesions on the hands of milkmaids who milked cows from cowpox led Jenner to believe that the cow disease was transmissible to man. Also noting that many of these persons did not develop smallpox when that disease was epidemic in the regions in which they lived, he was led to believe that they were protected from it by exposure to the cattle disease, and this led to his development of a vaccine.

The vaccinia lesion consists of a papule which quickly becomes a pustule. The lesion is reddened about its periphery. Although it itches, it is not particularly painful. The characteristic umbilication appears in most of the pustules. If not rubbed or scratched, the lesion becomes dehydrated after a few days and a scab forms which falls off after 10 to 14 days. The hand lesions usually are not numerous. If the individual suffers from eczema, the disease may spread over large areas of the skin, and there may be fever and illness lasting a few days.

## REFERENCES

1. Boerner. Jour. Am. Vet. Med. Assoc., 1923, *64*, 93.
2. Downie. Jour. Path. and Bact., 1939, *48*, 361.
3. Jenner. An inquiry into the causes and effects of the *variolae vaccinae*. S. Low, London, 1798.
4. Paschen. In: Kolle, Kraus, and Uhlenhuth. Handbuch der pathogenen Mikroorganismen. 3d. ed. G. Fischer, Jena, 1930, vol. *VIII*, part 11, p. 821.
5. Reece. Vet. Jour., 1922, *78*, 81.
6. Sayer and Amos. N.Y. State Jour. Med., 1936, *36*, 1163.

## Cowpox

The antigenic properties of this virus are close but distinct from vaccinia as determined by the use of complement-fixation, agar gel diffusion, and antibody-absorption tests (1). There is general agreement that the disease is distinct from vaccinia and pseudocowpox.

In general, the features of cowpox virus such as physiochemical properties, hemagglutination red cell spectrum, morphology, and cultivation in tissue culture and eggs are similar to vaccinia.

In cattle the virus affects the skin, particularly the teats and udders of cows. The papules develop into vesicles, followed by crusting which may persist for weeks. Lesions in man resemble those of primary vaccination and may be found on the hands, arms, face, and eyes of the milker (1). Man to man infection is rare.

The skin or testis are the sites of inoculation for experimental infection of rabbits, mice, guinea pigs, and monkeys (1).

**REFERENCE**

1.   Andrewes.   Viruses of vertebrates, Williams and Wilkins, Baltimore, 1964.

**Pseudocowpox**

SYNONYMS:   Paravaccinia, milker's nodules

This disease clinically resembles cowpox and vaccinia.

**Character of the Disease.** Pseudocowpox occurs in dairy herds in all parts of this country. The disease, *per se,* has slight effect upon cattle. The lesions re-

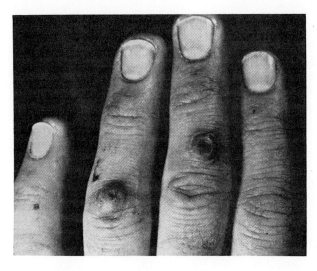

*Fig. 168.* Milker's nodules.

semble those of cowpox except that umbilicated pustules are seldom seen, the lesions progressing from papules to vesicles to raw areas that heal under a dry scab. The disease is very annoying because of the soreness of the teats, which makes the animals difficult to milk. The disease spreads to most of the cows that are milked, apparently on the hands of the milkers or through contamination of the milking machines. Dry cows, nonmilking heifers, and bulls rarely become involved. Mastitis sometimes results, apparently from secondary bacterial infections. Healing occurs after several weeks and the disease then disappears. Antiseptic ointments facilitate healing and make milking less painful.

**Properties of the Virus.** In 1963 it was shown to be caused by a virus (3). The dimensions are 190 by 296 m$\mu$. It has a spiral structure as in contagious ecthyma of sheep and bovine papular stomatitis. It is activated in 10 minutes by chloroform.

No cross-immunity has been demonstrated between this virus and cowpox or vaccinia. The virus is probably related to ORF and bovine papular stomatitis. It has been suggested that the immunity is transient in cattle.

**Cultivation.** The virus produces a cytopathogenic effect in bovine kidney cell cultures (3). After cultivation in bovine kidney cell culture, it grew in human embryonic fibroblasts but not in rabbit and rhesus monkey kidney cultures. The infection has not been successfully transmitted to rabbits, mice, guinea pigs, or chick embryos.

**The Disease in Man.** In man the milker's nodule lesion takes the form of hemispherical cherry-red papules (see fig. 170) which appear on the hands and sometimes on other parts of the body (1). The lesions begin as papules 5 to 7 days after exposure. They gradually enlarge into firm, elastic, bluish-red, smooth, hemispherical masses varying in size up to 2 cm in diameter. They are relatively painless but frequently cause an itching sensation. When fully developed they often show a dimple on the top, but they do not break down with pus formation. They are highly vascular. The tense grayish skin covering them remains intact. The granulation tissue that makes up the mass of the nodule gradually becomes absorbed. The lesions slowly flatten as this occurs and finally, after 4 to 6 weeks, they disappear. Sometimes there is slight swelling of the axillary nodes, but otherwise there is no evidence of any generalization of the disease.

### REFERENCES

1. Becker.   Jour. Am. Vet. Med. Assoc., 1940, *115*, 2140.
2. Berger.   Centrbl. f. Bakt. I, Abt. Orig., 1955, *162*, 363.
3. Friedman-Kiem, Rowe, and Banfield.   Science, 1963, *140*, 1335.

### Horsepox

SYNONYMS:   Contagious pustular stomatitis, "grease," "grease-heel"

Horsepox has not been reported from the United States and it seems to be much less common in Europe than it was a half-century ago.

**Character of the Disease.** The disease in horses takes two forms. The less important is an infection of the pastern region of horses, apparently spread by the hands of horseshoers and hostlers. This condition is known as *grease* or *grease-heel*. It is manifested by the appearance of a papular eruption on the flexor surface of the joints in the lower part of the leg. The papules change to vesicles, then to pustules, which finally dry up, forming crusts. The legs become somewhat painful but there is no general reaction as a rule.

The other form is manifested by the appearance of multiple lesions on the inside of the lips and the opposing surfaces of the gums, on the frenum of the tongue, and on the inside of the cheeks. These begin as papules, change to vesicles, and then become pustules. The animal may have some fever, and young animals may become very sick and occasionally die. Food is refused, saliva drools from the corners of the mouth, and the animal likes to dip its mouth in water. Beginning with a few lesions, new crops occur and finally nearly all the mucous membrane of the mouth will be involved. In some cases the lesions are found also in the nasal passages. Virus removed from the horse lesions will infect cattle and that of cattle will infect horses.

**Immunity.** Recovery from the disease leaves a substantial immunity. Because lesions on the skin are less severe than those on the mucosa of the mouth, some European authors have suggested vaccination of horses on the skin, claiming good results therefrom. The cow and horse diseases reciprocally immunize against each other, and both will transmit to persons who have not been vaccinated against smallpox and not to those who have been.

## REFERENCES

1.  De Jong.   Jour. Comp. Path. and Therap., 1917, *30*, 242.
2.  Zwick.   Berl. tierärztl. Wchnschr., 1924, *40*, 757.

### Swinepox

This disease has been reported in Europe, Japan, and the United States. It is very common in many of the swine-raising areas of the midwestern states of this country. It has been studied by McNutt, Murray, and Purwin (3), by Schwarte and Biester (6), and by Shope (7) in the United States. For detailed descriptions of this disease the reader is referred to these papers. As it occurs in this country it is not generally considered very important; however, some veterinarians believe that its importance is being underestimated.

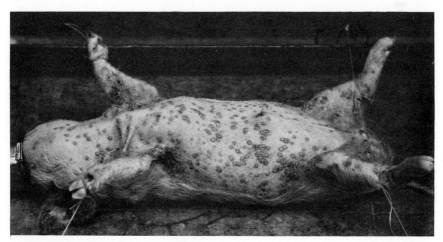

*Fig. 169.*   Swinepox. (Courtesy R. E. Shope.)

**Character of the Disease.** It affects principally young growing animals, suckling pigs being especially subject to it. McNutt and associates report that the lesions are usually found on the lower part of the abdomen and inside the thighs and arms, but in the outbreak in Iowa described by Schwarte and Biester the lesions were located on the backs and sides. Lesions are not located on the head or on the lower parts of the legs, as a rule.

The lesions, as described by Schwarte and Biester, consist of red papules that appear 4 or 5 days after virus is placed on the scarified skin. A slight fever and mild general reaction occur at this time. The lesions rapidly develop into raised, hard elevations, which may be from 1 to 3 cm in diameter. Hard crusts form on these areas, these drop off in a few days, and the whole process is completed in 12 to 14 days. Vesicles and pustules do not ordinarily appear in field cases, but they found typical lesions that passed through the papule, vesicle, and pustule stages on the abdomen of artificially inoculated pigs.

Two different diseases are known at present under the name of *swinepox*. One of them is caused by vaccinia, the other by an unrelated virus. Manninger, Cosontos, and Salyi (4) who have seen both diseases in Europe, propose to designate as swinepox the one caused by the vaccinialike virus and to call the other a poxlike disease of swine. Schwarte and Biester, who have dealt with the poxlike disease of Manninger, prefer to call the disease swinepox. We concur with Schwarte and Biester. So far as is known, all cases of swinepox occurring in the United States are caused by a virus that is unrelated to the pox viruses of other animals, and this includes vaccinia.

**Properties of the Virus.** The swinepox virus is 250 m$\mu$ with surrounding membranes (5). Crystalline bodies 800 m$\mu$ in diameter in the cytoplasm are seen only in this animal pox infection.

The virus is distinct from vaccinia and the other animal poxes, although a minor component common to vaccinia and cowpox was demonstrated by agar gel diffusion test with great difficulty (1).

**Cultivation.** The swinepox virus produces a cytopathogenic effect in porcine kidney, testes, embryonic lung, and embryonic brain cultures (2). Minute plaques are observed in an agar overlay system. Sera from hyperimmunized swine failed to neutralize the virus *in vitro*. Recovered pigs resisted infection to the virus.

Attempts to cultivate the swinepox virus in embryonated hens' eggs, horses, calves, sheep, dogs, cats, fowl, rabbits, rats, mice, and man failed. In contrast vaccinia has a wide experimental host spectrum.

**Immunity.** Pigs that have recovered from the disease appear to be solidly immune for life. Immunization is not generally practiced, the disease not being important enough for that. The elimination of lice probably would do a great deal to control the disease.

**Transmission.** Swinepox does not ordinarily pass from one animal to another directly. The transmitting agent usually is the hog louse, *Hematopinus suis*.

Since this parasite is found on the lower parts of the animal, on the belly, and in the armpits, and on the inside of the thighs, this explains why pox lesions usually are found in these locations. In a large herd studied by Schwarte and Biester, the pigs were free of lice and the lesions were found largely on the back and sides. This suggested that flies or other insects might be the transmitting agents, and this idea was supported by the fact that the disease disappeared as soon as cold weather eliminated the insects.

## REFERENCES

1. Datt and Orlans. Immunology, 1958, *1*, 81.
2. Kazka, Bohl, and Jones. Am. Jour. Vet. Res., 1960, *21*, 269.
3. McNutt, Murray, and Purwin. Jour. Am. Vet. Med. Assoc., 1929, *74*, 752.
4. Manninger, Cosontos, and Salyi. Arch. f. Tierheilk., 1940, 75, 12.
5. Reczko. Arch. f. die Gesam. Virusforsch., 1959, 9, 193.
6. Schwarte and Biester. Am. Jour. Vet. Res., 1941, *2*, 136.
7. Shope. Jour. Bact., 1940, 39, 39.

### Sheeppox

SYNONYMS: *Clavelie, Variola ovina*

Of all the animal poxes, sheeppox is the most damaging. Fortunately this disease does not exist in the Western Hemisphere. In past times it has done great damage in Europe, but it has now been controlled or eliminated from the greater part of that area. It continues to exist in southern and eastern Europe and in North Africa.

**Character of the Disease.** A generalized pox eruption occurs on the skin, and similar lesions often occur on the mucous membrane of the pharynx and trachea, sometimes even in the abomasum. Hemorrhagic inflammation of the respiratory passages and of the digestive tract occurs. Caseous nodules and areas of catarrhal pneumonia occur in the lungs. The mortality varies from about 5 percent to higher than 50 percent.

**Properties of the virus.** The virus is more elongated than other pox viruses and with a size of 115 by 194 $m\mu$ (1). It is inactivated in 15 minutes by 2 percent phenol.

All strains are serologically identical and goatpox virus protects against sheeppox. A complement-fixation test has been reported.

**Cultivation.** A cytopathogenic effect is produced in the cultures of skin, kidney, and testis of sheep, goats, and calves with no change in virulence for sheep after serial passage (3). An attenuated virus resulted after transfer in sheep embryo cultures (2).

The virus apparently can be adapted to embryonated hens' eggs with no apparent change in virulence for sheep (5).

**Control.** Vaccination is essential in areas where the disease is enzootic. Various vaccines are used. In Egypt a mild strain from Iran is used to immunize sheep (4). In Turkey a tissue-cultured attenuated vaccine is used with success (2).

## REFERENCES

1. Abdusalam and Coslett.   Jour. Comp. Path. and Therap., 1957, 67, 145.
2. Aygün.   Arch. Exp. Vet. Med., 1955, 9, 145.
3. Plowright and Ferris.   Brit. Jour. Exp. Path., 1958, 39, 424.
4. Sabban.   Am. Jour. Vet. Res., 1955, 16, 209.
5. Sabban.   Ibid., 1957, 18, 618.

### Goatpox

The disease is prevalent in North Africa and the Middle East. It also occurs in the Scandinavian countries and Australia. The virus causes generalized pocks on mucous membranes and skin of goats.

The virus produces a cytopathogenic effect and cytoplasmic inclusion bodies in cultures of lamb testis. It causes plaques on the choriollantoic membrane of embryonated hens' eggs (2). Elementary bodies are agglutinated by immune sera.

It is reported that goatpox immunizes against contagious ecthyma of sheep and sheeppox (2); the reverse is not true. It also protects against lumpy skin disease of cattle (1).

## REFERENCES

1. Capstick.   Quoted by Andrewes. Viruses of vertebrates, Williams and Wilkins, Baltimore, 1964.
2. Rafyi and Ramyan.   Jour. Comp. Path. and Therap., 1959, 69, 141.

### Virus Dermatitis in Goats

This disease was recently described in India by Haddow and Idnani (1). It is acute and highly fatal. It resembles goatpox but was considered sufficiently different to warrant another name. A virus is present in the local lesions and in the blood. The incubation period is between 7 and 10 days. Nonpustular, rubbery nodules, 4 to 12 mm in diameter, appear over the body surface and in the mouth. Pneumonia, which was invariably fatal, developed in most cases 1 to 2 days after the appearance of the skin eruption. The few animals that survived developed necrotic tissue in the skin nodules, and these changed into ulcers that healed very slowly. The scabs did not disappear for about 6 weeks.

## REFERENCE

1. Haddow and Idnani.   Indian Vet. Jour., 1948, 24, 332.

### Lumpy Skin Disease

SYNONYMS:  Lumpy disease, pseudourticaria, *knopvelsiekte*

This condition was first observed in Northern Rhodesia and Madagascar in 1929. It was recognized in Transvaal in 1945 and rapidly spread through South and East Africa. It may occur in buffaloes as well as cattle.

**Character of the Disease.** In cattle a fever develops accompanied by the production of multiple nodules in the skin, pathological changes in the mucous membranes and viscera, and also adenitis. Cytoplasmic inclusions are found in epithelial cells and histiocytes.

In past instances the clinical picture in cattle has been complicated by the presence of the Allerton virus, an agent possibly belonging to the herpesvirus group (1).

In rabbits it produces a transient local reaction with some generalized lesions.

**Properties of the Virus.** Several viruses have been isolated from cases of lumpy skin disease. The Neethling pox strain is closely related to African sheeppox which is comparable to goatpox (2). It is sensitive to 20 percent ether (3).

**Cultivation.** It multiplies in the chick embryo and chorioallantoic membrane producing pocks on the membrane.

After adaptation the virus produces spindle cells within 24 to 48 hours in tissue cultures of embryonic calf and lamb kidney and of calf and lamb testis.

**Control.** The main control measure is restriction in the movement of cattle from diseased to free areas. The Isiolo or Kedong strains of sheeppox have been used to protect cattle against Neethling virus (2).

Because of the serious economic importance of this disease, South African cattle should not be exported to other parts of the world until physical examinations and a study of their histories provide assurance that they are not infected.

## REFERENCES

1. Andrewes. Viruses of vertebrates. Williams and Wilkins, Baltimore, 1964.
2. Capstick. Quoted by Andrewes. *Ibid*.
3. Plowright and Ferris. Virology, 1959, 7, 357.

## Bovine Papular Stomatitis

This disease of cattle is probably the same as erosive stomatitis, stomatitis papulosa, ulcerative stomatitis, or pseudoaphthous stomatitis. There are many discrepancies in the literature so it is possible that more than one agent is involved in the syndrome (see p. 1349). It occurs in North America, Africa, and Europe.

The reported size of the virus varies from 125 to 150 m$\mu$ in diameter (1) to 207 by 215 m$\mu$ which are poxlike structures with single or double membranes (2). Two conflicting reports exist on its growth in embryonated hens' eggs. In cultures of calf testis the agent produces foci rapidly after adaptation.

The agent produces an ulcerative stomatitis in cattle. There may be crater-like ulcers 1 cm in diameter. The infection seems to be limited to the stoma. Cytoplasmic inclusions may be found in the infected cells. There is some question whether it can produce an infection in sheep and goats. Transmission to other animals has failed.

## REFERENCES

1.  Pritchard, Clafin, Gustafson, and Ristic. Jour. Am. Vet. Med. Assoc., 1958, *132*, 273.
2.  Reczko.   Centrbl. f. Bakt. I, Abt. Orig., 1957, *169*, 425.

### Contagious Ecthyma of Sheep

SYNONYMS:   Sore mouth, contagious pustular dermatitis of sheep, "scabby mouth," contagious pustular stomatitis, infectious labial dermatitis, ORF

This is a poxlike disease of sheep and goats. Occasionally infections of man occur. The disease is frequent on the western ranges during the spring and summer months, and it occurs occasionally in the farm flocks of the eastern part of the United States. It has been reported also in many other sheep-raising countries.

**Character of the Disease.** In areas where the disease has been well established, it is seen principally in the lambs and kids, the older animals being immune as a result of vaccination or of having suffered from the disease earlier in life.

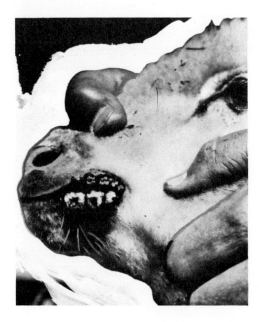

*Fig. 170.* Contagious ecthyma (sore mouth) in sheep. (Courtesy Jen-Sal Laboratories, Inc.)

It is characterized by the formation of papules and vesicles on the skin of the lips and sometimes around the nostrils and eyes. These rapidly change to pustules, and finally heavy scabs appear. With their thickened, stiff, sensitive lips, the affected lambs or kids can neither suckle nor graze, and rapid emaciation occurs. Healing usually is complete in about one month, the scabs having fallen off by this time leaving the lips smooth and without scars.

Fatalities are not numerous except in the presence of complications. In the more southerly states these are commonly the result of invasion of the lesions by the larvae of the flesh or screwworm fly (*Cochliomyia americana*). Where the screwworm does not exist, the only serious complication, according to Marsh and Tunnicliff (7), is the invasion of the lesions by the necrosis bacillus (*Spherophorus necrophorus*).

It is not uncommon for ewes, suckling infected lambs, to develop lesions on their udders.

In areas where the screwworm is prevalent, the losses in young lambs and kids frequently are very great. The disease in older animals is usually less severe, and such animals are better able to resist the damage from the fly larvae. The death rate from the uncomplicated disease is almost nil.

**Properties of the Virus.** By electron microscopy its size is 158 by 252 m$\mu$, with rounded ends and dense subpolar regions (2). It is an ether and chloroform resistant DNA virus.

Immune sera agglutinate elementary bodies, precipitate soluble antigen, and fix complement (1). The virus shows a small amount of cross-reaction with vaccinia and ectromelia as demonstrated by the complement-fixation and gel-diffusion tests; Contagious ecthyma antisera showed some neutralization of ectromelia (11). Goatpox will immunize against contagious ecthyma, but the converse is not true (3); the same situation prevails in the neutralization test. Strains of contagious ecthyma may not be serologically identical (6) but good immunity in sheep between strains from various countries occurs.

Boughton and Hardy (4) determined that the virus was destroyed by being heated to 58 to 60 C for one-half hour. It was not destroyed by the same exposure at 55 C.

Of the greatest practical importance is the resistance of this virus to natural conditions. The virus is able to retain viability for very long periods in the dried scabs which fall when the lesions heal. This is proved by the fact that premises have been known to harbor infection for more than a year after all animals had been removed. Boughton and Hardy showed that such scabs usually lost all virulence when placed on the surface of the ground during the hot summer period in western Texas for 30 to 60 days, but that if protected they retained their virulence much longer. Scabs placed outside in the fall of the year were found still virulent in the spring. Powdered, dry scab retained virulence for at least 32 months when it was kept in the refrigerator, but it lost it in from 54 to 120 days when stored in the dark at an average temperature of 83 F.

**Cultivation.** Greig (5) has reported success in cultivating the virus of this disease in monolayer cultures of embryonic sheep skin. Three strains were cultivated in this way.

The virus has also been cultivated in embryonic bovine kidney cells with no loss in pathogenicity for sheep (10). Mice, rabbits, guinea pigs, hamsters and chick embryos are refractory to inoculation.

**Relationship to Sheeppox.** There has been confusion in the past between this disease and pox of sheep and goats. There is no cross immunization between ecthyma and sheeppox; however, goatpox, which is a much milder disease, appears to give some protection against later exposure to ecthyma.

**Immunity.** Schmidt and Hardy (9) found that lambs and kids which had recovered from this disease were solidly immune thereafter. Some experiments conducted on a small group of sheep showed that it was possible to immunize them successfully with a technic similar to that used for vaccinating against smallpox in man. This method was successfully applied to large numbers of animals in the field by Boughton and Hardy (4). It has been widely and successfully adopted. Vaccination is best applied early in the season before the disease ordinarily appears, but it is useful in infected flocks and even on animals that are already showing signs. The normal course of the disease is usually shortened in such cases, and the signs are ameliorated.

The vaccine consists of the fully virulent material contained in the dried scabs. The scabs are ground and suspended in 1 percent concentration in a solution of equal parts of sterile physiological saline solution and glycerol. The suspension is applied with a stiff-bristled brush to one or more superficial scratches about 0.5-inch long on the skin. The scarification should be very superficial. If the area is too large or the scarifications too deep, the "takes" may be rather severe and attract the attention of the screwworm fly. Usually the site is in the inside of the flank where the wool is absent. Care should be taken to avoid areas that will rub against the abdomen. In old ewes and rams it is better to vaccinate in the armpit to avoid spreading the infection, by friction, to the udder and scrotum. A pustular lesion develops at the site of a successful inoculation. This becomes covered with a scab, which falls off after several weeks. Some of the lambs will nibble at the developing lesion because of itching and will thus convey the infection to their lips. This occurs in about 10 percent of those vaccinated. The disease in such animals is very mild and seldom causes trouble.

Animals that recover from the disease are immune thereafter for periods at least as long as 28 months, and perhaps much longer. As a practical matter, range animals that have had the disease or have been vaccinated are considered to be immune for life.

**Means of Transmission.** The evidence indicates that outbreaks are initiated by virus which persists in the soil from one season to the next or by contact with infected animals. Rapid spread, severe disease, and a high morbidity in an Australian herd was attributed to the concentration of sheep around a palatable scrub, *Templetonia retusa,* which caused extensive trauma to mucous membranes during grazing (5).

**Diagnosis.** The disease is recognized by its characteristic epithelial lesions that show ballooning of cells leading to degeneration, vesicle formation, and possible granulomatous formation. Type B cytoplasmic inclusion bodies are found. Absolute diagnosis is based upon the isolation and identification of the virus.

There are some similarities to bluetongue in the initial stages of the disease (5).

**Control.** In regions where this disease is prevalent, it is wise to vaccinate all lambs or kids each spring before the pasture season begins, because the disease tends to recur regularly each year on lands that are once infected.

**The Disease in Man.** Sheepherders are others who come in intimate contact with sheep infected with sore mouth are apt to develop lesions on their hands or face. In vaccinating lambs it is advisable, therefore, that those who handle the vaccine wear rubber gloves and that the vaccine not be spilled on clothing or disposed of carelessly when the task is completed.

The lesions begin in abrasions, as a rule. They consist of rather large vesicles that may be multiple in structure. The surrounding skin becomes reddened and moderately swollen. The individual may have some fever, there may be swelling of the axillary lymph nodes, and the local lesion is moderately painful. Secondary infection usually occurs and healing is often rather slow (8).

## REFERENCES

1. Abdusalam. Jour. Comp. Path. and Therap., 1958, 68, 23.
2. Abdusalam and Coslett. *Ibid.,* 1957, 67, 145.
3. Bennett, Horgan, and Hasseeb. *Ibid.,* 1944, 54, 131.
4. Boughton and Hardy. Texas Agr. Exp. Sta. Bul. 504, 1935.
5. Gardiner, Craig, and Nairn. Austral. Vet. Jour., 1967, 43, 163.
6. Greig. Canad. Jour. Comp. Path. and Vet. Sci., 1957, 21, 304.
7. Horgan and Hasseeb. Jour. Comp. Path. and Therap., 1947, 57, 8.
8. Marsh and Tunnicliff. Jour. Am. Vet. Med. Assoc., 1937, 91, 600.
9. Newsom and Cross. *Ibid.,* 1934, 84, 799.
10. Schmidt and Hardy. Texas Agr. Exp. Sta. Bul. 457, 1932.
11. Trueblood and Chow. Am. Jour. Vet. Res., 1963, 24, 47.
12. Webster. Austral. Jour. Exp. Biol. and Med. Sci., 1958, 36, 267.

## Other Animal Pox Diseases

Other mammals contract poxlike diseases that are quite important in their respective hosts. The known virus infections include rabbitpox, monkeypox, infectious ectromelia (mousepox), camelpox, Yaba monkey virus, molluscum contagiosum of humans, and canarypox. An agent with characteristics closely resembling a poxvirus causes avian arthritis (1). It is rather interesting that no poxlike infection has been observed in the dog or cat.

## REFERENCE

1.  Olson and Kerr.   Avian Dis., 1966, *10*, 470.

### Infectious Myxomatosis of Rabbits

*All rabbits*

This is a highly contagious and almost always fatal disease of domesticated rabbits which was first recognized in South America, later in Mexico, and the United States (California). The disease often destroys whole rabbitries. It was first described in 1898 by Sanarelli (13), who was working in Montevideo, Uruguay. Sanarelli ascribed the disease to a virus since he could not see or cultivate any organisms in the lesions. It is of interest to note that Sanarelli's paper appeared in the same year as that of Loeffler and Frosch, who determined the causative agent of foot-and-mouth disease of cattle to be a virus. The myxoma virus takes its place, historically, as the second animal disease virus to be recognized.

Myxomatosis affects ordinary domestic rabbits, Angora rabbits, Belgian hares, and Flemish giants, but the wild rabbit of Brazil, the common cottontail, and the jack rabbit of the United States are almost wholly resistant. The virus does not affect any animal species other than certain rabbits, and man is also resistant.

**Character of the Disease.** The disease begins with inflammation of the eyes. The eyelids swell and a copious discharge from the conjunctival mucous membrane appears. At first the discharge is serous but shortly it becomes purulent. Within 24 to 48 hours the eyes cannot be opened because of the swelling. A nasal discharge also appears, and swellings are noted involving the skin of the face and ears. The head may become very misshapen; then similar swellings may be noted on other parts of the body. The genital openings become inflamed and discharge a purulent exudate. Finally the tumorous masses may involve nearly the whole body; the affected animal appears very ill and almost invariably dies in from 7 to 15 days after the first signs are noted.

The tumorlike masses consist of tissue having a rubbery, gelatinous consistency. Usually the lungs, liver, and kidneys are normal in appearance, but the spleen is always swollen and the lymph nodes are enlarged and hemorrhagic. Although the external genitalia are inflamed, the testicles, uterus, and ovaries are generally free of lesions. The testicular swelling mentioned by many authors is usually caused by changes in the scrotum rather than in the testicle.

Sections of the myxomata show tissue characteristic of that type of tumor, that is, large stellate cells embedded in a homogeneous, gelatinous substance that is largely if not wholly mucin. In addition, however, there is evidence of inflammation manifested by engorgement and hemorrhages from the blood vessels and by collections of neutrophilic leukocytes. Rivers (11) was the first to call attention to another characteristic feature of these virus tumors, that is, a peculiar type of degeneration of the epithelial coverings. The epithelial cells are greatly swollen and vacuolated, and acidophilic bodies rapidly develop in

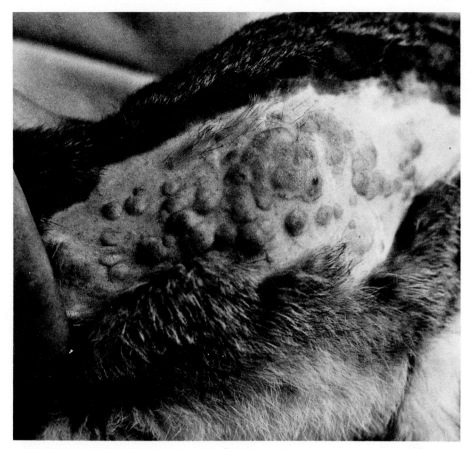

Fig. 171. Virus myxomatosis in the rabbit. Multiple primary tumors were induced by virus on the freshly shaved skin. (Courtesy Thomas M. Rivers, *Jour. Exp. Med.*)

their cytoplasm. These bodies contain blue-staining coccoid elements. The whole structure resembles the Bollinger bodies of fowlpox.

Rivers and Ward (12) have found it possible to obtain suspensions of these elementary bodies, which they regard as the virus, in a relatively pure form. Not only are such suspensions highly pathogenic, but the bodies are specifically agglutinated by the serum of recovered or immunized animals.

**Properties of the Virus.** Because this virus is indistinguishable from vaccinia virus by electron microscopy (4) and probably is a DNA virus, it is classified as a poxvirus (1) in subgroup E. The cytoplasmic inclusion bodies which presumably contain virus are Feulgen-positive.

It is a reasonably stable virus in glycerol and when frozen or dried. It is inactivated by heat in 25 minutes at 55 C. It survives many months in the skins of affected rabbits that are maintained at ordinary temperatures (8).

The virus is ether sensitive and in this respect unlike other poxviruses, but

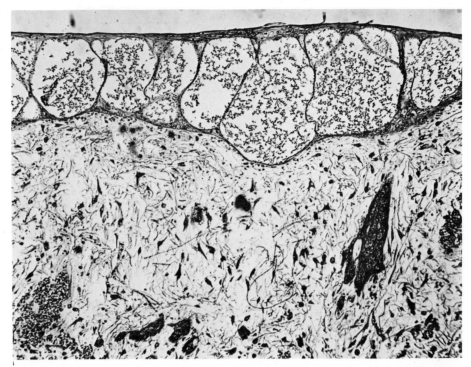

*Fig. 172.* Virus myxomatosis. The virus attacks epidermal cells as well as those of the subcutaneous tissue. In the lower part of the photograph the myxomatous tissue is seen. In the upper part is a series of vesicles—the end result of infection of epithelial cells. X 110. (Courtesy Thomas M. Rivers, *Jour. Exp. Med.*)

similar in that it is resistant to sodium desoxycholate (2). The specific gravity is estimated at 1.3.

The viral antigen produces complement-fixing, precipitating, and neutralizing antibodies. The virus is closely related to the rabbit fibroma.

**Cultivation.** Hoffstadt and Pilcher (7) have reported successful cultivation of myxoma virus on the chorioallantoic membrane of the developing chick embryo. The virus produces a cytopathogenic effect and grows in cell cultures from cotton-tail rabbits, squirrels, young rats, hamsters, guinea pigs, and certain human tissues (1). Plaques develop on cell monolayers.

**Immunity.** Among experimental rabbits the mortality from myxoma infection is so nearly 100 percent that only a few survivors have been available for studies on immunity. These have shown, however, a high grade of resistance to reinfection.

In Australia the initial mortality rates from the induced outbreaks was estimated to be 99.5 percent. It was found, however, in some regions that the mortality rate was not so high in successive seasons; hence a considerable number of survivors were available for study. According to Fenner, Marshall, and Woodroofe (6), these showed serum antibodies which persisted at least

18 months. Inoculation of such rabbits with virulent myxoma virus produced a small local lesion in some cases and no lesions at all in others. Fenner and Marshall (5) showed that the young of immune mothers were passively protected, at least in part. Such animals failed to develop infection with strains of greater virulence, some often survived, whereas there were no survivors among the progeny of nonimmune does.

Shope (14) discovered that the virus of the Shope fibroma, which is a benign tumor, immunized rabbits to the virus of myxomatosis. When first reported this interesting observation was thought to have little practical value. It has since been useful, however, as a means of protecting breeding stocks in Europe since 1953. Ritchie *et al.* (10) report that in England the method gives about 90 percent serviceable immunity, and that few problems have been occasioned by its use. On very young rabbits large tumors may be produced, but on older stock immunity often is obtained without the production of tumors.

**Transmission.** Myxomatosis spreads readily by contact or close cohabitation of domesticated rabbits. The incubation period is about 5 days.

In attempting to use the virus to destroy wild rabbits which had become a

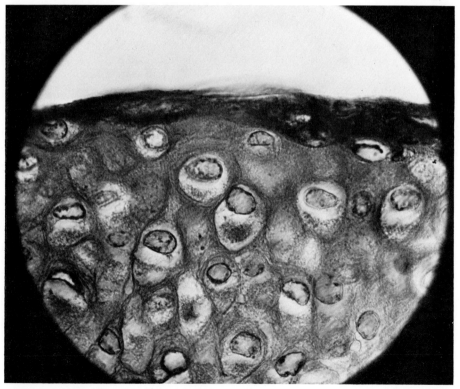

*Fig. 173.* Virus myxomatosis. Epidermis of a tumor shows cytoplasmic inclusion bodies. X 850. (Courtesy Thomas M. Rivers, *Jour. Exp. Med.*)

destructive pest in Australia it was learned that rapid spread of the disease occurred only when certain mosquitoes which fed freely on rabbits were present. After several trials had failed, an attempt to set up an epizootic succeeded brilliantly in one of the river valleys where there were many mosquitoes. The rabbit flea also is a transmitting agent, but unless rabbit populations are very dense flea transmission fails to produce epizootics. For papers dealing with the epizootiology of myxomatosis in wild rabbits, see papers by Myers, Marshall, and Fenner (9); Ritchie, Hudson, and Thompson (10); Bull, Ratcliffe, and Edgar (3); and Thompson (15).

**The Use of Myxoma Virus to Destroy Unwanted Rabbit Populations.** Reference has been made to the use of this disease to destroy rabbits in Australia. Because this disease is not pathogenic for man or any other species of animals, it had often been suggested as of possible service to destroy the rabbit pests of that continent. The wild Australian rabbit is a descendant of European rabbits imported many years ago. Because there are no natural enemies of rabbits in Australia, they thrived remarkably well. It is estimated that the number increased to a total somewhere between 1,000 and 3,000 millions. They ate up a huge amount of vegetation which could more profitably be used for feeding sheep and other animals.

In 1950 myxoma-infected animals were released in seven locations with the hope that the disease would spread from these centers in the form of a great epizootic. In six centers the attempt was a failure. In the seventh, in the Murray River Valley, large numbers of rabbits perished from the disease, and it was here that the importance of mosquito vectors was first appreciated. Hundreds of thousands of acres of land in this valley were cleared of rabbits. The following season, being hot and dry in the valley, mosquitoes were not numerous, and the disease did not flourish. In other areas, however, where there was more moisture and many mosquitoes, the disease spread rapidly. In later years the kill has been lower, and there is evidence that the host-parasite adjustment is occurring. Virus variants probably will have to be found if the rabbits are to be destroyed, because apparently a resistant population is now developing.

In 1952 a French physician who had retired to his country estate released some infected rabbits, hoping to destroy the rabbits which plagued his gardens. He not only destroyed his own rabbits but within 18 months the disease had spread through most of France, Belgium, Germany, and Holland; it had even crossed the English Channel into Great Britain. All attempts to stop the disease failed. Only the use of fibroma vaccine saved some of the domesticated species.

## REFERENCES

1. Andrewes. Viruses of vertebrates. Williams and Wilkins, Baltimore, 1964.
2. Andrewes and Horstmann. Jour. Gen. Microbiol., 1949, 3, 290.
3. Bull, Ratcliffe, and Edgar. Vet. Rec., 1954, 66, 61.

4.  Farrant and Fenner.   Austral. Jour. Exp. Biol. and Med. Sci., 1953, *31*, 121.
5.  Fenner and Marshall.   Jour. Hyg. (London), 1954, *52*, 321.
6.  Fenner, Marshall, and Woodroofe.   *Ibid.*, 1953, *51*, 225.
7.  Hoffstadt and Pilcher.   Jour. Bact., 1938, *36*, 286.
8.  Jacotot, Vallee, and Virat.   Ann. l'Inst. Pasteur, 1955, *89*, 290.
9.  Myers, Marshall, and Fenner.   Jour. Hyg. (London), 1954, *52*, 337.
10.  Ritchie, Hudson, and Thompson.   Vet. Rec., 1954, *66*, 796.
11.  Rivers.   Proc. Soc. Exp. Biol. and Med., 1926–27, *24*, 435.
12.  Rivers and Ward.   Jour. Exp. Med., 1937, *66*, 1.
13.  Sanarelli.   Centrbl. f. Bakt., I, Abt., 1898, *23*, 865.
14.  Shope.   Jour. Exp. Med., 1932, *56*, 803; Proc. Soc. Exp. Biol. and Med., 1938, *38*, 86.
15.  Thompson.   Agriculture (Gt. Brit.), 1954, *60*, 503.

## The Shope Fibroma of Rabbits

Shope (9) in 1932 described a type of fibrous tumor of the cottontail rabbit which proved to be transmissible to other cottontail rabbits and to the domestic species by the injection of cellular suspension and of Berkefeld filtrates. Although of interest on its own account, this virus has attracted much attention because of its relationship to the virus of myxomatosis.

**Character of the Disease.** The tumor occurs subcutaneously in naturally infected cases. There may be one or several in the same animal. They are firm, spherical masses which can be moved about under the skin because they are only loosely attached. Sections show that the masses are made up of spindle-shaped, connective tissue cells, without evidence of inflammatory reaction.

Filtrates of tumor tissue when injected into the testicles regularly cause the formation of similar tumors. Subcutaneous and intramuscular inoculations frequently, but not always, succeed. Intraperitoneal and intracerebral inoculations fail.

Inoculation transmits the tumors equally well in domestic and cottontail rabbits, but the behavior of the tumors in these species differs. In the cottontail rabbit growth is slow and continues over a long period of time. In the do-

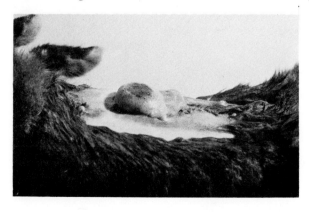

*Fig. 174.* The Shope virus fibroma. The tumor on the shaved skin of the abdomen of a rabbit was produced by experimental inoculation 11 days previously. (Courtesy R. E. Shope.)

mestic rabbit growth is rapid, but after about 10 days of active proliferation further growth does not occur and retrogression begins. The virus content of the cottontail tumors remains high for a long period (77 days at least) whereas in domestic rabbit tumors it is highest about 7 to 9 days after inoculation and disappears as retrogression occurs (10). Guinea pigs, rats, mice, and chickens proved refractory to inoculation. So far as is known, no animal other than rabbits can be infected with this virus.

**Properties of the Virus.** The virus in rabbit fibromatosis is found only in the tumors. It has not been demonstrated in the blood, visceral organs, or any of the secretions or excretions. In susceptible animals it stimulates a proliferation of the connective tissue at the point where it is deposited. There is no evidence of inflammation or of necrosis in the lesions.

This virus resembles vaccinia and myxoma viruses as determined by electron microscope studies. For this reason it is classified as a poxvirus in subgroup E. In thin sections its size is estimated at 200 to 240 millimicrons (2). It is ether sensitive and quite stable in glycerol and at low temperatures.

Rabbit fibroma virus is closely related immunologically to myxoma virus. There presumably are minor antigenic differences as determined by the com-

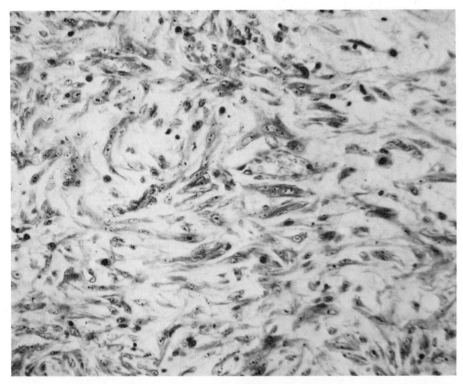

Fig. 175. The Shope virus fibroma, showing section of a testicular tumor produced by experimental inoculation of a rabbit. X 300. (Courtesy R. E. Shope.)

plement-fixation and agar gel diffusion tests. Interference is reported by virus III, Semliki forest virus, and Murray Valley encephalitis virus.

One strain of rabbit fibroma virus, after 18 passages in domestic rabbits, suddenly mutated and thereafter failed to produce tumors but instead caused inflammatory reactions in the injection sites. This change was detected by Andrewes (1) in England, to whom Shope had sent the material. Shope (13) was able to confirm Andrewes' findings. Passage through a series of cottontail rabbits restored part of the tumor-producing power. Other strains have not so changed. The changed strain continued to immunize against the tumor-producing strains.

**Cultivation.** The OA strain multiplies in the chorioallantoic membrane of embryonated hens' eggs without the production of lesions.

The agent produces a cytopathogenic effect and propagates in cell cultures of tissues from the domestic and cotton-tail rabbit and also in tissue cultures from the guinea pig, rat, and man (5). Foci appear on rabbit kidney monolayers (8).

**Immunity.** Shope (10) showed that domestic rabbits in which tumors had formed and retrogressed could not be reinfected with the same virus. To his surprise he found that such rabbits also had a high degree of resistance to the virus of myxomatosis. Whereas myxoma virus is almost always fatal to normal rabbits, it destroyed only 1 of a group of 15 fibroma-recovered animals. These animals then proved to be highly immune to myxoma virus as well as to fibroma virus. One rabbit that recovered from myxoma without having previously been affected with fibroma proved to be resistant to fibroma as well as myxoma (14).

Thinking that fibroma might be the natural reaction of cottontail rabbits to the virus of myxomatosis, Shope (11) attempted to pass the myxoma virus serially through these animals. Only minimal reactions were induced and these had the character of neither fibroma nor myxoma.

The unexpected finding of the immunological relationship between fibromatosis and myxomatosis suggested that the benign fibroma was caused by an attenuated strain of the malignant myxoma; however, Shope (12) expressed the opinion that such was not the case—that the viruses were qualitatively different.

In 1936 and 1937 Berry and Dedrick (4) and Berry (3) made certain observations on experiments conducted with fibroma virus that have come to be known as the Berry-Dedrick phenomenon. The virus of myxomatosis was heated to 75 C, which appeared to inactivate it completely. When the inactivated myxoma virus was mixed with active fibroma virus, the mixture produced typical myxomatosis in rabbits, and this disease could be transmitted to other animals in series indefinitely. It was suggested that something in the heated myxoma virus had acted as a hapten to lend greater virulence and malignancy to the fibroma virus. In the light of more recent knowledge of viruses, the phenomenon has been interpreted by some as meaning that the nucleic acid fraction of the myxoma virus, which carries the virulence factor and which is relatively heat-stable, had been preserved and needed only the protein fraction, which apparently is very much alike in myxoma and fibroma viruses, to make a complete, virulent myxoma virus.

**Transmission.** The mode of natural transmission is not known. Virus does not transmit from animal to animal by simple contact. Hyde and Gardner (7) found that it was not transmitted from mother to young either through the placenta or through the milk. Experimentally the disease has been produced only by inoculation. In view of what is now known about the transmission of myxoma, it seems to be fairly safe to assume that natural transmission occurs by means of biting insects (6).

**REFERENCES**

1. Andrewes. Jour. Exp. Med., 1936, 63, 157.
2. Bernhard, Bauer, Harel, and Oberling. Bul. Cancer, 1954, 41, 423.
3. Berry. Arch. Path., 1937, 24, 533.
4. Berry and Dedrick. Jour. Bact., 1936, 31, 50.
5. Chaproniere and Andrewes. Virology, 1957, 4, 351.
6. Dalmat. Jour. Hyg. (London), 1959, 57, 1.
7. Hyde and Gardner. Am. Jour. Hyg., 1939 (Sec. B), 30, 57.
8. Padgett, Moore, and Walker. Virology, 1962, 17, 462.
9. Shope. Jour. Exp. Med., 1932, 56, 793.
10. Ibid., 803.
11. Ibid., 1936, 63, 33.
12. Ibid., 43.
13. Ibid., 173.
14. Shope. Proc. Soc. Exp. Biol. and Med., 1938, 38, 86.

# XL | Infectious Canine Hepatitis and Other Animal Adenoviruses

The type species for the genus *Adenovirus* is *Adenovirus* h-1 of man. In 1971 33 serotypes of man were recognized. These are divided into four subgroups on the basis of their ability to agglutinate rhesus monkey and rat red blood cells (RBC). There is some correlation between this method of grouping and immunological groupings based upon cross-reactions with sera from volunteers inoculated with various members of the group. Hemagglutination-inhibition and neutralization tests have also demonstrated antigenic relationships among members of the four respective hemagglutinating groups, although cross-reactions are generally of low level and vary with the virus strain and the method employed. Other members of the genus include canine, simian, bovine, porcine, avian, and murine adenoviruses and other mammalian adenoviruses from sheep, horse, and opossum.

In general, the members of this genus have been well characterized, especially the human adenoviruses, and excellent reviews are available (1, 2, 3, 4). The virions contain double-stranded DNA with a molecular weight of 20 to 25 by $10^6$ daltons. Isometric nonenveloped particles have icosahedral symmetry, 70 to 90 m$\mu$ in diameter, with 252 capsomeres, each 7 m$\mu$ in diameter. Twelve vertex capsomeres are antigenically distinct from the other capsomeres and carry a fialmentous projection. The particles are ether-resistant. They have a buoyant density in RbCl of 1.34 g per ml and a sedimentation coefficient of 795 S. Viral assembly takes place in the nucleus of the cell where inclusion bodies are seen. A common antigen shared by all mammalian strains differs from the corresponding antigen of avian strains. Some viruses hemagglutinate cells of various species.

949

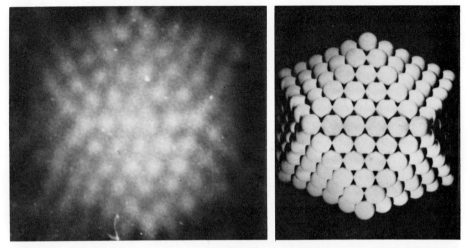

Fig. 176. (Left) Electron micrograph of an adenovirus, an icosahedral virus. It is embedded in phosphotungstate, magnified about one million diameters. (Right) A model of the figure on the left showing how the particles, 252 surface subunits or capsomeres, are arranged with icosahedral symmetry. (Courtesy R. W. Horne, S. Brenner, P. Wildy, and A. P. Waterson, Jour. Mole. Biol.)

Under certain conditions some are oncogenic. They produce a rather characteristic cytopathology in monolayer cell cultures with marked rounding of cells that form aggregates in grapelike clusters. The host specificity is relatively narrow and persistence of the virus in the natural host is quite common.

## REFERENCES

1. Cabasso and Wilner.   Adv. Vet. Sci. and Comp. Med., 1969, 13, 159.
2. Huebner.   Modern Med. (Minneapolis), 1958, 26, 103.
3. Pereira.   Brit. Med. Bul., 1959, 15, 225.
4. Sohier, Chardonnet, and Prunieras.   Prog. Med. Virol., 1965, 7, 253.

### Canine Adenoviruses (Infectious Canine Hepatitis)

SYNONYMS:–Hepatitis contagiosa canis, Rubarth's disease, fox encephalitis; abbreviation, ICH.

This disease has long been confused with canine distemper. It affects foxes as well as dogs and according to Chaddock (8), it also occurs in timber wolves, coyotes, and bears. Bolin, Jarnevic, and Austin (4) found neutralizing antibodies in the blood of a wild raccoon. Green (19) first described the disease in foxes, at which time it was thought to be a form of salmonellosis, but in 1930 Green, Ziegler, Green, and Dewey (21) published evidence which indicated that the causative agent was a virus. As early as 1927 Green and coworkers showed that the disease could readily be transmitted to dogs. The experimental disease in the dog was described in detail by Green and Shillinger (20) in 1934), and by Beckman and Torrey (3) in 1940. That the disease occurred naturally in dogs was soon recognized. DeMonbreun (14) in 1937 described the histological lesions accurately but assumed that the disease was canine distemper. Rubarth (30) in Sweden published a detailed account of the disease in 1947, and it was he who supplied the name by which it is now generally known. Rubarth recognized that the disease was the same as that which American authors had been discussing for some years under the name of fox encephalitis infection of dogs.

Canine adenovirus type 1 (strain Utrecht) is the only canine adenovirus officially recognized. There is a suggestion that the canine virus Toronto A26/21 of Ditchfield *et al.* (16) may soon be regarded as type 2 because biophysical data and differences in complement-fixing, hemagglutinating, and neutralizing antigens suggest a variation from type 1 and it has a marked predilection for respiratory tissue.

**Character of the Disease.** *Hepatic form in dogs.* This classical form is very widespread and probably occurs wherever dogs are numerous. Rubarth diagnosed 190 cases in Stockholm between 1928 and 1946, this number being 3.4 percent of all canine fatalities coming under his observation. The disease is very common in the British Isles, Denmark, Norway, Australia, and North America. Natural infections have been recognized in the United States by many; Storm and Riser (31) Riser (29), Coffin (11), and Chapman (10) were among the early reporters. It is now known that ICH is a common and destructive disease of dogs in the United States. Mixed infections with canine distemper (CD) may occur and such cases have an unusually high death rate.

The disease occurs at all times of the year. It is most frequent in young dogs but has been seen in all age groups. Young puppies, shortly after weaning, seem most susceptible and in them the mortality rate is highest.

The affected animal becomes apathetic and loses its appetitie but frequently shows an intense thirst. At this time the temperature is likely to be as high as 105 F or higher; later it may fall and become subnormal. Some cases exhibit edema of the head, neck, and lower portion of the abdomen. Vomiting and diarrhea are common. Many animals manifest pain by moaning, especially when pressure is brought to bear on the abdominal wall.

During the early temperature reaction, a blood count will disclose a leukopenia, the leukocytes usually falling to 2,500 per mm³ or less. Nervous signs usually are absent, and only rarely does icterus appear. A common sign is a transient opacity of the cornea (uveitis), which may appear in one or both eyes in from 7 to 10 days after the disappearance of the acute signs (1, fig. 177).

The mucous membranes are usually pale, and sometimes petechiae appear on the gums. The tonsils frequently are acutely inflamed and enlarged. The heart action is often accelerated, and the respiratory rate increased. Albuminuria occurs in many cases.

The incubation period is short. Baker *et al.* (1) report that after intravenous inoculation dogs showed signs on the 2nd or 3rd day; after subcutaneous inoculation, in 3 to 4 days; after being fed virus, in 4 to 6 days; and when suscepti-

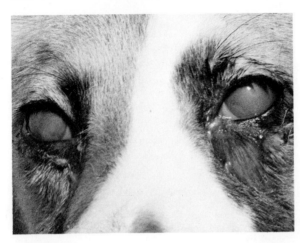

*Fig. 177.* Corneal opacity of both eyes of an experimental dog following intravenous inoculation of an attenuated canine adenovirus serotype 1 strain, classical ICH virus. (Courtesy L. Carmichael.)

ble dogs were allowed natural contact with infected ones, the susceptible usually developed signs from 6 to 9 days.

The progress of this disease is much more rapid than that of distemper. Most dogs have recovered or are dead within 2 weeks, and many succumb within a few days.

The mortality varies according to the age of the dog. Chaddock and Carlson (9) report about 25 percent mortality for artificially infected dogs. Baker *et al.* experienced only about 10 percent.

The autopsy findings of the hepatic form are rather characteristic. Because of the rapid progress of the disease, there is no evidence of emaciation. Edema of the subcutaneous tissues frequently occurs, and fluid is found in the peritoneal cavity in half or more of the cases. This fluid may be clear but more often it is blood-tinged, and usually it appears to consist almost wholly of pure blood. Upon exposure to the air this bloody exudate often coagulates. A fibrinous exudate is usually found among the intestinal loops even when no fluid is present in the cavity. Hydrothorax occurs only occasionally. Sometimes subserous hemorrhages are seen on the stomach, intestines, gall bladder, and diaphragm.

The liver may not be greatly changed in appearance but usually it is somewhat swollen and light in color. The capsule is tense, and the lobules appear more prominent than normal. The gall bladder generally shows a marked edema of its wall. The thickened wall may be hemorrhagic, in which case the whole sac may appear black or reddish black. The mucosa of the gall bladder is not changed in appearance, but fibrinous deposits are usually found in the vicinity of the organ. The spleen seems normal or slightly enlarged. The intestines may appear normal, but the contents are often mixed with blood. Edema of the lungs may occur, but pneumonia is absent.

The principal histological changes are found in the liver and endothelial cells (fig. 178). The blood content is increased and the larger vessels are

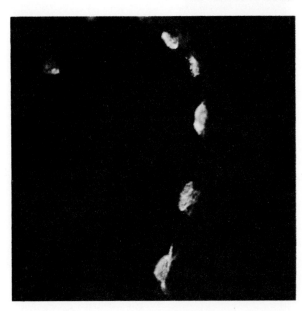

*Fig. 178.* Canine adenovirus serotype 1 (ICH) virus in vascular endothelial cells. FA. X 125. (Courtesy L. Carmichael and M. Appel.)

greatly dilated. The distended sinusoids cause pressure on the liver cells. The endothelial cells of the sinusoids and Kupffer cells are greatly swollen and undergoing degeneration. Nuclear inclusions occur to a varying degree in the liver cells, as well as in the lining cells of the sinusoids and the Kupffer cells and in the endothelial cells of the veins. Rubarth considers the primary damage to be in the endothelial cells, and the circulatory disturbances to be secondary. In the brain, serous effusions frequently occur under the pia mater, and there are cellular infiltrations around the blood vessels. The endothelial cells of the blood vessels often are swollen and undergoing degeneration, and many of the smaller veins are filled with such cells. Inclusion bodies are usually found in these cells. The picture is that of a nonpurulent encephalitis.

Inclusion bodies can be found readily in most cases, but sometimes they are not numerous. They occur in the endothelial cells of the sinusoids of the liver, of the spleen, of the lymph nodes, of the vascular system of the brain, and less commonly elsewhere in the hepatic form. They may be found in detached endothelial cells in the small blood vessels, especially in the brain and in the glomeruli of the kidneys. They are always intranuclear and acidophilic. The chromatic material of the affected nuclei breaks down and marginates, leaving a clear central area in which the inclusion bodies may be found. Usually there is but one inclusion body in each nucleus, but multiples are occasionally seen. They may be round or oval. The inclusion bodies may be found in tissue sections, or they may be demonstrated in touch preparations of fresh liver tissue (Davis and Anderson, 13).

The disease can be reproduced in dogs and foxes by inoculation. It is innocuous for ferrets, a fact which is utilized in differentiating this virus from that of canine distemper. It does not affect mink or the ordinary small laboratory mammals. Raccoons and ferrets do develop interstitial keratitis following injection of virus into the anterior chamber of the eye.

*Respiratory form in dogs.* The Toronto A26/21 strain of canine adenovirus was isolated from a dog with a respiratory illness (16). These original observations have been extended by others so it is accepted now that certain strains of canine adenovirus have a strict affinity for the epithelial cells lining the respiratory tract (fig. 179) and fail to produce hepatitis in dogs (37). Virus persisted in organ cultures from nasal mucosa for at least 12 weeks after oronasal exposure with A26/61 respiratory-type strain whereas cultures from dogs given hepatic-type virus were negative for virus (27). Conversely, virus was isolated from cell cultures derived from kidneys of these dogs but kidney cultures from dogs given A26/61 virus were negative.

The infection produced by the A26/61 was inapparent or quite mild (1, 19). In contrast, more severe respiratory signs of illness in dogs were described by Swango *et al.* (37) with their C955L strain which is serologically identical to A26/61. Certain bacteria, either pathogens or potential pathogens, were isolated singly or in various combinations from the lungs of dogs at necropsy. They probably contributed a great deal to the severity of the disease. The signs were observed in their contact dogs as well as the dogs infected by the aerosol method.

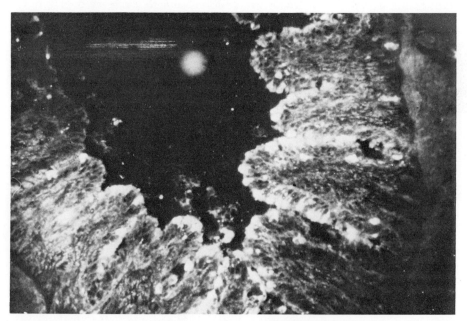

*Fig. 179.* Canine adenovirus serotype 2 virus (respiratory form) in bronchial epithelial cells of a dog, 6 days after aerosol exposure. FA. X 125. (Courtesy M. Appel and I. Parkinson.)

A fever usually persists for 1 to 3 days after an incubation period of 5 to 6 days for contact dogs. The disease may vary in severity from a harsh, dry hacking cough of 6 to 7 days duration to a fatal pneumonia. Other signs include depression, anorexia, dyspnea, muscular trembling, and serous nasal discharge. In some dogs the nasal discharge became mucopurulent. Vomition occurs in some animals and some have soft, mucoid feces. Dogs with a harsh and dry cough had less lung involvement than those dogs with a soft, moist, pulsating cough. The leukocyte counts were variable and inconclusive.

The gross lesions apparently are confined to the respiratory tract. There is atelectasis and congestion of lungs with varying degrees of consolidation sharply demarcated from normal tissue. Congestion and hemorrhages of the bronchial lymph nodes and congestion of mesenteric lymph nodes is seen in most dogs. There were no gross lesions in the liver or gall bladder as is characteristic of the hepatic form in dogs.

In histological studies moderate to severe pneumonic changes were observed in dogs infected with A26/21 type virus. Cowdry type A intranuclear inclusion bodies may occur in the bronchial epithelium, alveolar septal cells, and turbinate epithelium. Proliferative, adenomatous changes are seen in the lungs of dogs 10 days after infection ensues. The bronchial lymph nodes are congested and edematous. Similar but more severe histologic changes are seen in the lungs than in dogs infected with hepatic form, but centrilobular necrosis and intranuclear inclusion bodies in the liver and marked edema and hemorrhage in gall bladder were lacking in A26/21-type infections.

In studies with Toronto A26/61 strain, corneal opacities were not seen in 24 experimental dogs after infection (1). Corneal opacities are known to occur in a small percentage of dogs given attenuated vaccine produced with hepatic-type virus strains, or after natural disease with canine adenovirus type 1.

*Encephalitic form in foxes.* The disease occurs among wild animals, but the losses are seen principally on fur ranches. They may amount to 15 or 20 percent of the population of the ranch. The disease appears suddenly and the course in affected animals is very short. Loss of appetite may be noted for a day or two before other signs appear. In many cases animals are found dead without signs having been observed. Violent convulsions often initiate the signs. These are followed by a lethargic state in which the animal wanders about aimlessly and blindly. This may be interrupted by other convulsions. Usually the affected animal dies within 24 hours of the time when the first sign is seen. Toward the end various paralytic signs may be noted: paralysis of one leg, of the hind quarters, or of the entire body. A terminal coma may last for periods up to 24 hours. At the onset of the disease a watery nasal discharge is common, and sometimes there is a similar discharge from the eyes. The feces become soft and filled with mucus; sometimes there is a profuse diarrhea in which blood streaks are common.

Chaddock (1) says that the incubation period in artificially inoculated animals varies from 2 to 6 days depending upon the virulence of the strain.

The disease runs a very rapid course in foxes. It may be as short as 1 hour, and it usually is less than 24 hours, but a few cases may last as long as 3 days. Foxes that succumb to this disease generally remain in good physical condition because of the rapidity of its course.

Nearly all animals that show signs die. The spread of the disease in breeding pens is rather slow, and usually not more than 5 percent of the animals contract it. The disease persists for many years on fox farms, reappearing annually. The losses over a period of years may be great.

Gross lesions consist of hemorrhages in various parts of the body. These occur as rather large extravasations in some cases, and are small or absent in others. Large hemorrhages into the brain or into the cord serve to explain the paralytic signs often seen in this disease. Large hemorrhages into the lungs sometimes occur.

Although the name of this disease suggests that it is caused by a neurotropic virus, this is not the case. The disease in foxes is generalized, involving primarily the endothelial system, especially the endothelial linings of the smaller blood vessels. Injuries to these cells result in hemorrhages and in cellular degenerations. As the nervous system is very suceptible to this form of damage, the signs are largely referable to it.

Nuclear inclusion bodies may readily be demonstrated in endothelial cells of various organs and in epithelial cells of the liver. These are identical in appearance with those found in dogs.

**Properties of the Virus.** The negative staining technic has shown in electron photomicrographs that the virus particles are rigid icosahedra with 252 protein subunits (capsomeres) that comprise the overcoat (capsid) (12). The diameter is estimated at 75 to 80 m$\mu$. Some strains produce intranuclear virus crystals (23). The infectious particles in cesium chloride has a density of 1.35 per ml.

It is a stable, double-stranded DNA virus that survives well when frozen or dried. It is inactivated in 24 hours by 0.2 percent formalin but survives for days in 0.5 percent phenol (32). It is inactivated at 50 C after 150 minutes, or at 60 C in 3 to 5 minutes. It is ether and chloroform resistant and survives between pH 3 and 9 at room temperature.

The virus hemagglutinates chicken red blood cells at 4 C and pH 7.5 to 8 (17). It also hemagglutinates rat and human O cells at pH 6.5 to 7.5 (16). Viral hemagglutination is inhibited by antibody.

A group complement-fixing antigen is shared by ICH virus and other adenoviruses (6, 22). Complement-fixation and precipitin reactions are unilateral between ICH virus and human adenovirus types, since human adenovirus antiserums react with both human and canine virus types, but ICH antiserum fails to react with the human adenovirus antigens. No cross-neutralization occurs between ICH virus and certain other adenovirus types (22). Interferon is not produced by ICH virus in dog kidney tissue cultured cells, nor is the virus sensitive to interferon.

**Cultivation.** Up to the present little success has been realized in attempts to cultivate this virus in embryonated eggs. Miles *et al.* (24), in England, claim to have secure propagation in serial passage, but these studies have not been confirmed. Cabasso and co-workers (5) reported successful cultivation of this virus in roller-tube tissue cultures of dog kidney cells, in which specific cytopathogenic effects are produced. The virus can be carried indefinitely in such cultures. Independently and at about the same time, Müller and Thordal-Christensen (25), in Norway, also succeeded in propagating the ICH virus and demonstrating cytopathogenic effects in tissue cultures of canine kidney monolayer cells. Fieldsteel and Yoshihara (18) were the first to report success in propagating the ICH virus in tissue cultures consisting of cells other than those of dogs. They were successful with ferret kidney and swine kindney cells. Emery and York (15) likewise succeeded with swine kidney cell tissue cultures. They reported that the virus lost a substantial part of its virulence for dogs as a result of development in swine cells.

**Immunity.** Canine adenovirus type 1 protects dogs against itself and against Toronto A26/61 type virus and A26/21 type virus protects dogs against itself and against canine adenovirus type 1 virus (1). Consequently, presently available vaccines for ICH protect dogs against both types of canine adenovirus.

One attack of this disease confers a solid and permanent immunity. It has already been pointed out that immune animals may, nevertheless, be urine-virus shedders for long periods of time. There is no cross immunization between infectious hepatitis and canine distemper. Rubarth, in Sweden, and several workers in the United States have found that a considerable number of puppies having no history of the disease are, nevertheless, resistant to infectious hepatitis by virtue of neutralizing antibodies which they carry. This indicates that the virus is considerably more prevalent in our dog population than the recognized number of cases would indicate.

Poppensiek (26) showed that it was possible to protect susceptible puppies by passively immunizing them with homologous hyperimmune serum, and that solid, active immunization could be accomplished with serum and virus administered simultaneously. These dogs quite generally proved to be urine-virus shedders as in the natural disease; hence they were hazardous to non-protected puppies with which they came in contact.

As with canine distemper the virus-neutralization test is the only serological test that has been shown to indicate immunity. Other tests may be used for diagnosis but CF antibodies do not persist long after initial infection whereas neutralizing antibodies remain for a long period of time. Most dogs possess high levels of neutralizing antibodies at least 3.5 years after vaccination and at least 5.5 years after experimental infection.

The results obtained by Carmichael, Robson, and Barnes (7) with maternal immunity to ICH in puppies are remarkably similar to those obtained in distemper. Thus, active immunity cannot be induced until maternal immunity is lost. The age at which a puppy becomes susceptible depends upon the initial amount of antibody derived from its immune mother. The antibody half-life is 8.5 days. Unless the antibody titer of the mother or the progeny is measured by test, there is no way to predict when a puppy can be successfully immunized during its first 15 weeks of age.

In 1971, Appel *et al.* (1) suggested a practical way to overcome maternal immune interference. In their experiments, 4-week-old puppies with ICH maternal antibody titers ranging from $10^2$ to $10^{2.4}$ were inoculated with their respiratory strain $DK_{12}$ (closely related to Toronto A26/61) by the oronasal route. Virus was found in pharyngeal swabs 4 to 7 days after exposure but serum antibody titers continued to decline at a half-life rate of 8.5 days. When antibody titers of $10^1$ were reached a sudden increase in antibody occurred suggesting the production of an active immunity presumably due to persisting virus replication. These antibody levels remained and when some puppies were challenged at 14 weeks of age with canine adenovirus type 1 and the homotypic virus the puppies showed no signs of illness nor could virus be isolated from pharyngeal swabs or blood.

**Immunization.** Inactivated and attenuated virus vaccines, alone, or in combination with the distemper component, are manufactured in the United States and abroad. The ICH virus has been attenuated by transfer in dog, ferret, or pig kidney culture. The dual vaccine containing attenuated distemper and attenuated ICH viruses is used most commonly in the United States. On rare occasions the attenuated virus vaccine causes a corneal opacity, but this is the only sign of disease that ever occurs. The lesion disappears without treatment. Certainly cortisone therapy is contraindicated. Some manufacturers include *Leptospira canicola* bacteria so that immunization for three diseases can be gained at one time.

If the dual attenuated virus vaccine (or the triple vaccine) is given to puppies with an unknown maternal immunity for ICH or CD, it should be administered preferably at 9 weeks of age or whenever they are first presented, and then again at 15 weeks of age. This will cover the period of maternal insusceptibility for both diseases. Immunity acquired from the mother is likely to vary among litters of puppies because the mother will probably have a different antibody level of protection for each disease.

It is known that attenuated ICH virus is eliminated from the urine of vaccinated dogs. Susceptible dogs that come in contact with the attenuated virus will be immunized without signs of illness.

Foxes that recover from the natural infection are permanently immune thereafter, and it is possible to immunize with hyperimmune homologous serum and with vaccine (Chaddock, 1). Hyperimmune serum is used principally to stop outbreaks. Green, Ziegler, Green, and Dewey (3) failed in their attempts to immunize foxes with serum and virus used simultaneously. Animals treated in this manner did not sicken and die immediately as did the control animals, but most of them died about 5 weeks after treatment. It appeared that virus had persisted and produced disease only after the serum immunity had worn off.

Formalinized-tissue vaccines have been used successfully in foxes. Some of the commercial companies that make vaccine for canine use also recommend the vaccine for use on this animal.

**Transmission.** Baker and co-workers (1) have shown that this disease, unlike canine distemper, is not transmitted by droplet infection but requires more or less direct contact. Susceptible dogs, kept in cages separated from those of infected dogs by no more than 6 inches, remained uninfected. On the other hand, it was easy to infect through the mouth with infective materials. Transfer of saliva on the finger tips usually succeeded. More recently other investigators (37) suggested that the respiratory form of ICH, in contrast to the classical form, may be conveyed by aerosol transmission. Poppensiek and Baker (27) showed that virus is liberated in the urine during the acute phases and for many months afterwards in some dogs; this undoubtedly is the usual source of infection.

**Diagnosis.** Clinically, ICH is difficult to distinguish from other infectious diseases of the dog, principally, canine distemper (CD) and others which cause respiratory signs of illness. Because CD is the most serious malady of the dog the differentiation of ICH and other canine respiratory diseases from CD constitutes a major problem for the practitioner. ICH and CD vary in their signs of illness, but there is sufficient overlapping in the signs that a positive diagnosis is difficult. One major difference was cited by Poppensiek (26) who stated that the coagulation time of the blood is much increased in clinical cases of hepatic ICH while it is unchanged in CD.

At necropsy the hepatic form of ICH in dogs can be readily distinguished from CD. The characteristic liver and gall bladder lesions and the effusions which occur in the body cavities of hepatic ICH distinguish it from CD. Intranuclear inclusion bodies are found in tissues infected with ICH whereas CD has intracytoplasmic inclusion bodies—this readily differentiates the two viral diseases regardless of the disease form of ICH. ICH can be transmitted to suceptible dogs and foxes like CD, but unlike CD the virus of ICH is not transmissible to ferrets.

The methods that are used in dogs are applicable to the disease in foxes. In general, the acute course and the pronounced nervous signs make the clinical diagnosis easier in this species than in dogs.

Rubarth found that the complement-fixation test could be used successfully for diagnosing ICH. Extracts of the liver may be used as antigen, these being set up against a specific antiserum produced for the purpose. With such a test he reported that he was able to make specific diagnoses on dogs in which postmortem decomposition had made any other method of diagnosis impossible. The test was used in a survey of 100 dogs in the clinic at Stockholm which, at the time, were not suffering from hepatitis. Seventy percent of the animals were positive to the test, the incidence of reactors increasing with age. This would have to be taken into consideration when using the test for diagnostic purposes. In endeavoring to find a practical means of determining whether dogs of unknown history had, or had not, previously suffered from ICH, Prier and Kalter (28) compared the complement-fixation test with an in-

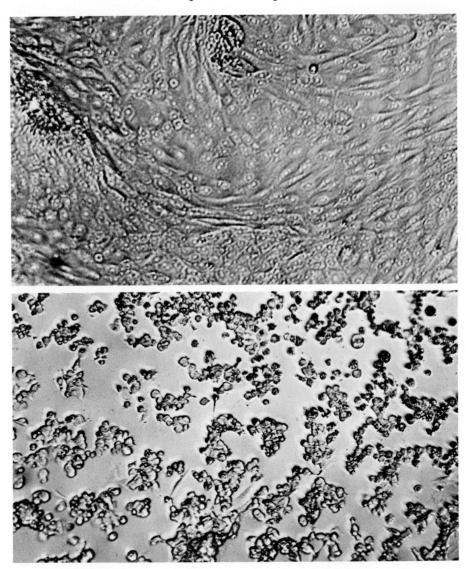

*Fig. 180.* Roller-tube cultures of canine renal cortex. (*Upper*) Uninoculated control showing solid sheet of epithelial cells. (*Lower*) Epithelial cells 3 days after inoculation with $10^4$ tissue culture inoculation doses of infectious canine hepatitis virus. X 100. (Courtesy Fieldsteel, *Am. Jour. Vet. Res.*)

tradermal test, using as antigen formalinized lymph node tissues from a dog acutely ill with ICH. They found the intradermal test much more accurate than the CF test.

Field strains of ICH virus readily produce a cytopathic effect in monolayer cultures of primary or secondary dog-kidney cells. This offers a convenient and excellent way of diagnosing the disease as the tissue-cultured virus can be readily recognized by its characteristic adenovirus type of cytopathic effect, by its ability to hemolyze and hemagglutinate erythrocytes from several animal species, by its production of intranuclear inclusion bodies in tissue-cultured cells, and by its neutralization with immune and convalescent ICH serum. The demonstration of a rising antibody titer utilized with paired sera from an active case is another means of diagnosing the disease.

**Control.** Because it appears that a high percentage of dogs harbor the virus of infectious hepatitis, it follows that most animals will come in contact with it sooner or later, unless they live an isolated and sheltered life. Apparently most cases are mild and they result in permanent immunity. The greatest mortality apparently occurs when hepatitis and distemper infections occur simultaneously. Because the distemper mortality is much greater than that from hepatitis, it is most important to protect good dogs against the former, but it is possible to vaccinate against both, and this probably is the best course.

**The Disease in Man.** The virus of canine hepatitis is not infective for man. The agent of a viral-induced infectious hepatitis of man was compared by Bech (2) with the ICH virus in many ways, and no antigenic relationship between them could be detected.

## REFERENCES

1. Appel, Pickerill, Menegus, Percy, Parsonson, and Sheffy.  Gaines Symposium, 1971.
2. Baker, Richards, Brown, and Rickard.   Proc. Am. Vet. Med. Assoc., 1950, p. 242.
3. Bech.   Proc. Soc. Exp. Biol. and Med., 1959, *100*, 135.
4. Beckman and Torrey.   North Am. Vet., 1940, *21*, 232.
5. Bolin, Jarnevic, and Austin.   Proc. Soc. Exp. Biol. and Med., 1958, *98*, 414.
6. Cabasso, Stebbins, Norton, and Cox.   *Ibid.*, 1954, *85*, 239.
7. Carmichael and Barnes.   *Ibid.*, 1961, *107*, 214.
8. Carmichael, Robson, and Barnes.   *Ibid.*, 1962, *109*, 677.
9. Chaddock.   Auburn Vet., 1948, *5*, 11.
10. Chaddock and Carlson.   North Am. Vet., 1950, *31*, 35.
11. Chapman.   *Ibid.*, 1948, *29*, 162.
12. Coffin.   Jour. Am. Vet. Med. Assoc., 1948, *112*, 355.
13. Davies, Englert, Stebbins, and Cabasso.   Virology, 1961, *15*, 87.
14. Davis and Anderson.   Vet. Med., 1950, *45*, 435.
15. DeMonbreun.   Am. Jour. Path., 1937, *13*, 187.
16. Ditchfield, MacPherson, and Zbitnew.   Canad. Vet. Jour., 1962, *3*, 238.
17. Emery and York.   Science, 1958, *127*, 148.

18.  Espmark and Salenstedt.    Arch. f. die Gesam. Virusforsch., 1961, *11*, 61.
19.  Fairchild, Medway, and Cohen.    Am. Jour. Vet. Res., 1969, *130*, 1187.
20.  Fastier.   Jour. Immunol., 1957, 78, 413.
21.  Fieldsteel and Yoshihara.    Proc. Soc. Exp. Biol. and Med., 1957, *95*, 683.
22.  Green.    *Ibid.*, 1925, *22*, 546.
23.  Green and Shillinger.    Am. Jour. Hyg., 1934, *19*, 343 and 362.
24.  Green, Ziegler, Green, and Dewey.    *Ibid.*, 1930, *12*, 109.
25.  Kapsenberg.    Proc. Soc. Exp. Biol. and Med., 1959, *101*, 611.
26.  Leader, Pomerat, and Lefeber.    Virology, 1960, *10*, 268.
27.  Menegus.    N.Y. State Vet. Col. Rpt., 1969–1970, p. 41.
28.  Miles, Parry, Larin, and Platt.    Nature, 1951, *168*, 699.
29.  Müller and Thordal-Christensen.    Nord. Vetmed., 1954, *6*, 767.
30.  Poppensiek.    Proc. Am. Vet. Med. Assoc., 1952, p. 288.
31.  Poppensiek and Baker.    Proc. Soc. Exp. Biol. and Med., 1951, 77, 279.
32.  Prier and Kalter.    *Ibid.*, 1954, 86, 177.
33.  Riser.    North Am. Vet., 1948, *29*, 568.
34.  Rubarth.    Acta Path. et Microbiol. Scand., Sup. 69, 1947.
35.  Storm and Riser.    North Am. Vet., 1947, *28*, 751.
36.  Surdan, Cure, Dumitriu, and Wegener.    Acta Virol., 1959, *3*, 115.
37.  Swango, Wooding, and Binn.    Jour. Am. Vet. Med. Assoc., 1970, *156*, 1687.

## Bovine Adenoviruses

Klein *et al.* (5) first isolated bovine adenoviruses from USA cattle and they now represent bovine adenovirus types 1 and 2. They were recovered from cattle during a search for viruses responsible for the production of poliovirus antibodies in cattle. A serotype antigenically distinct from types 1 and 2 was isolated in England from the conjunctiva of a healthy cow (4) and it is now recognized as bovine adenovirus type 3. Other strains have been isolated in Hungary from calves with diarrhea (1) and still others from calves with pneumoenteritis (1). In 1967 the first isolation of a bovine adenovirus in Japanese cattle was reported and it presumably is a new serotype. Some of these strains may be serotypes distinct from the above but insufficient comparative studies have been made with the three recognized serotypes to justify new serotype designations at this time. Reputedly there may be five additional new serotypes and it is reasonable to assume many other new bovine adenovirus serotypes will be recognized as studies progress.

**Character of the Disease.** Serological studies of small cattle-population segments in USA, Japan, Hungary, and England suggest that bovine adenovirus infection is common in the bovine species. Its true importance as a pathogen of economic significance remains to be determined. There is little doubt that some bovine adenoviruses produce a pneumoenteritis in colostrum-deprived calves and in calves 2 to 16 weeks of age under experimental conditions. The Hungarian workers who probably have had the greatest field experience repeatedly made isolations of bovine adenoviruses from natural cases of pneumoenteritis in calves where the mortality was a significant factor.

In the natural and experimental disease of calves the signs of illness and necropsy findings were similar (4). In experimental disease clinical signs referable to the respiratory and digestive tracts were observed 7 days after intranasal or intratracheal injection of virus. At necropsy, varying degrees of consolidation, collapse, and emphysema of the lungs were most prominent 7 days after viral exposure, but these lesions persisted for at least 3 months. Histologic features were proliferative bronchiolitis with necrosis and bronchiolar occlusion resulting in alveolar collapse. Nuclear inclusion bodies are found in the bronchiolar epithelium, septal cells, and bronchial lymph nodes.

**Properties of the Virus.** Several properties of bovine adenoviruses are known. Type 1 virus is a double-stranded DNA virus with a spherical diameter. The viruses are resistant to ether and possess a complement-fixing antigen common to the adenovirus group. Type 1 shows a two-way cross with human and canine adenoviruses (3).

Types 1 and 2 agglutinate rat erythrocytes and type 2 also agglutinates mouse erythrocytes. Neither serotype agglutinates red blood cells of chicks, guinea pigs, cattle, sheep, or human "O" (5).

Calf-kidney and calf-testes monolayers are the only cells which show a cytopathic effect after inoculation with bovine adenoviruses. The Hungarian workers made successful isolations only in bovine testicular cultures. The cytopathic effect is characteristic of the adenovirus group.

Type 3 virus induced tumors when inoculated into newborn hamsters, but the virus was not recovered (4). In contrast, types 1 and 2 failed to produce infection in suckling and adult hamsters, chicken embryos, guinea pigs, hamsters, or rabbits (5).

Adult hamster immunized with type 3 virus rejected tumor transplants from suckling hamsters with bovine adenovirus type 3 tumors whereas transplants were readily made in nonimmune adult hamsters.

**Immunity.** Calves inoculated with bovine adenoviruses develop neutralizing antibodies in 10 to 14 days reaching an approximate level of $10^{2.7}$ to 100 $TCID_{50}$ of homologous virus. Heterotypic responses were not observed. These antibody levels are maintained for at least 10 weeks. Precipitating antibodies appear in 3 weeks with no diminution of titer at 10 weeks (4).

Complement-fixing antibodies were not always present but CF antigen was found in various tissues of calves infected with type 3, particularly, in the upper respiratory tract (4).

Hemagglutinating antibodies reach a maximum level 7 days after intranasal exposure with type 1 virus which was maintained for at least 6 weeks (4).

The duration of immunity in cattle to the various serotypes of bovine adenovirus is unknown.

**Transmission.** From experimentally infected calves virus could be recovered from the conjunctiva, nose, and feces for periods ranging from 10 to 21 days after onset of infection. As carriers are typical of the adenovirus group more exhaustive studies may show that the virus persists for a longer period of time than 21 days. Present knowledge suggests that the virus is transmitted to susceptible cattle from acutely infected or infected cattle or their contaminated excretions.

**Diagnosis.** This is one of a number of bovine viruses which produces respiratory signs and, frequently, diarrhea as well. It is difficult to distinguish clinically for this reason. Consequently a positive diagnosis requires assistance from a laboratory that attempts virus isolation in monolayer cell cultures derived from calf testes, preferably, or calf kidney.

The best material for isolation is from exudate of nasal passages and conjunctiva and from feces of acutely ill cattle. Recovery of virus in tissue-culture cells was regularly accomplished from trachea and lung. The isolate can be identified by utilizing knowledge of its characteristics, given in the section on its properties. Particularly, the ability of most serotypes to hemagglutinate rat erythrocytes offers a convenient and quick method for identification. The demonstration of a rising titer with paired serums utilizing the serum neutralization, agar gel precipitation, passive hemagglutination, or hemagglutination-inhibition tests also is an excellent way to diagnose the disease.

In the serotyping of isolates no cross-reactions are noted in the neutralization test.

**Control.** At present no vaccines exist to assist in the prevention and control of bovine adenovirus infection. Present evidence suggests that cattle will also have a large number of serotypes with no cross protection between them. It seems unlikely that vaccination will ever play a prominent role in the control of the disease unless it is found that a very limited number of serotypes are the significant pathogens. A general characteristic of this adenovirus group is the persistence of virus and this feature also makes control of these diseases more difficult. The severity of the disease can be reduced by good management and proper facilities but prevention is difficult, if not impossible.

**The Disease in Man.** The relationship between bovine adenoviruses and infection in man has not been established. There is no reported evidence of disease in man but serum-neutralizing antibodies have been found in humans to bovine adenoviruses type 1 and 2. There is no cross-reaction between these two bovine serotypes with antiserums to human adenoviruses 1 through 18.

### REFERENCES

1. Aldasy, Csontos, and Bartha. Acta Vet. Acad. Sci. Hungarscae, 1965, *15*, 167.
2. Cabasso and Wilner. Adv. Vet. Sci. and Comp. Med., 1969, *13*, 199.
3. Carmichael. Quoted by Cabasso and Wilner, 1964.
4. Darbyshire. Jour. Am. Vet. Med. Assoc., 1968, *152*, 786.
5. Klein. Ann. N.Y. Acad. of Sci., 1962, *101*, 493.

### Porcine Adenoviruses

A porcine adenovirus first was isolated from a rectal swab of a 12-day-old piglet with diarrhea (3). Subsequently, porcine adenoviruses were derived from various tissues of normal pigs at slaughter, rectal swabs of healthy pigs, and from the brain of a 10-week-old pig with encephalitis (2, 5-8). During the passage of hog cholera virus in cell cultures from the kidneys of normal pigs taken at a slaughter house an adenovirus as well as particles similar in size to enteroviruses were isolated as latent viruses from the pig kidneys (4). The relationship of porcine adenoviruses to disease remains to be established.

By cross-neutralization tests with rabbit antisera, Clarke *et al.* (1) described three distinct serotypes of porcine adenovirus. Reference antisera against human adenoviruses types 1 to 31 failed to neutralize the three porcine adenovirus serotypes while neutralizing antibodies to the three porcine adenovirus serotypes were present in sera of normal sows.

Besides embryonic and piglet kidney-cell cultures, porcine embryonic lung- and testes-cell cultures and embryonic bovine cell cultures (after serial transfer) support the replication of porcine adenoviruses. The cytopathology of these cultures is characteristic of the genus *Adenovirus*.

## REFERENCES

1. Clarke, Sharpe, and Darbyshire. Arch. f. die Gesam. Virusforsch., 1967, *210*, 91.
2. Darbyshire, Jennings, Dawson, Lamont, and Omar. Res. Vet. Sci., 1966, 7, 81.
3. Haig, Clarke, and Pereira. Jour. comp. Path. and Therap., 1964, *74*, 81.
4. Horzinek and Uberschän. Arch. f. die Gesam. Virusforsch., 1966, *18*, 406.
5. Kasza. Am. Jour. Vet. Res., 1966, *27*, 751.
6. Kohler and Apodaca. Centrbl. f. Bakt., I. Abt. orig., 1966, *199*, 338.
7. Mahnel and Bibrach. Ibid, 329.
8. Mayer, Bibrack, and Bachmann. *Ibid.*, 1967, *203*, 60.

### Other Mammalian Adenoviruses

The murine adenovirus occurs in some mouse colonies. It is eliminated in the urine as it persists in the urinary tract and accounts for its maintenance in a colony. Suckling mice inoculated by various routes suffer fatal infection with disseminated pathological lesions particularly in the brown fat, heart, and adrenals.

The opossum adenovirus was isolated from a kidney-cell culture of this species. As adenoviruses commonly persist as latent viruses in the kidneys of various species, investigators who are using animal kidney-cell cultures must be aware of this situation. The ability of the opossum isolate to produce disease has not been determined.

Little is known about the equine adenovirus except that it exists.

Presently, there are 12 recognized serotypes of simian adenoviruses. Only a few instances of primate disease attributable to natural adenovirus infection of the respiratory tract or conjunctiva have been reported in the literature. Its physical and chemical properties are typical for the adenovirus group.

### Avian Adenoviruses

It appears that three distinct avian serotypes of avian adenoviruses and possibly six more exist. Included in type 1 are strains Gal 1, Gal 2, 65, and 95, while strains Gal 3, Gal 4, 93, and EV-39 compromise type 2. The CELO viruses are included in either type 1 or type 2. Consequently, the CELO and GAL virus groups, quail bronchitis virus, and strain 93 of chickens are known as distinct avian adenoviruses and probably will be given an arabic designation in due time.

The original type of quail bronchitis virus isolated many years ago, as well as a CELO virus, produce signs of illness in 4-week-old quail characteristic of quail bronchitis. The experimental disease also transfers readily to susceptible quail with the production of an acute, highly fatal respiratory disease. Quail that recover from experimental disease are resistant to the production of disease but reinfection does occur despite the presence of neutralizing antibody (3). At present this is the only disease in birds attributed to an avian adenovirus. By the oral route members of the avian adenoviruses produce infection but not disease in chickens (3). It has been suggested that *in ovo* transmission of certain avian adenoviruses may have an adverse effect on hatching and on chick survival after hatching (5).

The avian adenoviruses lack a common complement-fixing antigen shared by all mammalian adenoviruses. The physical and chemical characteristics are typical of the genus (1).

Chicken embryos infected with quail bronchitis virus or CELO virus become curled or dwarfed after one or a few serial passages (3). The cytopathic effects of avian adenoviruses in chicken embryo kidney (4) or liver (2) cell cultures are characteristic of the adenovirus group.

### REFERENCES

1. Cabasso and Wilner. Adv. Vet. Sci. and Comp. Med., 1969, *13*, 159.
2. Defendi and Sharpless. Jour. Nat. Cancer Inst., 1958, *21*, 925.
3. Olson. Proc. US Livestock San. Association., (Phoenix, Ariz.), 1950, *54*, 171.
4. Taylor and Calnek. Avian Dis., 1962, *6*, 51.
5. Yates, Chang, Dardiri, and Fry. *Ibid.*, 1960, *4*, 500.

# XLI | Infectious Bovine Rhinotracheitis, Feline Rhinotracheitis, Marek's Disease, and Other Animal Herpesviruses

The genus *Herpesvirus* contains many viruses responsible for important human and animal diseases. The type species is *Herpesvirus* h-1.

Herpesviruses have cuboidal symmetry. The particles are coated with an outer membrane which makes precise definition of their diameter difficult to ascertain. The particle is an icosahedral capsid with a diameter of 100 to 150 m$\mu$ and is constructed of 162 hollow capsomeres. Each capsomere is about 9 m$\mu$ across and 12.5 m$\mu$ deep; the central cavity is about 75 m$\mu$ in diameter and contains the double-stranded DNA molecule. The molecular weight of the nucleic acid for members of group varies from 52 to 92 by $10^6$ daltons which constitutes approximately 7 percent of the particle weight. The buoyant density in cesium chloride is 1.27 to 1.29 per ml. The particles are quite sensitive to lipolytic solvents such as ether and chloroform and readily inactivated.

The development of virus particles begins in the nucleus where it forms an intranuclear eosinophilic inclusion body and the particles become complete by the addition of protein membranes as the virus passes into the cytoplasm. Most viruses in the group have an affinity for epithelial tissue and tend to produce latent infections. In cell culture and on embryonating chicken membranes the members of the group for which information is available produce focal cytopathic effects in the form of plaques or pocks. Some members of the group are strongly cell-associated, requiring special procedures to release the virus into the tissue culture medium in appreciable titers; others readily release virus into the medium. These viruses are rather poor interferon producers.

Few serological relationships have been found among members of the genus, but rarely have investigations been done in this regard. Cross-neutralization reactions have been reported between herpes simplex virus and B-virus of monkeys and between herpes simplex virus and canine herpes virus. Infectious bovine rhinotracheitis and equine rhinopneumonitis viruses share a common antigen demonstrated by complement-fixation and agar-gel diffusion tests but reciprocal neutralization was not observed. Pseudorabies, herpes simplex virus, and B-virus share a common antigen as demonstrated by agar-gel test with no shared antigen from a neutralization standpoint. Pseudorabies virus when compared with other herpesviruses (such as infectious laryngotracheitis, equine rhinopneumonitis, virus III of rabbits, herpes zoster, and varicella), yielded negative results.

The herpesviruses presently included in this genus are as follows: infectious bovine rhinotracheitis, pseudorabies, feline rhinotracheitis, equine rhinopneumonitis, two other equine herpesvirus groups, canine herpesvirus, malignant catarrhal virus of cattle, bovine ulcerative mammillitis, Marek's disease, infectious laryngotracheitis, porcine inclusion body rhinitis virus, African clawed frog (*Xenopus*) lymphosarcoma, cytomegaloviruses of man and rodents, duck plague, mouse thymic virus; avian herpesviruses affecting pigeons, owls, parrots, and cormorants; and renal carcinoma of the leopard frog, snake herpesvirus, Epstein-Barr virus associated with infectious mononucleosis and Burkitt lymphoma of man, varicella, simian herpesviruses including B virus, virus III of rabbits, herpes zoster, and herpes simplex. The character of the diseases caused by this group vary from acute inflammatory conditions to the production of tumors.

### Infectious Bovine Rhinotracheitis and Infectious Pustular Vulvovaginitis

SYNONYMS:  Infectious bovine necrotic rhinotracheitis, necrotic rhinitis, "red nose" disease, bovine coital exanthema; abbreviations, IBR and IPV.

This disease affects cattle and perhaps mule deer. The respiratory form usually occurs in the colder months of the year. It was first recognized in beef cattle in feedlots of Colorado (17). It was then seen in California and other western states. The virus was recognized in the eastern part of the United States but manifested itself first as infectious pustular vulvovaginitis (11). On occasions it produces meningoencephalitis in calves (9), keratoconjunctivitis (1), or abortions of pregnant cows (7, 16) as the major herd disease manifestation. The disease causes marked economic loss in some outbreaks.

All forms of the disease now are recognized in the United States, Australia, many European countries, New Zealand, and Japan. In all likelihood it has a world-wide distribution. More than one form of the disease may be observed in a herd outbreak. In the United States the incidence of antibody in the bovine population in various states ranges from 10 to 35 percent.

**Character of the Disease.** The respiratory form (IBR) may occur in a very mild, unrecognized infection, or it may be very severe. The acute disease involves the entire respiratory tract with lesser damage to the alimentary canal. It begins with high fever (104.5 to 107.5 F), great depression, inappetence, and the development of an abundant mucopurulent nasal discharge. The nasal mucous membranes become very congested and shallow ulcers appear. Necrosis of the wings of the nostrils and of the muzzle occurs. The highly inflamed tissues gave rise to the name *red nose*. Manifestations of dyspnea and mouth breathing often appear as a result of closure of the nares by inflammatory exudate. Conjunctivitis and lacrimation may be seen, but necrosis of the lacrimal tissues does not occur. The breath usually becomes fetid because of the necrosis of the nasal mucosae. The respiratory rate usually is accelerated

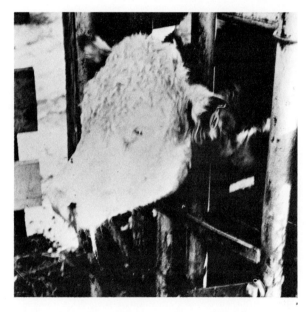

*Fig. 181.* Respiratory form of IBR with characteristic hemorrhagic exudate from the nose.

and a deep bronchial cough is frequent. A blood-stained diarrhea is sometimes observed.

Infectious pustular vulvovaginitis (IPV) occurs in heifers, dairy cows, and bulls (14, fig. 182). The degree of reaction varies greatly in an infected herd. Sometimes the disease spreads rapidly through a herd suggesting transmission by aerosol or by individuals handling the herd. The disease usually begins with a fever and severely affected cows show considerable anxiety and pain with frequent urination. There is swelling of the vulva and a sticky exudate may appear on the vulvar hair. The infection usually persists for 10 to 14 days in the herd. Bulls may have lesions on the penis and prepuce similar to those observed in the vulva of cows, and these may persist for 2 weeks or even longer if complications arise. Abortions are not always associated with the reproductive tract form.

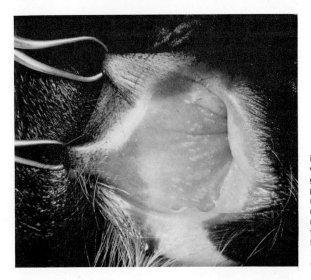

Fig. 182. The vulva of a heifer inoculated 48 hours previously with infectious pustular vulvovaginitis virus. The typical round pustules, some of which are in rows, are present on a reddened mucosa. Near the dorsal commissure the closely spaced pustules have coalesced to form a large plaquelike lesion. (Courtesy Kendrick, Gillespie, and McEntee, Cornell Vet.)

In calves this disease may manifest itself as a meningoencephalitis (9). This should not be surprising because it is a herpesvirus and other herpesviruses produce encephalitis in the young.

It also is recognized that this versatile virus has an affinity for mucous membranes and causes keratoconjunctivitis, usually without ulceration of the cornea (1); under certain circumstances field virus or attenuated virus vaccine (16) produce abortions, usually in first-calf heifers in any stage of gestation. Abortions occur sometimes with no signs of illness in the dam.

A rather interesting form of the disease was produced in experimental calves only a few days old by feeding, by intravenous injection, or by placing them in contact with infected calves (Baker, McEntee, and Gillespie, 3). The characteristic pustular lesions, intranuclear inclusion bodies, and necrosis were found in the oral cavity, esophagus, and forestomachs. Necrotic foci were observed in the liver, lungs, and kidneys. Calves that survived the acute infection developed a chronic cough with ensuing pneumonia, but virus could no longer be isolated at this stage. In 1964 Van Kruinigen and Bartholomew (23) described a fatal case in a calf that was associated with older animals suffering from the respiratory form of the disease. On postmortem examination the calf showed focal necrosis of the liver, necrosis of the suprapharyngeal lymph node, and necrosis of the rumen mucosa. IBR virus was isolated from this animal.

In the naturally transmitted disease the incubation period is from 4 to 6 days. By inoculation intratracheally or by nasal or vulvovaginal instillation this period can be shortened to 18 to 72 hours (10).

The course of the disease varies widely depending upon the severity of the infection. In the milder forms the disease may hardly be noticed. In the re-

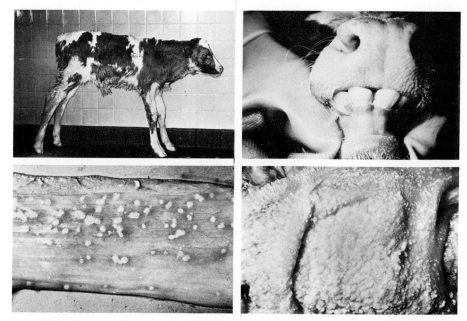

Fig. 183. IBR-IPV acute disease in infant calves. Calf in typical posture with excessive salivation (*upper left*). Pustular lesions on gum by margin of teeth (*upper right*). Necrotic foci, distal
portion of esophagus (*lower left*). Diffuse necrosis in the rumen (*lower right*). (Courtesy J. Baker,
K. McEntee, and J. Gillespie, *Cornell Vet.*)

spiratory or brain form some animals may die within a few hours after they
are first noticed to be sick; most of them will run a course of a few days.

The mortality varies widely depending upon the virulence of the virus, age
of cattle, the form of the disease, management conditions, and the condition
of the animals. In severe outbreaks in western feedlots 75 percent or more
may show respiratory signs with an average mortality of 10 percent.

In a susceptible group of calves mortality from the meningoencephalitis
form reached 50 percent. Calves that showed nervous signs seldom survived.

The characteristic lesions are the highly inflamed mucous membranes of the
respiratory tract, with shallow erosions, covered with a glary, fetid, mucopurulent exudate. These lesions may be found also in the pharynx, larynx, trachea, and larger bronchi. There may be a patchy, purulent pneumonia. Ulceration and inflammation of the abomasal mucosa is frequent, and there may be
a catarrhal enteritis involving both small and large intestines. Abscesses may
form in the lungs and liver of chronic cases.

Cheatham and Crandall (6) and Crandall, Cheatham, and Maurer (8) have
described intranuclear inclusion bodies in IBR. They occur in kidney cells in
tissue culture and in the epithelial cells of the respiratory tract. It seems that
these bodies appear quite early in the course of the disease and disappear before the disease is fully developed clinically.

In the vulva, circumscribed reddened areas become pustules that appear over the lymphatic follicles (14). Many pustules coalesce and a purulentlike exudate appears in the tract. Incomplete healing in some cows results in a condition known as granular vulvovaginitis. Histologically, there is a predominance of neutrophils and necrosis with a diffuse infiltration of lymphocytes in the connective tissue. Intranuclear bodies appear in the epithelial cells.

The brain lesions in cases of meningoencephalitis are quite characteristic of the viral type described by French (9). Aborted fetuses have some focal necrosis in the liver and spleen, and sometimes skin edema, but not consistent or severe enough to be pathogonomic (24).

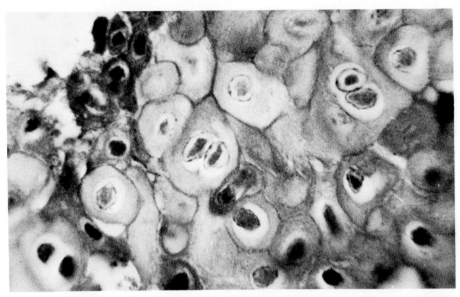

Fig. 184. Inclusion bodies in the vulvar epithelium 48 hours after inoculation with infectious pustular vulvovaginitis virus. Two of the inclusion-bearing cells contain double nuclei. Schleifstein's Negri body stain. X 800. (Courtesy Kendrick, Gillespie, and McEntee, *Cornell Vet.*)

**The Disease in Experimental Animals.** Cattle are susceptible to IBR virus. Young goats have been infected experimentally and develop a febrile reaction (15). Rabbits inoculated intradermally or intratesticularly developed local lesions (2), but serial passage of virus was unsuccessful.

**Properties of the Virus.** Tousimis *et al.* (22), who studied the virus by electron microscopy, determined that the IBR particles produced in bovine kidney cell cultures had a diameter of 145 to 156 millimicrons. In tissue fluids the diameter was determined to be 136±10 millimicrons. Griffin *et al.* (13) found this virus to be unusually stable when suspended in culture mediums at pH 7.0. The original titer was maintained for 30 days at 4 C. Only one log of infectivity was lost after 5 days at 22 C. Exposure of virus to equal parts of ether, alcohol, or acetone caused prompt inactivation. Calcium alginate wool swabs inactivate IBR virus.

Armstrong *et al.* (2) suggest that this is a DNA virus. It is antigenically homogeneous although slight differences between strains have been demonstrated by neutralization tests in tissue culture (25). Carmichael and Barnes showed some relationship to equine rhinopneumonitis by use of the complement-fixation and gel-diffusion tests (5). Other serological tests of value are fluorescent antibody test and an indirect hemagglutination test (24).

**Cultivation.** The IBR virus was first isolated by Madin, York, and McKercher (17) in 1956. In 1957 several groups of workers (10, 21) reported successful cultivation of the virus in bovine embryo tissue culture cells and in bovine kidney cells. The agent of IBR always exhibits strong cytopathogenic effect for practically all cells in which it is cultivated with an apparent cytopathology in 24 to 48 hours. It also grows and produces a cytopathogenic effect in pig, dog, sheep, goat, and horse kidney cells. Intranuclear inclusion bodies are produced in these cells and can be demonstrated by fixation with Bouin's and H and E stains. Plaques may be produced in bovine kidney monolayers and in many other cell cultures (24).

**Immunity.** Cattle that recover from natural disease are resistant to challenge by any strain of virulent IBR virus regardless of its place of origin in the body. The immunity is long-term in most instances. An animal with a neutralizing titer of $1 : 2$ against 100 $TCID_{50}$ of IBR virus is immune to challenge. Only occasionally will titers reach $1 : 256$, with the average falling into the range of $1 : 8$ to $1 : 64$.

Cattle that are immunized with attenuated virus are immune to challenge 3 to 4 weeks later with virulent virus by intranasal or intravaginal instillation. It has been observed that a few transient local lesions are produced after intravaginal installation of a massive dose of virulent virus but no febrile state results (14).

A modified IBR virus has served as a very effective vaccine for this disease (19). It was produced by rapid serial passage in bovine embryo kidney cell tissue culture. In this way the virulence of the virus is almost completely lost for cattle; yet it serves as an effective antigen which will protect against natural exposure and experimental inoculation. The virus probably does not spread from vaccinated to unvaccinated contact cattle. The duration of the immunity is not known; however, vaccine effectively protects cattle for more than the feedlot season, which is all that is required. It should be given, of course, before or at the time the animals are brought in from the range and to nonpregnant animals. Tissue-cultured vaccines produced in other cell cultures are now available.

Maternal antibodies are readily detected in calves from immune dams; the titers are low and sometimes persist until the calf is 4 months old. Maternal antibody interference must be taken into account in a herd vaccination program as it may interfere with active immunity production.

For complete discussion of the biologics for IBR and their recommended use in a herd health program the reader is referred to the Panel Report, American Veterinary Medical Association Symposium on Immunity to the Bovine Respiratory Disease Complex (12).

**Transmission.** The disease is readily transmitted by infected cattle. Evidence is now available that certain individuals remain carriers of the virus weeks after acute infection (21). All forms of the disease are transmitted by contact, especially under crowded conditions, and the venereal form can also be transmitted by coitus. The virus has been isolated from semen.

**Diagnosis.** Quite frequently diagnosis can be rendered on the basis of the history and character of the disease. To confirm the field diagnosis, isolation of the virus may be indicated.

For viral isolation the specimens should be collected from body systems displaying the signs and pathological lesions. Virus is most readily isolated in specimens taken during the febrile stage of the infection. In cases of abortion, virus has been isolated from the thoracic cavity fluid of the fetus and from cotyledons but not with high frequency.

IBR virus is readily isolated on bovine kidney cells in tissue culture. It may also be recovered on swine tissue-cultured kidney cells (4, 19) or other cells. The virus may be identified tentatively by its rapid and characteristic cytolytic effects, and also by neutralization and fluorescent antibody tests using tissue culture cells as indicators.

**Control.** Vaccination of young cattle before they are put into the feedlot in the fall will obviate losses from this disease.

**The Disease in Man.** The IBR virus is not pathogenic for man.

## REFERENCES

1. Abinanti and Plumer.  Am. Jour. Vet. Res., 1961, *22*, 13.
2. Armstrong, Pereira, and Andrewes.  Virology, 1961, *14*, 264.
3. Baker, McEntee, and Gillespie.  Cornell Vet., 1960, *50*, 156.
4. Cabasso, Brown, and Cox.  Proc. Soc. Exp. Biol. and Med., 1957, *95*, 471.
5. Carmichael and Barnes.  Proc. U.S. Livestock Sanit. Assoc., 1961, *65*, 384.
6. Cheatham and Crandell.  Proc. Soc. Exp. Biol. and Med., 1957, *96*, 536.
7. Chow, Molello, and Owen.  Jour. Am. Vet. Med. Assoc., 1964, *144*, 1005.
8. Crandell, Cheatham, and Maurer.  Am. Jour. Vet. Res., 1959, *20*, 505.
9. French.  Austral. Vet. Sci., 1962, *38*, 555.
10. Gillespie, Lee, and Baker.  Am. Jour. Vet. Res., 1957, *18*, 530.
11. Gillespie, McEntee, Kendrick, and Wagner.  Cornell Vet., 1959, *49*, 288.
12. Gillespie, McKercher, Jensen, Peacock, Bristol, Casselberry, Collier, Fox, Hejl, Mackey, Oberst, Pope, Jones, and Freeman.  Jour. Amer. Vet. Med. Assoc., 1968, *152*, 713.
13. Griffin, Howells, Crandell, and Maurer.  Am. Jour. Vet. Res., 1958, *19*, 990.
14. Kendrick, Gillespie, and McEntee.  Cornell Vet., 1958, *48*, 458.
15. McKercher.  Adv. Vet. Sci., 1959, *5*, 299.
16. McKercher and Wada.  Jour. Am. Vet. Med. Assoc., 1964, *144*, 136.

17. Madin, York, and McKercher.    Science, 1956, *124*, 721.
18. Miller.    Jour. Am. Vet. Med. Assoc., 1955, *126*, 463.
19. Schwarz, York, Zirbell, and Estela.    Proc. Soc. Exp. Biol. and Med., 1957, *96*, 453.
20. Schwarz, Zirbell, Estela, and York.    *Ibid.*, 1958, 97, 680.
21. Studdert, Wada, Kortum, and Groverman.    Jour. Am. Vet. Med. Assoc., 1964, *44*, 615.
22. Tousimis, Howells, Griffin, Porter, Cheatham, and Maurer.    Proc. Soc. Exp. Biol. and Med., 1958, *99*, 614.
23. Van Kruninigen and Bartholomew.    Jour. Am. Vet. Med. Assoc., 1964, *44*, 1008.
24. York.    *Ibid.*, 1968, *152*, 758.
25. York, Schwartz, and Estela.    Proc. Soc. Exp. Biol. and Med., 1957, *94*, 740.

## Bovine Ulcerative Mammillitis and Allerton Virus

Allerton virus was first isolated in 1957 from lumpy skin disease in South Africa by Alexander *et al.* (1). It is not believed now that the Allerton virus causes lumpy skin disease, because a pox virus has been incriminated in the production of that disease.

In 1960, Huygelen (3) isolated, from cattle with extensive erosion of the teats, a virus which was similar to Allerton virus. This occurred in Ruanda-Urundi. In 1966 Martin *et al.* (5) reported that bovine ulcerative mammillitis is caused by a herpesvirus which they called bovine mammillitis virus (BMV). This disease is believed to exist in England (8), in United States (9), and in Scotland (5). The Allerton virus and the BMV are indistinguishable antigenically and in physical properties.

**Character of the Disease.** *Bovine ulcerative mammillitis.* This condition assumes two forms (7) in a milking herd. In primary herd infections the morbidity rate is high affecting all ages of milking cows with no mortality. In previously exposed herds the disease is limited principally to first-calf heifers.

Ulcerative lesions appear on the teats and less frequently on the udders of affected milking cows (5). The infection usually causes gross swelling of the teat wall. Within 48 hours the skin over the affected areas become soft and sloughed, revealing an irregularly shaped, painful, deeply ulcerated area which heals slowly with formation of brown scabs within 5 or 6 days after skin lesions are observed. The scabs start shedding by day 14. Lymphadenitis occurs. Mastitis follows in approximately 22 percent of the cases.

Histologic changes (4) in the epidermis on the first day of the clinical reaction were severe inflammation accompanied by syncytia and inclusion bodies. Inflammatory changes rapidly became more intense in the next few days, with great numbers of polymorphonuclear and other leukocytes appearing in the epidermis and dermis. Syncytial masses containing many nuclei occurred in the lesions during the first few days as well as intranuclear inclusion bodies which varied somewhat in appearance depending on the age of the lesion.

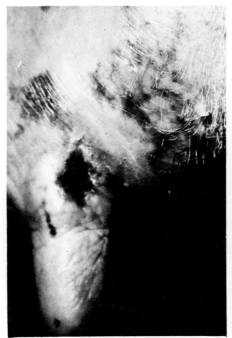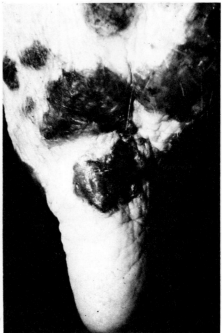

*Fig. 185.* Early lesions caused by bovine mammilitis virus (*left*) and later scabby lesions of same teat (*right*). (Courtesy W. B. Martin.)

More mast cells appeared in the dermis during the reaction. Viral particles were found in sections examined with the electron microscope and particles occurred within the nucleus with single limiting membranes either packed in crystalline array or dispersed irregularly. Particles in the cytoplasm usually had two limiting membranes, with the second one acquired at the nuclear membrane. Teat skin is not particularly susceptible to infection but skin damage does permit viral entry.

*Allerton virus infection.* When this virus strain is inoculated into cattle fever and eruption of skin nodules all over the body ensue. The nodules become necrotic. Lymphadenitis is another feature of the disease.

**The Disease in Experimental Animals.** One strain of Allerton virus produces skin nodules when inoculated into suckling mice and causes transient lesions when given intradermally to rabbits. It will also infect sheep and probably goats (2).

Day-old rats, mice, and Chinese hamsters are susceptible to BMV infection, characterized by stunting, with or without skin lesions, and high mortality, but older animals are not (8). In rabbits and guinea pigs, which are of lower susceptibility, no difference in age susceptibility was observed.

**Properties of the Virus.** The Allerton and BM viruses are members of the herpes group. They have all the biochemical and biophysical features of her-

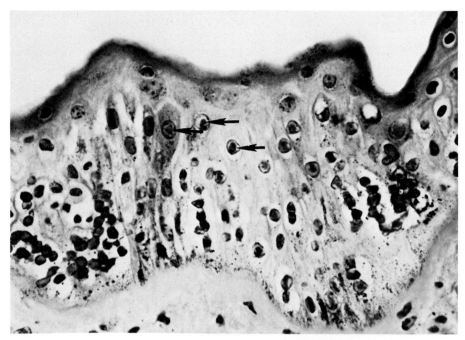

*Fig. 186.* Bovine mammilitis. Epidermal lesions from cow. Note hydropic degeneration and intranuclear inclusion bodies (*arrows*). H. and E. X 600. (Courtesy W. B. Martin.)

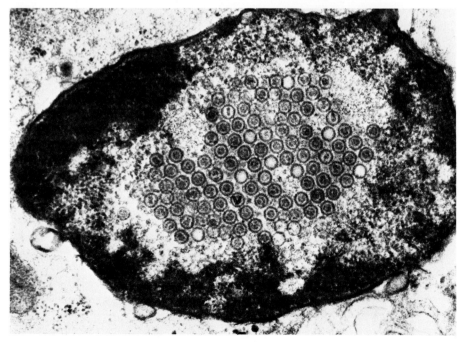

*Fig. 187.* Bovine mammilitis. Paracrystalline arrangement of virus particles (*V*) in the nucleus. X 38,010. (Courtesy W. B. Martin.)

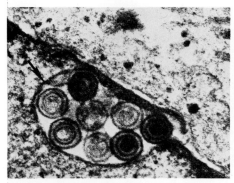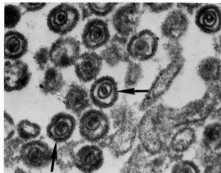

*Fig. 188.* Bovine mammilitis. Several enveloped viral particles within a vacuole formed by the nuclear membrane about to leave nucleus *(left)*. Extracellular viral particles *(right)*. X 48,000. (Courtesy W. B. Martin.)

pesviruses and have similar antigenic composition. Neutralizing antibodies are present in the sera of recovered animals.

**Cultivation.** The two virus strains replicate in calf kidney-tissue culture forming large syncytia which appear 8 hours after inoculation or as late as 8 days. Soon after formation, cell destruction is complete. Numerous large inclusions of Cowdry type A are present in the nuclei. Growth also occurs in baby hamster kidney cells and Allerton virus is known to multiply also in lamb testes.

**Immunity.** Neutralizing antibodies are found in the sera of recovered cattle. Complete protection results after experience with natural or experimental BMV disease. The duration of protection is unknown but it persists for at least 8 months (6). This was based upon challenge results. Maximal neutralizing antibody titers are achieved 3 weeks after inoculation but titers did not persist (4). In contrast, following recovery from natural disease, antibody titers persisted for at least 2 years (7).

**Transmission.** Transmission of BMV occurs mechanically by means of milkers or by biting flies (5, 8). Insects are known to transmit Allerton virus (2).

**Diagnosis.** In bovine ulcerative mammillitis the lesions are infective from the 1st to the 10th day. High infectivity titers of lesions and of exuding fluid were present during the first 4 days. With this material, virus readily produces a cytopathic effect in cell cultures (discussed in the section on cultivation). By the use of paired sera a rising neutralizing antibody titer can be demonstrated utilizing a cell-culture system.

Paravaccinia, a common cause of teat lesions, can be differentiated from BMV by use of biopsy material before scabbing occurs (8). Paravaccinia causes epithelial hyperplasia, intracellular edema of cells of the stratum spinosum, and cytoplasmic inclusions in the vesicular epithelial cells—this is in marked contrast to lesions described above for BMV.

**Control.** In a study of various experimental vaccine preparations with BMV the most practical virus vaccine was found to be an unaltered virus strain

(TV) administered intramuscularly (6). This vaccine was safe in pregnant animals and there was no evidence of excretion to susceptible contact animals. Protection lasted for at least 8 months. The use of an unattenuated vaccine must be viewed with reservations and only used in infected herds with the recognition that the disease may be perpetuating on the premises. Certainly a great deal of field study must be done to prove otherwise. Although viral carriers have not been demonstrated with either type of disease, latency is one of the prime characteristics of herpesviruses, so it is reasonable to assume that the carrier status may eventually be demonstrated.

**The Disease in Man.** There is no evidence that Allerton virus or BMV cause disease in man.

## REFERENCES

1.  Alexander, Plowright, and Haig.   Bul. Epizoot. Dis. Africa, 1957, 5, 489.
2.  Andrewes and Pereira.   Viruses of Vertebrates. 2d ed., Bailliére, Tindall, and Cassel, London, England, 1967.
3.  Huygelen.   Zentbl. f. Vet.-Med., 1960, 7, 664.
4.  Martin, James, Lauder, Murray, and Pirie.   Am. Jour. Vet. Res., 1969, 30, 2151.
5.  Martin, Martin, Hay, and Lauder.   Vet. Rec., 1966, 78, 494.
6.  Riveyemamu and Johnson.   Res. Vet. Sci., 1969, 10, 419.
7.  Riveyemamu, Johnson, and Laurillard.   Brit. Vet. Jour., 1969, 125, 317.
8.  Riveyemamu, Johnson, and McCrea.   Ibid., 1968, 124, 317.
9.  Weaver, Dellers, and Dardiri.   Jour. Am. Vet. Med. Assoc., 1972, 160, 1643.

### Malignant Catarrhal Fever

SYNONYMS:   Malignant head catarrh of cattle, *snotsiekte* (South Africa), bovine epitheliosis

Malignant catarrhal fever of cattle is, in Europe and America, a sporadic disease, characterized by a short febrile period, inflammation of the mucous membranes of the mouth, nose, and eyes, nervous signs, and a high death rate. The causative agent probably is a herpesvirus, which is not readily filterable. The disease that exists in Africa is believed to be the same as that occurring elsewhere, but there the disease occurs in epizootics and apparently it is more readily transmitted by inoculation. Differential diagnosis of this disease is very difficult, and it may be that more than one disease is now included in this category.

This is a disease of cattle. Sheep may be and African wildebeests are infected, but the signs in these species are vague or absent. Mettam (6) found that wildebeests carried virus without signs of illness and served as the source of outbreaks in cattle. Many Europeans have noted that outbreaks in cattle have frequently followed association with sheep and have thought that the latter carried the virus. Stenius (18), who made an extensive study of the disease in Finland is one of the latest workers to support the hypothesis that sheep often serve as the reservoir of infection for cattle. It is clear, however, that this disease occurs in cattle which have had no contact with sheep.

In North America the disease is generally seen in the late autumn and early spring months. Most cases occur sporadically—generally only one or two occur in any one herd during a single season. On some farms the disease appears regularly, season after season, occasioning severe losses over a period of years (1). Marshall *et al.* (5) described one outbreak in a large herd which began in the fall and continued until spring. A total of 31 animals died. The disease has been reported from most of the countries of Europe, from South. and Central Africa, and from North America.

**Character of the Disease.** The disease begins with a febrile reaction which lasts only 1 or 2 days. During this time the animal refuses feed and water and is greatly depressed. Inflammation of the mucous membranes of the mouth, nasal passages, and eyes appears early. Generally there is photophobia, lacrimation, injection of the sclera, cloudiness of the cornea, and even ulceration. The nasal mucosa becomes deep red, edematous, and covered with a fibrinopurulent exudate. Because of partial closure of the air passages the animals may have some difficulty in breathing. Ulceration of the nasal mucosa occurs occasionally with hemorrhage, and the breath becomes fetid. A similar process occurs in the mouth and pharynx. Fibrinopurulent pneumonia may occur, if the animal lives long enough.

Nervous signs develop early in most cases. Usually this takes the form of great depression or stupor, but sometimes there are signs of excitement. The animal may grind its teeth, bellow, and even charge other animals and human attendants. The victims become dehydrated and lose condition very rapidly.

According to Mettam (6), the incubation period of the African disease, experimentally produced by inoculation, varies from 10 to 34 days. Blood, Rowsell, and Savan (3) in 1961 made four successful transfers in cattle and the incubation period was 9 to 44 days.

The course of the disease varies greatly. Some of the peracute cases may result in death in 24 hours or less. In the "head and eye" form, the form that is most readily diagnosed and therefore reported most often, the course varies from 5 to 14 days, but a few cases (Rines and Barner, 16) may last much longer.

The mortality rate is always high. Goss, Cole, and Kissling (4) reported 16 deaths in 18 sporadic cases. Others report even higher rates.

Except the lesions referable to the general effects of fever, they are largely those of the mucous membranes of the head already described. The dark, swollen, glassy membranes of the turbinates and nasal sinuses are covered with shreds of fibrin and a dirty purulent secretion. Shallow ulcers generally are found on these surfaces. Similar lesions are found in the larynx, trachea, and the larger bronchi, and there may be areas of bronchopneumonia in the anterior lung lobes. The lymph nodes of the head are generally swollen.

The mucous membrane of the abomasum often is inflamed, edematous, and sometimes eroded, and there may be similar lesions in the small intestine.

The meninges of the brain often are congested and may show hemorrhages, but the brain itself is usually normal in appearance. Histologically, however, there are lesions of a nonpurulent encephalitis of the virus type, associated in some cases with acidophilic inclusion bodies. Some of the earlier workers reported the finding of inclusion bodies in the nerve cells of cattle dying from this disease. German workers found intranuclear bodies quite like those found in Borna disease in horses, and the suggestion was even made that this disease might be the same. This idea has not been confirmed elsewhere. Goss, Cole, and Kissling (4) reported the finding of acidophilic, cytoplasmic inclusions bodies in many of the epithelial cells. No confirmation of these findings has appeared. Stenius (18) reported the finding, in all of 50 cases examined, of acidophilic inclusions in degenerated motor neurons, especially in the vagoglossopharyngeal nucleus, and more sparsely in other areas in the medulla oblongata and elsewhere in the brain. These were seen by Schofield (13) and used to diagnose a case of the disease in which the clinical appearances were atypical.

Piercy (7, 8) and others in Africa apparently have had no particular difficulty in transmitting the disease to cattle, especially when lymph node material has been used for inoculation. Blood and other organ suspensions also usually transmitted the disease. In one experiment Piercy passed one strain through 19 generations of cattle. In 1961 Blood et al. in Canada made four serial transfers in cattle with infective blood (3). Of 41 cows inoculated, all but one contracted the disease. Stenius (18) inoculated a number of sheep with tissues from diseased cattle and a number of cattle with tissues from the infected sheep. In sheep, he produced an inapparent disease; however, characteristic lesions of a virus encephalitis were present. In cattle, mild lesions of catarrhal fever were produced with materials derived from the infected sheep. Piercy (10), although producing circumstantial evidence that sheep could carry the virus of this disease and serve as the source of bovine outbreaks, was not successful in finding the virus in sheep.

Piercy (10) reported that he had been successful on three separate occasions in adapting a bovine strain to rabbits. The response of this species was mild. Plowright (12), employing one of Piercy's strains, reports that in rabbits there was a febrile reaction followed by a mild leukocytosis in nine instances, a mild leukopenia in three, and no blood change in two. In all cases there was an increase in the nongranular cells during the reaction.

The experimental disease in the wildebeest was studied by Plowright (13, 14). A viremic state persisted in one wildebeest calf for 31 weeks and in the other one for 8 weeks. Neither calf showed signs of illness. Bovine calves maintained in contact with the first wildebeest calf during the early weeks of infection (2 to 12) developed typical malignant head catarrh. In conjunction with these studies cultural isolation was made from 7 percent (20) of 282 blood samples from wildebeests in Northern Tanganyika. Some calves were probably infected *in utero* as they were viremic during the first week of life. Transplacental infection occurs as virus was isolated from a fetal spleen.

**Properties of the Virus.** The virus of this disease is not readily filterable, and some authors, Mettam (6) for example, deny the filterability of the agent and yet believe it is a virus. In blood the virus is closely attached to the cells and cannot be washed off them. Piercy (8) believes the causative agent adheres to the leukocytes. Piercy (9) found it exceedingly difficult to preserve the agent of this disease for more than a few days. Storage at temperatures varying from 5 C to −60 C, lyophilization, and shell-freezing with dry ice and alcohol all failed to preserve viability for more than a very short time. All freezing methods actually seemed destructive to the virus. The best results were achieved with citrated blood stored at 5 C.

Armstrong (2) suggested that this virus was a herpesvirus after electron microscope studies of its structure.

No serological tests have been described.

**Cultivation.** Plowright, Ferris, and Scott (15) reported that the virus could be grown in thyroid or adrenal gland cultures. Cowdry's A-type inclusion bodies and syncytia are produced in these cell cultures. After several cell-culture transfers, the virus could be transferred to calf kidney cultures in which 19 successful passages were made. The adapted virus also grew in cultures of sheep thyroid, calf testis or adrenal gland, wildebeest and rabbit kidney.

**Immunity.** Nothing is known about immunity in the disease as it occurs in North America, since few animals survive the initial attack and survivors are unlikely to face new exposure. Unfortunately, no serological test is available for the study of immunity. With reference to the African disease, Piercy (11) reports that animals recovering from the natural or artificially produced disease are resistant to reinfection for periods as long as 4 to 8 months and even longer. He tried a formolized tissue vaccine and found that his vaccinated animals did not acquire sufficient immunity to resist inoculation of virus, but they appeared to resist field exposure better than others.

**Transmission.** Transmission occurred when cattle were placed in direct contact with wildebeests in the early stage of infection (14). Yet attempts to transmit the disease with nasal and other exudates from diseased animals have failed. No research has been conducted in North America or Europe in recent years, but with the advance of our knowledge of the disease in Africa, certain technics may be applied which should elucidate the means of transmission and the character of the infection in countries located in temperate zones.

Some of the African workers believe that arthropods may play a role in transmitting the disease, but infections in North America only occur during the cold months.

**Diagnosis.** The specific diagnosis of this disease offers a difficult problem. The clinical signs are similar to those of a composite of diseases that in recent years have been labeled "the mucosal diseases." The sporadic character of malignant catarrhal fever, the presence of eye lesions in most cases, and evidence of encephalitic changes tend to differentiate it from the other diseases which are characterized by mouth, nasal, and intestinal lesions, all much alike.

**Control.** The sporadic nature of the disease would make control measures difficult even if effective methods were known. In the present state of our knowledge nothing can be done to prevent the development of cases, and therapeutic treatment is hopeless. If multiple cases are occurring on the same premises, and if sheep are also kept, complete separation of the two species should be tried because the cattle may be acquiring the disease from the sheep.

**The Disease in Man.** No evidence has been found to indicate that man is infected with the agent of this disease.

## REFERENCES

1. Anonymous. 31st Ann. Rpt., N. Dak. Livestock San. Bd., 1937, p. 15.
2. Armstrong. Quoted by Andrewes. Viruses of vertebrates. Williams and Wilkins, Baltimore, 1964, p. 233.
3. Blood, Rowsell, and Savan. Canad. Vet. Jour., 1961, 2, 319.
4. Goss, Cole, and Kissling. Am. Jour. Path., 1947, 23, 837.
5. Marshall, Munce, Barnes, and Boerner. Jour. Am. Vet. Med. Assoc., 1919–20, 56, 570.
6. Mettam. 9th and 10th Rpts., Dir. Vet. Educ. and Res., Univ. South Africa, 1923, p. 393.
7. Piercy. Brit. Vet. Jour., 1952, 108, 35.
8. Ibid., 214.
9. Ibid., 1953, 109, 59.
10. Piercy. Proc. 15th Internat. Vet. Cong. (Stockholm), 1953, vol. I, p. 528.
11. Piercy. Brit. Vet. Jour., 1954, 110, 87.
12. Plowright. Jour. Comp. Path. and Therap., 1953, 63, 318.
13. Plowright. Res. Vet. Sci., 1965, 6, 56.
14. Ibid., 69.
15. Plowright, Ferris, and Scott. Nature, 1960, 188, 1167.
16. Rines and Barner. Mich. State Coll. Vet., 1955, 15, 108.
17. Schofield. Rpt. Ontario Vet. Coll., 1950, p. 104.
18. Stenius. Monograph, Bovine malignant catarrh. Inst. Path., Vet. Coll., Helsinki, 1952.

## Equine Rhinopneumonitis

SYNONYM: Equine virus abortion

Dimock and Edwards (9) reported a form of epizootic abortion in mares in Kentucky which was shown to be due to a virus. Their observations were confirmed by Miessner and Harms (26) in Germany, by Hupbauer (21) in Yugoslavia, and by Sedlmeier (30) in Austria. Manninger and Csontos (24) first called attention to the clinical relationship between the viruses of equine influenza and equine virus abortion. Doll and Kintner (14) in the United States made a comparative study of several strains of equine abortion virus with two strains of virus which had been isolated from horses suffering from respiratory infection and which had been regarded as influenza. These strains proved to be identical. Doll, Bryans, McCollum, and Crowe (13) encountered a severe outbreak of abortions in a large group of mares on a brood farm in Ohio, from which a viral agent different from that which had previously been regarded as the influenza virus was isolated. Doll, McCollum, Bryans, and Crowe (15) carried out serological comparisons of it with the viruses of human and swine influenza, among others, and found no relationships. Because equine abortion virus, is essentially a respiratory tract inhabitant and causes abortions secondarily, Doll *et al.* (13) proposed that it be called the virus of *equine rhinopneumonitis*. Now it is named equine herpesvirus 1.

During the past few years a number of equine herpesviruses have been isolated that show characteristics similar to those of the cytomegalovirus group. These isolates are serologically different from equine herpesvirus 1, have a slower growth rate in cell culture, and are more resistant to trypsin.

So far as is known, only horses are naturally affected by this virus. Experimentally, it has been possible to adapt equine herpesvirus 1 to several laboratory animals.

This disease not only has been reported in a great many areas of the United States but is known to exist in a number of European countries.

**Character of the Disease.** The disease appears in two different forms, the first in weanlings, the second in pregnant mares.

The weanling disease is manifested by a mild febrile reaction accompanied by a rhinitis or nasal catarrh which appears in the fall months. The disease is so mild as to cause little concern; however, Doll *et al.* (13) showed that it is accompanied by the development of antibodies for the virus of equine rhinopneumonitis. Whereas in September of each year, before the rhinitis appeared, all foals were free of antibodies for this virus, in each successive month while the disease was under way the number of positive animals increased until 80 to 100 percent were positive by December. Doll and associates (13) also showed the etiological connection between this virus and the disease by inoculating sucklings and weanlings with strains of virus obtained from aborting mares. The animals that were inoculated both intravenously and intranasally with virus in fetal tissue responded with a febrile reaction, a mild leukopenia, a mild mucopurulent nasal discharge, and the development of specific antibodies. There was no cough or development of pulmonary or conjunctival involvement.

The disease in mares consists only in abortions, which present differences from those caused by bacterial agents. According to Dimock, Edwards, and Bruner (11), the usual history of virus abortion is that the mare suffers practically no injury, and, after the fetus is expelled, its genital tract returns to normal as quickly as that of a normal animal. Characteristic lesions occur in the fetuses but none have been detected in the mare.

Virus abortions generally occur during the 8th, 9th, or 10th month of pregnancy, although some have been observed as early as the 6th month. Mares that become infected late in the period of pregnancy may produce either live or dead foals. Those born alive generally die within 36 hours.

In foals inoculated by intranasal instillation, the febrile response appears within 2 to 3 days, generally is diphasic in character, and persists for 8 to 10 days. In pregnant mares, abortions can be induced by experimental inoculations directly into the fetuses *in utero* in a few days, but inoculation of mares by other routes and observations on field outbreaks indicate that the usual period of incubation is approximately 3 to 4 weeks.

In foals the respiratory disease generally disappears, with complete recovery, within 8 to 10 days. In mares the abortions often occur with few or no premonitory signs. Except in those that are nearing the end of the gestation period, there is no enlargement of the udder or other signs of beginning lactation. The general health of the mare usually is not recognizably affected, and involution of the uterus ordinarily occurs in a normal manner. In a few bands of mares complications have appeared in the form of paralytic and other nervous signs, and deaths have occurred.

The mortality in sucklings and weanlings is negligible. In the abortion disease, mortality in the mares is low but the loss of foals through abortions may be high. The disease strikes from 10 to 90 percent of the pregnant mares living on the same premises. When the infection appears late in the foaling season after many of the mares have foaled, the incidence of abortion will naturally be much less than when it comes earlier. Good sanitary conditions, care taken to isolate aborting mares immediately, and separation of pregnant mares into small, isolated groups often have a marked effect upon the number of abortions that will occur on a particular farm.

In the weanling disease, the lesions consist only in reddening of the upper air passages and the collection of a mucopurulent exudate on the mucous membranes of the nasal passages.

In aborting mares, no lesions have been recognized in the dam but there are characteristic lesions in the fetuses. The most constant of these are multiple focal areas of necrosis in the liver. Many fetuses also exhibit petechial hemorrhages in the heart muscle and in the capsules of the spleen and liver. Edema of the lungs with excessive fluid in the chest cavity is also characteristic. Considered diagnostic of this disease are the inclusion bodies which in most cases are readily found in the liver and various other organs.

**Equine Venereal Vulvitis or Balanitis.** This condition also is known as genital horsepox, coital exanthema, and eruptive venereal disease. The disease is characterized by lesions on the vulva of the mare and the penis of the stal-

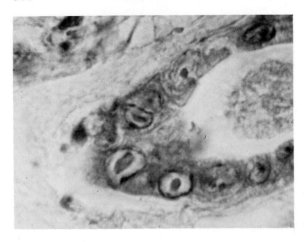

*Fig. 189.* Characteristic intra-nuclear inclusions of rhinopneu-monitis in the epithelium of a bronchus. X 900. (Courtesy Charles C. Randall, *Cornell Vet.*)

lion, and is spread in a stud by coitus. Gerard, Greig, and Mitchell (20) iso-lated a herpesvirus from two stud outbreaks which differed immunologically and culturally from equine herpesvirus 1.

Early lesions appear vesicular or pustular and occur in the vulva and peri-neal region in mares and on the penile mucosa of stallions (20). Later, un-complicated lesions appear circular and pocklike, and as healing progresses, affected areas are depigmented. In the absence of secondary bacterial infec-tion, healing was complete in 10 to 14 days. No effects on fertility are appar-ent but affected stallions are reluctant to cover mares until healing is com-plete. The incubation period is 6 to 8 days.

**Equine Rhinopneumonitis in Experimental Animals.** The injection or feeding of infective materials will sometimes cause susceptible mares to abort, but these methods are uncertain. Doll (12) reported abortion of only 5 in a group of 30 inoculations. He did not know how many of these mares might have ac-quired a naturally immune state and thus how many of these failures were due to this reason. He developed a technic of inoculating the fetuses *in utero* directly through the abdominal wall; this produced abortions in 100 percent of all cases, irrespective of whether or not the mare was immune to the virus.

The studies of Dimock, Edwards, and Bruner (10), Bruner, Doll, and Hull (2), and Kress (23) indicate that the virus will cause pregnant guinea pigs to abort. When virus material was injected into the fetuses of pregnant guinea pigs on the 35th day of gestation, the fetuses were aborted 7 to 9 days later. The injection of virus-free material into the fetuses of control animals did not cause abortions, and at birth the baby guinea pigs appeared entirely normal (2).

Doll, Richards, and Wallace (16) succeeded in adapting this virus to suc-kling hamsters, after Anderson and Goodpasture (1) had pointed the way by reporting the finding of intranuclear inclusions resembling those of virus abortion in sucklings of this species. Later Doll and associates succeeded in cultivating, in suckling hamsters, a number of strains of the abortion virus and the so-called *influenza virus,* which up to then was considered to be different. All of these strains produced identical lesions in the hamsters and resulted in their deaths (17). Typical acidophilic intranuclear inclusion bodies were found in the livers of all inoculated individuals, and horse tissues fixed complement with hamster antibodies and hamster tissues fixed complement with horse antibodies. It was this finding which first drew attention to the identity of the virus in the respiratory and the abortion disease of horses. Then it was demonstrated that the abortion virus was capable of producing a respiratory infection of a mild nature in young animals and sometimes in older ones, and that virus derived from these respiratory infections was capable of causing abortions when inoculated into pregnant mares.

**Properties of the Virus.** This is a DNA virus that produces intranuclear inclusion bodies. Particles have been described in the nuclei of affected hepatic cells of hamsters. The virus bodies are 92 millimicrons in diameter in and outside of the cytoplasm (33). Particles in the nuclei may be in crystalline array.

Virus survives for over 457 days at $-18$ C. The agent is labile in saline suspensions and it is inactivated by 0.35 percent formalin. Its density is 1.18.

Horse red blood cells are agglutinated by tissues of affected horses between 4 C and 37 C (25). The hemagglutinin is not neutralized by convalescent horse sera, but inhibition is produced by use of hyperimmune serum from horses given infected hamster tissue.

The virus has a complement-fixing antigen, and complement-fixing antibodies are present in horse serum for a few weeks after infection. It has been suggested that the equine herpesviruses may share a complement-fixing antigen. Carmichael and Barnes (8) showed that equine herpesvirus 1 and infectious bovine rhinotracheitis virus share common complement-fixing and precipitating antigens.

Erasmus (19) presently places equine herpesviruses into three groups based upon growth characteristics in cell culture and trypsin sensitivity until these viruses are examined for their guanine–cystosine ratio and their complete serological relationships. Equine herpesvirus 1 is listed as the classical rhinopneumonitis virus of Doll and is placed in Group I. It is pathogenic for horses; disease-related; rapidly cytopathic in cell culture, producing with high titers; markedly sensitive to trypsin; and known to replicate in many animal hosts. In Group II the viruses have the characteristics of cytomegaloviruses and thus differ markedly from the features described for Group I. Group III is a heterogenous group with characteristics common to Groups I and II, and includes such strains as $EHV_2$, $HK_2$, $HBM_7$, $HKV_4$, and possibly $EHV_3$. $EHV_2$ has been associated with respiratory illness in horses (23). A Japanese virus isolate also was associated with respiratory disease (18).

A good neutralization test exists for the comparison of equine herpesvirus 1 strains (19). The viruses in Groups II and III with strong cell-association characteristics present such a variety of problems in the neutralization test and in their poor antibody induction that comparative antigenic studies are difficult and less than satisfactory.

**Cultivation.** Strains of equine herpes 1 virus from the respiratory tract and also from tissues of aborted horse fetuses were adapted to hens' eggs by alternation between the hamster virus and the fertile egg (16).

Classical equine herpesvirus 1 and the viruses in Group II and Group III produced a cytopathic effect in cell cultures of fetal horse kidney, lamb kidney, and rabbit kidney (27), with the production of intranuclear inclusion bodies of varying types depending upon the virus isolate (19, 28). With equine herpesvirus 1 the cytopathic effect was rapid and complete. With the other two virus groups the cytopathic effect was slower and the cells usually remained attached to the glass and large syncytia were formed with $EHV_2$, $HKV_2$, and $HKV_3$ virus strains. All viruses except equine herpesvirus 1 appear to be strongly cell-associated. Equine herpesvirus 1 produces a cytopathic effect in a number of other cell culture types (19). Plaque-assay methods are available for equine herpesvirus 1, using monolayers of Earle's L cells (29) and horse kidney cells (32).

**Immunity.** Virus abortions are seldom if ever observed in the same mare in two successive seasons, although some have been known to have aborted a virus fetus several years after the first abortion. This would indicate the presence of an immune mechanism which gives a somewhat transitory resistance, or possibly infection with a heterologous type.

With equine herpesvirus 1, a serum-neutralizing titer of $10^2$ or greater (against 50 to 100 $TCID_{50}$ in a cell culture system) in a mare prevented reinfection by intranasal challenge (5, 6). Subcutaneous injection of virus produced viremia in immune mares regardless of the level of antibody. Virus was established in the leukocytes of some mares with neutralization titers lower than $10^2$, and it could be demonstrated in the buffy coats of blood samples from these animals for at least 3 weeks. The presence of viremia in a pregnant mare did not always result in an abortion. There seemed to be no apparent relationship between the occurrence and duration of viremia, except that abortigenic disease did not occur in any mare without viremia. Therefore it is speculated that the virus reaches the fetus fortuitously and the probability is related to the number of leukocytes carrying the virus. Because the incubation period for abortions varies markedly, it is assumed that the virus may persist in leukocytes or some other tissue of the dam for extended periods of time before invading the fetus, causing death and abortion within a few days after fetal infection.

**Transmission.** The respiratory disease is undoubtedly transmitted by droplet infection after outbreaks have once started. The source of the virus which initiates outbreaks is unknown. Aborted fetuses contain much virus, and aborting mares often bring infections to new premises. However, there is no evidence to indicate that virus is carried by an aborting mare very long after abortion occurs. Stallions are not known to have anything to do with the transmission of the disease except by ordinary contact. It is possible that dogs, foxes, and carrion birds may carry infection with fragments of aborted fetuses from one farm to another.

**Diagnosis.** Clinical diagnosis is usually not difficult. Autopsy of the aborted fetus generally will establish a precise diagnosis. In respiratory cases the lungs are usually edematous, there are hemorrhages on the pericardium and the typical liver lesions are most characteristic. The finding of the characteristic inclusion bodies is diagnostic. These are acidophilic, intranuclear, and usually numerous in the liver cells. Often from 50 to 80 percent of the liver cells are necrotic and contain these bodies. They may be found also in the epithelium lining the air passages and the bile ducts and in endothelial cells of the spleen, lymph nodes, and thymus. These were described by Westerfield and Dimock (34). Virus typing may be indicated in certain instances.

**Control.** Because the disease with equine herpesvirus 1 is highly contagious, isolation of the infected animals is recommended. Indiscriminate movement of infected foals or mares following an outbreak may result in spreading the disease. Following an abortion the stall of the aborting animal should be thoroughly disinfected. This is very important if other pregnant mares are kept in the same stable.

As a prophylactic measure in past years mares were vaccinated with a formalin-treated suspension of infected equine fetus liver (2, 3, 23). The equine tissue in the vaccine tended to cause complications in many mares by stimulating the formation of isoantibodies. Doll and Bryans have now prepared a hamster-adapted live-virus vaccine and with it have instituted a program of planned infections during periods when it is least likely to cause losses. They recommended that all horses on a farm be vaccinated late in June or early in July and again in October. The vaccine is administered by instilling 3 ml in one nostril. Mature horses do not show reactions, but weanlings often have a mild fever and a slight watery exudate from the nose following their first vaccination. This program has been successful as indicated by its use in more than 9,000 mares since 1959. In these mares 89 abortions occurred; half of this small percentage (0.93 percent) of abortions may have been due to field virus after a small percentage of immunization failures. By any biological standards this can be termed a reasonably safe and effective vaccine, but it is generally agreed that this immunization procedure should be improved, if possible, by the development of a safer and more effective vaccine.

If equine cytomegaloviruses are found in the United States as a cause of respiratory disease and abortion, the control program will require considerable modification (4).

**The Disease in Man.** This disease has not been reported in man. References to an obscure disease of the human fetus in which there are intranuclear inclusion bodies appears in the literature (4).

## REFERENCES

1. Anderson and Goodpasture. Am. Jour. Path., 1942, *18*, 555.
2. Bruner, Doll, and Hull. The Blood-Horse, 1949, *58*, 31.

3. Bruner, Edwards, and Hull.   *Ibid.*, 1948, *53*, 666.
4. Bryans.   Proc. Am. Vet. Med. Assoc., 1964, p. 112.
5. Byrans.   Jour. Am. Vet. Med. Assoc., 1969, *155*, 294.
6. Bryans and Prickett.   Proc. 2d Internatl. Conf. Equine Inf. Dis., S. Karger, Basel, Switzerland, 1969, p. 34.
7. Cappell and McFarlane.   Jour. Path. and Bact., 1947, *59*, 385.
8. Carmichael and Barnes.   Proc., U.S. Livestock Sanit. Assoc., 1961, *65*, 384.
9. Dimock and Edwards.   Ky. Agr. Exp. Sta., Sup. to Bul. 333, 1933.
10. Dimock, Edwards, and Bruner.   *Ibid.*, Bul. 426, 1942.
11. Dimock, Edwards, and Bruner.   Cornell Vet., 1947, *37*, 89.
12. Doll.   *Ibid.*, 1953, *43*, 112.
13. Doll, Bryans, McCollum, and Crowe.   *Ibid.*, 1957, *47*, 3.
14. Doll and Kintner.   *Ibid.*, 1954, *44*, 355.
15. Doll, McCollum, Bryans, and Crowe.   Am. Jour. Vet. Res., 1956, *17*, 262.
16. Doll, Richards, and Wallace.   Cornell Vet., 1953, *43*, 551.
17. *Ibid.*, 1954, *44*, 133.
18. Doll and Wallace.   *Ibid.*, 453.
19. Erasmus.   Proc. 2d Internatl. Conf. Equine Inf. Dis., S. Karger, Basel, Switzerland, 1969, p. 46.
20. Girard, Greig, and Mitchell.   Canad. Jour. Comp. Med., 1968, *32*, 603.
21. Hupbauer.   Deut. tierärztl. Wchnschr., 1938, *46*, 745.
22. Kawakawi, Kaji, Ishizaki, Shimizu, and Matumoto.   Jap. Jour. Exp. Med., 1962, *32*, 211.
23. Kress.   Wien. tierärztl. Monatschrift., 1946, *33*, 121.
24. Manninger and Csontos.   Deut. tierärztl. Wchnschr., 1941, *49*, 105.
25. McCollum, Doll, and Bryans.   Am. Jour. Vet. Res., 1956, *17*, 267.
26. Miessner and Harms.   Deut. tierärztl. Wchnschr., 1937, *45*, 685.
27. Plummer and Waterson.   Quoted by Andrewes. Viruses of vertebrates. Williams and Wilkins, Baltimore, 1964.
28. Randall.   Proc. Soc. Exp. Biol. and Med., 1957, *95*, 508.
29. Randall and Lawson.   *Ibid.*, 1962, *110*, 487.
30. Sedlmeier.   Münch. tierärztl. Wchnschr., 1938, *89*, 37.
31. Shimizu, Ishizaki, Kono, and Matumoto.   Jap. Jour. Exp. Med., 1958, 27, 175.
32. Shimizu, Ishizaki, and Matumoto.   *Ibid.*, 1963, *33*, 85.
33. Tajima, Shimizu, and Ishizaki.   Am. Jour. Vet. Res., 1961, *22*, 250.
34. Westerfield and Dimock.   Jour. Am. Vet. Med. Assoc., 1946, *109*, 101.

## Pseudorabies

SYMONYMS:   Aujezsky's disease, mad itch, infectious bulbar paralysis, (*Herpesivirus suis*)

This disease occurs naturally in cattle, sheep, dogs, cats, rats, and swine. Cases have been diagnosed clinically in horses, but in the absence of laboratory confirmation there is some doubt about the susceptibility of this species. In all but adult swine it is a highly fatal disease with few or no animals recovering. In adult pigs the signs are very mild and the mortality almost nil. The disease is usually transmitted from infected pigs to other hosts. Swine and dogs may become infected, however, from contact with carcasses of rats

and possibly other infected animals. By inoculation the disease can be produced in nearly all warm-blooded animals, including birds. The rabbit is especially suscepitble to inoculation and is commonly used in diagnostic work.

The disease was shown to be caused by a virus by Aujezsky (2) in Hungary
in 1902. It is known to occur in most European countries and in South America. It has been definitely diagnosed in North America in swine and cattle
(Shope, 19; McNutt, 14; Ray, 17; Shahan, Knudson, Seibold, and Dale, 18;
Morrill and Graham, 16) and in dogs (Eidson, Kissling, and Tierkel, 6).
Shope was the first to show that the disease was prevalent in swine in the
midwestern states of the United States and that cases in cattle stemmed from
the swine reservoir. A good review of the literature on this disease is that by
Galloway (7).

**Character of the Disease.** *In cattle.* The name *mad itch* has been applied to
the disease in this species. Intense pruritus of some portion of the skin is the
principal manifestation of the disease. This generally appears on one of the
flanks, or the hind legs, but it may be on any part of the body. If the part is
accessible, the animal begins licking it incessantly until it becomes reddened
and abraded. If the victim can reach a wall, post, or fence, it will rub the part
until the skin is broken and torn. The itching is so intense as to cause the animal to become frenzied. As the disease progresses, the medulla becomes involved, and this leads to paralysis of the pharynx, salivation, forced respiration, and cardiac irregularities. The animal remains conscious until death
approaches. There may be grinding of the teeth, bellowing, mania, and convulsions. Death usually occurs within 48 hours and sometimes much sooner.
Occasional cases die within several hours after signs are first observed and
without showing the pruritic signs.

*In dogs and cats.* Cases in these species seem to be common in some European countries; thus Galloway (7) reports that Marek, in Budapest, had seen
118 cats and 29 dogs in the period between 1902 and 1908. It is not clear why
more cases have not been seen in these species in North America. The signs
are essentially like those in cattle. The animals are driven into a frenzy because of the intolerable itching and do great damage to themselves by biting
and tearing at the affected parts. Bulbar paralysis is generally manifested
early; paralysis of the jaws and of the pharynx appears; plaintive cries and
howls are emitted; and saliva drools from the mouth. The appearance may
simulate rabies but, in contrast to the furious form of rabies, the affected animals show no tendency to attack other animals or man. As in cattle, consciousness is maintained until the end. At no stage is there any fever. In some
cases, especially in cats, the disease may progress so rapidly that death ensues
before pruritic signs have appeared. Death occurs usually within 24 to 36
hours after signs appear.

*In swine.* In this species pruritus does not occur. In adult animals the signs
may be vague and mild, and recovery is the rule rather than the exception.
There may be some fever and mental depression. Some animals vomit. The

animals generally recover completely in from 4 to 8 days. In some sows respiratory signs signal the onset of the disease (9). At this time the temperature is elevated and the sows stop eating on the third day after exposure. Constipation and depression may be accompanied by vomition during the next 2 days. If sows are pregnant about 50 percent will abort and the remainder will farrow. Some pigs will be macerated, others will be normal. Higher percentage of abortions occur in the first month of pregnancy. Late pregnancies may go as high as 17 days beyond the expected date of delivery. In suckling and recently weaned pigs the death losses may be very severe. According to McNutt (14), Ray (17), and Hirt (10), death losses in pigs less than 15 days old are frequently 100 percent. Such animals usually become prostrate within an hour or so from the time the first signs are observed, and they die in from 12 to 24 hours. McNutt says that the losses are directly proportional to the ages of the animals, varying from nil at maturity to 100 percent in the very young.

In experimentally infected animals, the incubation period varies according to the manner in which the virus is administered. When introduced through the skin, a route which probably is the natural one, the incubation period in swine and cattle is from 4 to 7 days, occasionally longer.

The course of the disease varies from 2 to 48 hours, except in swine, in which it may be as long as a week.

The mortality in dogs, cats, cattle, and very young pigs is 100 percent. As pigs become older, the mortality becomes less. In mature stock it is almost nil.

The lesions of this disease are not extensive. In those species in which pruritus occurs, the skin and underlying tissues at the point of infection usually are lacerated, torn, and covered with bloody exudate. The subcutaneous tissue of the region usually is very edematous. The lungs often show congestion and edema, and there may be fluid in the pericardial sac and hemorrhages on the epicardium. The other organs usually are normal. In swine, gross lesions generally are absent, but in adults subcutaneous edema may be found and even necrosis.

Infiltrations and necrosis of nerve elements can be seen by microscopic examination of various parts of the nervous system. These begin where the virus was introduced and proceed centripetally along the nerve trunks. Animals often die before the virus has reached the brain, or even the anterior part of the spinal cord. This should be taken into account when tissues are selected for laboratory diagnosis.

**The Disease in Experimental Animals.** The signs seen in naturally infected cases can be produced experimentally by the inoculation of animals with the virus. A little of the edematous tissue from the lesion in cattle injected subcutaneously in rabbits results in typical mad itch signs. These begin after an incubation period of about 2 days. The animal first licks the point of inoculation, later becomes more frenzied, and bites and tears the skin of this area.

This lasts for 4 to 6 hours, by the end of which time the animal is exhausted. It then lies on its side, shows clonic spasms and labored respiration, and dies. Material from cattle will not infect guinea pigs or mice when inoculated subcutaneously, but, curiously, virus that has been passed through a rabbit brain will cause mad itch signs in these animals (Shope, 21).

According to Hurst (11), who studied the distribution of the virus of pseudorabies in the rabbit, whether the animal is inoculated subcutaneously, intradermally, or intramuscularly, the virus reaches the central nervous system by passage through the peripheral nerves in spite of the fact that virus occurs for a time in the blood. After intracerebral inoculation, virus passes centripetally from the nervous system to the lungs. After intravenous inoculation, the virus rapidly disappears from the blood, forming multiple infective foci in the organs from which it passes through the nerves to the brain. When subcutaneous inoculation is done in an area deprived of its nervous supply, signs are delayed because the virus must then pass from the local area through the blood to establish visceral foci from which the infection of the central nervous system occurs secondarily. Hurst considers this a pantropic virus, that is, one that affects many cells derived from all of the embryonic layers.

When the virus is injected intracerebrally, it is uniformly fatal for rabbits, guinea pigs, rats, and mice. Pruritus of the skin does not occur in such cases. After an incubation period of 24 to 48 hours, signs of excitement are shown and blindness evidently occurs. The animals run about their cages wildly and injure themselves by running into the walls. Salivation and grinding of teeth frequently occur. Death follows after a short period of coma.

McNutt (14) studied the inoculation disease in swine. When virus was injected into the muscles of one leg, a characteristic behavior pattern was shown which varied according to the size and age of the animal. Those that weighed from 30 to 40 pounds usually became ill after an incubation period of 5 to 7 days and died about 2 days later. Larger pigs usually developed paralysis of the inoculated leg. Some of these died, others remained permanently paralyzed, and others recovered. The paralyzed pigs usually had good appetites, were active, had normal temperatures, and were not noticeably excitable. Virus was not found in the blood of most of these animals, or in the visceral organs. It was found regularly, however, in the nerve trunks of the affected legs, and frequently in the spinal cord and brain. Pigs weighing more than 80 pounds seldom showed any appreciable signs, but virus could be recovered from their nervous systems, and virus was discharged in their nasal secretions.

There is good evidence that natural infection in swine occurs by the nasooropharynx route. Gustafson (8) found that intranasal exposure to the virus results in a syndrome seen in natural infections as opposed to those resulting from intramuscular, intratracheal, or intragastric exposures. The primary site of viral multiplication was in the upper respiratory passages and tonsillar tissue. Virus isolations are made as early as 18 hours from olfactory epithelium and tonsils and at 6-to-12-hour intervals thereafter for at least 5 days. Similarly, virus was isolated from the medulla and pons at 24 hours, suggesting transmission from the nasal and oral cavities in the epineural lymph of the 5th and 9th cranial nerves. Virus was not found in the blood during this period.

**Properties of the Virus.** By ultrafiltration the particle size was estimated between 100 to 150 m$\mu$. By electron microscopy it resembles *Herpesvirus hominis* (herpes simplex). The development of the virus probably is completed within the nucleus and as mature particles have a diameter of 120 to 130 m$\mu$. The particle contains DNA with a relatively high content of guanine and cytosine (4). Both pseudorabies and herpes simplex viruses cause an increase of thymidine kinase *in vitro* which are immunologically distinct. It has been suggested that herpes simplex, pseudorabies, and monkey B-viruses share a common antigen that is not involved in the neutralization process.

Shope (19) reported that virus stored in 50 percent glycerol survives for 154 days with little loss of titer at refrigerator temperature. Virus survives on hay for 30 days in summer and 46 days in winter. It is stable between a pH of 4 and 9. One-half percent sodium hydroxide rapidly inactivates it, but 3 percent phenol is considerably less effective. Lyophilized virus survives 2 years; at low temperatures virus in tissue remains viable many years.

**Cultivation.** Traub (26) was the first to report success in cultivating the virus of this disease. He succeeded in obtaining multiplication in media containing minced testicular tissue of rabbits and guinea pigs, and also in minced chick emryo medium. Mesrobeanu (15) obtained growth in chick embroyos in 1938, and his work was quickly confirmed by a series of workers. The virus may easily be passed in series in egg embryos after it has once been adapted. Bang (3) called attention to the fact that the lesions which appear as whitish plaques on the chorioallantoic membrane after about 4 days' incubation are quickly followed by invasion of all parts of the central nervous system. Many strains produce hemorrhagic destruction of the nervous system, which leads to protrusion of the cranium of the embryo.

Tokumaru (25) was able to cultivate the virus in monkey kidney cells after it had first been adapted to eggs. Two cytopathogenic varieties were found; one produced typical cytopathogenic effects, the other a cell-rounding type of degeneration which had previously been described in certain other viruses. The virus also grows in cultures of chick, rabbit, guinea pig, and dog tissues. It causes a cytopathogenic effect and plaques are produced in agar overlays of pig kidney, rabbit kidney, and chick embryo cell cultures. It is suggested that the less virulent strains produce larger plaques. Intranuclear inclusion bodies are found in infected cultures and eggs.

**Immunity.** Practicable methods of immunization have not been developed. Shope (23) has shown that swine which have recovered from the disease have neutralizing antibodies in their sera. Using this technic, he was able to show that the European and the American diseases cross-immunized perfectly and

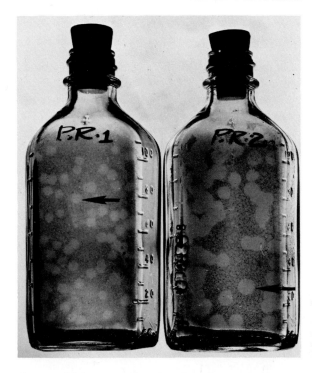

Fig. 190. Comparison of plaque size (*arrow*) and count of pseudo-rabies virus on porcine kidney (*PR1*) and rabbit kidney (*PR2*) monolayers 9 days after virus seeding. (Courtesy K. V. Singh, *Cornell Vet.*)

thus could be considered to be identical (20). The same method showed that swine on a farm where cattle had been lost from this disease had immunizing antibodies in their sera, and also that many swine originating in the midwestern states and being used for the production of anti-hog-cholera serum possessed neutralizing antibodies, whereas similar animals raised in the eastern states lacked them (24). Shahan, Knudson, Seibold, and Dale (18) showed that, after recovery from the disease, swine are thereafter immune to inoculation even by the intracerebral route. These workers were unable to immunize rabbits with formalin-treated brain virus.

**Transmission.** The principal natural reservoir of the virus of pseudorabies is in swine. Symptomless animals harbor and transmit the virus. A minor one, but perhaps important so far as its transmission from farm to farm is concerned, is in the brown rat. Other animal species contract the disease from one of these hosts, most often from swine, but the victims do not transmit it to other individuals. The recognition of the reservoir in swine was made by Köves and Hirt (12) and by Shope (24). The European workers assumed that the virus escaped from swine in the saliva and urine. Shope, however, showed that these fluids were not infectious and that the virus escaped only by way of the nasal secretions. Beginning about the 6th day after inoculation, when there is a concomitant temperature rise, and continuing for several days thereafter, virus is demonstrable in the scanty nasal discharge. Rabbits are easily infected by rubbing a slightly scarified skin surface on the snouts of the pigs during this time.

Shope (22, 24) also showed that the ordinary brown rat, which often frequents corn cribs and animal houses, readily develops pseudorabies by ingestion and suggested that such animals may be the means of carrying the disease from farm to farm. Cassells and Lamont (5) and Lamont and Gordon (13) have described cases in dogs (rat terriers) in Ireland in which it was believed that the infection was derived from killing rats on pig farms.

In the United States mad itch of cattle occurs most often on the feed lots in the midwestern states where range-raised beef cattle are fattened for market. Swine are commonly allowed to run with such cattle to salvage feed wasted by the cattle, and apparently these pigs infect minor wounds on the legs of the cattle.

In coitus, virus may be transmitted from the boar to the sow and vice versa (1). Evidence that this method of transmission takes place was made by the isolation of virus from the prepuce and vagina of infected swine. It is not known whether the virus is secreted with the sperm.

**Diagnosis.** In animals other than swine the clinical signs are quite characteristic and at least suggestive of the diagnosis. A definitive diagnosis may be made by recovering the virus. For this purpose, the edematous fluid of the local lesion, the nerve trunk of the region, parts of the spinal cord, and portions of the brain may be inoculated into rabbits. Virus may be detected as easily by subcutaneous as by intracerebral inoculation, and the former method has two advantages: intercurrent infections are not so apt to kill the rabbits and the characteristic local pruritus is an aid in recognizing the nature of the virus. For final recognition of the virus, virus-neutralization tests may be conducted using known antiserum against the newly recovered virus.

Acidophilic intranuclear inclusion bodies of the Cowdry A type are usually found in the spinal ganglia, in the posterior horn of the spinal cord, in the glia cells in various parts, and in a variety of cells in the local lesions in rabbits, according to Hurst (11). Such inclusions are found irregularly in cattle and do not occur in swine. The inclusions have little diagnostic importance. There are no cytoplasmic inclusions in any species.

**Control.** The available evidence indicates that this disease is transmitted principally by swine, and possibly also by rats. There is little to indicate that other animals are a source of danger. The destruction or control of rats is desirable for many reasons other than their relationship to this disease. Infected lots of swine should be segregated as much as possible, particularly from cattle.

**The Disease in Man.** The danger to man from this disease is apparently slight, but several human cases have been diagnosed in Europe, from some of which it is claimed that virus was isolated. These usually have involved contamination of skin wounds with tissues of infected animals. No fatalities have been reported, but severe pruritus has been noted in some of these cases. The fact that the disease can be produced experimentally in most warm-blooded animals should serve as a warning that some degree of human susceptibility is probable and that infected animals and their tissues should be handled with caution.

## REFERENCES

1. Akkermans. Jour. Am. Vet. Med. Assoc., 1963, *143*, 860.
2. Aujeszky. Centrbl. f. Bakt., I, Abt., Orig., 1902, *32*, 353.
3. Bang. Jour. Exp. Med., 1942, *76*, 263.
4. Ben-porat and Kaplan. Virology, 1962, *16*, 261.
5. Cassals and Lamont. Vet. Rec., 1942, *54*, 21.
6. Eidson, Kissling, and Tierkel. Jour. Am. Vet. Med. Assoc., 1953, *123*, 34.
7. Galloway. Vet. Rec., 1938, *50*, 745.
8. Gustafson. Diseases of Swine (ed. by H. W. Dunne), 2d ed., Iowa State Univ. Press, Ames, Iowa, 1970.
9. Gustafson, Claflin, and Saunders. Fed. Proc., 1968, *27*, No. 2, 425.
10. Hirt. Arch. f. Tierheilk., 1935, *70*, 86.
11. Hurst. Jour. Exp. Med., 1934, *59*, 729.
12. Köves and Hirt. Arch f. Tierheilk., 1934, *68*, 1.
13. Lamont and Gordon. Vet. Rec., 1950, *62*, 596.
14. McNutt. North Am. Vet., 1943, *24*, 409.
15. Mesrobeanu. Comp. rend. Soc. Biol. (Paris), 1938, *127*, 1183.
16. Morrill and Graham. Am. Jour. Vet. Res., 1941, *2*, 35.
17. Ray. Vet. Med., 1943, *38*, 178.
18. Shahan, Knudson, Seibold, and Dale. North Am. Vet., 1947, *28*, 440.
19. Shope. Jour. Exp. Med., 1931, *54*, 233.
20. Shope. Proc. Soc. Exp. Biol. and Med., 1932, *30*, 308.
21. Shope. Jour. Exp. Med., 1933, *57*, 925.
22. Shope. Science, 1934, *80*, 102.
23. Shope. Jour. Exp. Med., 1935, *62*, 85.
24. *Ibid.*, 101.
25. Tokumaru. Proc. Soc. Exp. Biol. and Med., 1957, *96*, 55.
26. Traub. Jour. Exp. Med., 1933, *58*, 663.

## Porcine Inclusion-Body Rhinitis

SYNONYM: Cytomegalic inclusion disease (CID) of pigs

This disease is caused by a cytomegalovirus or type B herpesvirus. It was first described by Done (1). From a clinical standpoint it is principally a disease of the respiratory tract accompanied by anemia in pigs less than 4 weeks of age.

It has been reported in most countries where pigs are raised. The incidence in Great Britain is about 50 percent while in Iowa a 12 percent attack rate has been reported. Infection is probably transmitted by infected sows, with no signs of illness, to piglets by the aerosol route.

The severity of the disease depends upon the age of the pig and the amount of colostrally acquired immunity (2). In the acute form of the disease, the signs of illness usually appear between 5 and 10 days after birth. Initial signs include sneezing, presence of nasal exudate, and inappetence probably due to obstructed nasal passages making suckling very difficult. This is followed by rapid loss of weight, paralysis, and death as early as 5 days later. Survivors are often stunted and secondary bacterial infections complicate the disease picture. Subacute infections generally occur in pigs over 2 weeks of age with clinical signs limited to the respiratory tract. In this age group the morbidity and mortality are low. A severe anemia occurs in clinically affected pigs despite iron therapy.

At necropsy there is a mucopurulent rhinitis, sinusitis, and sometimes turbinate atrophy. In severe cases piglets may show petechial hemorrhages in kidneys and myocardium. Microscopically, there are intranuclear inclusion bodies in enlarged cells in many organs, including the brain and especially in the tubuloalveolar glands of the nasal mucosa.

The virus is propagated in primary pig-lung cell cultures with the production of a cytopathic effect in 11 to 18 days postinoculation (3). Intranuclear inclusion bodies are formed in cell cultures.

There is no evidence that the virus causes disease in man.

**REFERENCES**

1.　Done.　Vet. Rec., 1955, 67, 525.
2.　Gustafson.　Personal communication, 1972.
3.　L'Ecuyer and Corner.　Canad. Jour. Comp. Med. and Vet. Sci., 1966, 30, 321.

### Feline Virus Rhinotracheitis

This virus possesses the properties of the genus *Herpesvirus*. The disease occurs in the Eastern and Western Hemispheres, principally, as a respiratory infection.

The virus was first isolated in 1957 by Crandell and Maurer (5) from young kittens with a respiratory disease. The first European isolation was made by Bürki in 1963 (3). It is now recognized that feline viral rhinotracheitis (FVR) is a very important disease of the domestic cat and one of a number of viruses involved in respiratory disease of this species.

An excellent short review of this disease is given by Crandell (4).

**Character of the Disease.** The respiratory disease varies markedly from an inapparent condition to severe respiratory involvement terminating in death. The disease principally affects the upper respiratory tract and is characterized by sudden onset; transient fever; neutrophilic leukocytosis; paroxsymal sneezing and coughing; nasal, turbinate, and conjunctival exudate; difficult breathing; and anorexia and weight loss (4, fig. 191). A similar picture is seen in germfree cats suggesting that the severity of FVR is not dependent on the secondary activity of respiratory microbes (8). Eosinophilic intranuclear inclusion bodies are associated with extensive nasal epithelial necrosis and

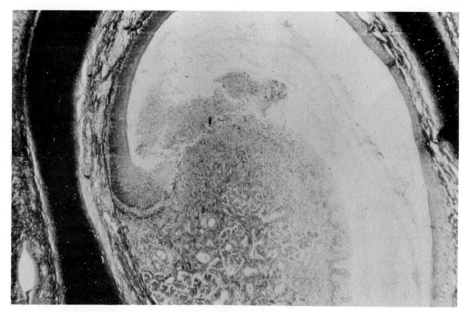

*Fig. 191.* Feline herpesvirus infection. Ulcerative area with cellular reaction in the turbinate. H and E. X 4. (Courtesy T. Walton and J. Gillespie, *Cornell Vet.*)

focal epithelial necrosis in the conjunctiva, tonsils, epiglottis, larynx, trachea, and rarely bronchi or bronchioles (8). Laryngotracheal lesions usually are mild and pulmonary lesions are rare with confinement to the bronchi and bronchioles. In natural cases pneumonia may occur as a result of secondary bacterial infection. In separate experimental studies in conventional cats (15) and in germfree cats (8), lingual ulceration was not observed, but it has been observed in feline calicivirus (picornavirus) infection (11).

In addition to resorption of turbinate bone in conventional cats (6) Hoover (8) observed severe osteolytic lesions simulating overt necrosis of bone in the turbinates of some germfree cats with FVR infection.

In experimental studies pathogen-free queens given FVR virus intravenously in the late stages of gestation (7th or 8th week) had stillborn fetuses (9). Other animal herpesviruses are known to have a similar effect under natural conditions and it is possible that feline herpesvirus may do likewise. Likewise, the inoculation of feline herpesvirus intracerebrally causes fatal encephalitis (8) so we may anticipate occasional natural cases, especially in neonatal kittens.

**Properties of the Virus.** The nuclear particles have an average diameter of 148 m$\mu$, consisting of a central dense core surrounded by a clear zone bounded by an outer membrane (4). Cytoplasmic particles vary in size from 128 to 167 m$\mu$ in diameter while extracellular particles are 164 m$\mu$ in diameter. The enveloped particle of cubic symmetry has 162 capsomeres. (fig. 192) It is a DNA virus (4) which is pH-labile and sensitive to ether and chloroform (1, 4).

The virus is highly species-specific, having been isolated only from the domestic cat. In all likelihood it causes infection in other members of the cat family.

Hemagglutinating and hemadsorbing properties of the virus have been demonstrated by utilizing feline red blood cells (7). A hemagglutination test was developed to detect feline herpes antibodies.

Many strains of feline herpesvirus have been compared by various investigators in the United States and Europe with the conclusion that only 1 sero-

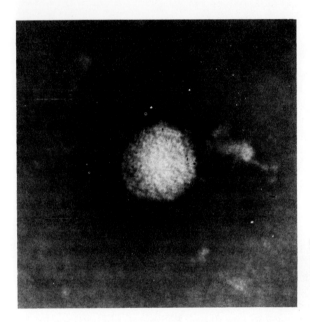

Fig. 192. Feline herpesvirus particle, stained with phosphotungstic acid, showing capsomeres and other structures characteristic of this genus. X 191,000. (Courtesy J. Strandberg, D. Kahn, P. Bartholomew, and J. Gillespie.)

type of feline respiratory herpesvirus is known to exist.° There is no serological relationship between FVR and feline panleukopenia, infectious bovine rhinotracheitis, pseudorabies, certain feline caliciviruses, and herpes simplex viruses as demonstrated by the neutralization test. By complement-fixation test, no antigenic relationship was demonstrated between FVR virus and certain feline caliciviruses (6) and the human adenovirus group.

**Cultivation.** The virus replicates and produces a cytopathic effect in cell cultures of feline origin (4) (fig. 193). Although tests have not been exhaustive in cell cultures, cytopathology of FVR virus is limited to cultures of feline origin (12).

---

° Recently, C. G. Fabricant and J. H. Gillespie isolated another feline herpesvirus serotype. Its significance as a feline pathogen is still to be determined.

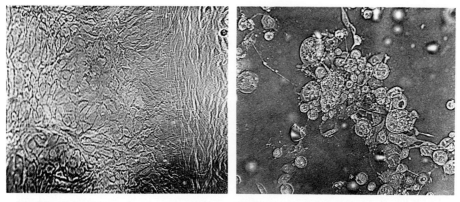

Fig. 193. Feline herpesvirus in feline kidney cell culture. Uninoculated monolayer (*left*) and inoculated culture showing characteristic CPE of a herpesvirus (*right*). (Courtesy T. Walton and J. Gillespie, *Cornell Vet.*)

The characteristic feature of its cytopathic effect is the formation of intranuclear inclusion bodies (fig. 194). Multinucleated giant cells or syncytia also are formed in cell cultures. Macroscopic plaques in cultures under agar are readily produced by many strains. The appearance of the cytopathic effect is dose-dependent but as a rule it is observed within 24 to 72 hours and reaches a maximum titer of $10^4$ to $10^6$ $TCID_{50}$ per 0.1 ml.

**Immunity.** Clearly, complete and undisputable knowledge about the immunity

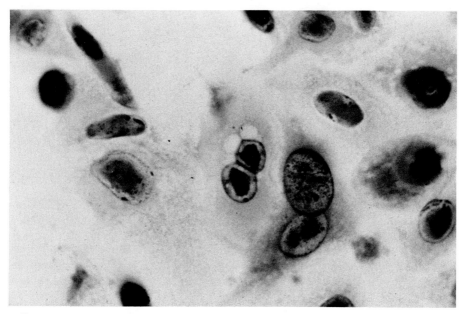

Fig. 194. Typical Cowdry type A intranuclear inclusion bodies caused by feline herpesvirus. May-Grünwald-Giemsa stain. X 430. (Courtesy F. Scott.)

to feline herpesvirus in cats is lacking. An evaluation of the present literature suggests that cats in the convalescent stage are completely immune even though some may lack neutralizing antibody at 21 days and a partial but significant immunity still exists after 5 months.

In experimental studies Walton and Gillespie (15) confirmed earlier reports that the initial antibody response after intranasal infection produced little or no neutralizing antibody (1, 4). In addition, the kitten challenged by aerosol route at 21 days did not respond clinically or excrete virus, but serum-neutralizing antibody titers increased significantly (1, 15). When challenged by the aerosol route at 150 days the serum titers of the kittens as a group were significantly lower, and the animals showed only mild signs of illness, with some kittens excreting virus for up to 6 days (15). Johnson and Thomas (10) have associated resistance to infection in older cats with and without detectable antibody levels. A transient antibody response was observed by Povey and Johnson (13) in recovered cats with the development of febrile reaction only upon challenge with virulent virus. They also reported a relatively persistent antibody response in cats that were resistant to challenge. Very little information is available in regard to the serological response following inoculations by routes other than intranasal.

**Transmission.** All evidence suggests that the infection is transmitted by cats to cats, presumably by the respiratory route. Cats that recover from disease may become carriers with localization occurring principally in the pharyngeal region (14).

**Diagnosis.** To distinguish respiratory disease in the cat caused by FVR virus from other respiratory conditions with other etiologies is difficult, if not impossible.

Successful isolation of the virus is achieved during the acute febrile stage of disease with sterile swabs applied to the pharynx, nasal passages, and conjunctiva in that order. This material is inoculated into cell cultures of feline origin, and with positive material a cytopathic effect is seen. The virus in a tissue-culture system can be quickly identified by a knowledge of its virus properties as described earlier and by the use of the fluorescent antibody test. The latter test can also be applied with good results (2) directly to smear preparations of the conjunctiva, and logically from other infected tissues as well.

**Control.** At present no vaccine is available for the control and prevention of this disease. There is a definite need for a good vaccine as an appreciable number of feline respiratory cases are caused by feline herpesvirus.

Herpesvirus infection in a cattery causes great problems. With the periodic appearance of susceptible kittens in the group that has carriers the disease remains endemic. Depopulation is often impossible so the disease persists as a major problem.

**The Disease in Man.** There is no evidence that feline herpesvirus causes disease in man.

## REFERENCES

1.  Bartholomew and Gillespie.   Cornell Vet., 1968, 58, 248.
2.  Bistner, Carlson, Shively, and Scott.   Jour. Am. Vet. Med. Assoc., 1971, 159, 1223.
3.  Bürki.   17th World Vet. Cong., (Hannover), 5/A/90, 1963, 559.
4.  Crandell.   Jour. Am. Vet. Med. Assoc., 1971, 158, 922.
5.  Crandell and Maurer.   Proc. Soc. Expt. Biol. and Med., 1958, 97, 487.
6.  Crandell, Rehkemper, Niemann, Ganaway, and Mauer.   Jour. Am. Vet. Med. Assoc., 1961, 138, 191.
7.  Gillespie, Judkins, and Scott.   Cornell Vet., 1971, 61, 159.
8.  Hoover and Griesemer.   Jour. Am. Vet. Med. Assoc., 1971, 158, 929.
9.  Johnson.   Jour. Exp. Med., 1964, 120, 359.
10.  Johnson and Thomas.   Vet. Rec., 1966, 79, 188.
11.  Kahn and Gillespie.   Cornell Vet., 1970, 60, 669.
12.  Lee, Kniazeff, Fabricant, and Gillespie.   Ibid., 1969, 59, 539.
13.  Povey and Johnson.   Vet. Rec., 1967, 81, 686.
14.  Walton and Gillespie.   Cornell Vet., 1970, 60, 215.
15.  Ibid., 232.

## Canine Herpesvirus Infection

A fatal septicemic disease of infant puppies caused by a herpeslike virus was described by Carmichael *et al.* (3). A virus with characteristics of herpesviruses also was recovered by Stewart (7) from young puppies that died of a hemorrhagic disease.

So far as is known, only dogs are susceptible, and fatal infections have been reported only in puppies less than 2 weeks of age. Mild rhinitis and vaginitis are the only signs of illness in older dogs inoculated with virus.

The disease has been observed in the United States, Great Britain, and Europe. Serologic studies indicate that the virus is widespread in the eastern and southeastern United States.

**Character of the Disease.** At the present time, severe disease has been recognized only in puppies less than 1 month of age. Fatal illness occurs in those less than 2 weeks of age. Signs in older dogs inoculated with virus were limited to mild rhinitis or vaginitis. The illness in infant puppies starts between the 5th and 14th day after birth with a soft, odorless stool that is yellowish-green in color, and with anorexia, labored breathing, abdominal pain, and painful crying as the principal signs.

The incubation period varies between 3 and 8 days in puppies inoculated by intranasal instillation or by intraperitoneal injection. The route of inoculation and virus dose does not appear to be related to the time of onset of signs or the severity of illness.

The course of the disease is short in puppies, most animals die within 24 to 48 hours after the onset of clinical manifestations. Signs of illness in older dogs are very mild, and the actual duration of the infection is not known.

Virus has been isolated from the nasopharynx of inoculated dogs for periods up to 21 days.

Pathologic changes are characteristic. Lesions in inoculated and naturally infected puppies consist of disseminated focal necrosis and hemorrhages. These lesions may be found in virtually all of the organs. Especially note-worthy changes occur in the kidneys, where subcapsular hemorrhages appear as bright red spots on the gray background of necrotic cortical tissue. The lungs are diffusely pneumonic. Focal necrosis and hemorrhages also are com-mon in the liver, intestinal tract, and adrenal glands. Spleens characteris-tically are enlarged. Meningoencephalitic lesions are frequently found and virus isolated even though clinical signs are lacking (5, 6).

In pathogenesis studies of the dog, Carmichael (2) suggested that virus en-ters the body by the oral or nasal routes with oral, nasal, vaginal excretions serving as the source of infection for susceptible dogs. Primary viral replica-tion takes place in the tonsils, nasal turbinate, mucosa, and pharynx. The virus is transported in the blood where it is associated with the leukocytes. Secondary viral replication takes place in blood vessels; reticuloendothelial cells of spleen, liver, and lymph nodes; parenchyma of liver, lungs, kidneys, spleen, and adrenal glands; lamina propria of intestinal tract; meninges; and brain.

Body temperature and its regulation is an important factor in the pathoge-nesis in infant pups (2, 5). By maintaining puppies that were inoculated with virus at 1 day of age in an environment that increased their body temperature from 38.4 to 39.5 C, survival was prolonged and viral growth was diminished (2). This phenomenon doesn't entirely explain the age resistance associated with canine herpesvirus (CHV) infection in their opinions.

The role of CHV in tracheobronchitis needs to be clarified (6), although it is unlikely that it is involved in the etiology of this disease (4).

**Properties of the Virus.** Virus particles in thin sections of dog kidney cells have an average diameter of 142 millimicrons. The particles contain a DNA core surrounded by two membranes. The protein coat is composed of 162 sub-units, a characteristic shared by other herpesviruses. The virus is inactivated by chloroform and ether, and is destroyed in less than 4 minutes at 56 C. In-fectivity is reduced by 50 percent after 5 hours at 37 C. Virus titers are main-tained for months at $-70$ C in virus stocks that contain 10 percent serum. Infectivity is lost below pH 4.5 after 30 minutes. Hemagglutination has not been demonstrated with erythrocytes from a variety of species. The virus is not related serologically to infectious canine hepatitis, distemper, infectious bovine rhinotracheitis, equine rhinopneumonitis, avian laryngotracheitis, or herpes simplex viruses.

**Cultivation.** This virus grows readily in dog kidney cell cultures. Characteris-tic cytopathic effects occur in susceptible cell cultures, beginning 12 to 16 hours after inoculation. Cytopathic effects consist of focal areas of rounded and degenerating cells that detach from the glass of the culture tube. Cells occasionally have faintly acidophilic intranuclear inclusion bodies. More typical intranuclear changes, however, consist of dissolution of chromatin and the formation of basophilic nucleoprotein bodies that are often most numerous adjacent to the nuclear membrane.

A plaque reduction test was developed by Binn *et al.* (1) for comparing antigenic relationships of various strains of CHV and no significant antigenic differences were noted in the comparison of four United States isolates.

**Immunity.** Puppies from inoculated pregnant females that had antibody titers at the time of inoculation did not develop illness. In contrast, susceptible pregnant females that were inoculated intravaginally with virus gave birth to puppies all of which died within 2 weeks. Virus was recovered from the dead puppies. It has been observed that females whose puppies died naturally of the disease gave birth 1 year later to normal puppies. Neutralizing antibodies develop in older dogs inoculated with the virus; however, the duration of immunity is not known. The need for a vaccine does not presently seem great, and none is available at the present time (2).

**Transmission.** The natural route of transmission is by inhalation or ingestion or both. Infections occurred in puppies whose mothers were inoculated intravaginally 2 weeks before whelping. Transmission by droplet infection has been observed between older inoculated dogs placed in close contact with uninoculated animals.

**Diagnosis.** The uncomplicated disease in older dogs is so mild that it probably is unnoticed, however, the disease-producing potential of this virus has not been fully explored. Pathological changes in affected puppies are characteristic. Necrotic and hemorrhagic lesions in the liver, lungs, and kidneys of dead puppies suggest this viral infection. Focal renal hemorrhages have not been reported in dogs infected with canine hepatitis or distemper viruses. Microscopic examination will reveal characteristic intranuclear inclusions in cells in areas of necrosis. These must be differentiated from canine hepatitis inclusions. Virus is isolated readily from tissues of dead puppies in dog kidney cell cultures.

The neutralization or complement-fixation tests can be used to demonstrate antibody (5), but CF antibodies are not present in sera of all convalescent dogs and they often disappear by 1 to 2 months after exposure. Neutralizing antibody titers are produced in low titer, which generally persist longer than CF antibody. Neutralizing titers can be increased two- to eight-fold by the addition of four units of guinea-pig complement ($C^1$).

**The Disease in Man.** There is no evidence that the canine herpesvirus is pathogenic for man.

## REFERENCES

1. Binn, Koughan, and Lazar. Jour. Am. Vet. Med. Assoc., 1970, *165*, 1724.
2. Carmichael, Squire, and Krook. Am. Jour. Vet. Res., 1965, *26*, 803.
3. Carmichael. Jour. Am. Vet. Med. Assoc., 1970, *156*, 1714.

4.  Gillespie, Carmichael, Gourlay, Dinsmore, Abbott, Binn, Cabasso, Fox, Gorham, Ott, Peacock, Sharpless, Decker, and Freeman.  Panel Members, Canine Symposium, AVMA. *Ibid.*, 1970, *156*, 1669.
5.  Huxsoll and Hemelt.  *Ibid.*, 1970, *156*, 1706.
6.  Percy.  *Ibid.*, 1970, *156*, 1721.
7.  Stewart, David, Ferreira, Lovelace, Landon, and Stock.  Science, 1965, *148*, 1341.

### Avian Infectious Laryngotracheitis

Until a few years ago a variety of diseases of the respiratory tract of birds were grouped together under the name *roup*. These have been differentiated during recent years into nutritional, bacterial, parasitic, and virus disorders. Infectious laryngotracheitis was shown, by Beach (1) in 1930, to be a specific virus diesase. First recognized in the United States, it is now known to exist in nearly all parts of the world where poultry are kept. The disease affects chickens and occasionally pheasants. Other types of birds are wholly immune. **Character of the Disease.** Infectious laryngotracheitis affects chickens of all ages. It is highly contagious, and when it enters a susceptible flock the disease does not stop until practically every bird has been attacked. Infection occurs through the respiratory tract. The incubation period is short, less than 48 hours as a rule. The course of the disease is acute, some birds dying within 24 hours of the time the infection is first detected, others running a course as long as 5 or 6 days. Birds that do not die during the first 5 days of signs practically always recover. Recovery generally is rapid. Although no single bird will show evidence of disease for as long as a week, the disease may require 3 or 4 weeks to run through a flock. An important fact is that a considerable number of recovered birds continue to harbor the virus, and such birds

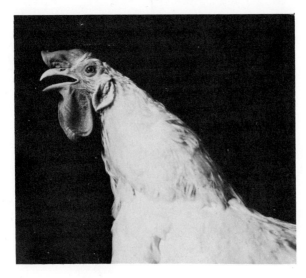

Fig. 195.  Infectious laryngotracheitis, showing the characteristic gasping type of respiration. (Courtesy E. L. Brunett.)

usually act as centers of new infections when transferred to new flocks, or when new birds are added, perhaps a season or more later (Gibbs, 9).

The signs depend upon the age of the birds and the season of the year. Young birds during the warm months usually are less severely affected, and the mortality rate is lower than in older birds during cold weather. Affected birds show respiratory embarrassment varying in degree. In severe cases the chickens extend their necks, open their mouths, and inhale in a gasping manner. Gurgling and rattling sounds are often heard. Sometimes they are best described as whistling. These sounds are due to partial obstruction of the air passages by exudate. Not all birds show marked respiratory embarrassment since the exudate sometimes is in the nasal passages or nasal sinuses. In mature birds in heavy production the mortality rate may be as high as 70 percent. Death appears to be due largely to suffocation.

The lesions are confined to the larynx, trachea, and bronchi. These are reddened, petechiated, and covered with a slimy exudate containing streaks of bright-red blood. Sometimes the exudate is of a caseous nature, and plugs of such material may wholly block the trachea.

In 1931 Seifried (11) described intranuclear inclusion bodies in the nuclei of the cells of the epithelium of tracheal lesions. Burnet (5) found similar bodies in the ectodermal cell lesions of the membranes of infected eggs.

**Properties of the Virus.** Beach (1), who first identified the virus of this disease, found that it could be filtered readily through Berkefeld V filters but not in every case through Berkefeld N filters. Gibbs (10) estimated the size of the virus elements as between 45 and 85 millimicrons. More recent evidence suggests that the particle is larger, and in size and structure it appears to resemble other herpesviruses (8). The virus is present only in the air passages and is infective only by introduction in this way, except that, rarely, infections can be established by intravenous inoculation. Injections subcutaneously, intramuscularly, and intraperitoneally are harmless.

The virus is moderately resistant. Premises do not retain effective quantities of virus for long after infected and carrier birds are removed. Beaudette and Hudson (4) reported that egg-propagated virus, when dried and kept in a refrigerator, retained its potency and immunizing properties for 421 days.

**Cultivation.** The virus of infectious laryngotracheitis was cultivated on the chorioallantoic membrane of developing chick embryos by Burnet (5) in 1934, by Brandly (7) in 1936, and by many others shortly afterward. The virus produces whitish plaques on the membrane. Two kinds of plaques have been described, but immunologically the viruses appear to be identical. Diluted viruses, according to Burnet (6), can be roughly assayed for virulence by counting the number of plaques produced per volume of virus.

**Immunity.** Birds that recover from this disease are solidly immune for the remainder of their lives. Many of these birds are virus carriers; hence when the disease has once occurred in a flock, annual recurrences of the disease must be expected in the young stock unless they are artificially immunized. In small flocks it is often simpler and less expensive to dispose of all old stock.

Beaudette and Hudson (3) developed a method of actively immunizing birds to infectious laryngotracheitis which has proved to be very successful. After trying modified viruses with unsatisfactory results, they hit upon the idea of using fully virulent material on the mucous membrane of the bursa of Fabricius, which is an outpouching of the cloaca. In this location the virus sets up a harmless inflammatory reaction that immunizes solidly. This method has been extensively employed. Its principal objection is that it utilizes a fully virulent disease-producing agent, which, if carelessly used, may do much damage. It should not be used until it is absolutely certain that the flock contains the infection. Full immunity is not developed until about 9 days after treatment (2).

The virus for the cloacal method of vaccination may be obtained directly from the trachea of diseased birds, or it may be virus that has been propagated on egg embryo membranes. Most of the commercially made vaccines are now manufactured by the chick embryo method. Commercially the virus usually is dried and shipped in sealed vacuum tubes with a separate container of glycerol-water mixture in which to suspend it prior to use. The virus mixture is applied with a stiff brush directly on the mucous membrane of the bursa, care being taken not to soil the feathers or to spill any vaccine. Five days later it is well to catch and examine a few birds to make sure that "takes" have occurred. If the vaccine has been potent and the work properly done, most of the birds will show swelling, inflammation, and a small amount of exudate at the point of inoculation. If the vaccine has not produced a high percentage of "takes," the flock should immediately be revaccinated with fresh vaccine, since virus has been introduced into the flock and a serious outbreak of tracheal infections is sure to develop otherwise.

In 1963 Shibley et al. (12) described the preparation and standardization of strain 146 for use as a conjunctivally administered vaccine. It causes conjunctivitis without production of permanent tissue damage. Neutralizing antibodies were still present 372 days postvaccination.

In flocks in which the disease has occurred in previous years, vaccination of the young stock should be done in the summer months after the birds are at least 6 weeks of age, preferably when they are about 4 months old. All birds on the premises must be vaccinated.

**Transmission.** The disease is transmitted naturally through droplet infection.

**Diagnosis.** Ordinarily after disease is well under way in a flock, a diagnosis can be made easily on the basis of signs and lesions. In individual birds it may not be so simple. If the question is sufficiently important to warrant the trouble, the answer can be obtained by swabbing the larynx of one or two susceptible birds with tracheal exudate from the suspected cases. These birds should develop signs some time between 2 and 5 days later if the disease is laryngotracheitis. If immunized birds are included in the test, they should prove resistant while the others sicken.

**The Disease in Man.** Infectious laryngotracheitis of poultry does not affect any mammals, including man, so far as is known.

## REFERENCES

1. Beach. Science, 1930, 72, 633.
2. Beaudette. Vet. Med., 1939, 34, 743.
3. Beaudette and Hudson. Jour. Am. Vet. Med. Assoc., 1933, 82, 460.
4. Ibid., 1939, 75, 333.
5. Burnet. Brit. Jour. Exp. Path., 1934, 15, 52.
6. Burnet. Jour. Exp. Med., 1936, 63, 685.
7. Brandly. Jour. Am. Vet. Med. Assoc., 1936, 88, 587.
8. Cruickshank, Berry, and Hay. Virology, 1963, 20, 376.
9. Gibbs. Jour. Inf. Dis., 1933, 53, 169.
10. Gibbs. Jour. Bact., 1935, 30, 411.
11. Seifried. Jour. Exp. Med., 1931, 54, 817.
12. Shibley, Luginbuhl, and Helmboldt. Avian Dis., 1963, 7, 184.

## Marek's Disease

SYNONYMS: Polyneuritis, neuritis, neurolymphomatosis gallinarum, range-paralysis, neural leukosis, skin leukosis, gray eye, fish eye, iritis, and uveitis.

There now is rather good proof that two viruses are involved in the production of the various forms of this avian leukosis complex (1). One group of isolates termed the leukosis viruses is now believed to produce visceral lymphomatosis, erythroblastosis, myeloblastosis, and possibly osteopetrosis (16). In 1962 it was proposed that the nephroblastoma produced by the BAI strain A should be considered as an additional type-tumor in this group (15). The virus strains of the Marek group cause neurolymphomastosis, ocular lymphomatosis, and to a lesser degree a form of visceral lymphomatosis. All the various forms included in the complex have been reproduced by experimental inoculation of filtrates.

The majority of the so-called avian leukosis cases are caused by the avian herpesvirus, a member of B-group of cell-associated herpesviruses. The chicken is the primary host for the virus, but it also is found in turkeys, pheasants, and possibly quail. Similar lesions are observed in the pigeon, duck, goose, canary, budgerigar, and sivan (17). The economic loss in chickens as a result of Marek's disease is extremely high, and it is the major disease of chicken flocks throughout the world. It is an acute fulminating type of oncogenic disease in young chicks that spreads quite rapidly.

**Character of the Disease.** Marek's disease is *lymphoproliferative*. It affects primarily the nervous system, but visceral organs and other tissues may also be involved. The disease is seen most often in young birds about the time they are turned out on the range, but it sometimes occurs as early as 3 or 4 weeks and sometimes after a year of age. The disease is manifested by a flaccid or spastic paralysis of a leg, wing, or, less commonly, the neck. Sometimes both legs or wings are affected but more commonly the disease is unilateral. The affected wing droops and may brush the ground as the bird walks. Affected legs usually are stretched forward or backward, and, when the disease has progressed far, the bird is unable to stand or walk. When the neck is affected, the head is depressed or there may be twisting (torticollis). The location and intensity of the paralysis varies widely in different birds in the same flock.

The gross lesions consist of a grayish-white swelling of localized areas of the principal nerve trunks of the region involved. When there is leg involvement, this swelling generally is found in the sciatic nerve on the inside of the thigh. By comparing the size of the nerve trunks on the two sides of the bird, even small tumors can be detected, but generally the growths are sufficiently great to be readily observed. Histological examination of the swollen nerve trunks shows extensive infiltration of small round cells, which generally cannot be distinguished from lymphocytes but sometimes appear like mononuclear cells or histiocytes. The lesion may be edematous, and there may be myelin degeneration of the nerve sheaths, but degeneration of the neuraxons is not conspicuous.

The Marek group of viruses are probably responsible for ocular lymphomatosis. The disease is manifested by a diffuse bluish-gray fading of the iris of one or both eyes. Depigmentation sometimes occurs in a spotty fashion and sometimes in the form of annular fading. The pupils frequently become irregular in outline. Histologically infiltrations of lymphocytic or mononuclear cells are found in the iris, and often there are similar infiltrations in the optic nerve. This form of the disease usually occurs in flocks affected with neurolymphomatosis, but the condition generally appears later in life. Many pathologists consider that it represents a latent form of neurolymphomatosis.

The visceral form of lymphoid tumors commonly involves the gonad, liver, lung, and skin. All degrees of severity are seen. In the most acute forms the disease may be observed in birds as early as 6 to 8 weeks of age. Morbidity and mortality may exceed 50 percent of the flock. The disease also may occur in older birds.

Pathogenic strains of virus produce signs of illness and lesions in genetically susceptible chicks, such as line 7 or Cornell 5, in 18 to 21 days when chicks are inoculated at 1 day of age.

**Properties of the Virus.** The herpesvirus of Marek's disease belongs to the cytomegalovirus or B-Group of cell-associated herpes viruses. All field isolates appear to be antigenically identical as they cross-react in the agar-gel precipitin and fluorescent antibody tests (4, 11), however, some are altered somewhat after cell culture passage (6). A herpesvirus isolated from turkeys is antigenically similar to Marek's disease virus and is nonpathogenic for chickens and turkeys (18).

The DNA virus particles are 85 to 100 m$\mu$ in diameter and the capsid has 162 hollow cylindrical capsomeres. The particles from feather follicles have a similar morphology but a loose irregular envelope up to 400 mμ in diameter. The extracted DNA has a high guanine-cytosine content characteristic of cytomegaloviruses.

Marek's disease virus is highly cell-associated and whole cells must be used as inoculum from all of the infected bird's tissues except from the feather follicles where the virus is excreted (2, fig. 196). Storage of virus-containing cells requires conditions essential for their preservation, utilizing the addition of dimethyl-sulfoxide, slow freezing, and holding preferably at 196 C. Viral preparations from feather follicles remain infectious after lyophilization and maintenance at room temperature.

Antibody can be demonstrated in serums of recovered birds by agar-gel precipitin (4), indirect fluorescent antibody (11) or passive hemagglutination tests (10). In the precipitin test up to 6 lines may form with the major line referred to as the precipitin line. This test is most widely used for the detection of antibody to Marek's disease. The indirect fluorescent antibody test is used to distinguish between Marek's disease and the herpes virus of turkeys.

**Cultivation.** Marek's disease virus produces CPE plaques in duck embryo fi-

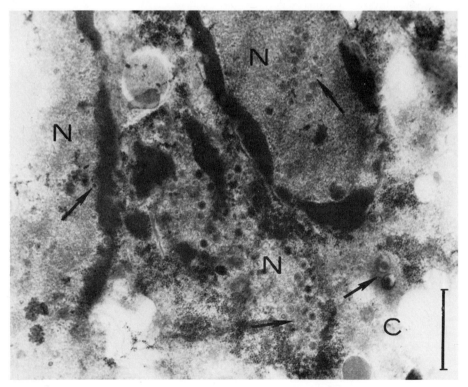

*Fig. 196.* Marek's disease. In the nucleus (*N*) naked, incomplete virions are found but in the cytoplasm (*C*) of the infected feather follicle numerous enveloped particles are observed. Scale—micron. (Courtesy B. Calnek.)

broblasts and in chick kidney cell cultures (5, 14). The plaques appear in 6 to 14 days consisting of rounded and fusiform cells and polykaryocytes containing Cowdry type A intranuclear inclusion bodies. Naked and occasionally enveloped virus particles are seen in the nucleus of the infected cells and occasionally in the cytoplasm.

The virus produces pocks on chorioallantoic membrane of embryonated hens' eggs when inoculated at 4 to 6 days of age by the yolk-sac route or at 10 to 11 days of age by the chorioallantoic membrane route. The yolk-sac route is preferred.

**Immunity.** Although there is no effective immunity to infection, resistance of chickens to tumor formation may be affected by the genetic line of the chicken (8, 9), age of infection (12), antibody status of the dam (3), and exposure to avirulent viruses (7, 13, 18). The resistance of chickens to tumor formation may be evaluated by intra-abdominal challenge with virulent virus or by exposure to infected chickens. To be a valid test, known susceptible controls must be challenged in a similar manner at the same time. A satisfactory challenge response is achieved in 6 to 20 weeks depending upon the virulence of the challenge virus, age of chicken, and the susceptibility of the chick line.

Passive immunity conferred by the dam may persist for 3 weeks after hatching. It will delay the onset and reduce the incidence of disease in birds chal-

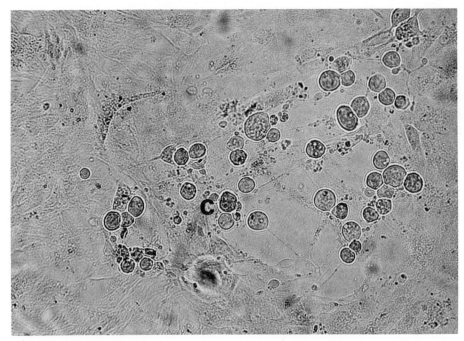

*Fig. 197.* CPE (*C*) caused by Marek's virus in chicken kidney cell culture, unstained. X 270. (Courtesy B. Calnek and S. Madin, *Am. Jour. Vet. Res.*)

lenged at 1 day of age by a natural route. It has little effect when birds are challenged intra-abdominally (3).

The indirect-hemagglutination antibody titer of chickens infected with Marek's disease virus suggests a direct relationship with the chicken's ability to survive the disease (10).

**Transmission.** Most birds have antibody to Marek's disease by the time of maturity. Infection persists in birds for long periods of time, possibly for life. Congenital (vertical) infection probably does not occur, so embryos and young chicks are free of virus and susceptible. Consequently, transmission of the disease occurs after the maternal immunity subsides by 3 weeks of age and by exposure to infected chickens or an environment with persisting virus in excreta, litter, and poultry house dust.

**Diagnosis.** Gross and/or microscopic lesions in nerves or viscera, presence of specific antigen in feather follicles demonstrated by immunofluorescence test, virus isolation in cell culture, or demonstration of antibody are all suitable methods of diagnosis.

Virus isolation can be made in cell culture with infected cells or with virus from feather follicles but it is 10-to-1,000-fold less sensitive than chicken inoculation (19). Direct cultivation of cells in culture from test chickens is more sensitive than inoculation of cell suspensions on monolayers of susceptible cell cultures.

If the passive hemagglutination test is used, a positive serum has a titer of 1:16 or greater (10). The agar-gel test is most widely used for detection of antibody and also for distinguishing between virulent and attenuated tissue cultured strains.

**Control.** Present knowledge makes it possible to develop a flock which is free of Marek's disease virus. Such flocks can be kept free of the infection by strict isolation, constant surveillance, and frequent monitoring for virus and antibody.

Commercial vaccines are now available that contain the herpesvirus of turkeys which is nonpathogenic for chickens and turkeys. This vaccine is effective in the prevention of the disease (tumor formation).

**The Disease in Man.** It is not known to occur.

## REFERENCES

1. Biggs.   Brit. Vet. Jour., 1961, *117*, 326.
2. Calnek and Hitchner.   Jour. Nat. Cancer Inst., 1969, *43*, 935.
3. Chubb and Churchill.   Vet. Rec., 1969, *85*, 303.
4. Chubb and Churchill.   *Ibid.*, 1968, *83*, 4.
5. Churchill and Biggs.   Nature, 1967, *215*, 528.
6. Churchill, Chubb, and Baxendale.   Jour. Gen. Virol., 1969, *4*, 557.
7. Churchill, Payne, and Chubb.   Nature, 1969, *221*, 744.
8. Cole.   Avian Dis., 1968, *12*, 9.
9. Crittenden.   World's Poultry Sci. Jour., 1968, *24*, 18.

10. Edison and Schmittle. Avian Dis., 1969, *13*, 774.
11. Purchase. Jour. Virol., 1969, *3*, 557.
12. Sevoian and Chamberlain. Avian Dis., 1963, 7, 97.
13. Rispens, VanUloten, and Moss. Brit. Vet. Jour., 1969, *125*, 445.
14. Solomon, Witter, Nazerian, and Burmester. Proc. Soc. Exp. Biol. and Med., 1968, *127*, 173.
15. Walter, Burmester, and Cunningham. Avian Dis., 1962, *6*, 455.
16. Walter, Burmester, and Fontes. *Ibid.*, 1963, 7, 79.
17. Wight. Vet. Rec., 1963, 75, 685.
18. Witter, Nazerian, Purchase, and Burgoyne. Am. Jour. Vet. Res., 1970, *31*, 525.
19. Witter, Solomon, and Burgoyne. Avian Dis., 1969, *13*, 101.

### Herpesvirus Infection in Pigeons

From racing pigeons with a disease resembling ornithosis isolates of a herpesvirus were made by Cornwell and Wright (1). Diphtheric foci were present in the pharynx or larynx of several birds and were associated with intranuclear inclusions in one of them. The herpesvirus produced pocks on the chorioallantoic membrane of the embryonated hen's egg and foci of necrosis in the embryonic liver.

The two strains were pathogenic for young pigeons, but not for chicks (2). Intraperitoneal inoculation of these strains caused pancreatitis, peritonitis, and in some birds hepatic necrosis. Eosinophilic intranuclear inclusions and specific viral antigen were seen in pancreatic acinor and in hepatitic parenchymal cells. Intranuclear inclusion bodies also were observed in the necrotic foci in the larynegeal epithelium after pigeons were given virus by the intralaryngeal route.

### REFERENCES

1. Cornwell and Wright. Jour. Comp. Path., 1970, *80*, 221.
2. Cornwell, Wright, and McCusker. *Ibid.*, 1970, *80*, 229.

### Duck Plague

SYNONYM: Duck virus enteritis

Duck plague is an acute, highly fatal disease of ducks caused by a virus, presumably a herpesvirus, that occurs in the blood and in all organs.

The disease has occurred in the Netherlands, Belgium, India, France, China, and more recently in the United States. The disease is limited to ducks and on one occasion it was diagnosed at necropsy in geese.

A recent article describing the disease was written by Jansen (1) who did much of the original work on the disease. Leibovitz and Hwang described the 1967 outbreak on Long Island, New York (3).

**Character of the Disease.** Naturally and experimentally infected ducks show similar signs of illness characterized by listlessness, ruffled and dull feathers, wet areas around the eyes, which later become mucoid; nasal discharge, labored breathing, inappetence, watery diarrhea; and nervous manifestations. Not all of these signs may be present and ducks frequently show temporary improvement before death occurs in 1 to 3 days. The mortality usually is high and disease often lasts on a premise about 3 weeks.

At necropsy the most striking lesions are multiple hemorrhages throughout the body, usually most pronounced in heart, serous membranes, and esophageal mucosa. Marked congestion occurs in the ovary that is in production. If the disease becomes subacute, diphtheric membranes may occur on the mucosa of the esophagus and cloaca. These membranes may extend to salpinx and rectum. In many cases there is peritonitis and the liver may be friable.

**Properties of the Virus.** Duck plague virus apparently is a member of the herpesvirus genus. There is only one serotype and one immunogenic type as complete cross-immunity has been demonstrated with various isolates by immunity tests in ducks and by neutralization tests in the embryonated duck egg.

Attempts to demonstrate a hemagglutinin have failed (1). The virus is quite stable at −20 C and in the lyophilized state.

**Cultivation.** The virus can be cultivated readily by inoculation on the chorioallantoic membrane of 12-day-old embryonated duck eggs. The embryos die in 4 days, showing extensive hemorrhage (1). Direct cultivation of the virus in the hen's embryonated egg is not possible. Duck-embryo-adapted virus can be established in the hen's embryo. Repeated passage in the latter host produces a virus that is attenuated for ducks (1). Cultivation of the virus in cell culture has been reported by Kunst (2).

**Immunity.** Ducks that survive the natural or experimental disease have a solid immunity that presumably persists for the lifetime of the bird.

The chick embryo adapted strain of duck plague virus that is avirulent for ducks produces an effective immunity in the duck. It also rapidly produces protection as a result of interference. Ducks given this vaccine 12 to 14 months were immune to challenge at this time despite the fact that the majority had no demonstrable neutralizing antibody (1).

There is evidence of parental antibody interference (4).

**Transmission.** Under natural conditions it is spread by contact because excretions from infected ducks contain virus. Free access to ponds, moats, and pools undoubtedly facilitates spread.

**Diagnosis.** Duck plague can be confused with fowl cholera, intoxication, or Newcastle disease. Inoculation of rabbits, chicks, and ducks should soon establish the diagnosis as duck plague virus causes disease in ducks only.

**Control.** Because free-flying birds are involved control is exceedingly difficult other than by a vaccination program.

**The Disease in Man.** The disease in man has not been reported.

## REFERENCES

1. Jansen.   Jour. Am. Vet. Med. Assoc., 1968, *152*, 1009.
2. Kunst.   Tijdschr. v. Diergeneesk, 1967, *92*, 713.
3. Leibovitz and Hwang.   Avian Dis., 1968, *12*, 361.
4. Newcomb.   Jour. Am. Vet. Med. Assoc., 1968, *152*, 1349.

### Pulmonary Adenomatosis in Sheep

SYNONYMS:   Ovine jaagsiekte (South Africa), progressive pneumonia of sheep, "lungers."

The disease has been recognized in certain parts of continental Europe, in Peru, in Iceland, in South Africa, in Israel, in India, and in the northern range states of the United States. In the United States herders refer to the disease as *lungers*.

The clinically diseased animals are usually breeding animals, 4 years old or older. Lesions may be found in younger animals, but in most cases they are not sufficiently advanced to cause signs. When a large portion of the air space of the lungs has been obliterated, the victims become dyspnoeic. These generally die within a few days to several weeks from anoxia. There are no recoveries from this disease, but many affected animals are marketed before it becomes advanced and general emaciation has occurred.

This is a chronic, progressive disease in which the lungs lose their elasticity due to proliferation of cells in the supporting tissue and gradually the alveoli become filled with proliferating cells causing consolidation of the pulmonary parenchyma; thus it is recognized as primary lung neoplasm that is transmissible and may be caused by a member of the herpesvirus group, although it has not been proved. The tumor is carcinomatous in nature and does metastize.

There is no known way of controlling this disease. Generally, the affected animals are removed from the flocks as soon as they are recognized, for such animals are never profitable to keep and they may serve to spread the disease.

## REFERENCES

1. Dungal, Gislason, and Taylor.   Jour. Comp. Path. and Therap., 1938, *51*, 46. (The disease in Iceland.)
2. Marsh.   Jour. Am. Vet. Med. Assoc., 1923, *62*, 458. (The disease in the United States.)
3. Robertson.   Jour. Comp. Path. and Therap., 1904, *17*, 221. (The disease in South Africa.)

# XLII | Equine Influenza, Swine Influenza, and Fowl Plague — Orthomyxoviruses

Members of the genus *Orthomyxovirus* contain 1 percent of single-stranded RNA. The molecular weight is approximately 2 to 4 by $10^6$ daltons. Its helical capsid is 9 to 10 m$\mu$, probably in six separate pieces. The enveloped particle, 90 to 120 m$\mu$, is spherical or elongated with numerous hollow and cylindrical spheres about 9 m$\mu$ long and 1.5 to 2 m$\mu$ wide. The virion contains lipid, carbohydrate, and neuraminidase. They are ether-sensitive, heat-sensitive, and acid-labile. Hemagglutination occurs at neuraminidase sensitive receptors. Replication is inhibited by actinomycin D. Nucleocapsids form in the nucleus and maturation takes place by budding at the cell surface. Genetic recombination is common and antigenic variation frequently occurs. There are three discrete antigenic types distinguished by the specificity of the ribonucleoprotein (or soluble) antigen. Antigenic crossing does occur between subtypes of the three types. The hemagglutinin subunits are likely composed of two different hemagglutinins in the viral envelope of influenza A viruses and constitute the main component of the spikes. They carry the specific receptors for the mucins and also the subtype and strain specific antigens commonly called "V" antigens. Antibodies are formed to these antigens and are demonstrated by serum neutralization, HI, and CF tests against homologous antigen.

The neuraminidase subunits are most likely located between the spikes of the envelope, a double-membrane that is 6 to 7 m$\mu$ thick. They represent the enzymatic activity of the virus and contain antigens which differ from the hemagglutinins. Antibodies to the enzyme inhibit neuraminidase activity but not viral infectivity although they do delay or even prevent liberation of infectious particles from cells.

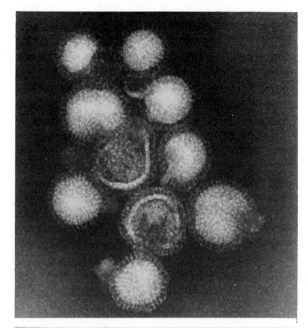

Fig. 198 (a). Influenza virus, A2/Hong Kong/1/68; negatively stained particles from chick embryo chorioallantoic fluid illustrating typical pleomorphism. All influenza virus strains are 90 to 120 mμ in diameter and have prominent surface projections or spikes covering a membranous envelope. X 140,000. (Courtesy F. Murphy.)

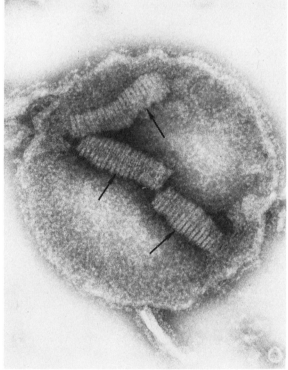

Fig. 198 (b). Influenza virus, A2/Aichi/2/68; an unusually large particle with three ribonucleoprotein (RNP) capsid coils (arrows). The RNP helix consists of a varying number of turns of a 9-mμ-diameter strand, which replicates as six separate pieces of RNA and thus makes genetic recombination (and antigenic variation) common. X 135,000. (Courtesy F. Murphy.)

The type species is *Orthomyxovirus* h-A (human influenza A). Other members are as follows:

Type A (1) Human influenza viruses ° = A/PR8/34, A1/Cam/46, and A2/Singapore/1/57. (2) Equine influenza viruses ° = A/Equi-1/Praha/56 and A/Equi-2/Miami/63. (3) Porcine influenza viruses °° = A/SW/Iowa/31, A/SW/Wis/61, and A/SW/Wis/68. (4) Avian influenza viruses °°° = Fowl plague, A/Duck/Czech/56, A/Duck/Eng/56, A/Chick/Scot/59, A/Turkey/Can/63, and A/Quail/Itally/11117/65.

Type B Human °° = B/Lee/40, B/Johannesburg/59, and B/Taiwan/62.
Type C Human = C/Taylor/1233/47.

The RNA genome is coated with basic proteins. They carry the type-specific antigen referred to earlier. This antigen can be detected by the complement-fixation or flocculation test. As a rule, antibodies against this antigen are developed only after infection. Consequently they are not produced in animals given inactivated or disrupted viruses unless a special procedure is used (4).

The principal diseases in domestic animals caused by members of the genus include equine influenza, swine influenza, and avian influenza occurring in chickens, turkeys, and ducks. In mammals the disease syndrome is largely confined to the respiratory tract, from which virus can be isolated in high titer and in low titer from bronchial lymph nodes.

Excellent review articles of orthomyxoviruses are available to the reader (1-3).

**REFERENCES**

1. Andrewes and Pereira. Viruses of vertebrates. 2d ed., Bailliére, Tindall, and Cassell, London, 1967.
2. Chanock and Coates. In: R. P. Hanson. Newcastle disease virus: An evolving pathogen. Univ. Wisconsin Press, Madison, Wis., 1964.
3. Wildy. Monographs in Virol., 1971, 5, 1.
4. Zavadova, Kutinova, and Vonka. Arch. f. die Gesam. Virusforsch., 1967, 20, 421.

**Equine Influenza**

SYNONYMS: Shipping fever, stable pneumonia, pinkeye, epizootic cellulitis of horses

The disease known as equine influenza resembles influenzas in swine and man. It is also included in the influenza A viruses and is a member of the orthomyxovirus group. Two immunological types are known to exist and they have been designated as A/Equi-1/Praha/56 and A/Equi-2/Miami/63 equine influenza viruses (4).

The disease spreads rapidly among susceptible horses. It affects animals of

° Distinct serotypes.　　°° No distinct serotypes.
°°° Wide range of antigenic variation but no distinct serotypes.

all ages but occurs mostly in young animals that have been moved into new surroundings, particularly when they come in contact with older animals. In the past it has given much trouble in sales stables, in dealers' herds, and in army remount stations (6). In centers where fresh "green" horses are arriving from time to time, the newly arrived, highly susceptible stock serves to keep the disease alive and in very virulent form. Under such conditions the death rate may be very high. Like influenza of man, this disease in the past has a history of great panzootics in which large areas have been involved, nearly every horse in these areas being a victim of the disease. The last one of this kind in the United States occurred in the winter of 1872–1873. At that time traffic in many of our large cities was nearly stopped because of the lack of horses well enough to do their normal work of drawing horsecars, drays, and delivery wagons. Like human influenza, the horse disease formerly occurred every year in a milder, less contagious form, and few horses escaped the disease.

As the horse population decreased in the cities and on the farms, equine influenza was less important as a disease in the horse. With increasing numbers of horses in recent years, its importance and incidence has increased, particularly as it affects the Thoroughbred and Standardbred horse populations.

At present only members of the equine family are known to be susceptible to the two equine serotypes.

**Character of the Disease.** The disease is highly contagious, practically every young horse and many of the older ones being attacked when the disease appears on the premises. Usually the mortality rate is moderate and the chief loss is from inability of the victim to work for periods varying from 1 to 3 weeks, occasionally even longer (7).

The disease affects only horses, asses, and mules. The onset is sudden and is manifested by a high temperature—103 to 106 F—which lasts about 3 days. Equine 2 virus causes higher temperatures than equine 1 virus (9). At the same time there is inappetence and great mental depression. The animal stands with head down and with ears depressed, taking little interest in its surroundings. Coughing is the most common sign of illness.

Photophobia and lacrimation are usually exhibited, and often the congested conjunctivae protrude from between the closed eyelids because of the infiltration of the tissues. A mucopurulent discharge from the eyes appears, the corneas often become clouded, and occasionally the function of one or both eyes is lost. Nasal catarrh is usually present, and the lymph nodes of the head may become swollen. Pneumonia occasionally occurs, in which case the victim usually dies, as a rule from secondary bacterial infection.

In some cases edematous swellings appear on the ventral parts of the trunk and especially in the legs, where the tendon sheaths often are inflamed. This form of the disease has been called epizootic cellulitis. Mild icterus is not infrequent. Catarrhal and even hemorrhagic enteritis occur in some cases, and kidney damage is not uncommon. Leukopenia appears in the early stages of the modern disease and presumably was present also in the classical disease.

In the accounts of the old classical equine influenza, abortions in mares are mentioned but one does not gain the impression that this was a frequent happening.

The period of incubation varies from 1 to 3 days with extremes of 0.5 days and 7 days. Its course varies greatly depending upon whether or not complications occur. Uncomplicated cases may be essentially well again within 1 week.

The general mortality of naturally occurring cases probably does not often exceed 5 percent. In some outbreaks the virulence becomes exalted and the losses may be very much higher.

The principal lesions in fatal cases are in the lungs, in which there may be extensive edema or a bronchopneumonia with pleurisy. The thorax is usually filled with fluid. Gelatinous infiltrations around the larynx and in the legs are common. Usually there is swelling of the lymph nodes.

**The Disease in Experimental Animals.** In experimental horses influenza virus is recoverable for 5 days after intranasal instillation (4). Edema of the throat and the intermandibular lymph nodes occurs in some animals. A thick purulent nasal discharge usually follows the acute stage, and it is associated with secondary bacterial infection.

Horses given equine influenza 2 virus by the intranasal route develop an elevated temperature 2 to 3 days later followed by coughing and other signs of illness referable to the lower respiratory tract 2 or 3 days after the onset of fever (3). A contact horse also developed the disease. Virus was readily recovered from the nasal mucosa during the first 5 days postinoculation and also from the contact horse. Other horses given the same virus intramuscularly did not develop signs of illness.

The virus has been adapted to produce pneumonia in mice after intranasal instillation, and encephalitis results after intracerebral inoculation of suckling mice. It causes inapparent infection of ferrets.

**Properties of the Virus.** All equine cases belong to type A and presumably have the main characteristics described for the type-species of the genus, human influenza A (11).

Based upon HAI tests equine influenza viruses are placed into two subtypes, A/Equi-1/Praha/56 and A/Equi-2/Miami/63. Variants showing slight antigenic differences are distinguished in A/Equi-2. No antigenic relationship has been demonstrated between the hemagglutinin and neuraminidase antigens of these two subtypes using antisera produced in laboratory animals. However, horses recovering from A/Equi-2 infections may have antibody rises to A/Equi-1 strains, to certain human A-2 strains, and to the infecting virus suggesting existence of shared minor antigens.

Certain antigenic relationships have been observed between the equine viruses, influenza A avian strains and strains of human origin. A/Equi-1 is antigenically related to fowl plague/27 and Turkey/England/63 viruses, including both hemagglutinin and neuraminidase antigens. A/Equi-2 virus shows some crossing with avian virus N and Quail/Italy/1117/65. A/Equi-2 shows some cross reaction with the human A-2/Hong Kong/1/68 hemagglutinin antigens.

Like other influenza viruses (14), both equine subtypes hemagglutinate erythrocytes of a wide range of species with the highest titers attained with pigeon cell suspensions (11).

**Cultivation.** Andrewes and Worthington (1) cultivated the Equine 1 virus in fertile eggs and in tissue cultures of bovine kidney, chick embryo kidney and fibroblasts, and rhesus monkey and human embryo kidney. Equine viruses are usually isolated and propagated in the hen's embryonated egg. A/Equi-2 is usually isolated in the egg without difficulty. In contrast, A/Equi-1 is rather difficult to isolate.

In general, isolation of virus in cell cultures is more difficult than isolation in the embryonated egg. A/Equi-2 viruses are isolated in primary cultures of monkey kidney cells but other primary kidney-cell cultures of bovine, equine, and human origin are not satisfactory for this purpose (11). Certain strains can be adapted to grow in chick and bovine cell cultures.

**Immunity.** Infected animals generally produce antibodies to the three major components of the viral particle. The horse given inactivated or disrupted virus only produces antibodies against the main envelop antigens (hemagglutinins and neuraminidase).

CF antibodies against type-specific S antigen may be detected as early as 4 to 6 days after illness has begun, reach their peak at 12 to 20 days, and usually are not detectable after 8 to 12 weeks. CF antibodies against strain-specific V antigen, serum-neutralizing antibodies, and HI antibodies develop later than S-specific CF antibodies but reach their peak at 15 to 20 days and decline until the 3rd month. The HI and SN antibodies level off at this time and remain constant for years. The V-specific CF antibody is no longer detectable as a rule at the 6th month.

It is generally agreed that antibody on the respiratory mucosa surface confers protection against this pneumotropic infection. The mucous titer is a good index for determining the level of protection. Although the mucous titer does not always parallel the serum titer, the serum titer gives an approximate idea of the measure of resistance in man and the same is likely to be true of equine influenza (2). This applies to vaccinated and unvaccinated individuals. Older horses that have had the disease earlier in life usually escape infection later. In times of past epizootics this immunity is frequently not adequate to protect horses completely. Information on the duration of immunity is based upon field observations; it is reported that natural infection produces a rather solid immunity that persists for 1 year (9).

**Transmission.** It is presumed that the respiratory form of the disease occurs as a result of droplet infection. Numerous reports have appeared of the transmission of this disease by stallions used for breeding purposes months after having recovered from influenza. Several reports of the demonstration of virus in the semen of such animals for periods varying from 1 to 6 years are in the literature (8). Schofield (13) in Canada observed two outbreaks apparently initiated by breeding stallions that had had the disease some months previously. The examination of the semen of one of these animals 6 months later failed to show the presence of the virus. A-Equi 2 virus has been isolated from a dead foal.

The pattern and incidence of infectious disease among horses is influenced by the immune status of the population, its concentration and the antigenic characteristics of the virus. Although natural resistance to influenza does not seem to be an important factor, it may account for a certain number of horses that show no signs of illness during epizootics (9).

When the disease occurs in a susceptible population it is explosive and the rapid aerosol spread is principally due to the strong and frequent cough. The short incubation period and the high concentration of virus in the respiratory tract also account for its rapid transmission from horse to horse.

**Diagnosis.** Equine influenza is generally diagnosed on clinical evidence. When the disease occurs in epizootic form, the signs of illness and high degree of contagiousness are generally sufficient to make a diagnosis. When brood mares abort as a result of this infection, they are sick at the time the abortions occur.

Positive diagnosis can only be assured by isolation of the virus or by the demonstration of a rising hemagglutination or by neutralizing antibodies with paired sera. In an initial outbreak there is a need to isolate the virus for typing. This information is essential to a vaccination program in an area, and also to a correct diagnosis. If a new type is involved serology alone will not give a satisfactory answer.

**Prevention and Control.** Two types of inactivated virus vaccine are available for use in horses (5, 12). They contain both subtypes of virus and are administered by parenteral injection. If young horses are vaccinated a second injection should be given 1 to 3 months later and it is advisable to vaccinate horses yearly.

In outbreaks, isolation and quarantine measures are advised in addition to vaccination.

**The Disease in Man.** There is a minor antigenic relationship between A/Equi-2 and A-2/Hong Kong (human) strains but there is no evidence that the A/Equi-2 produces infection in man; nor does the reverse occur (10).

## REFERENCES

1. Andrewes and Worthington. Bul. World Health Organ., 1959, 20, 435.
2. Beveridge. Proc. 2d Internatl. Conf. Equine Inf. Dis. S. Karger, Basel/Munich/New York, 1970, p. 119.
3. Blaskovic. *Ibid.*, p. 111.
4. Bryans. Proc. Am. Vet. Med. Assoc., 1964, p. 119.

5. Bryans, Doll, Wilson, McCollum. Jour. Am. Vet. Med. Assoc., 1966, *148*, 413.

6. Dale and Dollahite. *Ibid.*, 1939, 95, 534.

7. Doll, Bryans, McCollum, and Crowe. Cornell Vet., 1957, *47*, 3.

8. Gaffky. Zeitschr. f Vetkde., 1912, *24*, 209.

9. Gerber. Proc. 2d Internatl. Conf. Equine Inf. Dis. S. Karger, Basel/Munich/New York, 1970, p. 63.

10. McQueen, Kaye, Coleman, and Dowdle. Equine Dis. Sup., Jour. Am. Vet. Med. Assoc., 1969, *155*, 265.

11. Paccaud. Proc. 2d Internatl. Conf. Equine Inf. Dis. S. Karger, Basel/Munich/New York, 1970, p. 81.

12. Peterman, Fayet, Fontaine, and Fontaine. *Ibid.*, p. 63.

13. Schofield. Rpt. Ontario Vet. Col., 1937, p. 15.

14. Tumova and Fiserova-Sovinova. Bul. World Health Organ., 1959, *20*, 445.

## Swine Influenza

SYNONYM: Hog "flu"

Swine influenza is an acute disease of the respiratory organs which occurs in the colder months of the year. The onset of the disease is sudden and practically all animals in an affected herd show signs almost simultaneously. They are quite similar to those of epidemic influenza of man, and the virus of swine influenza is closely related to that of human influenza.

The disease was first recognized as an entity in the midwestern part of the United States in the fall of 1918, when a pandemic of human influenza was under way. The similarity of the diseases in man and pigs was recognized. Koen is credited by Dorset, Niles, and McBryde (2) as being the one who suggested the name *flu* or *influenza* for the disease, since he was convinced that it had been contracted from human cases. Much later, when the etiological agents of the two diseases were better understood, the concept that swine may have become infected from man, thus giving rise to a new disease in the species, became much more plausible than before. Three viral types are now recognized as the causative agents of human influenza. The virus of swine influenza is immunologically different from these, but the swine virus is more closely related to type A human virus than the human virus types are to each other. Many adult human beings carry antibodies which neutralize, in part at least, the virus of swine influenza. This has been regarded by some as evidence that these persons have been infected at some time in the past with the same type of virus that exists in pigs, but other explanations are possible. Because the influenza viruses were not known at the time of the last great pandemic in man, when the swine virus first appeared, it is not possible now to know whether the human virus of that outbreak was identical with any one of the viruses that now exist in man. It is possible, of course, that the 1918 virus in man was identical with that now current in swine, or the virus may have been modified by long-continued residence in swine. Work by Glover and Andrewes (5), in which they compared the antigenic structure of several swine strains and a human strain, indicated that there was as much difference among the swine strains as between human and swine strains.

**Character of the Disease.** Only swine appear to be naturally susceptible to the virus of swine influenza. The geographical distribution and economical importance of the disease is not well defined. In the USA it occurs primarily in the midwestern and north central states, but serological evidence for its existence in the eastern states exists (3). The virus has also been isolated in England, Russia, Poland, and Czechoslovakia. In 1959 Kaplan and Payne (6) found serological evidence for its existence in pigs in the United States, Germany and Czechoslovakia out of a total of 33 countries. It usually occurs in the fall and early winter months, rarely occurring as a disease during the warm months.

The disease usually appears suddenly in swine herds, and whole groups commonly develop signs of illness almost simultaneously. The development of the disease in many animals at almost the same time has commonly been attributed to an extreme degree of contagiousness, but Shope has put forward another conception; the disease-producing agent spreads widely without producing obvious disease and that a precipitating agent is responsible for the simultaneous development of many cases. It was suggested that the precipitating agent in this case might be the advent of cold, wet weather with consequent chilling of the animals.

The disease begins with fever, anorexia, extreme weakness, and prostration. The animals crowd together, lying down, and are moved only with difficulty. When moved or handled they exhibit evidence of muscular stiffness and pain. Other cases develop edema of the lungs and bronchopneumonia and usually die. At the height of the disease the animals exhibit a jerky type of respiration, caused by spasms of the diaphragm, which is commonly known as *thumps.* Bronchitis is indicated by coughing. When the animals are in good condition in the first place and are kept during the course of the disease in a dry, fairly warm place, well bedded with straw, the principal losses from this disease usually are in retardation of growth and decrease in weight.

The period of incubation is very short—from a few hours to several days. In uncomplicated cases the disease runs a course varying from 2 to 6 days, recovery occurring almost as suddenly as the disease begins. When pneumonia develops, the course will be longer. As a rule the mortality rate does not exceed 4 percent if the animals are given good care. In some instances it has been as high as 10 percent.

Animals killed at the height of the disease exhibit no significant lesions outside the chest cavity. The lung lesions are characteristic. They are limited, as a rule, to the cephalic, cardiac, and azygos lobes. Sometimes all five of these lobes are involved; sometimes only part of them. Usually the involvement is bilateral, but in some cases it is unilateral, the lobes of the right side being involved more frequently. These portions are collapsed, deep purplish red in color, and do not crepitate. They are not pneumonic. The condition is an atelectasis caused by a thick, mucilaginous exudate in the bronchioles and bronchi of the parts (15). The remainder of the lungs is usually pale because of interstitial emphysema. The cervical, bronchial, and mediastinal lymph nodes are swollen and filled with fluid. In the cases in which pneumonia occurs, the consolidated portions are the same as the atelectatic in the milder ones. The nonpneumonic lung portions in these cases are congested and edematous. The spleen often is moderately enlarged. There is hyperemia of the mucosa of the stomach in most cases. The other abdominal organs generally are normal.

Virus pneumonia of pigs presents lesions which can easily be confused with those of influenzal pneumonia. This was discussed more fully under the VP heading (see p. 522).

**The Disease in Experimental Animals.** Andrewes, Laidlaw, and Smith (1) demonstrated that the virus of swine influenza was pathogenic for mice when introduced by a special technic into the nasal passages. The virus also causes pneumonia in ferrets and lambs.

Mouse-passage virus retains its virulence for swine indefinitely (Shope, 17). The virulence of *Hemophilus* (*influenza*) *suis* may decline, however, in which case new cultures are needed to supply the necessary bacterial factors for producing a more severe form of the swine disease. The virus alone administered to normal pigs in an area where swine influenza does not exist produces a very mild, almost inapparent disease, which surely would be overlooked on the farm (9). *H. suis*, on the other hand, is virtually nonpathogenic for swine. When both agents are given simultaneously, however, typical influenza results. The experimental disease is a result of the concurrent action of two agents, a virus and a bacterium. In natural outbreaks *H. suis* is not always isolated. Scott (14) reported the isolation of *Pasteurella multocida* and virus and others (11, 20) reported the isolation of influenza virus only.

**Properties of the Virus.** Shope (16) isolated the virus in 1931 and at the same time determined that *H. suis* was regularly present (8). The virus is type A and possesses the characteristics of the influenza viruses described for the genus *Orthomyxovirus*.

It shares a common ribonucleoprotein (S) antigen with the human, equine, and avian members of the type A influenza viruses (3). Among the swine influenza viruses, insufficient antigenic differences have been observed to justify designation of subtypes. Three antigenic groupings have been made on the basis of HI and strain specific CF reactions (3, 9). The representative strains of the three groups are A/SW/Iowa/31 (the original Shope isolate), A/SW/Wis/61, and A/SW/Wis/68. Accumulated evidence suggests that swine influenza virus represents or is closely related to the 1918 pandemic virus of human influenza. More recently, an antigenic relationship between swine influenza virus and the A/Chick/Scot/59 virus of chickens has been described (19).

These viruses are stable at −70 C and in the lyophilized state for years.

Most are inactivated at 56 C for 30 minutes, but some require a longer period. Phenol, ether, and formalin inactivate the virus.

**Cultivation.** In affected pigs the virus is found in the nasal secretions, in the tracheal and bronchial exudate, in the lungs, and in the lymph glands draining the lungs. It is not ordinarily found in the blood, spleen, liver, kidneys, mesenteric lymph glands, and brain (Orcutt and Shope, 12).

Köbe and Fertig (7) and Scott (13) reported the successful cultivation of the virus of swine influenza on the chorioallantoic membrane of the developing chick. Scott reports that his cultures as far as the 50th generation were virulent for mice and swine, but that the 85th and later generations had lost their virulence. Intra-allantoic or intra-amniotic routes of inoculation into 10- to-12-day-old embryonated hens' eggs are the most commonly employed methods for cultivation of the virus. The virus is not lethal for the embryo, but it is readily detected by its hemagglutinating property.

Various tissue-culture monolayer systems involving primary or stable cell cultures have been used for propagation and assay (3). Depending upon the culture system, the virus is recognized by plaque-production or by hemadsorption of red cells in positive cultures. The virus also propagates in organ cultures of fetal pig tracheal, lung, or nasal epithelial tissue (11).

The immunofluorescence test has been used extensively in the study of influenza viruses, including swine influenza virus (11).

**Immunity.** Various serological methods, including the complement-fixation, hemagglutination-inhibition, serum-neutralization, and hemadsorption-inhibition tests have been used in swine-influenza immunity studies.

Based upon present evidence it is not clear whether swine recovered from influenza are refractory to subsequent infection. Shope has reported that swine fully recovered from swine influenza are immune. Subsequent respiratory outbreaks in a herd in a given season means that one of the outbreaks is caused by another pathogen. There is no unanimity of opinion on this point. According to Scott, experimental pigs with neutralizing antibody are not necessarily immune to challenge by the intranasal route with virus and *H. suis* combined. Pigs exposed to aerosols of virus 83 days after earlier intranasal and aerosol exposure all had HI titers of 80 or above at the time of challenge and resisted that challenge. Increasing evidence suggests that local antibody is very important in influenzal immunity, and subsequent studies centered around this concept may provide more information about the active immunity of this infection.

Maternal immunity plays a role in the epidemiology of the disease. Piglets from immune sows are protected as long as 13 to 18 weeks depending upon the serum titer level of the dam. In addition to providing protection, colostral antibody also inhibits propagation of the virus in the host and development of an active immunity.

**Transmission.** Swine influenza appears each autumn in midwestern United States. The epizootics coincide with the onset of autumn rains and marked fluctuating temperatures. The disease appears simultaneously on many farms, suggesting that the virus is widely seeded before the outbreak and then provoked by climatic conditions and management procedures. It appears that all pigs become ill at the same time on individual farms, but more astute owners often report that one or a few pigs are ill 2 to 5 days prior to the diffuse herd disease.

The ecology and epidemiology of swine influenza is complex and not completely understood. The question of how the disease is maintained through the nonepizootic portions of the year when the disease is not seen has possibly been answered by Shope (18), who has demonstrated that the lungworm and the earthworm can harbor the virus for long periods of time. Lungworms, living in the bronchi of affected pigs, ingest virus, and the virus is carried through the eggs and into the larvae of the parasite. These, hatching out in the air passages of the pig, are coughed up and swallowed, eventually reaching the ground in the feces. Here they are ingested by earthworms in which the larvae lodge, most of them being found in the heart and calciferous glands. They may remain in the worms from one season to the next. If the earthworms are fed to swine, as was done by Shope, the pigs show no ill effects. However, if the pigs are then given several intramuscular injections of *H. suis*, about one-half of them will suddenly develop typical swine influenza and both virus and bacterium will be found in the lungs. Shope regards the injection of the bacterium merely as a precipitating or provoking agent, since he was able to provoke a similar effect in a few cases by injecting calcium chloride into the pleural cavity. He has repeated these experiments successfully many times in the late fall, winter, and spring months but never in the summer. He speaks of the virus in the earthworms as existing in a "masked" form.

On the other hand, this complex association involving four species hasn't been entirely accepted. More recently it has been proposed that recovered animals become virus carriers and serve as a means of spread and perpetuation of the virus (11). This hypothesis is based upon epidemiological observations and serological testing. Virus was not isolated from pigs without signs of illness. With the newer means of identifying viruses in tissues perhaps this problem can be resolved.

**Diagnosis.** Swine influenza is suspected in a herd with respiratory disease in the fall or early winter. A clinical diagnosis is presumptive because influenza doesn't always follow the typical pattern and other respiratory diseases are similar (4).

A definitive diagnosis requires virus isolation or the demonstration of a rising titer with paired serum samples. In the past, intranasal inoculation of mice or ferrets was used but the generally accepted method is allantoic or amniotic inoculation of the 10-to-12-day-old embryonated hen's egg. Nasal exudate from a febrile pig or lung tissue usually contain virus. Proper treatment to eliminate bacteria and molds from test material is desirable to enhance viral isolation. After 72 to 96 hours of incubation the allantoic and amniotic fluids are tested for HA activity. If positive, the isolate is tested against influenza antisera for specificity.

The HI test is used most frequently in diagnosis when serology is applied. Paired sera are used. The first serum sample is taken during the acute phase of illness and the second one is obtained 2 to 3 weeks later. A rising titer constitutes a positive test. The serologist must be aware of the possible presence of nonspecific inhibitors of hemagglutination and the methods by which the sera can be treated to remove them (10).

**Prevention and Control.** There are no immunizing agents commercially available for swine influenza. Past vaccines have failed to protect. In addition, not all swine influenza strains protect against each other after parenteral inoculation. Although the economic aspects of the disease are not known, it would appear there is a need for a safe and efficacious vaccine which probably would be more effective if administered by the respiratory route. Furthermore, technics now are available for producing strains in the laboratory by recombinations that are safe and immunogenic (4).

There is no therapy for swine influenza. Careful nursing is important through the provision of comfortable and draft-free quarters with clean, dry, and dust-free bedding. Fresh, clean water and a good source of feed are essential. The animals should not be disturbed or moved during this period. Antibiotics and sulfonamides are useful on a herd basis to control secondary bacterial infections.

**The Disease in Man.** There is no evidence in recent years that a strain of swine influenza virus has infected man. Antibodies in the serum of aged persons suggests that they had an infection with a swine influenza virus many years ago or with a human influenza virus that shared a common antigen(s) with the early swine strain.

## REFERENCES

1. Andrewes, Laidlaw, and Smith. Lancet, 1934, 2, 859.
2. Dorset, Niles, and McBryde. Jour. Am. Vet. Med. Assoc., 1922, 62, 162.
3. Easterday, B. In: H. W. Dunne. Diseases of swine. 3d ed., Iowa State Univ. Press., Ames, Iowa, 1970, p. 127.
4. Easterday. Swine Disease Sup. Jour. Am. Vet. Med. Assoc., 1972, 160, 645.
5. Glover and Andrewes. Jour. Comp. Path. and Therap., 1943, 53, 329.
6. Kaplan and Payne. Bul. World Health Organ., 1959, 20, 465.
7. Köbe and Fertig. Centrbl. f. Bakt., I, Abt., Orig., 1938, 141, 1.
8. Lewis and Shope. Jour. Exp. Med., 1931, 54, 361.
9. Lief. CDC, Zoonoses Surveil., Rpt. 5, 1965.
10. Nakamura and Easterday. Bul. World Health Organ., 1967, 37, 559.
11. Nakamura and Easterday. Cornell Vet., 1970, 60, 27.
12. Orcutt and Shope. Jour. Exp. Med., 1935, 62, 823.
13. Scott. Jour. Bact., 1940, 40, 327.
14. Scott. Vet. Extension Quart., June, 1941, 1.

15. Shope. Jour. Exp. Med., 1931, *54*, 349.
16. *Ibid.*, 373.
17. *Ibid.*, 1935, *62*, 561.
18. Shope. Science, 1939, 89, 441; Jour. Exp. Med., 1941, *74*, 49.
19. Tumova and Pereira. Bul. World Health Organ., 1968, *38*, 415.
20. Urman, Underdahl, and Young. Am. Jour. Vet. Res., 1958, *19*, 913.

## Fowl Plague

SYNONYM: Fowl pest, avian influenza virus(es)

Fowl plague usually is an acute, highly fatal disease of chickens, turkeys, pheasants, and certain wild birds. Ducks, geese, and other waterfowl are less susceptible but develop the disease at times. Natural infection among pigeons is uncommon. Artificial infection of ducks, geese, and pigeons by the injection of large amounts of virus from naturally infected chickens often fails. The signs of illness and lesions of fowl plague are similar to those of fowl cholera. It is caused by a virus that occurs in the blood and all organs and is readily filterable.

Fowl plague has been known since about 1880, when it was recognized in Italy as a separate disease entity. Early in the present century it spread throughout the greater part of Europe. The virus was brought into the United States illegally in 1923 by a laboratory worker. In the fall of 1924 the virus escaped from the laboratory into the New York poultry market, where it has been estimated to have killed more than 500,000 birds (8). From this market it spread to a considerable number of eastern poultry farms, probably on the contaminated crates of dealers, causing large losses. The disease was stamped out within 1 year by rigid quarantine methods. In 1965 in Canada (6) and later in the United States (10, 11) it was reported as an acute respiratory disease in turkeys with a high morbidity and a low mortality (11). Apparently it still exists in these countries.

The disease has been reported in oriental countries, but it is probable that the diagnosis was confused with the pseudo fowl plague or Newcastle disease, which is known to be prevalent there. It has occurred in South America.

**Character of the Disease.** *In chickens.* The period of incubation is rather short—3 to 5 days as a rule. Inoculated birds may show signs within 24 to 36 hours. A high temperature rapidly develops (110 to 112 F), the appetite is lost, and the birds rapidly become lethargic. The comb and wattle commonly become bluish black. A mucoid nasal discharge appears, and often edema of the head and neck develops. The course of the disease is very rapid, death usually occurring within a few hours after the appearance of the first signs. The temperature commonly falls to subnormal shortly before death. The mortality rate sometimes is close to 100 percent.

The lesions generally are not numerous. They consist of petechial hemorrhages on the heart, on the fatty tissue around the gizzard, on the serosa of the body cavity, and on the mucous membranes of the proventriculus. In some cases a serofibrinous exudate appears in the pericardial sac. The principal organs may show petechiae and cloudy swelling. The nervous system appears normal, but microscopic examination shows a diffuse encephalitis with cuffing of the blood vessels, degeneration of nerve cells, and necrotic foci, around which there is proliferation of glia cells.

*In turkeys.* The first outbreaks in Canada occurred as an acute respiratory disease and a severe production problem in turkeys (6). The viral isolate designated A/Turkey/Canada/63 (Wilmot) was related to the influenza A group of viruses. In transmission experiments the virus regularly produced sinusitis in turkey poults under 4 weeks of age but was apathogenic for older turkeys and chickens of any age. In contrast, a later isolate designated A/Turkey/Ontario 7732/66 was highly pathogenic for turkeys and chickens (77).

A Massachusetts isolate produced an air-sac disease in semimature turkeys characterized by depression and sudden but slight mortality (10). Its antigenic relationship to the Canadian Wilmot virus was demonstrated by the HI test.

The Wisconsin isolate is a type A influenza virus that produced an acute respiratory disease in turkeys (11). The disease, with a high morbidity and low mortality, was seen in nine breeding flocks in northwestern Wisconsin and serologic evidence was demonstrated in 11 turkey flocks.

**Properties of the Virus.** The avian influenza viruses are members of the *Orthomyxovirus* Type A group. There is a wide range of antigenic variation but no distinct subtypes have been designated. Six avian influenza virus strains have been listed as representative of the group: fowl plague; A/Duck/Czech/56, A/Duck/England/56, A/Chick/Scot/59, A/Turkey/Can/63 (Wilmot), and A/Quail/Italy/65.

The virus particles are spherical, 80 to 100 millimicrons in diameter. Associated filaments average 80 millimicrons in diameter and are up to 8 microns in length (4). By electron microscopy Waterson *et al.* (12) showed that the avian virus resembled influenza A virus. It is an RNA virus.

The nucleoprotein is formed in the nucleus of the infected cells and hemagglutinin in the cytoplasm (2). Hemagglutination of red blood cells from fowl, rhesus monkeys, horses, and cattle has been demonstrated.

The avian viruses have a complement-fixing antigen common to the influenza–A virus group, but they are immunologically distinct from all other myxoviruses except there is minor crossing with equine influenza virus. Serological differences may occur between some avian strains.

**Cultivation.** The virus multiplies readily in embryonated hens' eggs. A cytopathogenic effect is produced in cell cultures of various fowl and mammalian tissues. Attenuation of virus for fowls is reported after transfers in chick, pigeon, and human cell cultures (5).

**Immunity.** Recovered birds are solidly immune for several months at least. The serum of recovered birds will give a considerable degree of immunity to susceptible fowls, but, because the immunity probably is short-lived and the amount of such serum which can be obtained from immune birds is small, the method has no practical value.

There is a rather large European literature on vaccines for fowl plague. Attempts have been made to produce vaccines from blood and from tissues. Treatment with heat, phenol, glycerol, ether, and formaldehyde will weaken and finally destroy the virus. Moses, Brandly, Jones, and Jungherr (9) obtained a high degree of immunity, which persisted for 18 to 21 weeks, following vaccination with whole-egg adjuvant vaccines (inactivated virus) and with living variant virus. Daubney, Mansi, and Zaharan (3), in experiments designed to improve the quality of the inactivated fowl plague vaccines, noted that serial passage of one strain of plague virus through pigeon embryos resulted in a mutant which is completely nonpathogenic for domestic fowls, turkeys, and young pigeons but which induces solid immunity against virulent fowl plague virus. They indicated that this variant gives promise of being a satisfactory immunizing agent against fowl plague.

**Transmission.** Fowl plague is somewhat self-limiting because the high mortality leaves few birds to serve as carriers. It is believed that ingestion of virus is the most common mode of infection, because the disease can easily be transmitted by feeding. Probably it is also transmitted by inhalation because the nasal discharges of affected birds contain virus. Some believe that insect vectors may play a role, because there is a viremia. A peculiar condition, often noted, is that the disease usually does not readily pass from one species of susceptible bird to another by ordinary contacts. Also, birds placed in uncleaned pens in which birds have just died from plague usually do not contract the disease. This is believed to be due to the rapid destruction of the virus by sunlight and drying.

**Control.** After the 1924–1925 outbreak, fowl plague was diagnosed in the United States by Beaudette, Hudson, and Saxe (1) in 1929. The second outbreak was a small one, involving only a few flocks in New Jersey. It was brought under control, as was the earlier, larger outbreak, by rigid quarantine measures. These involved controls for shipping birds and also the cleaning and disinfecting of poultry crates, egg crates, and other objects which might serve to carry virus from infected flocks to others. Vaccination methods were not used.

During the 1920's the disease was readily recognized by its characteristic signs and lesions and its high mortality in chickens. The infections in turkeys in the 1960's were clinically ill-defined and moderate in severity and in two instances occurred as inapparent flock infections. To eliminate the disease in its present form from Canada and the United States would be formidable in costs and effort.

**The Disease in Man.** There is no evidence that man, or any other mammal, can be infected with the virus of fowl plague.

## REFERENCES

1. Beaudette, Hudson, and Saxe.   Jour. Agr. Res., 1934, *49*, 83.
2. Breitenfeld and Schäfer.   Virology, 1957, *4*, 328.
3. Daubney, Mansi, and Zaharan.   Jour. Comp. Path. and Therap., 1949, *29*, 1.
4. Dawson and Elford.   Jour. Gen. Microbiol., 1949, *3*, 298.
5. Hallauer and Kronauer.   Arch. f. die Gesam. Virusforsch., 1959, 9, 232.
6. Lang, Ferguson, Connell, and Wills.   Avian Dis., 1965, 9, 495.
7. Lang, Narayan, Rouse, Ferguson, and Connell.   Canad. Vet. Jour., 1968, 9, 151.
8. Mohler.   Jour. Am. Vet. Med. Assoc., 1925, *67*, 764.
9. Moses, Brandly, Jones, and Jungherr.   Am. Jour. Vet. Res., 1948, 9, 399.
10. Olesuik, Snoeyenbos, and Roberts.   Avian Dis., 1967, *11*, 203.
11. Smithies, Radloff, Friedell, Albright, Misner, and Easterday.   *Ibid.*, 1969, *13*, 603.
12. Waterson, Rott, and Schäfer.   Ztschr. f. Naturforsch., 1961, *16*, 154.

# XLIII | Canine Distemper, Bovine Parainfluenza, Rinderpest Newcastle Disease, and Other Paramyxoviruses

In the genus *Paramyxovirus* there is a triad of important virus diseases, namely canine distemper, rinderpest, and measles, which are listed as possible members, but they lack neuraminidase in their envelope, a characteristic of other members of the genus. Other important possible members include respiratory syncytial virus of man and pneumonia virus of mice. Accepted members of the genus are parainfluenza virus 1 (human $HA_2$ and murine Sendai), parainfluenza virus 2 (human CA, simian $SV_5$, and avian), parainfluenza 3 (human $HA_1$ and bovine $SF_4$), parainfluenza 4, mumps virus, other avian parainfluenza viruses (turkey virus—Canada/68 and Yucaipa virus) and paramyxovirus a-1 (Newcastle disease virus). The syncytium-forming viruses of cats and cattle have some characteristics of the paramyxoviruses, so they are included in this chapter.

*Paramyxovirus* a-1 (Newcastle disease virus) is the type species for the genus. This virus contains 1 percent single-stranded RNA of a molecular weight 4 to 8 by $10^6$ daltons. The spherical-enveloped particles range from 150 to 300 m$\mu$ in diameter, with characteristic projections. The helical capsid is approximately 18 m$\mu$ in diameter and 1 micron long. Some particles contain more than one nucleocapsid. The particles are ether-sensitive, but they are antigenically stable. There are two main serological subgroups. Some viruses in the genus possess neuraminidase. All accepted members cause hemagglutination, but some possible members, such as canine distemper and rinderpest viruses, may not contain hemagglutinins. Mostly, the nucleocapsids develop in the cytoplasm and are resistant to actinomycin D. Genetic recombination does not occur.

## Canine Distemper

SYNONYM:   Carré's disease; abbreviation, CD

Distemper is a worldwide disease of young dogs. It is highly contagious and manifested by a diphasic fever curve, acute coryza, and later bronchitis and catarrhal pneumonia, severe gastroenteritis, and nervous signs. The initiating agent is a filterable virus, first described by Carré (15), but many of the pathological changes in naturally occurring cases are due to bacterial complications.

Carré's studies were not generally accepted until the classical reports of Laidlaw and Dunkin (21, 22, 36–38). Before that time most individuals accepted the proposition that *Bordetella bronchiseptica* was the primary cause.

Any classification of viruses should take into consideration the relationship of CD to human measles virus and bovine rinderpest virus. CD virus probably belongs in the paramyxovirus group.

Investigators (40) in England in 1948 described a disease in dogs which they termed *hard-pad disease*. This is simply one of the many manifestations that CD virus produces.

Many review articles exist on the subject of canine distemper (4, 6, 23, 29). The authors used these to good advantage in preparing this section as well as the AVMA canine distemper symposium proceedings (13).

**Character of the Disease.** CD causes the death or permanent disability of more young dogs than any other disease. The disease also occurs in wolves, foxes, jackals, badgers, stoats, weasels, grisons, letter pandas, kinkajous, coatis, coyotes, dingoes, raccoons, and mink. Ermine and martens are said to be susceptible by inoculation. Ferrets are exceedingly susceptible to distemper virus and almost always die of the disease. For this reason they are used frequently as experimental animals. There is an infectious disease of cats which is sometimes called *distemper* but this disease has nothing to do with the disease in dogs. None of the other domesticated animals or man is susceptible to the virus of canine distemper, although inapparent experimental infection has been produced in the domestic cat (4).

CD occurs in all parts of the world where dogs are raised. It is a disease of young dogs that is especially common in cities, dog colonies, or other situations where there are many contacts with other dogs. Puppies born of immune mothers acquire a passive immunity through the colostral milk which protects them until that immunity is lost. Unless the young dog is raised in relative isolation from other dogs it is likely to develop the disease at this time. Farm dogs, which often live in relative isolation, may escape distemper entirely, or perhaps have it when they are old. Old dogs are not immune to distemper because of age but only because they have had previous contacts with the virus.

The onset of the disease is usually manifested by a watery discharge from the eyes and nose, lassitude, inappetence, and fever, which may reach 105 F or higher. The lachrymal discharge may become purulent within 24 hours. The initial temperature rise lasts about 2 days and is followed by a period of 2 or 3 days in which the temperature may be nearly or quite normal. During this time the animal may feel better and may eat its food. This is followed by a secondary temperature rise which may last for several weeks. Again the dog feels badly, there is no appetite, vomiting usually occurs, pneumonia frequently develops, and in many cases a severe, fetid diarrhea appears. The feces are watery, mixed with mucus, offensive, and often bloody. Under these conditions the dog loses weight rapidly and usually becomes a sad spectacle. The death rate is high; hence the prognosis should be guarded.

In a few young dogs affected with distemper, a skin eruption appears with the initial temperature. This consists of pustules, which occur on the abdomen, the inside of the thighs, and elsewhere. As the animal recovers, these dry up and disappear. Because these lesions are not seen in the pure virus infections, they must be looked upon as secondary bacterial infections.

Nervous manifestations may occur. There seem to be enzootics, cyclic in nature, during which numerous puppies show nervous signs. On occasions catarrhal signs are not severe and the nervous signs predominate. Dogs with nervous manifestations have a syndrome characterized by several or all of the following signs: depression, myalgia, myoclonus, incoordination, circling, epileptiform convulsions, and coma. In general when dogs show convulsions, death results. In some cases chorea and paralysis may remain after other signs subside.

In the early febrile stage of the disease leukopenia occurs, but later if bacterial infection is not controlled by treatment, a marked leukocytosis appears.

Dunkin and Laidlaw (22), who worked with a pure virus and with dogs raised in strict isolation, were able to show that the uncomplicated virus infections produced severe signs in many cases but with a relatively low death rate. The high mortality usually seen in this disease was undoubtedly due, in most cases, to complications of bacterial infections to which the animal is predisposed by the action of the virus before the introduction of the sulfonamides and antibiotics. Now, mortality is usually the result of viral action on the central nervous system.

It has become obvious in recent years that another virus disease, *infectious canine hepatitis,* is often confused with distemper and that both diseases may occur in a dog simultaneously. There is no interference between the viruses of these two diseases, according to Gillespie, Robinson, and Baker (28). In experiments, dogs infected with both viruses develop a severer type of illness than is seen in others receiving only one virus. Both viruses are recovered from the blood of such dogs, and the typical inclusion bodies of both viruses are found in their tissues.

Dunkin and Laidlaw found the incubation period to be remarkably constant. In most dogs the febrile reaction began on the 4th day following exposure. Rarely it occurred on the 3rd day, occasionally on the 5th, and rarely on the 6th.

The course of the disease varies greatly, depending upon the character and severity of the secondary complications. In uncomplicated cases the dogs may show very mild signs, which may not be recognized, or the animal may suffer a febrile illness, which may last 2 weeks or longer. When complicated with catarrhal pneumonia and enteritis, the course may be much longer. Nervous signs may be evident for many weeks after recovery from all other signs.

The death rate varies widely depending upon the breed, age, kind of nursing care, and treatment given. It probably averages about 20 percent.

Distemper virus qualifies as a pantropic virus disease that has an affinity for epithelial cells. This accounts for the widespread appearance of lesions in the dog. In the skin a vesicular and pustular dermatitis may occur. These changes are confined to the Malpighian layer of the epidermis, but congestion of the dermis usually occurs and lymphocytic infiltration may occur. Proliferation of the keratin layer of the footpad epidermis results in a hardened pad which British investigators have termed *hard-pad disease*. The urinary epithelium may show vascular congestion with cytoplasmic and intranuclear inclusion bodies. These occur particularly in the bladder and renal pelvis. Few lesions are observed in the stomach and intestine; however, cytoplasmic acidophilic inclusion bodies may be found in the epithelial lining. Intranuclear acidophilic inclusions also may be seen occasionally in these cells. Excessive mucus is often seen in the large intestine. A catarrhal or purulent bronchopneumonia where bronchi and alveoli are filled with exudate was found more commonly before the introduction of the sulfa drugs and antibiotics. In other cases mononuclear cells lining alveolar walls or partially filling the alveoli are the only evidence of involvement. Epithelioid cells with fused cytoplasm (giant cells) line the bronchioles and alveoli adjacent to the pleura, and it appears microscopically as a giant-cell pneumonia. Inclusion bodies are found in giant cells, other mononuclear cells, and bronchiolar and bronchial epithelium. The spleen may be grossly enlarged, and congested necrosis of lymphoid cells in the splenic follicles may be observed microscopically. In uncomplicated cases the most significant change is a size reduction of the thymus gland, which may be gelatinous. Degenerative changes may occur in the adrenal, usually the cortex.

Intraocular lesions associated with CD were described by Jubb *et al.* (34). Leukocytes infiltrate the ciliary body. Exudative or degenerative changes are seen in retinal ganglion cells and proliferation in pigment epithelium. Edema causes focal retinal detachments. Ulcerative keratitis sometimes complicates a purulent conjunctivitis.

The urinary and reproductive organs may show lesions. The transitional epithelium of the urinary tract appears swollen and hydropic. Urinary bladder and kidney pelvis epithelium have many inclusion bodies. Mild interstitial epididymitis and orchitis are common.

Dogs with nervous manifestations may show perivascular cuffing, nonsuppurative leptomeningitis, and vacuoles in the white matter. Many Purkinje cells show degenerative changes. Numerous cells show pyknosis whereas other cells appear swollen and their Nissl granules are small and indistinct. Some Purkinje cells fade so that they are almost unrecognizable. Gliosis is seen in the cerebellum and is most marked in those dogs that develop nervous manifestations a considerable time after onset of infection. Degenerated myelin is not demonstrable in the cerebellum of experimental dogs that are destroyed after displaying nervous signs 7 to 16 days after intracerebral inoculation with Snyder Hill strain (27). Demyelinization accompanied by usual gitter cells and by intranuclear inclusion bodies in glial cells are found in the cerebellums of dogs with nervous manifestations observed at the longer intervals. These data lend support to the concept that demyelinization may be the response of a self-imposed antigen-antibody reaction. However, a direct effect by the virus on oligodendroglia cells that produce myelin has to be considered. By electron microscopy, crystallike structures similar to CD nucleocapsid are seen in the cytoplasm of endothelial and adventitial cells of meningeal veins and arteries, in the endothelium of cortical and plexus capillaries, in mononuclear cells within the lumen of blood vessels, in histiocytes and macrophages within the arachnoid space, in reactive microglia cells, and in ependymal cells (7).

**The Disease in Experimental Animals.** *In ferrets.* Ferrets are exceedingly susceptible to the virus of CD (21). Natural outbreaks of the disease often occur and the mortality is very nearly 100 percent. The disease is readily transmitted through the air. Dunkin and Laidlaw (21) found that they could not keep normal ferrets in the same building with those infected with virus, no matter how much care was used to prevent the spread of the virus. They concluded that the virus was air-borne.

The incubation period is about 10 days as a rule but may occasionally be 1 or 2 days shorter. A watery discharge from the eyes and the nose indicates the onset of the disease. This quickly becomes purulent, and the eyelids become swollen and pasted together. The chin becomes reddened and small vesicles form around the mouth where the hair meets the naked skin of the lips. The feet swell, the footpads become red, and sometimes the skin of the abdomen reddens. On the 3rd day the vesicles on the chin become pustules and the animal remains curled up in the cage, refusing all food. It becomes weaker and generally dies on the 5th or 6th day. Occasionally one lives longer and develops pneumonia or nervous signs, but ultimately it almost always dies.

Heath (33) has described a neurotropic strain of CD virus. After a few passages in ferrets in which typical signs were produced, the signs changed suddenly and nervous manifestations predominated in ferrets inoculated thereafter. The incubation period became longer (about 16 days). Some animals died suddenly without manifesting any signs. Others exhibited intermittent convulsions and died in from 2 to 4 days after the first spasms were seen.

*In dogs.* Susceptible dogs will exhibit the typical picture of acute distemper when inoculated with virus. Some virus strains develop neurotropic properties for dogs and will cause a high percentage of cases in which nervous signs are prominent (Mansi, 41; Gillespie and Rickard, 27). In susceptible puppies that are 1 to 2 weeks of age the only signs of illness are hemorrhagic diarrhea, dehydration, and inappetence, terminating usually in death 2 weeks after the onset of illness (25).

*In hamsters.* Cabasso, Douglas, Stebbins, and Cox (11) reported success in adapting a chick-embryo-adapted strain of CD virus to suckling hamsters. At the time of their report they had passed it through 16 generations. The infected animals died in from 4 to 7 days following inoculation. Proof of the identity of the strain was provided by serum-neutralization tests and by the successful immunization of ferrets.

*In suckling mice.* CD virus was first adapted to suckling mice by Morse, Chow, and Brandly (42). Intracerebral inoculation of chick embryo adapted strains into suckling mice produced nervous manifestations and death.

**Properties of the Virus.** Ultrafiltration experiments by Palm and Black (45) gave a particle size between 115 and 160 m$\mu$ in diameter. Subsequent electron-microscope photomicrographs of Cruickshank *et al.* (18) showed that most particles ranged between 150 and 300 m$\mu$. Electron-microscope photomicro-

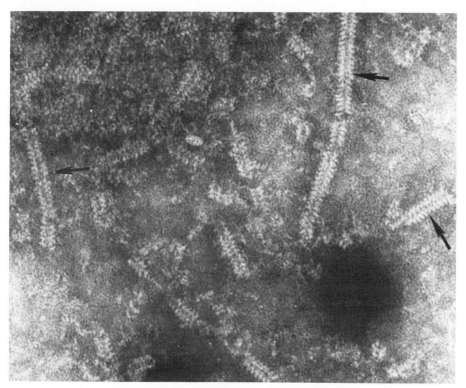

*Fig. 199.* Helical cores (*arrows*) of CDV. X 250,000. (Courtesy J. Almeida.)

graphs show that the central core contains helices that are 15 to 17 m$\mu$ in diameter (18, fig. 199). Filamentous forms of virus are described. It is an ether-sensitive RNA virus.

The virus remains viable for years at $-$ 70 C. Virus in dog spleen survives at 55 C for 30 minutes but not 1 hour. Egg vaccine virus is inactivated at 50 C within 10 minutes and cannot be detected after 7 to 8 days at 25 C. Egg virus survives between pH values of 4.4 and 10.4, with pH 8 as ideal (16).

Various chemical compounds have virucidal activity for CD virus, including 0.75 percent formalin (16). Hydroxylamine inactivates the virus under certain conditions. Beta-propriolactone in a final concentration of 0.1 percent inactivates CDV within 2 hours at 37 C (9).

Lyophilization provides a convenient method to preserve CDV in the laboratory and for commercial use. Large lyophilizers apply heat to remove residual moisture at the end of the process and this causes a reduction in titer, usually 0.5 to 1.5 $\log_{10}$ of virus. This may be critical for a commercial vaccine product depending upon its titer prior to lyophilization and subsequent treatment after reconstitution with sterile distilled water. The final product is quite stable, either as virulent or attenuated virus, provided the moisture content is low and it is maintained at approximately 6 C. Various tests have shown that the virus persists for years with little or no loss of titer.

A complement-fixing antigen can be demonstrated in infective spleen and in the chorioallantoic membrane of infected hens' eggs. Phillips and Bussell (46) separated three stable CF antigens by cesium chloride gradient centrifugation of the Onderstepoort egg-adapted strain of CDV. One antigen probably is a protein with a buoyant density of 1.289 and the other two probably are lipoproteins with densities of 1.234 and 1.140.

The plate and microscope slide procedures of the agar-gel diffusion test of Ouchterlony have been used to study CDV. Soluble antigens distinct from the infective particle precipitate specific antibody. Antigen can be derived from tissue fragments of mesenteric lymph node or spleen of infected animals or from supernatant fluid of infective tissue-culture fluids. An electroprecipitin test also has been reported for viral detection by Zydeck (55).

The immunofluorescence test has been used effectively in pathogenesis studies of the dog because viral antigen is readily demonstrated in tissue cells (4). It has been located in inclusion bodies of infected dog tissues (43). Yamanouchi et al. (54) claimed V and S antigen formed in cytoplasm because intranuclear fluorescence in tissue-cultured cells appeared only after 48 to 72 hours and a single growth cycle is approximately 18 hours. Complete virus on cell surfaces fluoresced indicating activity against V antigen. Activity against S antigen was not observed.

Vladimirov (52) has reported that CDV causes hemagglutination of human and frog erythrocytes at dilutions of 1:40 and 1:320. These results have not been confirmed. The blood cells from many other animal species including the dog are not hemagglutinated by CDV.

The virus of CD, like measles virus, is sensitive to light in fluid suspension and during viral replication. Calf serum or glutathione reduced the inactivation rate of CDV. Certain components of tissue-culture media enhanced light sensitivity but their presence was not essential for light inactivation. It has been suggested that a substance derived from the host cell that is incorporated into the viral overcoat serves to make CDV light-sensitive (4).

Neutralizing antibodies are formed and can be demonstrated in various systems such as the embryonated hens' eggs, suckling hamsters, suckling mice, ferrets, dogs, and various tissue culture systems. The chick embryo system has been used mostly for immunity studies in the dog. The agar-gel diffusion test has been used to study the viral antigenicity.

With various serological tests and protection tests in animals it has been possible to determine that the viruses of measles, canine distemper, and rinderpest of cattle share some common antigenic material. There is some similarity in the lesions which they produce in their respective susceptible hosts and in certain tissue-culture systems.

**Cultivation.** Haig (32) in 1948 reported success in cultivating a ferret-adapted strain of CD virus on the chorioallantoic membrane of embryonated chicks. The lesions appear as grayish-white thickenings. He had carried the strain through 30 generations at the time of his report. During the following year Cabasso and Cox (10) reported success with a dog-passage strain. This strain retained virulence for ferrets until the 24th to 28th serial passage, when it lost virulence but retained immunizing properties. This strain is the basis of a commercial vaccine.

In 1951 Dedie (20) reported successful cultivation of CD virus in tissue culture. Rockborn (51) propagated the virus in dog kidney monolayer cultures, and it produced syncytia, intranuclear and cytoplasmic inclusion bodies, and stellate cells. In chick embryo cell cultures, egg-adapted virus produced cellular granulation and fragmentation without the formation of syncytia (35). Isolation of virulent CDV in tissue culture is difficult although it has been done in various cell systems. Dog lung macrophages give good results. Once adapted to embryonating eggs or tissue culture the virus can be propagated in a large number of primary and stable cell cultures derived from canine, mustelid, avian, bovine, simian, and human tissues (4). Karzon and Bussell (35) used the plaque overlay method to quantitate virus or antibody.

**Immunity.** Dogs that recover from an infection with canine distemper virus usually are immune for life. The virus is so widespread that most dogs, except a few that lead sheltered lives, have had the infection before they are 1 year old and are immune. The duration of immunity persisted in dogs retained in isolation for at least 7 years (4). Occasionally older dogs with a history of previous vaccination that reside in an urban community develop clinical distemper. Immunity challenge in dogs is difficult to evaluate because contact-exposure to diseased dogs is unreliable and parenteral inoculation does not result in frank disease in some susceptible dogs. A more reliable

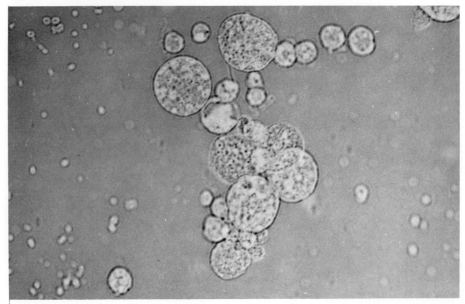

*Fig. 200.* The effects of Snyder Hill strain of CDV in dog macrophage culture. X 400. (Courtesy M. Appel.)

method is the intracerebral challenge with brain-adapted strains of CDV. Ferrets are often used as test animals as the mortality ranges between 90 and 100 percent. Ferrets given egg-attenuated virus vaccine are immune for at least 5 years.

Neutralizing antibody has been used as a means of evaluating the duration of immunity. Concurrent with protection in dogs neutralizing antibody appears which presently serves as the only *in vitro* method for measuring immunity. A maternal antibody titer of 1 : 100 or greater can be correlated with absolute protection against intracerebral or aerosal challenge with the Snyder Hill strain of CDV. Dogs with maternal titers of less than 1 : 20 are susceptible. On the other hand, dogs given inactivated CD virus or measles virus had little or no measurable neutralizing CD antibody. When these dogs are challenged no frank disease is produced and they react with an anamnestic antibody response. Consequently, the amount of neutralizing antibody is only a relative index of protection in the dog. Presently there is no good method for evaluating cell-mediated immunity.

At an American Veterinary Medical Association symposium on canine distemper, the Committee on Standardized Methods and Test Procedures made recommendations for the standardization of the neutralization test (13). These recommendations were based on the statistical evaluation tests of Robson *et al.* (50). Neutralization tests are performed in various tissue-culture systems; embryonated hens' eggs, mice, ferrets, dogs, and suckling hamsters with the properly adapted viral test strain used in each system. Neutralizing antibodies first appear in the circulation 8 to 9 days after aerosol exposure to virulent virus with maximal titers reached at 4 weeks with serum levels ranging from 1 : 300 to 1 : 3,000 when tested against approximately $10^2$ $EID_{50}$ (egg infective $dose_{50}$) of virus. Titers to vaccine virus are slightly lower. The main fraction of CD-neutralizing antibody is found in gamma globulin fraction of the serum. CD-neutralizing antibody is found in the cerebral spinal fluid of most dogs with demyelinating CD encephalitis. The majority of these dogs have a marked elevation of IgG and also an increase in IgM in the CSF.

Complement-fixing antibodies develop 3 to 4 weeks after initial infection but persist for only a few weeks thereafter. Consequently, this test offers a means by which a recent initial infection can be diagnosed. Dogs given inactivated virus develop CF antibodies that rapidly disappear. Upon challenge with virulent virus a few months later CF titers appear in 4 to 8 days which persist for at least 7 months at significant levels (26).

CD distemper antibody produced with the Rockborn strain of CDV inhibits the hemagglutination of monkey erythrocytes by Tween 80 ether-treated measles virus. In contrast, CD distemper antibody produced by the Snyder Hill strain of CDV failed, yet the serum-neutralization tests of both antiserums were similar.

Puppies, born of immune mothers, obtain an effective immunity from the mother, but this is passive antibody and disappears within a few weeks. This passive neutralizing antibody is transferred *in utero* (3 percent) and by combined placental and colostral antibody transfer equivalent to 77 percent of the mother's serum titer. The half-life of maternally transferred distemper antibody is 8.4 days (25).

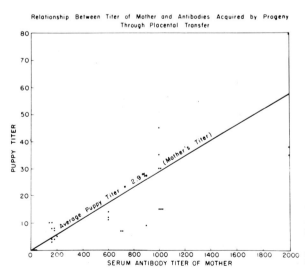

Fig. 201. Canine distemper. Relationship between titer of mother and antibodies acquired by progeny through placental transfer. (Courtesy J. Gillespie, J. Baker, J. Burgher, D. Robson, and B. Gilman, *Cornell Vet.*)

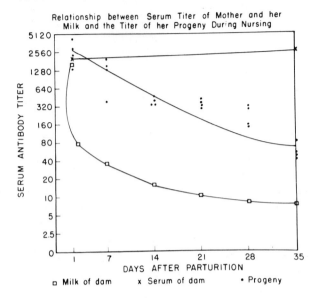

*Fig. 202.* Canine distemper. Relationship between serum titer of mother and her milk and the titer of her progeny during nursing. (Courtesy J. Gillespie, J. Baker, J. Burgher, D. Robson, and B. Gilman, *Cornell Vet.*)

Until recently it was believed that very young puppies were not capable of producing distemper antibodies. These failures now can be attributed to maternal immunity interference or improper immunization. No effect of age on distemper antibody was discernible when the nomograph was used to determine this age. Titers produced in puppies of any age group to egg-virus vaccine are identical (25). Puppies that do not suckle their immune mothers and receive no colostrum can be vaccinated at 2 weeks of age because the amount of antibody transferred *in utero* is relatively small.

**Transmission.** This disease is transmitted principally by droplet infection, virus being present in abundance in the serous excretions which run from the eyes and nose during the early febrile stage of the disease. Dunkin and Laidlaw found that it was impossible to keep susceptible dogs in the same room with infected dogs without the former becoming infected, no matter what precautions were taken. In their experimental work they set up individual kennels 100 to 150 feet apart, depending upon air dilution to prevent the passage of virus from one to another. This generally succeeded, but there were some instances when they believed that infected droplets had bridged these gaps.

The urine and fecal material contain virus and are capable of transmitting the disease. Kennels, runs, and other places haunted by dogs generally harbor virus. Arthropod carriers of this virus have not been found.

**Diagnosis.** A positive diagnosis is assured by the isolation of CD virus. The finding of typical cytoplasmic or intranuclear inclusion bodies in affected tissues is presumptive evidence for a definite diagnosis. The possible persistence of inclusion bodies could conceivably lead to a false positive diagnosis unless supported by serological or virological evidence.

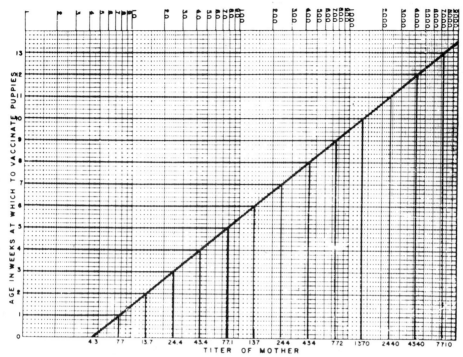

Fig. 203. A nomograph for CD showing relationship between serum titer of mother and the age in weeks at which to vaccinate her progeny. (Courtesy J. Baker, D. Robson, J. Gillespie, J. Burgher, and P. Doty, *Cornell Vet.*)

Distemper is a pantropic infection, so virus can be readily isolated from the blood, lymph nodes, spleen, lung, liver, and other visceral organs during the acute stage of infection by ferret or dog inoculation. It has also been isolated from the brain of dogs with epileptiform convulsions long after it was possible to isolate virus from the blood (27). No virus was isolated from the blood, urine, and brains of fully recovered dogs injected with virulent virus 30 days earlier.

The fluorescent antibody technic is used to demonstrate the presence of antigen in inclusion bodies observed in mononuclear cells in the blood (17). This method is used to diagnose distemper.

Generally, susceptible dogs or ferrets are used for the primary isolation of CD virus. The response in dogs can be slight, so the use of paired sera samples to demonstrate a rising antibody titer is essential in these instances. Less reliable results are obtained by isolation attempts in dog tissue culture systems unless dog macrophages are used. The use of hens' eggs, suckling mice, and suckling hamsters for primary isolation is inadvisable because these hosts only respond to adapted strains.

The clinical diagnosis of canine distemper has, in the past, been considered

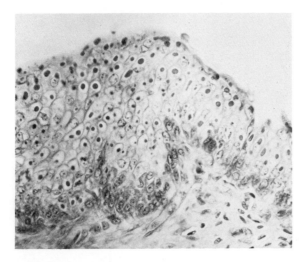

*Fig. 204.* Canine distemper inclusion bodies in the urinary bladder of a raccoon. The bodies are located in the epithelial cells. They are not always as numerous as in this case. X 600.

a relatively simple matter. It is now quite certain that under this single designation several different diseases of dogs have been included in the past. Probably the most important of these is infectious hepatitis. A specific diagnosis of distemper, obviously, is not simple. It has already been pointed out that neither signs of illness nor lesions are pathognomonic of the disease.

**The Relationship of the Virus of CD to Certain Other Viruses.** In 1957 Adams and Imagawa (1) found that a strain of the virus of human measles was neutralized by the serum of ferrets which had been actively immunized against CD virus. The serum of normal ferrets had no such effect. These neutralization studies were conducted in a tissue culture system. In animal studies, ferrets which had been immunized with measles virus showed partial protection when challenged with CD virus. Also, a mouse-adapted strain of CD virus was completely neutralized by measles antiserum prepared in ferrets.

Pursuing the matter further, Cabasso, Kiser, and Stebbins (12) found that puppies vaccinated against CD developed high levels of homologous antibodies but failed to develop either neutralizing or complement-fixing antibodies for measles virus. Similarly chickens, hyperimmunized against CD virus, did not develop antibodies for measles although their homologous titers were high.

Most dogs immunized with measles virus developed low distemper neutralizing titers and excellent homotypic antibody titers (26). On challenge with a brain-adapted strain of CD virus all dogs were protected, but the controls sickened and some died. The mechanism of protection depended upon a rapid secondary response of distemper antibody following the distemper challenge (26).

The relationship of measles virus (MV) and CDV in animal species is variable (4). Monkeys infected with MV react like humans and produce antibodies to both viruses. Infection of ferrets, rabbits, and guinea pigs with MV produce measles antibody titers but only low distemper neutralizing antibody titers in some of the animals, even after two infections with MV. Ferrets immunized with MV are partially protected against DV challenge. When CDV is inoculated into various species, production of MV antibody is found less frequently and protection against MV less effective.

Polding and Simpson (48) in East Africa, noting that a group of dogs which were constantly in intimate contact with cattle suffering from rinderpest remained free from CD, wondered if the apparent protection stemmed from exposure to rinderpest virus. They tested the hypothesis by injecting rinderpest virus into a group of CD-susceptible dogs and, after 25 days, inoculated these and a similar group of nontreated dogs with CD virus. Those injected with rinderpest virus remained healthy; those that were not so treated remained well also. Later, Polding *et al.* (49) inoculated cattle with CD virus. No clinically recognized response was elicited and all later proved susceptible to rinderpest when challenged with virus. Again, a group of dogs given a single dose of rinderpest virus later proved refractory to CD virus, but it was observed that other dogs, given large doses of antirinderpest immune serum, received only slight protection against a subsequent inoculation with CD virus.

For more information about this triad of paramyxoviruses the reader is referred to the monograph by Appel and Gillespie (4).

**Immunization.** At the American Veterinary Medical Association symposia (1965 and 1969) the Panels made recommendations for the immunization of dogs against canine distemper. These recommendations have led to a more standardized approach by the veterinary profession in the prevention and control of this most important disease. The panel recommendations are incorporated into this section on immunization.

*Passive immunization of dogs.* The first individuals to produce an antiserum for CD were Lockhart, Ray, and Barbee (39) in 1925. These workers hyperimmunized immune dogs by injections of virus-blood removed from susceptible dogs which had been injected with virus and were suffering a febrile reaction.

Laidlaw and Dunkin (36) prepared an immune serum by hyperimmunizing dogs that had recovered from an injection of virus about 1 month previously. The hyperimmunization was accomplished by making two subcutaneous injections, on successive days, of 20 ml of a 10 percent emulsion of spleen and lymph node tissue that were removed from distemper-affected dogs early in the course of the disease when the virus content of these organs is highest.

CD antiserum may protect susceptible dogs from the disease for a limited time. It is used in some animal hospitals for protecting young canine patients, which may not have had distemper, from infection which they are likely, otherwise, to contract there. If the animal comes in contact with the virus while protected by the serum, it may develop an active enduring immunity. Usually one 10-ml dose of serum is given for a few days' stay in the hospital or at a dog show. If the sojourn is prolonged, another dose is given about the 10th day. Immune serum sometimes is used to protect valuable puppies while they are susceptible. Puppies that are raised in relatively good isolation usually are untreated until they are old enough for the active immunization.

Some manufacturers immunize their serum-producing dogs with the bacteria commonly found as secondary invaders in distemper as well as with the virus of Carré, in the belief that antibodies against these organisms may be of assistance in combating the secondary infections. So far as we know there is no proof that these sera are better than those prepared against the virus alone, but there may be some merit in the idea, and certainly there are no objections.

One manufacturer in the United States (8) produced a canine globulin concentrate of distemper immune serum. It is claimed that the gamma globulin does not contain all of the immune bodies, that there are significant amounts in the beta fraction as well. Hence the product is a mixture of these two fractions. It is claimed that much extraneous material is eliminated and a more concentrated product obtained. It is freeze-dried for the trade and reconstituted just before use.

According to the AVMA panels (13, 14) there is evidence that the routine prophylactic use of agents that passively immunize pups against CD has less merit than multiple doses of attenuated live virus vaccines. Because it may block active immunization the use of antiserum or concentrated antiserum for short-term protection is to be discouraged. Antiserum or concentrated antiserum is of questionable value in the treatment of dogs with clinical signs of distemper.

*Active immunization of dogs.* Vaccination of animals represents the most effective means for the prevention of distemper. Seven vaccine methods are used in the dog: (1) formalin-treated virus vaccines, (2) ferret-passaged modified vaccine, (3) modified hen's egg virus vaccine, (4) combined use of distemper antiserum and virulent distemper virus (DV), (5) modified cell culture virus vaccines, (6) dual virus vaccine utilizing various combinations for distemper and infectious canine hepatitis (ICH), and (7) measles vaccine.

Immunization of dogs is a controversial subject, but most individuals including the AVMA panels feel that under normal conditions the modified virus vaccines of chick embryo or tissue culture origin are more desirable. Alone or in combination with modified infectious canine hepatitis virus and leptospirosis, the distemper component does not cause illness, is efficacious, does not spread to susceptible dogs, and gives a relatively long immunity. Immunity after vaccination with modified virus vaccines, but not with inactivated virus vaccines, can be tested by the serum-neutralization test.

The formalin-inactivated virus vaccines are usually made with infective dog spleen. Usually three injections at 2-week intervals are recommended for the dog. Neutralizing-antibody titers reach their maximum 30 days after the last injection. The titers seldom rise much above 100 and are no longer measurable 16 weeks after the first injection. Dogs are still sensitized to the distemper antigen 3 to 6 months later, and a secondary antibody response occurs which confers clinical protection when challenged with virulent virus (24). Some veterinarians still use inactivated virus vaccine, especially in the larger cities where repeated exposures are likely to occur assuring immunity—hopefully without the production of frank disease.

Ferret-passaged modified vaccine produces an immunity which is believed to be solid and enduring although serological studies have not been reported. Dogs should be in excellent condition at the time of vaccination. In some instances the dog has a reaction but usually it is mild. Some veterinarians use this product to treat early cases of distemper, although there are questions as to its validity. The procedure is based upon the virus interference studies of Green and Stulberg (31).

The combined use of distemper antiserum and virulent distemper virus is no longer employed in the United States.

As distemper virus causes the greatest mortality in young dogs, protection is desirable at an early age. Interference with active immunity by maternal antibody complicates a vaccination program because the immune status of a pup is variable. To overcome the problem, vaccination with MV seemed to be an ideal solution. Despite considerable research and field study the results are equivocal. Contrary to previous belief, the response to MV vaccination in dogs may be age-dependent with no definite information regarding the factor(s) involved. It has been shown that maternal measles antibody will interfere with an active immunity to that virus. Consequently the presence of maternally derived measles antibody must also be considered as well as distemper antibody in a distemper immunization program.

There has been much controversy in the past about the best age at which to immunize young animals. There are still differences of opinion, and it is not always possible to decide this for an individual animal with precision.

It has been pointed out that, when the mother is immune to CD, antibodies are stored in the colostral milk and these convey a passive immunity to the puppies. The concentration of antibodies in the colostrum varies in different immune bitches, however, and this affects the length of time the sucklings will have sufficient antibodies to protect them against natural exposure. If active immunization is attempted while the young animals retain substantial antibody levels derived from their mothers, enduring immunity will not result since the antigenic properties of the vaccines are wholly neutralized by the passively acquired antibody. On the other hand, if the mother is not immune to CD, there will be no antibody in her colostrum and her puppies will at once be highly susceptible to the disease.

Young dogs, therefore, may contract CD at any age, depending upon what level of colostral antibodies they possess. Because immunization will fail if done too early, and will fail also if it is deferred too long allowing natural infection to intervene, the selection of the best time for proceeding with artificial immunization is a difficult individual problem. Gillespie et al. (25) and

Baker *et al.* (5) have attempted to solve this problem by developing a nomo-graph which relates the serum antibody titer of the dam to the time after birth when, in most instances, the antibody titers of its offspring will have de-creased to the point that artificial active immunization is effective. The sys-tem predicts when the antibody loss of the young brings them into the period of susceptibility. The system is based upon sound scientific facts and gener-ally is quite effective, but it is more expensive than many dog owners will accept since it involves the taking of a blood sample from the dam before the birth of its offspring and having its virus-neutralizing titer determined by lab-oratory tests in infected eggs.

Then, too, individuals often purchase a puppy without the opportunity of determining the serum titer of its mother. Under these circumstances vaccina-tion of puppies at 9 weeks of age with egg or tissue culture virus vaccine im-munized approximately 82 percent of the puppies at this age (25). Revaccina-tion at 15 weeks of age took care of the other 18 percent that failed to respond earlier because of maternal antibody interference. One-third of these puppies have titers of less than 1:100 at 1 year of age (50). At 2 years of age another third have titers below this figure. A serum titer of 1:100 is used as the standard level for indicating immunity to CD, although it is recognized that some dogs with lower titers may be immune. It was recommended that dogs be vaccinated yearly with modified virus vaccine until a more sensitive test can be devised that will measure cellular immunity as well as neutraliz-ing antibody. In lieu of this procedure yearly blood tests can be performed. If the serum titer falls below 1:100, revaccination was indicated. Over 90 per-cent of vaccinated dogs will show a significant rise in titer above the 1:100 level; the absolute criterion that a dog will withstand challenge with virulent CDV.

*Recommended vaccination procedures by the AVMA panels.* (13) (14) Based on the knowledge available to the two panels concerned with Canine Distemper Immunization, the following recommendations were made as guidelines for the employment of professional judgment in canine distemper immunization. These recommendations have had general acceptance by the veterinary profession in the United States and are as follows:

The Panel recommends the use of modified live-virus vaccine of chicken embryo or tissue culture origin. There is no evidence that the vaccine will cause untoward reactions in parasitized, malnour-ished, or otherwise debilitated dogs, or interfere with the natural course of distemper in previously exposed animals.

The Panel recommends annual vaccination of all dogs. Although present evidence of untoward effects on the fetus is inconclusive, vaccination of pregnant bitches should be avoided.

When feasible, a nomograph should be used that predicts the age at which pups should be vaccinated against distemper.

Ideally, vaccinated dogs should be serologically tested 30 days after initial vaccination and revaccinated if so indicated by serologic test. Pups of unknown immune status and more than 3 months old should be given one dose of vaccine. If younger than 3 months, two or more doses should be administered; the first dose should be given after the pup is weaned and the last dose at 12 to 16 weeks of age. Administration of a dose of vaccine at 2-week intervals more nearly approaches the ideal.

Orphan pups that do not get colostrum can be vaccinated as early as 2 weeks of age with modified live-virus vaccine.

No dog should be admitted into an area of possible exposure to distemper without immediate vaccination with modified live-virus vaccine of chicken-embryo or tissue-culture origin, unless the dog has been given such a vaccination within the past 12 months.

Immunization of pups in the presence of homologous antibodies, either with modified canine distemper virus vaccine or attenuated measles virus vaccine, has not always been successful. Evidence indicates that measles vaccine was less effective in pups under 8 weeks old than in those over 8 weeks old. Consequently, the use of modified distemper vaccines may be preferred in pups under 8 weeks old.

*Immunization of foxes, mink, and ferrets.* Canine distemper virus causes natural epizootics among foxes, mink, and ferrets raised in captivity, the losses often being very great. The virus is the same as that which occurs in dogs, and the disease can be transmitted easily from any of these species to any other. In foxes the heavy losses occur in the fall when the animals are turned loose on the fur ranges.

For fox immunization, the process is best done shortly before the animals are turned on the range. The Laidlaw-Dunkin vaccine has been used successfully. Ott (44) reported success by using antiserum alone, but vaccines appear to be better and less expensive. Green and Carlson (30) were able to show that these losses could be greatly reduced by treating all animals with distemperoid, ferret-passage virus, and West and Brandly (53) had excellent success with formalin-inactivated vaccines made from virulent fox tissues (lungs, liver, spleen, kidneys, urinary bladder, and lymph nodes). A 20 percent suspension of these tissues was used, and the dose was 5 ml given subcutaneously or intramuscularly. Some of the vaccines that contained adjuvants (alumina gel and fatty agents) were somewhat more effective than those which did not contain them.

Distemper infection in foxes must be differentiated from that of fox encephalitis caused by infectious canine hepatitis virus and with which it may exist concurrently. Green states that this may be done by inoculating ferrets, which are susceptible to distemper but resistant to the other virus. He also points out that a search for inclusion bodies is helpful. Typical intracytoplasmic inclusion bodies, resembling those seen in dogs, may be found in the epithelial cells of the air passages and urinary bladder in cases of distemper, whereas they are not found in these cells in encephalitis infection.

Laidlaw and Dunkin (36) found it possible to immunize ferrets much more easily than dogs. A vaccine was prepared from the spleens of ferrets, removed on the 4th or 5th day of illness, by grinding them finely and making them into a 20 percent suspension. Formalin was added to these suspensions in a concentration of 0.1 percent, and the material was allowed to stand for at least 4 days, at which time viable virus had disappeared. When 2 ml of this suspension were injected subcutaneously into susceptible ferrets, they became solidly immune after a few days. After 2 weeks the immunity was made permanent by giving them a small dose of active virus, which they withstood without evidence of a physical reaction in most instances.

Pinkerton (47) reported satisfactory results in immunizing mink by the use of tissue vaccine made from lung tissue of infected mink. At the beginning of an outbreak on a ranch, some of the first animals were used as a source of vaccine virus. The finely ground tissue was made into a 10 percent emulsion, which was treated with 0.3 percent formalin. Several injections were given of from 2 to 4 ml at weekly intervals. One commercial company produces a 5 percent ferret spleen vaccine that has been inactivated with ultraviolet light.

The manufacturers of the egg-adapted vaccine claim that it has been used with complete satisfaction for immunizing ferrets and minks. They also say that gratifying results were obtained in stopping outbreaks of mink distemper with it.

**The Disease in Man.** So far as is known, the virus of CD is nonpathogenic for man.

## REFERENCES

1. Adams and Imagawa.   Proc. Soc. Exp. Biol. and Med., 1957, *96*, 240.
2. Appel.   Am. Jour. Vet. Res., 1969, *30*, 1167.
3. Appel, Percy, and Gaskin.   Personal communication, 1971.
4. Appel and Gillespie.   Handbook of virus research. Springer-Verlag, Vienna and New York, 1972.
5. Baker, Robson, Gillespie, Burgher, and Doughty.   Cornell Vet., 1959, *49*, 158.
6. Bindrich.   Kleintierpraxis, 1962, 7, 161 and 181.
7. Blinzinger and Deutschländer.   Verh. Deut. Ges. f. Path., 1969, *53*, 283.
8. Brueckner, Taylor, Schroeder, and Koehler.   Proc. Soc. Exp. Biol. and Med., 1959, *102*, 20.
9. Bussell.   Personal communication. (Quoted by Appel and Gillespie, ref. 4.), 1971.
10. Cabasso and Cox.   Proc. Soc. Exp. Biol. and Med., 1949, *71*, 246.
11. Cabasso, Douglas, Stebbins, and Cox.   *Ibid.*, 1955, 88, 199.
12. Cabasso, Kiser, and Stebbins.   *Ibid.*, 1959, *101*, 227.
13. Canine Distemper Symposium.   Jour. Am. Vet. Med. Assoc., 1966, *149*, part 2.
14. Canine Infectious Diseases Symposium.   *Ibid.*, 1970, *156*, part 1.
15. Carré.   Comp. rend. Acad. Sci., 1905, *140*, 689 and 1489.
16. Celiker and Gillespie.   Cornell Vet., 1954, *44*, 276.
17. Cello, Moulton, and McFarland.   *Ibid.*, 1959, *49*, 127.
18. Cruickshank, Waterson, Kanarek, and Berry.   Res. Vet. Sci., 1962, 3, 485.

19.  Cutchins and Dayhuff.   Virology, 1962, 17, 420.
20.  Dedie and Klopotke.   Arch. Exp. Vet. Med., 1951, 4, 137.
21.  Dunkin and Laidlaw.   Jour. Comp. Path. and Therap., 1926, 39, 201.
22.  Ibid., 213.
23.  Gillespie.   Ann. N.Y. Acad. Sci., 1962, 101, 540.
24.  Gillespie.   Cornell Vet., 1965, 55, 3.
25.  Gillespie, Baker, Burgher, Robson, and Gilman.   Ibid., 1958, 48, 103.
26.  Gillespie and Karzon.   Proc. Soc. Exp. Biol. and Med., 1960, 105, 547.
27.  Gillespie and Rickard.   Am. Jour. Vet. Res., 1956, 17, 103.
28.  Gillespie, Robinson, and Baker.   Proc. Soc. Exp. Biol. and Med., 1952, 81,
     461.
29.  Gorham.   Adv. Vet. Sci., Acad. Press, New York, 1960, p. 287.
30.  Green and Carlson.   Jour. Am. Vet. Med. Assoc., 1945, 107, 131.
31.  Green and Stulberg.   Science, 1946, 103, 497.
32.  Haig.   Onderstepoort Jour. Vet. Sci. and Anim. Indus., 1948, 23, 149.
33.  Heath.   Canad. Jour. Comp. Med., 1940, 4, 352.
34.  Jubb, Saunders, and Coates.   Jour. Comp. Path. and Therap., 1957, 67, 21.
35.  Karzon and Bussell.   Science, 1959, 130, 1708.
36.  Laidlaw and Dunkin.   Jour. Comp. Path. and Therap., 1926, 39, 222.
37.  Ibid., 1928, 41, 1.
38.  Ibid., 209.
39.  Lockhart, Ray, and Barbee.   Jour. Am. Vet. Med. Assoc., 1925, 67, 668.
40.  MacIntyre, Trevan, and Montgomerie.   Vet. Rec., 1948, 60, 635.
41.  Mansi.   Brit. Vet. Jour., 1951, 107, 214.
42.  Morse, Chow, and Brandly.   Proc. Soc. Exp. Biol. and Med., 1953, 84, 10.
43.  Moulton and Brown.   Ibid., 1954, 86, 99.
44.  Ott.   Jour. Am. Vet. Med. Assoc., 1939, 94, 522.
45.  Palm and Black.   Proc. Soc. Exp. Biol. and Med., 1961, 107, 588.
46.  Phillips and Bussell.   Personal communication, 1971.
47.  Pinkerton.   Jour. Am. Vet. Med. Assoc., 1940, 96, 347.
48.  Polding and Simpson.   Vet. Rec., 1957, 69, 582.
49.  Polding, Simpson, and Scott.   Ibid., 1959, 71, 643.
50.  Robson, Kenneson, Gillespie, and Benson.   Proc. Gaines Vet. Sympos., 1959,
     9, 10.
51.  Rockborn.   Arch. f. die Gesam. Virusforsch., 1958, 8, 485.
52.  Vladimirov.   Veterinariya (Moscow), 26 (7), 59. (Original not seen, Cited in
     Vet. Bul., 1951, 21, 77.)
53.  West and Brandly.   Cornell Vet., 1949, 39, 292.
54.  Yamanouchi, Kobune, Fuduka, Hayami, and Shishido.   Arch. f. die Gesam.
     Virusforsch., 1970, 29, 90.
55.  Zydeck.   Experientia, 1970, 26, 88.

## Rinderpest

SYNONYMS:   Cattle plague, oriental cattle plague (possible paramyxovirus)

Rinderpest is an acute, febrile disease of ruminants characterized by a rapid course and a high mortality rate (28). Excellent review articles have been prepared by Plowright (32) and Scott (37).

**Character of the Disease.** The disease affects principally cattle, hence its name. In the orient, water buffalo are frequent victims. Sheep, yaks, and goats are fairly resistant to natural infection and seldom are seriously affected, although a few large outbreaks have been reported. Some wild ungulates, swine, camels, and even wart hogs are said to be mildly susceptible.

The disease is enzootic in parts of Asia and Africa. It has spread from Asia on many occasions in the past, especially in times of war, to Europe, where it has affected cattle principally. The results of these epizootics have often been devastating. On some occasions a large portion of the entire cattle population has perished. Only once has the disease appeared in the Western Hemisphere. In 1921 it appeared in Brazil, where it apparently had been imported in zebu cattle. This outbreak was quickly recognized and stamped out after fewer than 1,000 cattle had developed the disease, and about 2,000 additional animals that had been exposed were slaughtered. Rinderpest could do great damage to the cattle population of North and South America should it ever gain a secure foothold. Veterinarians should constantly be on guard to detect it early if it should occur. Modern air travel has greatly increased the hazard of its bridging the oceans which have been our protectors in the past.

The virulence of rinderpest virus varies greatly from time to time and from place to place. The susceptibility of animals differs widely also. European and American cattle, which have had no contacts with the disease for many years, are generally highly susceptible. In Asia, where the disease is enzootic, the native cattle are much more resistant. Probably this is because the more susceptible strains of such cattle have gradually been weeded out through many years of exposure. Some breeds of cattle appear to be more susceptible than others. In India the so-called "hill cattle" are usually much more susceptible than the "plains cattle." In the same outbreak the mortality of the former may be high and that of the latter light or negligible. The carabao, or water buffalo, the common beast of burden in much of southern Asia, is susceptible to rinderpest, sometimes more so than the native cattle (23, 30).

When the resistance of the host is high and the virus comparatively mild, the signs may be so slight as to be overlooked. It is thought that such animals often are the means of importing the disease into new localities or countries. They acquire permanent resistance as a result of the experience. Young calves from immune mothers often suffer only slightly from rinderpest but acquire an immunity because of it.

Acute rinderpest is the most common form, and the only one that is likely ever to be seen in European cattle or in those of the Western Hemisphere, where this disease does not exist and where susceptibility is high.

Rinderpest is usually quite explosive; large numbers of animals are likely to exhibit signs almost simultaneously. High fever (104 to 108 F) is an early sign. This is seen about the 3rd day of the disease; later the temperature falls and usually becomes subnormal before death. Rumination is suspended; there is dullness and the coat becomes rough. The buccal mucosa becomes very congested. Early in the disease often there is constipation. The victim strains in defecating, and the bowel discharges are dry, often coated with mucus and sometimes with blood. Later there is severe diarrhea, the feces becoming quite fluid and very fetid. Frequently there is a profuse nasal discharge and lacrimation. The breath becomes very offensive because of the development of many shallow erosions on the lips, dental pads, and gums. The abdomen becomes very tender, the animal moans, becomes very dull, goes down, and is unable to rise; death usually occurs between the 2nd and 6th day after the first signs are exhibited.

The incubation period in naturally acquired rinderpest is from 3 to 8 days. Only occasionally is it a little longer.

Affected animals usually die in 1 week or less after signs are first observed. Some of the more resistant breeds may linger for 2 or 3 weeks. In some outbreaks the virulence of the virus is low, and many animals may show a longer course than usual. The mortality varies, although it is almost always high. In European and American cattle a mortality rate of 90 to 100 percent must always be expected. It is lower than this in regions where the disease is enzootic.

The gross and microscopic lesions of rinderpest are well described by Maurer, Jones, Easterday, and DeTray (21). The principal lesions are found in the digestive tract. Shallow ulcers are usually found in the mucosa of the mouth—in all parts except the dorsum of the tongue. Such ulcers may also be found in the pharynx and esophagus. These are shallow, have a "punched out" appearance, and are filled with whitish caseous material. The mucosa of the abomasum is usually deeply congested. The livid membrane has areas of blood extravasation and dark purplish stripes. Ulceration of the pyloric orifice and the folds is frequent. Sometimes the inflammatory exudate forms a false membrane which may easily be peeled off. The small intestines may exhibit similar lesions. The fluid content usually is very fetid. Lesions in the large intestines include hemorrhages (fig. 205) and the rectum often shows linear, bright-red stripes—the so-called *zebra striping*. The Peyer's patches are usually ulcerated, and ulcers may be found on other parts of the mucosa.

The respiratory tract shows deep reddening of the upper passages and often petechiation. A patchy pneumonia sometimes develops, a purely secondary lesion.

If the animal has lived more than a few days after becoming infected, there will be marked dehydration of all tissues and extreme emaciation.

Plowright (31) reported that degenerative changes in lymphoid tissues also occur. Formation of syncytia with cytoplasmic inclusion bodies has been demonstrated in the stratum spinosum of stratified squamous epithelia of the upper alimentary tract and in lymphoid tissues (31, 43). Intranuclear inclusion bodies *in vivo* have been described by Thiery (43).

**The Disease in Experimental Animals.** For many years it was thought that rinderpest could be transmitted only to cattle, water buffaloes, and a few

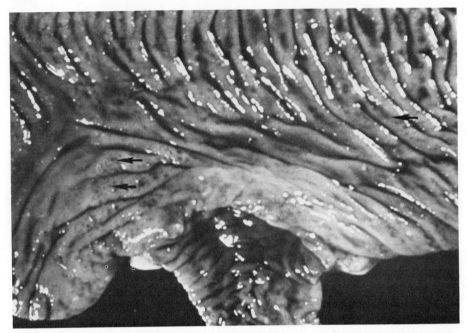

*Fig. 205.* Rinderpest. Petechial and ecchymotic hemorrhage areas in mucosal wall of gastrointestinal tract. (Courtesy J. J. Callis and staff, U.S.D.A.)

other species of ruminants. A few authentic outbreaks of rinderpest in sheep were recognized, but these animals and goats were known to be sufficiently resistant to the virus to enable them to escape the disease when it occurred in cattle kept in close association with them. Edwards (12) in 1930 adapted rinderpest virus to goats by serial passage and found that the goat virus could be used as a vaccine for cattle. In 1938 Nakamura, Wagatsuma, and Fukusko (27) succeeded in adapting several strains to rabbits so the virus could be propagated in that species. In the early passages there were no signs except a slight temperature rise which could easily be overlooked. After the virus has passed through several generations of rabbits, however, the animals show a sharp temperature rise during which they exhibit lassitude, inappetence, increased respiratory rate, and sometimes diarrhea. The febrile state lasts only about 36 to 48 hours, after which the signs subside and the animals again appear to be normal. Animals destroyed at the height of the temperature reaction often exhibit small necrotic areas in the intestinal mucosa, especially in the Peyer's patches. During this time there is a marked leukopenia. Further passage of the Nakamura III strain of lapinized rinderpest virus causes a very high mortality—greater than 95 percent. It is a very useful system to study rinderpest immunity.

In 1946 Baker also adapted a strain of rinderpest virus to rabbits (1) and guinea pigs (2). It also proliferates in mice, hamsters, dogs, ferrets, giant rats, and susliks (31).

**Properties of the Virus.** The morphological characteristics have been well described by Plowright (31) and Breese and de Boer (5, fig. 206). The particles are pleomorphic with an average diameter of 120 to 300 mμ. Like other paramyxoviruses it has an internal helical component and it is 17.5 mμ in diameter with a periodicity of 5 to 6 mμ. There is an enclosing membrane, and it has filaments that are similar to those observed for influenza A virus and Newcastle disease virus (Blacksburg strain, 31).

It is an ether-sensitive RNA virus. It does not hemagglutinate red blood cells. The virus attaches itself to the leukocytes in blood (9).

The virus is quite stable after lyophilization and at very low temperatures (−70 C or less). High passaged tissue-culture virus is relatively stable between pH 4 and 10 with the greatest stability between pH 7.2 to 7.9. Virulent strains are less stable under comparable conditions. The virus is stable in glycerol. Strong alkalis are the best disinfectants for its destruction. Certain chemicals, such as phenol, chinosol, formalin, and betapropiolactone, inacti-

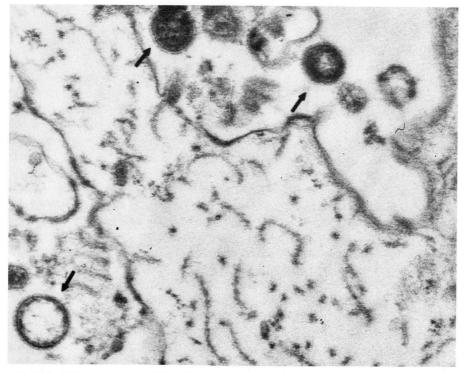

*Fig. 206.* Rinderpest virus particles. Two mature particles at top with *arrows* (dark center) and one immature particle at bottom with *arrow* (ghost particle) in cell vacuoles. X 53,400. (Courtesy S. Breese. U.S.D.A.)

vate rinderpest-infected tissues without loss of antigenicity. Trypsin and 1 M hydroxylamine also inactivate the virus. A small fraction of tissue-cultured virus survives heating at 56 C for 50 to 60 minutes and at 60 C for 30 minutes.

Virus is inactivated rather quickly (in 1 or 2 days) in dried secretions, but in the presence of moisture it retains its activity somewhat longer. Boynton (4) found that virus could never be detected by placing susceptible animals in corrals from which infected animals had been removed longer than 36 hours previously, even when water was present and parts of the area were shaded from the sun. He concluded that rinderpest virus does not survive long in pastures after affected animals are removed from them.

The virus contains antigens that produce neutralizing, complement-fixing and precipitating antibodies. Double diffusion in agar reveals a heat-stable and a heat-labile antigen. There is good evidence that the viruses of measles, canine distemper, and rinderpest share a common antigen (5). Rinderpest virus protects dogs against a challenge with virulent canine distemper virus. Interference with Rift Valley fever virus occurs, and attenuated rinderpest strains interfere with virulent ones. No hemagglutinin has been unequivocally demonstrated for rinderpest virus but it has been suggested by Provost and Borredon (35) that RV hemagglutinates erythrocytes of the monkey *Erythrocebus patas*. Infected cell cultures do not cause hemadsorption of erythrocytes.

**Cultivation.** Shope *et al.* (39, 40) succeeded in cultivating an African strain (the Kabete strain) on the chorioallantoic membranes of embryonating hens' eggs. They were not successful in adapting several other strains. Later Nakamura, Agric, and Miyamoto (24) reported success in the egg cultivation of a strain of lapinized virus. When the membranes were inoculated, the virus failed to infect the embryos, according to Shope. After several transfers on the membranes, the virus multiplied when inoculated into the yolk sac, and then could be maintained indefinitely in series by yolk-sac inoculation. In embryonated eggs inoculated into the yolk sac, the virus multiplied in the embryo, the fluids, and the egg membranes. Rinderpest virus of direct bovine origin injected into 7-day-old embryos by way of the yolk sac infected the embryos, but it was not possible to transmit this virus in series. Even the egg-adapted strain did not seriously damage the embryos since they regularly hatched. Chicks from such eggs never contained virus. Subsequently Furutani *et al.* (13), following the technic of Nakamura and Miyamoto, observed that the Nakamuru III strain of lapinized virus produced embryo deaths and reddening and swelling of embryonic spleens.

Kabete "O" strain of rinderpest virus multiplies and produces a cytopathic effect in primary monolayer cultures of calf and lamb testes; bovine embryonic kidney cells; bovine skin-muscle tissue; pig, goat, sheep, and hamster kidneys; calf thyroid; and dog kidney (31). Virulent field strains selected from tissues of infected cattle regularly produce a cytopathic effect in primary calf kidney cultures (31). Attenuated virus strains do not proliferate (31). The cytopathogenic strains in calf kidney monolayers produce syncytia or multinu-cleated giant cells together with eosinophilic cytoplasmic and type B intranu-clear inclusions. Recently isolated strains of low cattle virulence have a tendency to produce stellate-type cells, which are large and sometimes mul-tinucleated. There is more free virus in culture than cell-associated virus until the 9th day when the titers are comparable and rapidly dropping (31).

Initially, immunofluorescence antigen was not found in the nuclei except for a few granules in the later stages of infection. Using air-dried instead of acetone-fixed preparations, Leiss (20) showed fluorescent particles in the nu-cleus of infected cell cultures as early as 8 hours, often accompanied by peri-nuclear fluorescence. Cytoplasmic fluorescence was first noticed at 19 hours. It was concluded that the first synthesis of virus-specific materials probably oc-curred in the nucleus.

The Pendik strain of RV in primary monolayers of bovine kidney cells pro-duced plaques that become visible by 7 to 8 days and attain a diameter of 3 mm by day 12 and 5 mm by day 19 (22). The optimum concentration of Noble agar is 1 to 1.5 percent and a 1:5,000 dilution of neutral red or the lack of immune serum in the overlay had no effect on the results. Virus assay by plaque formation gives lower titers (approximately 2 $\log_{10}$ units) than 50 per-cent end points in monolayers. Plaque inhibition by specific immune serum is a usable system for virus identification.

Interferon produced in calf kidney cells by Sindbis virus suppresses the growth of a small amount of virulent RV in the same cell type (32). It sup-pressed the yield of released virus more than the cell associated virus replica-tion for which there is no explanation.

**Immunity.** Animals surviving an attack of rinderpest to a living virus prepara-tion are generally permanently immune thereafter. Nakamura *et al.* (25), however, claim that the immunity is not always permanent and that it is pos-sible to break it down in some animals by inoculation with highly virulent materials. Immunity to rinderpest is proved by the parenteral inoculation (usually subcutaneous) of $10^4$ TCID$_{50}$ or more of a strain which produces se-vere clinical reactions and high mortality in cattle. Production of significant levels of neutralizing antibody is indicative of resistance to test virus although a small percentage of resistant animals may have no detectable circulating antibody.

The hemagglutination-inhibition test, using measles virus hemagglutination, is applicable for detection of HI antibodies but its sensitivity is inferior to the neutralization test. Complement-fixing antibodies appear irregularly in the sera of recovered or vaccinated cattle and they persist for only a short period of time; thus the test is suitable as a diagnostic test on a herd basis but not for epidemiological surveys.

**Immunization.** Methods for artificially immunizing animals both actively and passively are available. The earliest method was by injecting nasal and ocular secretions under the skin of the dewlap. This method often served to propagate the disease, and the reactions usually were very severe. It is no longer used. Robert Koch in 1897 introduced a great improvement when he showed that cattle could be successfully immunized with bile obtained from animals killed on the 5th or 6th day of the disease. Normal bile is of no value. More than 2 million cattle in South Africa were successfully immunized by this method in a 2-year period. It has now been abandoned in favor of better vaccination procedures.

The methods used for artificially immunizing cattle against rinderpest today differ markedly in different parts of the world. Procedures which seem to be very satisfactory in one area often prove to be too drastic or ineffective in others. Obviously the virus strains in different regions differ greatly in virulence, and breeds of cattle differ greatly in susceptibility. For these reasons it appears that methods have to be adapted to the particular areas and breeds involved.

*Passive immunization.* Rinderpest antiserum. Serum from animals that have recovered from the disease possesses antibodies that are protective for susceptible animals. The value of such sera is greatly increased by hyperimmunization. Hyperimmune serum will give immediate protection, but the resistance can be expected to last only for 10 days to 2 weeks. Immune serum has no value in treating the disease. Its principal use is to protect cattle against transient exposure, such as when they are driven or shipped through infected regions, and to stop the progress of the disease in recently infected herds.

*Natural immunization of calves.* Calves born of immune mothers obtain transient immunity through the colostral milk of their dams. Such animals will resist infection. Active immunization of calves from immune mothers is unsuccessful because it tends to disappear within a few months.

*Active immunization.* Tissue vaccines containing inactivated virus. A number of these have been used with success. All are prepared by chemical treatment of tissue suspensions. They have the advantage of safety but the disadvantage that the immunity produced is not lasting. Generally they protect against ordinary exposure for periods up to 1 year. Because they did not give permanent immunity, these vaccines have been largely supplanted by attenuated virus vaccines.

Kakizaki, Nakanishi, and Ozumi (16) made a vaccine by treating spleen and lymphoid tissue pulp with glycerol, phenol, and eucalyptol. With this vaccine they successfully immunized thousands of cattle in Korea and Manchuria. Bennett (3) used a similar vaccine in the Sudan, with excellent results. This vaccine did not work so well in India, according to Edwards.

Boynton (4) made a vaccine in the Philippines by treating organ pulp with phenol and glycerol. The mixture was heated in a water bath at 42 C for 3 hours, then was kept in the refrigerator several months until tests indicated that the virus had been destroyed. The vaccine then had to be used rather promptly since old vaccines did not immunize successfully. This vaccine gave excellent success, but its method of manufacture was tedious and the keeping qualities were poor.

Kelser (17) prepared a vaccine by making a pulp of the spleen and lymphoid tissue of cattle, diluting the pulp with an equal quantity of saline solution, and adding 0.75 percent of chloroform. The chloroform rapidly destroys the rinderpest virus. After 48 hours the vaccine is ready for use. Kelser, Youngberg, and Topacio (18) used three doses given at weekly intervals. Rodier (36) later found that a single but somewhat larger dose was satisfactory. Excellent results were reported from the use of this vaccine.

A formolized spleen vaccine was developed and used by Daubney (9) in Africa. This vaccine was also used successfully by Keylock (19) in China.

Host-adapted vaccines. These vaccines contain living virus which has been altered in virulence by being serially passed through alien hosts. They cause mild, active infections which generally immunize cattle and carabao permanently, or at least for several years.

Caprinized (goat-adapted) vaccines. A serious disadvantage of using bovine blood and tissues for the immunization of cattle against rinderpest in most areas where the disease is enzootic is the fact that such materials often contain other disease-producing agents such as those of babesiosis and anaplasmosis. In an effort to propagate the virus in a host which would eliminate these extraneous infections, Edwards (12) in India discovered that goat-propagated virus gradually lost virulence for cattle and suggested that such virus be used as a vaccine for cattle. Stirling (41) used the material successfully in India in 1932. Pfaff (29), who worked in Burma, developed a goat-adapted vaccine, which was used extensively in that area. The earlier workers used citrated or defibrinated blood as the vaccine, but this material had poor keeping qualities. Later workers found that dried tissue vaccines, generally prepared from spleen pulp, were more stable.

The goat-tissue vaccine has been used with success on many millions of cattle and carabao and appears to be most popular in southern Asiatic countries. In some highly susceptible breeds the vaccine may cause too much mortality. This could be offset in some cases by administering a small dose of antiserum with the vaccine. Daubney (10), who tested the Indian strain of goat-adapted virus, found that it was too virulent in East Africa, especially for cattle with some European blood, in which the mortality rate was sometimes as high as 25 percent.

Lapinized (rabbit-adapted) vaccines. In 1938 Nakamura et al. (27) attenuated the rinderpest virus by 100 passages in rabbits. The vaccine was made from the mesenteric lymph nodes of the infected rabbits. No preservatives were added. This virus keeps its viability for a short time only; hence it must be used promptly. It was employed extensively in China and Korea. Korean cattle are more susceptible to rinderpest than those of Manchuria, where the disease is enzootic. The vaccine alone served satisfactorily on the latter, but for the Korean cattle it was necessary to give a small dose of antiserum simultaneously. This vaccine is claimed to be less virulent than goat vaccine. Nak-amura and Kuroda (26) were unable to transmit the infection by contact of normal calves with others that were sick and dying of lapinized virus infec-tion. Infected cows did not transmit the infection to their suckling calves.

Cheng and Fischman (8) vaccinated many cattle and carabao in China with a lapinized virus produced in the field. They reported excellent results. When vaccine was needed, the vaccine strain was inoculated into rabbits. On the 3rd or 4th day, when the temperature reaction was at its height, the rab-bits were bled to death from the heart. The spleen and lymph nodes were pooled, finely ground, and diluted with the defibrinated blood in the propor-tion of 1 : 4. Next the mixture was diluted 1 : 100 with saline solutions. It was then ready for use which was always within 8 hours of the time of its preparation. The vaccine was also made by lyophilization of tissues. This would keep satisfactorily for several months in the refrigerator.

Avianized (chick-embryo-adapted) vaccines. Jenkins and Shope (15) atten-uated the Kabete strain of rinderpest virus by adapting it to develop in egg embryos. After 19 to 24 passages by yolk-sac inoculation the strain had lost enough virulence for cattle while retaining antigenicity to make it useful as an immunizing agent for cattle. After 50 to 60 passages the strain lost its im-munizing properties. At the appropriate passage level, the strain solidly im-munized calves against inoculation with fully virulent spleen virus. Vacci-nated calves do not transmit the virus to susceptible animals, and thus this vaccine can be safely used in noninfected areas. The vaccine deteriorates very rapidly; thus lyophilization must be resorted to, and even then it must be stored and handled carefully. Hale and Walker (14) have described in detail large-scale production of the vaccine. Field tests in East Africa were satisfac-tory.

It has already been pointed out that not every strain of rinderpest virus will grow in eggs. Nakamura *et al.* (24) have succeeded in avianizing a strain which had already been lapinized, and with this strain they were successful in immunizing cattle in Asia. Brotherston (6) has propagated the Nakamura lap-inized strain of rinderpest virus in East Africa and has used it very success-fully on many thousands of cattle of many different breeds. Most cattle show very little reaction to the vaccine but are solidly immunized by it. Vaccinated cattle were tested by subcutaneous inoculation with virulent virus 8 to 15 months afterward and were found to be solidly immune. Natural exposure of 13 months likewise failed to break the immunity.

Tissue-culture vaccines. After 70 or more passages in calf kidney monolay-ers the virulent Kabete "O" strain produced no detectable clinical reaction in East African cattle and was stable on serial cattle passage. The duration of immunity was probably at least 4 years, and the infective titer for cattle with this modified strain was comparable to the tissue culture infectivity titer.

**Transmission.** Rinderpest can be transmitted to susceptible animals by feed-ing them with blood, urine, feces, nasal discharges, and perspiration. Natural

transmission apparently occurs through direct contact with these infected secretions and excretions. The urine is believed to be especially important in
the transmission of this disease. Some animals of the more resistant types may
suffer from the disease and eliminate virulent infectious material while showing only mild signs themselves. When these animals are driven to market, or
shipped to distant points, they may introduce the disease into new localities.
Because the virus is not very hardy, infected premises usually become free of
infection within a relatively short time after diseased animals have been removed from them. There is little evidence that droplet infection plays any
part in transmission, but infected meat may, since European pigs can acquire
the disease by ingestion of infected meat and the infected pigs spread the
virus by contact to other pigs or to cattle or vice-versa (11, 38). It has been
suggested that virus produces an exceedingly mild infection in pigs that may
be overlooked and presumably the virus may persist in this host for as long as
36 days.

In cattle the disease is usually found in yearlings with no maternal immunity. It is of a mild type, especially in the resistant native breeds. Control is
also made more difficult in Africa where large populations of susceptible
wildlife have the infection without any detectable mortality or morbidity.

Field experiments in Nigeria showed that recent isolates can spread, although irregularly, by close contact from cattle to sheep and goats and then
among small ruminants, but spreading from sheep to cattle was not demonstrable and there was infrequent transfer from goats to cattle (32). It is concluded that immunization of sheep and goats is not necessary once the disease is eliminated from cattle. Obviously, there is a slight element of risk,
but the economics involved warrant the risk in some countries.

**Diagnosis.** In areas where rinderpest in indigenous, the diagnosis usually
presents few problems. It is based upon signs and the lesions found at autopsy, and also upon the fact that the disease is evidently highly contagious.
In regions where the disease is not known, the diagnosis should be based
upon one or more of the following technics (32): (1) the isolation of the virus
from sick or dead animals; (2) the detection of virus specific antigens in the
tissues; (3) the demonstration of antibody production; and (4) histological
examination of tissues for virus-specific changes.

A tentative diagnosis is possible on the basis of gross examination and specific cytological changes including the formation of syncytia and the presence
of eosinophilic intracytoplasmic and perhaps intranuclear inclusion bodies as
well (32). The best tissues for histological examination are lymphoid-epi-
thelial such as the tonsil, Peyer's patches, and lymph nodes and also lesions
of the tongue, palate, and cheek papillae.

Studies in East Africa (33) show that naturally occurring strains can be
readily recovered from the blood of infected cattle or wild animals in primary
calf kidney cultures making this a simple, rapid, and excellent aid in the diagnosis of rinderpest. The neutralization of the isolate with rinderpest anti-

serum confirms the characteristic cytopathic effects if they are not considered to be adequate proof. The fluorescent antibody test also may be applied for the detection of rinderpest virus after its probable development.

It is possible to biopsy lymph nodes of infected cattle and test for antigen by the gel-diffusion agar technic (7). A rapid complement-fixation test for the diagnosis of rinderpest by the use of tissue extracts of biopsied lymph nodes from infected cattle gave excellent results (42).

The testing of paired serum samples by the neutralization tests in cell cultures and in embryonated hens' eggs are also useful in its diagnosis.

A disease which closely resembles rinderpest, except that the mortality rate is much lower, was first described in 1946. It is commonly called virus diarrhea of cattle (p. 1283). Virus diarrhea and malignant head catarrh (p. 979) may have lesions which resemble rinderpest.

**Control Measures.** In western Asia, India, and parts of Africa where rinderpest is indigenous, the disease is controlled principally by prophylactic vaccination. For this purpose the modified viruses seem to be the safest and most effective. In other parts of the world, including the Western Hemisphere, a complete embargo on the shipment of susceptible animals from infected areas is enforced and has generally succeeded in excluding this disease. Because the virus is a rather delicate one which does not remain viable very long outside the body of infected animals, there appears to be relatively little danger of infection being imported into areas remote from enzootic regions by means of meat, hides, or other contaminated objects. The principal danger appears to be in the importation of live animals of the more resistant types which sometimes suffer from rather chronic, almost inapparent infections.

If the disease should manage to reach the United States, or any other country that is remote from the enzootic regions, it would undoubtedly be dealt with as foot-and-mouth disease has been handled in this country. In countries free of the disease for long periods, or which have never been infected, rinderpest can be rapidly and completely eliminated by quarantine and vaccination as in the Philippines in 1955, by movement restrictions and slaughter as in Brazil and Australia, or by quarantine, slaughter, and antiserum as in Belgium (32).

**The Disease in Man.** There is no evidence that rinderpest virus causes disease in man.

## REFERENCES

1.  Baker.   Am. Jour. Vet. Res., 1946, 7, 179.
2.  Baker, Terrence, and Greig.   *Ibid.*, 189.
3.  Bennett.   Jour. Comp. Path. and Therap., 1936, *49*, 1.
4.  Boynton.   Philipp. Jour. Sci., 1928, *36*, 1.
5.  Breese and de Boer.   Virology, 1963, *19*, 340.
6.  Brotherston.   Jour. Comp. Path. and Therap., 1951, *61*, 289.
7.  Brown and Scott.   Vet. Rec., 1960, 47, 1055.

8.  Cheng and Fischman. Proc. F.A.O. Conference on Rinderpest, Nairobi, Kenya, 1948.
9.  Daubney. Jour. Comp. Path. and Therap., 1928, *41*, 228.
10. Daubney. Ann. Rpt. Vet. Dept., Kenya, for 1938, p. 70.
11. Delay and Barber. Proc. US Livestock Sanitary Assoc., 1962, *66*, 132.
12. Edwards. Imp. Inst. Agr. Res., Pusa (India), Bul. 199, 1930.
13. Furutani, Ishii, Kurata, and Nakamura. Bul. Nat. Inst. Anim. Health, Tokyo, 1957, *32*, 137.
14. Hale and Walker. Am. Jour. Vet. Res., 1946, 7, 199.
15. Jenkins and Shope. *Ibid.*, 174.
16. Kakizaki, Nakanishi, and Ozumi. Kitasato Arch. Exp. Med., 1918, *2*, 59.
17. Kelser. Military Surg., 1927, *61*, 31.
18. Kelser, Youngberg, and Topacio. Philipp. Jour. Sci., 1928, *36*, 373.
19. Keylock. Jour. Comp. Path. and Therap., 1933, *46*, 149.
20. Liess. Arch. f. Exp. Vet.-Med., 1964, *20*, 157.
21. Maurer, Jones, Easterday, and DeTray. Proc. Am. Vet. Med. Assoc., 1955, p. 201.
22. McKercher. Canad. Jour. Comp. Med., 1963, *27*, 71.
23. Naik. Indian Vet. Jour., 1946, *23*, 203.
24. Nakamura, Agric, and Miyamoto. Am. Jour. Vet. Res., 1953, *14*, 307.
25. Nakamura, Fukusko, and Kuroda. Jap. Jour. Vet. Sci., 1943, *5*, 455.
26. Nakamura and Kuroda. *Ibid.*, 1942, *4*, 75.
27. Nakamura, Wagatsuma, and Fukusko. Jour. Jap. Soc. Vet. Sci., 1938, *17*, 185.
28. Nicolle and Adil-Bey. Ann. l'Inst. Past., 1902, *29*, 429.
29. Pfaff. Onderstepoort Jour. Vet. Sci. and Anim. Indus., 1938, *11*, 263.
30. *Ibid.*, 1940, *15*, 175.
31. Plowright. Comp. virology. N.Y. Acad. Sci., 1962, *101*, 548.
32. Plowright. Virology monographs. Springer-Verlag, New York, 1968, *3*, 27.
33. Plowright and Ferris. Res. Vet. Sci., 1962, *3*, 172.
34. Provost, Borredon, and Queval. Rev. Elev., 1965, *18*, 385.
35. Provost and Borredon. *Ibid.*, 1968, *21*, 33.
36. Rodier. Philipp. Jour. Sci., 1928, *36*, 397.
37. Scott. Adv. Vet. Science, 1964, *9*, 113.
38. Scott, DeTray, and White. Bul. Off. Internatl. Epiz., 1959, *51*, 694.
39. Shope, Griffiths, and Jenkins. Am. Jour. Vet. Res., 1946, 7, 135.
40. Shope, Maurer, Jenkins, Griffiths, and Baker. *Ibid.*, 152.
41. Stirling. Vet. Jour., 1932, 88, 192; 1933, 89, 290.
42. Stone and Moulton. Am. Jour. Vet. Res., 1961, *22*, 18.
43. Thiery. Rev. d'Elevage., 1956, *9*, 117.

## Newcastle Disease

SYNONYMS: Pseudoplague of fowls, pseudo fowl pest, pneumoencephalitis, Ranikhet disease, *Paramyxovirus* a-1.

The disease was first encountered by Kraneveld (21) in Java and reported in 1926. In 1927 Doyle (9) described the disease in a flock of chickens in Newcastle-on-Tyne, England, and announced the cause to be a virus. By 1940

Newcastle disease had been recognized in the Philippines, Asia, Australia, and Africa. Later it appeared in continental Europe. Its identification in California in 1944 marked the first recognition of the malady in the Western Hemisphere (Beach, 2). It is widely scattered in the United States. Although the virus frequently produces grave epizootics and high mortality rates among fowls in the Eastern Hemisphere, the percentages of losses in the Western world have not been so great and usually have occurred only in young birds.

Chickens, turkeys, guinea fowl, ducks, geese, pigeons, pheasants, partridges, crows, sparrows, mayas, and martins, as well as unidentified species of free-flying birds, have been reported as affected during natural outbreaks (6). The virus sometimes causes conjunctivitis in man.

**Character of the Disease.** Outbreaks of Newcastle disease vary greatly in intensity. In some instances, particularly in adult birds, the signs may hardly be recognizable. In other cases, the disease may be very severe, resulting in deaths of the majority of those affected. All ages are susceptible, but young birds are usually more severely affected than older ones. The disease usually begins with respiratory signs; in fact, in the United States the disease is primarily a respiratory disease.

*In chicks* from a few days to a few weeks of age, the disease begins with respiratory signs. The infection spreads rapidly, and respiratory distress is evidenced by gasping, which may be accompanied by moist râles and crackling sounds. In many outbreaks nervous signs appear a few days after the onset of the respiratory syndrome. Very young chicks may show a profound stupor. They often rest on their hocks with toes slightly flexed, head depressed, and eyes closed, or they appear to be unable to use one or both legs and remain in lateral recumbency. Others may show signs of ataxia, such as staggering, torticollis, opisthotonos, and posterior propulsion. Handling them often intensifies the nervous manifestations. The death rate usually is high, and those that survive often are useless.

*In adult birds*, the disease also spreads rapidly and usually is first manifested by respiratory signs. In the laying flock there is a sudden depression in egg production. Frequently the flock will go from full production to almost zero production in less than 1 week, and resumption of egg laying is a slow process which begins after a week or so. The eggs that are laid after the non-laying period frequently are misshapen and usually have soft and imperfectly formed shells. The incidence of nervous signs in adult birds in the United States usually is low, and the mortality rate usually is low. There have, however, been reports, here and there, of heavy mortality rates among adult birds.

The lesions of Newcastle disease are not particularly striking. Fluid or mucus is usually found in the trachea, and the air sac membranes are cloudy. Sometimes the spleen is enlarged. When nervous signs have been prominent, microscopic lesions of mild encephalitis may be found. No inclusion bodies have been seen.

The incubation period varies from 4 to 14 days, with an average of about 5 days. The disease has been observed in 2-day-old chicks. Upon experimental inoculation chicks usually develop signs within 4 days.

Within 10 to 12 days after the onset of the disease the respiratory signs subside in recovering fowl. Nervous traits may or may not appear at that time, and survivors may show nervous damage for weeks or permanently. Flocks showing reduced egg production may not return to their former level for 4 to 8 weeks after apparent recovery from the infection.

In the United States the mortality in chicks has ranged from 5 to 90 percent. In adult chickens it usually is negligible, although instances of fairly heavy mortality have been reported. In turkey poults 50 percent mortality has been observed.

**The Disease in Experimental Animals.** The disease can be produced by inoculation in a wide series of wild and domesticated birds. Reagan, Lillie, Poelma, and Brueckner (23) successfully carried the virus through 12 Syrian hamsters by serial intracerebral inoculations. Brandly (5) cites Upton as having successfully achieved serial transfer of this virus in suckling mice.

**Properties of the Virus.** On the basis of filtration trials with graded collodion membranes, Burnet and Ferry (8) estimated the size of Newcastle virus to be 80 to 120 millimicrons. The virus will pass Seitz pads, Berkefeld N and W candles, and Chamberland $L_3$ and $L_5$ filters. It is destroyed by pasteurization and exposure to ultraviolet light. Pulp of infected organs dried *in vacuo* over $P_2O_5$ and stored in the refrigerator remains virulent for years. Allantoic-amniotic fluid from infected embryonated eggs retains its virulence for several years if stored in the moist or lyophilized state at $-70$ C. Boyd and Hanson (4) studied the survival ability of the virus in soils at varying temperatures and humidities. In the presence of some moisture the virus proved to be surprisingly resistant.

Newcastle virus is a member of the *Paramyxovirus* genus and is its type species. It has the same structural features as other members of this subgroup. It is also an RNA virus that is inactivated by formalin and by heating to 60 C for 30 minutes. It is immunologically distinct from other members of the genus except for a possible hemagglutination-inhibition test relationship with mumps virus of man. Immunological strain differences of Newcastle virus have been suggested.

Burnet (7) was the first to show that Newcastle disease virus has the property of agglutinating chicken erythrocytes and that antiserum will neutralize this property. The property of hemagglutination inhibition has proved to be valuable in diagnosis.

**Cultivation.** Newcastle disease virus is readily cultivated in embryonated chicken eggs. Bacteriologically sterile suspensions of virus-containing material are inoculated through the chorioallantoic membrane. The virus kills the embryo in about 2 to 6 days. In eggs dead on the 3rd day or later and occasionally in eggs dead on the 2nd day, a small opaque area is found on the chorioallantois at the point of inoculation. Sometimes the membrane is edematous. The yolk sac vessels are congested, and the embryo is reddened, especially in the feet and legs. The skin around the head often shows hemorrhages, and the liver is usually congested.

Newcastle virus produces a cytopathogenic effect in cell cultures of certain chick tissues. In some cell lines the cytopathogenic effect is only visible microscopically. Cultivation is also reported in monkey kidney cells, HeLa cells, and also calf kidney cells. Cytoplasmic inclusion bodies and multinucleated cells also occur in cultures.

**Immunity.** Fowls recovered from Newcastle disease are immune for years. The hemagglutination-inhibiting and serum-neutralizing antibodies are a criteria of immunity and they both persist for years.

Various vaccines have been used with varying degrees of success in the last 20 years. Formalin-inactivated vaccines were generally regarded as not conferring sufficient immunity and modified virus vaccines have been most popular in recent years. Hofstad (16) showed that two doses of an inactivated virus vaccine would confer a solid immunity, but he did not determine its duration.

In 1940 Iyer and Dobson (18) reported that certain English Newcastle strains had become avirulent by serial passage through embryonating eggs. They used these strains for immunization purposes and noted that only occasional fatalities occurred. Later it was shown by Komarov (19) that these vaccines could be used successfully to vaccinate day-old chicks from immune parents but produced high mortality when applied to chicks from susceptible parents. Further studies also showed that parental immunity usually interfered with immunity response and that chicks that gave no reaction to the vaccine soon became susceptible to infection.

Komarov and Goldsmit (20) modified Newcastle virus by serial passage in duck eggs. A vaccine prepared from infected eggs was used with apparent success in vaccinating young and adult chickens.

Beaudette, Bivins, and Miller (3) screened 105 strains of Newcastle disease virus to find one sufficiently nonpathogenic to be used for immunization purposes. The vaccine consisted of undiluted allantoic-amniotic fluid and was used to vaccinate chicks at 30 to 36 days of age by the "stick" and intramuscular methods. Losses from vaccination were very low and the chicks developed solid immunity. Vaccination of three successive lots of chicks, even after the disease had appeared in them, resulted in a marked reduction in the mortality as compared with previous nonvaccinated lots. A few adult birds vaccinated at the beginning of the period of egg production showed a decrease in production on the 5th or 6th day, but these returned to normal within 2 weeks after vaccination.

Hitchner (15) and Bankowski (1) have developed modified virus vaccines which have been used with success. Hitchner's vaccine was made from 20 percent suspensions of infected chick embryos. Given to chicks of less than 1 week of age, it produced no signs and the birds were solidly immunized for as long as 1 year. Bankowski's vaccine was made by growing an attenuated strain in minced chick embryo tissue cultures.

A nonavian tissue-culture-modified Newcastle disease vaccine developed by Gale *et al.* (12) had no detrimental effect on fertility and only a slight effect on hatchability and egg production. The vaccine virus did not spread to unvaccinated pen-contact control chickens. Upon challenge with the GB (intramuscular) and DK (intranasal) virulent test strains vaccinated hens showed only a slight decline in egg production, thus the vaccinated hens were well protected.

**Means of Transmission.** The disease spreads readily by direct contact. Chicks may carry the virus from an infected hatchery, or from contact with diseased fowl while en route, to the poultry farm. Susceptible birds will contract the disease from infected excretions or organs of diseased fowl, from water contaminated by such fowl, and from infected feed bags, feed containers, and the like. Eggs laid by hens during acute infection may contain virus; after a flock has returned to full production no virus is found in the eggs.

**Diagnosis.** Newcastle disease should be suspected when a respiratory disease in chicks is associated with or followed by nervous or paralytic signs and when there are tracheal exudates and clouded air sacs on autopsy. Since the disease is primarily a respiratory infection in this country, in the absence of nervous signs it is most likely to be confused with infectious bronchitis. Laryngotracheitis also exhibits respiratory signs, but gasping is more pronounced and respiration more rhythmical. Nervous signs appear in vitamin-deficiency diseases of chicks and in encephalomyelitis (epidemic tremor), but in these diseases no initial respiratory signs are seen. The fowl plague syndrome also simulates that of Newcastle disease and must be considered in the differential diagnosis in countries where it exists.

Virus-isolation and identification or serum-neutralization tests establish the identity of the Newcastle disease. Early in the course of the disease good sources of the virus are tracheal exudate, spleen, and brain. Within a few days after the onset surviving birds will show positive serum-neutralization reactions.

Fabricant (10) compared the results of hemagglutination-inhibition (HI) and serum-neutralization (SN) tests in infected chickens and found that the HI test reached a positive level sooner than the SN test. His studies indicated that the HI titer became positive from 2 days before to 5 days after (average 2 days after) the first appearance of respiratory signs. This test has proved to be quite satisfactory for rapid diagnosis of Newcastle disease.

**Control Measures.** Newcastle disease is highly contagious and spreads readily through direct contact. It appears to be scattered throughout the poultry-raising areas of the United States. In an outbreak of the disease, removal of the infected unit may eliminate the infection, but frequently it has spread so quickly that all units on the premises are exposed by the time it is diagnosed. Levine, Fabricant, Gillespie, Angstrom, and Mitchell (22) concluded that birds recovered from Newcastle disease do not harbor sufficient virus to infect susceptible birds 1 month after the flock recovers from respiratory signs.

It appears that the most effective vaccines contain live virus, and vaccination introduces this virus into the flock. Beaudette *et al.* (3) believed, however, that their nonpathogenic vaccine did not produce carriers but that the vaccinated flock was a source of infection for about 3 weeks.

Annual replacement of the laying flock at the end of the first laying year, with segregation of the replacement stock and the application of all sanitary precautions, has proved effective in controlling the disease on certain poultry farms.

Subtilin, a peptide antibiotic, inactivates Newcastle disease virus in allantoic fluid under well-defined conditions of subtilin concentration, pH, and the amount of allantoic fluid in the reaction mixtures (13). At present it has no application in the control of the disease.

Raggi and Lee state that viable infectious bronchitis (IB) virus interferes with Newcastle disease (ND) virus replication (14). The practice of combining IB and ND vaccine should be discouraged.

**The Disease in Man.** Although there are reports in the literature that Newcastle disease virus has caused generalized disease in man, it appears that this is not true. The virus causes conjunctivitis in man, and several reports of its isolation from this condition have been published (Freymann and Bang, 11; Ingalls and Mahoney, 17). Patients show acute, unilateral or bilateral conjunctivitis. No systemic symptoms appear and no ill effects are noted other than a mild irritation of about 3 to 7 days' duration.

### REFERENCES

1. Bankowski.   Proc. Soc. Exp. Biol. and Med., 1957, 96, 114.
2. Beach.   Science, 1944, 100, 361.
3. Beaudette, Bivins, and Miller.   Cornell Vet., 1949, 39, 302.
4. Boyd and Hanson.   Avian Dis., 1958, 2, 82.
5. Brandly.   In: Biester and Schwarte. Diseases of poultry. 3d ed. Iowa State College Press, Ames, Iowa, 1952, p. 541.
6. Brandly, Moses, Jones, and Jungherr.   Am. Jour. Vet. Res., 1946, 7, 243.
7. Burnet.   Austral. Jour. Exp. Biol. and Med. Sci., 1942, 20, 81.
8. Burnet and Ferry.   Brit. Jour. Exp. Path., 1934, 15, 56.
9. Doyle.   Jour. Comp. Path. and Therap., 1927, 40, 144.
10. Fabricant.   Cornell Vet., 1949, 39, 202.
11. Freymann and Bang.   Johns Hopkins Hosp. Bul., 1949, 84, 409.
12. Gale, Gard, Ose, and Berkman.   Avian Dis., 1965, 9, 348.
13. Lorenz and Jann.   Am. Jour. Vet. Res., 1964, 25, 1285.

14.  Raggi and Lee.   Avian Dis., 1964, 8, 471.
15.  Hitchner.   Cornell Vet., 1950, 40, 60.
16.  Hofstad.   Am. Jour. Vet. Res., 1956, 17, 738.
17.  Ingalls and Mahoney.   Am. Jour. Pub. Health, 1949, 39, 737.
18.  Iyer and Dobson.   Vet. Rec., 1940, 52, 889.
19.  Komarov.   Refuah Vet., 1947, 4, 96.
20.  Komarov and Goldsmit.   Cornell Vet., 1947, 37, 368.
21.  Kraneveld.   Hemera Zoa (N.I. Bl. v. Diergeneesk.), 1926, 38, 448.
22.  Levine, Fabricant, Gillespie, Angstrom, and Mitchell.   Cornell Vet., 1950, 40, 206.
23.  Reagan, Lillie, Poelma, and Brueckner.   Am. Jour. Vet. Res., 1947, 8, 136.

## Parainfluenza Infection in Cattle

Present evidence suggests that parainfluenza 3 (PI 3) virus of cattle plays an important role in acute bovine respiratory diseases commonly termed shipping fever, shipping pneumonia, stockyard fever, or the pneumonic or pectoral form of hemorrhagic septicemia. *Mycoplasma* and particularly *Pasteurella* species also are involved in the etiology with parainfluenza 3 virus. In some respiratory cases concurrent infection of PI 3 with bovine viral diarrhea-mucosal disease, infectious bovine rhinotracheitis, enteroviruses, hemolytic cocci, *Alkaligenes* species, *Actinobacillus actinoides* has been found.

The disease has been recognized for many years and has been the cause of heavy losses, especially in cattle shipped during the cold months. It formerly was believed to be caused by organisms of the *Pasteurella* group, particularly *Past. multocida*. Inasmuch as it was not possible to reproduce the disease with these organisms, it has long been suspected that other etiological agents are involved in the disease. Some think that this organism has nothing to do with the disease, and some cases have been reported in which it seemed to be absent; however, it is present in many cases and generally is found in great numbers in the fibrinous exudate in the alveoli of the lungs and in the pleural cavity. It is difficult to believe that *Pasteurella* species do not have an important role in the terminal lesions of the disease, if not in the initiation of the infection.

Collier, Chow, Benjamin, and Deem (2) suspected that some cases of shipping fever might be the result of a combined infection with the virus of infectious bovine rhinotracheitis (IBR) and *Pasteurella* organisms, particularly *Past. hemolytica*. Their experiments supported this belief to the extent that cattle were more severely affected when both agents were given simultaneously than when either was given alone. The disease produced was nonfatal, and while the authors say that the signs were typical of shipping fever, they are careful not to claim that they reproduced that disease.

Reisinger, Heddleston, and Manthei (9) also isolated the virus of IBR from cattle that were showing signs considered to be typical of shipping fever. They also isolated a hemagglutinating virus, a myxovirus belonging to the parainfluenza 3 group, which they identified as SF-4, and with this they were able to produce mild but typical cases of shipping fever. This agent was grown in bovine and porcine kidney cell cultures. It produced cytopathogenic changes in both types of cells, and intranuclear and intracytoplasmic inclusion bodies were observed in the bovine cells. There was no cross neutralization with IBR virus. These workers isolated *Pasteurella* organisms from 65 percent of the animals in herds where shipping fever occurred and in 50 percent of those that had not been affected. Recent studies by these same investigators indicate that perhaps *Pasteurella* spp. alone may cause respiratory infection in cattle under various stressing conditions.

**Character of the Disease.** Shipping fever seldom occurs naturally in calves. In adult cattle it takes the form of a fibrinous pneumonia. The animals cough, show very high temperatures (107 F and higher), and soon exhibit signs of great respiratory embarrassment. Often they stand with the forelegs held wide apart and the neck extended far forward. The breathing may become stertorous, and often through the mouth. Foamy saliva frequently is blown on the floor and walls before the animal. Such animals usually die within a few hours after the severe respiratory embarrassment is seen, and within 3 or 4 days from the time the first signs of illness are observed.

In typical cases of shipping fever the lesions are located in the respiratory tract, all others being secondary. The lungs often fill the thorax and are covered with a white fibrinous mass that may be peeled off the surface like coagulated egg albumen, the underlying surfaces being rough and congested. The lungs, especially the main lobes, may be very solid and heavy. Cut sections show deep-red lobules and grayish ones separated by interlobular tissue which has been greatly thickened by infiltration of coagulated exudate like that on the serous surface. Histologic examination reveals broncheolitis, alveolitis, serocellular exudate in the lung, intracytoplasmic acidophilic inclusion bodies in nasal and bronchial epithelium, and alveolar macrophages, together with marked fluorescence with specific antibody (13).

**The Disease in Experimental Cattle (13).** The first signs of illness occur in calves 24 to 30 hours after exposure. The signs may include increased temperature, lacrimation, serous nasal discharge, depression, and dyspnea followed by coughing. The signs may be mild and easily missed in some animals. A calf can have a marked pneumonia with meager clinical signs. A more severe disease results when *Pasteurella multocida* is given intranasally 24 to 48 hours following exposure to PI-3 virus. One strain produces diarrhea.

Colostrum-deprived calves have a mild illness after intranasal inoculation of PI-3 virus (15). *In utero* injection of virus into pregnant cows produces pathological changes in the fetus (11).

The PI-3 virus has been isolated from man, cattle, water buffalo, horses, and monkeys. Guinea pigs, hamsters, sheep, and swine are susceptible to experimental infection.

**Properties of the Virus.** The intact virus particles vary from 140 to 250 m$\mu$. It is an RNA virus that is labile at pH 3 and in the presence of ether or chloroform. The virion causes hemagglutination of red blood cells from birds, cattle, swine, guinea pigs, and human beings; guinea pig cells are most sensitive. Infected cell cultures show the phenomenon of hemadsorption. The virus produces interferon in fetal bovine kidney cell cultures (10). The human, bovine, and sheep PI-3 viruses are closely related but not identical. The human and bovine strains were differentiated by neutralization, hemagglutination-inhibition, and CF tests with guinea pig antiserum (7).

**Cultivation.** The virus replicates in many types of cultured cells including bovine, swine, equine, and rabbit kidneys, and also in cells from the chicken embryo. Multiplication in cell cultures usually produces syncytia and intracytoplasmic and intranuclear inclusion bodies. Plaques are produced in 3 to 5 days in agar overlay preparations. The virus also replicates and produces alterations in bovine fetal tracheal mucosa and bovine fetal lung organ cultures (8).

**Immunity (12).** The antibody level for bovine PI-3 in the cow increases prior to parturition and decreases to former levels during lactation. Antibodies are transferred in the colostrum resulting in blood levels equal to or greater than that of the mother. This passive antibody decreases with age and is no longer detectable by weaning at 6 to 8 months of age. This antibody presumably interferes with the production of active immunity.

Active antibody develops in calves with no colostral protection when the animal comes in contact with PI-3 virus and anamnestic responses presumably occur following re-exposure. It is not known if this antibody is long lasting or protective against subsequent exposure to virus. There are suggestions

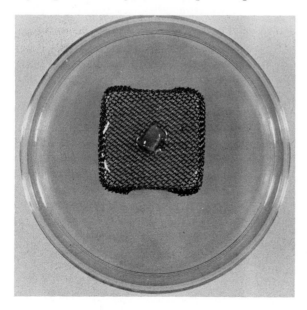

*Fig. 207.* Bovine parainfluenza virus 131. An organ culture of bovine fetal lung mounted on a wire grid and partially submerged in tissue culture media. (Courtesy J. Kita, R. Kenney, and J. Gillespie, *Cornell Vet.*)

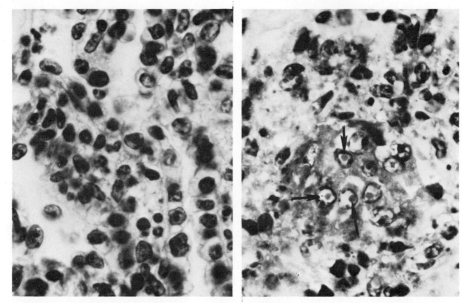

Fig. 208. (Left) Bovine parainfluenza 131. Bovine fetal lung organ culture, 14 days. Uninoculated. Note apparent cell viability with occasional large basophilic nucleoli and infrequency of pycnoses. Fixed in alcohol. H and E stain. X 850. (Right) Replicate culture, 13 days after inoculation with C3F-II strain of bovine parainfluenza virus. Note many intranuclear inclusion bodies (arrows), pyknosis, and karyorrhexis. Fixed in alcohol. H and E stain. X 850. (Courtesy J. Kita, R. Kenney, and J. Gillespie, Cornell Vet.)

that these antibodies do not always protect against aerosol challenge with virulent virus (5, 6). The active antibody must be constantly produced by latent virus or anamnestic responses occur as the majority of adult beef and dairy cattle have demonstrable HI antibody.

**Transmission.** Natural transmission in susceptible calves exposed to clinically ill calves excreting virus occurs in 5 to 10 days. Virus can be isolated from the nasal excretions for 7 to 8 days after infection and from the lungs for 17 days and perhaps longer despite the presence of serum antibodies. Infected cattle probably are the prime source for the continuity of the bovine PI-3 virus in nature.

PI-3 antibodies are found in man, horses (3), guinea pigs, swine, deer, and big horn sheep. Their role in the transmission of the disease is unknown but they may be involved in the ecology of the cattle disease which has a worldwide distribution and that has a very high incidence in the beef and dairy cattle populations.

**Diagnosis.** The virus can be readily isolated from the respiratory tract exudates in tissue culture. In tissue culture the virus can be identified by a combination of features: (1) the production of syncytia and cytoplasmic and intranuclear inclusion bodies, (2) a hemadsorbing virus, (3) fluorescence by a specific conjugate, and (4) neutralization of the isolate by specific antiserum.

The demonstration of a rising titer with paired sera is another method, although it doesn't eliminate the presence of a concurrent infection.

Certain clinical features may vary from those of other specific respiratory diseases of cattle, yet there is considerable overlap in the signs, making a positive diagnosis by this means often impossible (1).

**Prevention and Control.** The recommended procedures based upon our present limited state of knowledge for the prevention and control of bovine PI-3 in beef and dairy cattle was outlined by the Panel, Bovine Respiratory Disease Symposium, American Veterinary Medical Association, in 1968 (1). The reader is strongly urged to consult that reference for details, especially since the approach is different in dealing with dairy and beef herds.

In brief, the Panel recommended that beef calves be given PI-3 vaccine and *Pasteurella* bacterin at 4 months of age. One month later another injection of virus vaccine and *Pasteurella* bacterin should be administered. In open and closed dairy herds it is well to vaccinate the calves at 6 to 8 months of age with PI-3 and *Pasteurella* bacterin.

Studies by Woods *et al.* (14) and Gale *et al.* (4) show that 2 injections of inactivated virus vaccine are required to produce high HI titers. The vaccine produced by Gale *et al.* also contains *Pasteurella* bacteria as well as PI-3 inactivated virus. Some investigators have indicated that the vaccine does not always inhibit the disease in beef cattle but the disease in the vaccinates is less severe and weight loss, if any, is minimal. The unvaccinated cattle have a considerable loss in weight.

The shipping of cattle, inclement weather, and the associated stress have a marked influence on the severity of disease. Every effort should be made to make the cattle as comfortable as possible.

Clinical evidence indicates that animals sometimes may be successfully treated for shipping fever if treatment is begun early in the course of the disease. The tetracycline compounds appear to be useful, also several of the sulfonamides. Since these agents do not have any appreciable effect upon most viruses, their virtue probably lies in their effect on the bacterial agents, especially the *Pasteurella*, which are known to be especially susceptible to these compounds.

**The Disease in Man.** There is no evidence that the bovine strains of parainfluenza 3 virus produce illness in man, nor has the reverse been proved.

## REFERENCES

1. Bovine Respiratory Disease Symposium. Jour. Am. Vet. Med. Assoc., 1968, *152*, part 2.
2. Collier, Chow, Benjamin, and Deem. Am. Jour. Vet. Res., 1960, *21*, 195.
3. Ditchfield, Zbitnew, and MacPherson. Canad. Vet. Jour. 1963, *4*, 175.
4. Gale, Hamdy, and Trapp. Jour. Am. Vet. Med. Assoc., 1963, *142*, 884.
5. Gillespie. Unpublished data, 1957.
6. Hamparian, Washko, Ketler, and Hilleman. Jour. Immunol., 1961, 87, 139.

7.   Ketler, Hamparian, and Hilleman.   *Ibid.*, 1961, 87, 126.

8.   Kita, Kenney, and Gillespie.   Cornell Vet., 1969, *54*, 355.

9.   Reisinger, Heddleston, and Manthei.   Jour. Am. Vet. Med. Assoc., 1959, *135*, 147.

10.  Rosenquist and Loan.   Am. Jour. Vet. Res., 1967, *28*, 619.

11.  Sattar, Bohl, Trapp, and Hamdy.   *Ibid.*, 1967, *28*, 45.

12.  Sweat.   Jour. Am. Vet. Med. Assoc., 1967, *150*, 178.

13.  Woods.   *Ibid.*, 1968, *152*, 771.

14.  Woods, Mansfield, Segre, Holper, Brandly, and Barthel.   Am. Jour. Vet. Res., 1962, *23*, 832.

15.  Woods, Sibinovic, and Starkey.   *Ibid.*, 1965, *26*, 262.

## *SV-5* Respiratory Disease of Dogs

In 1967 a parainfluenza virus closely related to SV-5 parainfluenza virus of monkeys, a member of parainfluenza type II virus group, was implicated in an epizootic of respiratory disease in laboratory dogs (6). Two separate outbreaks occurred 1 year later in military dogs in the United States and these isolates were identical (7, 10).

**Character of the Disease.** The disease syndrome in field outbreaks is severe and probably involves other pathogens as well as SV-5 virus (1). The disease is characterized by sudden onset, copious nasal discharge, fever, and coughing in some dogs. Canine SV-5 virus can produce a disease that looks like "kennel cough" if *Mycoplasma* and certain bacterial organisms are also involved in the disease (2).

**The Disease in Experimental Animals.** With his original isolate, Crandell (10) produced mild respiratory signs in dogs exposed intranasally. The young dogs had tonsilitis and a slight nasal discharge but no fever. Others (8) observed similar signs in dogs exposed to Crandell's isolate by intranasal or intratracheal routes.

In a pathogenesis study Appel and Percy (1) inoculated dogs by various routes. Intramuscular and subcutaneous inoculation did not cause infection. In contrast, aerosol or contact exposure produced disease restricted to the respiratory tract. Virus inoculated into the urinary bladder directly resulted in local viral replication only and cystitis. By aerosol exposure to $10^4$ TCID$_{50}$ of virus a slight rise in temperature was noted in the majority of their experimental dogs (1) that occurred 2 to 3 days after exposure and persisted for 1 to 2 days. There was a slight nasal discharge in a few dogs and slightly less than 50 percent developed a slight nonproductive cough which could be forced by laryngeal palpation. The cough never persisted more than 1 week. At necropsy there were no lesions except for a few petechial hemorrhages in a few dogs sacrificed 4 days after exposure. Microscopic catarrhal changes are evident in the upper and lower respiratory tract and in regional lymph nodes. Virus is isolated from the oronasal specimens between the first and eighth day after exposure, but not from the blood. The highest titers are found from respiratory specimens occurring between the 3 and 6 days. Viral antigen as demonstrated by the immunofluorescence test is observed in the epithelial cells of nasal mucosa, trachea, bronchi, bronchioli, and peribronchial lymph nodes from 1 to 6 days after exposure, with considerable reduction in fluorescence by the 6th day.

When *Mycoplasma* and *Bordetella bronchiseptica* were given intransally after aerosol exposure to canine SV-5 virus the respiratory illness was more severe in all dogs with a dry cough, persisting in some dogs for several weeks (2). All dogs exposed to canine SV-5 virus developed serum-neutralizing antibody but levels declined thereafter with little or no antibody 3 to 4 months later.

**Properties of the Virus.** The canine strains are closely related to parainfluenza virus (2). The canine strains share a common complement-fixing antigen with SV-5 virus isolated from monkeys, but use of the hemagglutination-inhibition and serum-neutralization tests gave negative results (7, 10).

Other limited studies of properties place the virus in the *Paramyxovirus* genus. Its hemagglutinin and hemadsorbing properties are used in the study and diagnosis of the virus and disease.

**Cultivation.** The canine SV-5 virus replicates in cultures of primary dog kidney, of African green monkey kidney, of rhesus monkey renal, and of human embryonic kidney cells. The virus produces multinucleated giant cells and eosinophilic inclusion bodies in the cytoplasm of the renal cells.

Propagation of the virus in the amniotic cavity of the hen's embryonated egg was demonstrated by hemagglutination (10). No embryonic deaths were observed. Both amniotic and allantoic fluids contained virus with an HA titer of 1 : 128. The virus failed to replicate when inoculated into the allantoic cavity.

**Immunity.** Dogs which are infected by the respiratory route are fully immune to challenge by this same route 3 weeks later. There are no signs of illness and virus is not isolated from the respiratory tract. In contrast, dogs given virus parenterally develop good antibody titers but are not completely protected by an aerosol challenge (1).

Neutralizing antibody may persist for 3 to 4 months (2) and perhaps for 6 months (4). Its relationship to immunity has not been ascertained as yet. The serum-neutralization test is slightly more sensitive than the standard hemagglutination inhibition test (8).

The level and frequency of neutralizing antibody in the dog population is such that maternal immunity does not play a significant role in protection or in immunization (2).

**Transmission.** The infection is readily transmitted from dogs in the acute stage to susceptible dogs. It is an important disease where there is an assembly of dogs into a new environment such as laboratories or military service (5).

Virus cannot be recovered from the respiratory tract beyond 9 days after exposure. Natural infections in the dog seem to be limited to the respiratory tract. Serological evidence indicates that the incidence of the infection in the general canine population is quite low—less than 5 percent. Despite these two apparent facts, the virus persists in nature and under certain environmental conditions causes a severe disease in the dog.

The host range for SV-5 is unclear, but probably includes monkeys, man, and dogs. The present information suggests that monkeys are principally infected by man (3), or perhaps by dogs, as monkeys residing in the jungle lack antibody.

**Diagnosis.** To differentiate this viral disease from others in the dog at the clinical level is extremely difficult. There are many other canine viruses which produce comparable respiratory signs of illness.

Field strains from dogs grow quite readily and produce a cytopathic effect in cell cultures. A further distinguishing feature is its hemadsorbing effect. Consequently tissue culture is an excellent method for virus isolation and identification. The use of paired serums in the HI and SN test and the demonstration of a rising antibody titer serves as another means of diagnosis.

**Control.** More must be learned about the ecology of the disease before it can be controlled. Because secondary microorganisms often appear to be involved in the disease process, the use of antibiotics and sulfa compounds may aid in reducing the severity of the disease.

At the present time there is no vaccine available for dogs but there is an apparent need for an effective and safe biologic to prevent the disease (9).

**The Disease in Man.** In studies of the epizootiology in military dogs, handlers were not infected (10). The exact role of dogs in the epizootiology of SV-5 in other species, including man, is unknown.

## REFERENCES

1. Appel and Percy.   Jour. Am. Vet. Med. Assoc., 1970, *156*, 1778.
2. Appel, Pickerill, Menegus, Percy, Parsonson, and Sheffy.   Gaines Vet. Sympos., 1970, *20*, 15.
3. Atoynatan and Hsiung.   Am. Jour. Epidemiol., 1969, 89, 472.
4. Binn and Lazar.   (Quoted by Bittle and Emery. Jour. Am. Vet. Med. Assoc., 1970, *156*, 1771.)
5. Binn and Lazar.   *Ibid.*, 1970, *156*, 1774.
6. Binn, Eddy, Lazar, Helms, and Murnane.   Proc. Soc. Exp. Biol. and Med., 1967, *126*, 140.
7. Binn, Lazar, Rogul, Shepler, Swango, Claypoole, Hubbard, Asbill, and Alexander.   Am. Jour. Vet. Res., 1968, 29, 1809.
8. Bittle and Emery.   Jour. Am. Vet. Med. Assoc., 1970, *156*, 1771.
9. Canine Infectious Diseases Sympos.   *Ibid.*, 1970, *156*, 1661.
10. Crandell, Brimlow, and Davison.   Am. Jour. Vet. Res., 1968, 29, 2141.

## Paramyxovirus Infection in Other Domestic Animals

**Sheep.** Parainfluenza 3 virus was isolated from the pneumonic lungs of five sheep in three flocks in Australia (10). A mild pneumonia was produced in sheep when they were exposed to one of the isolates (CSL 6) under experimental conditions. It would appear that a PI-3 of sheep origin produces disease in sheep, probably playing a comparable role in the acute respiratory diseases of sheep that bovine parainfluenza viruses play in cattle respiratory diseases.

In the United States serological surveys utilizing the hemagglutination-inhibition and serum-neutralization tests show that PI-3 is a common infection in sheep and widespread in the United States. The CSL 6 strain is closely related antigenically to two bovine and one human PI-3 viruses, but not identical.

An epidemiological investigation in one sheep herd demonstrated that new lambs become infected in the Fall. In this herd the lambs showed no signs of illness. Lambs also acquire passive immunity from their mothers by colostral feeding.

Obviously, there is much work to be done before we understand the true economic and pathologic effects of this virus infection upon sheep.

**Horses.** Information about parainfluenza-3 virus in the horse is rather sparse. The virus was first isolated in 1961 from yearling Thoroughbred horses with acute upper respiratory disease (3). A serologic survey of the premises showed that a large number of horses 2 years or older had hemagglutinating inhibition antibodies to a virus isolate. In a reciprocal HI test with HA-1 (human type) and $SF_4$ (bovine type) PI-3 strains the equine PI-3 strain (RE 55) gave virtually identical results with the HA-1 strain and similar, but not identical, results with the $SF_4$ strain.

A PI-3 virus was isolated from four colts in Illinois (9) that had a disease diagnosed as strangles. All the animals in the herd of 10 horses had a mucopurulent discharge and/or a history of a recent respiratory disease. Significant serum HI titers were demonstrated in six of the colts.

Complement-fixing antibody apparently disappears about 4 months after infection. In contrast the HI and neutralizing antibody persisted for at least 1 year (2). Sibinovic et al. (9) tested 130 horse sera from 14 counties in Illinois and approximately one-half had high HI titers to equine PI-3 virus. Lief and Cohen (6) found CF antibodies in 20 percent of 129 Philadelphia (SSA) area horses. Although Todd (11) had negative test results for PI-3 neutralizing antibodies in his serological survey, it is likely that PI-3 infection is common in horses. However, its significance as a pathogen is yet to be ascertained as it relates to horses, human beings, and other animals.

**Pigs.** The hemagglutinating virus of Japan (HVP), or Sendai virus, is a parainfluenza I virus that infects mice and perhaps swine and man. In swine,

Sendai virus reputedly causes bronchopneumonia in young pigs, although there is no serological evidence in the swine population in Japan to support this contention. In pregnant sows inoculation of the virus early in pregnancy produces mummified fetuses and stillborn pigs (7, 8).

Greig *et al.* isolated a parainfluenza III virus from the brain of a pig (5). It crosses antigenically with parainfluenza II virus. Its pathogenicity for swine has not been ascertained.

**Chickens.** A hemagglutinating agent designated Yucaipa (MVY) virus was isolated from chickens with a mixed respiratory infection (1). It is immunologically and serologically distinct from other known avian viruses and the paramyxoviruses of mammals. This paramyxovirus causes a mild respiratory disease in chickens by the intratracheal route.

The virus can be propagated in chicken embryos and in tissue cultures (1). Infected fluids from embryos hemagglutinate chicken erythrocytes. Chickens produce a specific hemagglutination-inhibiting antibody distinct from Newcastle disease virus and other agents of the paramyxovirus group.

### REFERENCES

1. Bankowski and Corstvet.   Avian Dis., 1961, 5, 251.
2. Ditchfield.   Jour. Am. Vet. Med. Assoc., 1968, *155*, 384.
3. Ditchfield, MacPherson and Zbitnew.   Canad. Vet. Jour., 1963, *4*, 175.
4. Fischman.   Am. Jour. Epidemiol, 1967, 85, 272.
5. Greig, Johnson, and Bouillant.   Res. Vet. Sci., 1971, *12*, 305.
6. Leif and Cohen.   WHO Informal Meeting on Coordinated Study of Animal Influenza, 1964 (July), Geneva.
7. Sasahara, Hayashi, Kumagai, Yamamoto, Hirasawa, Munakata, and Okaniwa. Virus, 1954, *4*, 131.
8. Shimuzu, Kawakami, Fukuhara, and Matomoto.   Jap. Jour. Exp. Med., 1954, 24, 363.
9. Sibinovic, Woods, Hardenbrook, and Harquis.   Vet. Med., 1965, *60*, 600.
10. St. George.   Austral. Vet. Jour., 1969, *45*, 321.
11. Todd.   Jour. Am. Vet. Med. Assoc., 1968, *155*, 387.

### Mumps Virus Infection In The Domestic Cat And Dog

Clinical observations by veterinary practitioners (4) suggest that both cats and dogs are susceptible to human mumps virus. A number of cases of parotitis have been seen in pet cats or dogs at the same time that members of the household were infected with mumps virus (4).

Mumps virus was isolated from the saliva of two dogs with swollen parotid glands (6). Both cases occurred during outbreaks of mumps in two households. These isolates produced a cytopathic effect in HeLa cells and the hemagglutinating properties of the virus were inhibited by human mumps antiserum. Stone (8) reported that mumps virus may produce meningoencephalitis in the dog without involvement of the parotid gland. Morris *et al.* (5) reported that 38 of 209 dog sera collected at random from a population fixed complement in the presence of mumps virus. In another study Cuadrado (2) found that the sera of 20 dogs had HI titers greater than 1 : 20 against mumps virus. Mumps virus given to dogs by the intraparotid route failed to produce signs of illness and virus was not recoverable from the saliva, but dogs did develop mumps antibody. Binn (1) suggests that observations on mumps virus should be viewed with caution especially because SV-5 virus antigens are commonly noted in monkey kidney cell cultures and SV-5 antibodies are often seen in guinea pig serum used as a source of complement in the CF test (3).

Wollstein published two reports (9, 10) which reported on the infectiousness of human mumps virus for the domestic cat. When bacterial sterile saliva from infected humans was inoculated into the parotid salivary gland and the testes of half grown cats orchitis and parotitis resulted. The experimental cats had a febrile response, leukocytosis, tenderness, and swelling of the injected glands and histological lesions similar to human mumps.

More recently Scott, Schultz and Gillespie (7) showed that mumps virus replicated in feline kidney and feline lung cells *in vitro*. They also demonstrated that direct inoculation of virulent mumps virus into the parotid salivary gland and testes of an adult male cat resulted in parotitis and orchitis. Infection spread to the opposite gland, and virus was recovered from the parotid 59 days after inoculation. Oral and intravenous inoculation of pregnant cats with mumps virus resulted in viral replication within the fetuses, indicating that virus had crossed the placenta.

Present evidence would suggest that mumps virus infection does occur as a natural infection in dogs and cats. Its true significance as a pathogen and its incidence in these hosts is yet to be ascertained as well as their importance in the transmission of this virus to man.

### REFERENCES

1. Binn.  Canine Infectious Diseases Sympos., Am. Vet. Med. Assoc., 1970, *156*, 1672.
2. Cuadrado.  Bul. WHO, 1965, *33*, 803.
3. Hsuing, Isacson, and McCollum.  Jour. Immunol., 1962, *88*, 284.
4. Kirk.  Personal communication, 1970.
5. Morris, Blount, and McCown.  Cornell Vet., 1956, *46*, 525.
6. Noice, Bolin, and Eveleth.  Jour. Dis. Child., 1959, *98*, 350.
7. Scott, Schultz, and Gillespie.  Unpublished findings, 1972.
8. Stone.  Jour. Small Anim. Pract., 1969, *10*, 555.
9. Wollenstein.  Jour. Exp. Med., 1916, *23*, 353.
10. *Ibid.* 1918, *28*, 377.

### Syncytium-Forming Viruses

The syncytium-forming viruses detected by their characteristic cytopathic effect in tissue-cultured systems have been isolated from tissues of many different species, including cattle and domestic cats. The isolates, in many instances, came from cats or cattle with disease, but at present they cannot be viewed as pathogens with one possible exception (2). Based upon preliminary evidence it appears that syncytium-forming viruses most closely resemble members of the genus *Paramyxovirus*.

### Feline Syncytium-Forming Viruses

At least 30 isolations have been made by research workers in California, Ohio, and New York (8). Isolates have come from cats with respiratory infections (3), urolithiasis (2), feline infectious peritonitis (3), neoplasms (5-7), ataxia (1), and no illness (1). Most isolates are made by direct cultures from feline tissue, but some have been made from nasal or pharyngeal swabs or urine.

**Character of the Infection.** The syncytium-forming viruses are associated with various diseases of the cat but experimental inoculation in cats has not produced clinical signs of illness (1, 5, 6). Virus was recovered from all of the numerous tissues examined by direct cell culture from cats sacrificed at 14, 29, and 56 days' postinoculation (1) and also readily from the blood of carrier cats by cocultivation of infected leukocytes with feline fibroblastic cells (3).

The role of syncytium-forming virus in urolithiasis is unknown, but their presence in natural and experimental cases is very interesting. Further studies in disease-free cats under isolation is required to assess its real importance in this most important disease of cats.

Limited studies suggest it is ubiquitous in nature and can persist in the tissues of cats for long periods of time. Utilizing the agar-gel technic, Gaskin (3)

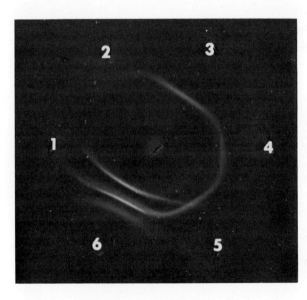

*Fig. 209.* Immunodiffusion test depicting the development of precipitating antibody in a cat inoculated with the feline syncytium-forming virus. Serial weekly serum samples starting with the 3rd week postinoculation (*1*) are reacted with antigen (*center well*) prepared from infected tissue cultured cells. Precipitating antibody develops during the 4th week postinoculation (*2*) and forms a line of identity with one of three lines characteristically formed by the serum of a chronically-ill cat (*6*). (Courtesy J. Gaskin.)

has shown that there is a close relationship between the persistence of precipitating antibody and infectious virus in the cat. Consequently, a single test is now available to test for antibody and virus in cat populations.

**Properties of the Virus.** The feline syncytium-forming viral isolates are sensitive to ether, chloroform, heat, and acid (5, 6). The viral particle contains RNA and the infectious virion appears to be cell-associated (6). Naked viral particles in the cytoplasm are approximately 45 m$\mu$ in diameter with an electron-lucent center (1, 7, 8). As the particles bud through the cell membrane into vacuoles they acquire an outer protein coat with projections in the process. The complete particles are 110 m$\mu$ in diameter. The feline syncytium-forming isolates may be confused with feline leukemia-sarcoma viruses. They are about the same diameter but the syncytium-forming virus particles show initial formation as a core in the cytoplasm, lack C-type particles, and they display studs or spikes that are absent on the outer membrane of feline leukemia-sarcoma particles. In mixed infections of cell cultures containing both viruses, one finds particles with characteristics of both—in addition, fragments and abnormally constructed particles are common (4). Thus, one must proceed with care when relying entirely on electron microscopy for identification and differentiation (4).

All isolates except one fail to hemagglutinate or hemadsorb cat, chicken, guinea pig, or human O erythrocytes (6, 7). The exception occurred when one of the isolates caused some hemagglutination after sonication (2).

Riggs *et al.* (7) has tested about 10 isolates with the serum-neutralization test. Seven isolates were similar, one was clearly different, and two others may be different (4).

Feline syncytium-forming isolates appear to contain an RNA polymerase common to RNA type C oncogenic viruses and visna virus. There is great interest in this finding as the syncytium-forming viruses could conceivably act in concert with these viruses that have oncogenic capabilities.

**Cultivation.** Feline syncytium-forming viruses replicate in cell cultures derived from cat, dog, chicken, horse, pig, monkey, and man (7, 8). Most of the iso-

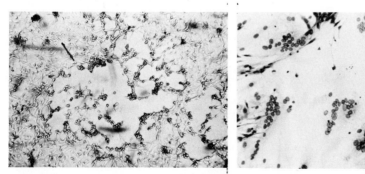

*Fig. 210.* The production of syncytia in feline cell cultures by a feline syncytium-forming virus. Unstained (*left*). X 65. Stained with May-Grünwald-Giemsa. (*right*). X 185. (Courtesy C. Fabricant.)

lates produce characteristic syncytium-formation in these cultures. Multinucleated cells may contain 80 or more nuclei (1). Many cultures do not contain
syncytia until 7 and 10 days, with maximum titers attained at 10 to 14 days
(7). Occasionally 3 to 4 weeks are required before syncytia become evident.
The use of direct cell cultures enhance success of viral isolation.

**Immunity.** Antibody persists after exposure to the virus, but the virus apparently also persists in most, if not all, cats. At present this causes no concern,
as the viruses are not known pathogens.

**Transmission.** The mode of transmission of this agent is not definitely known
(3). Although virus can be isolated from pharyngeal swabs from carrier cats,
the infection does not seem to spread readily to uninfected cats housed in the
same quarters. Feline syncytium-forming virus is associated with leukocytic
cells, and it seems likely that infection may occur early in life by movement
of such cells from dam to offspring either in the uterus or via the milk.

**The Disease in Man.** At present there is no evidence that the feline syncytium-forming viruses cause disease in humans.

### REFERENCES

1. Csiza.   Cornell Univ. Thesis, 1970.
2. Fabricant, Rich, and Gillespie.   Cornell Vet., 1969, *59*, 667.
3. Gaskin.   Cornell Univ. Thesis, 1972.
4. Hackett and Manning.   Jour. Am. Vet. Med. Assoc., 1971, *158*, 948.
5. Kasza, Hayward, and Betts.   Res. Vet. Sci., 1969, *10*, 216.
6. McKissick and Lamont.   Jour. Virol., 1970, 5, 247.
7. Riggs, Oshiro, Taylor, and Lennette.   Nature, 1969, *222*, 1190.
8. Scott.   Jour. Am. Vet. Med. Assoc., 1971, *158*, 946.

### Bovine Syncytium-Forming Viruses

In the course of studies with bovine leukemia Malmquist *et al.* (1) isolated
a syncytium-forming virus from a case of bovine lymphosarcoma. Paccaud
and Jacquier (2) isolated a respiratory syncytium-forming virus from cattle in
two herds with respiratory disease. Scott *et al.* (3) isolated syncytium-forming
viruses from the lung and kidney of a cow with winter dysentery, from the
uterus of a cow, and from the buffy coat of a cow with respiratory signs of illness. Gaskin has also isolated the virus from the buffy coat of cattle (personal
communication, 1971).

To date, none of the bovine isolates have been compared with each other
by serological means. The virus isolates of Paccaud and Jacquier are antigenically related to human respiratory syncytial viruses, yet the evidence is strong
that they are of bovine origin as evidenced by seroconversions of bovine field
cases and by some differences in biological traits between the viruses of
human and bovine origin.

None of the above isolates are known pathogens for cattle, but experimental trials in cattle for pathogenicity are extremely limited. Paccaud and Jac-

quier anticipate that their respiratory syncytial viruses will produce disease in cattle when tested. This assumption is based upon their antigenic relationship to the human virus which is a common cause of respiratory illness in children. Apparently they assume the same unknown role in cattle that the feline syncytium-forming agents take in cats. Consequently, they are principally known for their ubiquitous nature persisting in tissues despite the presence of antibody. As such they present some difficulties in the diagnosis of other viral diseases such as bovine leukemia and in the use of bovine tissues for the tissue culture where they may be found as contaminants.

## REFERENCES

1.  Malmquist, Van Der Matten, and Boothe.    Cancer Res., 1969, 29, 188.
2.  Paccaud and Jacquier.    Arch. f. die Gesam. Virusforsch., 1970, 30, 327.
3.  Scott, Shively, Gaskin, and Gillespie.    Submitted for publication, 1973.

# XLIV | Feline Panleukopenia and Other Parvoviruses

The parvoviruses formerly were called picodnaviruses as an analogy to the RNA picornaviruses. The parvoviruses contain single-stranded DNA with a molecular weight of 1.2 to 1.8 by $10^6$ daltons. In members of the subgroup B the single strands are complementary and band together *in vitro* to form a double strand. The isometric nonenveloped particles, 18 to 22 m$\mu$ in diameter with icosahedral symmetry probably have 32 capsomeres, 2 to 4 m$\mu$ in diameter. The buoyant density in cesium chloride is 1.4 g per ml. The particles are heat-stable and ether- and acid-resistant. The Subgroup B members which are the adenoassociated viruses, replicate only in the presence of an adenovirus which serves as the "helper" virus (fig. 211). All members multiply in the nucleus of the dividing cell.

The type species for the genus is *Parvovirus* n-1 (Kilham rat virus). Other members of Subgroup A are the H viruses ($H_1$ and $X_{14}$), minute mouse-viruses, and porcine parvoviruses. The Subgroup B includes the types 1, 2, 3, and 4 adeno-associated (satellite) viruses. Other possible members in the genus are feline panleukopenia, mink enteritis, hemorrhagic encephalopathy, and densonucleosis (Galleria) viruses and also the avian parvovirus and bovine parvovirus.

The most significant pathogen of domesticated animals is feline panleukopenia virus. For information about members of this genus that will not be given treatment in this chapter the reader is referred to articles by Kilham (1) and Toolan (2).

## REFERENCES

1. Kilham. Viruses of laboratory rodents. Natl. Cancer Inst. Monograph no. 20, 1966, pp. 117.
2. Toolan. Internatl. Rev. Exp. Path., 1968, 6, 135.

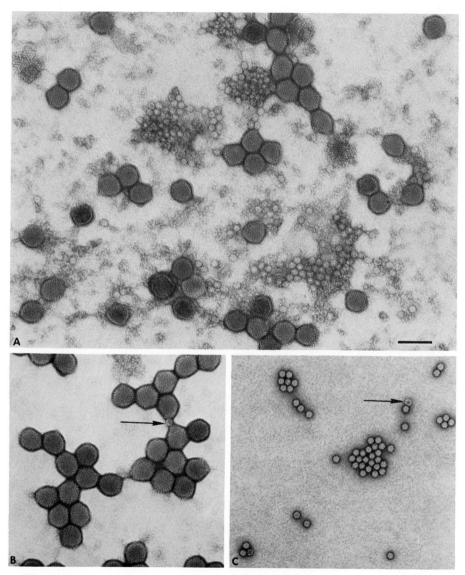

*Fig. 211.* (A) Crude tissue culture harvest showing many empty and full 22-nm AAV particles as well as many 80-nm ICH virions; (B) ICH virions from the adenovirus band after 48 hours of centrifugation in an isopycnic CsCl gradient, *arrow* shows a single empty 22-nm particle; and (C) Micrograph showing 22-nm AAV virions in AAV band of 48-hour-old isopycnic CsCl gradient, *arrow* again points out empty AAV capsid. Each preparation stained with 1 percent uranyl acetate. X 94,000. (Courtesy M. David Hoggan and Gunter F. Thomas, NIH.)

### Feline Panleukopenia

SYNONYMS: Feline distemper, feline agranulocytosis, cat plague, cat fever, feline infectious enteritis, feline ataxia, FPL.

This disease is highly contagious and often the mortality rate is high. It occurs in many parts of the world and has been described in France, England, India, Brazil, Canada, and the United States. A disease which may be the same but which is manifested a little differently was described by Seifried and Krembs (34) in Germany. The disease destroys many pet animals and formerly was a scourge in catteries and in animals that had been exposed in cat shows. In the past the disease has been ascribed by various authors to different bacterial agents. The true cause, a virus, was first identified by Verge and Cristoforoni (36) in 1928. The findings of the French workers were confirmed by Hindle and Finlay (12) in England in 1933 and by Leasure, Lienhardt, and Taberner (24) in the United States in 1934. In 1938 Lawrence and Syverton (22) studied a disease that occurred spontaneously in cats kept for laboratory purposes. The disease was manifested by signs that will be described below, but the most striking characteristic was the rapid disappearance of white blood cells from the blood during the early stages of the illness. It was shown to be caused by a virus. The following year Hammon and Enders (11) described the disease independently. They gave it the name *panleukopenia,* because of the almost total disappearance of leukocytes from the blood. There is no doubt that these workers were dealing with the disease known in veterinary circles at that time as *infectious enteritis.* The panleukopenia had not been previously recognized.

**Character of the Disease.** The disease is seen most often in domestic cats; however, zoological parks have suffered losses in their wild cats. Cockburn (3) reports deaths in the London zoo in tigers, leopards, lynxes, servals, ocelots, cheetahs, and some others. He believed the majority of wild *Felidae* to be susceptible, excepting lions, civets, and genets. Torres (35) found this virus in a fatal disease of caged wild cats. Hyslop (13) transmitted the virus from a domestic cat to two lynxes, then to a cheetah, and then back to a domestic cat in which the typical disease was produced. The signs in the wild cats were very similar to those seen in the house cat.

Schofield (30) in 1949 described a highly fatal disease of mink in Canada which could be readily transmitted with bacteria-free filtrates. In 1952 Wills (37) studied this disease more fully and came to the conclusion that its causative agent was the same as that of feline enteritis. This was confirmed by Gorham and Hartsough (10) in 1955, although Burger *et al.* have some reservations about it (2). Thus, all members of the cat family (*Felidae*) are susceptible as well as the raccoon, coati mundi, and ringtail in the family *Procyonidae* and also mink.

The disease infects young cats especially, although older ones are susceptible if they have had no previous contact with it. The affected animal develops lassitude, inappetence, and fever. In animals that are closely watched following natural exposure, a diphasic fever curve usually occurs. The first febrile reaction may reach a peak of 104 to 105 F within a few hours and remain at this level for about 24 hours. It then usually falls to normal, or near-normal, for 36 to 48 hours, at the end of which time it again rises. By the time of the second rise the cat is very ill. It is depressed, has a rough unkempt coat, lies on its abdomen with its head on its front paws, and is indifferent to its owner or surroundings. Death usually occurs shortly after the peak of the second temperature curve is reached, or the temperature will fall precipitously and the animal recover. Animals lose weight rapidly because of dehydration. Vomiting is common. Many of the cases develop a profuse watery diarrhea which is often blood-tinged. Most of them exhibit mucopurulent discharges from the eyes and nose. Gochenour (9) has seen cases in which there was no temperature rise.

Intrauterine infection with FPL virus may result in abortions, stillbirths, early neonatal deaths, or cerebellar hypoplasia (fig. 212) manifested by ataxia first seen at 2 to 3 weeks when the kittens become ambulatory (5, 6, 20, 21).

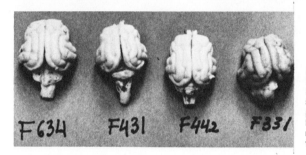

Fig. 212. Cerebellar hypoplasia caused by feline infectious panleukopenia virus. Infected neonatal kittens F634, F431, and F442 showing varying degrees of hypoplasia. The brain labeled F331 has a normal-sized cerebellum removed from an uninfected kitten. (Courtesy C. Csiza.)

In artificially inoculated animals the incubation period may be as short as 48 hours, but it usually is about 4 days. By natural contact it is generally longer—sometimes as long as 9 days but usually not over 6 days. The disease progresses to its crisis very rapidly in most instances. According to Riser (28), the average duration is about 5 days, but some animals may die within 3 days and others may last more than a week. Animals that survive as long as 9 days practically always recover.

The incidence, morbidity and mortality may vary considerably under field conditions. The morbidity is usually high, but the mortality may run from low to high, in some instances 90 percent. Subclinical infections must occur, as most unvaccinated adult cats have antibody and many cats have never exhibited clinical disease.

Lesions of enteritis are found, usually in the terminal portion of the ileum, where the mucosa may be only slightly inflamed or there may be severe pseudomembranous inflammation. In some cases the inflammation may be more extensive, involving much of the small intestine. The mesenteric lymph nodes

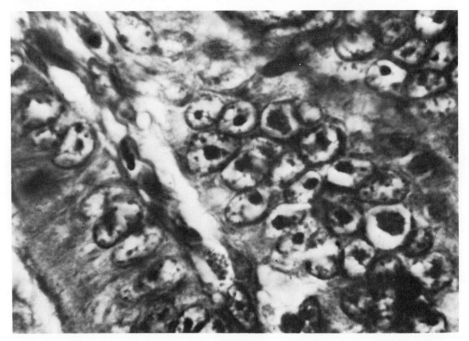

*Fig. 213.* Feline infectious panleukopenia. Intranuclear inclusion bodies in small intestine. X 1,120. (Courtesy C. Csiza.)

may be swollen and petechiated. The red marrow of the long bones is greasy and gelatinous. Microscopically the epithelium of the villi of the affected portions of the intestine shows degeneration, and intranuclear inclusion bodies (fig. 213) may be found in these cells. The intestinal wall is thickened with edematous fluid. Degeneration of the liver cells and of the tubular epithelium of the kidney is found, and these cells also contain the intranuclear inclusion bodies. If the animal dies quickly, or is killed early in the course of the disease, the blood-forming tissue of the bones is inconspicuous, having been replaced by fat cells.

The blood reaction in this disease is exceedingly interesting. Lawrence, Syverton, Shaw, and Smith (23) divided their cases into two classes according to the manner in which the leukocytes disappeared from the peripheral circulation under the influence of the virus. In the first group the leukocytes gradually diminished from the time of exposure until the time of the temperature peak. In the other there was little change in the leukocyte count for 5 to 6 days; then during the febrile reaction there was a precipitous drop. From a normal of about 15,000 leukocytes per mm $^3$ the count usually dropped to 2,000 or less, and not infrequently to zero. In about 20 percent of their cases the count varied from 0 to 200 cells per mm $^3$. During this time there was only a slight decrease in the red cell count and the percentage of hemoglobin.

The virus obviously has a severely destructive effect upon the hemopoietic centers.

**The Disease in Experimental Cats.**   In a pathogenesis study of newborn kittens, every tissue in the body contained virus following intranasal or oral inoculation (5, 6). It appears that the virus first establishes itself in the oral pharynx at 18 hours and then a viremia develops. At 48 hours every tissue has significant amounts of virus and high titers persist through day 7. As serum antibody appears, virus titers drop precipitously with little or no virus by day 14 in most tissues. Small quantities of virus may persist for 1 year in some tissues such as the kidney (4).

The pathogenesis in the cat is dependent largely upon the mitotic activity of various tissues within the body. In the newborn cat the thymus and external granular layer of the cerebellum are undergoing rapid development and these tissues are severely affected at this stage. In older kittens the infection occurs primarily in the lymphoid tissues of the oropharynx, epithelium of the intestinal crypts, and bone marrow.

In a pregnant cat the virus readily infects the uterus and crosses the placental barrier to the fetus where it invades the brain. The type of teratogenic effects depend upon the stage of gestation at the time of infection.

Mink affected with mink enteritis virus are anoretic, have abnormal enteric mucoid discharges often with blood streaks and intestinal casts. The mortality varies between 10 and 80 percent (7, 29).

The neonatal ferret inoculated intracerebrally is the only animal known to be susceptible other than those previously mentioned (20).

**Properties of the Virus.**   The virus has the principal characteristics of the type species for the genus *Parvovirus.* This DNA virus which is probably double-stranded (16, 18, 36) resists ether, chloroform, heat (56 C for 30 minutes), acid, phenol, and trypsin but can be inactivated by 0.2 percent formalin (14). Its size by electron microscopy is 20 to 25 m$\mu$ and the specific gravity is 1.33 g per ml (16, 19). At low temperatures or in 50 percent glycerol the virus is infective for long periods of time.

Reciprocal serum-neutralization tests with many isolates and their antisera resulted in equivalent titers in all cases (31). The same results were obtained with mink enteritis, feline ataxia, and feline panleukopenia isolates (15, 17). This is rather good evidence that FPL virus is a single antigenic serotype.

The complement-fixation test has been used by employing a purified mink enteritis virus antigen (19). There is no evidence that FPL virus contains a hemagglutinin (27).

There is no evidence of cross-reaction between FPL virus and other members of the genus, but complete cross testing has not been done. The Kilham rat virus inoculated into neonatal kittens produces degeneration of the cerebellum similar to FPL virus (27).

**Cultivation.** Cell cultures of feline kidney origin are preferred for the isolation and cultivation of FPL virus. The virus has a selective affinity for the mitotic

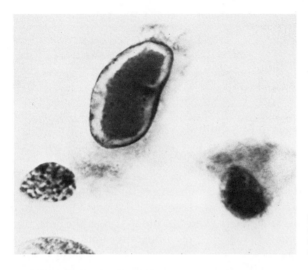

*Fig. 214.* Feline infectious pan-leukopenia. Cowdry type A inclusion bodies in feline kidney cell culture. May-Grünwald-Giemsa stain. X 880. (Courtesy F. Scott.)

cell so the best results are obtained when cultures are inoculated with virus 2 to 3 hours after cell seeding. The maximum cytopathic effects are observed after 4 to 5 days at 37 C. Unless the cultures are inoculated with a high viral content the use of May-Gruenwald-Giemsa stain, hematoxylin-eosin stain, or specific fluorescein isothiocyanate conjugate is required to identify the virus in culture as the CPE in unstained cultures is negligible. With the dye stains Cowdry type A intranuclear inclusion bodies can be detected. The virus also replicates in cell cultures of a feline-tongue diploid line, of a feline-thymus diploid line, and of cell lines of feline kidney (Crandell), lion kidney, and a feline neurofibrosarcoma (25).

No multiplication of virus occurs in the embryonated hen's egg (8).

**Immunity.** Neutralizing antibodies appear in the circulation of cats about 3 days after the onset of illness. The titers develop rapidly to reach 1,000 to 10,000 about 10 to 11 days after onset of illness (32). Neutralizing antibody presumably persists in the cat for years, and such cats are protected against a subsequent exposure to virulent challenge virus by various routes of inoculation or by contact exposure to cats acutely ill with FPL infection.

Maternal antibody conferred from the immune dam to its progeny interferes with vaccination and also protects against virulent virus (33). The serum-neutralizing antibody titer of the progeny is equivalent to the dams' 24 to 48 hours after birth, then gradually declines with an antibody half-life of approximately 9.5 days. Maternity titers of 30 or greater (tested against 100 $TCID_{50}$ of virus) usually protect kittens against challenge with 1,000 to 3,000 $TCID_{50}$ of virulent challenge virus, and seroconversion does not occur. Attenuated virus vaccines will replicate in kittens with titers of 10 or less and produce an active immune titer at a high level; any demonstrable maternal antibody interferes with inactivated virus vaccines.

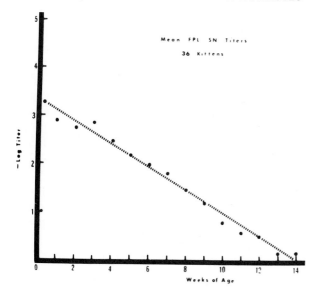

Fig. 215. The mean maternal immunity to feline panleukopenia in a group of kittens born to immune queens. (Courtesy F. Scott, C Csiza, and J. Gillespie, *Jour. Am. Vet. Med. Assoc.*)

Most field strains produce frank disease in experimental cats purchased from the field sources. Subclinical or mild infections occur frequently in susceptible cats with some strains so the investigator must be selective in his choice of test strain used for challenge (31). Subclinical or mild infections occur in gnotobiotic cats given virulent virus (29).

**Transmission.** Viral transmission usually occurs by direct contact of susceptible cats with infected cats in the acute stage of illness when the virus is excreted in the feces, urine, saliva, and vomitus. It may also occur mechanically by contact with contaminated food dishes, bedding, infected cages, or by humans. Recovered cats may shed the virus in their feces or urine for considerable periods of time with virus known to persist for several weeks in the kidney of recovered cats and for at least one year in the kidneys of neonatally infected cats (4). Recovered mink may shed the virus in their feces for at least one year (1).

During acute stage of illness fleas may transmit the disease (16) and it seems likely that biting insects may do likewise.

The virus is extremely stable and probably survives for a considerable period of time in the environment of infected premises.

The facts cited above readily explain how this virus maintains itself in nature.

**Diagnosis.** A presumptive diagnosis of FPL can be made on basis of the clinical signs, and the presence of leukopenia. The diagnosis can be confirmed by pathological lesions, viral isolation, demonstration of immunofluorescence of infected tissues with a specific FPL conjugate, or demonstration of a rising serum titer. The direct immunofluorescent test can be used for detection of virus in cell culture or in tissues.

The serum-neutralization test is generally used to detect antibody (33). Serum dilutions are mixed with an equal volume of virus (100 to 300 TCID $_{50}$ per 0.1 ml). Aliquots of the serum-virus mixtures are incubated at room temperature for 1 hour and 0.2 ml of each is inoculated into secondary feline kidney cells in Leighton tube coverslip cultures 2 to 3 hours after transfer. After 4 days at 37 C the coverslips are stained and examined for intranuclear inclusion bodies as outlined in the section on cultivation. The metabolic inhibition test or direct examination of unstained cultures can be used if the cultures are good and the proper amount of virus is used in the respective tests. Nonspecific degeneration of cultures often makes the end point difficult to ascertain with these latter methods.

**Prevention.** There are several excellent biologics for the prevention of feline panleukopenia. Inactivated and attenuated virus vaccines produced an immunity which presumably persists for years although there is no definite information on this point. Because the disease can be prevented by immunization, clinicians should emphasize the importance of proper vaccination. An evaluation of the types of biologics was made and various guidelines for their use were recommended by the Panel of the American Veterinary Medical Association Colloquium on Selected Feline Infectious Diseases (7). The Panel made the following recommendations for vaccination based upon information presented at the colloquium.

The Panel recommends the use of tissue culture origin (TCO), inactivated or modified live-virus (MLV) vaccines, although tissue-type vaccines have been known to be efficacious for years. However, The Panel notes that, according to the information provided at the colloquium, TCO vaccines appear to have a slight advantage for the following reasons: These vaccines tend to break through a low level of maternally derived immunity and hence may be effective in cats of a slightly younger age. They contain less organic material and cause less discomfort at the time of administration. The antigenic content of TCO vaccines is easier to monitor.

Due to varying degrees of maternal antibody in kittens, the Panel recommends administration of two doses of vaccine starting at 9 to 10 weeks of age. For the MLV vaccines, the second vaccination should be given at 14 to 16 weeks of age. If the kittens are older than 12 weeks at the time of the first vaccination with MLV vaccines, a second vaccination is not necessary.

For the inactivated vaccines, the second dose should be given 2 weeks later. For maximum protection, a third vaccination should be given when the cat is 16 weeks old.

Annual revaccination is recommended for maximum protection. Unvaccinated kittens should not be admitted to an area of possible exposure to FPL without immediate vaccination or administration of antiserum. Colostrum-deprived kittens should be given antiserum for immediate protection followed by repeated doses of vaccine as indicated.

The Panel recommendations for the use of antiserum are as follows: There are two specific indications for the use of antiserum (or normal serum). First, susceptible cats that have been exposed to FPL should be given antiserum immediately at the rate of 1 ml per pound of body weight. Second, colostrum-deprived kittens should be given antiserum as soon after birth as possible. Vaccines should be given later at appropriate intervals.

**Control.** The disease is difficult to control in a group of cats once the infection starts. Antiserum is quite effective in outbreaks where certain cats have not shown signs of illness at the time of its administration. After signs are observed the antiserum has little or no benefit.

The stability of this virus dictates thorough cleansing and disinfection of infected premises before the introduction of infected cats. Unless several months have passed, new cats should be vaccinated approximately 2 weeks before introduction into infected premises.

**The Disease in Man.** There is no evidence that FPL virus causes disease in humans.

## REFERENCES

1.  Bouillant and Hanson.   Canad. Jour. Comp. Med. and Vet. Sci., 1965, *29*, 183.
2.  Burger, Farrell, and Gorham.   West. Vet., 1958, 5, 68.
3.  Cockburn.   Vet. Jour., 1947, *103*, 261.
4.  Csiza, Scott, de Lahunta, and Gillespie.   Am. Jour. Vet. Res., 1971, *32*, 419.
5.  Csiza, Scott, de Lahunta, and Gillespie.   Jour. Inf. and Immunity, 1971, *3*, 838.
6.  de Lahunta.   Jour. Am. Vet. Med. Assoc., 1971, *158*, 901.
7.  Feline Infectious Diseases Colloquium.   *Ibid.*, 1971, *158*, 835.
8.  Gillespie.   Unpublished observations, 1971.
9.  Gochenour.   North Am. Vet., 1943, *24*, 104.
10. Gorham and Hartsough.   Am. Fur Breed., 1955 (Apr). (Abstract in: Jour. Am. Vet. Med. Assoc., 1955, *126*, 467.)
11. Hammon and Enders.   Jour. Exp. Med., 1939, *69*, 327.
12. Hindle and Finlay.   Jour. Comp. Path. and Therap., 1932, *45*, 11.
13. Hyslop.   Brit. Vet. Jour., 1955, *111*, 373.
14. Johnson.   Res. Vet. Sci., 1966, *7*, 112.
15. Johnson.   Jour. Small Anim. Pract., 1967, *8*, 319.
16. Johnson and Cruickshank.   Nature, 1966, *212*, 622.
17. Johnson, Margolis and Kilham.   *Ibid.*, 1967, *214*, 175.
18. Judkins and Gillespie.   Unpublished observations, 1968.
19. Kääriäinen, Kangas, Keränen, Sirkka, Nyholm, and Weckström.   Arch. f. die Gesam. Virusforsch, 1966, *19*, 197.
20. Kilham, Margolis, and Colby.   Lab. Invest., 1967, *17*, 465.
21. Kilham, Margolis, and Colby.   Jour. Am. Vet. Med. Assoc., 1971, *158*, 888.

22. Lawrence and Syverton. Proc. Soc. Exp. Biol. and Med., 1938, 38, 914.
23. Lawrence, Syverton, Shaw, and Smith. Am. Jour. Path., 1940, 16, 333.
24. Leasure, Lienhardt, and Taberner. North Am. Vet., 1934, 15, 30.
25. Lee, Kniazeff, Fabricant, and Gillespie. Cornell Vet., 1969, 59, 539.
26. Lust, Gorham, and Sato. Am. Jour. Vet. Res., 1965, 26, 1163.
27. Margolis and Kilham. Chapter 8, Internatl. Acad. Path. Monograph no. 9. Williams and Wilkins Co., Baltimore, 1968.
28. Riser. North Am. Vet., 1943, 24, 293.
29. Rohovsky and Griesemer. Path. Vet., 1967, 4, 391.
30. Schofield. North Am. Vet., 1949, 30, 651.
31. Scott. Feline panleukopenia. Cornell Univ. Thesis, 1968.
32. Scott, Csiza, and Gillespie. Cornell Vet., 1970, 60, 183.
33. Scott, Csiza, and Gillespie. Jour. Am. Vet. Med. Assoc., 1970, 156, 439.
34. Seifried and Krembs. Arch. f. Tierheilk., 1940, 75, 252.
35. Torres. North Am. Vet., 1941, 22, 297.
36. Verge and Cristoforoni. Comp. rend. Soc. Biol. (Paris), 1928, 99, 312.
37. Wills. Canad. Jour. Comp. Med., 1952, 16, 419.

## Porcine Parvovirus

SYNONYMS: PPV, porcine picodnavirus

Pathologic changes generally are not attributed to the porcine parvovirus although a small DNA virus has been described in England (1) which may be responsible for abortions, stillbirths, and infertility in swine. This English isolate has properties similar to PPV but its relationship has not been determined.

Infected swine develop antibodies without production of clinical disease or pathological lesions (2). No pathological changes are produced in newborn hamsters or rats with PPV (4). The virus has been isolated in Europe (3-5) and a large percentage of pigs in New York State (6) and Germany (2) have antibodies. The pig is the only species known to be susceptible to PPV.

This virus was isolated from several stocks of tissue-cultured hog cholera virus (2, 4) and from primary monolayer cultures of kidneys from healthy piglets (4). The virus produced a cytopathic effect characterized by a diffuse granulation, by rounding and detachment of cells from the glass of primary and cell line pig kidney cell cultures. Intranuclear inclusion bodies occur. Maximum virus yields of $TCID_{50}$ $10^4$ to $10^5$ per 0.1 ml are attained by inoculating cultures before they become confluent and harvesting the fluid at 72 to 108 hours later (4).

The virus contains a hemagglutinin. The HA test is performed at 4 C using erythrocytes of the guinea pig, mouse, rat, cat, chicken, or human type O but not hamster, pig, rabbit, dog, sheep, horse, or goose (4). Its virus particles are 20 to 22 m$\mu$ in diameter with a morphology comparable to other parvoviruses (4). It has a buoyant density of 1.38 g per ml (4).

## REFERENCES

1.  Cartwright and Huck.   Vet. Rec., 1967, *81*, 196.
2.  Bachman.   Zentbl. f. Vet.-Med., 1969, *16B*, 341.
3.  Horzinek, Mussgay, Maess, and Petzoldt.   Arch. f. die Gesam. Virusforsch., 1967, *21*, 98.
4.  Mayr, Bachmann, Siegl, Mahnel, and Sheffy.   *Ibid.*, 1968, 25, 38.
5.  Mayr and Mahnel.   Centrbl. f. Bakt., I Abt. Orig., 1966, *199*, 399.
6.  Sheffy.   Personal communication, 1969.

## Bovine Parvovirus

A hemadsorbing enteric virus (HADEN) was isolated from the gastrointestinal tract by Abinanti and Warfield (1) and later classified as a parvovirus by Storz and Warren (4).

The bovine parvovirus has not been established as a pathogen for cattle, although very little work has been done in this regard.

The HADEN strain has all the characteristics of a parvovirus (2, 4). Its size is approximately 23 m$\mu$ and resistant to ether and sodium deoxycholate (3). It is stable over a pH range of 3 to 9. Intranuclear inclusion bodies of the Cowdry type A are produced in bovine embryonic kidney cells. The virus produces hemagglutination and hemadsorption of human, dog, and guinea pig red blood cells and elution of virus does not occur (1, 2). Actinomycin D, and also bromo- and 5-fluoro-$2^1$ deoxyuridine (BUDU and FUDR) inhibited the replication of virus in cell culture.

Comparative HI serological investigations revealed no relationship between the bovine parvovirus and RV, H-1, MM, PPV and FPV (2).

## REFERENCES

1.  Abinanti and Warfield.   Virology, 1961, *14*, 288.
2.  Bachmann.   Zentbl. f. Vet.-Med., 1971, *18B*, 80.
3.  Spahn, Mohanty, and Hetrick.   Canad. Jour. Microbiol., 1966, *12*, 653.
4.  Storz and Warren.   Arch. f. die Gesam. Virusforsch, 1970, *30*, 271.

## Canine Parvovirus

A canine virus was isolated from the feces of four adult dogs. The recovered isolates had many of the properties of the *Parvovirus* genus so it was proposed that this canine virus be designated a member of the genus and called the minute virus of canines.

The isolates were recovered in a continuous canine cell line, WRCC. Each isolate produced a similar type of CPE characterized by infected cells becoming rounded, developing distinct cell membranes and cytoplasmic strands and, finally, detaching from the glass. In this system viral titers of TCID$_{50}$ $10^7$ usually were achieved. The isolates failed to induce CPE in cell cultures of primary dog kidney, of human embryonic kidney, of African green monkey kidney, of feline kidney, and of kidneys from many other animal species. Attempts to produce overt signs of illness in newborn and weanling mice, hamsters, and guinea pigs failed.

The minute virus of canines has a different hemagglutinating spectrum for red blood cells than the rodent, feline (feline panleukopenia), and pig parvoviruses. The canine virus agglutinates simian erythrocytes but not guinea pig, human O, rat, or pig red blood cells. Furthermore, the canine virus produces a cytopathic effect only in the continuous canine cell line, WRCC.

The pathogenicity of the canine parvovirus for dogs is unknown. Based upon limited serological studies it appears that the virus infection may frequently occur in canine populations.

**REFERENCE**

1.   Binn, Lazar, Eddy, and Kajima.    Inf. and Immunity, 1970, *1*, 503.

# XLV | Avian Infectious Bronchitis, Transmissible Gastroenteritis of Pigs, and Other Coronaviruses

The coronaviruses probably contain RNA. The enveloped particles vary in size from 70 to 120 mμ in diameter. The nucleocapsid is probably helical and loosely wound, either 7 or 9 mμ in diameter. The surface has characteristic pedunculated projections (fig. 216). The buoyant density in cesium chloride is 1.15 to 1.16 g per ml. The particles are ether-sensitive.

Replication occurs in cytoplasm and the virus is unaffected by DNA inhibitors. Maturation occurs by budding into cytoplasmic vesicles (fig. 217). The viruses in the genus are antigenically heterogenous and there is some relationship between certain human and murine strains.

The type species for the genus is *Coronavirus* a-1 (avian infectious bronchitis virus). Other members of the group are mouse hepatitis virus, human respiratory virus, transmissible gastroenteritis virus, and possibly an equine coronavirus and hemagglutinating encephalitis virus of pigs.

This chapter will include sections on avian bronchitis, transmissible gastroenteritis of pigs, and the hemagglutinating virus of pigs.

## Avian Infectious Bronchitis

SYNONYMS:   Chick bronchitis, gasping disease, *Coronavirus* a-1.

This disease was first described by Schalk and Hawn (18) in 1931. These authors did not determine its cause. In 1933 Bushnell and Brandly (3) carried on some filtration studies and decided that a filterable agent was its cause. More extensive studies were reported by Beach and Schalm (1) in 1936 which showed that the causative agent was a virus which differed in several respects

1099

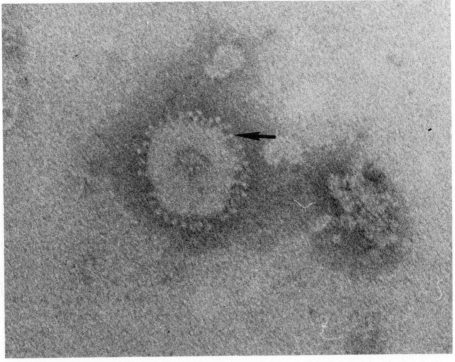

*Fig. 216.* Avian bronchitis virus. Stained with phosphotungstic acid (negative-staining). Note pedunculated projections (*arrow*) at the surface of the virion. (Courtesy B. Cowen.)

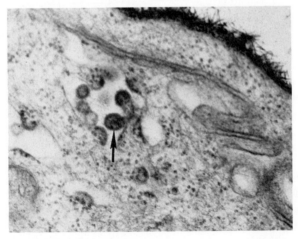

*Fig. 217.* Maturation by budding of avian bronchitis virus into cytoplasmic vesicles of an embryonated hen's egg cell. (Courtesy B. Cowen.)

from that of infectious laryngotracheitis. This disease has been reported from North America, where it frequently causes serious losses, and also from England, Holland, and Japan.

**Character of the Disease.** This disease occurs in chicks from 2 days to 3 or 4 weeks of age. In some sections of the country it has become of great importance as a disease of partly grown and laying pullets and hens. The disease occurs often in hatcheries selling "started" chicks and from them is spread to flocks through the sale of the infected chicks. It causes large losses in establishments engaged in raising birds for the broiler trade, since in these plants large numbers of young birds are raised in very crowded conditions. Affected laying birds show a sharp decline in egg production, which may persist for several weeks. There is a marked loss of shell firmness and a deterioration in the internal quality of the egg. Virus may be present in the eggs from some hens during this period.

The disease is characterized by listlessness, depression, gasping, and râles, and by such rapidity of spread that nearly all exposed birds develop the disease at almost the same time. The outbreak runs a rapid course, and the mortality rate is from 25 to 90 percent in young chicks. The effect on birds from the age of 6 weeks up to shortly before the first egg is laid is not likely to be more than slight retardation in their development. In the laying flock the damage is due to depression of egg yield rather than to death losses. Exudate that may be mucoid or caseous is regularly found in the bronchi and sometimes in the nasal passages. In chicks that die, plugs of fibrinopurulent exudate often are found in the lower part of the trachea or in the larger bronchi. No inclusion bodies are found. Chicks that are inoculated into the trachea develop the disease after an incubation period of 24 to 48 hours as a rule, occasionally as long as 4 days, and death or recovery occurs in from 6 to 18 days.

**Properties of the Virus.** Particles in cytoplasm are 200 millimicrons in diameter and others in infected egg fluid 60 to 100 millimicrons (7). Heat stability at 56 C varies with the strain but none consistently survive more than 30 minutes at that temperature. A 1:10,000 dilution of $KMnO_4$ and 1 percent formalin inactivates the virus. It is ether labile and resistant to pH 2 for 1 hour at room temperature.

Low-passaged egg virus treated with trypsin will hemagglutinate chicken red blood cells at pH 7.2 in 45 to 60 minutes at room temperature. Egg-adapted strains were less active. No elution occurred (4).

By the use of the neutralization test in hens' eggs Hofstad (11) showed the presence of two antigenic types, Connecticut and Massachusetts, but with some cross-reaction. Iowa strains 97 and 609 represent additional serotypes. There are also additional field isolates that cannot be identified with existing recognized serotypes. The field strain most commonly isolated is the Massachusetts serotype.

By means of agar diffusion analysis antigen-antibody complexes of virus and antisera may be detected. None of the precipitating antigens can be specifically ascribed to infectious bronchitis virus (IBV) (8).

Suckling mice are susceptible by intracerebral inoculation to certain strains of IBV.

**Cultivation.** In 1937 Beaudette and Hudson (2) found that bronchitis virus can be propagated in chicken embryos. Characteristic dwarfing (9) and curling (10) of the embryo has been described.

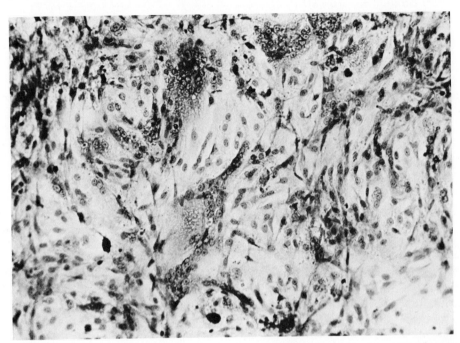

*Fig. 218.* Syncytia with necrosis induced by viral replication of avian bronchitis virus in chicken kidney cell culture. Giemsa stain. X 85. (Courtesy B. Cowen.)

Virus titration may be performed in chicken embryo-kidney cultures with chicken egg adapted strains by using cytopathic effects as revealed by the formation of large syncytia followed by necrosis and by the plaque technic (8).

**Immunity.** Chickens that recover from natural infection are solidly immune for at least 6 to 8 months. Challenge of immunity is done by aerosol exposure, by intranasal inoculation, or by natural exposure. With adequate controls the natural exposure to virus is preferred. Challenge is evaluated by production of tracheal râles and by attempted isolation of virus from tracheal swabs.

Inactivated virus vaccines for infectious bronchitis have been unsuccessful. Active strains which have lost their virulence for chickens have also proved worthless.

For some years in the northeastern part of the United States a method of immunization recommended by Van Roekel *et al.* (19) was used with excellent success. This involved deliberately inoculating a small portion of flocks with active virus when the birds were from 7 to 15 weeks of age. At this stage of their development birds are not seriously damaged by the disease. The mortality of younger birds and the disruption of production in laying flocks are not experienced in birds of this age. The method served very well but had the disadvantage that active virus perpetuated the disease in the flock and in the community. This procedure has now been given up in favor of modified virus vaccines (6, 13). These vaccines are not avirulent and trouble sometimes results from their use, but generally they are safer and apparently just as effi-

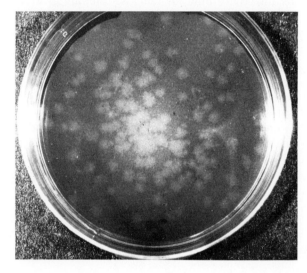

*Fig. 219.* Necrosis of syncytia in figure 218 manifested as plaques by the agar overlay method. (Courtesy B. Cowen.)

cient as the active virus. Vaccines are generally administered to flocks *en masse* by aerosol or sprays (5) or dusts (15), or they are given in the drinking water (14). Satisfactory immunity is not always attained by the use of these products (17). Successful vaccination has been further complicated by demonstration of multiple antigenic serotypes.

**Transmission.** Infections can readily be induced by inoculating minute amounts of virus into the respiratory apparatus. Natural infections, it seems certain, are contracted through inhalation of infective droplets. Levine and Hofstad (12) demonstrated experimentally that the infection can be air-borne for a distance of at least 5 feet. Virus carriers have been demonstrated for periods longer than 35 to 49 days. Outbreaks have been traced to hatcheries which deal in "started chicks." Infection established in these chicks is carried to the farm of the purchaser. Egg-borne transmission is another possibility.

**Diagnosis.** In the absence of any nervous signs coughing and gasping suggest infectious bronchitis in young chicks. Because nervous signs are not always apparent in Newcastle disease in chicks, a differential diagnosis is necessary.

In older birds infectious bronchitis must be differentiated from laryngotra-cheitis, Newcastle disease, infectious coryza, and *Mycoplasma* infections.

Respiratory tissues are most useful for viral isolation. It is not usually possi-ble to isolate virus after 10 to 14 days. Lung and trachea placed in 50 percent glycerol may be shipped to the laboratory without refrigeration. Inoculation of an infective-tissue suspension into the allantoic sac of a 9-to-11-day-old em-bryo causes stunting of the embryo. In initial passages stunting may not be prominent but on continued passage all embryos will be stunted and some embryos die after 5 to 6 days of incubation.

Certain features of the virus can be used in its identification such as its stunting effect on embryos, its infectivity only for chickens among all avian species, its resistance at pH 2 for 1 hour at room temperature, its heat and ether-sensitivity, and its neutralization by specific bronchitis antiserum. Its antigenic variation does limit the usefulness of the serum-neutralization test in the diagnosis.

The fluorescent-antibody test has been used in detecting IBV in tracheal smears of acutely affected chickens with reasonable success.

**Control.** The disease is best controlled by disposing of entire flocks, cleaning and disinfecting the premises, and beginning over with clean stock. If infec-tion occurs, resort must be made to vaccines unless the more radical proce-dure of disposing of all stock is feasible.

**The Disease in Man.** The virus of avian infectious bronchitis is not infective for man or other mammals.

## REFERENCES

1.  Beach and Schalm.   Poultry Sci., 1936, *15*, 199.
2.  Beaudette and Hudson.   Jour. Am. Vet. Assoc., 1937, *90*, 51.
3.  Bushnell and Brandly.   Poultry Sci., 1933, *12*, 55.
4.  Corbo and Cunningham.   Am. Jour. Vet. Res., 1959, *20*, 876.
5.  Crawley.   Proc. Am. Vet. Med. Assoc., 1953, p. 342.
6.  Crawley.   *Ibid.*, 1955, p. 343.
7.  Cunningham.   Am. Jour. Vet. Res., 1957, *18*, 648.
8.  Cunningham.   *Ibid.*, 1960, *21*, 498.
9.  Delaplane.   Proc. 19th Ann. Northeastern Pullorum Conf., 1947.
10.  Fabricant.   Cornell Vet., 1949, *39*, 414.
11.  Hofstad.   Am. Jour. Vet. Res., 1958, *19*, 740.
12.  Levine and Hofstad.   Cornell Vet., 1947, *37*, 204.
13.  Luginbuhl and Jungherr.   Poultry Sci., 1952, *31*, 924.
14.  Luginbuhl, Jungherr, and Chomiak.   *Ibid.*, 1955, *34*, 1399.
15.  Markham, Hammar, Gingher, and Cox.   *Ibid.*, 442.
16.  Mohanty and Chang.   Am. Jour. Vet. Res., 1963, *101*, 822.
17.  Raggi and Bankowski.   *Ibid.*, 1956, *17*, 523.
18.  Schalk and Hawn.   Jour. Am. Vet. Med. Assoc., 1931, 78, 413.
19.  Van Roekel, Bullis, Clarke, Olesiuk, and Sperling.   Mass. Agr. Exp. Sta., Bul. 460, 1950.

## Transmissible Gastroenteritis of Pigs

SYNONYM:   Gastroenteritis in young pigs; abbreviation, TGE

This is a readily transmissible gastroenteritis of swine. The disease is highly fatal to pigs less than 10 days old. Older animals usually recover. In adult swine the disease is almost negligible. The viral agent is a member of the *Coronavirus genus.*

**Character of the Disease.** No animals other than swine are known to show signs of illness from this virus.

The disease was first reported in Indiana by Doyle and Hutchings (8) in 1946, although it is clear that it had existed much earlier. It occurs throughout the swine belt of the United States (northcentral states) and sporadically in other areas where swine are kept. A disease like TGE was described in England by Goodwin and Jennings (10) in 1959. It has since been reported in Canada, Taiwan, and many European countries.

The disease generally spreads rapidly when it first enters a herd, involving animals of all ages. The older breeding animals generally show relatively mild signs varying from none at all to inappetence, vomiting, profuse scouring, severe weight loss, and even death in rare instances. The older animals generally recover within a week, although the decrease in weight in feeder pigs may be a serious loss to the owner. Death losses are in young pigs under 2 weeks of age, reaching close to 100 percent. These suffer severe diarrhea, the bowel discharge being watery and whitish or whitish green in color. The animals suffer from severe thirst and frequently collect around the watering troughs, from which they drink excessively. Some die within 2 days, but most of the deaths are on the 4th or 5th day. Most piglets over 3 weeks of age survive but often remain stunted afterward for a long period of time.

The period of incubation is relatively short—within 12 to 18 hours in many cases. The clinically sick animals in most instances are either well on the road to recovery or are dead within 1 week from the onset of signs. Some, especially very young pigs, may die within 2 or 3 days, and some survivors may show the effect of the disease for weeks afterward.

Besides gastroenteritis, there are few lesions in this disease. Emaciation and dehydration occur in animals that have lived long enough. Sometimes there are evidences of nephritis and hepatic degeneration. The stomach and intestines may exhibit severe enteritis. These lesions are nearly always found in older animals that die from the disease. In the young pigs, however, there may be little evidence of inflammation but the intestines are distended with liquid ingesta (14). The wall of the intestinal tract is thin and almost transparent as a result of villi atrophy. The absence of chyle in the mesenteric lymphatics is a constant feature.

**The Disease in Experimental Animals.** The pathogenesis of TGE in newborn pigs has been studied to a certain degree by Lee (15), Young *et al.* (26), and Hooper and Haelterman (13). Ingestion and airborne infection constitute the means by which TGE virus enters the body to initiate the infection. The gastrointestinal route probably is the most important one but virus replicates to high titer in the nasal mucosa and lungs so the question hasn't been resolved. When the virus reaches the highly susceptible epithelial cells of the small intestine, infection causes destruction of columnar epithelial cells with an accompanying marked shortening or contraction of the villi resulting in malabsorption. The shortened villi of the small intestine, particularly the jejunum, viewed through a dissecting microscope (X10) are quite characteristic of the disease (13). Other morphologic changes include vacuolation (10) and a loss (or decrease) in the height of their brush border, no vesicles in the apical cytoplasm, accumulation of fat globules in the cytoplasm, and abundance of polyribosomes (24). There is a reduction in these cells of alkaline and acid phosphatase, adenosine triphosphatase, succinic dehydrogenase, and nonspecific esterase (24). Lactose activity is not detected in the atrophic villi of the small intestine (7).

Dogs given TGE infected pig intestinal tissue develop a serological response and virus is isolated from rectal swabs of dogs by inoculation of composite samples into susceptible piglets (19).

**Properties of the Virus.** Various investigators (4, 6, 22) have studied certain biochemical and biophysical properties of the virus. This is an RNA virus which is ether labile and trypsin resistant. There are conflicting reports on its stability at pH 3, although the virus is entirely stable at pH 4 to 8. Amantadine-HCl and puromycin reduce viral replication at least 98 percent as determined in a tissue-culture system (18). The virus is relatively heat-labile and also photosensitive. Phenol at 0.5 percent level destroys the virus held at 37 C for 30 minutes.

The virus is quite stable when stored in the frozen state, particularly in the tissue state. There is only a one-log drop in titer after storage at −18 C for 18 months.

TGE virus has the morphological characteristics of a typical coronavirus, varying in size between 75 and 120 m$\mu$. Most particles are located in the cytoplasmic vacuoles with some budding from intracytoplasmic membranes. Concentrated viral preparations examined by negative staining have spherical particles with indistinct clublike projections.

The virus apparently does not contain a hemagglutinin nor does it cause hemadsorption of bovine, porcine, guinea pig, or human erythrocytes (3, 22).

**Cultivation.** Lee (16) was able to grow the virus in porcine kidney cells but did not note any cytopathogenic effects. More recently, Harada *et al.* (12) described strains that had the ability to destroy cells in pig kidney-cell cultures. Likewise, porcine thyroid and salivary gland cultures support viral replication. Virus also is propagated in canine kidney-cell cultures. The CPE produced by field strains usually is transient or slight in early passages, consequently, the piglet probably is a more sensitive experimental subject for detecting field virus. The plaque technic is more sensitive, achieving titers of $10^6$ and $10^7$ PFU per ml of tissue-cultured virus, and reliable for the assay of TGE virus than the conventional fluid cell culture procedure (3, 18).

The interference phenomenon utilizing bovine viral diarrhea-mucosal disease virus (17) or pseudorabies virus (20) has been used to demonstrate non-cytopathogenic strains of TGE virus in monolayer cultures.

Eto *et al.* (9) have propagated TGE through 20 transfers in the amniotic cavity of embryonated hens' eggs.

In piglets, the highest titers of virus are achieved in the jejunum and duodenum, usually $10^6$ PID (pig infectious doses) per gram of infective material. Relatively high titers also are found in respiratory tissue and kidney early in the disease. The piglet is still commonly used for the cultivation of virus that is utilized for various purposes.

**Immunity.** There are many facts lacking about passive and active immunity to this disease. It is generally agreed that swine recovered from TGE usually are clinically protected when challenged with virulent test virus. However, immunity to reinfection or even to disease is probably not complete. It depends upon the challenge dose, and swine infected as piglets have a lesser degree of immunity than older animals.

It has been observed that pigs that are born several weeks after the subsidence of an outbreak frequently escape the disease, also that when sows that have lost their litter of pigs from the disease are bred back immediately the second litter escapes the disease. It appears that the immunity of such animals is passive, but the protection transmitted to piglets by immunized sows is not conferred by the absorption of globulin from the colostrum—rather it depends on a continuous supply of antibody in the milk from the dam (11). The mechanism of active immunity is less clear. Is local humoral antibody or cellular immunity responsible for protection? What is the nature of immunoglobulin if antibody plays a role in protection? Certainly, the mechanism of maternal immunity is unique and involves a new concept in protection of progeny.

Some large swine farms that have suffered heavily from the disease follow the practice of feeding stored, frozen intestines from infected animals to their bred sows about a month before the farrowing date. The sows suffer from a mild diarrhea but recover, and their litters acquire enough immunity from their dams to protect them from the disease.

Neutralization tests can be done in piglets and in cell culture. The test in piglets was used for some period of time before cytopathic strains were described with limited and varying results by various investigators. The piglet test is seldom used now. In cell-culture systems neutralization is determined in one of three ways: inhibition of CPE, plaque reduction, or stained monolayer test (25).

Sibinovic *et al.* (23) developed a bentonite agglutination test based upon the agglutination of TGE-treated bentonite particles by specific antibody. The test is complicated and of limited value in the diagnosis of TGE and does not correlate well with the neutralization test (2).

A ring-precipitation test has been described using concentrated TGE antigen and antiserum in small glass tubes (5). A fluorescent-antibody test (17) is used for detection of antigen in cell culture and in infected tissues of swine.

Inactivated TGE virus produces an immunity in sows which is inadequate to confer sufficient protection to their progeny through the colostrum. TGE virus strains that were attenuated through serial transfer in pig kidney-cell cultures (1, 22) gave similar results as suckling pigs from immunized sows were not adequately protected. Hopefully, research and development will ultimately produce vaccines that will confer protection to the piglets.

**Transmission.** The virus is present in all organs and fluids of the body as well as in the discharges. Because infection is readily produced by ingestion it seems certain that normal transmission is by contact, directly or indirectly, with the diarrheal discharges of the victims. Virus may persist in feces of recovered pigs for 10 weeks (16). The disease usually does not remain for long periods on farms unless there is a program of more or less continuous farrowing.

The disease usually occurs during the colder months of the year. This may be due to the fact that the virus is more stable in the frozen state and less subject to sunlight in the winter. In some instances the virus may be transferred by people from an infected premises to a clean area. Starlings may also be involved in its spread as starlings fed TGE virus have infective droppings for 32 hours postfeeding (21). Furthermore, these birds are observed in large numbers among swine in the midwest.

**Diagnosis.** The diagnosis of this disease is easier than many others. The main features in differentiation from other swine enteric disorders are as follows: (1) rapidity of spread through all age groups, (2) lack of response to antibiotics, and (3) high mortality only in very young piglets and rapid recovery of older stock. Additional differences that separate it from swine enteric diseases include its lack of skin lesions, nervous signs, abortions, and stillbirths.

Laboratory confirmation is accomplished by the use of virus isolation or by the demonstration of a rising titer of neutralizing antibodies. These procedures involve the use of tissue-culture and also of immunofluorescence tests in certain instances.

**Control.** Apparently little can be done to stop outbreaks after they begin. Treatment of infected pigs has little or no value, especially in piglets under 10 days of age. Fortunately, on farms with an interval of several months between spring and fall farrowing periods, the disease seldom carries over into the next period. When farrowings are frequent on a farm where TGE has occurred two procedures might be considered to reduce the losses of newborn pigs: (1) infect sows which will farrow in more than 2.5 weeks so they will be immune at farrowing and (2) susceptible sows should be isolated prior to and following farrowing in an area where they are least likely to be exposed to TGE virus.

**The Disease in Man.** There is no evidence indicating that the virus of TGE is pathogenic for man.

## REFERENCES

1. Bohl. Proc. World Vet. Cong., 1967, *18*, 577.
2. Bohl. In: Dunne. Diseases of swine. Iowa State Univ. Press, Ames, Iowa, 3d ed. 1970, pp. 158–176.
3. Bohl and Kumagai. Proc. U.S. Livestock Sanit. Assoc., 1965, *69*, 343.
4. Bradfute, Bohl, and Harada. Quoted by Bohl in ref. 2.
5. Caletti and Ristic. Jour. Am. Vet. Med. Assoc., 1968, *29*, 1603.
6. Cartwright, Harris, Blandford, Fincham, and Gitter. Jour. Comp. Path., 1965, *75*, 386.
7. Cross and Bohl. Jour. Am. Vet. Med. Assoc., 1969, *154*, 266.
8. Doyle and Hutchings. *Ibid.*, 1946, *108*, 257.
9. Eto, Ichihara, Tsunoda, and Watanabe. Jour. Jap. Vet. Med. Assoc., 1962, *15*, 16.
10. Goodwin and Jennings. Jour. Comp. Path. and Therap., 1959, *69*, 87 and 313.
11. Haelterman. 17th Internat. Vet. Cong. (Hanover), 1963, p. 615.
12. Harada, Kumagi, and Sasahara. Natl. Inst. Anim. Health, 1963, *3*, 166.
13. Hooper and Haelterman. Jour. Am. Vet. Med. Assoc., 1966, *194*, 1580.
14. Hutchings. Vet. Med., 1947, *42*, 297.
15. Lee. Ann. N.Y. Acad. Sci., 1956, *66*, 191.
16. Lee, Moro, and Baker. Am. Jour. Vet. Res., 1954, *15*, 364.
17. McClurkin. Canad. Jour. Comp. Med. and Vet. Sci., 1965, *29*, 46.
18. McClurkin and Norman. *Ibid.*, 1967, *31*, 299.
19. McClurkin, Stark, and Norman. *Ibid.*, 1970, *34*, 347.
20. Phel. Arch. f. Exp. Vet.-Med., 1966, *20*, 909.
21. Pilchard. Am. Jour. Vet. Res., 1965, *26*, 1177.
22. Sheffy. Proc. U.S. Livestock Sanit. Assoc., 1965, *69*, 351.
23. Sibinovic, Ristic, Sibinovic, and Alberts. Am. Jour. Vet. Res., 1966, *27*, 1339.
24. Thake. Am. Jour. Path., 1968, *53*, 149.
25. Witte and Easterday. Am. Jour. Vet. Res., 1968, *29*, 1409.
26. Young, Ketchell, Luedke, and Sautter. Jour. Am. Vet. Med. Assoc., 1955, *126*, 165.

## Hemagglutinating Encephalomyelitis Virus (HEV) of Pigs

In 1962 Greig *et al.* (2) described three natural outbreaks in Ontario, Canada, of encephalomyelitis in baby pigs. The affected animals were 4 to 7 days of age when signs of illness first appeared and death occurred usually within 3 days (4). The morbidity and mortality in infected litters approached 100 percent. The infection was characterized by depression, loss of condition, hyperesthesia, inco-ordination, and occasionally vomition. Concurrent illness in sows and older pigs characterized by inappetence, wasting, and vomition was seen in several instances, but its association with HEV infection was not proved. The exact incidence and distribution of the disease has not been determined. The HEV has been recovered from swine in England that showed vomiting and wasting disease. A similar virus also has been isolated in the United States.

The three strains of virus derived from the three original outbreaks were isolated in cultures of pig kidney cells from the feces and brains of infected piglets causing the formation of multinucleated giant cells. These strains and subsequent isolates appear identical except for one (HEV-18) which is probably a parainfluenza 3 virus (3). The six strains that have been examined by electron microscope consist of spherical bodies ranging from 100 to 130 m$\mu$ in diameter surrounded by a fringer of club-like surface projections 20 to 30 m$\mu$ long (3). Consequently HEV probably is a coronavirus but with no apparent antigenic relationship to transmissible gastroenteritis virus of pigs. The HEV virus causes hemagglutination of chicken erythrocytes with a more permanent attachment to the red blood cells (3). There is no evidence of neuraminidase and thus no spontaneous elution. Red cells treated with neuraminidase are agglutinated equally well as nontreated cells.

The HEV virus is quite heat-labile but reasonably stable at refrigerator and freezer temperatures and in the lyophilized state (1). Ether and chloroform remove its infectivity and hemagglutinating activity.

The disease was reproduced in baby pigs that received colostrum when administered infective material orally or by parenteral injection. In experimental studies unqualified success in the reproduction of clinical disease was only achieved with pigs 7 days of age or less. The signs of illness and histological lesions of encephalomyelitis were closely similar to those observed in natural cases (1). Pigs from natural or experimental studies developed hemagglutinating antibodies. Pigs with hemagglutinating antibodies are immune.

Preliminary immunological studies suggest that this virus is not immunologically related to Teschen disease, but histologically it is impossible to distinguish between HEV and Teschen disease (1).

## REFERENCES

1.  Greig and Girard.   Res. Vet. Sci., 1963, *4*, 511.
2.  Greig, Mitchell, Corner, Bannister, Meads, and Julian.   Canad. Jour. Comp. Med. and Vet. Sci., 1962, *62*, 49.
3.  Greig, Johnson, and Bouillant.   Res. Vet. Sci., In press, 1971.
4.  Mitchell.   *Ibid.*, 1963, *4*, 506.

# XLVI | The Family *Togaviridae* (Arboviruses)

At present two genera are included in this proposed family. They are *Alphavirus* and *Flavovirus*. The genus *Alphavirus* is a new designation for the arbovirus A group and the genus *Flavovirus* formerly was called the arbovirus B group. There are over 200 recognized arboviruses. Biologic and serological diversities characterize the arboviruses. As the arboviruses are better characterized more definitive genera can be devised. Most arboviruses replicate in an arthropod host as well as vertebrates.

Although Rift Valley fever is not included in either the genus *Alphavirus* or *Flavovirus* it seemed reasonable and logical to include the disease in this chapter as it is an arbovirus.

## THE GENUS *ALPHAVIRUS*

The type species for the genus is *Alphavirus sindbis*. Other members in the group are as follows: Aura virus, Chikungunya virus, Eastern equine encephalitis virus, Getah virus, Mayaro virus, Middelburgh virus, Mucambo virus, Ndumu virus, O'Nyong-nyong virus, Pixuna virus, Ross River virus, Semliki Forest virus, Una virus, Venezuelan equine encephalitis virus, Western equine encephalitis virus, Whataroa virus.

These viruses contain 4 to 6 percent of single-stranded RNA with a molecular weight of approximately 3 by $10^6$ daltons. They are spherical enveloped particles, with a diameter between 25 to 70 m$\mu$. They contain lipid and are sensitive to ether. The buoyant density in cesium chloride is 1.25 g per ml. Trypsin does not destroy the infectivity of the particle. Hemagglutination is not inhibited by phospholipids. The hemagglutination reaction occurs over a rather narrower range of temperature and pH than with group B viruses. The A group viruses are less inhibited by bile salts than B members. The virion replicates in the cytoplasm and maturation occurs by budding. All members of A group show cross-reactions in the hemagglutination-inhibition test but not with B group members. All A members replicate in arthropod vectors including the mosquito.

Three viruses in this genus are pertinent to a discussion of infectious diseases of domestic animals—eastern equine encephalomyelitis (EEE), western equine encephalomyelitis (WEE), and Venezuelan equine encephalomyelitis (VEE).

### Western and Eastern Equine Encephalomyelitis

It appears certain that an enzootic encephalomyelitis of horses of virus origin has occurred in the United States for many years. In the late summer and early fall of 1912 large numbers of horses were lost in Kansas, Nebraska, Colorado, Oklahoma, and Missouri from what was most certainly virus encephalitis, although it was not recognized as such at the time. The outbreak and the characteristic lesions were described by Udall (61). It is estimated that 35,000 horses died of the disease from midsummer until heavy frosts in October put an end to the outbreak. In later years small outbreaks of the malady have appeared in many of the western states.

In July 1930 the disease appeared among horses in the San Joaquin Valley in California. The outbreak continued through August, reached its peak in September, and disappeared with the advent of cool weather in November. It was studied by Meyer, Haring, and Howitt (43), who estimated that 3,000 horses and mules perished from this disease, this number being about one-half the total of recognized cases. These workers isolated and studied the virus of the disease. The following year the disease reoccurred in the same area and appeared for the first time in several of the neighboring states. The disease reappeared each successive summer, spreading over a larger and larger area. In 1937 the disease was recognized in every state west of the Mississippi River and in several east of it. The peak in the disease incidence occurred in 1938, when 184,000 horses were estimated by the United States Bureau of Animal Industry to have died from it. By this time every state lying west of the Appalachian Mountains had cases.

In 1933 an isolated focus of the disease appeared along the coastal plains of Delaware, Maryland, Virginia, and southern New Jersey, and at least 1,000 horses died of the disease in that year. The signs of illness of affected animals were much like those exhibited by horses in the western parts of the country, but the mortality rate was much higher, approximating 90 percent. It was generally believed at first that the disease was identical with that which prevailed in the country west of the Appalachian Mountains, but TenBroeck and Merrill (58) pointed out that the virus was immunologically different, because animals immunized to the virus of the eastern disease were not protected against the virus of the western disease, and vice versa. These results were quickly confirmed by others, and it was generally accepted that there were two types of the disease in the country, these being differentiated under the names of the *western type* and the *eastern type*. Both types produce encephalomyelitis in horses, the signs of illness and pathological changes being practically identical. The principal differences are that the eastern type is much more virulent for horses, most experimental animals, and man, and that there is little or no cross immunity between the two types.

The U.S. Department of Agriculture has collected statistics on the yearly occurrence of equine encephalomyelitis since 1935. It is recognized that these figures are not complete, nevertheless they give an indication of the importance of this disease in the United States. The latest figures are given in Table XXXV.

**Character of the Disease.** Although these viruses are named for the horse be-

Table XXXV. THE REPORTED ANNUAL MORBIDITY AND MORTALITY FOR INFECTIOUS EQUINE ENCEPHALO- MYELITIS FOR THE PERIOD 1935 THROUGH 1970*

| Year | Animals affected | Deaths |
|---|---|---|
| 1935 | 23,512 | — |
| 1936 | 3,929 | — |
| 1937 | 173,889 | — |
| 1938 | 184,662 | — |
| 1939 | 8,008 | 2,471 |
| 1940 | 16,941 | 4,187 |
| 1941 | 36,872 | 8,210 |
| 1942 | 4,939 | 1,334 |
| 1943 | 4,768 | 1,622 |
| 1944 | 19,590 | 4,779 |
| 1945 | 3,212 | 1,165 |
| 1946 | 2,805 | 957 |
| 1947 | 8,716 | 5,086 |
| 1948 | 1,796 | 635 |
| 1949 | 4,037 | 2,426 |
| 1950 | 1,023 | 417 |
| 1951 | 762 | 274 |
| 1952 | 2,226 | 898 |
| 1953 | 2,813 | 827 |
| 1954 | 1,075 | 357 |
| 1955 | 1,236 | 663 |
| 1956 | 1,284 | 493 |
| 1957 | 1,525 | 639 |
| 1958 | 2,054 | 494 |
| 1959 | 817 | 324 |
| 1960 | 813 | 252 |
| 1961 | 781 | 245 |
| 1962 | 734 | 141 |
| 1963 | 1,386 | 162 |
| 1964 | 3,950 | 392 |
| 1965 | 4,391 | 705 |
| 1966 | 2,123 | 291 |
| 1967 | 965 | 163 |
| 1968 | 1,617 | 317 |
| 1969 | 1,767 | 681 |
| 1970 | 1,211 | 321 |

* Compiled by the U.S. Department of Agriculture.

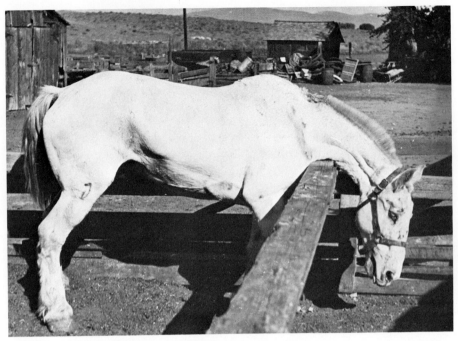

*Fig. 220.* Equine encephalomyelitis. (Courtesy Edward Records.)

cause it was first found in that species, it is evident that horses are not their natural reservoir. Because of the relatively low virus titers in the blood of affected horses, it is believed that horses are comparatively unimportant in the natural history of the disease. That these viruses might have their reservoir in birds was first suggested by TenBroeck, Hurst, and Traub (57) in 1935. The truth of this suggestion has been amply demonstrated by a series of workers in recent years. In 1938, during an outbreak in horses and man in Massachusetts, Tyzzer, Sellards, and Bennett (60) isolated the eastern-type virus from dead and dying wild pheasants in the infected area. In 1945 Hammon, Reeves, Benner, and Brookman (16), while studying a severe outbreak in the Yakima Valley in the state of Washington, discovered that from 30 to 50 percent of all chickens in the area possessed neutralizing antibodies for the western-type virus. There had been no sickness in these birds which could be attributed to the prevalence of this virus. Sooter, Howitt, and Corrie (52), in 1949, found neutralizing antibodies for the western-type virus in 11.6 percent of migratory birds trapped in Kansas, which at the time was epidemic-free. In Colorado, at a time when there was disease in horses, 25 percent of the migratory birds showed evidence of having been infected. In 1950 Kissling *et al.* (31) recovered eastern-type virus from an apparently healthy purple grackle which was shot in flight in Louisiana. Holden (19) recovered western-type virus in sparrows in New Jersey and at the same time demonstrated neutralizing antibodies in chickens in the same area. No cases of virus encephalitis were recognized in any species of mammals living in the area at that time. In fact the western-type virus has never been found in mammals in New Jersey.

It is obvious that many species of wild and domesticated birds may be asymptomatic carriers of this virus and thus serve as reservoirs. Not all birds escape the damaging effects of the virus. The Chinese pheasant raised in captivity is highly susceptible to damage by the eastern-type virus, and many outbreaks have been described in which the death rates have been as great as 25 percent (Beaudette, Black, Hudson, and Bivins, 4). A study of the pathogenicity of the eastern virus for various kinds of wild birds was made in Louisiana by Kissling, Chamberlain, Sikes, and Eidson (30). High-titer viremias were produced in all species. Purple grackles, ibises, and several species of egrets showed slight or no signs. Red-winged blackbirds, cardinals, cedar waxwings, and sparrows nearly always developed fatal infections. Other workers have shown that ordinary barnyard fowls and turkeys rarely show any signs, but these species later have high virus-neutralizing titers in their blood. WEE has been isolated from an opossum in the USA.

The virus of equine encephalomyelitis, western type, has caused outbreaks in horses and man in all states of the United States west of the Appalachian Mountians, and outbreaks have also been recognized in western Canada. The western-type virus was not recognized on the eastern seaboard until 1954, when it was isolated from sparrows in New Jersey by Holden (19) and later in Florida chukars. Late in 1955 the North Carolina State Board of Health reported the finding of virus of this type in a number of mosquitoes trapped in that state. Up to the present time no cases of the disease caused by the western-type virus have been recognized in either horses or man along the eastern seaboard.

Equine encephalomyelitis occurs in Argentina. According to Meyer, Wood, Haring, and Howitt (44), the Argentina virus is very closely related, or perhaps identical, to the western-type virus of North America.

In 1941 Randall and Eichhorn (45) recognized a small outbreak in the vicinity of Brownsville, Texas, as caused by eastern-type virus. More recently the eastern-type virus has been found in Michigan, Wisconsin, Missouri, and other midwestern states. Large and severe outbreaks have occurred in Louisiana.

An encephalomyelitis of horses occurs in Brazil. According to Carneiro and Cunha (7), the virus is closely related, if not identical, to the eastern type of North America. Livesay (35) and Mace, Ott, and Cortez (37) have reported the eastern-type virus in native Philippine monkeys (*Macacus philippensis*) suffering from a disease which resembled poliomyelitis. This disease has not been recognized in Philippine horses, but Mace and coworkers found neutralizing antibodies for eastern-type virus in 26 of a series of 86 horses.

In the United States and Canada this disease is distinctly seasonal. In all but the most southerly parts of the United States it occurs from June to November; in the warmer states sporadic cases may be seen during the winter months. As a rule, the disease is sporadic during the early summer, assumes epizootic proportions during August and September, and diminishes in intensity afterward. In most of the country all outbreaks cease by the middle of November, because the mosquito population has been killed by frosts.

Horses of all ages may succumb to the disease, but younger animals appear somewhat more susceptible than older ones. It is unusual for more than 20 percent of the horses on any one place to become affected, and considerable periods often elapse between cases on the same farm.

It is known from observations on experimental animals that a febrile reaction is the first manifestation of the infection. The depression that occurs at this time may be so mild as to be unnoticed. At this stage there is a viremia —an opportunity for bloodsucking insects to obtain virus. Invasion of the nervous system does not occur in all animals. If it does not occur, the animal is not observed to be ill but will possess neutralizing antibodies in its blood serum for some time thereafter. When involvement of the nervous system occurs, the signs are, in general, those of deranged consciousness. The fever has disappeared by this time and the blood is no longer infective. In the early stages of neural involvement, the victim may show signs of restlessness and mild excitement. The animal may walk in circles or crash through fences or walk aimlessly into obstacles of any kind. It may shy at low doorsills and jump high in clearing them. It refuses food and water. Later a sleepy attitude develops and it stands with head depressed, resting it on the manger or on a fence. It can be aroused, but it quickly relapses into the sleepy posture when not prodded into activity. It may sit on its hind quarters, or stand with its front legs crossed, or assume other unusual and unnatural postures. Finally evidence of paralysis of portions of the body may become evident: its lower lip often becomes pendulous, its tongue may be protruded, or it has difficulty in walking because of lack of full control of its hind legs. Finally the paralysis may become general: it lies on the ground and is unable to rise. Death usually occurs within a day or two after the nervous signs begin. The horses that recover frequently show permanent cerebral damage, manifested by loss of ability to react to normal stimuli. Such animals are often called *dummies* by horsemen.

The incubation period is from 1 to 3 weeks. In this respect the American forms of encephalomyelitis differ markedly from the German Borna disease, in which it is from 4 to 7 weeks or more.

The course of the disease varies widely. In some cases animals die within a few hours from the time that the first signs are noted. At the height of outbreaks most deaths occur within 2 to 4 days. Animals that survive the effects of the virus may develop terminal pneumonia and die from this after a week or more. Others may recover completely, or show various paralytic effects for many weeks, or permanently.

The eastern-type virus is considerably more virulent for horses than the western type. In the former the death rate generally exceeds 90 percent; in the latter it may be as high as 50 percent but averages from 20 to 30 percent.

There are no characteristic gross lesions in animals dying of this disease. Hurst (24), who studied the histology of the lesions in the central nervous system, says that the gray matter is affected to a greater extent than the white and that the lesions are most marked in the cerebral cortex, thalamus, and hypothalamic regions, with the brain stem and spinal cord as a rule being less involved. The lesions consist of degeneration of the nerve cells, perivascular cuffing with mononuclear and polymorphonuclear cells in varying proportion, polymorphonuclear leukocyte infiltrations into the gray matter, and proliferation of glial cells. The lesions produced by the western-type virus are, as a rule, less intense than those caused by the eastern type.

**The Disease in Experimental Animals.** Meyer, Haring, and Howitt (43) found that guinea pigs were highly susceptible to intracerebral inoculation with virus of equine origin, and these animals were the most suitable for diagnostic work. Death occurs in 4 to 6 days, as a rule, being preceded by an early febrile reaction followed by muscular tremors, flabbiness of the abdominal muscles, salivation, and trotting movements after the animal becomes prostrate. Rabbits are much less susceptible. A febrile reaction occurs and virus exists in the blood, but signs are very mild or absent, and recovery generally occurs. White mice are very susceptible. They may be infected by intracerebral inoculation and also through the undamaged nasal mucosa. According to Mediaris and Kebrick (39), suckling mice are even more susceptible to this virus than hens' eggs and constitute the most sensitive means of detecting virus. Calves can be infected by intracerebral inoculation. These animals display marked nervous signs beginning about the 5th day. By the 14th day recovery usually is complete, according to Giltner and Shahan (12). These authors found that sheep, dogs, and cats were refractory to inoculation. The common ground squirrel of the western states (*Citellus richardsoni*) may readily be infected by intracranial inoculation.

Karstad and Hanson (27) showed that swine were highly susceptible to infection with the virus of eastern encephalomyelitis, either naturally or by inoculation. No signs were exhibited by the infected animals but high antibody titers were quickly developed. Inasmuch as they were unable to demonstrate a viremia in swine, it was concluded that this species probably has little or nothing to do with the natural propagation of this virus.

The eastern-type virus generally produces fatal infections when inoculated into pheasants, quail, pigeons, blackbirds, cardinals, cedar waxwings, sparrows, juncos, thrushes, young chicks, ducklings, chukar partridges, and young turkey poults. Adult domesticated fowl, turkeys, and some wild birds are resistant to inoculation. Ordinarily these birds do not show recognizable signs, but high-titer viremias generally develop for a day or two and these are followed by high antibody titers.

**Properties of the Virus.** Eastern equine encephalomyelitis (EEE) virus is a spherical particle (56) with size estimates from 20 to 30 mμ by ultrafiltration. Its RNA central core is infectious. Its specific gravity is 1.13, and the particle is inactivated in 10 minutes at 60 C. The virus withstands freezing and thawing and is readily maintained at low temperatures. Ether and desoxycholate inactivate the agent. The virus disappears rapidly in tissues after death probably because of the acidity. The virus is readily destroyed by formalin but not phenol. A hemagglutinin has been demonstrated, and a hemolysin also exists. By the use of CF tests and with neutralization tests in mice by intracerebral inoculation and with plaque inhibition in tissue culture the virus is distinct from other arboviruses. In hemagglutination-inhibition tests some common antigenic components are demonstrated with other group A arboviruses. Some slight antigenic variations are demonstrated between strains of EEE virus coming from different areas. Interference, probably through the production of interferon, occurs between this virus and certain other arboviruses, myxoviruses, and picornaviruses.

Western equine encephalomyelitis (WEE) virus is essentially the same size as EEE and shares most of its physical-chemical characteristics. It has been estimated that 100 infectious particles are released from an infected cell, but only a few at a time. It is more closely related to Sindbis virus than other group A arboviruses as determined with the plaque inhibition test. In addition, this has been established by the use of the hemagglutination-inhibition test which also shows some crossing with other A arboviruses. This virus also produces interferon in appreciable amounts so that it is commonly used to study this nonspecific protein substance produced in tissue culture by many viruses.

**Cultivation.** In 1935 Higbie and Howitt (18) reported successful cultivation of both eastern and western types of equine encephalomyelitis virus in chick embryos. Minute amounts of brain virus placed on the chorioallantoic membrane resulted in deaths of the embryos in from 15 to 24 hours, the embryonic tissues being saturated with virus of a very high titer. The sensitivity of chick embryos to the virus of this disease is very great; less than 0.1 MLD for the guinea pig is frequently sufficient to infect. Both viruses produce a cytopathogenic effect in hamster kidney cell cultures (29). They also grow in cell cultures from many species. Plaques are produced on monolayers of chick embryo cells. A color test in tissue culture depending on a change of pH has been used as means of titration of WEE virus.

A method for the germ-free cultivation of the mosquitos *Aedes aegypti* and *Aedes trisbriatus* was developed so primary tissue cell cultures could be prepared from minced larvae of both insect species (26). The Louisiana strain of EEE grew in larval tissue cultures of both mosquitoes. There was some evidence of a virus-inactivating substance in the cultures of both mosquito species.

**Immunity.** Live virus vaccines were used experimentally for a time (Records and Vawter, 46). Traub and TenBroeck (59), for example, produced a vaccine with a virus strain that had been passed through many generations of pigeons until it had lost much of its virulence for horses. In 1934 Shahan and Giltner (49) opened the way for a safer vaccine when they showed that horses could be effectively immunized with brain virus that had been inactivated with formalin. The formalinized brain vaccine was used in the field for several years but with only partial success. A highly successful vaccine was introduced in 1938 by Beard, Finkelstein, Sealy, and Wyckoff (3). This is made from infected chick embryo tissues.

The *chick embryo vaccine* is made by inoculating the chorioallantoic membrane of developing embryos about 10 days old (incubation time) with virus. The virus multiplies very rapidly, reaching a high titer in about 15 hours, and the embryo usually dies from the virus reaction in from 15 to 24 hours. The vaccine is made by harvesting the virus-containing embryos, grinding them into a paste, suspending them in a saline buffer solution in a 10 percent concentration, and treating the suspension with 0.4 percent formalin. Undoubtedly the greater effectiveness of the chick embryo vaccine over the horse brain or guinea pig brain vaccines lies in the fact that the concentration of virus is very much greater. The virus content of the chick embryo is from 1,000 to 10,000 times as great as that of infected mammalian brains. The eastern-type virus regularly attains 3 by $10^9$ mouse infective units per gram, whereas the western type attains 3 by $10^8$ and sometimes 3 by $10^9$ units.

This vaccine is best administered intradermally, the usual dose being 1 ml for the monovalent vaccines and 2 ml for the bivalent (Schoening, Shahan, Osteen, and Giltner, 48). The latter is used only in those areas where either eastern- or western-type virus may be implicated. The dose should be repeated within a week or 10 days. The immunity induced is established in about 2 weeks from the time of the initial dose, is very solid, and lasts long enough to protect during the current epizootic season. Annual vaccination is practiced in those areas where the disease is expected. This is best done in early summer before the disease has appeared.

Before the intradermal method of administration was introduced, the vaccine was given subcutaneously in 10-ml doses. This gave good protection, but at times there were complications, which are seldom or never seen with the intradermal method. These were described by Shahan, Giltner, Davis, and Huffman (50). The nature of the malady, which was dubbed *X-disease of horses*, is not clear. It was characterized by icterus, constipation, and nervous signs and was highly fatal. Parenchymatous degeneration of the liver and kidneys was commonly found. No lesions were noted in the nervous system, and virus was never demonstrated in the tissues. The disease never developed immediately after vaccination but usually 30 days afterward or even later. It was thought to be some type of toxic reaction. Similar reactions were observed in South Africa following the administration of horse-sickness vaccines (Theiler's disease). Isolated cases have been observed after the injection of other biological products containing foreign proteins.

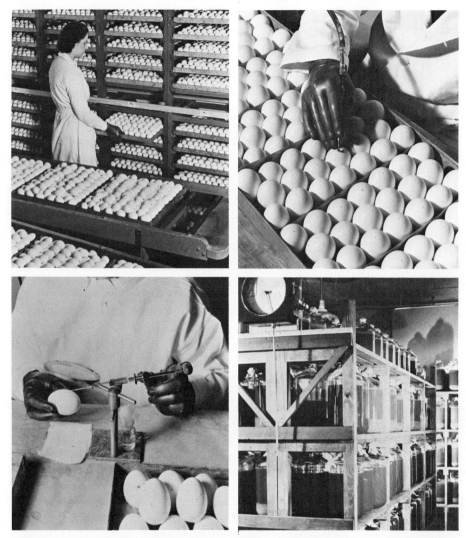

*Fig. 221.* Commercial manufacture of equine encephalomyelitis vaccine from egg-embryo-prop-agated virus. (*Upper left*) Trays of fertile hens' eggs in an incubating room. The eggs must be incubated until the embryos are about 10 days old. After inoculation they are incubated for an additional 24 hours, at which time most of the embryos have died from the effects of the virus. (*Upper right*) Making holes in the shells to permit inoculation. This is being done with a power-driven dental drill. (*Lower left*) Inoculating the embryo with virus. A small amount of virus is de-posited on the chorioallantoic membrane. From this point it quickly invades the embryo. (*Lower right*) The virus-containing embryos are ground to a paste, which is suspended in saline solu-tion. Formalin is added in 0.4 percent concentration, and the suspensions are placed in large bottles, which are kept in an incubator room until the virus has been inactivated. It is then packaged and stored in refrigerators until needed. (Courtesy Lederle Laboratories Division, American Cyanamid Co.)

At one time an encephalomyelitis antiserum was available, but apparently its manufacture has been discontinued by American biological supply companies. Large doses of such sera will protect horses for a short time against homologous viruses. After nervous signs have appeared, antisera have little or no value.

The tissue-cultured virus produces an immunity in guinea pigs as effective as the chick embryo propagated virus. Attenuation of WEE virus was achieved by selection and transfer of a clonal variant in a chick embryo culture system. Hughes and Johnson (23) reported an attenuated WEE virus vaccine that failed to produce any signs of illness in 367 horses and 1 donkey —69 were pregnant and there was no evidence of abortion or disease in the foals from these mares. Because maternal antibody may interfere with vaccine virus, foals vaccinated during first 8 months of life should be vaccinated again at 1 year of age.

An inactivated tissue-cultured origin vaccine for WEE and EEE was evaluated for safety and antigenicity in 17 pregnant mares and 16 foals (14). Two intradermal 1-ml doses of vaccine given 2 weeks apart caused no reaction. The HI antibody response to both viral antigens compared favorably with titers in horses recovered from acute disease. There was no significant difference in the antibody response of foals and adults to vaccine virus.

Foals of dams which have had an exposure to WEE are temporarily protected by colostral antibody. There is a suggestion that an active immunity is produced by inactivated virus despite the presence of colostral antibodies in the foal.

The immunity to both viruses persists for years after natural infection and after vaccination with modified (attenuated) virus.

**Transmission.** Vawter and Records (62) showed in 1933 that horses could be readily infected by intranasal instillation of virus, and transmission in this way probably occurs at times. The epizootiology of the disease indicates, however, that this cannot be the usual way. Transmission by bloodsucking insects, particularly by mosquitoes, had previously been suspected, but Kelser (28) was the first to show, in 1933, that mosquitoes could be infected and could convey the disease from animal to animal. In his work he used yellow-fever mosquitoes (*Aedes aegypti*), which, 6 to 8 days after they had been allowed to feed on infected guinea pigs, were capable of infecting other guinea pigs and a horse. This finding was confirmed by several workers. Merrill, Lacaillade, and TenBroeck (40) in the following year showed that the ordinary salt marsh mosquito (*Aedes sollicitans*) was capable of transmitting both the eastern and western types of virus. Another salt marsh mosquito (*Aedes cantator*) proved capable of transmitting the eastern-type virus but not the western. *Anopheles quadrimaculatus* and *Culex pipiens* were incapable of transmitting either type. Madsen and Knowlton (38) in 1935 showed that local species of *Aedes* mosquitoes in Utah, *Aedes dorsalis* and *A. nigromaculis*, were capable of transmitting the western-type virus. Others have shown that

*Aedes albopictus, A. taeniorynchus,* and *A. vexans* were able to transmit the western-type virus. Merrill and TenBroeck (41) proved that the virus multiplies in the affected *A. aegypti* by feeding starved individuals upon previously infected mosquitoes that had been ground into a paste. In this way they propagated the disease through ten lots of mosquitoes, in each of which it was estimated that there had been a dilution of at least 1 : 100. They concluded that the results could be explained only on the basis that the virus had increased in the insects.

In all of the mosquito experiments mentioned above, the insects were infected by being fed upon artificially infected animals or brain material. It was not until the summer of 1941 that naturally infected wild mosquitoes were detected. In that year Hammon, Reeves, Brookman, Izumi, and Gjullin (17) demonstrated the western-type virus in one lot of mosquitoes (*Culex tarsalis*) caught in the Yakima Valley in Washington during the course of an outbreak of the disease in horses. This species is widely distributed in the states west of the Mississippi River. It is known to feed upon man, horses, mules, cattle, and various birds.

A number of other species of mosquitoes have been found naturally infected with the western-type virus. Hammon, Reeves, Benner, and Brookman (16) found *Culiseta inornata* and *Culex pipiens,* besides *Culex tarsalis,* infected in the Yakima Valley, but *C. pipiens* proved incapable of transmitting the virus. The first isolation of eastern-type virus from naturally infected mosquitoes was reported by Howitt, Dodge, Bishop, and Gorrie (22) in 1949. The species was *Mansonia perturbans,* and the mosquitoes were captured in Georgia. During the previous year the same workers (21) reported the finding of naturally infected chicken mites (*Dermanyssus gallinae*) and chicken lice (*Menapon pallidum* and *Eomenacanthus stramineus*) taken in Tennesee. The virus was the eastern type. Neutralizing antibodies for this virus were found in one cow and a few chickens in the locality where the strain originated.

Although equine encephalomyelitis can be transmitted by a considerable number of species of mosquitoes, it has become obvious that the western type is transmitted to both birds and mammals principally by *Culex tarsalis,* and the principal vector of the eastern type to birds but not to mammals is the fresh-water swamp mosquito, *Culiseta melanura.* It is not yet clear whether there is a principal transmitter of the eastern-type virus from the bird reservoir to horses and man, but it cannot be *C. melanura,* since this species attacks only swamp-inhabiting birds (8).

In 1940 Kitselman and Grundmann (32) demonstrated the western-type virus in a large bloodsucking insect known as the *assassin bug* (*Triatoma sanguisuga*) captured in a pasture in Kansas. Since this insect is common in many parts of the west and is known to feed upon horses, it is possible that it sometimes plays a part in the transmission of the virus.

In 1944 Smith, Blattner, and Heys (51) and in the following year Sulkin (54) reported the recovery of western-type virus from the chicken mite (*Dermanyssus gallinae*). Since chicken mites will feed upon horses stabled near chicken houses, they may be of some importance in conveying the disease. Furthermore, it is possible that this virus may be harbored from one season to the next in this mite, as has been found to be true of the virus of St. Louis encephalitis.

Syverton and Berry (55) showed, in 1937, that the spotted fever tick, *Dermacentor andersoni*, could serve as a vector for the western type of equine encephalomyelitis virus. Adult and nymphal stages of this tick were allowed to feed on recently infected guinea pigs. At intervals varying from 32 to 80 days thereafter, successive stages in the developmental cycle of these ticks were allowed to feed on normal guinea pigs and ground squirrels. The disease was conveyed to these animals. Continuity of the virus through all stages, including the eggs, was demonstrated. At the time of the report virus had remained in these ticks for 130 days, a period sufficiently long to suggest that this might be one way by which the virus was preserved from one season to the next. The essential details of this work were confirmed by Gwatkin and Moore (15).

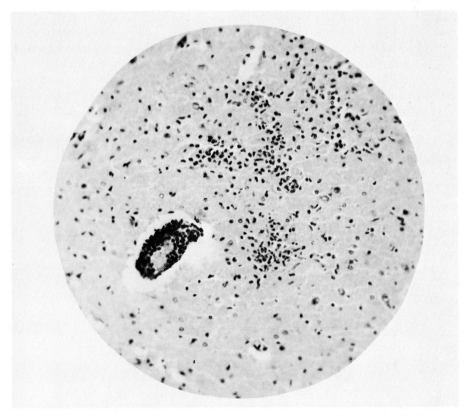

*Fig. 222.* Equine encephalomyelitis, showing brain of a guinea pig inoculated with the western-type virus. There are cellular infiltrations of both gray and white matter and perivascular cuffing. X 200. (Courtesy S. H. McNutt.)

Through the work of many it is clear that this disease is transmitted primarily by mosquitoes of various kinds. Transmission by direct contact and by other arthropods undoubtedly occurs, but this is of slight importance in the total picture. There is experimental proof that the disease may be transmitted from infected horses to others by mosquitoes, but many workers believe that the virus reservoir in horses is much less important than that in various wild and domesticated birds. The known presence of virus in hibernating *Culex tarsalis* in all months except December and the experimental over-wintering of virus in garter snakes appears to be important in setting the stage for epidemics in horses and man. Moreover, the transmission of WEE to snakes by infected *Culex tarsalis* takes place quite readily (11).

**Diagnosis.** Although the clinical signs are characteristic, they are not always diagnostic, especially in isolated cases. Several cases thought to be equine encephalomyelitis have turned out to be dumb rabies.

For a specific diagnosis, the virus must be isolated. This is best done by intracerebral injection of animals, preferably guinea pigs, or of embryonated eggs. Fresh brain material should be used for this purpose. The virus is not always isolated, even when other indications make it clear that virus encephalitis is present, for virus often disappears from the tissues very quickly after death. For laboratory confirmation it is best to destroy the animal when it is obvious that it is not going to survive, rather than to let it die naturally. The brain should be removed promptly, cooled quickly, and delivered to the laboratory as soon as possible.

If the virus is isolated, it often becomes desirable to determine whether it is of the eastern or western type. This is most readily accomplished by inoculating several guinea pigs that have been previously immunized with eastern-type vaccine and several more that have received vaccine of the western type. Since there is relatively little cross immunization between these virus types, the homologous animals should survive and the heterologous die. Another approach is to incubate the unknown virus in antisera specific for each viral type and inject the mixtures into a susceptible laboratory animal or a susceptible tissue culture system to establish which of the two specific antisera cause virus neutralization.

The microscopic lesions in the brain are characteristic of virus encephalitis. In diagnostic work it is well to fix material for sectioning, in case virus isolation fails. The histological changes never prove the precise type of virus involved, but the findings can be strongly indicative of this disease.

Meyer, Haring, and Howitt (43) were unable to find inclusion bodies in this disease and made a point of this fact in differentiating it from the Borna disease of Germany. During the Kansas horse plague of 1912 a number of workers, including Joest, sought unsuccessfully to demonstrate inclusion bodies similar to the Joest bodies of Borna disease. Hurst (24), on the other hand, has described acidophilic intranuclear bodies in some of the degenerated neurons.

**Control.** So far as horses are concerned, annual vaccination with inactivated virus vaccine is highly satisfactory. Because the transmitting agents are a number of species of mosquitoes, antimosquito measures undoubtedly help to reduce the incidence of the disease.

**The Disease in Man.** In 1932 Meyer (42) reported three cases of encephalitis in persons who had associated with horses suffering from the western type of encephalomyelitis. One proved fatal. Virus was not isolated from any of these cases. The author suggested that these might have been human infections with the virus of the horse disease and advised workers to be on the lookout for such cases. The first human cases proved to be caused by the equine encephalomyelitis virus were described by Fothergill, Dingle, Farber, and Connerley (10) in the late summer of 1938. Shortly afterward others were reported by Wesselhoeft, Smith, and Branch (64). These cases occurred in eastern Massachusetts during the height of the outbreak in horses. At least 40 human cases occurred, and the nature of the virus was established in nine cases. Webster and Wright (63) proved by neutralization tests on laboratory animals that the virus was of the eastern type, and Schoening, Giltner, and Shahan (47) showed that the human virus would kill unprotected horses as well as one immunized to the western-type virus but was innocuous to horses immunized against the eastern-type virus. The persons affected were mostly children. There were no multiple cases in families, and none had had any contact with horses. The season had been very wet, however, and mosquitoes were common.

The onset of EEE was sudden and was characterized by high fever, convulsions, vomiting, and drowsiness, which rapidly progressed to a comatose condition. Nearly all patients died. The high death rate distinguishes this illness from other forms of virus encephalitis in man which ordinarily have a much lower mortality rate.

In 1938 Howitt (20) reported the first proved case of equine encephalomyelitis virus infection in man caused by WEE virus. This was in a 20-month-old infant who died after an illness of 5 days. In 1941 the most extensive outbreak of human encephalitis ever recorded was reported by Leake (34) in the north-central part of the United States. Nearly 3,000 human cases were recognized. In general, the cases were mild; however 195 deaths occurred. During the same period Jackson (25) reported numerous human cases in the Province of Manitoba, Canada, which lies just north of the epidemic area in the United States. Most of these were in infants under 1 year of age and in old persons. Cox, Jellison, and Hughes (9) isolated the western type of equine encephalomyelitis virus from eight fatal cases and virus neutralizations with sera of recovered cases leave no doubt that the equine virus was the cause of the outbreak. The disease in horses at the time of the human outbreak was not nearly so prevalent as it had been in several preceding years when human cases were not recognized. It was a rather damp summer, however, and mosquitoes were unusually numerous. An interesting feature of this outbreak was that cases were more than twice as numerous among males as in females, which means, presumably, that men working in the harvest fields were more exposed to mosquitoes than were women.

Following the demonstration that an effective vaccine could be made for protecting horses from the virus propagated in developing chick embryos, a number of laboratories began manufacturing the vaccine in 1939. Very soon several fatal human infections occurred in these laboratories. The manufactures then began to immunize their workers with a somewhat refined vaccine of the type used on horses (Beard, Beard, and Finkelstein, 2). This has proved effective and has not caused unusual discomfort or resulted in undesirable sequelae. The vaccine is recommended for persons unusually exposed to danger of infection. Laboratory workers who are exposed to both western and eastern types of virus should use a mixture of both types of vaccine.

In the epidemic area in Manitoba in the summer of 1941, Jackson (25) reported the vaccination of more than 3,000 adult humans with the chick embryo vaccine. There were no untoward results, although more than one-half suffered from mild vaccine reactions.

### Venezuelan Equine Encephalomyelitis

A virus encephalomyelitis of horses occurs in Venezuela. It is a member of the genus *Alphavirus*. Beck and Wyckoff (5) studied the virus and compared it with the North American types. They found it considerably more virulent for guinea pigs and chick embryos than either the eastern or western types of North America. A vaccine made of formalinized tissue of the Venezuelan virus protected against the homologous virus but not against the North American types. Animals immunized to the North American types succumbed to the Venezuelan virus, but those immunized with the eastern-type virus showed evidence of partial protection.

In 1943 an explosive outbreak of equine encephalomyelitis appeared on the island of Trinidad, which lies off the coast of Venezuela. Gilyard (13) isolated the virus, which proved to be of the Venezuelan type, and vaccine made from this type of virus brought the outbreak under control. The virus was obtained from a local mosquito, *Mansonia titillans*, but other types were not excluded as vectors. A seaman of the United States Navy stationed on the island died of encephalitis about 6 weeks before the animal outbreak. The Venezuelan type of virus was isolated from his brain. This is the first reported case of human infection with virus of this type. Later experiences showed that this type of virus is very highly infectious for man.

In 1962–64 there was a severe epidemic by VEE subtype 1 B in Venezuela and Colombia causing innumerable cases in horses and 30,000 cases in humans with 300 deaths. In 1960–64 VEE antibodies were found in Seminole Indians of Florida and virus later was isolated from rodents, mosquitoes, and three human cases. This strain causes a mild disease in horses but it produces an immunity.

In 1968 the VEE subtype 1 B appeared in Central America where it spread rapidly and caused severe disease in horses and man. This subtype then appeared in Mexico in 1970 and by midsummer of 1971 was diagnosed in Texas horses and in human patients residing in that state. The disease moved northward into the United States despite an effort to control the disease in Central America and Mexico by the use of a modified VEE vaccine (developed for man) in horses, and the use of a spraying program. In certain localities these efforts were begun too late or with logistical problems that decreased the effectiveness of the planned control procedures. The disease moved very fast and it was essential to move well ahead of the disease front and vaccinate most, if not all of the horses, and also spray with effective insecticides to control the mosquito population. Obviously, the introduction of this disease into the United States caused considerable havoc in the horse population, and marked concern on the part of public health authorities. With its multiple-host distribution among mammals, reptiles, and insects, the elimination of this disease from a given area is extremely difficult. Consequently, the disease usually must be controlled by vaccination and by mosquito control.

**Character of the Disease.** The signs of illness in horses are similar to WEE and EEE. The fever is accompanied by a viremia for approximately 5 days. Marked diarrhea and nuerological manifestations usually occur on the 5th or 6th day and fatal cases usually die 1 or 2 days later. Not all fatal cases show nervous manifestations. Survivors have detectable antibodies within the first 2 weeks after the onset of illness.

The gross and microscopic lesions are typical of a viral encephalitis with no distinguishing features that separate it from WEE, EEE, and most other encephalitides.

**Properties and Cultivation of the Virus.** In general, properties of the VEE virus are similar to WEE and EEE viruses. There is evidence that VEE virus is not inactivated by the same treatment with formalin as EEE and WEE viruses (33, 65). In each situation safety tests indicated there was no residual VEE virus, but the use of the inactivated vaccine resulted in clinical disease. This problem lead to the development of an attenuated virus vaccine for man.

VEE virus has essentially the same mammalian host range and tissue-culture cell range as WEE and EEE viruses, so comparable methods are used for its cultivation and assay.

**Immunity.** VEE virus produces a solid and long-lasting immunity.

An attenuated viral vaccine produced by U.S. Army scientists (6, 36) for use in man was used to control the 1969 Central America epizootic (53). Vaccination of the horse population at the periphery of the epizootic was performed to create an artificial barrier to limit the spread of VEE. Vaccination of horses was also practiced within the epizootic area. Within 7 to 10 days after vaccination, even on ranches where the disease was rampant, all equine cases subsided. Complete protection occurred in areas where horses were vaccinated and also prevented the spread of VEE into Guatemala by an immune

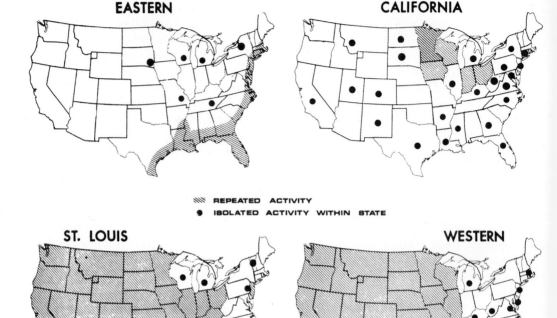

Fig. 223. Encephalitis in the United States. (Courtesy R. Chamberlain, CDC, USPHS.)

barrier of vaccinated horses, 50 kilometers wide, established on the Pacific Coastal Plain. In 1970 this virulent strain somehow breached the immune barrier and became established in Costa Rica, then Mexico, and reaching the USA in 1971; yet no epizootic occurred in 1970 or 1971 in either Guatemala or Nicaragua, evidence which strongly supports the view that the attenuated virus vaccine gives a lasting protection against the disease. Vaccination of pregnant mares may have undersirable effects on the developing fetus.

There is no evidence that vaccination against EEE or WEE provides protection against VEE. Previous claims that the combination of EEE and WEE vaccines, or multiple doses, will provide protection probably are not correct, so it is advisable to use a VEE vaccine to protect horses and man against this specific virus.

**Transmission.** The culicine mosquitoes *Aedes taeniorhynchus* and *Masonia titillans,* and Tabanid flies, are known field vectors of VEE, and there may be others. Experimental horse transmission of VEE with *Aedes triseriatus* has been accomplished. *Masonia indubitans, Masonia perturbans,* and *Psorophora ferox* are susceptible to laboratory infection with VEE virus. The genus *Aedes* is very abundant in the United States; *M. perturbans* and *P. ferox* are common in southeastern United States; and *M. indubitans* and *M. titillans* occur in Florida. Tabanid flies are found throughout the United States.

Many birds are susceptible to VEE, including migratory birds. Birds generally have lower virus levels than certain mammals (such as rodents) which suggests that the natural cycle more likely occurs in mammals and insects than birds.

Direct-contact transmission occurs between horses, presumably by the respiratory route. VEE virus is found in mouth, nasal, and eye excretions and in milk and urine of infected horses.

The disease coincides with mosquito activity so it is a seasonal disease in colder climates.

**Diagnosis.** The disease is identifiable as one of the viral encephalitides by the typical neurologic signs in horses; however, fatal cases can occur without neurologic signs.

A specific diagnosis can be made only by laboratory procedure, either by the isolation of the virus from central nervous tissue, blood, or nasopharyngeal washings or by the demonstration of a rising serum-neutralization or complement-fixing antibody titer. Serological confirmation is difficult or impossible to achieve since animals often die before a convalescent serum can be obtained. Because the virus is hazardous to humans, few laboratories are willing to attempt viral isolation unless special facilities and vaccinated personnel are available.

Certain other diseases can be confused with VEE. Toxic encephalitis causes similar nervous manifestations but occurs commonly in the fall and winter as the result of eating moldy corn or fodder. Purpura head swellings are similar in appearance, but VEE fails to cause respiratory distress or hemorrhages common to purpura. Rabies may be confused with VEE but the history often aids in differentiating the two diseases. African horsesickness (AFS) virus produces head swellings and it is very difficult to differentiate from the encephalitides, including VEE, because AFS has many immunologic types. Mineral poisoning and botulism can be differentiated from VEE chiefly by their non-seasonal nature and history.

**Control.** Vector control should be given first consideration but to be effective it must be complete. If vaccination of horses is permitted then it should be a part of the control program.

Suspected cases should be immediately reported to the proper control agencies so early typing of the virus as well as immediate quarantine can be instigated. Isolate acutely ill animals in separate stalls that are mosquito-proof, if possible.

**The Disease in Man.** Naturally-occurring epidemics of VEE in man have been reported in Columbia, Panama, Venezuela, Mexico, and the State of Texas in the United States. Serological evidence indicates that the infection has occurred in Brazil and in the State of Florida.

Numerous infections in laboratory workers attests to the marked susceptibility of man to this agent. Further evidence is the production of disease in man with inactivated virus vaccines which pass the safety tests in animals. The isolation of VEE virus from the upper respiratory tract of an infected laboratory worker has important epidemiological implications. There is strong field evidence that the disease can be transmitted from man to man.

## REFERENCES

1. Bauer, Cox, and Olitsky. Proc. Soc. Exp. Biol. and Med., 1935, 33, 3.
2. Beard, Beard, and Finkelstein. Science, 1938, 88, 530.
3. Beard, Finkelstein, Sealy, and Wyckoff. Ibid., 87, 2265.
4. Beaudette, Black, Hudson, and Bivins. Jour. Am. Vet. Med. Assoc., 1952, 121, 478.
5. Beck and Wyckoff. Science, 1938, 88, 530.
6. Berge, Banks and Tigertt. Am. Jour. Hyg., 1961, 73, 209.
7. Carneiro and Cunha. Arch. Inst. Biol., São Paulo, 1943, 14, 157.
8. Chamberlain. Ann. New York Acad. Sci., 1958, 70, 312.
9. Cox, Jellison, and Hughes. Pub. Health Rpts. (U.S.), 1941, 56, 1905.
10. Fothergill, Dingle, Farber, and Connerley. New Eng. Jour. Med., 1938, 219, 411.
11. Gebhardt, Stanton and St. Jeor. Proc. Soc. Exp. Biol. and Med., 1966, 123, 233.
12. Giltner and Shahan. Science, 1933, 78, 63.
13. Gilyard. Bul. U.S. Army Med. Dept., 1944, 75, 96.
14. Gutekunst, Martin and Langer. Vet. Med., 1966, 61, 348.
15. Gwatkin and Moore. Canad. Jour. Comp. Med. and Vet. Sci., 1940, 4, 78.
16. Hammon, Reeves, Benner, and Brookman. Jour. Am. Med. Assoc., 1945, 128, 1133.
17. Hammon, Reeves, Brookman, Izumi, and Gjullin. Science, 1941, 84, 328.
18. Higbie and Howitt. Jour. Bact., 1935, 29, 399.
19. Holden. Proc. Soc. Exp. Biol. and Med., 1955, 88, 490.
20. Howitt. Science, 1938, 88, 455.
21. Howitt, Dodge, Bishop, and Gorrie. Proc. Soc. Exp. Biol. and Med., 1948, 68, 622.
22. Howitt, Dodge, Bishop, and Gorrie. Science, 1949, 110, 141.
23. Hughes and Johnson. Jour. Am. Vet. Med. Assoc., 1967, 150, 167.
24. Hurst. Jour. Exp. Med., 1934, 59, 529.
25. Jackson. Am. Jour. Pub. Health, 1943, 33, 833.
26. Johnson. Am. Jour. Trop. Med. and Hyg., 1969, 18, 103.
27. Karstad and Hanson. Jour. Inf. Dis., 1959, 105, 293.
28. Kelser. Jour. Am. Vet. Med. Assoc., 1933, 82, 767.
29. Kissling. Proc. Soc. Exp. Biol. and Med., 1957, 96, 290.
30. Kissling, Chamberlain, Sikes, and Eidson. Am. Jour. Hyg., 1954, 60, 251.
31. Kissling, Rubin, Chamberlain, and Eidson. Proc. Soc. Exp. Biol. and Med., 1951, 77, 398.

32. Kitselman and Grundman. Kan. Agr. Exp. Sta. Tech. Bul. 50, 1940.
33. Kubes. Science, 1944, 99, 41.
34. Leake. Pub. Health Rpts. (U.S.), 1941, 56, 1902.
35. Livesay. Jour. Inf. Dis., 1949, 84, 306.
36. McKinney, Berge, Sawyer, Tigertt, and Crozier. Am. Jour. Trop. Med. and Hyg., 1963, 12, 597.
37. Mace, Ott, and Cortez. Bul. U.S. Army Dept., 1949, 9, 504.
38. Madsen and Knowlton. Jour. Am. Vet. Med. Assoc., 1935, 86, 662.
39. Mediaris and Kebrick. Proc. Soc. Exp. Biol. and Med., 1958, 97, 152.
40. Merrill, Lacaillade, and TenBroeck. Science, 1934, 80, 251.
41. Merrill and TenBroeck. Jour. Exp. Med., 1935, 62, 687.
42. Meyer. Ann. Int. Med., 1932, 6, 645.
43. Meyer, Haring, and Howitt. Science, 1931, 74, 227.
44. Meyer, Wood, Haring, and Howitt. Proc. Soc. Exp. Biol. and Med., 1934, 32, 56.
45. Randall and Eichhorn. Science, 1941, 93, 595.
46. Records and Vawter. Jour. Am. Vet. Med. Assoc., 1934, 84, 784.
47. Schoening, Giltner, and Shahan. Science, 1938, 88, 409.
48. Shoening, Shahan, Osteen and Giltner. Vet. Med., 1940, 35, 377.
49. Shahan and Giltner. Jour. Am. Vet. Med. Assoc., 1934, 84, 928.
50. Shahan, Giltner, Davis, and Huffman. Vet. Med., 1939, 34, 354.
51. Smith, Blattner, and Heys. Science, 1944, 100, 362.
52. Sooter, Howitt, and Corrie. Proc. Soc. Exp. Biol. and Med., 1952, 79, 507.
53. Spertzel. US Anim. Health Assoc., Proc. 74th Ann. Mtg., 1970, p. 18.
54. Sulkin. *Ibid.*, 1945, 101, 381.
55. Syverton and Berry. Jour. Bact., 1937, 33, 60.
56. Taylor, Sharp, Beard, and Beard. Proc. Soc. Exp. Biol. and Med., 1942, 51, 332.
57. TenBroeck, Hurst, and Traub. Jour. Exp. Med., 1935, 62, 677.
58. TenBroeck and Merrill. Proc. Soc. Exp. Biol. and Med., 1933, 31, 217.
59. Traub and TenBroeck. Science, 1935, 81, 572.
60. Tyzzer, Sellards, and Bennett. *Ibid.*, 1938, 88, 505.
61. Udall. Cornell Vet., 1913–14, 3, 17.
62. Vawter and Records. Science, 1933, 78, 41.
63. Webster and Wright. *Ibid.*, 1938, 88, 305.
64. Wesselhoeft, Smith, and Branch. Jour. Am. Med. Assoc., 1938, 111, 1735.
65. Young and Johnson. Am. Jour. Epidemiol., 1969, 89, 286.

## THE GENUS *FLAVOVIRUS*

In this genus there are a number of arthropod-borne viral encephalitides of man in which domestic animals are involved. The viral encephalitides included in this section include St. Louis encephalitis, Japanese B encephalitis, California encephalitis, Louping-ill of sheep, Central European tick-borne fever, Murray Valley encephalitis, Wesselsbron disease, Israel turkey meningoencephalitis, and Nairobi disease of sheep.

The type species for the genus is *Flavovirus febricis*, otherwise known as yellow fever virus. A typical member of the group contains approximately 7 to 8 percent of single-stranded RNA. Its molecular weight is 3 by $10^6$ daltons. Spherical enveloped particles, 20 to 50 m$\mu$, have a buoyant density in cesium chloride of 1.25 g per ml. The particles contain lipid and are sensitive to ether and trypsin. The particles contain a hemagglutinin. The virions multiply in the cytoplasm and mature by budding. Not all viruses in this genus are proved to replicate in arthropods but all are serologically related.

### St. Louis Encephalitis

This is a warm-weather disease which occurs sporadically in the central and western parts of the United States. It was first identified as the cause of a rather large outbreak in and around St. Louis, Missouri, in the summer of 1933, hence its name. It occurs in the late summer and early fall. A number of species of mosquitoes, including many of those that transmit western equine encephalomyelitis, are known to be transmitting agents, and it is believed that they ordinarily convey the disease to man. Hammon and Reeves (5) isolated this virus from eight pools of *Culex tarsalis* captured in the Yakima Valley in 1941, 1942, and 1944, and from other species elsewhere. It is a member of the B group of arboviruses. They found that chickens were easily infected with this virus, a viremia of 2 to 3 days' duration being induced. The infected birds showed no clinical signs. Neutralizing antibodies were found in large numbers of chickens in areas where the disease was occurring in man. Smith, Blattner, Heys, and Miller (13) showed that certain mosquitoes could easily be infected by being fed on virus-containing materials and that such insects could transmit the infection to chickens and hamsters for periods of several weeks thereafter, a viremia but no encephalitis being produced. They also demonstrated that the chicken mite (*Dermanyssus gallinae*) could be infected with the virus and that this could be transmitted through the eggs from generation to generation. Infection in these mites could continue indefinitely. It was suggested that this may be the way the virus is maintained from one season to the next.

In an epidemiological study of the 1962 epidemic of St Louis encephalitis in Florida involving four counties, 222 laboratory-confirmed cases occurred in humans with 43 deaths (1). The virus was recovered from four human beings and from 42 mosquito pools of which 40 were *Culex nigripalpus*. All fatal cases occurred in persons over 45 years of age and death rate was unusually high in persons 65 years of age and over. Widespread viral activity in nature was demonstrated by mosquito collections and serologic findings in wild or domestic birds in these four counties.

Whenever this disease appears in man, neutralizing antibodies may be found in horses and some other mammals. Hammon, Carle, and Izumi (4) inoculated horses with virus freshly isolated from mosquitoes. No signs were produced but viremias occurred in some of the animals and high antibody titers in all. There is no evidence that horses ever suffer from a clinically recognizable disease as a result of infection with this agent or that they play any significant role in the propagation of the human outbreaks. The virus was isolated from the brain of a California gray fox, *Urocyon cimereoargenteus* (2). It was also isolated from the Mexican free-tailed bat, *Tadarida b. mexicana*, during an outbreak in Texas in 1964 (14).

## Japanese B Encephalitis

This is a virus-induced encephalitis which occurs in man in Japan, Korea, Manchuria, Malaya, China, Indo-China, and Sumatra; it has been classified as a member of the B group of arboviruses. It is probable that a disease called Australian X-disease is identical with it. Large outbreaks with high mortality rates have occurred from time to time. A milder form evidently exists since large numbers of people in the Orient carry neutralizing antibodies for this virus. It is reported, for example, that more than 90 percent of all Koreans exhibit antibodies. The attention of western workers was called to this infection when American military personnel went into the infected regions during the recent war. The disease was found in Guam in 1948.

The disease is mosquito-borne. Hammon, Tigertt, Sather, and Schenker (9) confirmed earlier Japanese findings that *Culex tritaeniorhynchus* and a local variety of *Culex pipiens* were capable of transmitting the virus, and they captured virus-carrying mosquitoes of the first species in the wild in areas where the disease was endemic. In Japan and neighboring regions the disease occurs only during the summer months. In Guam and other tropical regions the disease may occur the year round.

Hodes, Thomas, and Peck (10), Sabin (12), and Hammon (3), working at different times on the island of Okinawa, showed that most of the horses, pigs, and cattle carried neutralizing antibodies. They all agreed that chickens rarely had such antibodies; apparently these birds do not play the same role that they have in the dissemination of the western equine encephalomyelitis and the St. Louis viruses. Hammon, Reeves, and Sather (6) found that certain wild birds (finches and red-wing blackbirds) circulated more virus following inoculation than did chickens and thus conclude that some wild birds have at least a potential importance in the propagation of this disease.

The various surveys in the endemic areas showing the high incidence of horses, cattle, and swine with high antibody titers indicate that the infection must occur frequently in a mild form. There is evidence, however, that this virus may produce fatal disease in all of these species. Patterson *et al.* (11) describe deaths of a number of race horses in Malaya, and Japanese authors have described fatal cases in cattle and swine. By intracerbral inoculation all of these species show fatal susceptibility.

## California Encephalitis

In 1952 Hammon, Reeves, and Sather (7) isolated a new virus from mosquitoes (*Aedes dorsalis* and *Culex tarsalis*) in Kern County, California. Encephalitis, sometimes fatal, developed in mice, cotton rats, and hamsters following inoculation, especially when the inoculum was introduced intracerebrally. The signs and lesions in the experimental animals were indistinguishable from those induced by the equine encephalomyelitis and St. Louis viruses. Guinea pigs, rabbits, ground squirrels, a calf, and a monkey gave serological responses to the injection of the virus, but these animals exhibited no signs. Squirrel and rabbit reactions were of particular interest since both developed viremias which could infect mosquito vectors. Chickens proved to be wholly refractory.

Both species of mosquitoes which had been found to harbor this virus in nature could readily be infected by feeding, and they maintained the virus for at least 7 or 8 days. In one instance it was established that the artificially infected *Aedes dorsalis* could transmit the infection to a rabbit. More recently a virus of this group was isolated from the mosquito, *Culex inornata*.

A case of nonfatal encephalitis in man was suspected to have been caused by this virus, since neutralizing antibodies were demonstrated after recovery. The authors believed that the evidence at hand indicated that this virus has a natural reservoir in wild and perhaps also in domestic mammals, the infection being propagated by mosquitoes. Cross-neutralization tests indicated a close relationship with a virus that caused an outbreak of human encephalitis in Barnes County, North Dakota, in the summer of 1949. This outbreak was described by Wenner, Kamitsuka, Cockburn, Krammer, and Price (15).

Other viral isolates have been made which are closely related to the original California isolate. In addition to the five previously recognized viruses in the group, two of which were from the United States, there now appear to be at least seven antigenic types in the United States (8). A member of this group has been isolated from a pool of 23 *Aedes cenerus* mosquitoes in New York State that was antigenically different from the prototype BFS-283 strain for the group (16).

## REFERENCES

1. Bond, Quick, Witte, and Oard. Am. Jour. Epidemiol., 1965, *81*, 392.
2. Emmons and Lennette. Proc. Soc. Exp. Biol. and Med., 1967, *125*, 443.
3. Hammon. Proc. 4th Internat. Cong. Trop. Dis. and Malaria, 1948, p. 568.
4. Hammon, Carle, and Izumi. Proc. Soc. Exp. Biol. and Med., 1942, *49*, 335.
5. Hammon and Reeves. Am. Jour. Pub. Health, 1945, *35*, 994.
6. Hammon, Reeves, and Sather. Am. Jour. Hyg., 1951, *53*, 249.
7. Hammon, Reeves, and Sather. Jour. Immunol., 1952, *49*, 493 and 511.
8. Hammon and Sather. Am. Jour. Trop. Med. and Hyg., 1966, *15*, 199.
9. Hammon, Tigertt, Sather, and Schenker. Am. Jour. Hyg., 1949, *50*, 51.
10. Hodes, Thomas, and Peck. Science, 1946, *103*, 357.
11. Patterson, Ley, Wisseman, Pond, Smadel, Diercks, Hetherington, Sneath, Witherington, and Lancaster. Am. Jour. Hyg., 1952, *56*, 320.
12. Sabin. Jour. Am. Med. Assoc., 1947, *133*, 281.
13. Smith, Blattner, Heys, and Miller. Jour. Exp. Med., 1948, 87, 119.
14. Sulkin, Sims, and Allen. Science, 1966, *152*, 223.

15.  Wenner, Kamitsuka, Cockburn, Krammer, and Price.  Pub. Health Rpts. (U.S.), 1951, *66*, 1075.
16.  Whitney, Jamnback, Means, Roz, and Rayner.  Am. Jour. Trop. Med. and Hyg., 1969, *18*, 123.

## Louping-III

SYNONYM:   Infectious encephalomyelitis of sheep

Louping-ill has occurred in the highland sheep of Scotland and the northern part of England for more than a century. It also exists in Ireland. Only recently has it been tentatively identified with a disease of man occurring in Czechoslovakia and Russia known as spring-summer encephalitis. It is not known to occur in the Western Hemisphere. The disease receives its name from the peculiar leaping gait of the ataxic animals. It was shown to be inoculable by intracerebral injection by Pool, Brownlee, and Wilson (11) in 1930. Greig, Brownlee, Wilson, and Gordon (8) proved, the following year, that the causative agent was a filterable virus.

The disease is primarily one of sheep but it occasionally affects cattle pastured on the same lands with affected sheep. Human infections also occur. **Character of the Disease.** Under conditions of natural exposure, the incubation time is from 6 to 18 days. The earliest signs are dullness and a high temperature, which may be 107 F or more. At this stage virus is present in the blood. The temperature generally falls after a day or so and the animal appears better, but improvement is only temporary for a second temperature rise usually occurs about the 5th day. At this time involvement of the nervous system may occur. If it does not, the animal recovers rapidly and thereafter is strongly immune. Those that develop nervous signs begin with muscular inco-ordination, tremors, cerebellar ataxia, and finally paralysis. A high percentage of those that show nervous signs eventually die; those that do not die usually are permanently damaged. The disease resembles poliomyelitis of man in that it is always a generalized infection in the beginning which may, or may not, be followed by invasion of the central nervous system.

In very acute cases death may occur within a day or two of the time the first signs are observed. In chronic cases paralytic changes may exist for months.

If only generalized or viremic changes occur, without nervous system involvement, the death rate is practically nil. In the highly infected areas of the British Isles it has long been recognized that sheep more than 1 year old seldom develop the disease; they are immune as a result of unrecognized infections. This disease is seen mostly in young lambs.

The lesions are typical of a virus-type encephalomyelitis and meningitis. Degeneration of neurons, and particularly of the Purkinje cells of the cerebellum, is characteristic. There are no typical gross lesions.

**The Disease in Experimental Animals.** By intracerebral inoculation of brain virus the disease can be produced in sheep, cattle, swine, mice, hamsters, and monkeys. Rabbits and guinea pigs do not appear to be susceptible. According to Galloway and Perdrau (6), monkeys and mice can be readily infected by instilling virus in their nostrils. The incubation period in these cases varied from 13 to 22 days, averaging 17 days. Hurst (9) found characteristic cytoplasmic inclusion bodies in the brain of mice, but he could not find them in monkeys, and others have not been able to find them in other species. Edward (3) was able to produce encephalitis in only 44 percent of susceptible lambs by inoculating virus subcutaneously. The injection of sterile starch solution intracerebrally 3 days after inoculation of the virus subcutaneously increased the number of cases of encephalitis to nearly 100 percent.

**Properties of the Virus.** Like the other five members in the family of tick-borne B arboviruses (2) the virus particle is spherical with an estimated diameter of 15 to 20 m$\mu$ (5) and an infectious RNA has been reported. The virus hemagglutinates rooster red blood cells. Crossing occurs with the other B arboviruses in the hemagglutination inhibition tests but not to the same degree as with other members of tick-borne B viruses. The agent is well preserved by freezing and glycerol but deteriorates rapidly in saline or broth, especially in dilute and somewhat acid suspensions.

A complement-fixation test is available, but CF antibodies are transient, so the test has limited value in diagnosis and research (14).

**Cultivation.** Rivers and Ward (13) were successful in obtaining artificial cultures of the virus on minced chick embryo medium. The virus also grows in cultures of pig kidney. Edward (4) grew it in embryonated eggs by inoculating either the yolk sac or the embryo.

**Immunity.** Recovery from natural or artificial infections always results in a solid and enduring immunity. Young suckling lambs whose dams are immune are protected by colostral antibody until after weaning time. A vaccine developed by Gordon (7), consisting of formalinized nerve tissue, provides effective protection to young lambs. Vaccinated lambs will succumb if inoculated with virus intracerebrally because the protection is due to circulating antibodies, which prevent the initial build-up of virus in the blood stream.

**Transmission.** Experimentally it has been shown that monkeys and man can contract infection by inhaling infective droplets. This may sometimes happen in sheep, but most transmissions occur through the agency of bloodsucking arthropods. McLeod and Gordon (10) in 1932 showed that in the louping-ill districts of the British Isles the principal transmitter was the castor bean tick, *Ixodes ricinus*. The larval ticks, feeding on infected sheep, convey the infection to new hosts when they next feed as nymphs; or if the tick becomes infected as a nymph, it conveys the disease to a new host as an adult. The disease is prevalent in the early summer, subsides during midsummer, and reappears in early fall. These periods correspond to the seasons of tick activity in the area.

**Diagnosis.** Diagnosis from the clinical signs may be difficult unless the animals are in a louping-ill district. Virus may be most readily demonstrated by inoculating mice intracerebrally with nerve tissue. Serological tests may be necessary to make a definitive diagnosis in many cases.

**Control.** Louping-ill may be controlled in two ways: (*a*) by immunizing all newborn lambs with nerve-tissue vaccine shortly after weaning, and (*b*) by dipping the flocks to remove all castor bean ticks.

**The Disease in Man.** Although louping-ill has occurred for many years, human infections were not recognized until recently. The first cases, described by Rivers and Schwentker (12), were three laboratory workers engaged in research work on the disease in the Rockefeller Institute in New York City in 1933. The illness was of an influenzal nature. Virus was not recovered from these patients, but neutralizing antibodies appeared in their sera shortly after recovery.

More recently several cases have been recognized in the British Isles. One described by Brewis, Neubauer, and Hurst (1) is typical. A young shepherd whose flock was affected by the disease was the victim. His disease was biphasic. An initial febrile illness of short duration was followed by apparent recovery. About 1 week later, he became delirious and comatose for a period of 36 hours. Virus was recovered by the inoculation of mice with cerebrospinal fluid, intracerebrally and intramuscularly, and neutralizing antibodies later appeared in his blood. He recovered almost completely except for some mild symptoms of ataxia.

## REFERENCES

1. Brewis, Neubauer, and Hurst.   Lancet, 1949, *1*, 689.
2. Clarke.   Symposium on biology of viruses of the tick-borne encephalitis complex. Academic Press, N.Y., 1962.
3. Edward.   Brit. Jour. Exp. Path., 1947, *28*, 368.
4. *Ibid.*, 1947, *28*, 237.
5. Elford and Galloway.   Jour. Comp. Path. and Therap., 1933, *37*, 381.
6. Galloway and Perdrau.   Jour. Hyg. (London), 1935, *35*, 339.
7. Gordon.   Vet. Jour., 1936, *92*, 84.
8. Greig, Brownlee, Wilson, and Gordon.   Vet. Rec., 1931, *11*, 325.
9. Hurst.   Jour. Comp. Path. and Therap., 1931, *44*, 231.
10. McLeod and Gordon.   *Ibid.*, 1932, *45*, 240.
11. Pool, Brownlee, and Wilson.   *Ibid.*, 1930, *43*, 253.
12. Rivers and Schwentker.   Jour. Exp. Med., 1934, *59*, 669.
13. Rivers and Ward.   Proc. Soc. Exp. Biol. and Med., 1933, *30*, 1300.
14. Williams.   Am. Jour. Vet. Res., 1968, *29*, 1619.

## Central European Tick-Borne Fever

SYNONYMS:   Diphasic milk fever, Russian spring-summer encephalitis (Western form)

This member of the tick-borne encephalitis complex produces a diphasic disease in man. The initial phase is influenzalike and the second stage, after a 4- to 10-day afebrile period, is characterized by meningitis or meningoencephalitis. Virus may be present in the milk of infected goats and thus infect man (2). Experimentally virus may localize in the mammary glands of infected goats, cows, and sheep and be present in the urine. The vector is *Ixodes ricinus,* and it probably is the most important reservoir of infection for man. An attenuated virus vaccine is being tested for immunization of cattle, sheep, and goats (1).

### REFERENCES

1.  Blaskovic.   Symposium on biology of viruses of the tick-borne encephalitis complex. Academic Press, N.Y., 1962.
2.  Van Tongeren.   Arch. f. die Gesam. Virusforsch., 1955, *6,* 158.

### Murray Valley Encephalitis

SYNONYM:   Australian X disease

This virus is a group B arbovirus with the usual characteristics attributed to this group. The encephalitis in man resembles Japanese B encephalitis and occurs in certain areas of Australia and Papua. Horses may be infected but do not develop encephalitis (1). The important vector is *Culex annulirostris* (2).

### REFERENCES

1.  Anderson.   Jour. Hyg. (London), 1954, *52,* 447.
2.  McLean.   Austral. Jour. Exp. Biol. and Med. Sci., 1953, *31,* 481.

### Wesselsbron Disease

This virus is a member of group B arboviruses, and the disease occurs in South Africa, Rhodesia, and Mozambique. The virus may infect man producing fever and muscular pains. It is known to cause epizootics in sheep, with abortions and death of newborn lambs and pregnant ewes a characteristic feature. Jaundice and hemorrhages may occur and meningoencephalitis in fetuses. It probably causes abortion in cattle as well. The virus has a diameter of 30 m$\mu$ (2), grows in the chick embryo after yolk-sac inoculation, and propagates in cultures of lamb kidney. The mosquitoes *Aedes caballus* and *A. circumluteolus* (1) are primarily responsible for virus transmission.

### REFERENCES

1.  Kokernot, Smithburn, Patterson, and Hodgson.   So. African Jour. Med. Sci., 1960, *34,* 871.
2.  Weiss, Haig, and Alexander.   Onderstepoort Jour. Vet. Res., 1956, *27,* 183.

### Turkey Meningoencephalitis

In 1960 Komarov and Kalmar (1) described a disease of turkeys in the Shomron area of Israel. It was characterized by a progressive paralysis associated with a nonpurulent meningoencephalitis. The agent is a filterable virus, cultivable in embryonated hens' eggs, and produced plaques on chick embryo cell culture monolayers. Turkeys and mice were susceptible to the virus, whereas chickens, ducks, pigeons, hamsters, and guinea pigs were resistant. Turkeys which recovered were resistant to reinfection.

Following serial passages of the virus in chicken eggs, modification of its virulence for turkeys and mice resulted without loss of antigenicity.

Preliminary studies suggest that a species of mosquito may be involved in its transmission. Mice immune to the turkey virus were susceptible to representative members of groups A and B arboviruses. In 1961 Porterfield (2) showed that this virus falls in the group B arboviruses.

## REFERENCES

1. Komarov and Kalmar. Vet. Rec., 1960, 72, 257.
2. Porterfield. *Ibid.*, 1961, 73, 392.

### Nairobi Disease of Sheep

This arbovirus disease occurs in British East Africa. It affects sheep which each year are brought down from the northern districts into Nairobi to be offered for sale. It has been described by Montgomery (2).

The disease is characterized by acute hemorrhagic gastroenteritis. The mortality varies from 30 to 70 percent. The causative agent is a virus that is readily filterable. The blood and tissues are always infective during the temperature reaction. The urine is said to be infective at this stage, but the feces ordinarily contain no virus.

The disease is transmitted by the adult forms of a tick, *Rhipicephalus appendiculatus,* which have fed as nymphs upon infected sheep.

Recovered animals possess a lasting immunity. Artificial immunization has been attempted only on a small scale. Control depends upon eradication of the transmitting agent. This tick also transmits East Coast fever of cattle; hence dipping of both sheep and cattle should be done, with benefit to both species. The virus was propagated in tissue-cultured cells of goat testes, goat kidney, and hamster kidney (1). A cytopathic effect of a consistent and uniform nature occurred only with hamster kidney cells.

## REFERENCES

1. Howarth and Terptra. Jour. Comp. Path., 1965, 75, 347.
2. Montgomery. Jour. Comp. Path. and Therap., 1917, 30, 28.

### Spontaneous Virus Diseases of the Nervous System of Experimental Animals

No attempt will be made here to describe the spontaneous encephalitides that occur in animals commonly used for the isolation and study of viruses of man and animals. It is desired merely to call attention to the fact that such viruses exist and that workers must be on their guard, when using such animals, not to confuse these disease with ones believed to be in the material inoculated. Viruses causing spontaneous encephalitis have been found in rabbits, guinea pigs, and mice, and probably they occur occasionally in all species. These viruses often are latent, or masked, and become evident only when inoculations containing foreign material act as a local irritant to the nerve tissue. Having been activated in this way, such viruses may then be passed readily from animal to animal in series. Römer (4) has described a virus of guinea pig paralysis, and Traub (5) demonstrated that the virus of lymphocytic choriomeningitis may sometimes occur spontaneously in colonies of white mice. The virus of herpes of man has been found occurring spontaneously in rabbit colonies. When viruses are recovered from experimental animals, it is important to make sure, either by a study of the specific histological changes and of the action of the virus on other animal species or by immunological procedures, that the virus is not one that occurred spontaneously in the experimental animal.

In the study of neurotropic viruses it sometimes happens that two or more viruses exist in the same material, or a virus may become contaminated with another that existed spontaneously in some animal through which the original material was passed. While studying the etiology of St. Louis encephalitis in man, Armstrong and Lillie (1) first encountered the virus that is now known as that of lymphocytic choriomeningitis. In another instance Dalldorf, Douglass, and Robinson (3) produced a nervous disease in monkeys by injecting them with canine distemper virus. This surprising discovery was explained later when Dalldorf (2) found that the distemper virus had been contaminated with the virus of lymphocytic choriomeningitis, the type species for the genus *Arenavirus,* and that the signs were caused by the latter rather than by the virus of distemper.

### REFERENCES

1. Armstrong and Lillie.   Pub. Health Rpts. (U.S.), 1934, *49,* 1019.
2. Dalldorf.   Jour. Exp. Med., 1939, *70,* 19.
3. Dalldorf, Douglass, and Robinson.   *Ibid.,* 1938, *67,* 323.
4. Römer.   Centrbl. f. Bakt., 1911, *50,* Beihefte, p. 30.
5. Traub.   Jour. Exp. Med., 1936, *63,* 533.

### Rift Valley Fever

SYNONYM:   Infectious enzootic hepatitis of sheep and cattle

This disease takes its name from a geographic area in Kenya, British East Africa, where the disease was first described.

It occurs primarily in sheep and cattle. Outbreaks in goats have been described. It is highly contagious to man, and human cases invariably occur where the disease exists in animals.

So far as is known, this disease occurs only in Africa, except for human laboratory infections which have appeared in Europe, the United States, and Japan. It was first described by Daubney, Hudson, and Garnham (3) in 1931 in Kenya, but there is much evidence that the disease had occurred for many years previously in the French and Anglo-Egyptian Sudan and other parts of equatorial Africa. In 1951 it suddenly appeared in South Africa (Alexander, 1). Outbreaks occur during warm humid periods, because mosquitoes are the principal transmitting agents.

**Character of the Disease.** The disease is most acute and causes the heaviest losses in sheep. Very young lambs often die in large numbers. The mortality rate in ewes is less but still serious. In the original outbreak described by Daubney, 3,500 lambs and 1,200 ewes died in a 2-week period.

*In lambs,* the disease is characterized by a high fever, prostration, and a rapid course which leads to death generally within 24 hours.

*In ewes,* abortions frequently are seen before lamb losses occur. Ewes are observed to be sick only a few hours before they die, or they are simply found dead in the corrals. Some vomit. Many have thick purulent nasal discharges. Some pass stools that consist of almost pure blood. Some show no signs other than abortion.

*In cattle,* the disease resembles that in sheep in every way but the losses are not so high.

The incubation period of Rift Valley fever is very short. It may be no more than 24 hours in some cases and generally is not longer than 3 days.

In young lambs the course of the disease is rarely longer than 24 hours. In older animals it may be longer. After a short period of obvious illness pregnant ewes appear well but often abort a few days later. In young lambs the mortality often is from 95 to 100 percent. In ewes it probably does not exceed 20 percent. In cattle of all ages the losses from death average about 10 percent, but many pregnant cows abort.

The most characteristic lesion in ruminants is focal necrosis of the liver. In many lambs the necrosis is so complete that sections are hardly recognizable. Findlay (4) and others have described inclusion bodies of an intensely acidophilic character in the nuclei of the liver cells. Other lesions consist principally of hemorrhages—in the lymph nodes, subendocardial and subepicardial, and in the gastric and intestinal mucosa. Blood examinations show severe leukopenia. In lambs especially it is sometimes difficult to find any mature leukocytes in blood films.

**The Disease in Experimental Animals.** The disease is readily produced in cattle and sheep by inoculation. White mice of the Swiss type are very easily infected. They die within 2 or 3 days after inoculation by any parenteral route. Infections can be produced by inoculation in monkeys, ferrets, hamsters, white rats, and possibly rabbits. Horses, swine, guinea pigs, and domestic and wild birds are not susceptible.

**Properties of the Virus.** This ungrouped member of the arbovirus group is about 30 m$\mu$ and relatively resistant. Infective virus persists for 3 months at room temperature and almost 3 years in serum kept at $-4$ C. It withstands lyophilization, but inactivation occurs in a 1 : 1,000 dilution of formalin.

The virus has a hemagglutinin for red blood cells of day-old chicks at pH 6.5 and 25 C. The observation of interference between yellow fever and Rift Valley fever viruses was the first reported for serologically unrelated viruses.

**Cultivation.** The virus grows in cell cultures of the chick, rat, mouse, human, and lamb. Binn *et al.* (2) described its propagation and plaque formation in primary cell cultures of lamb kidney and of hamster kidney.

It produces a thickening of the chorioallantoic membrane of embryonated hens' eggs. Inoculation by the yolk-sac route is also successful.

**Immunity.** Animals and men that recover from a natural infection are solidly resistant thereafter. Sabin and Blumberg (6) have shown that neutralizing antibodies appear in the blood of man within a few days after recovery from infection and that these persisted, in one case, for as long as 12 years.

Smithburn (7) passed strains of Rift Valley fever virus serially in white mice by intracerebral injection and found that as they acquired neurotropic properties they lost viserotropism. He used these strains for immunizing ewes, finding that when injected subcutaneously virus did not appear in the blood and the animals suffered no damage from them. By this means the newborn lambs were protected during the period of greatest susceptibility.

Both neurotropic and field strains of Rift Valley fever virus have been adapted to embryonated eggs by Kaschula (5). The neurotropic strains are used successfully for field immunization. The immunity conferred is not as lasting or as solid as that conferred by actual infection.

Vaccines cannot be used on very young lambs or on pregnant ewes or cows. Safe protection of such animals can be conferred only by the use of convalescent serum.

Recently Weiss (9) suggested that the 102nd intracerebral mouse passage level virus is a safe vaccine for 1-day-old lambs. Formalin-inactivated virus vaccines are also available for animals (2).

**Transmission.** Daubney and Hudson, in their original investigations, found that Rift Valley fever could be easily transmitted by the inoculation of blood or tissue extracts. They, and all others who have worked with this disease in the field or laboratory, discovered that all persons who had intimate contact with infected animals developed the disease within 5 days after exposure. On the other hand, infected and susceptible sheep might be kept together and, in the absence of certain transmitting agents, the disease would not be transmitted. It was even shown that infected ewes did not infect their suckling lambs, and that infected lambs did not infect their mothers. This made it seem probable that an invertebrate vector played an important role in the disease.

Smithburn, Haddow, and Gillett (8) in 1948 succeeded in isolating the virus from six different lots of mosquitoes in the Semliki Forest in an uninhabited part of Uganda. These mosquitoes included several species of the genus *Eretmapodites*, and it was later shown that some of these could transmit the disease. The present evidence points strongly to these and perhaps other species of mosquitoes as the principal transmitting agents. Because there were no cattle or sheep in the Semliki Forest, the presence of infected mosquitoes strongly suggests the existence of a reservoir of virus in wild animals.

**Diagnosis.** The clinical behavior of the disease in sheep and cattle is at least highly suggestive. The presence of extensive liver necrosis should serve to confirm the suspicion. Inoculation of white mice results in prompt fatal infections. Final confirmation must come from serological tests, using known antisera. These may be neutralization tests, using mice for the test species, or the complement-fixation, gel-diffusion, or hemagglutination-inhibition tests may be employed.

**Control.** The original outbreak described by Daubney *et al.* was controlled promptly when the flocks were driven into ranges at a higher altitude. Presumably this put the animals above the mosquito range. Immunization by means of the neurotropic vaccines is well tolerated by adult animals, and this offers a way to protect flocks and herds that must remain in regions inhabited by the vectors.

**The Disease in Man.** It has already been pointed out that veterinarians, laboratory workers, and herd and flock attendants almost invariably become infected when the disease appears. Butchers and housewives have also suffered from handling fresh meat which came from infected animals. The infections in these cases are obviously the result of direct contact with infected tissues. It is not clear whether human infections occur as a result of mosquito transmission.

The disease is almost never fatal. The attacks occur within a few days after exposure. The symptoms resemble those of influenza or dengue. The onset is sudden, with malaise, headache, and a feeling of chilliness. Fever develops quickly and joint pains, often rather extreme, soon appear. Nausea and vomiting sometimes occur and often there is some abdominal distress. The disease lasts only a few days and recovery is complete. A formalin-inactivated virus vaccine is available for immunization of humans.

## REFERENCES

1.  Alexander.   Jour. So. African Vet. Med. Assoc., 1951, *22*, 105.
2.  Binn, Randall, Harrison, Gibbs, and Aulisis.   Am. Jour. Hyg., 1963, *77*, 160.
3.  Daubney, Hudson, and Garnham.   Jour. Path. and Bact., 1931, *34*, 545.
4.  Findlay.   Brit. Jour. Exp. Path., 1933, *14*, 207.
5.  Kaschula.   Personal communication, 1957.
6.  Sabin and Blumberg.   Proc. Soc. Exp. Biol. and Med., 1947, *64*, 385.
7.  Smithburn.   Brit. Jour. Exp. Path., 1949, *30*, 1.
8.  Smithburn, Haddow, and Gillett.   *Ibid.*, *29*, 107.
9.  Weiss.   Onderstepoort Jour. Vet. Res., 1962, *29*, 3.

# XLVII | Rabies and Other Rhabdoviruses

The most important animal pathogen in this genus is rabies virus, although the type species is *Rhabdovirus* b-1, commonly known as vesicular stomatitis virus. Other members include Cocal, Hart Park, Kern Canyon and Flanders viruses. Some possible members are hemorrhagic septicemia virus of trout (Egtved), Sigma virus, *Drosophila* virus, Lagos bat virus, Mount Elgon bat virus, shrew virus (Iban 27377), bovine ephemeral fever virus, and perhaps the Marburg (monkey) virus. The latter virus is unique in that particles occur as filaments as much as 1 m$\mu$ long. There also are a large number of plant viruses that are placed in this genus.

A typical member of this genus contains 2 percent single-stranded RNA with a molecular weight of 3.5 by 10$^6$. There is a helical nucleocapsid surrounded by a shell with an envelope containing 10 m$\mu$ spikes. The whole particle is bullet-shaped, measuring 175 (130 to 220) m$\mu$ by 70 m$\mu$. In cesium chloride it has a buoyant density of 1.20 g per ml. Infectivity is destroyed by lipid solvents and a low pH. Some members of the genus contain a hemagglutinin. Maturation of virus particles occurs at the cytoplasmic membrane. Most members multiply in arthropods as well as vertebrates. Antigenic relationships occur between some members.

## Rabies

SYNONYMS: Hydrophobia, *Tollwut* or *Wut* (German), *le Rage* (French)

Rabies has been known since ancient time in Europe and Asia. Apparently its principal reservoir for many centuries was in wild animals, although dog infections were well known. For the last 200 years in western Europe the principal reservoir has been in dogs. It was introduced into America by dogs brought along by some of the early colonists and it has spread widely. It was first reported in Virginia, North Carolina, and New England in the middle of the 18th century.

**Character of the Disease.** The virus of rabies will usually produce fatal disease, by inoculation, in all warm-blooded animals. In the more densely populated parts of the world the disease occurs principally in dogs and cats. It is widespread over the world in wildlife. Foxes, wolves, skunks, mongooses, bats, and other wild carnivora are the principal host reservoirs in various parts of the world. Cases in man are never very numerous in terms of the whole population, but the fear of the disease, instilled by general knowledge of the dreadful signs and its uniform fatality, makes it of far greater importance to mankind than the incidence suggests.

*Table XXXVI.* INCIDENCE OF RABIES IN THE UNITED STATES BY TYPE OF ANIMAL, 1953–1969 *

| Year | Dogs | Cats | Farm animals | Foxes | Skunks | Bats | Other animals | Man | Total |
|---|---|---|---|---|---|---|---|---|---|
| 1953 | 5,688 | 538 | 1,118 | 1,033 | 319 | 8 | 119 | 14 | 8,837 |
| 1954 | 4,083 | 462 | 1,032 | 1,028 | 547 | 4 | 118 | 8 | 7,282 |
| 1955 | 2,657 | 343 | 924 | 1,223 | 580 | 14 | 98 | 5 | 5,844 |
| 1956 | 2,592 | 371 | 794 | 1,281 | 631 | 41 | 126 | 10 | 5,846 |
| 1957 | 1,758 | 382 | 714 | 1,021 | 775 | 31 | 115 | 6 | 4,802 |
| 1958 | 1,643 | 353 | 737 | 845 | 1,005 | 68 | 157 | 6 | 4,814 |
| 1959 | 1,119 | 292 | 751 | 920 | 789 | 80 | 126 | 6 | 4,083 |
| 1960 | 697 | 277 | 645 | 915 | 725 | 88 | 108 | 2 | 3,457 |
| 1961 | 594 | 217 | 482 | 614 | 1,254 | 186 | 120 | 3 | 3,470 |
| 1962 | 565 | 232 | 614 | 594 | 1,449 | 157 | 114 | 2 | 3,727 |
| 1963 | 573 | 217 | 531 | 622 | 1,462 | 303 | 224 | 1 | 3,933 |
| 1964 | 409 | 220 | 594 | 1,061 | 1,909 | 352 | 238 | 1 | 4,784 |
| 1965 | 412 | 289 | 625 | 1,038 | 1,582 | 484 | 153 | 1 | 4,584 |
| 1966 | 412 | 252 | 587 | 864 | 1,522 | 377 | 183 | 1 | 4,198 |
| 1967 | 412 | 293 | 691 | 979 | 1,568 | 414 | 250 | 2 | 4,609 |
| 1968 | 296 | 157 | 457 | 801 | 1,400 | 291 | 210 | 1 | 3,613 |
| 1969 | 256 | 165 | 428 | 888 | 1,156 | 321 | 307 | 1 | 3,522 |

* Data prior to 1960 from USDA, ARS. Subsequent data from CDC, USPHS.

Rabies occurs on all the continents of the world, except Australia, from which it has been successfully excluded by rigid quarantine requirements. Many islands such as New Zealand, Hawaii, and Great Britain are now free of the disease, also the Scandinavian countries of Europe. It is a very common disease in Mexico. It occurs in varying degrees in most parts of the United States, but Canada appears to be free from it, except possibly in the frigid Northwest Territory where it was quite prevalent a few years ago among sled dogs. There is an old belief that rabies in dogs is much more prevalent in late summer ("dog days") but this is not true. In general, the incidence is highest in late winter or early spring. A possible reason for this may be the more promiscuous mixing of animals at that time because of the urges of the breeding season. The disease occurs, it will be noted, in all climates from tropic to frigid.

NUMBER OF RABIES CASES REPORTED BY STATE, 1970

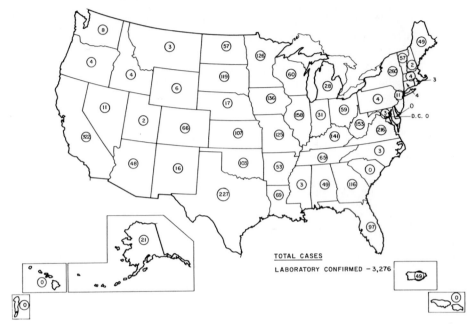

*Fig. 224.* Rabies reported in each state of the United States, 1970. (Courtesy Public Health Service, CDC.)

The signs of illness of rabies are similar in all species, but those in individuals vary widely. Two forms are generally recognized: (*a*) the furious form, and (*b*) the paralytic or dumb form. Actually, most cases exhibit some manifestations of both forms. When the stage of excitation is very marked, the first term is applied; when it is not, the second is used. The paralytic is always the terminal stage. Some animals die in convulsive seizures during the furious stage and do not exhibit the final stage. Many exhibit few or no signs of excitement, the clinical signs consisting wholly of paralytic signs. Rarely, affected animals die suddenly, exhibiting few or no signs.

In the stage of excitation many animals become aggressive and dangerous. While in this stage, carnivorous animals may snap at imaginary objects and bite other animals and man. In this way the disease is transmitted. Within a few hours these signs give way to those of the final stage, which usually lasts only a day or two and terminates in death.

An earlier stage is recognized in the disease in man, and this may also be recognized in pet animals that are well known and closely observed. This is called the prodromal stage, since it precedes the other signs described. In this stage vague changes in temperament occur. In man, the individual feels restless, uneasy, and apprehensive. Dogs that are normally affectionate may hide away and shun company; others may become unusually attentive and affectionate, a manifestation probably of a feeling of insecurity. This stage, if it occurs in other species, is not recognized.

*In dogs* furious rabies is manifested by restlessness, nervousness, and a developing viciousness. At first this is more apt to be manifested toward strangers, but later the animal apparently does not recognize its human friends and is as apt to injure them as others. If the animal is free, it may often leave home and travel great distances, biting and snapping at anything that attracts its attention. If restrained, it will chew viciously on metal chains or the bars of the cage which confines it. The dog may inflict severe bite wounds on itself; it often breaks its teeth, lacerates its lips and tongue, and froths at the mouth, the frothy saliva usually being tinged with blood. The dog seems quite oblivious to pain. It frequently utters strange cries and hoarse howls because of partial paralysis of its vocal cords. Usually it shows no interest in food at this stage, and frequently it is unable to swallow because of paralysis of the muscles of deglutition. The lower jaw often hangs for the same reason. The eyes are usually staring because of dilatation of the pupils. Sometimes the dog is unable to close its eyes, and the cornea becomes dry and dull. It often swallows pieces of wood, stones, its own fecal material, and other foreign bodies. There does not seem to be any real hydrophobia (fear of water) as there is in man. Convulsive seizures often precede the appearance of muscular inco-ordination, which is the first sign of the final stage of the disease.

The dumb form of rabies in dogs is much less spectacular and often is not diagnosed. Paralysis usually appears first in the muscles of the head and neck. The victim cannot chew its food; it cannot swallow water or does so with much difficulty. Its lower jaw hangs; it cannot close its mouth. A ropy saliva drools from its mouth. The owner often thinks that a bone or other object has become lodged in the dog's throat. In trying to examine the animal's mouth for an object that is not there, the animal's human friends often expose themselves to the disease by scratching their hands on its teeth, or by merely bathing hands that are abraded in the copious saliva. The signs of local paralysis are quickly succeeded by more general signs of like nature, and the animal usually dies within 48 hours of the time the original signs were observed.

*In cats* the disease generally takes the furious form and the signs are similar to those in dogs. Rabid cats are very dangerous animals for human attendants because of their viciousness and quickness of action.

*In horses* the first manifestation frequently is evidence of itching at the site where the bite wound occurred. The animal rubs and bites the part and often tears the flesh. Frequently it is unusually alert and tense, its ears being held erect and moved quickly back and forth as if to listen to sounds from many directions. Genital excitement often is evident. The horse may try to break or bite through its halter rope and may attack the manger with such force that it breaks its teeth or even its lower jaw. It refuses food but may swallow bits of wood, manure, or other foreign bodies. The first signs of paralysis usually appear in the throat. The horse may try but cannot swallow food and water. Generally it drools saliva. Locomotor difficulties then appear, and finally it becomes recumbent. Death follows in a few hours.

*In cattle* the signs often are particularly vague and confusing until late in the course of the disease. If the furious form occurs, the animals bawl, paw the earth and, if not restrained, may attack attendants or other animals. More often they show no evidence of exitement. Salivation is seen in many but not all cases, depending on whether or not pharyngeal paralysis develops. Perhaps the most common sign is tenesmus. Many cattle will strain more or less constantly for many hours as if to defecate. Usually air is aspirated into the rectum when there is relaxation between the straining periods. Beginning paralytic signs are often seen in locomotor difficulties. A frequent sign is knuckling over of the hind fetlocks. The tail often becomes paralyzed. In bulls, the penis may be protruded in a flaccid state. Cases diagnosed as indigestion, milk fever, and acetonemia when first seen often turn out to be rabies. The form of rabies that is transmitted by the vampire bat in Central and South America is almost invariably the paralytic type in all species (Metevier, 41).

*In sheep* rabies is not often encountered. One outbreak was described by Darbyshire (11) in Rhodesia. A large number of Merino sheep were bitten by a rabid ratel (honey badger). Clinical signs were exhibited by 44 animals. The first case appeared on the 19th day, 19 on the 25th, 7 on the 27th, and the others later. The course was usually 5 or 6 days. The signs were twitching of the lips, restlessness, and excitement. Many showed sexual excitement. Some developed wild and staring eyes. Only one animal exhibited marked salivation, and only one became aggressive.

The incubation period in rabies varies widely in all species. Experimentally it has been shown that the period of incubation varies inversely with the size of the inoculum, and this, no doubt, is also a factor in the natural disease. In man, it has long been recognized that bites in the region of the head and neck, particularly those which result in severe lacerations, are likely to have a higher rate of infectivity and a shorter period of incubation than those which occur on other parts of the body. *In man* the incubation period may vary from 10 days to 6 months or more. Nearly half of all cases develop signs during the 2nd month after exposure. *In the dog* the incubation period averages somewhat shorter than in man although the extremes are about the same. The majority of exposed dogs develop signs within 3 to 6 weeks and very few after 4 months.

Data on other farm animals are rather meager. *In cattle* considerable experience with a fox-borne outbreak in central New York indicates that the incubation period may be as short as 13 days and as long as several months, but the average is about 3 weeks. *In horses and swine* it is believed that the period is about the same as for cattle.

In contrast to the frequently long incubation periods are the generally short periods of signs of illness. In dogs and other carnivorous animals, the course of the disease is rarely longer than 5 days, though a few may linger a day or two longer. There have been reports of periods as long as 11 days in dogs, but these are very exceptional. The course of the disease in cattle is about the same as in dogs. Most animals die by the 5th day but some may longer as long as 9 days.

A peculiar situation exists as to rabies in vampire bats, which may have the disease in latent form for many months. Pawan (45) has shown that inoculated and naturally infected vampires alike may harbor rabies virus and be active transmitters of the disease for many months while apparently living a normal existence. He showed conclusively that many of these bats were capable of transmitting rabies several months before they died. Those of this type that were held in captivity generally died suddenly without showing any signs of rabies. Negri bodies and virus could usually be demonstrated in their brains. On the other hand, many of these creatures have been observed showing signs of furious rabies, and these generally died within a few days. Those affected in this way flew about in bright sunlight, attacked animals and man in the daytime and, when captured, were unusually vicious and aggressive.

When rabies virus is inoculated into one of the body extremities, it may be demonstrated several to many days later in the nerve trunks of that extremity even though no virus then exists in the spinal cord or the brain. Sometimes it may be demonstrated in the posterior part of the cord when it is absent in the anterior portion and in the brain. Apparently virus travels from the bite wound, not through the blood and lymph, but through the nerve trunks to the central nervous system. No matter when the examination is made, virus is very seldom demonstrable in the blood or the principal body organs. It is a true neurotropic virus. The relatively long and variable period of incubation may be due, in part at least, to the peculiar and relatively slow way in which the infective agent travels from its introductory point to vital centers.

It is generally considered that rabies is invariably fatal in all species. It is true that there have been no proved cases of human recoveries but there is evidence that animals may sometimes recover. (55). These cases are so rare as to be negligible. For practical purposes we may consider rabies in man and the domesticated animals as invariably fatal.

There are no pathognomonic gross lesions in rabies. The finding of foreign materials such as stones, wood, and fecal material in the stomach of dogs is suggestive. There may be some congestion of the meninges of the brain, and the brain tissue itself may be unusually pink because of congestion. Microscopic evidence of encephalitis is present, but this cannot be distinguished from some other virus infections except by identifying the characteristic inclusion body of rabies. This will be discussed under "Diagnosis."

**The Disease in Experimental Animals.** Rabies may be transmitted by inoculation to all warm-blooded animals. Virus is found with greatest certainty in the central nervous system, particularly the brain. It is found less frequently in the salivary glands except during the latter stages of the disease. It is rarely found in other organs and tissues although it is sometimes present in the kidney and adrenal glands of animals in the terminal stages.

The most certain way to infect an experimental animal is to inject virus directly into nerve tissue, i.e., intracerebrally. Inoculation into the posterior chamber of the eye, into the muscles, or under the skin are decreasingly effective in the order named. The dosage factor is important.

When inoculated intracerebrally, experimental animals nearly always develop the paralytic form of the disease. The incubation period generally is short, but if the dose is small, the period may be prolonged. These factors will be considered more fully under "Diagnosis."

**Properties of the Virus.** By use of filtration the virus particle size is estimated

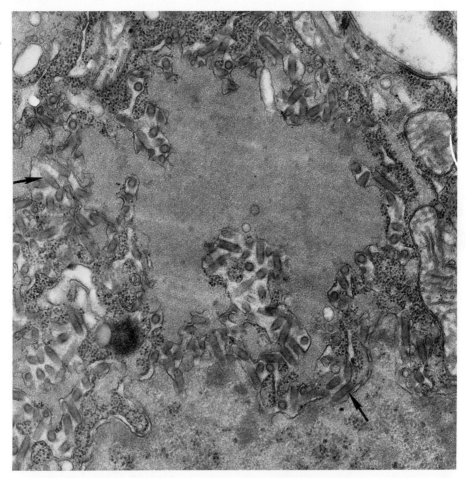

*Fig. 225.* Rabies virus. Note fibrillar nature of cytoplasmic inclusion body in a mouse neuron with bullet-shaped virions, 75 X 180 m$\mu$ (*arrows*), at its periphery. X 28,500. (Courtesy F. Murphy, CDC, USPHS.)

to be between 100 to 150 mμ; rods, 110 to 112 mμ, have been observed in nerve cells. By electron-microscope studies the virus particle clearly is bullet-shaped and its size is typical for this genus. The antigen can be located in Negri bodies and other particulate matter in the cytoplasm of nerve cells by the fluroescent-antibody technic (15). Virus bodies resembling those of myxo-viruses have been observed (2). The Negri bodies consist of a DNA matrix containing RNA granules (54). It is inactivated by ether.

Neutralizing and CF antigens are present in the virus particle. In gel-diffusion agar tests two lines of precipitate develop when fixed virus and specific sera are used.

Interference with poliomyelitis has been observed and also with western

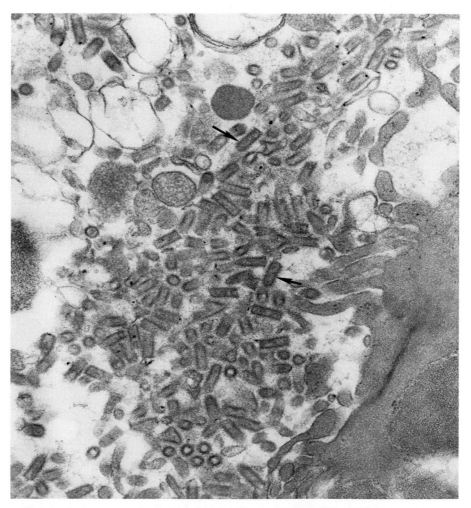

*Fig. 226.* Rabies virus in fox salivary gland. Higher magnification (X 45,866) showing more detail of the numerous bullet-shaped virions. (Courtesy F. Murphy, CDC, USPHS.)

equine encephalitis virus in a tissue culture system, interferon being responsible in the latter instance. The virus in aqueous suspension is readily destroyed by acids, alkalies, phenol, formalin, chloroform, bichloride of mercury, and many other disinfectants. In very thin layers it is readily inactivated by ultraviolet light. It is destroyed by pasteurization. It deteriorates rather rapidly in suspensions, particularly dilute suspensions, at room temperature. Lyophilized virus may be kept for relatively long periods. Pieces of nerve tissue preserved in 50 percent glycerol solution will retain virulence for months at refrigerator temperatures. Virus in dried saliva loses virulence within a few hours at ordinary temperatures.

**Cultivation.** The virus of rabies can be cultivated in tissue cultures containing viable nerve cells. Webster and Clow (63) obtained multiplication in a medium consisting of embryonic mouse or chicken brain suspended in Tyrode's solution. Kligler and Bernkopf (28) and Dawson (12) showed that the virus could be propagated in chick embryos. Koprowski and Cox (34) were able to cultivate in chick embryos a virus strain which Harald N. Johnson had passed through a long series of day-old chicks by intracerebral passage. This strain is of special interest since it was passaged directly from the human patient into chicks, and it has proved to be useful in immunizing animals. It is known as the Flury strain. Virus has also been grown in duck eggs and is now in use for immunization (46).

Kissling (27) cultivated rabies virus in hamster kidney cell cultures without a cytopathogenic effect. Fixed virus in cultures of human diploid and canine cell cultures produced a cytopathogenic effect. Subsequently, it was found that rabies virus could be grown in many cell types from various animal species (1, 26, 65).

**Immunity.** Because recoveries from rabies are so rare, little is known about the immunity that a natural attack confers. Experience with vaccines makes it quite certain, however, that such animals would have a high degree of immunity for at least 9 months. No biological or other form of treatment is known which influences the course of the disease, or its fatal outcome, after signs have developed. Taking advantage of the fact that the period of incubation is relatively long, Pasteur devised a vaccine that can be given after an individual has been exposed to the disease and before signs have appeared. This vaccine and its modifications have reduced human mortality from this disease to a small fraction of what it used to be. The vaccine can also be used to immunize animals. Pasteur demonstrated its safety and efficacy on dogs before it was used on man. Pasteur vaccine has never been extensively used on animals, principally because of its cost, but some of the newer vaccines have been so employed with a large measure of success.

**Immunization.** The vaccines that are used to protect against rabies are of two kinds: (a) those that contain attenuated but active virus, and (b) those that contain inactivated virus. All vaccines of both types, except the recently introduced avianized and duck types, are related to the original one of Pasteur in that they are made from a lapinized (rabbit-adapted) strain of virus. Its production will be discussed under the Pasteur vaccine.

Rabies vaccines have only prophylactic value. They are used on man only when individuals have been exposed by the bite of an animal or otherwise and are presumed to be in the incubative stage of the disease since there are some hazards in the use of the vaccine which should not be risked except as a means of avoiding the greater risk of the disease itself. These risks, which are not very great and usually consist of paraplegias of a transitory nature, are warranted in animals, particularly in dogs. In areas where rabies is prevalent, the practice is well established in the United States of encouraging antirabic vaccination of all dogs before thay are actually exposed. Such vaccines may be used on animals after they have been exposed, but their efficacy is not so great under these circumstances. Furthermore, owners of dogs and cats, animals that are likely to become dangerous if the disease develops, should be encouraged to destroy their pets when it is known that they have been exposed rather than run the risk of having them develop the disease and perhaps infect other animals or persons. If they are not willing to do this, whether or not they have been vaccinated, they should cause such animals to be securely confined under close observation for a period of from 4 to 6 months before thay are again allowed to run at large.

Large numbers of rabies vaccines have been made and used with variable success. No attempt will be made here to discuss or even name all of them. Those who wish further details should consult more comprehensive texts such as that of Van Rooyen and Rhodes (60). It should be emphasized that none of the present vaccines are successful in all cases. In man, deaths from rabies have occured in individuals who have received all types of vaccine, and the same is true in dogs. Mass immunization of dogs, however, has proved a very valuable means of controlling outbreaks in this species, a fact which proves that the degree of immunity conferred is significant.

*Rabies vaccines containing active virus.* The Pasteur vaccine. The basis of this vaccine is a virus modified by long serial passage through rabbits (Pasteur, 44). The first rabbits die in about 15 to 18 days following inoculation into the brain of nerve tissue of a dog affected with the naturally acquired disease (street virus). As the process of serial inoculations in rabbits continues, the period of incubation becomes shorter and shorter. Eventually the inoculated animals die on the 6th or 7th day; then, no matter how long the serial inoculations are continued, the incubation period will not become shorter. This means that a stage of maximum and stable virulence for rabbits has been reached. Pasteur called such a virus his *virus fixe*, and the term *fixed virus* continues to be used for it. Whereas fixed virus is much more pathogenic for rabbits than street virus, its pathogenicity for dogs, man, and other animal species has decreased so greatly that it will not ordinarily produce rabies when injected into them by routes other than into the brain itself.

In the making of the Pasteur vaccine, the fixed virus in the spinal cords of rabbits is further attenuated, or perhaps only reduced in amount, by drying the cords suspended in the air in large bottles over caustic potash. Fresh cords are obtained every day, so that tissues which have been dried for periods varying from 1 to 14 days are on hand. Treatment of man is begun by injecting suspensions of cords that have been dried for 14 days. Gradually, day by day in successive doses, suspensions of cords that have been dried for shorter periods are used until finally those that have been dried only 2 or 3 days are given. In the older treatments, 21 days were required for the full course of treatments, but more recently they have been completed in 14 days. Two injections are made per day in the beginning, particularly if the bite happens to be on the face, in which case it is desirable that immunity be built up as rapidly as possible because of the short incubation period of such cases.

The original Pasteur-type vaccine is no longer used for human or animal immunization in most parts of the world. It has been replaced, for human immunization, with inactivated vaccines. Inactivated vaccines are also widely used for animals, but they are rapidly being replaced by the avianized vaccine. The latter is now widely used for dogs. It and the duck-embryo vaccine are recommended for the immunization of man.

The avianized (Flury) vaccine. Although a number of strains of rabies virus have been cultivated in series in embryonated eggs, only one of these strains has been widely used as an immunizing agent. This strain was isolated by Leach and Johnson (38) from a child whose name was Flury. The strain was isolated by direct inoculation of the child's brain tissue into the brain of a day-old chick and was then carried by Johnson through 136-day-old chicks by serial intracerebral inoculation. By that time the pathogenicity for laboratory animals and dogs had been greatly reduced. The strain was then given to Koprowski and Cox (34), who carried it through another series of passages in chick embryos. After 40 to 50 passages the strain had lost its neutrotropic properties for the embryos; the virus now occurred in high concentration in all tissues, including the blood. This attenuated strain was then tested by Koprowski and Black (31) as a vaccine for dogs. It produced a solid immunity and there were no undesirable reactions. Extensive field trials in several parts of the United States, Israel, and Malaya showed that the vaccine was a very good one. Not only is a high level of protection conferred on dogs by a single injection, but this immunity persists for at least 3 years in most dogs (Tierkel *et al.*, 57). Comparative experiments with inactivated vaccine (Semple, see below) by Koprowski and Black (32) showed that the immunity produced by the Flury vaccine was better at 1 year, and very much better at 2 years, than that produced by the other vaccine.

An additional advantage of the Flury vaccine over the brain-tissue vaccines is the absence of paralytic phenomena following its use. This will be discussed below.

Schroeder *et al.* (49) used this vaccine in Central America on more than 6,000 cattle living in an area where rabies (*derriengue*) transmitted by the vampire bat was prevalent. They reported no untoward results attributable to the vaccine itself and no reports of rabies in vaccinated animals although the incidence in the unvaccinated controls was great. In the United States, however, a few cases of vaccine paralysis have occurred, indicating that this vaccine is probably a little too potent for cattle. Koprowski and Black (33) have produced what they call a high-egg passage (HEP) Flury vaccine by continuing chick embryo serial passage to the 178th generation. This strain has lost almost all pathogenicity for laboratory animals and seems to be innocuous for domesticated animals, although it appears to have retained much of its antigenicity. It is recommended for use on cattle. Deterioration of some lots of commercially produced low-egg-passaged (LEP) vaccines for dogs has been experienced. The U.S. Department of Agriculture now requires that samples of all lots of vaccine on the market be collected from distributors and retested 5 months after the original potency test.

Tissue-cultured attenuated vaccines. Two virus strains of rabies virus have been adapted to tissue culture systems for use as virus vaccines. Both the low-egg passage (LEP) and high-egg passage (HEP) of the Flury strain were cultivated in cell culture and now used as articles of commerce. The tissue-cultured ERA strain also is given intramuscularly as an attenuated virus vaccine for cats, cattle, dogs and other domestic animals. This strain was isolated from the brain of a rabid dog. Subsequently it was passaged in mice, hamster kidney tissue culture, chick embryo, and finally in porcine kidney cell culture.

The attenuated virus vaccines of chick embryo and tissue-culture origin are tested for efficacy by a single vaccination of guinea pigs with a specified fraction of an animal dose. Both the vaccinated and control guinea pigs are given a challenge dose of fixed or street virus calculated to infect 80 percent of the control guinea pigs; 80 percent of the vaccinated guinea pigs must survive.

*Rabies vaccines containing inactivated virus.* Several vaccines containing inactivated virus have been used in the past. A vaccine inactivated with chloroform (Kelser, 25) proved to be effective. Others were inactivated with phenol, ether, and formalin. In 1937, Hodes, Lavin, and Webster (22) described a vaccine inactivated with ultraviolet light. Habel (20) confirmed the finding that such vaccines were somewhat more potent than chemically altered vaccines made from the same materials. Irradiated vaccines have been used to some extent on people but not on animals.

Phenol-"killed" vaccines. Semple (50) working with the British Army in India as early as 1911 used fixed virus inactivated with phenol as a vaccine for rabies in man. In recent years the Semple vaccine has been used in the United States and many other parts of the world for human protection. It has given protection which appears to be as good as that conferred by the Pasteur method. Since the Semple vaccine can be made up in lots and kept for considerable periods of time without deterioration, and since it can be shipped and administered by local physicians, its use is much simpler, more convenient, and less expensive than the Pasteur vaccine, which has to be freshly made and used almost immediately. Treatment with the Semple vaccine consists, in man, of multiple doses, each dose consisting of the same material as the preceding ones.

Interest in the use of a phenol-inactivated fixed virus for preventing rabies in dogs stems from the work of Umeno and Doi (59) in Japan, who published their results in 1921. These workers immunized large numbers of dogs in Tokyo, where rabies was rampant at the time, with a single dose of their vaccine, which was made from the brains and cords of rabbits dead of fixed-virus infection, the virus being inactivated with 1.25 percent phenol. Of 215,000 dogs which they immunized, only 175 (0.76 percent) later died of rabies, whereas in the same region 2,860 cases of rabies were diagnosed in nonimmunized dogs.

A phenol-inactivated vaccine for dogs to be given in a single treatment was introduced into the United States by Eichhorn and Lyon (13) in 1922. Commercial vaccines of this type were soon on the market and were rather widely used. Mass immunization of dogs was required by many local governments. It soon became apparent that the results were not uniform; in some instances they were good, in others they appeared to be largely ineffective. The reason for these discrepancies was first suggested by Webster (62) in 1939. Using laboratory mice, Webster was able to show that most of the commercial phenol-treated vaccines were lacking in antigenicity. This was true of those prepared for human use as well as of those made for dogs.

Habel (18) confirmed Webster's findings and devised a method of assessing the antigenicity of rabies vaccines. This method, which has become known as the Habel test, was applied to all inactivated commercial vaccines with interesting results. This test involves the use of 48 white (Swiss) mice for each lot of vaccine tested. Thirty mice, at 2-day intervals, are given six doses of 0.25 ml of a 0.5 percent brain emulsion of the vaccine, intraperitoneally. Fourteen days after the first dose of vaccine is given, the mice are divided into smaller groups of six each. Both vaccinated and unvaccinated mice are now inoculated with a strain of fixed virus, the different groups receiving different dilutions. The $LD_{50}$ dose of the virus is that which kills three out of six mice of the unvaccinated group. This is called the MLD of the virus strain, since it is very close to it. The immunity end point of the immunized mice is determined by the largest dose of virus that is successfully resisted by three out of six mice. The protective value of the particular vaccine is judged by the ratio existing between the $LD_{50}$ doses of virus for the protected and the unprotected mice. Using vaccines of his own manufacture, Habel found that he could induce protection against as much as 50,000 MLD. He suggested that a requirement of at least 1,000 MLD for all commercial products was reasonable. This standard is now enforced for all inactivated vaccines sold in the United States.

In his studies on commercial vaccines, using the procedure just described, Habel (17) found that only 12 of 31 protected against as much as 100 MLD, and some gave no protection whatsoever. Of these 31 strains, 25 originated from the old Pasteur fixed-virus strain. Some of the potent strains originated from ones which were now found to be impotent. It was apparent that in the course of propagating these strains by different people, using different animals and slightly different methods, unsuspected changes had occurred affecting their usefulness. Government control agencies immediately required all manufacturers to acquire satisfactory virus strains and to test each lot henceforth for antigenicity.

The phenol-inactivated vaccines, as already noted above, have been widely used with very satisfactory results. Johnson (23) carried out experiments with dogs which showed clearly that a single dose of phenol-inactivated vaccine would give strong protection when challenged at 1 month, and very satisfactory protection when challenged after 1 year. Using 52 vaccinated and 52 control dogs, he challenged all after 1 year by injecting a potent street virus strain intramuscularly. Only 6 of the vaccinated succumbed as against 41 of the controls. He also tried three injections on 25 dogs to learn whether better protection could be engendered. Upon challenge 1 year later, 17 of the 25 control dogs died but none of the vaccinated.

Inactivated duck-embryo vaccine. A strain of rabies virus has been adapted to embryonated ducks' eggs. After beta-propiolactone inactivation it is then used as a vaccine which elicits a good antibody response in humans (46). At present it is the vaccine of choice for humans.

Inactivated tissue-cultured vaccine. The CVS strain is propagated in hamster kidney cell cultures. The phenolized vaccine contains virus that is propagated on primary hamster kidney cells. In the formolized vaccine product virus is propagated in serum-free medium. Although the titer is lower due to the absence of serum the use of an oil-in-water adjuvant reputedly enhances the immune response to the virus.

Passive immunization. As early as 1889 Babes and Lepp (15) showed that it was possible to prevent the development of rabies in animals by injecting a specific antiserum simultaneously with, or shortly after, a dose of active virus. The use of antiserum in field practice is a comparatively recent development. Interest in the United States in this approach was stimulated by a paper by Habel (19) in 1945. He and others who have studied the subject more recently have shown that antiserum will give better results in protecting inoculated animals than multiple doses of phenol-inactivated vaccine, and that antiserum and vaccine will give better results than either alone. To be effective it appears that the serum must be given as soon as possible after the exposure. When given after the 3rd day, it is not effective in saving the life of the animal but it generally results in a considerable lengthening of the period of incubation.

Rabies antiserum is at present used for prophylaxis in people who have been exposed after a skin test for serum sensitivity is performed. It appears to be particularly useful in those cases in which the incubation period is likely to be short and in which vaccines are generally useless since their effect is too belated. In such cases antiserum is first given followed immediately by a course of vaccine treatments. Up to the present there has been little or no use of antiserum on animals.

*Interferon.* There is evidence accumulating that interferon inducers produce interferon levels in laboratory animals such as the rabbit which protects them against challenge with lethal doses of rabies virus. To be protective the inducer must be given to the animals before virus challenge or within a few hours after injection of virus. These results suggest that interferon inducers may be used as a future means of treating individuals immediately after a bite by a rabid animal.

*Recommended vaccination procedures.* Various agencies have been involved in the development of recommended vaccination procedures, notably the World Health Organization and the United States Public Health Service. More recently, through colloquia conceived and cosponsored by the American Veterinary Medical Association, recommended procedures for vaccination of domestic animals, particularly the dog and cat, have emerged in the last 3 years. American Veterinary Medical Association Panels (3, 4), while recognizing that local rabies statutes must be given preference, suggest the following guidelines to veterinary practitioners for their rabies vaccination programs.

*Dogs.* The low-egg passage (LEP) Flury rabies vaccine should be used only in dogs. It should be administered only intramuscularly in the hindlimb. High-egg passage (HEP) chicken-embryo origin rabies vaccines are not recommended for dogs. The general guidelines for the dog are given in Table XXXVII.

Table XXXVII.  SUMMARY OF CANINE RABIES VACCINES AND USES

| Vaccine | Strain | Dosages available | Route of administration | Age to vaccinate |
|---|---|---|---|---|
| Inactivated | | | | |
|   Nerve tissue | Fixed | 5 ml * | sc | 4 months |
|   Cell-culture origin | Fixed | 2 ml and 5 ml | sc or im | 4 months |
| Attenuated | | | | |
|   Chicken-embryo origin | Flury LEP** | 2 ml and 3 ml | im | 4 months |
|   Cell-culture origin | Flury LEP** | 1 ml and 2 ml | im | 4 months |
| | Flury HEP | 1 ml | im | 4 months |
| | ERA | 2 ml | im | 4 months |

* Increase dose if large dog.   ** Administer only to dogs, in hindlimb.

Limited data indicate that many attenuated vaccines confer immunity in most dogs for about 3 years. However, some dogs fail to respond adequately to the initial vaccination. A few dogs are immunized but become susceptible to rabies again in 1 or 2 years. Consequently, annual revaccination will provide the greatest assurance that an individual dog is continually immune to rabies, but in 1973, the AVMA panel recommended vaccination every 3 years.

The ability of pups to respond to rabies vaccine increases with time up to 4 months of age. The immune response in younger pups is variable, and immunization may be unsuccessful in pups less than 3 months old. All pups vaccinated when younger than 4 months old, regardless of the type of vaccine used, should be revaccinated when 1 year old.

*Cats.* The vaccines listed in Table XXXVIII are safe and efficacious for the cat. They should be used only for cats or other species as specified on the manufacturer's label instructions. Because there is limited data on the safety of live virus for pregnant animals, its use in pregnant animals is not recommended at this time.

*Table XXXVIII.* SUMMARY OF RABIES VACCINES AVAILABLE FOR USE IN CATS

| Vaccines | Strain | Dosages available | Administration route |
|---|---|---|---|
| Modified live-virus, chicken-embryo origin, high-egg passage | Flury | 1 ml | im |
| Modified live-virus, tissue-culture origin, high-egg passage | Flury | 1 ml | im |
| Modified live-virus, tissue-culture origin | ERA | 2 ml | im |
| Killed virus, tissue-culture origin* | Fixed | 1 ml | im |
| | | 1 ml | sc or im |
| | | 3 ml | sc or im |
| | | 2 ml | sc or im |
| Killed virus, caprine origin* | Fixed | 3 ml | sc or im |
| | | 3 ml | sc |

im = intramuscular; sc = subcutaneous.
* The various doses and routes of administration represent recommendations by different producers for their products.

The Panel concurred generally with recommendations of the U.S. Public Health Service (52) reported at the Colloquium:

All cats should be vaccinated annually with a rabies vaccine licensed for use in cats. Cats should be vaccinated initially when they are between 5 and 6 months of age. Any of the vaccines other than those containing low egg passage (LEP)-Flury strain of virus may be used. LEP-Flury vaccine may produce clinical rabies in cats.

Limited data indicate that some vaccines confer immunity for longer than one year. However, some animals fail to respond adequately to initial vaccination. Annual revaccination will provide the greatest assurance that an individual cat is continually immune to rabies.

The ability of kittens to respond to rabies vaccine is variable. Immunization may be unsuccessful in kittens less than 4 months old. If a kitten is vaccinated when less than 4 months old, regardless of vaccine type used, it should be revaccinated when 5 to 6 months old.

Rabies is infrequently diagnosed in cats. However, their hunting and prowling habits bring them into contact with many wild animals which serve as reservoirs for rabies. Vaccination of cats allowed to roam outside should therefore be encouraged.

*Other domestic animals.* Cattle are occasionally vaccinated against rabies in the United States. The HEP-CEO vaccine is safe and efficacious in this species. The ERA vaccine also is safe in cattle and produces an immunity which persists for at least 4 years (36).

Phenolized rabies vaccine produces an immunity in horses (39). Horses of various ages were given two subcutaneous injections of 5 ml of the inactivated vaccine 1 week apart and all had neutralizing antibody when tested 40 days later. Revaccination with a 3 ml subcutaneous injection of the same vaccine 18 months after the initial vaccination caused a significant increase in titer. In unusual situations where rabies immunization of horses is indicated the above procedure should protect horses against rabies.

There is little satisfactory information on the rabies immunization of other species. Perhaps the wisest procedure would be the use of inactivated virus vaccine. Certainly, the manufacturer of the biologic should be consulted regarding its safety, efficacy, dosage, and age of vaccination before use in these species.

**Transmission.** Rabies is usually transmitted when the virus reaches and is eliminated by the salivary glands. Infections are set up in other individuals by the entrance of this infected saliva into their tissues through wounds or abrasions. Usually this is accomplished through bite wounds, but infections may also occur through contamination of existing wounds with salivary virus. Persons have been infected through scratch wounds or by contaminating existing abrasions on the hands while endeavoring to find the "bone in the throat" of dogs with rabic pharyngeal paralysis. Constantine also suggests that rabies transmission can occur by aerosol (9).

Because of its unusual mode of transmission the disease is very seldom transmitted by herbivorous animals. Of the domestic animals only the dog and cat are of any importance in this respect. Insectivorous and fruit-eating bats also play important roles in rabies transmission. It should be kept in mind, however, that virus is eliminated through the saliva by all species of animals, and such animals should be handled by human attendants with due care.

It has been demonstrated by several workers that virus sometimes appears in the saliva before recognizable signs of the disease have appeared. Nicolas (43) demonstrated salivary virus in one dog on the 5th day prior to the appearance of signs; others have reported the 2nd and 3rd days. In dogs and most animals, virus has never been found in the salivary gland when it was absent from the brain. This finding has been reported, however, in vampire bats.

Virus does not invariably appear in the saliva of rabid animals. Whether it does or not, or the frequency with which it appears, apparently depends upon the strain of virus and the animal species in which it develops. Fixed virus (see p. 1153) strains apparently never appear in the saliva of any animal. In the vampire bat, virus apparently has a strong predilection for the salivary glands, since in this species the saliva may be infectious for long periods while no nervous signs are exhibited. In studies reported by Johnson (24), 21 of 28 dogs in which virus had been demonstrated in the brain showed virus in their salivary glands (75 percent). In rabid foxes, salivary virus was demonstrated in 130 of 150 animals (87 percent); in rabid cattle, the ratio was 16 : 34 (53 percent).

The natural reservoir of rabies is in wild carnivora. In the United States wild foxes are reservoir hosts in many parts of the eastern portion of the country. In the north-central states skunks have been the main offenders. In the prairie states ground squirrels, ordinary squirrels, and coyotes harbor the disease. In South Africa (53) and many other areas the mongoose is the principal reservoir. Wolves (40) are the principal hosts in many undeveloped areas of the world. In Trinidad and much of South and Central America, the vampire bat (*Desmodus rotundus*) is the principal host. In areas where the vampire bat occurs, rabies has been recognized in fruit-eating and insectivorous bats, but it was supposed that these infections had been contracted from the blood-eating vampire. In 1953 a case of rabies was diagnosed in an insectivorous bat in Florida (48). This area is far outside the range of the vampire. Shortly afterward incidents and surveys brought to light the fact that rabies occurred in bats in a great many parts of the United States (8, 66). Cases have been recognized in about 40 states so situated as to suggest that the disease probably occurs in all. They have been found in three Canadian provinces (Beauregard, 6) and in several countries of Europe (56).

It has been presumed that the nonhemophagous bats constitued a reservoir of infection for man and animals, but this has not yet been satifactorily proved. These bats, when rabid, often attack man and animals. There have been no proved natural transmissions to animals, but there appear to be several well-documented cases in people. Certainly it seems that the disease is not very frequently transmitted to other species of animals by bats other than the vampires.

Domestic animals and man have often been infected by these wild animal hosts. In large cities and in densely populated areas where wild animals have been driven out, dogs constitute the host species. In many ways these animals are more dangerous for man than wild animals, because of their intimate relationships with him.

It has long been recognized that not all bite wounds made by animals suffering from rabies result in the disease. As a matter of fact, it is estimated that before prophlyactic treatment for rabies was developed, not more than one-fifth of all persons bitten actually developed the disease. We know that many rabid animals do not have virus in their saliva and thus are incapable of transmitting the disease, even though the disease causes them to attack and bite others. Also it is known that the dosage factor is important and that many minor bite wounds and scratches do not become contaminated with enough virus to establish infection. This is particularly true of bites through thick hair coats or, in the case of people, through clothing both of which undoubtedly soak up much of the saliva and prevent its entering the wound.

Rabies virus has been detected by a few workers in mammary tissue and in milk. Even if milk were regularly and heavily infected, and apparently this is not the case, there is practically no danger of the transmission of the disease by the ingestion of milk. In the past, various individuals failed to transmit rabies by ingestion. More recently, Fischman and Ward (14) reported that oral transmission was routinely observed in mother mice following cannibalism of their infant mice previously infected with virus. Transmission of virus to infant mice from an infected mother was demonstrated on rare occasions. This was not readily reproducible so this mechanism of transmission from mother to offspring is unclear.

Remlinger and Bailly (47) fed dog ticks (*Rhipicephalus sanguineus*) on two inoculated dogs and later were able to demonstrate rabies virus in the ticks. They did not determine whether or not these ticks could transmit the disease naturally. Konradi (30) claimed to have demonstrated rabies virus in the fetuses of pregnant, rabid dogs. These findings indicate that the virus of rabies occurs in the blood at times. Generally, attempts to demonstrate virus in the blood fail.

**Diagnosis.** The signs of rabies are so characteristic in most instances that a diagnosis may be made from the clinical signs. This is not always true, however, especially in animals that are not commonly affected by the disease. In several instances, diseases that have been diagnosed as encephalitis, both in man and animals, were proved to be rabies. The nature of the disease, when the clinical diagnosis is not clear, can be confirmed only by laboratory examinations. The most important of these are:

1. *By mouse inoculation.* Swiss mice are regularly susceptible when inoculated intracerebrally with test suspensions. Leach (37) suggests that a 27-gauge needle one-fourth inch long be used and that this be forced directly into the brain at right angles with the external surface at a point a little off the median line and about halfway between the eyes and the ears. The mouse should be etherized before the injection is made. The material for injection is prepared by grinding a part of the Ammon's horn in a sterile mortar, suspending it in sterile broth in a proportion of one part of brain to nine of broth, and then centrifuging the mixture at 2,000 rpm for 5 minutes. The opalescent supernatant fluid is used for inoculation. For the mouse the standard dose is 0.03 ml injected with a 0.25-ml tuberculin syringe.

Paralysis of the hind legs of inoculated mice may occur as early as the 7th day or as late as the 25th day, and this is followed by death within 24 hours. Convulsions may be observed just before the paralytic signs occur. Although the incubation period is variable, the majority of inoculated mice show signs and die between the 8th and 14th days. When several mice are inoculated with the same material containing rabies virus, it is unusual for none of them to show within 10 days. It is not unusual, however, for one or two of them to exhibit longer incubation periods, and even for some of them to escape the infection entirely. This emphasizes the fact that several animals should always be inoculated with suspected material.

Wilsnack and Parker (64) stated that the mouse-inoculation test is not accurate in detecting the presence of rabies antigen in the salivary glands and brains of infected animals because such tissues contain a material termed rabies-inhibiting substance (RIS), which renders the rabies virus nonlethal for mice by the intracerebral route. RIS does not impede detection of rabies antigen by immunofluorescent staining. Guinea pigs and rabbits usually exhibit longer incubation periods than mice, and some periods are much longer. Occasionally these species pass through a siege of convulsions before paralytic signs develop. Negri bodies can be found in the brains of animals inoculated with street virus (see p. 1153) by the time that signs are evident. Leach (37) states that they may sometimes be found in white mice as early as the 5th day after inoculation. When several animals have been inoculated and it is important that an early diagnosis be given, it is recommended to sacrifice one or two of them as soon as signs are seen in order to hurry the search for Negri bodies.

If it has been demonstrated satisfactorily that an encephalitis-producing virus is concerned in a particular disease but it is not clear whether the virus is that of rabies or not, the specific identification can be made by conducting a virus-neutralization test. With an antiserum for rabies virus, tests may be conducted on Swiss mice to determine whether the questionable virus is, or is not, neutralized by it *in vitro*. Inasmuch as there is no plurality of viruses in this disease, so far as has been demonstrated, neutralization with a known antirabies serum indicates that the unknown virus is that of rabies.

2. *By the demonstration of Negri bodies.* In 1903 Negri (42) described the inclusion bodies which now bear his name. These bodies are specific for rabies; thus their identification makes it possible to diagnose the disease very quickly and with certainty. If they are not found, it is not permissible, however, to assume that the disease is not rabies, since a certain number of cases of the disease do not exhibit recognizable Negri bodies, and in others they are sparse and may be overlooked. Koch and Jahn (29) in Berlin reported that of 4,682 positive laboratory diagnoses, 4,125 (88.1 percent) disclosed Negri bodies and 557 (11.9 percent) failed to show them but were positive on animal inoculation. Damon and Sellers (10) in the United States found 189 (12.3 percent) of 1,531 cases positive by inoculation but negative microscopically. Hagan and Evans (21) in a fox-borne outbreak in New York found only 3.1 percent of rabid fox brains negative for Negri bodies but positive on inoculation, but the percentage amounted to 12.6 percent in cattle and 19.3 percent in dogs.

Negri bodies are not found in fixed virus infections in any species; hence these can be diagnosed only by the signs induced in experimental animals and confirmed by neutralization tests.

Negri bodies occur in the cytoplasm of nerve cells in all parts of the brain and spinal cord. They are usually numerous in the hippocampal convolution, or Ammon's horn, of the cerebrum and this part is usually chosen for examination. Smears, impression preparations, or sections may be made. Near the periphery of the convolution large triangular motor nerve cells are found, forming an almost continuous line. In these cells the Negri bodies are found. Similar cells are found also in the cerebellum at the juncture of the white and gray matter, and these also usually contain Negri bodies. In many cattle and horse brains Negri bodies may be found in the cerebellum when they are absent in Ammon's horn.

Negri bodies are found in the cytoplasm, never in the nucleus. They are spherical or oval bodies that vary in size from less than 1 micron in diameter to as much as 30 microns. From one to a half-dozen may be found in a single cell. The smaller bodies may be a hyaline appearance, but the larger ones often show a number of poorly staining "inside" bodies. The Negri bodies are acidophilic. They may be differentially stained by a number of methods.

3. *By fluorescent antibody technic.* This method is supplanting the use of mice in the diagnosis of rabies. The correlation between this procedure and mouse inoculation is remarkably good, but the immunofluorescence staining test is more sensitive and accurate than the other two methods for diagnosis. Consequently it is the test of choice for the diagnosis of rabies. It is advisable

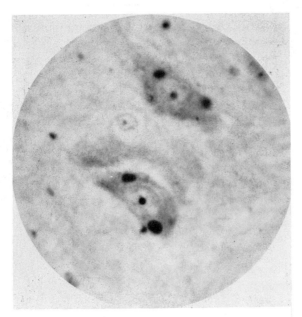

*Fig. 227.* Negri bodies in motor cells of Ammon's horn in a dog. The clear vesicular nuclei with sharply stained nucleoli occupy the center of the cells. The Negri bodies are located outside the nuclei in the cytoplasm. X 1,200. (Courtesy S. H. McNutt.)

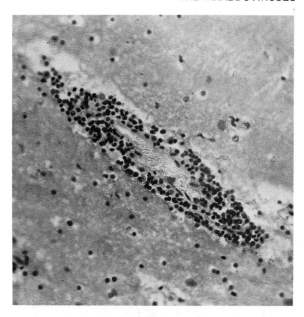

*Fig. 228.* Rabies, showing peri-vascular cuffing in Ammon's horn in a rabbit's brain. X 320. (Courtesy S. H. McNutt.)

to run the mouse inoculation test in conjunction with this method to detect the odd case that is positive by mouse inoculation and is negative by the im-munofluorescence test.

The immunofluorescence test detects rabies antigen present in the tissues under inspection. Like the Negri body procedure a diagnosis can be made the same day the suspect brain is presented at the laboratory, but the fluorescent antibody diagnostic procedure is more accurate and sensitive. Residual virus may be found on slides after fixation unless the smear preparation is exposed to a fixative such as ethanol at 4 C for 4 hours. Ethanol fixation provides for excellent conjugate staining.

**Control Measures.** Because rabies is transmitted almost exclusively by the bites of rabid animals, its control depends upon the success achieved in controlling the activities of the species that is acting as the resevoir in a particular area. If the reservoir is in wild animals—in foxes, wildcats, bats, mongooses—the disease can be eliminated only by destroying these animals or by greatly reducing the population. This often is a very difficult and even an insoluble problem in some parts of the world.

When the dog is the principal reservoir host, the problem is simple in theory but often difficult in practice. England has eliminated rabies on several occasions by simple quarantine measures. Owners are required to keep their dogs under control at all times, and ownerless dogs are caught and impounded until owners are found for them, or they are destroyed. When the co-operation of the people can be obtained so that these measures can be made effective for 6 months, rabies will disappear. England and Australia have been successful in preventing the entrance of the disease over long periods by requiring a 6-month quarantine on all imported dogs. Hawaii has been equally successful with a 4-month period.

Muzzling of dogs has been employed as a means of rabies control. It is of limited value. Effective muzzles are hard to keep in place on certain dogs, some types are not effective, and many sympathetic people object to them and will not co-operate in their use.

In the United States vaccination of dogs has come to be an important factor in the control of rabies. If the reservoir of the infection is in dogs, the method is very effective. This has been demonstrated in many localities by the rapid subsidence of the disease after mass vaccination of dogs (Brueckner, 7). When the reservoir is in animals other than dogs, vaccination of dogs is effective in preventing the establishment of a secondary reservoir in that species (Korns and Zeissig, 35).

Most of the dog and other animal immunizations are carried out on individuals that have not been known to have been exposed, and the recommended procedures outlined above are based on this assumption. If a dog or cat has been bitten by an animal known to have had rabies, it is generally best to urge the owner to consent to destroying the animal, since one cannot be sure that rabies will be prevented and one may risk human exposure if the animal becomes rabid. If the owner insists on keeping the animal, it may be given multiple injections of vaccine and kept under secure control for at least 4 months. Other farm animals may be treated with multiple injections of vaccine in the same way, but there is no reliable data on whether enough animals will be saved to pay for the cost of the vaccine.

Compulsory vaccination of dogs has been found difficult to administer effectively in the United States because of lack of co-operation by many dog owners. New York State has found it better to carry out a well-organized educational program among dog owners, to provide free vaccination clinics in all involved areas, and to offer inducements to owners to have their dogs immunized. The inducement is that all dogs that carry special tags on their collars indicating that they have been vaccinated are allowed to be at large, whereas those who do not have such tags, when found at large, are retained by dog catchers and impounded. Owners may reclaim their pets only after paying a fine, and if the animal is not claimed within a reasonable time, it may be destroyed or a new owner found for it. In an infected district such freedom is not permitted until 30 days after attendance at the vaccination clinic in order that the dog may be fully protected before it is allowed to risk exposure.

**Postvaccinal Paralysis.** In a small percentage of individuals, both human and animal, who have been vaccinated with antirabic vaccines made from nerve tissue, postvaccinal paralysis develops. In man, one serious case occurs in several thousand vaccinations. Cases are probably somewhat more numerous than this in dogs; nevertheless the incidence is very low. At first when the

Pasteur vaccine was commonly used, it was thought that these might be cases of fixed-virus rabies infections, or perhaps street virus infections that had been modified by the use of vaccine. Some fixed-virus infections have been found. When only inactivated vaccines were used and there had been no natural exposure, other explanations had to be sought. It is now believed that these effects are due to reactions, probably of an allergic nature, to constituents of the nerve tissue.

Many of these reactions in animals are mild and transient, but others may result in permanent damage. The signs generally do not appear sooner than 5 days after vaccination and sometimes considerably later. The paralysis may involve only a few muscles. Frequently this occurs in the extremity in which the vaccine was injected. Sometimes the paralysis gradually extends and death finally results. The signs are the result of a demyelinating process which occurs in the brain or spinal cord, or both.

The proponents of the avianized vaccines, tissue-culture origin vaccines, and the duck-embryo vaccine claim that they do not cause postvaccinal paralysis.

**The Disease in Man.** Rabies in man presents essentially the same picture as that seen in animals. Both furious and paralytic forms of the disease occur, the latter being the most common. The incubation period varies within wide limits—from about 12 days to 6 or more months, but the average is between 30 and 60 days. Bites on the face generally have a short incubation period. The course of the disease is short—only a few days—and the mortality is practically 100 percent. There are no records of rabies being transmitted by a human case, but the saliva is often infective and attendants should be cautious in handling bed clothing and other materials contaminated with it. The number of cases of rabies diagnosed in man in the United States averages about 30 a year; hence it is not a very significant disease statistically. It has already been pointed out, however, that the mental anguish caused those who have been exposed to it and the discomfort of some thousands of persons who each year take prophylactic treatments for it make it a far more important public health hazard than statistics indicate.

Mass vaccination of people is not done. This is partly because of the postvaccinal accidents which, even though rare, must be considered. Vaccine generally is given only when an exposure, or a possible exposure, has occurred. In these cases, the best course is to first give one dose of antirabic serum followed immediately by a regular course of vaccine treatments. In this country the Semple type of vaccine was most commonly employed, although irradiated vaccines were used to some extent. Antiserum is particularly indicated for severe bites and especially for those around the head, since these usually have a short incubation period. In such cases vaccine therapy alone fails more frequently than it succeeds. It has been shown in experimental animals that serum has a decided tendency to prolong incubation periods. It is probably this effect that enhances the vaccine when it is used with serum; i.e., the serum prolongs the incubation period giving the vaccine time to stimulate the protection needed.

A comparison by Greenberg and Childress in 1960 (16) was made of general and local reactions and the antibody titers produced in 123 patients given an injection of duck-embryo vaccine and 127 patients given Semple vaccine. Duck-embryo vaccine stimulated an earlier production of antibodies, but the range of titers between the 11th and 15th day was not significantly different. Booster effects were obtained with both vaccines. The complication of encephalomyelitis did not occur after the use of duck-embryo vaccine but did occur in two patients given the brain tissue vaccine. Tierkel and Sikes (58) made a comparative study of vaccines of chick and duck origin and concluded that the most practical regimen consists of two subcutaneous injections of 1 ml of duck embryo vaccine given 1 month apart followed by revaccination again at 7 months after the second injection. Shipley and Jubelt (51) recommended that all known human exposures should be given at least 1 booster injection of duck-embryo vaccine. On the basis of these studies duck-embryo vaccine has supplanted brain tissues vaccine for the prophylaxis of rabies is high risk groups. For more complete information about rabies prevention in man the reader is referred to the report of the WHO Expert Committee on Rabies (61).

## REFERENCES

1. Abelseth.    Canad. Vet. Jour., 1964, 5, 279.
2. Almeida.    Virology, 1962, 18, 147.
3. American Veterinary Medical Association.    Panel Rpt., Canine Inf. Dis. Symposium, Jour. Am. Vet. Med. Assoc., 1970, 156, 1664.
4. American Veterinary Medical Association.    Ibid., 1971, 158, 840.
5. Babes and Lepp.    Ann. l'Inst. Past., 1889, 3, 384.
6. Beauregard.    Canad. Jour. Compar. Med., 1969, 33, 220.
7. Brueckner.    Proc. U.S. Livestock San. Assoc., 1944, 48, 78.
8. Burns and Farinacci.    Science, 1954, 120, 548.
9. Constantine.    Pub. Health Rpts. (U.S.), 1962, 77, 287.
10. Damon and Sellers.    Vet. Med., 1942, 37, 253.
11. Darbyshire.    Vet. Rec., 1953, 65, 261.
12. Dawson.    Am. Jour. Pub. Health, 1941, 17, 177.
13. Eichhorn and Lyon.    Jour. Am. Vet. Med. Assoc., 1922, 61, 38.
14. Fischman and Ward.    Am. Jour. Epidemiol., 1968, 88, 132.
15. Goldwasser, Kissling, Carski, and Host.    Bul. World Health Org., 1959, 20, 579.
16. Greenberg and Childress.    Jour. Am. Med. Assoc., 1960, 173, 333.
17. Habel.    Pub. Health Rpts. (U.S.), 1940, 55 (II), 1473.
18. Ibid., 1619.
19. Ibid., 1945, 60, 545.
20. Ibid., 1947, 62, 791.
21. Hagan and Evans.    Proc. 14th Internat. Vet. Cong., London, 1949, II, 457.

22.  Hodes, Lavin and Webster.   Science, 1937, *86*, 447.
23.  Johnson.   Proc. U.S. Livestock San. Assoc., 1945, *49*, 99.
24.  Johnson.   In: Virus and rickettsial infections of man. 2d ed. Lippincott, Philadelphia, 1952, p. 267.
25.  Kelser.   Jour. Am. Vet. Med. Assoc., 1930, 77, 595.
26.  King, Croghan, and Shaw.   Canad. Vet. Jour., 1965, *6*, 187.
27.  Kissling.   Proc. Soc. Exp. Biol. and Med., 1958, *98*, 223.
28.  Kligler and Bernkopf.   *Ibid.*, 1938, *39*, 212.
29.  Koch and Jahn.   In: Kolle and Wassermann. Handbuch der pathogenen Mikroorganismen. 3d ed. G. Fischer, Jena, 1930, vol. *III*.
30.  Konradi.   Centrbl. f. Bakt., I, Abt., Orig., 1908, *47*, 203.
31.  Koprowski and Black.   Jour. Immunol., 1950, *64*, 185.
32.  Koprowski and Black.   Proc. Soc. Exp. Biol. and Med., 1952, *80*, 410.
33.  Koprowski and Black.   Jour. Immunol., 1954, *72*, 503.
34.  Koprowski and Cox.   *Ibid.*, 1948, *60*, 533.
35.  Korns and Zeissig.   Am. Jour. Pub. Health, 1948, *38*, 50.
36.  Lawson, Walker, and Crawley.   Vet. Med., 1967, *62*, 1073.
37.  Leach.   *Ibid.*, 1938, *28*, 162.
38.  Leach and Johnson.   Am. Jour. Trop. Med., 1940, *20*, 335.
39.  Marx and Sikes.   Jour. Am. Vet. Med. Assoc., 1966, *149*, 1159.
40.  McMahon.   Vet. Rec., 1935, *15*, 1464.
41.  Metevier.   Jour. Comp. Path. and Therap., 1935, *48*, 245.
42.  Ñegri.   Zeitschr. f. Hyg., 1903, *43*, 507.
43.  Nicholas.   Comp. rend. Soc. Biol. (Paris), 1906, *60*, 625.
44.  Pasteur.   Comp. rend. Acad. Sci., 1881–1886. A series of papers.
45.  Pawan.   Ann. Trop. Med. and Parasitol., 1936, *30*, 401.
46.  Peck, Powell, and Culbertson.   Jour. Am. Med. Assoc., 1956, *162*, 1373.
47.  Remlinger and Bailly.   Ann. l'Inst. Past., 1939, *62*, 463.
48.  Scatterday and Galton.   Vet. Med., 1954, *49*, 133.
49.  Schroeder, Black, Burkhart, and Koprowski.   *Ibid.*, 1952, *47*, 502.
50.  Semple.   Sci. Mem., Off. Med. and San. Depts., Govt. India, Calcutta, n.s. 44, 1911.
51.  Shipley and Jubelt.   Jour. Am. Vet. Med. Assoc., 1968, *153*, 1771.
52.  Sikes.   *Ibid.*, 1971, *158*, 1006.
53.  Snyman.   Jour. So. African Vet. Med. Assoc., 1937, 8, 126.
54.  Sokolov and Vanag.   Acta Virol. (Eng. ed.), 1962, *6*, 452.
55.  Starr, Sellers, and Sunkes.   Jour. Am. Vet. Med. Assoc., 1952, *121*, 296.
56.  Tierkel.   In: Brandly and Jungherr.   Advances in veterinary science, Academic Press, New York, 1959, vol. V, p. 183.
57.  Tierkel, Kissling, Eidson, and Habel.   Proc. Am. Vet. Med. Assoc., 1953, p. 443.
58.  Tierkel and Sikes.   Jour. Am. Med. Assoc., 1967, *201*, 911.
59.  Umeno and Doi.   Kitasato Arch. Exp. Med., 1920–21, *4*, 89.
60.  Van Rooyen and Rhodes.   Virus diseases of man. 2d ed. Thos. Nelson and Sons, New York, 1948.
61.  WHO Expert Committee on Rabies.   WHO Tech. Rep. Series no. 321, WHO, Geneva, Switzerland, 1966.
62.  Webster.   Jour. Exp. Med., 1939, *70*, 87.

63. Webster and Clow. *Ibid.*, 1937, *66*, 125.
64. Wilsnack and Parker. Am. Jour. Vet. Res., 1966, *27*, 39.
65. Witkor, Fernandes, and Koprowski. Jour. Immunol., 1964, *93*, 353.
66. Witte. Am. Jour. Pub. Health, 1954, *44*, 186.

### Lagos Bat Virus and Shrew Virus

The Lagos bat virus and an isolate from shrews (Ib An 27377), both from Nigerian hosts, showed a relationship to rabies virus (3).

Both viruses were bullet-shaped, a characteristic of the genus *Rhabdovirus*, and they matured intracytoplasmically in association with a distinct matrix. By the use of reciprocal complement-fixation tests, rabies, Lagos bat, and the shrew viruses clearly were shown to share a common CF antigen. The same reagents employed in reciprocal CF tests with other members of the genus *Rhabdovirus* gave negative results. Reciprocal neutralization tests in mice between the three viruses further demonstrated the relationship as there was neutralization to all three viruses but the three agents were readily distinguishable by this test.

Minor antigenic differences among rabies strains have been reported (1, 2), but the magnitude of these differences was not comparable to those observed for the Lagos bat virus, shrew virus, and rabies virus. The authors suggest that the degree of cross-reactivity between the three viruses substantiates a distinct subgrouping within the genus *Rhabdovirus* (3).

### REFERENCES

1. Crandell. Proc., Natl. Rabies Sympos, Natl. Commun. Dis. Center, Atlanta, Ga., 1966, 37.
2. Johnson. Am. Jour. Hyg., 1948, *47*, 189.
3. Shope, Murphy, Harrison, Causey, Kemp, Simpson, and Moore. Virology, 1970, *6*, 690.

### Vesicular Stomatitis

SYNONYMS: Sore mouth of cattle and horses, possibly the same as mycotic stomatitis, *mal de yerbe* (Mexico); abbreviation, VS

The disease occurs naturally among horses, cattle, and swine. Formerly it was recognized most often among horses; in more recent years it has occurred chiefly in cattle. Until very recently the disease was rarely recognized in swine, but it is now known that the disease is enzootic in swine in some regions (17). Serological evidence that the disease occurs in feral swine, raccoons, and deer in the southeastern part of the United States has been obtained, and the susceptibility of deer has been confirmed by inoculation tests (8).

A number of human infections have been recognized, mostly in laboratory workers. It is probable that such cases occur naturally in the field. By experimental inoculation the disease has been produced in sheep, hamsters, ferrets, and chinchillas. Dogs appear to be resistant.

VS is said to have occurred in Europe and South Africa before the time of World War I, but if so it attracted little attention. Undoubtedly it had also occurred in the United States at an earlier date, but it is not clearly recognized as a distinct entity until 1916. At that time a great many horses were purchased from farms in the midwest for the use of the armies in Europe. The disease was observed in France and then was traced back to the collection centers and the eastern shipping ports in the United States. Outbreaks occurred also in cattle, in which it was first thought to be foot-and-mouth disease. The disease was recognized to be contagious, but the causative virus was not determined until 10 years later.

VS occurs sporadically in the United States and Canada. Outbreaks are seen only during the months of July, August, September, and October with the highest incidence rate falling in September. The disease disappears promptly after killing frosts in the fall.

During the foot-and-mouth outbreak in Mexico (1946–1954) it was discovered that VS was prevalent in the more tropical parts. It occurred at all times of the year. Disease outbreaks have occurred in Argentina and Brazil (5). Hanson (7) suggests that the sporadic outbreaks in the United States and Canada may have their origin in this permanent reservoir.

**Character of the Disease.** As a rule this disease, *per se,* is not very serious. When it occurs in cattle or swine, its principal significance is that it may not be distinguished readily from foot-and-mouth disease. If naturally infected horses are found, or if horses are successfully infected by artificial inoculation, FMD can definitely be ruled out, because horses are not susceptible to the virus of that disease.

The signs of this disease have been described by Mohler (12). In horses and cattle the principal lesions are found in the mouth. Vesicles that may not be distinguished from those of FMD may be found on the tongue of the mucosa of the oral cavity. Apparently in many outbreaks in cattle vesiculation of the mouth cavity is not common, the lesions appearing only as papules. Vesicles, when present, appear early in the course of the disease and disappear quickly. Before these appear the animals suffer from a febrile reaction, and there may be some inappetence. When the vesicles appear, the animals champ their jaws, drool a clear, ropy saliva from their lips, and generally refuse feed but eagerly accept water. Horses often rub their lips on the edges of the mangers, or other objects, manifesting itchiness. Unlike FMD, secondary lesions on other parts of the body are uncommon in horses and cattle in most outbreaks. Hanson (7) reports, however, that in one outbreak foot lesions occurred in cattle in about 50 percent of all cases. In swine, foot lesions apparently are quite common (16, 18). Teat lesions occur rather rarely in cattle in most outbreaks, yet Strozzi and Ramos-Saco (20) report an extensive outbreak in Peru in which the lesions were almost exclusively on the teats.

Apparently this is about the same as for FMD. Inoculated animals usually show signs within 24 hours of the time of inoculation.

In all species the course of the disease is short. After 3 or 4 days the animals usually resume normal eating habits and rapidly regain lost weight. The mouth lesions heal quickly without complications, and since these are the only lesions in most cases, the effects of the disease are much less severe than those of FMD. When foot lesions occur, bacterial complications may prolong the recovery time. In the uncomplicated cases, and most of them are of this type, the death loss is almost nil.

The lesions consist only of the vesicles that appear on the tongue and other parts of the oral mucosa, on the snouts of pigs, occasionally in the interdigital space of swine and cattle, rarely in the coronary band of horses, swine, and cattle, and sometimes on the surface of the udder and especially the teats of cattle. These vesicles cannot be distinguished from those of FMD.

**The Disease in Experimental Animals.** Horses, cattle, swine, and sheep are easily infected by inoculating them with virus into the epithelium of the dorsum of the tongue (intradermal lingual injection). Lesions generally appear within 24 hours. Only in rare instances do secondary lesions appear in the feet or elsewhere. Olitsky, Traum, and Schoening (13) pointed out that this virus differs from that of FMD in that it is not infective for cattle when inoculated intramuscularly.

Cotton (4) showed that the virus would cause infections in guinea pigs when it was injected into the footpads. The lesions cannot be distinguished from those of FMD. Kowalczyk and Brandly (11) showed that ferrets, chinchillas, and hamsters could be infected with the virus of VS but dogs proved resistant by all routes tested. The susceptible species were infected by intranasal instillation and by intracerebral injection. Ferrets survived inoculation by the intranasal route and sometimes by intracerebral injection but usually exhibited secondary lesions in the footpads. Hamsters and chinchillas succumbed the inoculation by both routes and never showed evidence of secondary lesions.

**Properties of the Virus.** The virus particles are rods, 176 by 69 m$\mu$, with the suggestion of a coiled headed filament capped by a spherical granule (2). Electron photographs by Reczko (15) showed rods, 154 by 57 m$\mu$, with one rounded and one truncate end, suggesting that the core consists of a helix with a hollow center. This virus is the type species for the genus *Rhabdovirus*.

It is an RNA virus inactivated in 30 minutes at 58 C and also by visible light as well as ultraviolet light. The virus is stable between a pH 4 or 5 and 10. It survives in the soil for many days at 4 to 6 C and for long periods of time an exceedingly low temperatures. It is ether sensitive because it contains considerable phospholipid. Interferon is produced in cell culture by the virus. It is somewhat more resistant to chemicals than FMDV. It is quickly destroyed by 1 percent formalin and by a number of ordinary commercial disinfectants. VSV resists normal pasteurization temperature.

Cotton (4) showed that there are two immunogenic types of VSV—New Jersey and Indiana. They are separable by neutralization and CF tests. There is one antigen, and possibly a second, common to the two serotypes. The more virulent New Jersey type occurs more frequently than the Indiana type in United States outbreaks.

A third type called Cocal virus was reported in 1964 (10). The agent is related to, but different from, type Indiana as determined by complement-fixation and neutralization tests. No relationship to the New Jersey type was detected. Its structure is similar to the Indiana and New Jersey types. Other variants have been isolated from birds in South Africa and Egypt and several genera of arthropods in the Caribbean and in Central and South America (1). In comparative studies with strains of VSV isolated in South America with Indiana C serotype, Federer et al. (5) demonstrated that the Argentina and Cocal strains were identical antigenically, but each differed considerably from Indiana C to the same degree as from the Brazil strain based upon complement-fixation tests and cross-neutralization tests. It was proposed that the three antigenic groups represented by these strains be referred to as subtypes.

**Cultivation.** Burnet and Galloway (3) cultivated VSV on the chorioallantoic membrane of the embryonated hens' eggs. The embryos die within 1 or 2 days, or survive showing proliferative and necrotic changes on the membrane. There is also good growth in the allantoic cavity.

The virus has a rapid cytopathogenic effect in fluid cell cultures of chick embryo or chick kidney, and on epithelial cultures of cattle, pig, rhesus monkey, and guinea pig. In the agar overlay system plaques are produced in the monolayer of kidney cells.

**Immunity.** Antisera can be prepared to neutralize this virus (21), but there are no practical uses for it. Horses and cattle that have recovered from natural infections maintain a serviceable immunity of at least 1 year's duration.

**Transmission.** It has long been recognized that VS does not spread nearly so readily as FMD. Because the virus is present in the saliva of affected animals, it has long been assumed that the disease was transmitted in a manner similar to FMD. This probably is correct for the New Jersey type, since there is no evidence to the contrary. On the other hand Ferris, Hanson, Dicke, and Roberts (6) have demonstrated the ability of a number of insects to transmit this virus. The stable fly (*Stomoxys calcitrans*), six species of tabanids, three species of *Chrysops,* and four species of mosquitoes were shown to be mechanical carriers of the virus. Indiana type virus has been isolated on four occasions from *Phlebotomus* sandflies collected in the tropical rain forest of Panama (19). While both types of spread probably occur, direct contact with infected animals appears to be more important than by arthropods.

**Diagnosis.** The problem in diagnosis is to distinguish this disease from foot-and-mouth disease. In a country like the United States where the latter does not occur, every outbreak has to be carefully examined with respect to the possibility of its being FMD. A mistake in one direction might lead to disastrous conditions; in the opposite direction it might lead to serious and expensive restrictions that are unnecessary.

When the disease affects horses, there is no serious diagnostic problem because horses are not susceptible to FMD. The disease has some resemblance to contagious pustular stomatitis, but the mouth lesions are quite different.

Differentiation of the VS virus from that of FMD can be accomplished by animal inoculation tests or by the complement-fixation test. These tests will be described under "Differentiation of the Viruses of Foot-and-Mouth Disease, Vesicular Stomatitis, and Vesicular Exanthema" (p. 1230). In laboratories equipped for the test, the complement-fixation test is much more rapid and at least as accurate as the animal tests. The only laboratory in the United States now able to make this test is the Plum Island Laboratory of the U.S. Department of Agriculture.

**Control.** Drastic control methods are not justified in view of the mildness which the disease usually exhibits. Infected premises should be quarantined and infected animals not moved until all signs have disappeared.

**The Disease in Man.** Clinical reports have been published from time to time suggesting human infections with VS virus. Hanson *et al.* (9) furnished satisfactory proof that human infections occur although they did not recover virus. During a period of 7 years while laboratory work and animal inoculation tests were going on at the Beltsville laboratories of the U.S. Department of Agriculture on this disease, 54 cases of human infections were recognized (14). These were observed in laboratory workers and animal handlers. The disease is comparatively mild and influenzalike. Characterized by sudden onset, fever, chills, malaise, the muscle soreness in most instances, mild stomatitis and tonsillitis are seen in some cases. A few show a diphasic fever curve, the second peak appearing 4 to 5 days after the first. Except for some malaise and weakness most victims completely recover within 1 week. After recovery neutralizing antibodies develop. A survey of the Beltsville situation showed that 96 percent of all personnel who had been associated with the VS project during the 7-year period carried neutralizing antibodies for the virus, but only 57 percent of these recalled any clinical symptoms which could be related to their period of infection. It appears that VS is a much more common disease of man than has previously been suspected.

**REFERENCES**

1. Andrewes.  Viruses of vertebrates. Williams and Wilkins, Baltimore, 1964.
2. Bradish, Brooksby, and Dillon.  Jour. Gen. Microbiol., 1956, *14*, 290.
3. Burnet and Galloway.  Brit. Jour. Exp. Path., 1934, *15*, 103.
4. Cotton.  Jour. Am. Vet. Med. Assoc., 1926, *69*, 313.
5. Federer, Burrows, and Brooksby.  Res. Vet. Sci., 1967, 8, 103.
6. Ferris, Hanson, Dicke, and Roberts.  Jour. Inf. Dis., 1955, *96*, 184.
7. Hanson.  Bact. Rev., 1952, *16*, 179.
8. Hanson and Karstad.  Proc. U.S. Livestock San. Assoc., 1958, *62*, 309.
9. Hanson, Rasmussen, Brandly, and Brown.  Jour. Lab. and Clin. Med., 1950, *36*, 754.
10. Jonkers, Shope, Aitken, and Spence.  Am. Jour. Vet. Res., 1964, *25*, 236.

11.   Kowalczyk and Brandly.   *Ibid.*, 1954, *15*, 98.
12.   Mohler.   U.S. Dept. Agr. Bul. 662, 1918.
13.   Olitsky, Traum, and Schoening.   Jour. Am. Vet. Med. Assoc., 1926, *70*, 147.
14.   Patterson, Mott, and Jenney.   *Ibid.*, 1958, *133*, 57.
15.   Reczko.   Arch. f. die Gesam. Virusforsch., 1961, *10*, 588.
16.   Sanders and Quin.   North Am. Vet., 1944, *25*, 413.
17.   Schoening.   Proc. U.S. Livestock San. Assoc., 1954, *58*, 390.
18.   Schoening and Crawford.   U.S. Dept. Agr. Cir. 734, 1945.
19.   Shelokov and Peralta.   Am. Jour. Epidemiol., 1967, *86*, 149.
20.   Strozzi and Ramos-Saco.   Jour. Am. Vet. Med. Assoc., 1953, *123*, 415.
21.   Wagener.   *Ibid.*, 1932, *81*, 160.

## Ephemeral Fever

SYNONYMS:   Three-day sickness, stiff sickness, bovine epizootic fever

Ephemeral fever is an acute febrile disease of cattle characterized by high temperature, stiffness, and lameness. The mortality is low. The disease is widespread in Africa, and similar diseases have been reported in many tropical and subtropical regions of the Eastern Hemisphere (1, 5).

**Character of the Disease.** The incubation period is about 2 to 3 days, and the disease begins suddenly with a high temperature accompanied by rigors, rough coat, running eyes and nose, swollen eyelids, and drooping ears. A characteristic feature of ephemeral fever is the presence of pain in the throat region. The animal shows it by refusing to swallow. Feeding and rumination are suppressed and milk production is reduced. Spontaneous recovery is usual and rapid.

Prevalence of infection varies from 10 to 50 percent. Fatal cases in Africa are rare, but this was not true in an outbreak in Australia in 1936.

The usual postmortem lesion is "foreign-body" pneumonia. The mucous membranes of the respiratory and alimentary systems may be congested. The lymph glands may be swollen. Effusions into the pericardium and hemorrhages of the epicardium and myocardium are usually present. Secondary infections may mask the true lesions of the disease.

**Properties of the Virus.** The blood of infected animals contains the virus. It appears to be host-specific and cell-specific. It is associated with the leukocytic-platelet fraction of the blood and probably with the platelets.

The virus is cone-shaped, 88 by 176 m$\mu$ by electron microscopy (3), and has been classified as a possible member of the genus *Rhabdovirus*. It is readily inactivated by ether and desoxycholate (6). The virus is rapidly inactivated at high and low pH and within 10 minutes at 56 C. It retains its infectivity for long periods at −70 C, but declines readily at −20 C.

**Cultivation.** Mackerras *et al.* (4) propagated a strain of virus for 2.5 years by 81 serial passages in cattle, administering it by the intravenous route.

After passage in suckling mouse brains the virus readily propagates in monolayers of baby hamster kidney-cell line (BHK 21) (6) and also in monkey kidney-cell lines, MS, and Vero (2). Cytopathology usually becomes visible after three to four passages and develops in 48 to 72 hours after inoculation. Plaque formation occurs under agar overlay in Vero and MS cells (2).

**Immunity.** It has been reported that an attack of the disease confers an immunity for about 2 years, but repeated attacks have been recorded in the field (4). The latter observation suggests that more than one serotype exists but this has not been proved.

Cell-culture or mouse-adapted viruses in oil adjuvant given as multiple subcutaneous inoculations to cattle stimulate high neutralizing antibody titers. These cattle usually are resistant to challenge with virulent virus.

**Transmission.** The disease has not been transmitted in cattle by contact. Ceratopogonid gnats have been incriminated as important vectors of the disease.

The infection was not established in horses, sheep, goats, dogs, rabbits, guinea pigs, rats or mice by inoculation (4).

**Diagnosis.** The drooling and lameness associated with EF suggest vesicular disease but there are no vesicular mouth or foot lesions. Inflammatory lesions of the joints and nasal and oral mucosa, and edematous lymph nodes are the usual lesions observed in fatal cases or sacrificed cattle during acute disease.

The virus is associated with the leukocyte-platelet fraction of the blood (4). Virus from this source can be adapted to suckling mice by intracerebral inoculation (6). Between the sixth and ninth intracerebral transfer in suckling mice the virus causes paralysis and death between 2 and 4 days after inoculation (6).

Neutralizing antibodies can be demonstrated in serum of cattle by virus neutralization in suckling mice or in cell culture.

Other serological tests used in the diagnosis are the agar double-diffusion technic (2) and the complement-fixation test (4, 6).

**Treatment.** The benign nature of the disease obviates the necessity of medical treatment, and there is danger in administering drugs by mouth because paralysis of the pharyngeal muscles may allow the fluids to pass down the trachea into the lungs and cause pneumonia.

**The Disease in Man.** It does not appear that this virus causes disease in man.

## REFERENCES

1. Henning. Animal diseases in South Africa. 2d ed. Central News Agency, South Africa, 1949, p. 797.
2. Heuschele. Proc., 73rd Ann. Meet., US Anim. Health Assoc., 1969, p. 6.
3. Lecatsas, Theodoridis, and Erasmus. Arch. f. die Gesam. Virusforsch., 1969, 28, 390.
4. Mackerras, Mackerras, and Burnet. Austral. Council Sci. and Indus. Res. Bul. 136, 1940.
5. U.S. Livestock Sanitary Association. Foreign animal diseases. U.S. Livestock Sanit. Assoc., Trenton, N.J., 1954, p. 60.
6. Van der Westhuizen. Onderstepoort Jour. Vet. Res., 1967, 34, 29.

# XLVIII | African Swine Fever

## African Swine Fever

SYNONYMS: East African swine fever, wart hog disease, Montgomery's disease; abbreviation, ASF

African swine fever (ASF) is a possible member of a new genus called *Iridovirus*. At present ASF is the only animal virus included in this genus that causes disease in a domestic animal. Other members as well as probable and possible members of the genus include *Tipula iridescent* (type species), *Sericesthis iridescent*, *Aedes iridescent*, *Lymphocystis* (fish), *Amphibian cytoplasmic*, and Gecko viruses. Some possible members such as ASF have a lipid envelope.

Montgomery (11) first described ASF from Kenya Colony, where it was recognized as an entity in 1910. Later it was studied by Steyn (13, 14) and Walker (15). The disease is an acute, highly fatal disease of domesticated swine of European breeds imported into several areas of East Africa. The signs and lesions are much like those of hog cholera. Montgomery viewed the disease as a hyperacute form of swine fever (hog cholera), but others regard it as a different malady. It is caused by a virus distinct from hog cholera, and it differs immunologically from European hog cholera. Montgomery was unable to protect against the disease with anti-hog-cholera serum, and he had very little success with East African virus and antiserum. Steyn confirmed these results. When the disease appeared on isolated ranches, almost all pigs died. In several survivors Steyn was able to show that virus was detectable in the blood up to 2 months afterward.

Until 1957, African swine fever was not known to occur in any part of the world other than East Africa. In that year the disease was found in Portugal (12). At first thought to be hog cholera, it was finally recognized to be ASF. Before it was stamped out, 433 herds had become infected comprising more than 16,000 pigs. In 1959 the disease was found in Spain and in 1960 it reoc-

1177

curred in Portugal. In 1964 the disease appeared in the Paris, France, area. Its presence in Europe constitutes an ominous threat to the swine industry of that continent and this, in turn, represents a serious hazard to the industry in North America. The disease reputedly occurred in Cuba in 1971 and this constitutes an even greater risk to the swine industry in the U.S. if it is not successfully eradicated.

**Character of the Disease.** ASF is quite similar to hog cholera in some respects. The incubation period is 5 to 9 days and the onset of illness is characterized by a sudden rise in temperature. Death usually occurs 4 to 7 days later with an exceedingly high mortality as a rule. A day or two prior to death the temperature falls rapidly. At this time the animal may show some or all of the following signs: labored breathing, depression, weakness, bloody feces, incoordination, reddish discolorations on ears, snout, fetlock, and flanks, coughing, and occasionally a sticky ocular discharge. Unlike swine with hog cholera, swine with ASF may continue to eat until death.

It was difficult to account for the sudden appearance of this disease on isolated establishments. Because wild pigs of the wart hog variety were common in some affected areas and these frequently visited the farms in search of food at night, it was thought that they might be the means of transmission. Montgomery obtained a few of these and found that they were quite refractory to the action of the virus, although they usually developed a thermal reaction 3 or 4 days after inoculation. Much later Steyn was able to confirm these observations with the wart hog and with another species, the bush pig. Finally he was able to show that some wart hogs, shot in the area where the disease occurred in domestic pigs, carried virus in their blood, whereas such virus was not demonstrable in the same species in other regions where the disease did not exist. Thus it appears to have been satisfactorily established that the reservoir of this disease is in certain wild animals in which the virus is relatively harmless.

DeTray (4) has shown that African swine fever sometimes behaves in European swine in about the same way as it does in native African swine in that surviving animals have a persisting viremia for long periods of time even though they appear well. Two European pigs which showed no signs of the disease after inoculation nevertheless became virus carriers and had viremia. Two animals had protective antibodies and viremia simultaneously. The antibodies were demonstrated in the serums of these animals on the 27th and 33rd day, respectively. Virus was demonstrated simultaneously and for a long period afterward. Antibodies could not be demonstrated later. Immunity to the homologous virus strain seems transient.

Maurer, Griesemer, and Jones (9) studied the pathology of ASF. In comparison with hog cholera they found few differences. The primary lesions are in the lymphatic tissues and in the walls of arterioles and capillaries. A marked difference was a severe karyorrhexis of the lymphocytes, which occurs in ASF but not in hog cholera. DeTray and Scott (5) confirmed the work of Montgomery by finding that hyperimmune hog cholera antiserum had virtually no effect upon the ASF virus *in vitro* or *in vivo*.

**Properties of the Virus.** In electron micrographs of thin sections of cells the mature viral particles have a hexagonal outer membrane, 175 to 225 m$\mu$ in diameter, separated by a clear region from a dense nucleoid, 72 to 89 m$\mu$ (3). In negatively stained cell-spread preparations, collapsed particles appear to be icosahedral capsids suggesting cubic symmetry (2). Extraction of infectious nucleic acid from ASFV and direct characterization by ultraviolet light and by reaction with RNase and DNase have proved that it is a DNA virus (1). The virus contains a lipid membrane and is ether-sensitive. It is inactivated in 30 minutes at 55 C and in 10 minutes at 60 C, thus it is less heat resistant than hog cholera virus. The virus survives for years when dried at room temperature or frozen in skin or muscle. It is resistant to most disinfectants but is inactivated by 1 percent formaldehyde in 6 days, by 2 percent NaOH in 24 hours, and by chloroform and other lipid solvents.

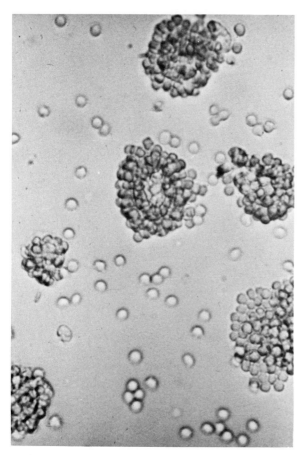

*Fig. 229.* Hemadsorption of red blood cells in virus-infected cell cultures used for diagnosis of ASFV. (Courtesy J. J. Callis and staff, USDA.)

The viral particles appear to be formed in the cell cytoplasm and they bud out from the cell membrane, many acquiring an added layer (3). Hemagglutination of red blood cells is not reported but hemadsorption of pig red blood cells is seen in cultures of pig marrow or "buffy coat" (8) (fig. 229).

There are several serotypes in Africa, but probably only one in Europe. Specific and group antigens are demonstrated by the complement-fixation, gel-diffusion, and other tests. The CF test is group reactive but hemadsorption-inhibition test is specific (7).

**Cultivation.** McIntosh (6) was able to cultivate the ASF virus in chick embryos through 12 transfers by inoculating them into their yolk sacs. The virus is lethal to the embryos, deaths generally occurring on the 6th or 7th day following inoculation. Malmquist and Hay (8) were successful in cultivating the virus in tissue cultures consisting of bone marrow cells or of cells from the buffy coat of swine blood. Cytopathogenic effects and hemadsorption were observed. More recently Malmquist showed that the Hinde strain produced a cytopathogenic effect in cultures of pig kidney cells.

**Immunity.** Immunity to homologous strains seems to be transient. Pigs that recover from the disease often remain carriers of the virus in the blood stream for months. Attenuated strains have been used as vaccines in Spain and Portugal but vaccinated pigs may carry the virus.

**Transmission.** Domestic pigs in Africa may contract the infection from wart hogs and these animals may liberate the virus, particularly during farrowing and other periods of stress. Thereafter infection is by contact and through fomites. Infected premises remain infective for long periods.

A different cycle of transmission has developed in Europe, where the disease became less virulent, and chronically infected pigs perpetuated the infection.

Virus has been recovered from the argasid tick, which may be a factor in the pig disease.

**Diagnosis.** Of most importance is the differentiation of ASF from hog cholera. This must be done by virus isolation or by the demonstration of a rising serum titer utilizing the hemadsorption-inhibition or complement-fixation test.

**Control.** As yet a satisfactory vaccine has not been developed despite a concerted research effort in several places around the world. Present control of the disease is based upon early reporting and a rapid diagnosis followed by immediate slaughter of all infected and exposed swine coupled with a strict quarantine in the infected area. This is likely to be the approach if the disease is ever introduced into the United States. Success has been achieved in certain European countries in recent years by this approach.

**REFERENCES**

1.  Adldinger, Stone, Hess, and Bachrach.   Virology, 1966, 30, 750.
2.  Almeida, Waterson, and Plowright.   Arch. f. die gesam. Virusforsch., 1967, 20, 392.

3.  Breese and DeBoer. Virology, 1966, *28*, 420.
4.  DeTray. Am. Jour. Vet. Res., 1957, *18*, 811.
5.  DeTray and Scott. Jour. Am. Vet. Med. Assoc., 1955, *126*, 313.
6.  McIntosh. Jour. So. African Vet. Med. Assoc., 1952, 23, 217.
7.  Malmquist. Am. Jour. Vet. Res., 1963, *24*, 450.
8.  Malmquist and Hay. *Ibid.*, 1960, *21*, 104.
9.  Maurer, Griesemer, and Jones. Ibid., 1958, *19*, 517.
10. Mendes. Bul. Off. Internatl. Epiz., 1962, *58*, 699.
11. Montgomery. Jour. Comp. Path. and Therap., 1921, *34*, 159.
12. Ribeiro, Azevedo, Teixeira, Braco Forte, Ribeiro, Noronha, Pereira, and Vigario. Bul. Off. Internatl. Epiz., 1958, *50*, 516.
13. Steyn. 13th and 14th Ann. Rpts., Dir. Vet. Educ. and Res., Union So. Africa, Part I, 1928, p. 415.
14. Steyn. 18th Ann. Rpt., *Ibid.*, 1932, p. 99.
15. Walker. Proc. 11th Internatl. Vet. Cong. (London), 1930.

# XLIX | African Horsesickness, Bluetongue, and Other Reoviruses

The genus *Reovirus* includes some important animal pathogens. The type-species for the genus is *Reovirus* h-1 (human type), one of the three mammalian serotypes. Other members are five avian serotypes and also simian and canine reoviruses. Other possible members are feline reoviruses, epizootic diarrhea of infant mice, infectious pancreatic necrosis of trout, rice dwarf virus, clover-wound tumor virus, Colorado tick fever virus (man), the virus of epizootic hemorrhagic disease of deer, bluetongue virus (18 serotypes), African horsesickness virus (9 serotypes), Corriparta virus, Kemerova and related viruses, Changuinola and related viruses, and Eubenangee virus.

Viruses in this genus are characterized by double-stranded RNA in several pieces that vary in content from 10 to 20 percent in the virion. Its total molecular weight is about 15 by $10^6$ daltons. The particle is an isometric capsid with icosahedral symmetry, usually naked; but a pseudomembrane, probably of host origin, is seen. The capsid diameter is 75 to 80 m$\mu$. The buoyant density in cesium chloride is 1.31–1.38 per ml. The virion resists treatment with lipid solvents. Virus synthesis and maturation occurs in cytoplasm with the formation of inclusions sometimes containing virions in crystalline arrays. Most viruses in this genus have two layered capsids but bluetongue, African horsesickness, and Eubenangee viruses are reputed to have single-layered shells.

As it relates to the definite members of this genus a striking feature exists with the mammalian reoviruses as they are indistinguishable from each other. The occurrence of these three serotypes in different species naturally suggests transmission from one animal species to another in nature. Although this has not been demonstrated it is reasonable to assume that it does occur on occa-

1182

sion. At present, the importance of these reoviruses as a cause of disease is still largely unknown. This same statement cannot be made for such possible members of the genus as African horsesickness or bluetongue of sheep, for they are exceedingly important animal diseases that cause mortality and heavy economic losses.

Other characteristics of reoviruses that help to distinguish them from other mammalian viruses include: (1) the rather distinctive cytopathic effects including intracytoplasmic inclusion bodies in cell cultures from a variety of animal species; (2) a common complement-fixing antigen; and (3) ability to agglutinate human group O and bovine erythrocytes, but not chick or guinea pig erythrocytes.

The importance of reoviruses as pathogens in humans is still largely unknown. It is obvious that most infections are inapparent or mildly symptomatic (1).

An excellent review of the accepted mammalian and avian reoviruses was written by Rosen (1).

**REFERENCE**

1. Rosen. In: Gard, Hallauer, and Meyer. Virology monographs, 1968, *1*, 74.

**African Horsesickness**

SYNONYMS: Equine plague, *pestis equorum*

This is an acute or subacute infectious disease of solipeds which occurs principally in Africa, although it has raged through the Middle East and parts of Asia since 1944. It is unknown in the Western Hemisphere.

Horses are most susceptible and the principal losses occur in them. Mules are considerably more resistant than horses. Donkeys in most parts of Africa are quite resistant, but Alexander (3) found donkeys of the Near East to be fairly susceptible. Outbreaks have been reported in zebras, but generally this species is highly resistant. There have been a few reports of sickness in dogs, the disease generally being attributed to the feeding of infected horse meat. In such districts dogs are not often infected by insects. Angora goats are known to be susceptible.

The disease occurs principally in south and central Africa and along the Nile Valley in Egypt. In 1944 cases of horsesickness were diagnosed in Palestine, Syria, Lebanon, and Transjordan. The disease occurs in warm, humid regions, particularly during unusually wet seasons. It is said to be found mostly in relatively flat coastal plains, but it also occurs in level valleys lying at considerable altitudes. It is definitely a seasonal disease, occurring mostly in the late summer and disappearing quickly after frosts come.

The disease remains as an immediate threat to Europe and Soviet Russia. With modern transport systems no country is safe from the disease as the vector may survive journey by aircraft.

**Character of the Disease.** Some cases are very mild, recovery occurring in from 3 to 5 days. There is fever (105 F or higher), inappetence, redness of the conjunctivae, and labored breathing. The highly acute form which accounts for most of the deaths is the pulmonary type in which there is severe edema of the lungs and the victims literally drown in their own fluids. There is coughing, severe dyspnea, fever, and copious foamy discharges from the nostrils. A somewhat more chronic form is characterized by the presence of heart lesions and edema of the tissues of the head and neck. Many of these cases recover. A mixture of both forms is most commonly observed in field cases.

In the experimental disease the incubation period generally is about 7 to 9 days, but occasionally it is much shorter or longer. It has been noted that in the natural disease no new cases are seen 9 days after the time of the first severe frost.

In the severe forms of the disease the course is rarely longer than 5 days, since the animal generally dies by that time. In the milder forms the course may be several weeks. The mortality varies considerably. In some outbreaks in which the agent is highly virulent the death rate may be as high as 90 to 95 percent. In others the death rate may be as low as 25 percent.

The lesions depend upon the severity of the case. In the acute type the thorax generally contains several liters of fluid, and the lungs are distended with fluid. The interlobular tissue generally is separated from the alveolar portions by infiltration of a yellowish fluid. Upon section the lungs do not collapse; the surface is wet, and fluid runs out of the cut surface. The pericardial sac may have some fluid in it, and subendocardial hemorrhages generally are present. Some fluid is usually present in the abdominal cavity, the liver is swollen, and the intestines are reddened.

In the more chronic form, characterized by edema of the head, neck, and sometimes the shoulder region, a hydropericardium generally is found and there is hydropic degeneration of the myocardium, but the lungs and pleural cavity show only moderate edema.

**The Disease in Experimental Animals.** Horses can readily be infected by the injection parenterally of small amounts of blood, tissue emulsions, and bronchial secretions. The urine is infective only occasionally. By feeding, the disease is transmitted irregularly, and only with large amounts of material.

In addition to the animals that are naturally susceptible, the disease can be transmitted by inoculation to goats, ferrets, rats, guinea pigs, and mice.

**Properties of the Virus.** That the disease was caused by a virus was first shown by McFadyean (10) in 1900. Polson and Madsen (15) suggested that there were 2 different-sized particles, 50.8 m$\mu$ and 31.2 m$\mu$ in diameter.

According to Breese et al. (6) the spherical particle has an average diameter of 49 m$\mu$ in negative-stained preparations and about 71 m$\mu$ with an inner core diameter of 36 m$\mu$ in thin sections. The core of AHSV contains RNA (11) and may be double-stranded. The particle has 92 capsomeres.

The virus is stable between a pH of 6 and 10 and it survives for years in the cold in an oxalate-phenol-glycerol mixture (1). It is ether-stable and resistant to sodium desoxycholate but readily inactivated by a 1 : 1,000 dilution of formalin in 48 hours. The virus is relatively resistant to heat. The neurotropic virus is destroyed at 60 C within 15 minutes, but infective virus in tissue-culture medium persists after heating at 50 C for 3 hours or at 37 C for 37 days. At 4 C the cultured virus retains its infectivity for long periods of time. The best method of storage is to freeze-dry the virus with lactone and peptone or to maintain viral suspensions or infected tissues at −70 C.

There are nine immunological virus types as determined by crossneutralization tests in mice (9). Each virus strain possesses a common CF antigen which has a diameter of 12 m$\mu$ (15). The virus in mouse brain tissue also hemagglutinates horse cells at pH 6.4 at 37 C for 2 hours (14).

**Cultivation.** Various cell lines such as Vero, MS (monkey kidney), baby hamster kidney (BHK) and primary cultures of BHK support replication of AHSV (12). Not all serotype viruses produce a cytopathic effect on first passage of field specimens, but on subsequent passages characteristic CPE may be produced in 48 to 96 hours. The onset of CPE is shortest in MS cell line and occurs within 24 hours after infection with some strains (11). Plaques are produced in Vero and MS cell cultures (11).

Infected cell cultures have multiple inclusion bodies in the cytoplasm. The inclusions are near the nucleus and these bodies show immunofluorescence (11). AHS virus propagated in suckling mouse brains may be readily adapted to adult mice and chick embryos.

**Immunity.** Animals that have recovered from horsesickness are not always permanently immune to the disease. Immune mares convey a passive immunity to their foals, usually protecting them until they are 6 months old. Cases have been reported of animals having the disease a second time. These have been explained by the finding that there are at least 9 types of virus, and immunization against one type does not fully protect against all others. Usually second attacks of the disease are mild.

An immune serum serves to provide passive protection from the disease for a limited time. This serum is made by hyperimmunizing recovered horses by transfusing them directly with blood from horses in the febrile stage of horsesickness. To obtain a lasting immunity, horses formerly were given simultaneous injections of large doses of immune serum and small doses of virus. About 85 percent of such horses developed fever, in which case another dose of immune serum was given. A considerable number always developed severe disease and about a 4 percent mortality was expected. The method has been abandoned in favor of vaccines.

Du Toit, Alexander, and Neitz (8) reported in 1933 on a vaccine for horsesickness made from formolized spleen pulp emulsion. Four doses were given, the first having been treated by formalin in a concentration of 1 : 1,000, the second in 1 : 2,000, the third and fourth in 1 : 3,000 and 1 : 4,000. The results were generally satisfactory but the resulting immunity was not permanent.

Alexander and Du Toit (4), Alexander (2), and Alexander, Neitz, and Du Toit (5) have reported successful immunization of horses with a living vaccine made by modifying the virulence of the horsesickness virus by intracerebral passage through mice. As the virus became adapted as a neurotropic strain for mice, its virulence for mice increased but that for horses decreased. After it had gone through more than 100 passages in mice, the virulence became fixed for this species and was no longer capable of producing the disease in horses. Because of the several immunological types, it was necessary to make fixed virus from each type. The field vaccine is manufactured from a mixture of 9 types, because it was found that a polyvalent vaccine made from 9 selected virus strains usually protects against all the types found in South Africa. A single dose of 100 mouse-infecting doses of each type is enough to afford protection.

The mouse brain vaccines have now displaced all others for protecting horses against this disease. The immunity conferred may not be permanent; hence exposed animals should be vaccinated annually before the horsesickness season.

**Transmission.** Horsesickness is not directly transmissible from animal to animal. Affected animals placed in stables with susceptible horses do not cause outbreaks of the disease. Outbreaks usually occur in warm, damp weather, on swampy, low-lying farms, and only in horses that are pastured at night. These facts indicate that night-flying insects are the probable vectors. Certain species of *Culicoides* (midges) have been shown to harbor the virus of horsesickness and to be capable of transmitting the infection by bite (7). These insects feed at night and are believed to be the main and perhaps the only vector of the disease. Multiplication and persistence of the virus in *Aëdes* mosquitoes has been demonstrated experimentally (13). Mules, asses, and dogs, which are not as susceptible to the disease as are horses, have been suggested as possible reservoirs of virus.

**Diagnosis.** When AHS first appears in a country free of the disease the condition is frequently diagnosed as equine infectious arteritis, equine infectious anemia, trypanosomiasis, or anthrax as these diseases exhibit similar clinical signs and postmortem findings. Consequently, a field diagnosis should be confirmed by viral isolation and identification or by serological means using paired serums.

Suckling mice are most commonly used for viral isolation from infectious blood or tissues. They are inoculated intracerebrally with 0.03 ml of each preparation. The incubation period may vary from 4 to 20 days and the mortality may reach 100 percent in the first passage. Serial passages of brain virus shortens the incubation period and suckling mice die within 2 to 7 days after inoculation. Tissue-cultured cells also may be used for field isolations but these cells are not as susceptible as suckling mice or horses.

The demonstration of a rising titer utilizing paired serums is ample proof that the disease is AHS. The complement-fixation, agar-gel diffusion, and the immunofluorescence tests are disease specific as all nine serotypes share a common antigenic component. There are at least two precipitating antigenic components common to the nine serotypes.

Viral typing is usually done by the serum-neutralization test but the hemagglutination test also may be used. The neutralization tests are performed in mice (1) or in tissue culture. Some cross-neutralization occurs among some of the nine serotypes with greatest level occurring between types 6 and 9.

**Control.** Vaccination is the best means of control in infected regions, but nonvaccinated animals can be given protection by stabling them at night in insect-proof stables.

**The Disease in Man.** This virus has not been reported to cause disease in man.

## REFERENCES

1. Alexander.  Onderstepoort Jour. Vet. Sci. and Anim. Indus., 1935, 4, 349.
2. Ibid., 1936, 7, 11.
3. Ibid., 1948, 23, 77.
4. Alexander and Du Toit.  Ibid., 1934, 2, 375.
5. Alexander, Neitz, and Du Toit.  Ibid., 1936, 7, 17.
6. Breese, Ozawa, and Dardiri.  Jour. Am. Vet. Med. Assoc., 1969, 155, 391.
7. Du Toit.  Onderstepoort Jour. Vet. Sci. and Anim. Indus., 1944, 19, 7.
8. Du Toit, Alexander, and Neitz.  Ibid., 1933, 1, 25.
9. Howell.  Onderstepoort Jour. Vet. Res., 1962, 29, 139.
10. McFadyean.  Jour. Comp. Path. and Therap., 1900, 13, 1.
11. Ozawa.  Arch. f. die Gesam. Virusforsch., 1967, 21, 155.
12. Ozawa and Hazrati.  Am. Jour. Vet. Res., 1964, 25, 505.
13. Ozawa, Shad-Del, Nakata, and Navai.  Proc. First Internatl. Conf. on Equine Inf. Dis. (Stressa, Italy), 1966, 196.
14. Pavri.  Nature, 1961, 189, 249.
15. Polson and Madsen.  Biochem. Biophys. Acta, 1954, 14, 366.

## Bluetongue

SYNONYMS:  Catarrhal fever of sheep, sore muzzle of sheep, range stiffness in lambs

Bluetongue is an infectious viral disease of ruminants transmitted by the insect vector, *Culicoides variipennis*. In sheep the disease is characterized by fever, emaciation, oral lesions, lameness, and a substantial death rate with the heaviest losses in lambs.

The heaviest losses are in sheep, but infections of cattle have been reported. It has been suspected that cattle may sometimes be the source of infection for sheep. In certain areas of South Africa sheep have developed the disease after being brought into areas where no sheep or cattle have existed previously; hence it is highly probable that other natural hosts of this virus exist such as goats, wild ruminants, and possibly certain wild rodents.

In 1966 Howell (10) reported that at least 18 immunologic serotypes exist on a world-wide basis. Also using the neutralization test at least six antigenic types were recognized in 1967 in the United States (15) and additional types are likely to emerge with further study of new field isolates.

Bluetongue was first reported in South Africa by Theiler (28) in 1905. The disease has constituted a serious disease problem there throughout the years up to the present. In recent years it has been identified in Palestine and on Cyprus. In 1952 a clinical diagnosis of bluetongue in sheep was made in California by McGowan (18) and in the following year the virus was isolated by McKercher, McGowan, Howarth, and Saito (20). These authors sent a strain of their virus to South Africa, where it was compared immunologically with South African strains and the identification confirmed. Soon afterward a disease which had been described by Hardy and Price (8) in Texas under the name of *sore muzzle* was identified as bluetongue. According to Price (23), by 1954 bluetongue had been identified in sheep by laboratory means, not only in California and Texas, but also in Arizona and Colorado. Since then it has been identified in Kansas, Missouri, Nebraska, New Mexico, Oklahoma, Oregon, and Utah. Because of its wide distribution it is obvious that the disease was not recently introduced. Apparently it has existed for many years unrecognized on our western sheep ranges.

**Character of the Disease.** The disease is seen only in midsummer and early fall, and is especially prevalent in wet seasons. It disappears abruptly with the onset of frosts.

In sheep, the principal losses are in feeder lambs but losses in older animals occur. There is an early temperature reaction which reaches 105 F or higher and which lasts only a short time. The victims are greatly depressed, they do not feed, and they lose weight rapidly. Edema of the lips, tongue, throat, and brisket develops in many animals. The buccal mucosa sometimes becomes flushed or even cyanotic. Erosions usually appear on the dental pad, tongue, gums, margins of the lips, and corners of the mouth. The lips bleed easily. Frequently there is a thick, tenacious nasal discharge which dries and crusts on the muzzle. There may be an eye discharge, and edema of the lungs and pneumonia sometimes occur. Occasionally there is a diarrhea, especially in young animals. Abortions may occur in pregnant ewes.

A characteristic sign is stiffness or lameness due to muscular changes and also, in many cases, to the development of laminitis. Examination of the feet often shows a reddish or purplish line or zone in the skin of the coronet, and the hemorrhages frequently extend into the horny tissue. Following recovery, a definite ridge, which persists for many months, may be seen in the horn of the hoof. If animals survive the acute attack, many will need months to reacquire thriftiness.

It should be pointed out that virulence of the causative agent varies widely, and there are differences in susceptibility in different breeds of sheep. Very young lambs suckling immune ewes are protected by colostral antibodies. Price (23) believes that the syndrome which has long been known in Texas

under the name of *range stiffness in lambs* is a mild form of bluetongue contracted by lambs before they have wholly lost their colostral immunity. In
most outbreaks many of the older animals have only very mild attacks, manifested principally by a short febrile period.

Experimental studies indicate that the incubation period in bluetongue is
relatively short—from 3 to 10 days. Death seldom occurs before 8 to 10 days
following the appearance of the first signs. In many animals the course is
much shorter, the mild signs having disappeared after several days. Animals
that are severely affected, if they survive, are apt to have a prolonged period
of convalescence.

The mortality varies widely. In Africa, where the disease obviously is much
more virulent than in this country, it is said to range from 2 to 30 percent. In
California the mortality in 1952 was estimated to be about 5 percent. In
Texas the mortality has been considerably less.

The principal lesions in sheep are cyanosis, edema, and erosions found in
the oral mucosa and tongue, edema and hemorrhages in the musculature,
hemorrhages on many of the serous membranes, and hyperemia of the mucous
membranes of the rumen, abomasum, and intestines. Frequently there are hyperemic areas of the skin, and these may develop into localized areas of dermatitis. The congestion and hemorrhages in the coronary band have already
been mentioned. Leukopenia is found in the early stages of the disease. Later
there may be leukocytosis and anemia.

The foregoing description of bluetongue has been of the disease as it occurs
in sheep. The picture in cattle is quite similar except that cattle generally suffer only mild infections and have a low mortality rate (3, 16). In Africa infections have been confused with foot-and-mouth disease. In many other instances the disease in cattle has been diagnosed only by inoculating sheep.
Sometimes there may be frank signs and well-developed lesions. The mouth
lesions, the crusts and excoriations on the muzzle, the nasal discharge, the
laminitis which is often severe, and an acute dermatitis of a patchy nature
involving the flanks, groin, perineum, udder, and teats are characteristic. Necrosis of the skin in the interdigital spaces often occurs. In certain instances
a suggested carrier status was established (16).

**The Disease in Experimental Animals.** The disease may be produced by inoculation of blood or tissues in sheep producing a disease similar to the one observed in nature. The mutton breeds are more susceptible than the wool
breeds and native African sheep are resistant to the disease.

Goats are susceptible to virus but there is no evidence of clinical signs experimentally or during natural outbreaks. The experimental infection in cattle
also is inapparent.

Experimental disease of wild ruminants has been produced in the blesbok
and white-tailed deer. Naturally occurring cases have been observed in a
bighorn sheep and a captive deer herd. Based upon a serological survey for
bluetongue in wild ruminants of North America (29) elk, antelope, big horn

sheep, Barbary sheep, moose, and 3 species of deer should be susceptible to the virus. Experimental bluetongue disease in white-tailed deer usually terminates in death (31). The signs of illness and lesions of bluetongue and epizootic hemorrhagic disease are similar. In fatal cases of bluetongue the lesions are subendocardial hemorrhages, hemorrhages in the tongue, and enteritis in the small and large intestine. The predominant histological changes are extensive thrombosis with hemorrhages, degenerative changes, and necrosis in affected tissues and organs. Bluetongue virus is readily recovered from the blood and a variety of tissues. Neutralizing antibodies are detected in all convalescent sera.

Cabasso *et al.* (4) have succeeded in propagating this virus in suckling hamsters, and Van den Ende and coworkers (30) were successful in transmitting it in series in mice by intracerebral inoculation.

**Properties of the Virus.** Polson and Decks (22) estimated the bluetongue virus to be a sphere 70 to 80 mµ with 92 rod-shaped capsomeres which has been generally acceptable. Recent information by Els and Verwoerd (6) suggests that bluetongue virus consists of 32 capsomeres rather than the 92 accepted for reoviruses. There is a difference of opinion regarding the presence or absence of a true envelope—it apparently depends upon the degree of purification. The virus has a hemagglutinin.

The virus is resistant to ether, chloroform, and deoxycholate. The virus is sensitive to trypsin and has a narrow zone of pH stability between 6 and 8. It is extraordinarily resistant to influences which destroy most viruses quickly. It will withstand, for example, a considerable amount of putrefaction. The virus has been recovered unchanged by filtering highly decomposed blood. Neitz (21) was able to isolate virulent virus from a lot of infective blood which had been preserved more than 25 years at room temperature in a glycerol-oxalate-phenol mixture. Air-dried virus keeps unusually well, and freeze-dried material remains viable for many months. McCrory, Foster, and Bay (17) found the virus comparatively resistant to several common disinfectants, such as sodium hydroxide, sodium carbonate, and ethyl alcohol. The most effective chemical disinfectant tried was a proprietary preparation known as Wescodyne.

In Africa 18 different antigenic strains of bluetongue virus have been recognized. Price and Hardy (24) compared American virus strains and found that not all were alike; however, they were not sure whether the differences were great enough to warrant considering them as distinct types. In 1967 there were six recognized serotypes in the United States (16).

**Cultivation.** Alexander (1) in South Africa showed that bluetongue virus could readily be propagated in chick embryos providing the temperature did not exceed 33.5 C. This is considerably below the optimum temperature for development of the embryo. Serial passage in egg embryos rapidly reduces the virulence of the virus. The yolk sac or intravascular route of inoculation are satisfactory, but the latter method is more sensitive and more time-consuming (16).

Haig *et al.* (7) demonstrated that egg-adapted strains of virus could be cultivated on monolayers of sheep kidney cells and that cytopathogenic activity was exhibited. This activity could be neutralized with homologous antiserum. Cytolytic phenomena were not seen with virulent, unmodified virus on the same cells. Two adapted strains produce a cytopathogenic effect in bovine kidney cells. Since the original studies it has been demonstrated that the virus propagates in various primary and established cell lines including the baby hamster-kidney cell line. Using egg-adapted strains of virus it was possible to plaque the virus in a mouse fibroblast cell line under agarose (11).

**Immunity.** Sheep that have recovered from an attack of bluetongue are solidly resistant for a period of months to infection by inoculation with the same virus strain. If more than one type of virus exists in the same locality, second infections may occur within a short time, but this does not happen often since some different types partially immunize against each other. Because there is a plurality of viral serotypes and variability in susceptibility of sheep breeds, no clear pattern of the duration and degree of immunity has been ascertained. Active immunity in sheep produced by virulent virus is associated with the formation of neutralizing and CF antibodies (9). Neutralizing antibodies at a high level persist for over 2 years. In contrast, CF antibodies are detectable for 6 to 8 weeks postinfection but barely detectable at 1 year (9).

In South Africa a vaccine was used for many years that had been produced by inoculating virus serially in sheep, without intervention of the natural vector. Attenuation was obtained in this way, and a serviceable vaccine developed. A more uniform, better vaccine was developed by Alexander, Haig, and Adelaar (2) in 1947. The new vaccine was a strain of bluetongue virus attenuated by serial passage through chick embryos until it no longer produced signs in sheep. Generally it is necessary to combine several types of strains in a single vaccine in order to give protection against the multiple types found in the field. In 1957 McKercher and coworkers (19) introduced a modified virus vaccine for use in the United States. American strains also were attenuated by serial passage in fertile hens' eggs. A freeze-dried product was tested in the laboratory and field and was found to be very successful. This vaccine produces only nominal reactions when injected into sheep, it does not regain virulence by sheep passage, and it immunizes solidly against massive challenges with virulent virus. When stored under good refrigeration, the vaccine deteriorates very slowly.

In 1968 Leudke and Jochim (15) reported a variation in the clinical and immunologic response of sheep to vaccination. An egg vaccine produced fairly good SN indices but a tissue-culture vaccine produced little or no antibody response in a 21 day exposure period. A poor correlation also was apparent between the clinical response of sheep after challenge and its serum-neutralization index. Obviously, more research must be done in this area. There also was evidence of immunologic nonspecificity for one of the serotypes.

**Transmission.** This disease is not transmissible by simple contact. It has long been known that an insect vector must be involved. Mosquitoes were suspected but largely acquitted by experimental work. Du Toit (5) in 1944 showed that gnats (*Culicoides*) were natural transmitters. In this country Price and Hardy (25) found the virus in *Culicoides variipennis*, which happened to be the most common gnat in the infected regions of Texas. If there are any other natural insect carriers of this disease, they have not yet been identified.

Because of the need for a vector, the disease occurs only in warm weather, generally in midsummer or later when the insect population has built up to maximum heights, and it is generally worst in wet seasons. In California it occurs on irrigated pastures where conditions for insect development are ideal.

The probable carrier status of cattle after infection and the susceptibility of domestic and wild ruminants, and possibly of rodents, must be considered in the ecology of the disease.

**Diagnosis.** In regions where the disease commonly occurs, the diagnosis is usually based upon the clinical signs. Bluetongue resembles, but must be differentiated from, such diseases as foot-and-mouth disease, mycotic stomatitis, infectious bovine rhinotracheitis, bovine viral diarrhea-mucosal disease, rinderpest, and vesicular stomatitis. In newly infected regions, confirmation should be obtained by transmission experiments, serological tests, or serum-protection tests.

Viral isolation from blood or tissues can be done by inoculation of susceptible sheep, of embryonated hens' eggs (14); of susceptible cell cultures (9, 10), and of suckling mice and hamsters (9). The system of choice at present for field isolations is the inoculation of the embryonated hen's egg. If blood is used quantitation of virus is dependent upon ultrasonic disruption of blood samples. The use of the glycerol-oxalate-phenol preservative mixture is an excellent stabilizer for the virus and enhances its isolation.

Five separate serological tests can be used in aiding a diagnosis of bluetongue. They are the serum-neutralization (SN) test done in cell culture, microagar-gel diffusion (AGP) test (12), fluorescent-antibody direct and indirect tests (13), complement-fixation test (16), and the modified complement-fixation test (MCF). The serum-neutralization test has been used most widely in diagnosis and viral typing and is based upon inhibition of cytopathic effects in a cell culture by specific antibody. Because the AGP test is simple, sensitive, and economical it is the *in vitro* test of choice for study of group-specific antigens. The direct FA test can be used for detecting antigen in bovine labile mucosa tissues and chicken embryonic membranes.

**Control.** Ordinary isolation measures will not stop the spread of bluetongue in regions infested with *Culicoides*. Control must be aimed at reduction of the gnat population, moving the lambs out of the gnat-infested regions, using repellent sprays on the lambs to discourage gnat bites, keeping the lambs indoors from the late afternoon until well into the next day, or immunizing the lambs shortly after they are weaned and before the advent of the gnat season.

South African workers claim that gnats, unlike mosquitoes, will seldom enter buildings at night, even though unscreened, unless they are attracted by lights.

Immunization is the most practical scheme, but pregnant ewes must not be vaccinated during early pregnancy (particularly 4 to 8 weeks) because vaccine virus produced stillborn, spastic "dummy or crazy," putrified, and de-

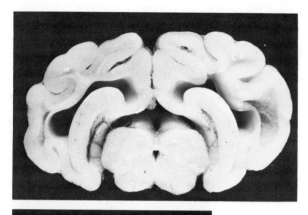

Fig. 230. Subcortical cavitation (hydranencephaly) in lamb brain following *in utero* bluetongue virus infection. (Courtesy D. Cordy.)

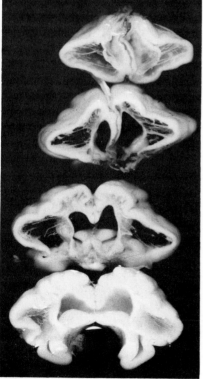

Fig. 231. Severe hydranencephaly in lamb following *in utero* infection. Secondary hydrocephalus *ex vacus* also is present. (Courtesy D. Cordy, Jour. Neuropath. and Exp. Neurol.)

formed lambs (26). Sheep should be vaccinated after shearing as wool fiber breaks occur in severely reacting sheep (9). Maternal immunity protection persists for 3 to 6 months and this fact must be considered in any immunization program.

**The Disease in Man.** There is no evidence that the virus causes disease in man.

## REFERENCES

1. Alexander. Onderstepoort Jour. Vet. Sci. and Anim. Indus., 1947, *22*, 7.
2. Alexander, Haig, and Adelaar. *Ibid.*, *21*, 231.
3. Bekker, DeKock, and Quinlan. *Ibid.*, 1934, *2*, 393.
4. Cabasso, Roberts, Douglas, Zorzi, Stebbins, and Cox. Proc. Soc. Exp. Biol. and Med., 1955, *88*, 678.
5. Du Toit. Onderstepoort Jour. Vet. Sci. and Anim. Indus., 1944, *19*, 7.
6. Els and Verwoerd. Virology, 1969, *38*, 213.
7. Haig, McKercher, and Alexander. Onderstepoort Jour. Vet. Sci., 1956, *27*, 171.
8. Hardy and Price. Jour. Am. Vet. Med. Assoc., 1952, *120*, 23.
9. Howell. Bluetongue. Emerging diseases of animals. FAO, Dept. Vet. Sci., Onderstepoort, 1963, *61*, 111.
10. Howell. Bul. Off. Internatl. Epizoot., 1966, *66*, 341.
11. Howell, Verwoerd, and Oellermann. Onderstepoort Jour. Vet. Res., 1967, *34*, 317.
12. Jochim and Chow. Am. Jour. Vet. Res., 1969, *30*, 33.
13. Livingston and Moore. *Ibid.*, 1962, *23*, 701.
14. Luedke. *Ibid.*, 1969, *30*, 499.
15. Luedke and Jochim. *Ibid.*, 1968, *29*, 841.
16. Luedke, Jochim, Bowne, and Jones. Jour. Am. Vet. Med. Assoc., 1970, *156*, 1871.
17. McCrory, Foster, and Bay. Am. Jour. Vet. Res., 1959, *20*, 665.
18. McGowan. Cornell Vet., 1952, *42*, 213.
19. McKercher, McGowan, Cabasso, Roberts, and Saito. Am. Jour. Vet. Res., 1957 *18*, 310.
20. McKercher, McGowan, Howarth, and Saito. Jour. Am. Vet. Med. Assoc., 1953, *122*, 300.
21. Neitz. Onderstepoort Jour. Vet. Sci. and Anim. Indus., 1944, *20*, 93.
22. Polson and Decks. Quoted by Andrewes. Viruses of vertebrates. Williams and Wilkins, Baltimore, 1964.
23. Price. Proc., U.S. Livestock Sanit. Assoc., 1954, *58*, 256.
24. Price and Hardy. Proc. Am. Vet. Med. Assoc., 1954, p. 65.
25. Price and Hardy. Jour. Am. Vet. Med. Assoc., 1954, *124*, 255.
26. Schultz and Delay. *Ibid.*, 1955, *127*, 224.
27. Shone, Haig, and McKercher. Onderstepoort Jour. Vet. Sci., 1956, *27*, 179.
28. Theiler. Ann. Rpt., Dir. Agr., Transvaal, 1904–1905, p. 110.
29. Trainer and Jochim. Am. Jour. Vet. Res., 1969, *30*, 2007.
30. Van den Ende, Linder, and Kaschula. Jour. Hyg. (London), 1954, *52*, 155.

31.  Vosdingh, Trainer, and Easterday.  Canad. Jour. Comp. Med. and Vet. Sci.,
     1968, 32, 382.

## Feline Reoviruses

Reovirus 3 was isolated from a cat in 1968 by Scott *et al.* (6), which was suspected of having died from feline infectious panleukopenia. Cell cultures inoculated with a suspension of intestinal tract from this cat developed intracytoplasmic inclusion bodies. These inclusions were subsequently shown to be produced by reovirus 3. Three subsequent isolations of reovirus 3 from cats were made by Csiza *et al.* (1). Hong (2) also made three isolations of reovirus from feline neoplasm cell cultures and all were typed as reovirus 1 as determined by the hemagglutination test.

**Character of the Disease.** The experimental disease produced by feline reovirus 3 is mild (4, 6). The experimental disease is characterized by conjunctivitis, photophobia, gingivitis, serous lacrimation, and depression. A majority of contact cats developed similar signs of illness 4 to 19 days after exposure and signs persisted from 1 to 29 days. Virus is isolated from the pharynx, eye, and rectum of the experimentally infected cats with 6 to 10 days being the optimal times for isolation. Cytoplasmic reovirus inclusion bodies are found in the bronchiolar epithelium of severely stressed neonatal experimental kittens (2).

**Properties of the Virus.** Feline reovirus 3 particles in negatively stained preparations have a diameter of 75 m$\mu$ and exhibit prominent hollow-cored capsomeres (6) (see fig. 232). The hexagonal-shaped particle has icosahedral symmetry and is composed of 92 capsomeres. With acridine staining, infected cell cultures have green-staining inclusion masses and the borders of the cytoplasm fluoresced reddish orange. Viral particles in infected cell cultures examined by electron microscopy were either arranged as closely packed, highly ordered paracrystalline arrays or spread rather diffusely through osmophilic reticular masses (see fig. 233). A few cells contain masses of viral particles in membrane-bound cytoplasmic vesicles within their cytoplasm.

The virus is quite thermostabile as there is no loss of virus after heating for 30 minutes at 56 C.

**Cultivation.** The virus was propagated in primary cultures of feline kidney cells and of bovine fetal kidney cells (6). The feline kidney-cell cultures give a titer of approximately $10^6$ TCID$_{50}$ per ml whereas the titer is about 1 log less in the bovine kidney cultures. The virus produces a typical cytopathic effect in unstained cultures (see fig. 234). In May-Gruenwald-Giemsa-stained preparations large, irregularly shaped, blue-staining intracytoplasmic inclusions begin to appear on the 3rd or 4th day after inoculation (see fig. 235).

**Immunity.** Little is known about the immunity. Neutralizing antibodies are produced in cats to the homotypic virus. The high incidence of neutralizing antibody in a small population of cats suggests that it is a common disease

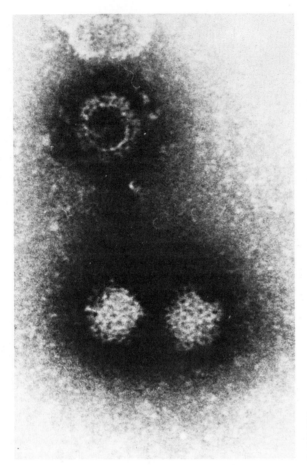

*Fig. 232.* Feline reovirus particles. Prominent capsomeres with
hollow cores are evident in a
negatively-stained     preparation.
(Courtesy F. Scott, D. Kahn, and
J. Gillespie, *Am. Jour. Vet. Res.*)

and the majority of cats are immune. Obviously, considerably more work
must be done in this regard.

It is not practical at this time to develop a vaccine against the feline reoviruses until we have more information about the immunity, pathological effects, and pathogenicity of these viruses in cats.

**Transmission.** The virus is readily transmitted from infected cats to susceptible cats maintained in the same room. At present this is the only known
means of transmission.

The incidence of the disease is not known, although it probably is widespread (5). The virus has been isolated from cats in California and New York,
and neutralizing antibodies are present in a significant percentage of cats in
the Ithaca, New York area (50 percent for reovirus 3 and 71 percent for reovirus 1).

**Diagnosis.** Reovirus infection in the cat can be confused with other feline re-

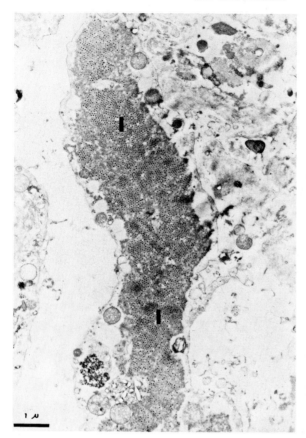

*Fig. 233.* Single cytoplasmic inclusion (*I*) of feline reovirus particles in a closely packed paracrystalline array. (Courtesy F. Scott, D. Kahn, and J. Gillespie, *Am. Jour. Vet. Res.*)

spiratory diseases. Its importance as a feline pathogen is still undetermined. Scott (5) has made the following observations which help to differentiate it from the others. The clinical disease is mild and usually of short duration. The signs of illness are restricted primarily to the eyes; a nasal discharge usually is associated with other respiratory infections. A febrile response, leukopenia or leukocytosis, and anorexia generally are not observed.

Certain ground rules must be observed in attempts to isolate feline reoviruses from feline tissues in cell culture. Since the cytopathic effect in unstained cell cultures may go unnoticed for up to 10 days, cultures must be retained for this period of time. Although not proved, it may be necessary to make blind passages before declaring a test sample negative. At present the cell-culture method would appear to be the method of choice for viral isolation.

Serological methods such as the neutralization and hemagglutination tests can be used to demonstrate a rising titer with paired sera from active cases. **The Disease in Man.** The occurrence of reovirus 1 and 3 in cats and humans

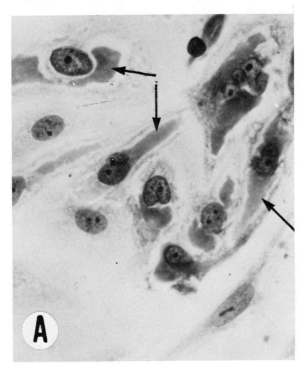

Fig. 234. Note production of large cytoplasmic inclusion bodies in a 4-day-old feline kidney cell culture. May-Grünwald-Giemsa stain. X 600. (Courtesy F. Scott, D. Kahn, and J. Gillespie, *Am. Jour. Vet. Res.*)

naturally suggests the possibility of transmission in nature between these species and others which harbor these viruses. Such transmission has not yet been demonstrated but it is almost inconceivable that it does not occur on occasion (3).

### REFERENCES

1.  Csiza, Scott, and Gillespie.   Quoted by Scott. Jour. Am. Vet. Med. Assoc., 1971, *158*, 944.
2.  Hong.   Cornell Univ. Thesis, 1970.
3.  Rosen.   In: Gard, Hallauer, and Meyer. Virology monographs, 1968, *1*, 74.
4.  Scott.   Cornell Univ. Thesis, 1968.
5.  Scott.   Jour. Am. Vet. Med. Assoc., 1971, *158*, 944.
6.  Scott, Kahn, and Gillespie.   Am. Jour. Vet. Res., 1970, *31*, 11.

### Bovine Reoviruses

Reoviruses 1, 2, and 3 were recovered from the feces of naturally infected cattle (4). Their importance as important pathogens in the respiratory syndrome is still undetermined. Bovine reoviruses are widespread in nature and their incidence in the cattle population is significant.

**Character of the Disease.** Present evidence strongly suggests that it causes an inapparent infection in nature (2, 4) although one group (6) reported the production of a mild respiratory disease in calves with a strain (Lang) of reovirus 1 of human origin.

Although no clinical signs of illness were produced in colostrum-deprived calves with reovirus 1 strains of human and bovine origin macroscopic and microscopic lesions of interstitial pneumonia were seen 4 and 7 days after a combined regimen of intranasal and intratracheal routes of inoculation (1, 2). There also was a nonspecific lymphadenitis of the retropharyngeal, bronchial, mediastinal, and mesenteric lymph nodes and some congestion and degenerative changes in the liver. Virus in low titers was recovered up to day 5 from nasal swabs and for 7 days from rectal swabs. In a viral distribution study, suspensions of respiratory tissues had higher titers than other body tissues (2).

It has been suggested that a strain of *Pasteurella multocida* did not enhance reovirus infection in calves (6). *Pasteurella hemolytica* did enhance reovirus 1 infection in day-old calves deprived of colostrum (2).

**Properties of the Virus.** Properties of the 3 reovirus types recovered from cattle are indistinguishable from these same serotypes isolated from other species.

**Cultivation.** Bovine reoviruses 1, 2, and 3 have been propagated in bovine kidney-cell cultures (4, 5) and also in pig kidney, monkey kidney and mouse fibroblast (L strain) cell cultures (2). The three bovine serotypes cause a cytopathic effect in these cell cultures, but the bovine kidney-cell cultures seem to be more resistant to pathological change (2).

**Immunity.** Maternally acquired immunity does not appear to protect calves from infection under natural conditions (5) and perhaps under experimental conditions as well (2).

The degree and duration of protection of cattle after active infection is unknown, but neutralizing antibodies are formed and presumably persist for a period of time.

**Transmission.** Bovine reoviruses may be detected in the feces of naturally and experimentally infected cattle for as long as 1 month although they usually are present for a shorter period of time (3-5). Virus also is discharged from the nasal passages and conjunctiva, probably for a comparable period of time. Through contact with these infected sources susceptible cattle may become infected. Although it has not been demonstrated, the possibility exists that cattle may become infected with the three serotypes which are common to many animal species.

**Diagnosis.** As a potential respiratory pathogen, reoviruses must be distinguished from numerous other microbial respiratory pathogens of cattle. This is a difficult, if not an impossible task unless one resorts to viral isolation or serology.

The only practical means for viral isolation and identification is in a tissue-culture systen. The neutralization or hemagglutination-inhibition test (HI) can be used for demonstrating a rising serum titer with paired sera. With the HI test a rise in titer of four-fold or greater between the acute and convalescent samples is considered positive (2).

**The Disease in Man.** Although not proved, it is conceivable that the bovine reoviruses may infect man.

## REFERENCES

1.   Lamont.   Proc. Roy. Soc. Med., 1966, 59, 50.
2.   Lamont.   Jour. Am. Vet. Med. Assoc., 1968, 152, 807.
3.   Moscovici, LaPlaca, Maisel, and Kempe.   Am. Jour. Vet. Res., 1961, 22, 852.
4.   Rosen and Abinanti.   Am. Jour. Hyg., 1960, 71, 250.
5.   Rosen, Abinanti, and Hovis.   Ibid., 1963, 77, 38.
6.   Trainor, Mohanty, and Hetrick.   Am. Jour. Epidemiol., 1966, 83, 217.

### Canine Reovirus

Rovirus 1 was isolated from dogs with respiratory signs of illness (2). Studies by these investigators with their isolate showed that interstitial pneumonia was produced in naturally and experimentally infected dogs. The inoculation of this same isolate into germ-free and specific pathogen-free dogs failed to produce signs of illness or pathological changes but it did cause infection as virus was isolated and seroconversion occurred (1). Massie and Shaw (3) recovered reovirus 1 from 4 of 133 dogs. In four experimental puppies one of their isolates produced signs of illness referable to the respiratory and enteric tracts. It is obvious that further studies in conventional and pathogen-free dogs are essential to determine the factors responsible for the pathogenicity of reovirus 1 in dogs.

## REFERENCES

1.   Holzinger and Griesimer.   Am. Jour. Epidemiol., 1966, 84, 426.
2.   Lou and Wenner.   Am. Jour. Hyg., 1963, 77, 293.
3.   Massie and Shaw.   Am. Jour. Vet. Res., 1966, 27, 783.

### Infectious Bursal Disease

SYNONYMS:   Gumboro disease; avian nephrosis

The virus that causes infectious bursal disease appears to possess properties most closely related to the genus *Reovirus*.

The disease entity was described as a specific entity by Cosgrove in 1962 (3) and is termed avian nephrosis. As it was first observed in the neighborhood of Gumboro, Delaware and Gumboro disease became another name for the condition. Winterfield and Hitchner (11) soon confirmed the original observations of Cosgrove and also successfully propagated the virus in chicken embryos. The disease is prevalent in the United States and in other parts of the world in concentrated poultry-producing areas.

**Character of the Disease (8).** The natural infection occurs in chickens only, and White Leghorns show a more severe reaction than the heavy breeds. The disease is principally limited to young chickens with the greatest incidence in chicks 3 to 6 weeks of age. The initial outbreak is usually the most severe.

Subsequent outbreaks in succeeding broods are less severe and often are unnoticed.

The incubation period is short, as clinical signs are detected in 2 to 3 days.
The birds display ruffled feathers and a droopy appearance. Other signs include soiled vent feathers, whitish or watery diarrhea, anorexia, depression,
trembling, severe prostration, and finally death. In affected flocks the morbidity approaches 100 percent and mortality begins 3 days after inoculation and
recedes 5 to 7 days later. The mortality varies from negligible to 30 percent.

Birds that die are dehydrated, with discoloration of pectoral muscles that
also may show hemorrhages. There is increased mucus in the intestine, and
the kidneys are enlarged from the accumulation of urates. The bursa of Fabricius is the target organ for this virus and, initially, it is edematous, hyperemic, and cream-colored with prominent longitudinal striations; by the time
of death it is atrophied and gray. The bursa often show necrotic foci and may
have hemorrhages on the serosal surface. The spleen may be enlarged with
small gray foci on the surface. On occasion, hemorrhages are seen in the mucosa at the junction of the proventriculus and gizzard. The condition is regarded as an infectious lymphocidal disease with the principal histologic lesions appearing in the lymphoid structures such as the bursa of Fabricius,
spleen, thymus, and cecal tonsil (5).

**Properties of the Virus.** Information about the physicochemical characteristics
is rather limited (2) so its classification as a reovirus is provisional. It is resistant to ether and chloroform and also to pH2. It is quite resistant to heat,
being viable after treatment for 5 hours at 56 C. The virus is unaffected by
exposure for 1 hour at 30 C in 0.5 percent phenol or 0.125 percent merthiolate
solutions. There is a marked reduction in virus titer when exposed to 0.15
percent formalin for 6 hours. Chloramine in 0.5 percent concentration destroyed the virus in 10 minutes.

By electron-microscope studies the virus particle is 58 to 65 m$\mu$ (4, 8).

**Cultivation.** Isolation and serial propagation of the virus in 10-day-old embryonated hens' eggs is not difficult if eggs are purchased from a flock free of
the disease. Infected chorioallantoic membranes of embryos are used as the
source of virus for passage, and the eggs are inoculated on the chorioallantoic
membrane (6). Embryo adaptation of the virus by serial passage can result in
increased virus titers in amniotic-allantoic fluid (10). Embryo mortality occurs
between the 3rd and 7th days after inoculation (6). The dead embryos show
edematous distension of the abdominal region, cutaneous congestion and petechial hemorrhages on toe joints and in the cerebral region, occasional necrosis and hemorrhages in the liver, a pale "parboiled" appearance of the
heart, congestion and necrosis of the kidneys, congestion of the lungs, and
pale spleen, sometimes with necrotic foci. The chorioallantoic membrane may
have hemorrhagic areas, but the bursa of Fabricius does not undergo marked
changes.

Landgraf *et al.* (7) reported on the propagation of the virus in monolayer cultures of chick embryo fibroblasts. Petek and Mandelli (9) observed cyto-pathic changes in chick embryo kidney cell cultures. These tissue-cultured vi-ruses were not inoculated into chicks, so their effect in the natural host is un-known.

**Immunity.** Antibodies are transferred from immune dams to their progeny through the yolk sac of the egg. These chicks with parental antibody are pro-tected for a minimum of 4 to 5 weeks after hatching.

Four-week-old susceptible birds develop an excellent neutralizing antibody response to chicken-embryo-adapted virus with a mean titer of $10^{3.5}$ (10). In contrast 3-day-old chicks had titers between $10^{1.5}$ to $10^{2.0}$. Hitchner (6) ob-served excellent titers in 12-week-old birds that were above $10^{3.8}$ after 27 weeks. Adult birds usually do not respond as well to virus. The delayed and poor response is probably due to the absence of an active bursa of Fabricius.

**Transmission.** The disease is highly contagious and spreads readily on an in-fected farm. The virus is resistant to heat, acids, and many chemicals, so it may remain viable on infected premises for at least 122 days after removal of the infected birds (1).

The existence of carrier birds is unknown. The lesser mealworm, *Alphito-bius diaperinus*, taken from infected premises 8 weeks after an outbreak, was infectious for susceptible chickens. Conceivably, insects may play a role in its transmission.

**Diagnosis.** In acute outbreaks in susceptible flocks the high morbidity, the rapidity of onset and recovery from clinical signs (5 to 7 days) in 3 to 6-week-old chicks, and the spiked mortality curve should make the diagnosti-cian consider infectious bursal disease. Pathological confirmation can be made by the examination of the bursa of Fabricius and other organs for le-sions typical of this disease.

Isolation of the virus can be readily accomplished in the embryonated hen's egg for identification by the use of a known positive antiserum against the isolate in the neutralization test. The use of paired serums for demonstration of a rising neutralizing antibody serum could be used as a method of diagno-sis but is rarely done because the history, signs of illness, and gross pathologi-cal changes, particularly of the bursa, are sufficient to render a correct diag-nosis as a rule.

**Control.** Once infection occurs on premises, control is often accomplished in a natural way because chicks exposed at an early age develop an active immunity without showing signs of illness. The resulting infection without disease may be the result of natural resistance of chicks at an early age or the effect of parental antibody. Vaccination with a lyophilized virus vaccine is recommended in flocks where management practices do not control the dis-ease.

**The Disease in Man.** It has not been reported in man.

## REFERENCES

1. Benton, Cover, and Rosenberger. Avian Dis., 1967, *11*, 430.
2. Benton, Cover, Rosenberger, and Lake. *Ibid.*, 1967, *11*, 438.
3. Cosgrove. *Ibid.*, 1962, *6*, 385.
4. Cheville. Am. Jour. Path., 1967, *51*, 527.
5. Helmboldt and Garner. Avian Dis., 1964, 8, 561.
6. Hitchner. Personal communication, 1971.
7. Landgraf, Vielitz, and Kirsch. Deut. tierärztl. Wchnschr., 1967, *74*, 6.
8. Mandelli, Rinaldi, Cerioli, and Cervio. Atti della Soc. Italiana delle Scienze Vet., 1967, *21*, 1.
9. Petek and Mandelli. *Ibid.*, 1968, 22, 875.
10. Winterfield. Avian Dis., 1969, *13*, 548.
11. Winterfield and Hitchner. Am. Jour. Vet. Res., 1962, *23*, 1273.

## Deer Hemorrhagic Fever

This disease occurs in the Virginia white-tailed deer (*Odocoleus virginianus*) and is caused by a virus which is tentatively classified as a reovirus.

Shope *et al.* (4) first described the natural disease. It was characterized by an incubation period of 6 to 8 days, severe shock, multiple hemorrhages, and associated edema in various tissues, serous sacs, coma, and death. Prothrombin deficiency may cause the hemorrhages (1).

Mule deer and other species are insusceptible to the virus. An arthropod vector is suspected of transmitting the disease because infection does not occur by direct contact. Intracerebral inoculation of suckling mice causes 100 percent mortality and after four transfers in this host the virus produced an inapparent infection in deer (2).

Two antigenic strains of virus, New Jersey and South Dakota, cross-react in the complement-fixation test but only partially in the neutralization test. Its diameter is probably 20 to 30 millimicrons (3), markedly different in size from other reoviruses. The New Jersey strain produces a cytopathic effect in HeLa cells (2) and a similar effect is produced by the South Dakota strain in embryonic deer kidney cells (3).

## REFERENCES

1. Karstad, Winter, and Trainer. Am. Jour. Vet. Res., 1961, 22, 227.
2. Mettler, MacNamara, and Shope. Jour. Exp. Med., 1962, *116*, 665.
3. Pirtle and Layton. Am. Jour. Vet. Res., 1961, *22*, 104.
4. Shope, MacNamara, and Mangold. Jour. Exp. Med., 1960, *111*, 155.

## Other Avian Reoviruses

Most chicken reoviruses have been recovered from the rectal contents or rectal swabs but on two occasions reoviruses were isolated from the trachea (6). More recently (1968), reoviruses were obtained from the intestinal tracts of turkeys with bluecomb disease from widely separated geographic areas of the United States and Canada (1).

Three reoviruses which are related to the human reoviruses 1, 2, and 3, as demonstrated by hemagglutination-inhibition, complement-fixation, serum-neutralization, and agar-gel diffusion tests, were isolated from chicks showing severe cloacal pasting (2). No clinical signs were seen in chickens inoculated orally or intravenously with three chicken serotypes isolated by Kawamura (5). Attempts to reproduce cloacal pasting in chicks maintained under isolation with two reovirus isolates from cloacal chick disease were successful but inconsistent (3). The chicks that developed cloacal pasting were depressed and lost weight. In contrast, germ-free chicks failed to develop cloacal pasting. Day-old turkey poults also failed to show signs or lesions after viral inoculation of these cloacal isolates. Generally speaking, it would appear that avian reoviruses are not significant pathogens in chicks or in poults, although future studies of natural and experimental infections may prove otherwise.

The properties of avian reoviruses generally are consistent with reoviruses isolated from other species (6). A major difference is the lack of hemagglutinins that is a characteristic of mammalian reoviruses. Avian reoviruses produce pocks on the chorioallantoic membrane of embryonated chicken egg. The 7-day-old eggs are killed when inoculated by the chorioallantoic membrane, yolk-sac, and allantoic cavity routes. These observations were extended by Deshmukh and Pomeroy, who observed embryo stunting and necrosis of the liver with two of their strains (2).

Two reovirus strains associated with chick cloacal disease produced a syncytial type of cytopathic effect in whole chicken embryo primary-cell culture, although the viral titer was not high (3). Plaques also are produced in this type of culture. A similar type of CPE was produced in chicken embryo kidney-cell culture. CPE was not observed in cultures of bovine fetal kidney, liver, endocardial, and corneal cells.

Studies with these viruses suggest that avian reoviruses are egg-transmitted, an important finding, because it relates to reovirus infection in birds (3).

## REFERENCES

1. Deshmukh and Pomeroy.   Jour. Am. Vet. Med. Assoc., 1968, *152*, 1346.
2. Deshmukh and Pomeroy.   Avian Dis., 1969, *13*, 239.
3. *Ibid.*, 427.
4. *Ibid.*, 16.
5. Kawamura.   Quoted by Rosen. In: Gard, Hallauer, and Meyer. Virology monographs, 1968, *1*, 74.
6. Kawamura, Shimizu, Maeda, and Tsubahara.   Natl. Inst. Anim. Health Quart., 1965, *5*, 115.

### Reovirus Infection in Mice

Spontaneous disease caused by reovirus type 3 has been observed in laboratory mice and is commonly called epizootic diarrhea of infant mice. As suckling mice may be used for isolation of reoviruses, this fact must be kept in mind. Reovirus types 1 and 2 also cause inapparent infections in mice. Reovirus infections in mice are reviewed in Rosen's monograph.

# L | The Family *Picornaviridae*, Including Foot-and-Mouth Disease Viruses, and Teschen Disease Virus

The viruses in the *Picornaviridae* family are placed in three genera: (1) *Rhinovirus*, (2) *Enterovirus*, and (3) *Calicivirus*. This is a rather large family with a primary affinity for superficial tissues and contains many important animal virus diseases, particularly foot-and-mouth disease (FMD).

The viruses that have been well studied in these three genera share certain biochemical and biophysical characteristics. They contain single-stranded RNA with a comparable molecular weight. All are nonenveloped isometric particles of small size, which are ether-resistant and which are synthesized in the cytoplasm of cells.

## The Genus *Rhinovirus*

The type-species for the genus *Rhinovirus* is *Rhinovirus* h-1A of man. Other members in the genus are additional human rhinoviruses (>90), equine rhinoviruses, and bovine rhinoviruses, including seven FMDV serotypes and the CO-7 strain. The particles contain 30 percent of single-stranded RNA with a molecular weight of 2.4 to 2.8 by $10^6$ daltons. Isometric nonenveloped particles are 20 to 30 m$\mu$ in diameter, probably with icosahedral symmetry. Thirty-two capsomeres seem to form a symmetrical capsid for the RNA core. Ether-resistant particles are labile at pH 3 and some viruses are stabilized by $MgCl_2$. They have a sedimentation rate of 140 to 150 S and a buoyant density in cesium chloride of 1.38 to 1.43 g per ml. The viruses multiply in the cytoplasm and normally reside in respiratory and ancillary structures.

1205

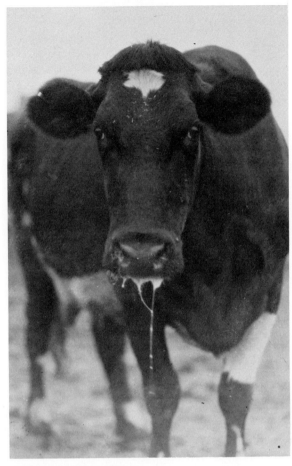

*Fig. 235.* Foot-and-mouth disease, showing the characteristic drooling of saliva. Affected animals do not eat because of the soreness of their mouths. They champ their jaws, making a smacking sound. (Courtesy L. M. Hurt.)

**Foot-and-Mouth Disease**

SYNONYMS: Aphthous fever, epizootic aphthae, infectious aphthous stomatitis, *Maul- und Klauenseuch* (German), *fièvre alphtheuse* (French), *aftosa* (Italian and Spanish); English abbreviation, FMD, (*Picornavirus*)

Foot-and-mouth disease occurs in most of the cattle-raising regions of the world. It has never obtained a firm foothold in Australia, New Zealand, and North America, regions which have long used drastic means of preventing its establishment. The disease is exceedingly contagious. On at least nine occasions it has broken out in the United States, but all of these outbreaks were successfully stamped out without excessive cost. At the time this is written (Jan 1972) there have been no outbreaks in this country since 1932. The disease has been of great interest to animal disease control authorities because of the great outbreak that occurred in Mexico between 1946 and 1954. In 1951–1952 a small outbreak in western Canada, very close to the international border, caused considerable concern in this country.

Foot-and-mouth disease affects cloven-footed animals, especially cattle and swine. Sheep and goats are also affected, and there have been outbreaks in wild ruminants, particularly deer. Naturally infected hedgehogs have been found in England. Human cases occasionally occur, but these are rare and rather trivial in nature. Carnivorous animals are resistant, and solipeds are completely resistant.

**Character of the Disease.** FMD is the most feared disease of cattle the world over. From time to time the disease spreads over the entire continent of Europe. These great panzootics usually run a year or two and then disappear. The disease never completely disappears, however, for infected centers always remain somewhere, from which it again spreads when a new, highly susceptible cattle population has been developed. The disease causes its greatest losses in cattle, it may be serious in swine, but in sheep and goats it usually is not very important.

The importance of FMD lies not so much in its killing power, for the mortality usually is not great. The importance lies in the moribidity losses—the loss of milk and of flesh, the long periods in which the affected animals are not productive.

FMD spreads most rapidly during the summer months because of the greater traffic in animals during those months. The disease is especially difficult to handle in the United States because of the highly developed transportation system and the practice of shipping animals long distances—from range to feed lots, from feed lots to slaughtering centers, from farms to marketing centers, and back to other farms.

*In cattle* the disease is characterized by depression, fever, and the appearance of vesicles filled with clear fluid in certain mucous membranes and portions of the skin. The essential pathological change in the tongue is necrosis of epithelial cells in the stratum spinosium, intercellular edema, and granulocytic infiltration (43). Circumscribed, slightly elevated, blanched areas termed "initial lesions" develop in the lingual mucosa. Separation of the mucosa from the underlying tissue causes much of this initial lesion to develop into vesicles. Some initial lesions fail to separate from the underlying tissue with the result that the desiccating necrotic mucosa becomes discolored without vesicle formation. Failure to vesiculate in the interdigital skin is exceptional, but the initial lesion is similar to the lingual process.

The vesicles appear principally on the mucous membranes of the mouth (tongue, cheeks, dental pad, and gums), on the skin of the muzzle, of the interdigital space, and around the tops of the claws, and on the teats and occasionally the surface of the udder. More rarely they may be seen around the base of the horns and in the pharynx, larnyx, trachea, esophagus, and wall of the rumen, especially around the esophageal groove.

Within 24 to 48 hours after multiplying in the epithelium, which is first invaded, the virus escapes into the blood stream, by which it is carried to all organs and tissues. This often results in the appearance of secondary vesicles in epithelium remote from the point of entry of the virus. The virus does not

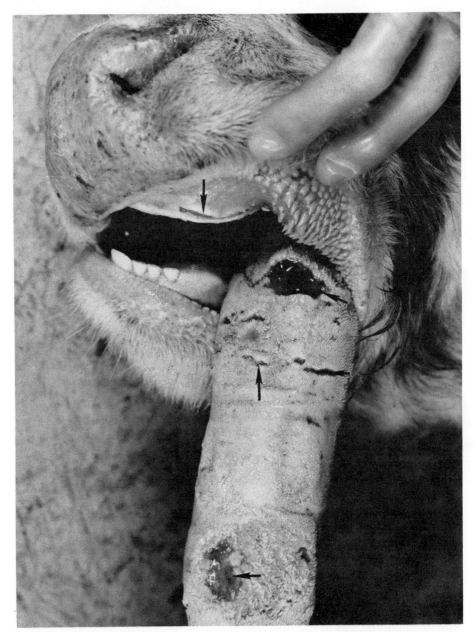

*Fig. 236.* Ruptured vesicles (*arrows*) of the tongue epithelium in a steer infected with FMDV. Note ruptured vesicle (*arrow*) on dental pad. (Courtesy J. Callis and staff, USDA.)

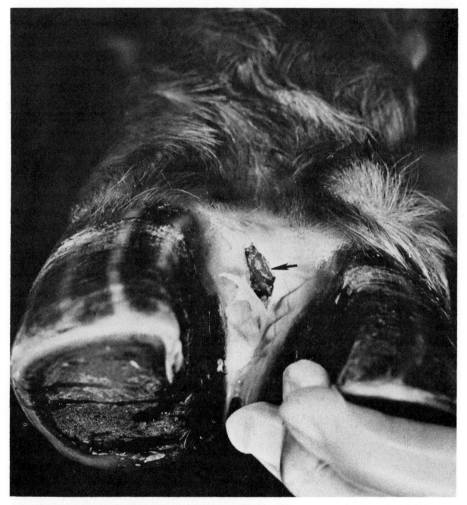

*Fig. 237.* Ruptured vesicle (*arrow*) in the interdigital region of a steer infected with FMDV. (Courtesy J. J. Callis and staff, USDA.)

multiply in the blood, but presumably does in certain organs. It produces degenerative changes in the muscular tissues, particularly those of the heart. Yellowish streaks and foci of parenchymatous degeneration are the manifestations of this damage. Severe damage of this type is seen most often in young calves and pigs, and this accounts for the greater mortality in young stock than in adult animals. In some outbreaks, the heart damage is greater than usual and the mortality of adult as well as young stock may be much higher than usual. This is said to be the malignant form of FMD. In these outbreaks many of the deaths occur early in the course of the infection and are attributed to the specific action of the virus.

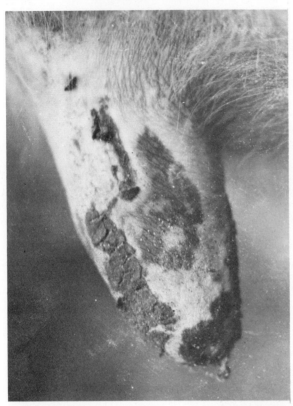

*Fig. 238*. Foot-and-mouth disease, showing lesions on the teat of a cow. Beginning as papules which change to vesicles, the latter rupture leaving raw surfaces. These become infected with bacteria, and mastitis often develops as a result of extension of the infection into the teat canal. The surface lesions finally heal under scabs. The lesions here depicted are healing. (Courtesy L. M. Hurt.)

Affected cattle become lame as a result of the foot lesions, and they champ their jaws and drool from the mouth because of the mouth soreness. They lie down as much as possible and move with great reluctance. They do not eat, and as a result they lose flesh rapidly and milk secretion diminishes greatly. The vesicles in the mouth rupture within a few hours of the time they are formed, leaving large flaps of whitish, detached epithelium under which are raw, bleeding surfaces. Many times a large part of the tongue is denuded. Secondary bacterial infections of the denuded areas between the claws usually occur, and these result in deep necrosis of tissue and suppurations that frequently undermine the claws, causing them to be loosened from the soft tissues and eventually to be cast off. The mouth lesions usually heal quite promptly so that the soreness disappears within a week, but the foot lesions often require much longer to heal.

Much of the damage in most outbreaks of FMD is caused by bacterial complications. The foot infections have been mentioned. These often require slaughter of the animal. In the few cases in which vesicles develop in the upper respiratory tract, pneumonia may occur. A common and serious complication in dairy cattle is udder infection. Early in the course of the disease, acute swelling of the udder is often noticed and the milk becomes thick and viscid, assuming the appearance of colostrum. Whether this is a result of virus action is not clear, but many European workers have so regarded it. In any case streptococcic, staphylococcic, and other bacterial infections often develop, resulting in mastitis.

*In swine* lameness is usually the most conspicuous sign and the first noticed. The animals have little appetite, have fever, and move with great reluctance. The lesions in the mouth and between the claws (fig. 239) are much

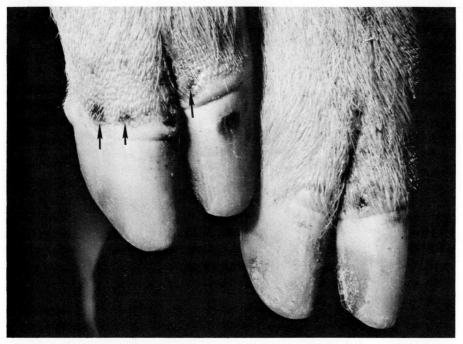

Fig. 239. Ruptured vesicles (*arrows*) on the coronary band of the feet of a pig infected with FMDV. (Courtesy J. Callis and staff, USDA.)

like those seen in cattle. Large vesicles not uncommonly develop in the snouts of pigs.

*In sheep and goats* also lameness is usually the most conspicuous sign. As a general rule, these animals are not severely affected by FMD. There are exceptions to this rule, however. There have been outbreaks in Europe in which sheep and goats were more severely affected than cattle.

The incubation period in FMD is very short. Inoculated animals develop lesions at the point of inoculation in less than 24 hours, and generalization with fever in less than 48 hours. When cattle and swine are exposed naturally, the incubation period is usually not longer than 4 days and may be shorter than 48 hours.

Cases without complications with pyogenic bacteria usually recover completely within 2 to 3 weeks, although milk production may be depressed much longer and recovery of the original body weight may not have occurred at that time. Complications are very common, however, and these may cause trouble for many weeks or months.

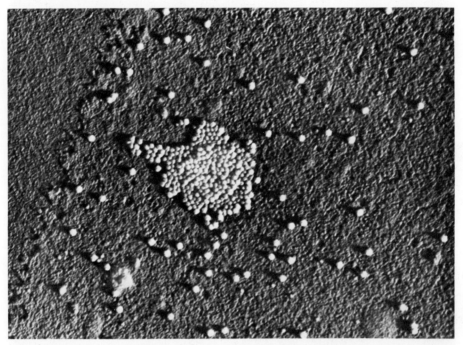

*Fig. 240.* Foot-and-mouth disease virus, 23 millimicrons. (Courtesy H. L. Bachrach and S. S. Breese, *Proc. Soc. Exp. Biol. and Med.*)

In most outbreaks of FMD the mortality is not high. It seldom averages more than 3 percent and often is less than 1 percent. Occasionally it may be much higher, even as great as 50 percent (29). The death rate among young stock is higher than among adults, and somewhat greater in young pigs than in calves. It is usually very low in sheep and goats.

**The Disease in Experimental Animals.** FMD may be readily produced in naturally susceptible species by inoculation parenterally. Cattle are easily infected by rubbing virus-containing material on the mucous membrane of the mouth. When cattle are used to detect virus in suspected materials, the most sensitive procedure is to inoculate intradermally into the dorsum of the tongue. After inoculation vesicles appear at the point of injection within 10 to 12 hours and fever and viremia occur within 20 to 24 hours. Secondary vesic-

ulation generally appears in the interdigital space within 2 to 4 days following this method of inoculation.

For many years research studies on this disease were greatly hampered by
the fact that infections of small laboratory animals could not be produced;
thus swine and cattle, which are very expensive, had to be used. Another handicap was the great contagiousness of the disease in these species, a fact that required elaborate equipment and housing facilities to prevent the infection
from escaping from the laboratory and from spreading uncontrolled to all susceptible stock brought to the laboratory. The discovery by Waldmann and
Pape (56) in 1921 that guinea pigs could be infected with the virus of foot-
and-mouth disease by the utilization of a special technic was an advancement
of great importance. These animals can be used to detect virus in animal tissues, and in materials that have been in contact with cases. Furthermore, the
disease in guinea pigs is not naturally transmissible, and thus the problem of
keeping susceptible animals on the premises for experimental work was immediately solved.

Very young and very old guinea pigs are not satisfactory for work with this
virus. Half-grown animals weighing about 350 g are best. Inoculation is done
by introducing the virus intradermally into the foot pads of the hind feet either with a fine hypodermic needle or by scarification. A primary vesicle
usually appears at the point of inoculation within 24 hours, occasionally
longer. At the time the primary vesicle appears, virus can be demonstrated in
the blood. Within 18 to 36 hours later, secondary vesicles appear in the
mouth, and the virus disappears from the blood. Complete repair of the lesions requires several weeks. Only an occasional animal dies of the disease.
There is no evidence that the virus multiplies elsewhere than at the site of the
lesions. Recent studies show that intralingual injection is more sensitive than
foot-pad inoculation (28). It is not known why the disease in this animal is not
naturally transmissible.

In 1951 Skinner (46) showed that unweaned white mice are very sensitive
to foot-and-mouth disease virus and that these animals constitute the best laboratory species for detecting small amounts of virus in suspected materials.
The mice are inoculated intraperitoneally. Those from 7 to 10 days old prove
most suitable. A spastic paralysis of the hind legs generally appears after several days, but some mice die before this sign is exhibited. Those that die or
are destroyed after several days show a marked degeneration of the musculature of the hind quarters and often of the lumbar and intercostal regions. Half
or more of all animals exhibit myocardial degeneration.

It was shown by Skinner and confirmed by others that unweaned mice
were 10 to 100 times as sensitive to foot-and-mouth virus as the guinea pig,
by foot-pad inoculation, and always fully as susceptible, and occasionally
more so, than cattle inoculated intralingually.

Other animals such as armadillos, cats, dogs, hamsters, wild and white rats,
and rabbits have been infected artificially.

Various investigators have succeeded in cultivating the virus in birds and chick embryos. In 1954 Gillespie (22) infected day-old chicks with tissue-cultured adapted types A, O, and C FMD viruses and 6-week-old birds with the type A virus. Degenerative gizzard muscle lesions were produced in most chicks and heart lesions in a small percentage. With some cattle strains Skin-

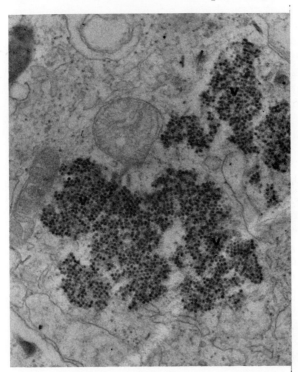

*Fig. 241.* Note cytoplasmic crystalline array of FMDV particles(*V*) in a bovine kidney tissue culture cell. X 35,000. (Courtesy S. Breese, USDA.)

ner (47) infected day-old chicks and observed lingual lesions. Injection of FMDV in the tongue or foot pads results in the development of characteristic lesions in bantams, ducks, geese, guinea fowl, and turkeys.

In 1948 Traub and Schneider (50) adapted guinea pig virus to the hen's egg but this virus was no longer pathogenic or immunogenic for cattle. With chick embryos Skinner (47) succeeded in passing several cattle strains for many generations by intravenous injection. Gillespie (23) did likewise with chick-adapted type C virus by inoculation on the chorioallantoic membrane and noted some attenuation for cattle with the 25th egg transfer. Embryos usually died in 2 to 6 days. Infected embryos showed edema and hemorrhages in the skin, hemorrhages in the liver and kidneys, serous or blood-tinged fluid in the body cavity and pericardial sac and, occasionally, enlarged white areas in the heart muscle. The greatest concentration of virus was in the heart muscle.

**Properties of the Virus.** In their excellent review articles on FMD Shahan (30) and Bachrach (1) covered the biochemical and biophysical properties of FMDV. In early investigations two complement-fixing antigens were demonstrated in infected guinea pig and cattle vesicular fluids with two different sedimentation coefficients (s rates). The infectious virion (particle) has an s rate of 140 S and a diameter of $23 \pm 2$ m$\mu$ and the smaller particle, without infectivity, has an s rate of 12 S with a diameter of 7 to 8 m$\mu$. This smaller particle has the properties of an euglobulin and more stable to heat, acids, and enzymes than the infective particle.

More recently, two additional virus-specific antigens have been identified in infected tissues. Graves *et al.* (26) described empty viral capsids with an s rate of 75 S and Cowan and Graves (17) reported a virus infection-associated antigen (VIA antigen) with an s rate less than 4.5 S. Empty capsids are precipitated by antibody to virions as well as by antibody to 12 S viral subunit. The VIA antigen is probably enzymatically inactive FMDV-specific RNA polymerase, because its antibody inhibits polymerase activity. The VIA-RNA polymerase antigen is formed prior to virions and only when virus replicates in cells of animals indicating translation from noncapsid cistrons of the virus genome. Consequently, animals vaccinated with inactivated virus do not produce VIA antigen or its antibody. The test of VIA antibody is a powerful tool in determining whether an animal has ever replicated virus. Thus it is useful in epidemiological studies, in safety evaluation of inactivated virus vaccine preparations, and in detection of infection in an animal population in eradication programs. All VIA antigens are immunologically identical regardless of virus type. VIA antigen as well as 12 S protein subunits interfere with the specificity of complement-fixation tests used for typing FMDV. The adverse effect of these two antigens in this test can be minimized by the use of a short high-temperature test at 37 C for 30 to 90 minutes and by the use of high dilutions of antiserum.

All four antigens of the FMD system are active in CF and agar-gel precipitation tests. Only antibodies to 140 S virion are known to be type-specific. The 140 S and 75 S antigens only appear to produce neutralizing antibody and immunity. As little as 0.2 $\mu$g of purified 140 S antigen is required to produce measurable neutralizing antibody in guinea pigs. The immunogenic potency of purified 75 S empty capsids has not been determined but it is anticipated that it would be comparable to infective virus.

The agar-gel diffusion test coupled with acridine orange staining differentiates the 140 S RNA containing virions from the other RNA-free 75 S, 12 S, and VIA antigens since the 140 S antigen only fluoresces under ultraviolet light. In contrast the fluorescein-labeled antibody (FA) probably is determined by antibody to VIA antigen. Labeling is not type-specific and occurs only with antiserum from animals in which virus replicates. Direct and indirect FA tests detect FMD infection.

The outer protein coat of the infectious virus may be removed with phenol, freeing its infective ribonucleic acid (RNA) core. The spherical infectious particle is quite readily inactivated by heat, but its stripped RNA core remains infectious after boiling for 5 minutes. RNA is more stable than intact virus in the presence of acid. The virus may be preserved at low temperatures for long periods of time. Practical experience over a long period of time has shown that the power to transmit the disease is removed from milk by ordinary pasteurization. Experimentally, however, it has been shown that a minute fraction of active residual virus remains in fluids subjected to much more than pasteurization temperatures for periods up to as much as 7 hours (3). Although it has been possible to produce infections in unweaned mice and cattle with such undamaged residual virus, it appears that the amounts are too small to initiate infections in cattle by ordinary exposures.

Resistance to drying varies according to the way it is done. If the virus is contained in albuminous material, is dried quickly and completely, and is kept dried, it will persist for very long periods. Virus in epithelial fragments appears to be more resistant than when free in fluids. Schoening (41) found that virus dried on hay and on soil particles remained viable for about a month, and Trautwein (51) found epithelial fragments still infective after being exposed to winter weather for more than 2 months. Gailiunas and Cottral (21) found that virus persisted in bovine skin for varying periods of time after treatment by one of four conventional methods for preservation of hides. The shortest period for viral inactivation was 21 days and the longest was 352 days. It was indicated that FMDV may survive even longer under field conditions. The virus types isolated from hides stored under experimental conditions were virulent and occasionally highly pathogenic for cattle. The present practice of cattle-hide importation into the United States from countries with FMD obviously poses a potential hazard, despite the fact that the importation of hides from these countries has continued since 1930 and no outbreak has occurred.

The resistance of the virus of FMD to drying and its persistence in infected tissues are matters of great importance, since they have a distinct bearing on the possibilities of new outbreaks being established in distant regions from accidental transfer of the virus. There is no evidence, for example, that any of the last half-dozen outbreaks of this disease in the United States were the result of importing infected animals. At least two had their origin in imported meat scraps that found their way into garbage and then into native swine (Mohler, 30, 31), and at least one originated in vaccine virus imported from a foreign country (Mohler and Rosenau, 32). The origins of several of these outbreaks were never discovered, but they may well have begun with virus dried on straw packing materials or on other objects contaminated with dried virus.

FMDV is quite sensitive to acid pH. At pH 6.5 there is a 10-fold loss every 14 hours at 4 C and at pH 6 and pH 5 inactivation rises to 90 percent per minute and second, respectively. It is quite stable at 4 C at pH 7 to 7.5 and only slightly less stable at pH 8 to 9. Purified FMDV-RNA is more stable at pH 4 than crude virus preparations. The RNase present in the latter serves to inactivate the RNA released by acidification of virions.

Many strains of FMDV have been characterized by their resistance to thermal inactivation (5). There is an initial rapid first-order inactivation of tissue-cultured virus followed by tailing, which suggests the presence of a small heat-resistant population of virus. The heating of virus yields infectious RNA in absence of RNase. The thermal stability of the FMDV is largely determined by the nature of its protein capsid.

Phenol and hexylresorcinol release single-stranded infectious RNA from FMDV by stripping the protein coat. The RNA has an s rate of 37 S. RNA extracted from crude virus still contains some RNase to cause slow inactivation so storage at $-196$ C or in 70 percent ethanol at $-20$ C is required to retard inactivation. The FMDV protein is recovered from the phenol phase in pure form by precipitation with methanol and resuspension in phenol, formic acid, or 0.1 percent sodium dodecyl sulfate (6).

Viruses containing RNA, such as FMDV, are inactivated by ultraviolet light through changes in their uracil components. FMDV retains its antigenicity and ability to attach to cells after ultraviolet treatment with the maximum rate of inactivation at 265 m$\mu$.

The FMD virion has a molecular weight of 6.9 by $10^6$ daltons and contains 69 percent protein and 31 percent RNA. There are 32 capsomeres which form a symmetrical icosahedral (20 sides) capsid for the RNA core. During replication in tissue culture cytoplasmic crystalline arrays of complete virus (fig. 241) and empty capsids may be observed. Its RNA base composition is G.24:A.26:C.28:U.22. Its isodensity in CsCl$_2$ is 1.43 g per ml.

FMDV induces the production of interferon in cell culture (18). Medium from infected cultures interferes with heterotypic FMD viruses, as well as parainfluenza, pseudorabies, and bovine enteroviruses. It has been suggested that FMDV with low virulence, or with many defective particles, is a better inducer of interferon than highly virulent strains. Synthetic polyribonucleotide duplexes which produce interferon presumably cause interference with FMDV replication in tissue culture cells. Bögel (10) has found a thermostabile inhibitor of FMDV in normal pig serum which is probably a beta-macroglobulin and not interferon.

**The Carrier Problem.** Most animals that recover from FMD become free of infectivity for other animals within a very short time after complete clinical recovery from the disease. The fact that many outbreaks of FMD have occurred in isolated areas, where it has been difficult to explain the origin of the infection, has caused many to believe that recovered animals may continue to harbor virus long after all signs of the disease have vanished, and that such animals often were the cause of new outbreaks. Most attempts to demonstrate

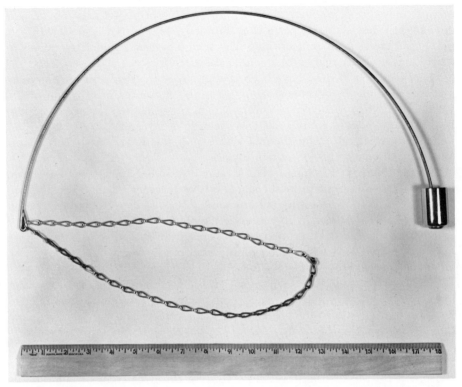

*Fig. 242.* Cup probang used for collecting saliva and mucus samples for FMDV isolation from the posterior pharynx and esophagus of the bovine. (Courtesy J. J. Callis and staff, USDA.)

virus in recovered animals failed, but van Bekkum (7) demonstrated virus in the saliva of cattle several months after recovery, the virus being capable of infecting unweaned mice and cattle upon inoculation (fig. 242). It did not pass naturally to susceptible contact cattle. These studies have been confirmed by many other investigators. Burrows (14) reported on the persistence of FMDV in the tonsils, pharynx, and dorsal surface of the soft palate of sheep for 1 to 5 months. Cattle become carriers after infection with attenuated or virulent virus and the virus recovered from carriers is more virulent for pigs than cattle (49). In a field study, 1-year-old calves from cows immunized with rabbit-attenuated virus became carriers with the majority lacking demonstrable antibody. Carrier virus in esophageal-pharyngeal fluid may be partially masked by antibodies or other inhibitors, because fluorocarbon treatment increases the infectivity of the test fluid by 10- to 100-fold. It has also been demonstrated that cattle immunized with inactivated virus vaccine may become carriers after exposure to virulent test virus without showing clinical signs of illness. Cattle may be carriers for at least 15 months.

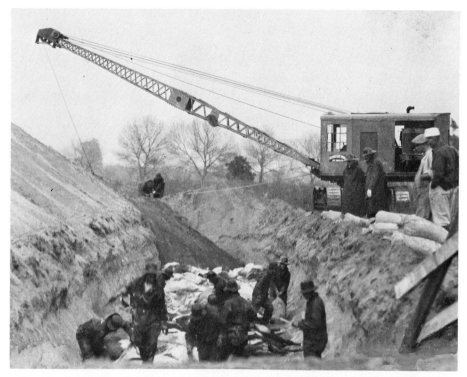

*Fig. 243.* Foot-and-mouth disease eradication in the United States. Outbreaks of this disease in this country are stamped out by the drastic method of slaughter and burial on the premises of all infected and all exposed animals. Great trenches are dug, the cattle are driven into them, slaughtered there, and covered with a deep layer of soil. Before the soil is returned to the trench, the hides of the carcasses are slashed and they are covered with a layer of quicklime. The photograph shows the burial of a herd of infected cattle. (Courtesy L. M. Hurt.)

Many unsuccessful attempts to transmit FMDV from carrier to contact cattle under experimental conditions suggest the existence of unknown factors accountable for successful transmission. Carrier cattle undoubtedly contribute to changes in virulence and antigenicity of FMDV, and probably account for the emergence of new viral subtypes where the disease is enzootic and vaccination is practiced. New variants often are available for selection since the mutation rate of some FMDV strains is 1 : 10,000 (35).

**Resistance to Chemical Disinfection.** For many years it has been customary to use 2 percent commercial lye (KOH) as a disinfectant for premises where FMD has occurred. Sometimes a 4 percent solution of soda ash ($Na_2CO_3$) has been used, since it was considered to be as efficient and was much less corrosive than lye. In this country it has also been customary to allow at least 30 days to intervene before fresh cattle are brought back to the formerly infected premises. These methods have given complete satisfaction, and are regarded as efficient as well as cheap.

Studies (3) have now shown that FMD virus is more sensitive to acids than to alkalies. The effectiveness of the long-accepted procedures appears to have been due to (*a*) the time interval the premises were left vacant, and (*b*) the detergent or cleansing effect of the alkali which tended to remove protective coatings in which virus particles were embedded. In spite of the fact that alkali is not nearly so virucidal as has been thought, the time-tested procedures probably will continue to be used.

For disinfecting small objects contaminated with FMD virus, ethylene oxide gas is quite effective and noninjurious to the objects. Formalin, vaporized with steam, is an effective fumigant for destroying virus in rooms.

The virus is resistant to alcohol, ether, chloroform, and other fat solvents. Glycerol has a preservative effect, especially if it is mixed with a buffer solution, which prevents the development of acidity. Infected lymph and tissues may be stored for long periods in such a solution without loss of virulence, especially if the solution is kept cold.

**Cultivation.** *In embryonated hens' eggs.* Reference has already been made to the studies in adapting a number of FMDV strains to chick embryos. More recently other investigators have used chick-adapted strains for successful transfer in hens' eggs. Some of these egg-adapted and chick-adapted strains have undergone a marked loss of pathogenicity for cattle.

*In tissue cultures.* Frenkel and co-workers (19, 20) of Amsterdam have developed a method by which the virus of FMD may be propagated in tissue culture indefinitely. The method has been perfected to the degree that it is now used for the commercial production of vaccine.

The cultures consist of epithelial tissue from cattle suspended in a solution of peptone, glucose, and salt with small amounts of a number of other substances known as Baker's solution (34). The epithelial tissue is obtained from the tongues of freshly slaughtered cattle. Small amounts of penicillin and streptomycin are added to the medium, since these do not influence the development of virus but restrain the growth of bacterial contaminants. After inoculation with virus, the flasks are incubated at 37 C, a stream of sterile air being bubbled through the medium during incubation. The flasks are harvested after 24 hours' incubation, at which time the virus titer is usually $10^5$ to $10^6$.

Propagation of FMDV in monolayer cultures of bovine and porcine kidney origin was first reported in 1955 (4, 44). Some other cell cultures that have been used include embryonic bovine skin and muscle, embryonic heart and lung, lamb kidney, fetal rabbit kidney, and murine mammary carcinomatous tissue. The stable line of baby hamster-kidney cells (BHK-21) is now commonly used in monolayers and in suspension cultures for research and vaccine virus production, since it is highly susceptible to FMDV and the cells grow exceedingly well and are readily maintained in culture.

By the use of the plaque overlay method or the production of a cytopathogenic effect, certain cell cultures can be used to assay for virus. The sensitivity and precision of plaque assays for FMDV depends upon the virus-strain cell-substrate system, and on environmental factors (1).

**Immunity.** Cattle that have recovered from FMD generally have enough immunity to protect them from the same type of virus for a year or more, but the resistance is not lifelong. Natural immunity in cattle and swine is negligible, although some individuals have greater resistance than others. Little is known about duration of immunity in swine except it is shorter than in cattle. Even less is known about such other animals as sheep and goats.

Antibodies which develop in immunized or convalescent animals are of two types—early and late (11). The early antibody is present 7 days after inoculation but persists for 30 days only. It is a 19 S beta$_2$ or gamma$_1$ macroglobulin which adsorbs strongly to DEAE-cellulose and is sensitive to 2 M mercaptoethanol. This antibody neutralizes and precipitates homo- and heterotypic FMDV but has little or no CF activity. The late-appearing antibody appears in 10 to 14 days and may persist for several months. It is a low molecular weight 7 S gamma$_2$ globulin which adsorbs weakly to DEAE- cellulose and is resistant to 2 M mercaptoethanol. The 7 S antibody possesses neutralizing, precipitating and complement-fixing activities which are type specific. Two or three other late-appearing classes of antibody exist in convalescent cattle sera which have not been fully characterized.

Immunity in animals, particularly cattle, is challenged by qualitative and quantitative means. Various qualitative technics, such as contact exposure, "cloth infection," intranasal or intrapharyngeal instillation, and arbitrary dose of virus on the tongue, are employed. Quantitative methods are more accurate, and include (1) intralingual titration of virus; (2) tongue, intramuscular, or subcutaneous inoculation of a standardized dose of virus.

*Plurality of viruses.* The French workers Vallée and Carré (54) in 1922 discovered the existence of two immunologically different types of FMD virus. Waldmann and Trautwein (57) in 1926 confirmed the French findings and added a third type. The original French types are now designated A (*Allemand*—French word for "German") and O (for the Oise Valley, from which it came). The German type is known as C. Thus we have three types, O, A, and C, which are known as the European types. Several years ago three new types were found in South Africa. These are designated SAT$_1$, SAT$_2$, and SAT$_3$. The English FMD laboratories reported on a 7th type found in widely separated parts of Asia which they designated the Asiatic type 1.

In addition to the seven basic types, 53 subtypes have been recognized. Some of these have been designated by exponents such as A$^5$ and O$^3$. Some of these field subtypes are sufficiently different immunologically from the parent strains to make successful immunization dependent upon the use of specific variant vaccines.

The virus of FMD appears to be unusually variable. In later stages of outbreaks in Europe new types or variants appeared which seemed to be derived from the original one rather than introduced from outside. Ramon (36) suggests that such variations may be arising as a result of vaccines which imperfectly immunize animals, thus setting up within them the means for forcing variations in the field strains.

Animals which have recovered from FMD caused by one type generally are sufficiently resistant to that type to withstand additional exposure for 6 months to 1 year. Such animals may be immediately infected with one of the other types and exhibit typical signs however.

The differentiation of types is a laboratory procedure. It may be done with guinea pigs or unweaned mice or by the complement-fixation test. In the animal tests it is necessary to have on hand high-titer immune serum of a known type. The unknown virus is mixed in appropriate dilutions with the known antisera, and the mixtures are injected into the animals. The virus is typed to correspond to the type of antiserum which proves to be able to neutralize it. The complement-fixation test for virus typing has been highly developed and in competent hands has a high order of reliability in differentiating between FMD and other vesicular diseases, with slightly less efficiency in differentiating between the foot-and-mouth virus types. The technic has been extensively studied by Brooksby (12) in England. Confirmation of CF typing results are made by cross neutralizations between virus strains and strain-specific antisera.

*Maternal immunity.* In 1963 Graves (25) reported that the transfer of neutralizing antibody to calves born of dams vaccinated against foot-and-mouth disease was by colostrum only. Immunoelectrophoretic study showed that calves were born with no gamma globulin in the serum, but it was present 2 hours after the ingestion of colostrum. Transfer of antibody could be blocked by prior feeding of skim milk or immune bovine serum. A passively immune calf did not respond to vaccination until the serum antibody reached low levels, whereas calves of the same age from nonimmune mothers could be vaccinated as evidenced by the production of neutralizing antibody. Piglets derive their maternal immunity through the colostrum.

**Immunization.** *Passive.* Susceptible animals can be protected against some of the damages of FMD by injecting them with immune serum just before or simultaneously with the exposure to virus. The protection is short-lived—only 1 or 2 weeks—and often it is not sufficient to prevent infection.

*Active.* Beginning in 1934, however, Schmidt and Hansen (40) began experiments on the use of adjuvants with inactivated foot-and-mouth disease virus to enhance its immunizing power. These culminated in success in 1936 (Schmidt, 38, 139). Waldmann and Kobe (55) in 1938 reported the successful use of this vaccine in the field. It is now known as the *Waldmann* or *Schmidt-Waldmann vaccine* and has been used very successfully in many European countries and in Latin America. A variation known as the *Rosenbusch vaccine* (37) was developed in Argentina. The vaccine used to control the Mexican outbreak was of the Rosenbusch type. Inactivated and attenuated vaccines of tissue-culture origin are also frequently used now.

Inactivated vaccines. The production of the Schmidt-Waldmann vaccine differs somewhat from one laboratory to another, but the principles are the same. Virus is obtained by inoculating susceptible cattle with diluted virus. The inoculum is injected in many places over the surface of the tongue, the virus being deposited in the deeper layer of the tongue epithelium. In about 18 hours large confluent vesicles should be present, loosening practically all of the epithelium of the dorsal surface of the tongue. If they have reached a satisfactory stage of development, the animals are slaughtered. If necessary the animals are allowed to live longer, their mouths being examined hourly until the disease has progressed to the desired stage. The tongues are now carefully removed and saved for the harvest of virus. The processed viral suspension is mixed in about 1.5 percent concentration in a colloidal suspension of aluminum hydroxide [$Al(OH)_3$], to the particles of which it is believed that the virus particles are adsorbed. Formalin is added to a concentration of 0.1 percent, and the suspensions are held at 26 C for 24 hours. This constitutes the vaccine. After being appropriately tested both for innocuity and immunizing ability, it is ready to be bottled for field use. The finished vaccine is an opalescent fluid, the appearance being due to the aluminum hydroxide. The material must be kept cold but it is spoiled by freezing and by heat. It is injected subcutaneously in a dose of 30 ml.

Immunity develops after 7 to 10 days but does not reach its peak until 21 days. European workers consider that a serviceable degree of immunity lasts for 1 year in cattle. In Latin America, where management practices are different, cattle must be vaccinated three times per year for maximum protection. In 1963 van Bekkum, Fish, and Dale (8) stated that the serum titers of Dutch dairy cattle given two or more annual vaccinations remained high for at least 2 years.

The Rosenbusch vaccine differs from the Schmidt-Waldmann only in that it contains much more virus material, i.e., about 5 percent instead of 1 to 1.5 percent. It is used intradermally, and the dose is 2 ml. The injections are made in the thick skin of the neck just back of the ears. Rosenbusch claims that immunity develops earlier and that it is as solid and lasting as that of the European type.

The method devised by Frenkel (19) of Holland for cultivating the virus of FMD has been described in an earlier section. Frenkel and his co-workers were successful in adapting their methods to mass production of high-titer virus. From this virus, vaccine is made by the same procedures as are used for making the Schmidt-Waldmann vaccine (Frenkel, 20). Henderson (27) checked several vaccines made in this way and found them fully as good and perhaps better in some instances than those made from cattle tongues.

Other inactivated virus vaccines have utilized FMDV produced in primary calf-kidney cell cultures in Roux flasks and later in large roller bottles (52). Cell production is limited by the difficulty of processing kidneys and the relatively low cell density reached in the monolayers. The stable baby hamster-kidney (BHK) cell line is a vast improvement, as its cell population in roller bottles is eight times greater than primary bovine kidney monolayers, and it can also be grown in 30- to 100-liter submerged cultures with automatic control of temperature and pH (15). Vaccines prepared with BHK cells are as potent as other inactivated vaccines, lack other latent kidney viruses, such as bovine virus diarrhea virus and bovine adenoviruses, and are apparently free of tumorigenicity.

Brown, Hyslop, Crick, and Morrow (13) reported that vaccines prepared by the inactivation of virus with acetylethyleneimine were as potent as the corresponding formalin vaccines. By adding an oil adjuvant, vaccines become more efficient than the standard formalin—Al (OH)$_3$ vaccines because the duration of immunity is lengthened in cattle and pigs.

Modified live-virus vaccines. The adaptation of FMDV to unweaned mice by Skinner (46) and to chick embryos and day-old chicks by Skinner (47) and by Gillespie (22, 23), to other small animals (45), and to tissue cultures, led to the development of modified live virus vaccines. Virulent virus was transferred through one or more of these hosts until the virulence for cattle was markedly reduced. Attenuation for one host does not imply reduction of virulence for another host, or even avirulence for the same host under conditions of stress. There is also a suggestion that in a combined vaccine, two serotypes may interfere with each other to some degree, although this is not true in all instances since it is possible for certain subtypes within serotypes to cross-protect (33). Although modified live-virus vaccines undoubtedly confer longer lasting immunity than inactivated vaccines and show considerable promise under field conditions in certain areas of the world, many problems (33) remain to be solved, such as undesirable effects in young cattle, possible activation of other infectious latent agents, the role of this type of vaccine in carrier cattle, and the production of postvaccinal teat lesions leading to mastitis.

**Transmission.** The greater part of the virus in affected animals is localized in the epithelial lesions, but during the early febrile period all tissues and organs and all secretions and excretions contain virus. Transmission to susceptible animals near at hand probably occurs through infected saliva. The disease spreads very rapidly to all susceptible animals on infected farms.

Cottral *et al.* (16) demonstrated FMDV in semen before clinical signs appeared and for 10 days after inoculation, and showed that the disease could be transmitted by artificial insemination. This fact should be borne in mind by artificial breeder organizations. No biological insect vector has been identified as important in the spread of FMD. However, there are a few reports that ticks transmitted the disease to cattle. FMD can occur in any season and often seems to be related to the movement of livestock.

Long experience has made it clear that within a comparatively short time after an outbreak on a farm has subsided, or after all infected animals have been removed, the virus disappears. Residual virus may remain in dark damp areas for a long time, however; hence it is very necessary to clean and thoroughly disinfect premises where infection has existed before they are re-stocked with susceptible stock. It is also wise to allow the premises to remain unstocked for a considerable time after disinfection.

It is the practice of the U.S. Department of Agriculture (53) to permit grad-ual restocking of premises 30 days after disinfection. A few yearling calves or hogs are first introduced. These are carefully inspected every second day for 10 days, and then semiweekly until the end of the 2nd month. Additional stock may be introduced at this time, but the herd is kept under quarantine and surveillance for a 3rd month. If at the end of 90 days after disinfection there is no evidence of the disease on the premises and no active infection ex-ists on any farms in the immediate neighborhood, the farm is released from quarantine.

It has long been recognized that FMD virus can be shipped to distant parts of the world in infected meat. England has had much experience with this source of infection since it has had to import most of its fresh meat from countries where the disease is enzootic.

The last two outbreaks of FMD in the United States occurred in California in 1924 and 1929. They began in swine fed on ships' garbage that contained scraps of meat from infected areas of the Orient and South America, respec-tively. The evidence is very strong that the virus was imported in this way. As a result of this experience, ships coming from countries where this disease occurs are no longer allowed to land garbage in any of our ports.

Stockman and Minett (48) studied the survival of FMD virus in carcasses of animals slaughtered while suffering from this disease. They showed that the acidity which develops in muscular tissue after the onset of *rigor mortis* rapidly destroys any virus it contains. Usually virus cannot be demonstrated after a few days even when the meat is refrigerated normally. Virus in vis-ceral organs, however, and in the marrow of the long bones is not subject to the action of tissue acids, and virus was often demonstrated in such materi-als for 40 days, and longer when they were kept under refrigeration.

Under a provision of the Smoot-Hawley Tariff Act of 1930, the Secretary of Agriculture of the United States is required to maintain an embargo against the importation of fresh meat, fresh hides, and fresh offal from countries in which FMD is known to exist. This has resulted in the exclusion of meat from these countries, except that which has been canned, dried, or otherwise pro-cessed in a way that destroys the virus.

There has been much speculation about the possible role of wild birds in the spread of FMD. Since birds are not naturally susceptible to the virus of this disease, they would have to be mechanical carriers of the virus if they carried it at all. Many species of birds associate closely with farm livestock, and it seems reasonable to believe that they might have some importance in spreading the disease, particularly since no practical quarantine measures have been devised to control their movements. More recently, winds have been incriminated in the spread of FMD by the aerosol route. The initial patterns of outbreaks in England in 1967 suggested that spread was airborne.

The carrier status of FMD in the epidemiology was alluded to in an earlier part of this section of FMD. In all likelihood, carrier animals are stressed under field conditions by various unknown factors, and by the release of virus from the oral cavity and subsequent transmission to susceptible or partially immune animals in the herd, with active disease as the result.

**Diagnosis.** In countries like the United States where FMD does not exist, it is of the utmost importance that cases caused by imported virus be quickly recognized. The stamping-out method is not costly if the disease has not spread far from the initial site.

Veterinarians and others should always be suspicious of this disease when a number of animals of susceptible species develop stomatitis or lameness about the same time. In these cases the mouths of a number of animals should be examined for evidences of the characteristic vesicles or the denuded areas that follow rupture of the vesicles. The feet should be examined for similar lesions. The epithelial coverings of unruptured vesicles of tongue and feet are the best source of virus (42).

Two other diseases of farm livestock present mouth vesicles and sometimes foot lesions that are not distinguishable from those of foot-and-mouth disease. These are *vesicular stomatitis* and *vesicular exanthema*. Differentiation of these diseases from FMD is discussed on page 1230. Although the tests are relatively simple, it should be strongly emphasized that the importance of an accurate, early diagnosis is so great that those who have had no experience with them should not ordinarily attempt them. *When a disease is seen in any part of the United States that resembles foot-and-mouth disease, it should be reported promptly to the chief disease-control officer of the state, who will act promptly to have experts assigned to the diagnostic problem.*

**Control.** Two general methods of control are used:

1. *The slaughter method.* This method is the one that has been used in the United States and in other countries sufficiently isolated to make it economically feasible. It has been used successfully and often in the British Isles. It has not been used so often, or with so much success, on the mainland of Europe.

When this procedure is followed, drastic quarantine measures must be established immediately and enough quarantine officers placed on duty to enforce the regulations. Not only the affected farms but those in a radius of several miles are included in the quarantine. On all the farms of the area the cattle are confined to their stables or corrals, swine are restricted to buildings or small pens, sheep are restrained, and even dogs and cats are confined to the premises. It is no less important that people be confined and allowed to move from one place to another only by special permission, and then only after thorough disinfection if it is thought that they may have been in contact with infectious materials. The affected animals and all other susceptible stock that may have been in contact with them, whether or not they show any evidence of the disease, are slaughtered as quickly as possible and buried on the premises. The infected premises are then thoroughly cleaned and disinfected with a strong alkali solution. The U.S. Department of Agriculture uses a whitewash made of 5 pounds of hydrated or water-slacked (*not air-slacked*) lime, 1 pound of concentrated lye or caustic soda, and 10 gallons of hot water to disinfect floors, stanchions, walls, fences, and any other objects that may have been contaminated with virus. If lime is not available, the lye or soda is used alone at the rate of 2 pounds to each 10 gallons of water. This should be applied with a power spray. In any case, all objects should be well soaked with the solution. A 4 percent solution of formaldehyde is considered suitable for harness, blankets, ropes, and finished surfaces that would be damaged by the alkali. Dwellings, milkhouses, and other tight buildings may be fumigated with formaldehyde gas.

Persons whose work requires them to come in contact with infected animals are required to wear rubber clothing—hats, coats, pants, boots, and gloves. These may be disinfected with a 2 percent lye solution or with one of the cresylic acid disinfectants. The lye is caustic and will burn the skin if it is permitted to remain on it. Immediate washing with water is usually sufficient to prevent this; the lye may also be neutralized with vinegar. The alkali solutions may be stored in wooden, earthenware, or metal containers made of any of the common metals except aluminum. Hay stacks that may be infected can be made safe by removing the surface layers and spraying the remainder with a 4 percent solution of formalin. Old straw, dried manure, and old wooden structures of small value should be burned. Manure piles may be burned, if sufficiently dry, or the material may be thinly spread on fields to which cattle will not have access and buried by being plowed underground. All procedures must be done very thoroughly.

In the United States the owners of destroyed animals are indemnified from government funds to facilitate the control of FMD. They may also be indemnified for losses of feed, hay, or any other materials destroyed in the course of the cleaning and disinfecting.

All susceptible livestock on farms in the vicinity of infected premises are frequently and thoroughly inspected for evidence of the disease. Milk-receiving stations drawing from the quarantined area are inspected to see that they have suitable equipment, and that it is properly used, to insure that all milk cans returned to farms will be adequately sterilized.

2. *The quarantine and vaccination method.* This method has never been used in the United States. It is unlikely that it ever will be employed in this country unless FMD should become so widespread that the slaughter method would be impracticable. It has been used successfully in some of the countries of continental Europe, and it appears to have contributed to the success of the campaign to stamp out a very extensive outbreak in Mexico.

The method consists of rigid quarantine of infected premises with immediate use of inactivated vaccine in all susceptible animals in a zone several miles in width around the center of the infection. This should be done as quickly as the virus type has been determined and vaccine can be procured. When large areas become involved, as in Mexico, all susceptible animals in the entire infected area should be injected.

When vaccines are used, the importance of strict quarantine measures should not be ignored. So far as possible the movement of livestock and of the people who are in contact with livestock should be restricted. The feeding of garbage to swine in such regions should be prohibited unless it is cooked, and unpasteurized milk should not be fed to calves. In 1951–1952 an exceptionally virulent and widespread outbreak of foot-and-mouth disease occurred in Europe. Efforts to control this outbreak by vaccination were not very successful as the disease spread faster than animals could be vaccinated. Also, a number of variant types appeared against which the current vaccines were not potent. According to Ramon (36), too little attention was paid to sanitation and quarantine—the old accepted methods—since the opinion existed that these were no longer necessary when the cattle had been vaccinated.

**The Disease in Man.** Human beings are only slightly susceptible to the virus of FMD. There have been no recognized cases of human infections in any of the more recent outbreaks of the disease in the United States, and none in the recent one in Mexico, although countless people have had close contact with active virus. Many of the early reports of foot-and-mouth disease in man must be discounted because of lack of critical evidence that the conditions described were caused by this specific virus.

There are some clear-cut records of the disease in man, however. Gins (24) describes the case of a worker in one of the vaccine laboratories who cut his hand in an accident in which a flask containing vesicular fluid was broken. In this case foot-and-mouth disease virus was identified in the fluid of vesicles that developed along with other symptoms in the individual. There are other authentic cases on record but the number is less than fifty. The susceptibility of man to the virus of FMD has recently been reviewed by Betts (9), who concludes that "the number of credible cases in relation to the number of persons exposed is infinitesimal."

The symptoms in man are fever, vomiting, a sense of heat and dryness in the mouth, and the appearance of small vesicles on the lips, tongue, and cheeks. Lesions on the hands have also been described. The course of the disease is short, and there are no records of serious complications or deaths.

FMDV infection in man may be confused with a vesicular exanthema of the hand, foot, and mouth of human beings caused by certain serotypes of Coxsackie virus group A, a subgroup of the genus *Enterovirus*.

## REFERENCES

1. Bachrach.   Ann. Rev. Microbiol., 1968, 22, 1508.
2. Bachrach and Breese.   Proc. Soc. Exp. Biol. and Med., 1958, 97, 659.

3. Bachrach, Breese, Callis, Hess and Patty. *Ibid.*, 1957, 95, 147.
4. Bachrach, Hess, and Callis. Science, 1955, 122, 1269.
5. Bachrach, Patty, and Pledger. Proc. Soc. Exp. Biol. and Med., 1960, 103, 540.
6. Bachrach and Vande Woude. Virology, 1968, 34, 282.
7. Van Bekkum, Frenkel, Fredericks, and Frenkel. Tijdschr. v. Diergeneesk., 1959, 84, 1159.
8. Van Bekkum, Fish, and Dale. Am. Jour. Vet. Res., 1963, 24, 77.
9. Betts. Vet. Rec., 1952, 64, 641.
10. Bögel. Zentbl. f. Vet.-Med., 1966, 14, 79.
11. Brown and Graves. Nature, 1959, 183, 1688.
12. Brooksby. Agr. Res. Council (Gt. Brit.), Rpt. Series no. 12, 1952, H.M. Stationery Office, London.
13. Brown, Hyslop, Crick, and Morrow. Jour. Hyg. (London), 1963, 61, 337.
14. Burrows. Jour. Hyg., 1968, 66, 633.
15. Capstick, Telling, Chapman, and Stewart. Nature, 1962, 195, 1163.
16. Cottral, Gailuinas, and Cox. Arch. f. die Gesam. Virusforsch., 1968, 23, 362.
17. Cowan and Graves. Virology, 1966, 30, 528.
18. Dinter and Philipson. Proc. Soc. Exp. Biol. and Med., 1962, 109, 893.
19. Frenkel. Bul. Off. Internat. des Epizooties, 1947, 28, 155.
20. Frenkel. Am. Jour. Vet. Res., 1951, 12, 187.
21. Gailuinas and Cottral. *Ibid.*, 1967, 28, 1047.
22. Gillespie. Cornell Vet., 1954, 44, 425.
23. Gillespie. *Ibid.*, 1955, 45, 170.
24. Gins. Klin. Wchnschr., 1924, 3, 1135.
25. Graves. Jour. Immunol., 1963, 91, 251.
26. Graves, Cowan, and Trautman. Virology, 1968, 34, 269.
27. Henderson. Proc. 15 Int. Vet. Cong. (Stockholm), 1953, 1, 191.
28. Hyde and Graves. Am. Jour. Vet. Res., 1963, 24, 642.
29. McFadyean. Vet. Rec., 1926, 6, 358.
30. Mohler. U.S. Dept. Agr. Cir. 400, 1926.
31. Mohler. Rpt., Chief, Bur. Anim. Indus., U.S. Dept. Agr., 1929.
32. Mohler and Rosenau. U.S. Dept. Agr. Cir. 147, 1909.
33. Palacios. Rpt. Mtg. Res. Group Standing Tech. Comm., European Comm. Control FMD, Rome, Italy, Paper 8, 1967.
34. Parker. Methods of tissue culture. Paul B. Hoeber, New York, 1938.
35. Pringle. Bul. Off. Internat. des Epizoot., 1964, 61, 619.
36. Ramon. *Ibid.*, 1952, 37, 625.
37. Rosenbusch. Jour. Am. Vet. Med. Assoc., 1948, 112, 45.
38. Schmidt. Zeitschr. f. Hyg., 1936, 191, 1.
39. Schmidt. Zeitschr. f. Immunol., 1936, 88, 91.
40. Schmidt and Hansen. Comp. rend. Soc. Biol. (Paris), 1935, 120, 1150.
41. Schoening. Jour. Bact., 1927, 13, 21.
42. Scott, Cottral, and Gailuinas. Am. Jour. Vet. Res., 1966, 27, 1531.
43. Seibold. *Ibid.*, 1963, 24, 1123.
44. Sellers. Nature, 1955, 176, 547.
45. Shahan. N.Y. Acad. of Sci., 1962, 101, 444.
46. Skinner. Proc. Royal Soc. Med. (Gt. Brit.), 1951, 44, 1041.

47.  Skinner.   Nature, 1954, *174*, 1052.
48.  Stockman and Minett.   Second Progress Rpt., Foot and Mouth Dis. Research Comm. H.M. Stationery Office, London, 1927.
49.  Sutmöller, McVicar, and Cottral.   Arch. f. die Gesam. Virusforsch., 1968, *23*, 227.
50.  Traub and Schneider.   Zeitschr. Naturforsch., 1948, *3b*, 178.
51.  Trautwein.   Arch. f. Tierheilk., 1926, *54*, 273.
52.  Ubertini, Nardelli, Prato, Panina, and Santero.   Zentbl. f. Vet.-Med., 1963, *10*, 93.
53.  U.S. Dept. Agr., Bureau of Animal Industry.   Instructions for employees engaged in eradicating foot and mouth disease. Washington, 1943.
54.  Vallée and Carré.   Comp. rend. Acad. Sci., 1922, *174*, 1498.
55.  Waldmann and Kobe.   Berl. tierärztl. Wchnschr., 1938, *22*, 317 and 349.
56.  Waldmann and Pape.   *Ibid.*, 1921, 37, 349.
57.  Waldmann and Trautwein.   *Ibid.*, 1926, 42, 569.

### Differentiation of the Viruses of Foot-and-Mouth Disease FMD, Vesicular Stomatitis (VS), and Vesicular Exanthema (VE)

In countries where the slaughter method of dealing with foot-and-mouth disease is followed, it is of paramount importance to establish a positive diagnosis at the earliest possible time. When the natural disease occurs in horses, there is no difficulty, for horses are naturally susceptible to only one of these viruses, that of vesicular stomatitis. When it occurs in cattle, the question to be decided is whether it is FMD or VS; when in swine it may be any of the three viruses.

Both field and laboratory methods are used to reach a decision. If a suitably equipped laboratory is available, not only may these three viruses be quickly differentiated from each other by the complement-fixation test, but the virus types may be determined (Brooksby, 1; Camargo, Eichhorn, Levine, and Giron, 3; Camargo, 2). In experienced hands the tests are not only much more rapid than the field or inoculation tests, but they are more accurate and more sensitive.

The field methods of differentiating these viruses depend upon animal inoculation. The procedures, as recommended by Traum (5), are as follows:

1. Inoculate at least two cattle using fresh vesicular fluid. One should be injected intravenously or intramuscularly; the other should be injected in the mucosa of the tongue, lips, or dental pad, or the fluid may be rubbed into scarified areas.

If the virus is that of FMD, both animals should develop the disease.

If it is VS, the animal injected intravenously or intramuscularly will fail to develop the disease; the other should do so.

If it is VE, both animals will fail to develop the disease.

2. Inoculation of swine is useless because the animals usually will develop disease when any of the three viruses are present.

3. Inoculation of horses is very helpful in differentiating between FMD and VS. The horse is susceptible to the virus of VS but is entirely resistant to that of FMD. The virus of VE is mildly pathogenic for horses. Some animals develop small vesicles near the point of inoculation, others do not. Horses should be injected in the mucous membrane of the dorsum of the tongue, or the virus may be introduced through scarification at this site.

4. Guinea pigs are helpful in differentiating between the virus of VE and the other two viruses, since the former does not cause infections when introduced through the footpad, whereas FMD and VS quite regularly produce vesicular lesions.

In 1968 Nardelli *et al.* (4) described a vesicular viral disease in Italian pigs which is clinically indistinguishable from FMD, VE, and VS. The Italian virus is classified as an enterovirus, as it has all the characteristics of that genus. By careful study of its properties one can distinguish it from the other vesicular viral diseases of the pig (see section on enteroviruses).

*Table XXXIX.* TABULAR REPRESENTATION OF THE RESULTS OF INOCULATING ANIMALS WITH THE VIRUSES OF FOOT-AND-MOUTH DISEASE, VESICULAR STOMATITIS, AND VESICULAR EXANTHEMA

|  | FMD | VS | VE |
|---|---|---|---|
| Horse (intradermal-lingual) | — | + | — * |
| Cow (intradermal-lingual) | + | + | — |
| Cow (intramuscular) | + |  | — |
| Guinea pig (intradermal-footpad) | + | + | — |

\* Small local lesions often produced; no generalization.

## REFERENCES

1. Brooksby. Jour. Hyg. (London), 1950, *52*, 394.
2. Camargo. Proc. U.S. Livestock San. Assoc., 1954, *58*, 379.
3. Camargo, Eichhorn, Levine, and Giron. Proc. Am. Vet. Med. Assoc., 1950, p. 207.
4. Nardelli, Lodetti, Gualandi, Burrows, Goodridge, Brown, and Cartwright. Nature, 1968, *219*, 1275.
5. Traum. Jour. Am. Vet. Med. Assoc., 1936, *88*, 316.

## Bovine Rhinovirus

Bovine rhinovirus is one of a number of viruses isolated from the respiratory tract of cattle and it was first described by Bögel (1). Its significance as a pathogen is still unclear, but fragmentary evidence suggests that it is a widespread infection in the cattle population (2). Limited serological surveys have always found antibodies to rhinovirus in test cattle populations in rather high percentages (2, 5). The virus appears to be highly specific for cattle, with a strict affinity for mucous membranes of the respiratory tract, principally the nasal mucosa.

**Character of the Disease.** Field experience with respiratory disease caused by bovine rhinovirus is limited, and only a few isolations have been made. It is rarely isolated from bovine respiratory outbreaks but this failure may be due in part to the difficulties associated with isolating the virus.

In natural and experimental cases the disease is usually characterized by a serous nasal discharge that is seen 2 to 4 days after exposure (2). Other signs of illness may be a rise in temperature, depression, coughing, anorexia, hyperpnea, and dyspnea (6). A pneumonic condition may occur in some experimental calves without other signs of illness (6, 7). In their experiments Mohanty *et al.* (6) observed pneumonia in calves inoculated intratracheally but not in calves exposed to their isolate by the intranasal route. Mayr *et al.* (4) failed to produce disease in calves with their isolate of bovine rhinovirus. Thus, virulence of a strain may play an important role in the production of disease, but, a great deal more needs to be learned about host susceptibility and immunity. The principal pathological changes occur in the nasal passages.

Apparently the morbidity in affected herds is high, but the morality is negligible. The infection has been reported in Western Germany (2), Great Britain (3), and the United States (2, 6).

**Properties of the Virus.** Bovine rhinovirus is an RNA virus less than 30 m$\mu$ in diameter. It is resistant to lipid solvents such as chloroform, ether, and sodium dodecyl-sulfate. It is inactivated at pH 4 to 5.

The few isolates of bovine rhinovirus now available are serologically related or identical (2, 3). In comparative studies with 11 human rhinovirus serotypes no serological relationship was found. Over 90 rhinovirus serotypes have been described in man so it will not be surprising if additional serotypes are subsequently described in cattle.

Attempts to demonstrate a viral hemagglutinin utilizing red blood cells from various species failed (3).

**Cultivation (2).** The only known host systems available for the cultivation of bovine rhinovirus are bovine kidney-cell cultures. Cytopathogenic effects are observed in monolayer cultures maintained at 33 C 1 to 3 days after inoculation. At 33 C viral replication leads to more marked cytopathic changes and a higher infectivity yield than incubation at 37 C. At 33 C viral titers usually are approximately $10^5$ TCID$_{50}$, and disruption of cells produces higher virus yields. Virus plaques are visible in this cell-culture system 4 days after inoculation.

Bovine rhinovirus failed to produce a cytopathic effect in cell cultures of other bovine tissues and kidney cells from other species. Clinical signs were not observed in various aged mice inoculated by various routes. No alterations were observed in guinea pigs or in embryonated hens' eggs injected with bovine rhinovirus.

The virus is quite stable at −60 C for long periods of time. It is readily inactivated by heat.

**Immunity.** Cattle with low titers of serum-neutralizing antibodies can be infected with challenge virus of the same serotype and maternal immunity in calves is never complete (2). These experimental observations suggest that cattle may be reinfected with the same serotype if the titer drops to a low level, but this is mere speculation.

In cattle with no serum-neutralizing antibody, active immunity is accompanied by the production of serum-neutralizing titers that range from 1 : 2 to 1 : 100 against 100 $TCID_{50}$ of rhinovirus (2). The mean antibody titer seems to increase with age, possibly as a result of reinfection with some serotype (2).

There is no evidence that recovered cattle are carriers of the virus although exhaustive studies have not been done. Virus carriers have been detected in other animal species recovered from *Picornaviridae* infections.

**Transmission.** Virus can be isolated from the nasal exudate of cattle only for a few days after inoculation. It is obvious that our knowledge of the transmission and maintenance of this virus in the cattle population is extremely limited. Somehow the virus is maintained in nature and commonly transmitted to cattle, as the morbidity in this host is high.

**Diagnosis.** Clinically, diagnosis of rhinovirus infection from other respiratory pathogens of cattle is difficult if not impossible. The demonstration of a rising serum-neutralizing titer with paired sera is a sound basis for a positive diagnosis. Isolation of the virus in tissue culture is rather difficult, but is the only method available at the present time. Its identification as a rhinovirus includes resistance to chloroform, sensitivity to acid media (pH 4 to 5), optimum growth at 33 C, and a lack of demonstrable pathogenicity for embryonated hens' eggs or small laboratory animals.

**Vaccination.** Until we have further information regarding the economic importance of this disease there is no need for a vaccine.

**The Disease in Man.** There is no evidence that bovine rhinovirus causes disease in man.

## REFERENCES

1. Bögel. Zentbl. Bakt., 1962, *187*, 2.
2. Bögel. Jour. Am. Vet. Med. Assoc., 1968, *152*, 780.
3. Ide and Darbyshire. Brit. Vet. Jour., 1969, 125, Initial Rpt. VII, No. 1.
4. Mayr, Wizigmann, Wizigmann, and Schliesser. Zentbl. f. Vet.-Med. 1965, *12B*, 1.
5. Mohanty. Jour. Am. Vet. Med. Assoc. 1968, *152*, 784.
6. Mohanty, Lillie, Albert, and Sass. Am. Jour. Vet. Res., 1969, *30*, 1105.
7. Wizigmann and Schiefer. Zentbl. f. Vet.-Med., 1966, *13B*, 37.

### Equine Rhinovirus

Equine rhinovirus infection occurs in North America, South America, and Africa. In most instances the infection in horses is inapparent, but it may cause a mild to severe upper respiratory disease. Plummer first characterized the virus and disease in horses (4, 5). All subsequent isolates from horses are serologically related to the first isolate of Plummer except one isolated and described in Canada (3).

**Character of the Disease.** The incubation period is 3 to 7 days. The signs of illness in natural outbreaks include fever, anorexia, and a copious nasal discharge (3). The discharge is initially serous but later mucopurulent in nature. There may be a mild cough and a marked pharyngitis. Lymphadenitis and abscessation of the submaxillary lymph nodes is sometimes observed as a result of secondary bacterial infection, usually with *Streptococcus equi* or *Streptococcus zooepidemicus,* and this prolongs the disease beyond a few days. Infected stables have a high morbidity but a negligible mortality. Virus is recovered from nasopharyngeal swabs taken from horses with high antibody levels (1, 6).

**The Disease in Experimental Animals.** Plummer and Kerry (6) described the clinical signs and virological findings of experimental infection in horses. The clinical signs were similar to those observed in natural disease. The majority of susceptible horses developed a viremia which lasted 4 to 5 days, terminating with the appearance of serum-neutralizing antibodies. Virus was recovered from the pharyngeal tissues of slaughtered horses but not from the intestinal tract. It was estimated that virus persisted for at least 1 month in the pharyngeal tissues on the basis of virus recovery from the feces.

Equine rhinovirus differs from human and bovine rhinoviruses in its pathogenicity for other animal species (5). Rabbits, guinea pigs, monkeys, and man are susceptible to intranasal instillation of rhinovirus type 1 (5). Virus was isolated from blood of man and monkeys, and from rabbits, for a few days after virus instillation and from the upper respiratory tract and associated lymph nodes of the laboratory animals for as long as 10 days after infection. Virus also was isolated from the urine and kidneys of some laboratory animals. Neutralizing antibody appeared in the serum of all species about 7 days after exposure.

Unsuccessful attempts to infect mice, hamsters, chickens, and embryonated hens' eggs have been reported (1). A Canadian strain also failed to produce infection in the guinea pig (10).

**Properties of the Virus.** The physicochemical properties are similar to those of bovine rhinovirus (1). Its particle diameter is 25 to 30 m$\mu$ with an RNA genome. Its sedimentation coefficient in sucrose is 160 S and its density in cesium chloride is 1.40. It is reasonably heat-stable, with little loss of infectivity over several days at 37 C, and with no appreciable loss of titer of two virus strains maintained at 50 C for 1 hour (7). The virus is not stabilized against inactivation at 50 C with 1 M MgCl$_2$.

All isolates except one are serologically identical. The other serotype occurs in Canada and awaits confirmation of its distinct antigenicity by another research group.

No hemagglutinin has been demonstrated for this virus. The only serological test presently available is the serum-neutralization test (2).

**Cultivation.** The equine rhinovirus strains differ from human and bovine rhinoviruses since they will grow in cultures prepared from several animal species (1). A cytopathic effect is produced by equine rhinovirus in primary kidney cultures prepared from the horse, monkey, rabbit, dog, and hamster, in diploid cells of equine origin, and in stable cell lines such as HeLa and HEP-2 from the human, LLC-MK$_2$ from the monkey, and RK-13 from the rabbit. Field isolations have been made in several of these cell culture types. The cytopathic changes in cell culture are typical of rhinoviruses and plaques are present under suitable cultural conditions. A temperature of 33 C and the special requirement of low bicarbonate for human and bovine rhinoviruses are not essential for optimum growth with known strains of equine rhinovirus.

**Immunity.** Our knowledge of immunity to equine rhinovirus is rather limited and some of our present ideas are based upon our general knowledge of immunity as it pertains to other rhinovirus infections of animals and man.

Neutralizing antibody to equine rhinovirus is detected 7 to 14 days after infection and some horses develop maximum serum titers ($>$log 10 $^3$) which presumably persist for long periods of time. The persisting titers are based upon field observations, so reinfection cannot be excluded as the factor accounting for persisting antibody. The relationship of antibody level and protection against disease is not known for equine rhinovirus infection. There probably is a relationship as established for rhinovirus infections of other species since a low level of antibody ($<$log 10 $^{0.5}$) does not protect against infection, whereas higher levels do. There is indirect evidence that maternal neutralizing antibody protects, as 22 foals less than 6 months of age had no antibody (3). It is assumed these foals were protected against this common infection without the development of an active immunity and by 5 to 6 months of age lost their maternal antibody. This speculation was confirmed in a study of 5-month-old foals from immune mares that had no antibody (1). In contrast, a high percentage of Thoroughbreds in training had antibody (6). Other small serological surveys have demonstrated that it is highly contagious and common infection in the horse population.

**Transmission.** Rhinovirus infections of horses are spread mainly by direct or indirect contact with nasal excretions from infected horses and by aerosol inhalation over limited distances (1). Horses can carry the virus for at least 1 month after infection so carrier horses as well as horses in the acute stage of infection with or without signs of illness are good sources of virus for perpetuating the disease on a premises. The virus is also quite stable and conceivably could survive on inanimate objects of an infected premises for a long period of time.

**Diagnosis.** Isolation of the virus from the blood or from the nasal excretions during the acute stage of disease can be readily made in a tissue-culture system. Virus can also be isolated from the pharynx of some horses for as long as 30 days after onset of infection. The virus has the characteristics of a typical rhinovirus being a small RNA virus with resistance to lipid solvents, with susceptibility to pH 4 to 5, lack of demonstrable pathogenicity for embryonated hens' eggs and typical *Picornaviridae* cytopathic effect in cell culture.

The demonstration of a rising serum titer with paired sera is another excellent means of diagnosis.

**Vaccination.** Present knowledge suggests that a suitable vaccine could be developed that would protect horses against this disease (1). If a number of serotypes are subsequently found it may not be feasible. This is the problem in man where at least 90 serotypes are known to exist.

**Disease in Man.** Plummer's studies (4, 5) suggest that man can acquire infection from contact with diseased horses but he found no evidence of man-to-man transmission or from laboratory-animal-to-laboratory-animal transmission.

## REFERENCES

1.   Burrows.   Proc. 2d Internatl. Conf. Equine Inf. Dis. Paris, 1969. S. Karger, Basel, Munich, and New York.
2.   Ditchfield.   Jour. Am. Vet. Med. Assoc., 1969, *155*, 384.
3.   Ditchfield and MacPherson.   Cornell Vet., 1965, *55*, 181.
4.   Plummer.   Nature, 1962, *195*, 519.
5.   Plummer.   Arch. f. die Gesam. Virusforsch., 1963, *12*, 694.
6.   Plummer and Kerry.   Vet. Rec., 1962, *74*, 967.
7.   Wilson, Bryans, Doll, and Tudor.   Cornell Vet., 1965, *55*, 425.

## THE GENUS *ENTEROVIRUS*

The type-species for the genus *Enterovirus* is *Enterovirus* polio 1. Other members of the genus are at least 63 human enteroviruses including polio-, coxsackie-, and echoviruses; bovine enteroviruses; porcine enteroviruses including Teschen virus; simian enteroviruses; Nodamura virus; murine encephalomyelitis virus; and encephalomyocarditis virus. Other possible members are duck and turkey hepatitis viruses, avian encephalomyelitis virus, and acute bee-paralysis virus.

The particles contain 20 to 30 percent single-stranded RNA with an approximate molecular weight of 2.5 by $10^6$ daltons. Nonenveloped isometric particles with icosahedral symmetry are 20 to 30 m$\mu$ in diameter. The particles have a sedimentation rate of 150 to 160 S and a buoyant density in cesium chloride of 1.34 to 1.35 g per ml. Naturally occurring protein shells have a sedimentation rate of 80 S. The particles are naked (no envelope) and inactivated at 50 to 60 C after 30 minutes. The virions are acid-stable at pH 3 and are resistant to ether and other lipid solvents. The virus is synthesized in the cytoplasm and principally resides in the intestinal tract.

## Porcine Enteroviruses

Porcine enteroviruses are cytopathogenic agents isolated from the feces, alimentary tract, and the nasopharynges of pigs in cell cultures. The prototype porcine enterovirus is the virus of Teschen disease.

The physicochemical characteristics of porcine enteroviruses are typical of the genus *Enterovirus*. Multiplication of the viruses take place principally in the alimentary tract but it can also be recovered from the brains of colostrum-deprived pigs that develop nervous manifestations as a result of experimental infection. All porcine enteroviruses grow well on primary porcine kidney cells. Most isolates replicate well on the PK 15 stable kidney-cell line but isolation is more difficult to achieve in this line than in primary cultures. The viruses produce two different types of cytopathogenic effect and most strains will cause plaque formation. The viruses are host-specific, as attempts to adapt them to other hosts have failed except those of Moscovici *et al.* (5), who reported pathogenicity for the hen's embryonated egg.

There are many porcine enterovirus serotypes and some are pathogenic for the natural host. Most pathogenic strains produce polioencephalomyelitis although others called SMEDI (Stillbirth, Mummification, Embryonic Death, Infertility) viruses are implicated with reproductive disorders. One strain of porcine enterovirus reputedly causes severe pneumonia when instilled into the nostril (4) and other strains produce mild pneumonitis by the same route (1). Pericarditis and myocarditis have been observed in experimentally infected germ-free pigs who also developed encephalomyelitis (2).

The porcine enteroviruses have been divided into serological groupings by various investigators (1). More detailed studies now in existence, and close collaboration between working investigators, should soon lead to a single serological classification of porcine enteroviruses acceptable to the International Commission on Nomenclature of Viruses. Serological surveys have shown that porcine enteroviruses are world wide in distribution and the infection rate among pig populations is high. It is extremely difficult to prevent the spread of these agents and it is rare indeed to find a pig herd without antibodies to one or more of the porcine enteroviruses. The antibody response of the pig to various enteroviruses varies, but in general, higher neutralizing-antibody titers are produced by the pathogens. In some inapparent cases of Teschen disease only low titers of neutralizing antibody are produced and precipitating antibodies are absent (3). Perhaps these infections were limited to the gastrointestinal tract and high titers are associated with those cases in which a viremia is part of the infectious process.

Only vaccination against Teschen disease is presently indicated for any of the porcine enteroviruses. If virulent strains of Teschen disease virus are not known to exist in a country or territory, there is every justification to guard against introduction of virulent strains.

These viruses are not known to cause disease in humans or in animals other than the pig.

## REFERENCES

1. Betts. Porcine enteroviruses. Diseases of swine, 3rd ed., H. W. Dunne, ed. Iowa State Press, 1970.
2. Long, Koestner, and Kasza. Lab. Invest., 1966, *15*, 1128.
3. Mayr and Wittman. Zeitschr. f. Immunoforsch., 1959, *117*, 45.
4. Meyer, Woods, and Simon. Jour. Comp. Path., 1966, *76*, 397.
5. Moscovici, Ginevri, and Mazzaracchio. Am. Jour. Vet. Res., 1959, *20*, 625.

### Teschen Disease

SYNONYMS: Porcine poliomyelitis, Talfan disease, infectious porcine encephalomyelitis.

This is a virus-induced encephalomyelitis of swine which has caused serious losses in Czechoslovakia, southeastern Germany, Hungary, Yugoslavia, and Poland. It has also been reported in Switzerland, France, Sweden, Denmark, Great Britain, and Madagascar. In England it became known as *Talfan disease* before its identity became established as a milder form of the disease. This disease has not been recognized in Asia. Mild strains are present in Canada (12), United States (7), and Australia. A condition described by Thordal-Christensen in Denmark as *benign enzootic paresis of swine* may be a mild form of Teschen disease (13).

The disease was first accurately described in 1929. The word *Teschen* is the name of a town in Czechoslovakia where the disease was first recognized. So far as is known, natural infection with this virus occurs only in swine.

**Character of the Disease.** The incubation period averages about 14 days, though it may be considerably longer or shorter. Sometimes the disease is sporadic, affecting only a few individuals in a herd; at other times it may affect nearly the whole herd. The disease may be acute or chronic, and apparently there is an inapparent form. The prodromal signs are fever, lassitude, and inappetence. This may be followed by a variety of nervous signs—irritability, convulsions, prostration, stiffness, and then paralysis of the legs, particularly of the hind legs. Opisthotonos is frequent. Often the animals lie on their sides and make running motions with their forelegs. Sometimes they squeal when disturbed. The mortality averages about 70 percent, varying from 50 to 90. Animals that recover from the acute stages frequently have residual paralysis. If such animals are carefully nursed, they may live a long time, in which case atrophy of affected muscles may occur. Animals that live more than 1 week often develop pneumonia and succumb.

There are no gross lesions with the possible exception of myocardial lesions. The microscopic lesions are confined to the central nervous system, in which they are typical of a diffuse encephalomyelitis. Cytoplasmic masses occur in nerve cells. With minor exceptions the lesions are confined to the gray matter. Dobberstein (2) was so impressed with the similarity of these lesions to those of poliomyelitis of man that he insisted upon calling the disease *porcine poliomyelitis.* Horstmann, Manuelidis, and Sprinz (6), while admitting that the cord lesions have a resemblance to those of poliomyelitis, think that the diffuseness of the lesions and especially their great concentration in the cerebrum make them very different from those of the human disease.

**Properties of the Virus.** Being an enterovirus, the virus particles are approximately 20 to 25 m$\mu$ in diameter (5). The viral antigen has been demonstrated in the cytoplasm and to a lesser degree at the periphery of the nucleus (11). Cold phenol has been used to extract the infectious RNA.

It has a wide range of pH stability and shows ether resistance, and it survives well at icebox or low temperatues. A temperature of 60 C for 20 minutes or 0.15 percent formalin inactivates the virus.

Immunologically distinct strains have been described, but in general, virulent strains are serologically similar (14). Strains can be separated into three antigenic subtypes (8). The neutralization test in pig kidney cell cultures and the gel-diffusion test both demonstrate antibodies.

**Cultivation.** Fortner was able to obtain growth of the virus in chick embryos. Horstmann obtained survival in tissue cultures for 17 days but was unable to prove that multiplication had occurred. Mayr and Schwobel (10) were successful in cultivating the virus in swine kidney cell tissue cultures. After some passages the virus grew well, produced cytopathogenic effects, and retained irs virulence for swine. It also produces plaques on monolayers.

**Immunity.** Animals that have recovered from this disease are solidly immune thereafter, at least for a few months. Several attempts have been made to make a brain-virus vaccine. Fortner (3, 4) had only indifferent success with a formalin-treated vaccine. Single injections failed completely. Better but unsatisfactory results were obtained with two injections. Zarnic (15) reported somewhat better results with a formol-treated brain vaccine.

Rapid passage in pig kidney cultures attenuates the virulence of the virus for piglets. This attenuated virus vaccine or formalin-inactivated vaccine using culture virus gave 80 to 86 percent protection (9). Fortner found that the blood serum of recovered pigs had little effect in protecting against virus exposure.

**Transmission.** The disease apparently is transmitted by direct contact. Experimentally it was shown that it can be transmitted by feeding and by intranasal instillation. Fortner, however, was not able to demonstrate virus in the nasal secretions. The virus is usually a harmless inhabitant of the intestinal tract. Seldom does the disease spread rapidly in a herd. Fortner obtained infection by pen contact in only 3 out of 29 trials.

It was suggested that the disease might be due to the virus of cholera, but Diernhofer (1) found that animals immune to cholera can be infected with the Teschen virus and that animals that have recovered from the latter can be infected with cholera. It seems to be clearly established that the Teschen virus is unique and not related to any other disease-producing agent.

Virus has been inoculated by various workers into mice, rats, guinea pigs, sheep, cattle, and monkeys, generally intracerebrally, with negative results.

## REFERENCES

1. Diernhofer.   Deut. tierärztl. Wchnschr., 1940, 48, 213.
2. Dobberstein.   Zeitschr. f. Infektionskr. Haustiere, 1942, 49, 54.
3. Fortner.   Deut. tierärztl. Wchnschr., 1941, 49, 43.
4. Fortner.   Zeitschr. f. Infektionskr. Haustiere, 1942, 59, 81.
5. Horstmann.   Jour. Immunol., 1952, 69, 379.
6. Horstmann, Manuelidis, and Sprinz.   Proc. Soc. Exp. Biol. and Med., 1951, 77, 8.
7. Koestner, Long, and Kasza.   Jour. Am. Vet. Med. Assoc., 1962, 140, 811.
8. Mayr.   Bul. Off. Internat. Epizoot., 1961, 56, 106.
9. Mayr and Correns.   Zentbl. f. Vet-Meds., 1959, 6, 416.
10. Mayr and Schwoebel.   Monatsh. f. Tierheilk., 1956, 8, 49.
11. Mussgay.   Centrbl. Bakt. I, Abt. Orig., 1958, 171, 231.
12. Richards and Savan.   Cornell Vet., 1960, 50, 132.
13. Thordal-Christensen.   Monograph, Royal Vet. and Agr. College, Copenhagen, 1959.
14. Whitman.   Zentbl. f. Vet-Med., 1958, 5, 505.
15. Zarnic.   Jugoslav. veterinarski glasnik, 1947, 11–12, 600. (Abstract in: Jour. Am. Vet. Med. Assoc., 1948, 113, 181.)

## Porcine SMEDI Group of Enteroviruses

In 1965 Dunne et al. (2) reported on two serologically distinct groups of swine enteroviruses that are associated with stillbirth, mummification, embryonic death, and infertility in swine. These groups were designated as SMEDI A and SMEDI B. More recently, Wang and Dunne (4) reported that the SMEDI virus strains fell into 4 of their 10 serological group designations for porcine enteroviruses.

**Character of the Disease.** The three problem herds from which these viruses were isolated had similar disease syndromes and epizootiological pictures. The most consistent observation was a decrease or absence of living pigs at birth and the passage of 1 to 12 mummified fetuses of varying sizes. Many pigs alive at birth died a few hours later. The number of live pigs farrowed by infected sows was less than one-half the average number of unaffected sows. Some infected sows that were bred returned to heat but never farrowed. Repeat breedings were more frequent. At no time during the course of infection did sows show signs of illness. No other diseases were observed in these herds and certain ones such as brucellosis and leptospirosis were eliminated on the basis of serological testing. Both Yorkshire and Berkshire breeds were involved. In one herd two serological types of SMEDI viruses were isolated in kidney cells from fetal or newborn pigs.

At necropsy the gross lesions in experimental and field stillborn pigs were limited to mild edema, particularly of the spiral colon, hydrothorax, and hydropericardium. Preliminary histological studies of a few stillborn pigs included cellular infiltration, edema, and hemorrhage. These lesions were in most but not in all of the stillborn pigs examined. Encephalitic lesions were seen in a number of the animals.

In England, swine herds affected with similar reproductive disorders were studied by Cartwright and Huck (1). Fifteen enteroviruses were isolated and five were placed in the SMEDI A group, three in the SMEDI B group, two in the SMEDI C group, and one in the T80 group of porcine enteroviruses. A parvovirus also was isolated from many of their test materials. The pathogenic significance of the porcine parvovirus has not been determined as yet, but parvoviruses in other species are responsible for fetal defects and abortions. Steck and Addy in Switzerland (3) isolated 30 enteroviruses from 47 aborted fetuses. Their isolates fell into two serological groups with some cross reaction with SMEDI B and SMEDI C groups.

**Properties of the Virus.** By electron microscopy Dunne *et al.* (2) estimated the particle size to be 30 millimicrons, and it appeared to be icosahedron in shape. The virus was resistant to heating at 56 C for 2 hours and it was ether resistant.

By the use of the tissue culture neutralization test the SMEDI group A and B viruses were compared with many other viruses of swine. The SMEDI group A appears somewhat related to a group of swine enteroviruses not yet fully classified but designated as Group II. The SMEDI group B show some relationship to edema disease virus and the virus of Ontario (Canada) polioencephalitis of swine. There was no relationship of either group with Ontario (Canada) hemagglutinating, Teschen (Talfan), hog cholera, or transmissible gastroenteritis viruses.

Hemagglutination and hemadsorption trials were negative.

**Cultivation.** The SMEDI viruses were isolated from infected fetuses, still alive or dead for only a short period of time, in kidney cell cultures from healthy fetuses or newborn pigs. The viruses produced a cytopathogenic effect in these cultures.

**Immunity.** After infection, sows develop a significant neutralizing antibody titer. The importance of these antibodies in terms of protection or its duration have not been ascertained.

**Control.** No control measures can be suggested because the means of transmission of this disease are not definitely known.

**The Disease in Man.** There is no evidence that it occurs in man.

## REFERENCES

1. Cartwright and Huck.   Vet. Rec., 1967, *81*, 196.
2. Dunne, Gobble, Hokanson, Kradel, and Bubash.   Am. Jour. Vet. Res., 1965, *26*, 1284.

3.  Steck and Addy.   Personal communication, 1968.
4.  Wang and Dunne.   Personal communication, 1969.

### A Porcine Enterovirus Causing Vesicular Disease (1)

In 1966 a disease appeared on two farms in large numbers of pigs that was indistinguishable from other porcine vesicular diseases including foot-and-mouth disease, vesicular stomatitis, and vesicular exanthema. Present evidence suggests that it is a porcine enterovirus.

**Character of the Disease.** The clinical signs include a fever and vesicular lesions on the coronary band and bulbs of the heel and in the interdigital spaces. Vesicles are found also on the snout and on the skin overlying the metacarpals and metatarsals of some animals. Vesicles rupture after 2 to 3 days and healing is rapid in most animals without secondary bacterial infection.

**Transmission.** The disease appeared on two farms at the same time, both receiving pigs for fattening from a common source. All introduced pigs on both farms were afflicted and approximately 25 percent of the resident pigs in the same pens on both farms showed signs of illness. No new cases were seen after 3 weeks later.

**Properties of the Virus.** This porcine virus has all the characteristics of an enterovirus. It is stable at pH 5 and it is stabilized by 1 M $MgCl_2$ at 50 C. Its buoyant density in cesium chloride is 1.34 g per ml. The virion is resistant to ether. The sedimentation rate is 150 S in sucrose gradients. Viewed with the electron microscope it is roughly spherical, 30 to 32 m$\mu$ in diameter, thus further assisting in differentiation from FMD, VS, and VE viruses.

**Cultivation.** The virus produces a cytopathic effect in primary and secondary pig-kidney monolayer cultures and in cultures of pig-kidney cell lines PR 15 and IB-RS-2. No effect was observed in primary calf-kidney or in calf-thyroid monolayer cultures or in first-passaged baby hamster kidney cell-line cultures.

**The Disease in Experimental Animals.** The disease is reproduced in susceptible pigs by inoculation of infected epithelial suspensions or infective tissue culture suspensions into the coronary band or bulb of the heel or by contact with infected pigs. Experimental disease is less severe than field infection and only 50 percent of experimental pigs develop clinical signs.

The injection of the tongue dermis of a donkey, two cattle, rabbits, and chickens with infective vesicular epithelium failed to induce frank disease. Injection of the foot-pads of guinea pigs or of the abdominal skin of hamsters failed to elicit an inflammatory reaction. Large doses of tissue-cultured virus given intracerebrally or intraperitoneally in day-old mice produced nervous signs 4 to 5 days after inoculation and death in 5 to 10 days. Virus was distributed in the brain, spinal cord, and muscular tissues. No signs of illness were produced in 7-day-old mice with the same inoculum by the same routes.

**Immunity.** Little is known. Neutralizing antibodies are formed in the pig but their relationship to protection is not known.

**The Disease in Man.** Unknown.

## REFERENCE

1. Nardelli, Lodetti, Gualandi, Burrows, Goodridge, Brown, and Cartwright. Nature, 1968, *219*, 1275.

## Bovine Enterovirus

Bovine enteroviruses (BE) have been isolated from normal cattle, and from cattle showing various signs of illness. Numerous strains (>60) isolated in various parts of the world have failed to produce disease in experimental cattle although Van Der Matten and Packer claim that some of their strains caused diarrhea (3).

The bovine enteroviruses have the same physicochemical properties as other members of the genus *Enterovirus*. BE are present in feces and produce a characteristic enterovirus cytopathic effect in cell cultures of embryonic bovine kidney, calf testicle, embryonic lamb kidney, human kidney, rhesus monkey kidney and testes, rabbit kidney, established bovine kidney, and diploid embryonic bovine trachea (2). Embryonic bovine kidney or calf testicle cell cultures are recommended for initial isolations.

Neutralizing antibody can be produced in various laboratory animals. The rooster and goat are preferred to produce hyperimmune antisera. Rabbits should be avoided because their sera contain a naturally-occurring inhibiting substance.

Various systems have been employed by investigators to classify the numberous isolates including the plaque-reduction test. LaPlaca has divided BE into 2 major groups based on the hemagglutination of rhesus monkey RBC and sensitivity to HBB (1). A comparison of 13 BE strains in North America by plaque-reduction test yielded four major antigenic groups (4). Comparative studies of strains isolated in various parts of the world are now in progress and should lead to a satisfactory nomenclature of BE.

## REFERENCES

1. LaPlaca. Arch. f. die Gesam. Virusforsch., 1964, *17*, 98.
2. Moll and Davis. Am. Jour. Vet. Res., 1959, *20*, 27.
3. Van Der Matten and Packer. *Ibid.*, 1967, *28*, 677.
4. York. Personal communication, 1970.

## Avian Encephalomyelitis

SYNONYMS: Epidemic tremor of chicks

This avian enterovirus disease was first described by Jones (7) in Massachusetts in 1932. In a more complete description of the disease and the virus that causes it, Jones (8) in 1934 called the disease *epidemic tremor* because of the peculiar vibration of the head and neck which characterizes many cases. Because this sign is not so frequently seen as others referable to damage of the nervous system, Van Roekel, Bullis, and Clarke (15) proposed that it be named *infectious avian encephalomyelitis*. The word *infectious* is now generally dropped from the name.

The disease has been recognized only in very young chickens. It generally makes its appearance when the chicks are from 2 to 3 weeks of age, but it may appear earlier or later. Van Roekel and associates have observed signs in chicks as they were removed from the incubator within 24 to 48 hours after they had been hatched. Others have reported cases as late as 42 days after hatching.

**Character of the Disease.** The disease was first diagnosed in the northeastern part of the United States and for some years was believed to be confined to this region. In later years, according to Feibel, Helmboldt, Jungherr, and Carson (5), it has been identified in many states across the country, and it has been reported also from Canada, Great Britain, Sweden, South Africa, Korea, and Australia. The disease has a seasonal prevalence in the United States, being seen more frequently in the winter and spring months than in the summer.

The first sign noted is an ataxia or inco-ordination of the muscles of the legs. The signs become more obvious as the disease progresses, and finally the bird may lose all control of its legs and be unable to stand. Before this stage is reached the bird is reluctant to move and may walk on its shanks. The characteristic vibration of the muscles of the head and neck usually appears well after the ataxic signs have been noticed. This tremor is periodic, continuing for varying lengths of time. Finally the victim is unable to feed, becomes somnolent, and dies. In many cases the course of the disease is very rapid, somnolence appearing within 24 hours after the first signs are noted.

Chicks artifically infected by intracerebral inoculation rarely show signs in less than 9 or 10 days. There are no data on the incubation period in natural infections; however, it probably is 2 weeks or more.

The course of the disease varies greatly. Many birds become incapacitated so they cannot reach food and hence die of starvation; others are killed by being trampled by other birds. If separated and given individual care, many severely affected birds will live for a long time, and some even recover.

The losses may be very high, in excess of 50 percent in some cases. The average mortality is about 10 percent.

There are no gross lesions. Microscopically, the islands of lymphatic tissue which, in birds, are scattered throughout the organs, show evidence of marked hyperplasia. The most characteristic lesions, however, are found in the central nervous system. Exceptionally large masses of lymphocytes and monocytes surround all of the blood vessels. Extensive neuronal degeneration occurs especially in the anterior horn of the cord, in the medulla, and in the pons. No specific inclusion bodies have been identified in this disease.

**The Disease in Experimental Animals.** Avian encephalomyelitis has not been observed naturally occurring in species other than chickens and pheasants; however, ducklings, turkey poults, and young pigeons may be infected by inoculation. All mammals are refractory. All workers have found that the most certain way of reproducing the disease is by intracerebral injection. Injection of virus peripherally—intravenously, intraperitoneally, or intramuscularly—induces signs in only a small proportion of those inoculated. Chicks from hatching time to 3 weeks of age are most susceptible to inoculation, but Van Roekel (15) and others have succeeded in producing the disease in birds up to 3 months of age, and Feibel (4) has infected birds more than 6 months of age by intraperitoneal injection. Ingestion, even of large amounts of virus, has uniformly failed to produce disease. Some infections have been produced by intranasal instillation.

**Properties of the Virus.** Virus is regularly present in the nervous system of infected birds. Virus suspensions regularly pass V and N Berkefeld filters and Seitz disks. Olitsky and Bauer (12) showed by filtration through Gradocol membranes that the particle size of this virus is about 20 to 30 millimicrons in diameter. The virus is readily preserved for long periods by rapid freeze-drying, and it has retained viability for at least 80 days when suspended in 50 percent neutral glycerol. Olitsky (11) found no relationship between the virus of avian encephalomyelitis and that of equine encephalomyelitis. The chick virus proved innocuous for mice, guinea pigs, and monkeys, which are susceptible to the equine virus; furthermore, there were no cross-immunological reactions between the two viruses.

**Cultivation.** Jungherr, Sumner, and Luginbuhl (9) successfully propagated the virus in embryonated eggs by inoculating them into the orb of the eye. Wills and Moulthrop (17) succeeded by inoculating into the yolk sac and into the allantoic cavity. Kligler and Olitsky (10) failed with chick embryos but succeeded in obtaining growth in a medium consisting of minced chick embryos suspended in a mixture of rabbit serum and Tyrode's solution. Neutralizing antibodies are demonstrable by the use of the cytopathogenic effect produced in monolayers of chick fibroblast cultures (6) and in monkey kidney cell cultures.

**Immunity.** Schaaf and Lamoreux (13) observed that after a flock had suffered from an outbreak of this disease, generally there was very little further trouble from it; apparently the flock has become immunized. Following this observation they injected virus into the birds of the breeding flock when they were from 16 to 20 weeks of age. Birds at this age react very mildly to the virus but they become solidly immune thereafter and they apparently do not lay infected eggs when they come into production. They claim to have eliminated the disease from a flock by following this procedure. Chicks which have recovered from this disease are resistant to reinoculation, and neutralizing antibodies can be demonstrated in them.

**Transmission.** Rather convincing information now exists which shows that horizontal and vertical transmission of the disease takes place. The disease is transmitted from infected chickens of various ages to susceptible birds or by placing susceptible birds in a colony house that previously housed infected chickens (2). Virus has been recovered from the feces of normal chicks. Vertical transmission occurs via infected eggs from carrier birds which produces clinical infection in the progeny (2). Transmission of virus occurs when egg-infected chicks are placed with susceptible contact chicks following exposure within the incubator during hatching (3, 15) or in batteries following hatching with an incubation period of 11 to 16 days following contact (2). Because the disease usually occurs during the winter months, it is unlikely that insect vectors play a role in its transmission.

**Diagnosis.** Clinical diagnosis of avian encephalomyelitis in young chicks is not difficult. In doubtful cases other chicks may be inoculated intracerebrally with brain tissue. This procedure is not always successful since the viral content of brain tissue of diseased chicks sometimes is below an infectivity level. The presence of blood vessel cuffing, gliosis, and neuronal degeneration points toward a viral encephalitis but does not necessarily indicate this disease. The demonstration of rising antibody titer with paired sera is also useful.

**Control.** A simple test that is based upon the failure of embryos produced from immune hens to support the growth of virus can be used to select resistant-breeder flocks as a means of avoiding disease in their progeny (14).

It is possible to produce an immune breeder flock by the use of live and inactivated vaccines when used under the appropriate circumstances (1).

**The Disease in Man.** It is not known to occur in man.

## REFERENCES

1. Calnek, Luginbuhl, McKercher, and Van Roekel.   Avian Dis., 1961, 5, 456.
2. Calnek, Taylor, and Sevoian.   *Ibid.*, 1960, 4, 325.
3. Doll, Bruner, and Hull.   Rpt. of the Director, Ky. Agr. Exp. Sta., 1948, p. 48.
4. Feibel.   Thesis, Univ. Conn., 1951. (In: Biester and Schwarte. Diseases of poultry. 3d ed. Iowa State Press, Ames, Iowa, 1952, p. 621.)
5. Feibel, Helmboldt, Jungherr, and Carson.   Am. Jour. Vet. Res., 1952, *13*, 260.
6. Hwang, Luginbuhl, and Jungherr.   Proc. Soc. Exp. Biol. and Med., 1959, *102*, 429.
7. Jones.   Science, 1932, 76, 331.
8. Jones.   Jour. Exp. Med., 1934, 59, 781.
9. Jungherr, Sumner, and Luginbuhl.   Science, 1956, *124*, 80.
10. Kligler and Olitsky.   Proc. Soc. Exp. Biol. and Med., 1940, *43*, 680.
11. Olitsky.   Jour. Exp. Med., 1939, 70, 565.
12. Olitsky and Bauer.   Proc. Soc. Exp. Biol. and Med., 1939, *42*, 634.
13. Schaaf and Lamoreux.   Am. Jour. Vet. Res., 1955, *16*, 627.
14. Taylor and Schelling.   Avian Dis., 1960, 4, 122.
15. Van Roekel, Bullis, and Clarke.   Jour. Am. Vet. Med. Assoc., 1938, *93*, 372.
16. Van Roekel, Bullis, and Clarke.   Vet. Med., 1939, *34*, 754.
17. Wills and Moulthrop.   Southwest. Vet., 1956, *10*, 39.

## Virus Hepatitis of Ducklings *Picorna*

This disease was first recognized and described by Levine and Fabricant (7) in 1950. The disease had not been seen previously by experienced observers in the duck-raising area on Long Island, where many ducklings have been raised annually for many years. Dougherty (4) has reported finding the disease in Massachusetts and in the western part of New York State. Hanson and Alberts (6) reported an outbreak in Illinois. Asplin and McLauchlin (3) reported the presence of the disease in England. Virus isolated from English birds was neutralized by antiserum obtained from New York. The disease was recognized in Canada in 1957 and the virus isolated (8). It has since been recognized in Michigan and also in various other countries of the world.

This virus affects only young ducklings. There are no signs in adult birds, although such birds often harbor infection. Young chicks and turkey poults have been raised in close association with infected ducks without developing the disease.

**Character of the Disease.** In the earlier outbreaks, losses occurred only among ducklings between 2 and 3 weeks of age, but later losses were incurred on many farms on birds as young as 3 days. The disease is very acute with a short incubation period of about 2 to 3 days. In most instances signs were not observed longer than 1 hour before death. The affected birds were observed to lag behind the remainder of the hatch; they quickly became somnolent, fell on their sides, and died after a brief struggle. Nearly all deaths in a particular hatch occurred within 4 days, the peak of the death rate usually occurring on the 2nd day. The mortality varies from flock to flock, and from hatch to hatch in the same flock. Sometimes it is as high as 85 to 95 percent of large hatches. In other cases it may be as low as 35 percent.

The principal lesions are found in the liver. Usually it is enlarged and contains petechiae and ecchymotic hemorrhages. Mottling of the parenchyma is commonly seen. Focal necrosis of liver cells occurs. The spleen and kidneys often are swollen. The microscopic changes (5) consist of necrosis of the parenchymal cells and proliferation of bile duct epithelium. These changes are accompanied by varying degrees of inflammatory reaction and hemorrhages. In ducklings that do not die, successful regeneration of liver parenchyma occurs.

In 1969 Toth (11) reported the isolation of an agent from liver suspensions from ducks that died under 2 weeks of age with hepatitis despite a parenteral immunity to duck hepatitis virus. These agents caused hepatic disease in susceptible ducks and in duck hepatitis virus immune ducks. The clinical signs and lesions were similar but not completely identical to typical virus hepatitis of ducks. Present evidence suggests that the agent is a new serotype of duck hepatitis virus or an entirely different infectious agent, probably the former.

No species other than that in which the disease naturally occurs has been found to be susceptible.

**Properties of the Virus.** Electron photomicrographs showed the virus to be spherical and quite small, 20 to 40 millimicrons. It is an RNA virus which is ether resistant. Inactivation occurs in 30 minutes at 62 C, but not at 56 C. It resists 0.1 percent formalin for 8 hours at 37 C. It is classified as an enterovirus.

Attempts to demonstrate hemagglutinins have failed. Two lines of precipitate have been demonstrated in the gel-diffusion test. In 1963 Sueltenfuss and Pollard (10) described a technic for the cytochemical assay of interferon produced by duck hepatitis virus.

**Cultivation.** The virus can be propagated in developing chick embryos, killing most of the embryos in 4 days without observable lesions. Later deaths showed characteristic lesions consisting of stunting of growth; severe edema; greenish discoloration of the embryo liver, egg fluids, and yolk-sac; and necrotic foci of the liver (7).

In cultures of chick embryo tissues propagation of the virus occurs without production of a cytopathic effect (9).

**Immunity.** Ducks recovering from the natural disease or from inoculation with egg-propagated virus are resistant to reinoculation, and their sera contain neutralizing antibodies for the virus.

Artificial immunization of ducklings has been attempted. Active immunization with vaccines made from allantoic fluid and embryo livers, inactivated with formalin, and from living virus of egg origin did not give satisfactory results. The failure apparently was due to the fact that the disease usually struck before the tissues had had time to produce a protective antibody level. Much better results were obtained with antiserum from ducks that had recovered from the disease. This was secured at the slaughterhouse at the time the birds were dressed for market. This serum, administered intramuscularly in 0.5-ml doses, protected most of the ducklings from the disease when administered at ages varying from 3 to 11 days. In eight trials the treated ducklings showed mortality rates varying from 0 to 19 percent, whereas control ducklings, raised in the same pens, had mortality percentages varying from 26 to 80.

This procedure has been used with success on many thousands of ducklings during the last 10 years in the concentrated duck-raising area of eastern Long Island, New York.

Asplin (1) has reported success in preventing losses of ducklings by actively immunizing the breeder ducks with virulent virus. He has also reported the successful use as a vaccine of an attenuated strain of virus which had been modified by growth in chick embryos. Ducklings were vaccinated with a needle which was thrust through one of the foot webs after being dipped in virus (2).

The new variant agent of Toth (11) is now included in the immunization program for prevention of virus hepatitis in ducks on Long Island. This program now has fewer immunization problems since the variant agent has been recognized and included.

**Transmission.** The means of transmission is not entirely clear. The high incidence of the disease in infected flocks indicates a high rate of transmissibility; yet many instances have occurred in which hatches with a high mortality rate have been kept in the same buildings, and sometimes in the same rooms, with other hatches in which the disease has failed to develop. Transmissibility through eggs has not been proved, and considerable evidence is at hand to indicate that this does not occur. Hatches, and parts of hatches, which have been removed to other premises directly from the incubators have failed to develop the disease, whereas the remainder, kept on the premises, have exhibited a high mortality rate. Present evidence indicates that the disease spreads during the brooding process by contacts other than through droplets.

**Diagnosis.** The diagnosis is based upon clinical signs and by inoculation of chick embryos. Inoculations succeed when organ suspensions, blood, or brain material is used for injection.

**The Disease in Man.** There is no evidence to connect this disease with illness in man. Comparisons of the virus of duck hepatitis with those of virus hepatitis of dogs and man show no serological relationships (5).

## REFERENCES

1. Asplin.  Vet. Rec., 1956, 68, 412.
2. Asplin.  *Ibid.*, 1958, 70, 1226.
3. Asplin and McLauchlan.  *Ibid.*, 1954, 66, 456.
4. Dougherty, III.  Proc. Am. Vet. Med. Assoc., 1953, p. 359.
5. Fabricant, Rickard, and Levine.  Avian Dis., 1957, 1, 257.
6. Hanson and Alberts.  Jour. Am. Vet. Med. Assoc., 1956, 128, 37.
7. Levine and Fabricant.  Cornell Vet., 1950, 40, 71.
8. MacPherson and Avery.  Canad. Jour. Comp. Med., 1957, 21, 26.
9. Pollard and Starr.  Proc. Soc. Exp. Biol. and Med., 1959, 101, 521.
10. Sueltenfuss and Pollard.  Science, 1963, 139, 595.
11. Toth.  Avian Dis., 1969, 13, 834.

## Virus Hepatitis of Turkeys

Two groups of workers in the eastern part of the United States (1, 2) independently and almost simultaneously described a hitherto-unknown viral-induced hepatitis of turkey poults. Both were successful in propagating the virus in the yolk sacs of embryonating eggs and in producing the disease in day-old poults by inoculating them into the unabsorbed yolk sacs.

The virus is classified provisionally as an enterovirus. It is resistant to penicillin, streptomycin, and tetracycline. Baby chicks are resistant to inoculation with the virus.

The disease is very contagious and produces a high death rate in poults under 2 weeks of age. Turkeys which recover from infection developed resistance to reinfection but no serum-neutralizing antibodies were demonstrated in the sera of these birds or in the serum of chickens, turkeys, or rabbits repeatedly inoculated with this virus (3). A common antigen between turkey and duck hepatitis viruses was demonstrated by the agar gel diffusion test but other characteristics of the two viruses are dissimilar (3). Attempts to infect ducklings, quail, and pheasants proved unsuccessful (3).

### REFERENCES

1.  Mongeau, Truscott, Ferguson, and Connell.   Avian Dis., 1959, 3, 388.
2.  Snoeyenbos, Basch, and Sevoian.   *Ibid.*, 377.
3.  Tzianabos and Snoeyenbos.   *Ibid.*, 1965, 9, 578.

### Human Enteroviruses in Dogs

It was reported that the human enteroviruses: echovirus type 6, Coxsackie virus $B_1$, $B_3$, and $B_5$ were isolated from nasopharyngeal and rectal specimens of Beagle dogs without signs of illness (2, 3). Low neutralizing antibody titers against Coxsackie virus $B_3$ and $B_5$ were present in some of the sera collected from these dogs. No titers were demonstrated for Coxsackie virus $B_1$ or echovirus type 6. There was no correlation between virus isolation and serum titers.

Feeding echovirus type 6 to dogs produced signs of enteric disease (4). Although virus was recovered from fecal samples of 5 of the 6 dogs antibody was not demonstrated.

Neutralizing antibody to poliovirus types 1 and 3, Coxsackie virus A9 and $B_2$, and echovirus types 6, 7, 8, 9, and 12 has been found in dog serums (1). Replication of these viruses and the production of disease in the dog by them has not been ascertained.

### REFERENCES

1.  Gefland.   Progr. Med. Virol., 1961, 3, 193.
2.  Lundgren, Clapper, and Sanchez.   Proc. Soc. Exp. Biol. and Med., 1968, *128*, 463.
3.  Pindak and Clapper.   Am. Jour. Vet. Res., 1964, 25, 52.
4.  Pindak and Clapper.   Texas Rep. Biol. and Med., 1966, *24*, 466.

### Equine Enterovirus

An equine enterovirus was isolated from the liver and spleen of an aborted foal (1). The RNA virus is less than 28 m$\mu$. It is resistant to ether, chloroform, and trypsin, relatively stable to cations at normal temperatures, and over a wide pH range.

Its significance as a pathogen is yet to be ascertained.

### REFERENCE

1.  Böhm.   Zentbl. f. Vet.-Med., 1964, *11*, 240.

## THE GENUS *CALICIVIRUS*

This is a newly characterized genus that includes the vesicular exanthema viruses and also a large group of feline viruses formerly called feline picorna-viruses.

The type species for the genus *Calicivirus* in the family *Picornaviridae* is vesicular exanthema type A virus. The particles in this genus contain single-stranded RNA with a molecular weight of approximately 2 by $10^6$ daltons. The isometric nonenveloped particles with 32 capsomeres and with probable icosahedral symmetry are 30 to 40 m$\mu$ in diameter. Their buoyant density in cesium chloride is 1.37 to 1.38 g per ml. The particles are unstable at pH 3 and have variable stability at pH 5. The virions are resistant to ether and chloroform. Replication takes place in the cytoplasm of susceptible cells.

### Vesicular Exanthema

SYNONYMS: None; abbreviation, VE

**Species Susceptible.** VE occurs naturally only in swine. Even by inoculation it is difficult to produce more than local lesions in experimental animals other than swine.

**Occurrence.** VE has been recognized only in the continental United States, Hawaii, and Iceland, where it undoubtedly was carried in American pork. The disease was eradicated in the United States in 1959. Despite this fact it can be confused with FMD, so we should have a knowledge of this disease as it may reappear.

Early in 1932 an outbreak of what was regarded as foot-and-mouth disease (FMD) appeared in a number of swine herds in southern California. Seventeen premises eventually became infected and about 18,000 hogs were slaughtered and buried in an effort to stamp out the disease. It reappeared the following year, but on a much smaller scale, and was again handled in the belief that it was FMD. Investigations conducted during these outbreaks led to the conclusion that the disease was not what it had been thought to be, but a hitherto-unknown virus-induced malady. The disease was first differentiated from FMD by Traum (9), who proposed the name by which it is now known.

VE continued to occur in California year after year since little effort was made to control it after it was recognized not to be FMD. In 1952, just 20 years after it had first been recognized, the disease suddenly spread eastward in the United States. Within a few months outbreaks had been reported in 42 states and the District of Columbia. Vigorous control measures were then initiated, with the result that the disease was eliminated by 1959.

**Character of the Disease.** In VE, as in FMD, vesicles of varying size occur on the snout, lips, tongue, footpads, and skin between the claws, around the coronary bands and dew claws, and also on the teats of nursing sows. About 12 hours before the lesions appear a febrile period occurs in most animals.

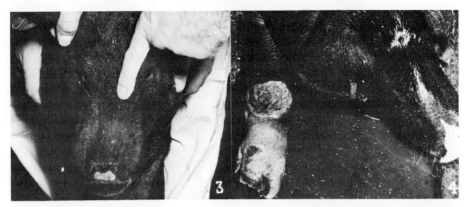

Fig. 244. Vesicular exanthema, showing ruptured vesicles on the snout (3) and on the forelimb (4). These lesions cannot be distinguished from those of foot-and-mouth disease. (Courtesy L. M. Hurt.)

Failure of the animals to come for feed when called is frequently the first sign noted. It is then noticed that the animals are lame. This is generally more severe in heavy animals than in those of lighter weight. The foot soreness causes most of the animals to lie down, and they protest by squealing when they are forced to rise to their feet and walk. Sometimes animals will walk knuckled over on their fetlocks to remove weight from their feet. During this time rapid loss in body weight usually occurs. It has been estimated that the weight loss in growing pigs as a result of this disease amounts, on the average, to the equivalent of one month's feeding. All experienced observers agree that the lesions of VE cannot be distinguished from those of FMD by gross inspection.

According to White (10), the incubation period in this disease usually is about 48 hours, though sometimes it may be as short as 18 hours. In a few instances it has been reported to be very much longer. Apparently it is about the same, as a rule, as that of FMD.

The course of the disease in individuals is relatively short. The mouth lesions heal quickly, but the foot lesions may cause lameness of several weeks' duration because of secondary bacterial infections. The disease in an infected herd may last several weeks to several months, because it does not spread as rapidly as FMD. Some animals may escape infection even though they are susceptible.

The death rate among adult animals is very low, but heavy losses often occur among suckling pigs. The baby pigs are believed to die from suffocation because of vesicles that form in their nostrils or from starvation because of failure of lactation in the sows.

The lesions of VE consist of the vesicles on the skin and mucous membranes already described. As in FMD, these vesicles rupture very easily leaving raw surfaces with ragged margins to which whitish flaps of partially detached epithelium often adhere.

**The Disease in Experimental Animals.** The disease may readily be produced in swine by inoculation with virus-containing materials or by feeding organs or tissues containing virus. All attempts to infect cattle, calves, sheep, goats, rabbits, rats, mice, hedgehogs, and chick embryos have failed. In horses, intradermal lingual injection gives variable results. Some strains produce vesiculation at the points of injection; others do not. Crawford (3) found that two strains with which he worked regularly produced such lesions and two others did not. Since those that succeeded were of a different serological type than those that failed, it was his belief that the difference was a type characteristic. This has not been confirmed. It may be only a question of relative virulence without reference to serological grouping.

Unlike the viruses of FMD and vesicular stomatitis (VS), the virus of VE does not ordinarily infect guinea pigs. Traum claims that he has seen vesiculation in a few cases at the point of injection. His attempts to adapt some such strains to continued passage in this species have always failed after a few passages.

Bankowski and Wood (2) reported occasional successes in infecting dogs by intradermal lingual injection. The lesions produced at the point of inoculation were mild and characterized by erosion of epithelium and blanching. Often the animals showed some fever. Virus was recovered on one occasion from the spleen of a dog 16 hours after inoculation. It was not recovered from several others that did not become febrile. Dogs were successfully infected with strains belonging to the three types of virus then known.

Madin and Traum (6) report success in infecting hamsters with VE virus. With one strain they succeeded in making six serial passages by intradermal inoculation of the skin of the abdomen. The strain then lost its ability to cause further infections. Another strain proved to be regularly pathogenic for hamsters. Secondary lesions were never found. The development of local lesions was definitely associated with a fever curve.

**Properties of the Virus.** Crawford was the first to show that there was a plurality of viruses in VE. He identified four serological types, which were designated A, B, C, and D. Unfortunately the strains with which he worked have been lost, so they cannot be identified with relation to present-day strains. Madin and Traum (6) proposed that three types found in southern California be named A, B, and C, and to these Bankowski *et al.* (1) added a fourth, D. More recently at least 9 more types were identified in California, making a total of 13. As in FMD, all of these types are immunologically distinct from each other. As to pathogenicity for swine, no differences have been recognized among the several types.

Multiple-virus types have been found only in California. In all other areas where the disease has been found after the 1952 spread, only the B type was identified.

Electron micrographs showed that the virus bodies were 35 m$\mu$ across. Resistance is similar to FMDV. It is inactivated in 60 minutes at 62 C, or in 30 minutes at 64 C. The virus survives 6 weeks at room temperature and 2 years in the refrigerator in 50 percent glycerol. Two percent sodium hydroxide is recommended for its destruction.

This virus is provisionally placed with the caliciviruses.

**Cultivation.** The types grow with considerable ease in kidney, skin, or embryonic tissue cultures of swine, horse, dog, and cat with the production of CPE (5). On monolayers of pig kidney cultures plagues of two sizes occur, the larger ones being more virulent for swine (4).

**Immunity.** Swine inoculated with any of the types of VE virus develop, within 3 weeks, a solid immunity to that type which lasts for at least 6 months and perhaps much longer. Animals recovering from infection with one type may, however, almost immediately develop the disease again as a result of infection with one of the other types of virus. Madin and Traum (6) made a formalin-killed vaccine adsorbed to an aluminum gel, by essentially the same technic as that used for the Schmidt-Waldmann vaccine for FMD, and found that it would create a solid immunity. No attempt has been made to make such a vaccine for field use.

**Transmission.** It has been pointed out that nearly all outbreaks of VE have occurred in herds of swine that were fed garbage. White (10) reported that in the 1939–1940 outbreak in California, only 8 of the 123 herds involved had not been fed raw garbage, and four of these had had some contact with herds that had been fed garbage. Throughout their entire experience with this disease, it has been recognized that new herd infections are initiated in one of two ways: (a) by the introduction of infected animals into the herd, or (b) by the feeding of uncooked garbage which originated off the premises.

Garbage-fed swine undoubtedly become infected from pork scraps and trimmings derived from carcasses which contained virus at the time of slaughter. Meat-inspection authorities make efforts to prevent the use of meat from any slaughtered animals that are infected, but it is known that such animals often cannot be detected, and their flesh enters trade channels. It is such meat that, finding its way uncooked into garbage, eventually sets up outbreaks in swine herds.

Mott, Patterson, Songer, and Hopkins (7) found that it was not easy to infect susceptible pigs placed in uncleaned pens which had previously contained infected ones. These findings accord with field experience that the disease is not so easily transmitted as FMD.

**Diagnosis.** As with VS, the matter of greatest importance is to make sure that the disease outbreak is not, in fact, FMD. In California during the many years when little was done to control VE, the precaution was taken of requiring garbage feeders to keep a few young calves in the same pens with the swine. When a vesicular disease struck the herd, authorities felt safe in assuming the disease to be VE rather than FMD if the calves remained free of infection. The differentiation of FMD, VE, and VS is discussed in the section on FMD (page 1230).

**Control.** Since this disease does not have the high level of infectivity that FMD possesses, it has not proved so difficult to control. For the 20 years the disease was confined to a single state and very little effort was made to control it after it became known that it was not FMD. When it was thought to be FMD, two attempts were made to stamp it out by the drastic methods employed for that disease. On both occasions all herds in which the disease was recognized were slaughtered and buried, and yet the disease reappeared in other herds the following year. Undoubtedly the virus had been carried over in refrigerated pork. Had the drastic method of control been in force for a few years, it is probable that the disease would eventually have been stamped out, because infected pork would eventually have been eliminated.

Experience has shown that VE is more readily controlled than FMD. The methods used since 1952 in the United States are as follows:

1. *The quarantine of infected herds.* Animals from infected herds should not be permitted to go to slaughter until at least 2 weeks (8) after all evidence of active disease in the herd has disappeared. Even this time period may not be safe in all instances. A better procedure is to allow animals from recently infected herds to go only to processing plants where all meat is cooked or otherwise processed by methods which will destroy the virus.

2. *The enactment and enforcement of garbage-cooking laws.* This is undoubtedly the most effective single procedure. If such laws were universally enforced, they would quickly eliminate the disease. They would also remove part of the danger of infection with FMD, would greatly reduce the trichinosis hazard in man, and would help in the control of hog cholera. All states but one have enacted such laws and are endeavoring to enforce them, and these have certainly helped greatly in bringing the disease under control. The Federal government has assisted by banning the interstate shipment of pork from pigs fed uncooked garbage at any time in their lives unless the meat has been processed in such a way as to destroy any virus which it might contain.

**The Disease in Man.** There is no evidence that VE is infective for man.

## REFERENCES

1. Bankowski, Keith, Stuart, and Kummer. Jour. Am. Vet. Med. Assoc., 1954, *125*, 383.
2. Bankowski and Wood. *Ibid.*, 1953, *123*, 115.
3. Crawford. Proc. U.S. Livestock San. Assoc., 1936, *40*, 380.
4. McClain, Hackett, and Madin. Science, 1958, *127*, 1391.
5. Madin. Vesicular exanthema. In: Dunne. Diseases of swine. 2d ed. The Iowa State University Press, Ames, Iowa, 1964.
6. Madin and Traum. Vet. Med., 1953, *48*, 395.
7. Mott, Patterson, Songer, and Hopkins. Proc. U.S. Livestock San. Assoc., 1953, 57, 334.
8. Patterson and Songer. Proc. U.S. Livestock San. Assoc., 1954, *58*, 396.
9. Traum. Jour. Am. Vet. Med. Assoc., 1936, *88*, 316.
10. White. *Ibid.*, 1940, *97*, 230.

### Feline Caliciviruses

SYNONYM: Feline picornaviruses.

Until 1971 the feline caliciviruses were called feline picornaviruses. In most instances the infection is limited to the upper respiratory tract but it may also produce pneumonia. In 1957 Fastier (10) first isolated and studied a virus representative of this group. Other investigators then made isolations characteristic of the group and it soon became apparent that many serotypes exist.

**Character of the Disease.** The disease is characterized by a diphasic temperature reaction, serous and mucoid rhinitis, conjunctivitis, profound depression, and in some cats, râles, and ulcerative glossitis. Cats that survive 4 to 5 days of illness fully recover in 7 to 10 days. The incubation period is estimated at 2 to 3 days.

Present evidence suggests that this is a common disease in many cats and often is a major disease problem in catteries. In these circumstances the morbidity is high and the mortality usually is low.

**The Disease in Experimental Animals.** Information about experimental disease in cats with the feline caliciviruses is rather limited but the signs of illness are similar to those observed in cats with natural infection. Kittens show marked and acute signs including dyspnea, depression, and pulmonary râles. Pneumonia was detected by radiography (13).

A pneumotropic strain was used by Kahn and Gillespie to study the pathogenesis of a feline calicivirus (15). At necropsy, pneumonia was the most consistent lesion found at death or when kittens were sacrificed at various times after aerosol exposure to virus. During first days after exposure, the lungs were mottled with reddish-gray areas of congestion and edema. Kittens examined after acute inflammatory response contained slightly elevated, firm areas in the lung, pink gray to pale red in color. The lesions had a patchy distribution and by day 10 the pneumonia was resolving and by day 34 the lungs were normal. In the oral cavity glossal and palantine ulcers, 2 to 5 mm, were irregular with well-defined margins. The most common site of ulcer formation was the rostrodorsal epithelium of the tongue. Ulcers also were seen on lateral margins of tongue, base of tongue, and beneath the tonsillar folds. The spleens of most kittens had irregular transverse bands, 5 to 10 mm in width. The tissues of experimental kittens were studied further by histopathological examination and by immunofluorescence. Some kittens had a mild fibrinous rhinitis but lesions in the upper respiratory tract and eye were minimal. Ulceration of tongue epithelium and the hard palate was a necrotic process accompanied by a neutrophilic reaction beneath the lesions. Viral antigen was demonstrated at the base of a tongue ulcer by fluorescent antibody technic (13). The acute inflammatory response in the lungs was maximal by the second day and was followed by hypertrophy of alveolar macrophages which had desquamated into the alveolar spaces. Small accumulations of mononuclear cells were seen in some bronchi. At this stage viral antigen was seen in the cytoplasm of alveolar macrophages. Fluorescence also was observed in bronchial and bronchiolar epithelial cells. Mild hypertrophy and hyperplasia of the epithelium of these air passages also were apparent. By the 5th day, neutrophils are replaced largely by lymphocytes and plasma cells. Specific fluorescence was seen in the cytoplasm of columnar epithelial cells lining bronchiolar passages. The proliferation of mononuclear cells was accompanied by a proliferation of macrophages lining the alveoli resulting in adenomatoid formations. These reactions seemed most prominent between the 7th and 10th days and thereafter slowly resolved. Resolution was still incomplete at 34 days. The spleens had well-developed foci of hematopoiesis and also a reticuloendothelial hyperplasia. Diffuse fluorescence may occur in some kittens. Fluorescence in the tonsillar cells is confined to the epithelium of the tonsillar crypts and the staining was not intense.

The original isolations of some feline caliciviruses by various investigators were made from visceral tissues so it is apparent that a viremia does occur in some feline calicivirus infections. In this regard it differs from human rhinovirus infections, which are limited to the respiratory tract.

Experimental evidence exists that one feline calicivirus is probably involved in the etiology of feline urolithiasis (8, 18). The disease has been reproduced in a significant percentage of experimental cats by the inoculation of this virus. Present studies suggest a complex etiology (8, 9). Certain interesting facts are emerging, but considerable research work is essential to define the role of this virus and others in the pathogenesis of feline urolithiasis.

Attempts to produce disease in such laboratory animals as rabbits, mice, and guinea pigs have failed.

**Properties of the Virus.** Estimation of the virus particle size has been done by filtration (5, 6) and by electron-microscopic examination (2, 19, 21), and it is generally agreed that its diameter is 37 to 40 m$\mu$. The 32 hollow capsomeres are arranged hexagonally to match a rhombic triacontahedron (2, 21) although Strandberg (19) described the capsomeres as thin and rod-like, 5 m$\mu$ long and 2.5 m$\mu$ wide (fig. 245). The virions are naked and this is in accord with their resistance to lipid solvents such as ether, chloroform, and desoxycholate (3, 10). The virus is a single-stranded RNA particle (1, 13). The members of this group exhibit a pH sensitivity that is intermediate between enteroviruses and rhinoviruses. In general, the feline caliciviruses are inactivated at pH 3 and stable at pH 4 and pH 5 (5, 6, 14). The virus is resistant to HBB (hydroxybenzylbenzimiazole), guanidine HCl and 0.2 percent sodium deoxycholate (5). These viruses are inactivated at 50 C in 30 minutes. The presence of $MgSO_4$ or $MgCl_2$ does not stabilize the agents; in fact $MgCl_2$ enhances thermal inactivation (14).

No hemagglutinin has been associated with feline picornaviruses (7, 11).

The neutralization test is utilized for the determination of serotypes in this virus group. A number of investigators in the United States and Europe (4, 5, 6, 17) have studied the serological relationship of many isolates of feline cali-

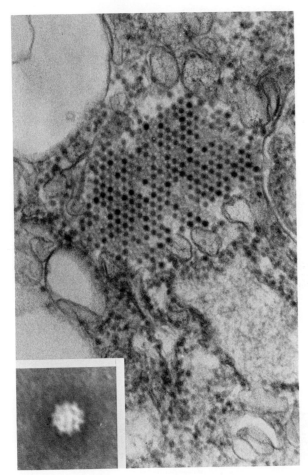

*Fig. 245.* Feline calicivirus. Virus crystals (V). X 69,000. (*Inset*) A single virion of stain KCD showing thin and rodlike capsomeres. Negative stain. X 230,000. (Courtesy J. Strandberg, D. Kahn, P. Bartholomew, and J. Gillespie.)

civirus. There are many problems, such as antigenic crossings, that exist in the development of a satisfactory nomenclature for these viruses; but there is little doubt that innumerable serotypes exist. Limited comparative studies also suggest that protection is induced to the homotypic serotype but not against heterotypic serotypes.

**Cultivation.** These viruses originally were isolated in monolayer cultures of feline kidney cells (7, 10). All serotypes tested produce a cytopathic effect, usually within 48 hours, in monolayer cultures of primary and secondary feline kidney cells, of diploid feline tongue and feline thymus cell lines (16), and of established cell lines from feline kidney cells (Crandell) and from embryonic feline lung.

Attempts to cultivate a few serotypes in monolayer cultures of established cell lines from selected tissues of various hosts other than domestic cat or lion failed (16).

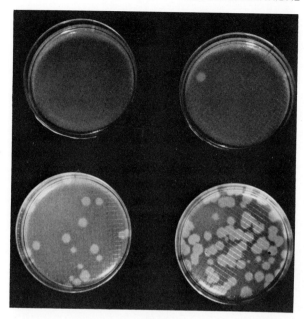

*Fig. 246.* Agar overlay monolayer cell cultures with clearly defined plaques showing results of a virus titration of a feline calicivirus (strain C14). (*Top left*) An uninoculated control. (*Top right*) A $10^{-7}$ dilution of virus (0.1 ml of inoculum). (*Lower left*) A $10^{-6}$ dilution. (*Lower right*) A $10^{-5}$ dilution.

In susceptible cell cultures overlayed with agar or methyl cellulose, feline caliciviruses produce plaques (3, 5, 6). It is sometimes difficult to obtain suitable plaques in successive transfers for plaque purification with certain serotypes (12).

The cytopathology in a tissue-culture system at the ultrastructural level showed that the virus replicated within the cytoplasm of infected cells, forming large crystalline arrays of closely packed particles (20), similar to poliovirus. (fig. 247). The infected cells develop large numbers of small, membrane-bound vesicles, myelin figures, and other membraneous structures within their cytoplasm. Changes occurring within the nucleus, although secondary to viral infection, included the formation of dense nuclear masses of clumped chromatin.

**Immunity.** Limited knowledge suggests that a specific feline calicivirus protect cats against itself but not against other serotypes. The degree of neutralizing-antibody response varies markedly depending upon the serotype. The relationship of the neutralizing antibody to protection in the cat is not known with certainty.

**Transmission.** The feline caliciviruses appear to be limited in nature to the cat family. The virus may persist in the pharyngeal area after acute respiratory disease and conceivably carriers play a role in the transmission of the infection (13).

**Diagnosis.** The diagnosis of the respiratory disease is difficult for the clinician as a number of other respiratory pathogens produce similar signs of illness in the cat. After the technic is refined it should be possible to detect the

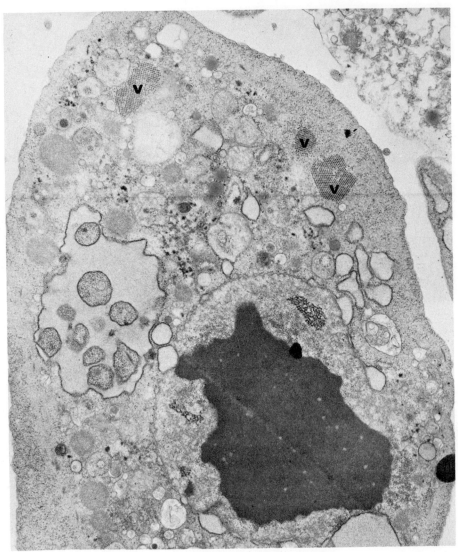

*Fig. 247.* Feline calicivirus. Note crystalline array of virus particles (*V*) in the cytoplasm. X 13,660. (Courtesy J. Strandberg, D. Kahn, P. Bartholomew, and J. Gillespie.)

viral antigen in conjunctival scrapings or in tonsillar biopsies by the use of immunofluorescence. A conjugate prepared with antiserum against a single serotype will be sufficient to make a diagnosis for most, if not all, as the feline caliciviruses share a common antigen that is demonstrable by this test (12).

Isolation of the virus can be made in cell cultures of feline origin from nasal excretions, pharyngeal swabs, or conjunctival scrapings during acute stages of respiratory illness. Virus may be found in blood during the acute stage but it is not a tissue of choice for this purpose. It is not difficult to establish the identity of a tissue-cultured feline calicivirus isolate as a member of that group by utilizing our knowledge of its physicochemical properties and the immunofluorescence test. Its identity as a specific serotype is cumbersome, time-consuming, and expensive and is presently done only by investigators specifically interested in a research study of these viruses. An International Working Team under the World Health Organization is in the process of producing viral and serum reagents to many serotypes in an effort to learn more about the nature of these viruses and their effects on members of the cat family.

**Control.** Feline calicivirus infections in the cat population are exceedingly difficult to control and treat because of their contagious nature, many serotypes, and refractiveness to specific therapy. The husbandry practices used to maintain cat colonies tend to encourage the dissemination of respiratory illnesses. The existence of carriers and the relative stability of feline caliciviruses further complicates the control. Unless depopulation of a colony and proper disinfection of the premises is done the infection is likely to persist in cat colonies for an indefinite period of time.

At present the development and use of vaccines for feline caliciviruses is impractical.

**The Disease in Man.** There is no evidence that feline calicivirus causes disease in man.

## REFERENCES

1. Adldinger, Lee, and Gillespie. Arch. f. die Gesam. Virusforsch., 1969, *28*, 245.
2. Almeida, Waterson, Prydie, and Fletcher. *Ibid.*, 1968, *25*, 105.
3. Bartholomew and Gillespie. Cornell Vet., 1968, *58*, 248.
4. Bittle, York, Newberne, and Martin. Am. Jour. Vet. Res., 1960, *21*, 547.
5. Bürki. Arch. f. die Gesam. Virusforsch., 1965, *15*, 690.
6. Crandell. Proc. Soc. Exp. Biol. and Med., 1967, *126*, 240.
7. Crandell, Nieman, Ganaway, and Maurer. Virology, 1960, *10*, 283.
8. Fabricant, Rich, and Gillespie. Cornell Vet., 1969, *59*, 667.
9. Fabricant, Gillespie, and Krook. Jour. Inf. and Immunity, 1971, *3*, 416.
10. Fastier. Am. Jour. Vet. Res., 1957, *18*, 382.
11. Gillespie, Judkins, and Scott. Cornell Vet., 1971, *60*, 159.
12. Gillespie, Judkins, and Kahn. *Ibid.*, 172.
13. Kahn. Cornell Univ. Thesis, 1969.
14. Kahn and Gillespie. Cornell Vet., 1970, *60*, 669.
15. Kahn and Gillespie. Am. Jour. Vet. Res., 1971, *32*, 521.
16. Lee, Kniazeff, Fabricant, and Gillespie. Cornell Vet., 1969, *59*, 539.
17. Prydie. Vet. Rec., 1966, *79*, 729.
18. Rich and Fabricant. Canad. Jour. Comp. Med., 1969, *33*, 164.
19. Strandberg. Cornell Univ. Thesis, 1968.
20. Strandberg, Bartholomew, Kahn, and Gillespie. Unpublished information, 1971.
21. Zwillenberg and Bürki. Arch. f. die Gesam. Virusforsch., 1966, *19*, 373.

# LI | Hog Cholera, Bovine Viral Diarrhea-Mucosal Disease, and Equine Arteritis

There are three small RNA-enveloped viruses, probably helical, that are of considerable importance as animal pathogens and are treated as a separate group at the present time. Hog cholera virus (HCV), bovine viral diarrhea-mucosal disease virus (BVD-MDV), and equine arteritis virus (EAV) share many characteristics yet do not fit into any presently recognized genus established by the International Committee on Nomenclature of Viruses. They do share some common properties with members of the arbovirus subgroup B, but there are enough differences that they are not included in this genus.

Hog cholera virus and bovine viral diarrhea-mucosal disease virus are closely related to each other biophysically, biochemically, and biologically (see page 1280). The equine arteritis virus shares most of the biophysical and biochemical characteristics of the other two. A difference in this regard is the resistance of EAV towards 0.5 mg per ml of trypsin whereas HCV and BVD-MDV are trypsin-sensitive. HCV and BVD-MDV share a common soluble antigen with each other, but not with EAV. There seems little doubt that HCV and BVD-MDV are more closely related to each other than to EAV.

## Equine Arteritis

SYNONYMS: Epizootic cellulitis-pinkeye syndrome, *rotlaufseuche;* abbreviation, EA

It may be the same disease that was described by German scientists as *Rotlaufseuche* and by English writers as epizootic cellulitis-pinkeye syndrome or typhoid fever. In 1953 the virus was isolated from outbreaks in Ohio, (U.S.) that were characterized by illness in horses and abortions in the mares (4). Since then virus has been isolated from three other epizootics in the United

1262

States by these same investigators. The first isolation of EAV in Europe was made in Switzerland (3) and later in Vienna, Austria (3). There is serological evidence for the disease in India (3).

In the past this disease has been confused with equine influenza and equine rhinopneumonitis. The horse is the only susceptible animal and the principal natural infections have been observed only on breeding farms (2).

**Character of the Disease.** The horses develop a fever, stiffness of gait, edema of the limbs, and swelling around the eyes. The disease spreads rapidly to susceptible horses on the premises. Pregnant mares abort, and this was the essential feature of the disease in the four natural outbreaks. Stallions may also contract the disease. It usually occurs on breeding farms and no fatalities are observed, nor does it cause residual damage.

**The Disease in Experimental Horses.** Inoculation of the virus into pregnant mares or young horses causes death in almost 50 percent of the animals (4). Abortions were produced in the mares. These experimental effects suggest that this virus conceivably could cause mortality under favorable circumstances.

The incubation period is 3 to 5 days (4). Fever is a constant sign, and the other signs were dependent upon the site and amount of damage to the arteries. Other signs in fatal cases included pronounced conjunctivitis, palpebral edema and edema of the nictitating membrane, and excessive lacrimation. The nasal membrane became congested, and a serous nasal discharge was noted. Pulmonary dyspnea was frequent, and there was marked depression and muscular weakness. Mild or severe colic may be accompanied by watery diarrhea. There was edema of the limbs. On occasions keratitis, hypopyon, icterus, edema of the abdomen, and marked loss of weight were observed. Panleukopenia characterized by lymphopenia occurs in affected horses.

The basic lesions involve small arteries about 0.5 mm in diameter, and these arteries are the smallest vessels that possess well-developed muscular coats (6). The arterioles (less than 0.3 mm in diameter) and the large muscular and elastic arteries are free of specific lesions. Veins and lymphatics are often distended with blood or lymph, respectively, but were neither inflamed nor necrotic. The specific lesions in small arteries are distributed at random in segments of the arterial system throughout the body. Arterial lesions were found in every organ, but more conspicuously in the cecum, colon, spleen, lymph nodes, and adrenal capsule.

The specific microscopic lesion starts with necrosis of muscle cells in the arterial media (6). Edema and a few leukocytes then appear in the adventitia. The arterial media becomes edematous and infiltrated by lymphocytes, some with karyorrhectic or pyknotic nuclei. Initially, these changes may be limited to one microscopic segment of the artery viewed in cross section. As the lesion progresses, most of the arterial media is involved and replaced by edema and leukocytes. At this stage the artery is tortuous and the intact endothelium becomes surrounded by leukocytes and edema which replaces the media and adventitia. The lumen usually is empty and contains a few erythrocytes. In the large intestine and spleen, frank thrombosis and infarction occurs. Consequently, the effect of these arterial changes is most often edema and hemorrhage. The mechanism of death is not definitely known, but the probable changes in electrolytes in cells and tissue fluids might be important (6).

The gross lesions are explained entirely on the basis of distribution of the lesions in small arteries (6). Edema and petechiae are conspicuous in adult animals and fetuses. Fetuses are particularly edematous but no distinct microscopic lesion is found in the arteries. Edema is found in the subcutis of the legs and abdomen, adjacent to the injection site, and in the adjacent fascia. Edema and petechiae are also found in the omental, mesenteric, and perirenal fat, subpleural and interlobular septums of the lungs, in the intra-abdominal lymph nodes, the broad ligament, and the adrenal cortex. Similar hemorrhages and edema are evident along the course of the ileocecocolic and anterior mesenteric arteries. The intestines, especially the cecum and colon, are severely involved with sharply demarcated segments, 1 to 2 meters long. The entire wall is edematous and the mucosa markedly hemorrhagic. These lesions are related to typical changes in submucosal arteries with thrombosis in most vessels. Sharply demarcated, often elevated hemorrhagic infarcts are seen in the spleen, particularly in younger horses.

**Properties of the Virus.** The incorporation of 5-iodo-2-deoxyuridine in tissue cultures does not inhibit the replication of virus, presenting indirect evidence that EVA is an RNA virus (3). The virus is readily inactivated by lipid solvents and by sodium deoxycholate. It survives 20, but not 30, minutes at 56 C (10). The virus is quite stable at low temperatures. It is resistant to trypsin. In sucrose gradients its density is 1.18 to 1.20 g per ml (7).

By Millipore filtration the particle size is estimated from 50 to 100 m$\mu$ (3). Virus was concentrated and purified by ultracentrifugation and again by zonal centrifugation in sucrose gradients (7). This preparation was treated with uranyl acetate and phosphotungstic acid. The negatively stained particles observed in the electron microscope were spherical and had an average diameter of 60±13 m$\mu$. The inner core of the virion had an average diameter of 35±9 m$\mu$. In the cytoplasm of infected tissue-cultured cells virus particles located in the cytoplasmic vacuoles are 43±2 m$\mu$, with a core diameter of 35±2 m$\mu$ (1). These particles are observed at 18 hours postinoculation but not at 12 hours. The viral particles are found in increasing concentration and in increasing numbers of cells at 24, 30, 34, and 43 hours postinfection.

The virion apparently lacks a hemagglutinin but does contain a complement-fixing antigen component. Only one immunogenic type of virus is known to exist and it produces neutralizing antibodies. The prototype virus is the Bucyrus strain (4).

**Cultivation.** Attempts to propagate EAV in the hen's embryonated egg and in laboratory animals have failed (4). It produces a cytopathogenic effect in cultures of horse kidney cells and becomes attenuated so it can be used for immunization (10). It also grows in hamster kidney cells (11) and in rabbit kidney cells (9). This virus produces plaques in overlay cultures. Thus far, only cells of equine origin show a CPE upon inoculation with material from infected horses. Adapted strains replicate in tissue cultures from other species. In cell culture the Bucyrus strain usually yields $10^6$ TCID$_{50}$ per ml. Sonified tissue-culture preparations are used as a good source of CF antigen (3).

**Immunity.** Horses that recover from infection or immunization with a modified live virus have a solid immunity. Vaccinated horses are immune for at least 1 year to virulent virus challenge and presumably for many years (8). Antibodies against EAV can be demonstrated by the CF and neutralization tests.

The Bucyrus strain was modified by transferring it 131 times in primary cell cultures of horse kidney followed by 111 transfers in primary cell cultures in rabbit kidney. As little as 200 TCID$_{50}$ of virus by the intramuscular route protected horses against challenge with virulent virus. Vaccine administered by the intranasal route failed to immunize horses effectively. The virus protected pregnant mares without causing any ill effects on their fetuses. Newborn foals from two vaccinated mares were not protected by colostrum when they were challenged at 5 and 9 days of age. These studies should be expanded to include greater numbers and also serology correlated with challenge before any definite conclusion on maternal immunity can be ascertained.

Serial passage of the vaccine virus did not restore its virulence. The vaccine virus did not spread to susceptible horses maintained in direct contact with the vaccinated horses.

**Transmission.** The virus is spread by aerosol and contracted by inhalation (2). The virus is in the nasal secretions for 8 to 10 days. The tissues and fluids of infected aborted fetuses contain virus.

**Diagnosis.** Arteritis occurs sporadically, and in the typical outbreak mortality does not occur, but abortions occur in 50 to 80 percent of pregnant mares. The aborted fetuses often are autolyzed in contrast to the fresh aborted fetuses usually associated with rhinopneumonitis virus infection.

For diagnosis by virus isolation samples may be taken from the nostrils, blood, or conjunctival sac. The nasal or conjunctival exudate is placed in Hanks' balanced salt solution with antibiotics and 1 percent bovine albumin. These specimens can be stored at $-20$ C for weeks. At necropsy, many different organ tissues can be used for virus isolation. Virus isolation attempts are made in primary cell cultures of horse origin or by horse inoculation. The demonstration of a rising antibody titer by the use of the complement-fixation test or neutralization test is another suitable means for making a diagnosis.

**Control.** According to the Panel of the American Veterinary Medical Association Symposium on Immunity to Selected Equine Diseases (5) the disease may be prevented and controlled by good management practices and vaccination. It was their recommendation that the attenuated HK-131 RK-111 Bucyrus virus vaccine be licensed when justified by supplementary data received by the Veterinary Biologics Division, U.S. Department of Agriculture from potential commercial producers (5). The Panel also recommended continued research of an inactivated virus vaccine.

**The Disease in Man.** It is not known to occur.

## REFERENCES

1. Breese and McCollum.   Proc. 2d Internatl. Conf. Equine Inf. Dis., S. Karger & Co., Basel, Switzerland, 1969, 133.
2. Bryans.   Proc. Am. Vet. Med. Assoc., 1964, p. 112.
3. Bürki.   Proc. 2d Internatl. Conf. Equine Inf. Dis., S. Karger & Co., Basel, Switzerland, 1969, 125.
4. Doll, Bryans, McCollum, and Crowe.   Cornell Vet., 1957, 47, 3.
5. Equine Disease Symposium.   Panel Report. Jour. Am. Vet. Med. Assoc., 1969, 155, 237.
6. Jones, Doll, and Bryans.   Cornell Vet., 1957, 47, 3.
7. Maess, Reczko, and Böhm.   Proc. 2d Internatl. Conf. Equine Inf. Dis., S. Karger & Co., Basel, Switzerland, 1969, 130.
8. McCollum.   Jour. Am. Vet. Med. Assoc., 1969, 155, 318.
9. McCollum, Doll, Wilson, and Cheatham.   Cornell Vet., 1962, 52, 454.
10. McCollum, Doll, Wilson, and Johnson.   Am. Jour. Vet. Res., 1961, 22, 731.
11. Wilson, Doll, McCollum, and Cheatham.   Cornell Vet., 1962, 52, 200.

### Hog Cholera

SYNONYM:   Swine fever (English); abbreviation, HC

Hog cholera is an acute, highly contagious disease of swine characterized by degeneration in the walls of the smaller blood vessels, which results in multiple hemorrhages, necrosis, and infarctions in the internal organs. Affected animals are prone to suffer from the effects of bacterial agents that frequently accompany the virus, but these secondary agents are not necessary for the production of the disease. The cause of the disease is a virus.

The history of HC was reviewed by Kernkamp (32). Hog cholera was first recognized as a separate disease entity by Salmon and Smith (46) in 1885, but it was erroneously believed to be caused by the bacterium which they called *Bacillus cholerae-suis*, now known under the name *Salmonella choleraesuis*. The error was corrected in 1903 when DeSchweinitz and Dorset (16) proved that the disease was caused by a virus and that the "hog cholera bacillus" played a secondary and nonessential role in the disease.

Hog cholera is a tremendously destructive disease which, despite fairly satisfactory immunization procedures, causes large losses in the United States and most other parts of the world where swine are raised. The disease seems to have been first seen in the state of Ohio in 1833; from there it spread to all parts of the United States through the shipment of stock. Its greatest prevalence in the United States is in the northcentral states, the so-called *corn belt*, where the greatest concentration of the swine population occurs. Cholera was not seen in England until 1862 and on the continent of Europe until 1887. There is an eradication program now in progress in the United States.

**Character of the Disease.** Present knowledge suggests that hog cholera virus produces natural disease only in domestic and wild pigs. Outbreaks of the disease in swine have been recorded in nearly all European countries, in Africa, Asia, Australia, and the United States. The disease occurs only sporadically in Canada.

The disease is first manifested by fever (104 F or higher), although often the first sign noticed is loss of appetite. In a fully susceptible herd the disease generally begins in a few animals, then gradually spreads to others until finally practically all are sick. The affected animals appear dull and drowsy; they crowd together in corners or under haystacks or in any other protected place as if chilled. Vomiting is common, a mucopurulent discharge from the eyes frequently is seen, and many suffer from diarrhea. Sometimes the diarrheal attacks alternate with periods of constipation. In white-skinned animals a livid coloring of the skin frequently appears, especially on the abdomen and the inside of the thighs and flanks. Cutaneous hemorrhages may also appear in these areas. If the course of the disease is prolonged beyond 1 week, as it often is, bacterial complications usually occur, principally in the form of pneumonia and ulcerative enteritis.

Nervous signs occur quite commonly in hog cholera. These may be manifested by grinding of the teeth, evidence of local paralyses, locomotor disturbances, and occasionally lethargy and convulsions. These are manifestations of an encephalomyelitis which occurs in a large percentage of all cases. Seifried (51) found brain and cord changes in 33 out of 39 cases, although most of the animals had not manifested unusual nervous signs. Macroscopically, hemorphages are often found in the meninges and in the brain substance. Microscopically, besides the hemorrhages, the usual evidence of encephalomyelitis is found, i.e., perivascular "cuffing" with lymphocytes, mononuclear cells, and a few plasma and eosinophilic cells. The glial cells show proliferation both diffusely and in the form of compact nodes. There is degeneration of nerve cells and some neuronophagia. Changes of this type are found in some pigs very early in the disease and before recognizable signs have occurred. They represent a true virus type of reaction.

Inclusion bodies have been recognized in hog cholera. Boynton, Woods, Wood, and Castleberry (7) believed that certain bodies that they saw in the nuclei of epithelial cells of the gall bladder in cholera were of this type. Intranuclear inclusion bodies were observed in reticuloendothelial cells of various organs from more than half of the pigs given three different strains of virulent virus, but inclusion bodies were not found in pigs injected with various strains of modified HC virus (61).

Congenital infections of the dam cause small litters, fetal deaths, premature births, stillbirths, cerebellar ataxic piglets, and tremors. Congenital disease may occur in immune pregnant sows as well as susceptible dams (8, 62). Some piglets that survive are unthrifty and remain as viral carriers. Those piglets that fail to survive beyond a few weeks have a disease totally different from classical hog cholera (23).

Lewis and Shope (34) called attention to a reaction in hog cholera which apparently had first been noted by Dinwiddie (18) as early as 1914. This is the precipitous fall in the number of circulating leukocytes in the blood—a severe leukopenia. Within 48 hours after the inoculation of the hog cholera virus, the leukocytes, which vary between 14,000 and 24,000 per $mm^3$ in normal pigs, fall to a level below 4,000 and sometimes no leukocytes can be found. So far as is known, no other common disease of pigs exhibits this reaction. Late in hog cholera, when secondary bacterial action plays a prominent part in the disease picture, the leukopenia is replaced by a leukocytosis.

Animals that die within 1 week after first showing signs usually exhibit lesions which are purely of virus origin. The pure virus disease is best seen in inoculated animals held under good hygenic conditions. When these are destroyed at the height of the temperature reaction, which occurs generally on the 5th or 6th day, many will have practically no lesions visible to the naked eye. If lesions are found, they consist only of petechia hemorrhages in the kidney cortex and in the mucosa of the urinary bladder, larynx, and trachea. Sometimes they are found also on some of the serous membranes. Larger hemorrhages often are found in the intestinal mucosa, in the lungs, in the spleen, and especially in the cortex of many of the lymph nodes. These hemorrhages are caused by the rupture of capillaries in which retrogressive changes have occurred as the result of virus action (fig. 248). The endothelial linings of the vessels commonly show swelling and proliferation, and many lymphatic channels are plugged with such cells which have desquamated. Many small vessels degenerate into hyaline tubes, which readily rupture allowing blood to leak into the lymph channels. These changes have been minutely described by Seifried and Cain (52).

In the cases which run a longer course, fibrinous pheumonia, often with necrotic foci in the consolidated portions, and fibrinopurulent enteritis with ulceration are commonly found. In these cases the "button" ulcers of the mucosa may appear, especially in the region of the ileocecal valve. Because of the deposition of concentric layers of fibrin over the mucosal perforations, raised, buttonlike deposits are formed—hence the name. These lesions may be associated with the activities of the "hog-cholera bacillus" (S. choleraesuis) and the necrosis bacillus (Spherophorus necrophorus). The latter lives saprophytically in the alimentary canal of most swine and causes damage only when the way for it is paved by some other agent such as S. choleraesuis.

Following inoculation with virulent virus, pigs remain apparently well for at least 3 days. Field exposures to much smaller quantities of virus by natural routes may cause this incubation period to be prolonged to 6 or 7 days.

Most swine die within 7 to 10 days from the time signs first appear. Some-

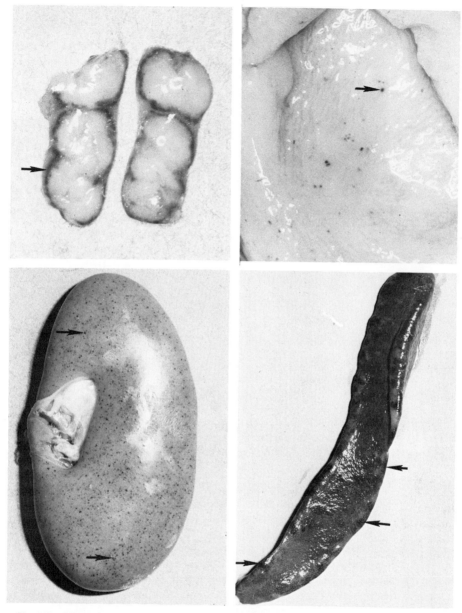

*Fig. 248.* Gross lesions in swine associated with hog cholera virus emphasizing the production of hemorrhages. (*Upper left*) Peripheral hemorrhage in cervical lymph node. (*Upper right*) Submucosal hemorrhages in urinary bladder. (*Lower left*) Subcapsular petechiation of kidney. The white areas are photographic artifacts. (*Lower right*) Hemorrhagic areas along margin of the spleen. (Courtesy D. Gustafson.)

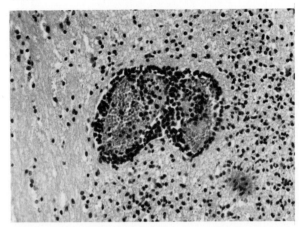

*Fig. 249.* Hog cholera, showing lesions of encephalitis, which commonly occur in this disease. Perivascular cuffing and infiltrations of round cells into the nerve tissue are shown. X 200. (Courtesy S. H. McNutt.)

times individuals will live longer, in which case pneumonia and enteric complications are apt to appear.

The mortality in some natural outbreaks is close to 100 percent. Since the introduction of the attenuated virus vaccines, many outbreaks of HC have occurred where the mortality is low. Some individuals suggest that these outbreaks represent strains of attenuated virus that have increased in virulence by transfer in nature.

**The Disease in Experimental Animals.** Only swine show clinical signs of illness with HC virus. The virus has been adapted to rabbits, and after several passages, the only sign of illness is a slight rise in body temperature (3). Growth of virus has been demonstrated by serial transfer in cattle, goats, sheep, and peccaries (32). Significant antibody production was detected in peccaries, calves, goats, sheep, and deer after inoculation with HCV. The inoculated animals failed to transmit the virus by contact to penmates of the same species and calves failed to transmit the infection to susceptible cohabiting pigs (37). Antibody production was not detected in wild mice, cottontail rabbits, sparrows, wild rats, raccoons, or pigeons after HCV inoculation (37).

In experimental studies in pigs, the virus is introduced into the body either by the respiratory system or by the upper digestive tract (24). According to Lin *et al.* (35) the tonsil is a prime target area because the greatest concentration of virus is found there. Infectious virus is present in the blood stream 24 hours after respiratory or tonsillar exposure. Leukocytes of the peripheral blood are infected and capable of viral replication. Regional lymph nodes are the first tissues to show edema and hemorrhage. After intravenous inoculation of HCV, infective virus could not be demonstrated at 0.5, 5, 8, and 13 hours after injection, but blood samples at 16 and 18 hours contained infective virus (24). Apparently many reticuloendothelial cells become infected. Many internal organs contain virus, but not until 48 hours after infection.

**Properties of the Virus.** The particle size of HCV is generally believed to be approximately 38 to 44 m$\mu$ (22). Small particles ranging from 3 to 23 m$\mu$ have

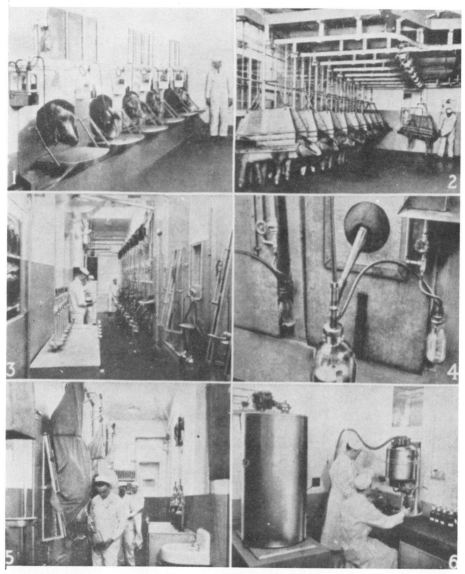

*Fig. 250.* The production of antihog cholera serum. (*1*) "Hypering." Large quantities of highly virulent blood are injected into the ear veins of immune pigs. (*2*) Preparing the hyperimmunized pigs for tail bleeding. The animals are restrained in special crates which lift their feet off the floor. Their tails are cleaned and shaved. (*3*) Tail bleeding. The tails of the pigs shown in the previous picture pass through small openings in the wall into the bleeding room. (*4*) Detail of the vacuum bleeding apparatus. After it has been thoroughly cleaned and disinfected, the end of the tail is amputated and the stump placed in a metal tube connected with the bleeding jar. Suction created by the vacuum line seen at the right of the picture hastens bleeding and tends to prevent clotting in the caudal arteries. A flexible shaft operates an agitator in the blood jar, which defibrinates the blood as it is drawn. (*5*) "Bleeding out." After the hyperimmunized pig has been tail-bled a number of times, it is finally bled out. This is done by thrusting a large cannula through the base of the neck into the large blood vessels at the base of the heart. (*6*) Bottling the serum. The large tank is used for mixing the sera of many animals. (Courtesy Pitman-Moore Co.)

been observed in many tissue-cultured HCV virus preparations (22). In some instances they are known to be a parvovirus. A ring of light particle projections observed at the particle surface probably represent the soluble antigen of HCV (44). This RNA virus is spherical with an envelope (17). It is sensitive to ether and chloroform. In a sucrose density gradient the particles are seen as a visible bond at a density of 1.13 to 1.14 (11). It is a relatively stable virus. It survives 50 C for 3 days, 37 C for 7 but not 15 days, and −70 C for many years without appreciable loss of infectivity. After an initial drop upon lyophilization it remains viable at 6 C for years. Greatest pH stability of virus in defibrinated blood occurs at pH 5 to 5.5. The virus is inactivated by Roccal, cresol, sodium hypochloride, sodium-o-phenylphenate, and beta proprolactone.

There is only one serotype. A number of serological methods have been described to study HC antigen and antibody. A conglutination-complement-absorption test for the detection of HC antibody was described by Millian (41). A hemagglutination test was used to measure hog cholera virus and antibody (50). This latter test is based upon the linkage of formolized erythrocytes through diazo bonds with either HC virus or HC antibody. The agar-gel method of Ouchterlong is used to demonstrate a specific antigen-antibody precipitation. The neutralization test in pig kidney cultured cells is possible since the isolation of a cytopathic strain of HC virus by Gillespie et al. (26). An indirect neutralization test called the *END method* was developed by Japanese workers (33) and its cytopathogenicity is based upon the exaltation effect of Newcastle virus on HC virus in a tissue culture system. A complement-fixation test is available and was used to demonstrate that HCV and viral diarrhea-mucosal disease virus share a soluble antigen (29).

**Cultivation.** Virus was found to multiply in embryonated hens' eggs only when freshly minced testicular tissue was placed on the chorioallantoic membrane (60).

HCV was first grown in cell culture by Hecke in Maitland plasma cell type cultures (22). Frenkel et al. (22) cultivated the virus in suspended porcine spleen tissue. In general, HC viruses have grown most successfully in primary or stable cell cultures derived from swine tissues. The tissues used include bone marrow, lymph node, lung, leukocytes, kidney, testicle, and spleen. In most instances no cytopathic effect was observed following inoculation with HC virus. A slight cytopathology in spleen cultures was reported by Gustafson and Pomerat (28). A strain (PAV-1) was described in 1960 (26) that produced marked cytopathology in primary swine-kidney cells. This virus also grows in swine testicular cells. Subsequent studies by a Munich group (2) with this cytopathic strain (PAV-1) have shown that it contains no adenovirus, bovine viral diarrhea-mucosal disease virus or *Mycoplasma* agents (6, 31). The Munich group (53) also reported that their viral preparations of PAV-1 had particles of two sizes, 39 to 40 m$\mu$ and 14 to 16 m$\mu$, which both banded in cesium chloride fractions between 1.14 and 1.20 g per ml. The larger ones are believed to be the principal HCV particle since the smaller particles were not found in the Ames or Strain A HC pig virus strain preparations (53). The exact nature of the smaller particle or its relationship to the larger HCV particle, if any, has not been ascertained (2). It is unlikely that it is a *Parvovirus* as members of this genus band at 1.4 g per ml in a cesium chloride gradient. Whether the larger particles of the PAV-1 strain have unique cytopathic properties by themselves, or whether the combined efforts of both particles are required for the cytopathic effect in cell culture remains to be determined.

The production of cytopathogenesis by the exalted effect of Newcastle virus on hog cholera was described in 1961 (33). Any strain of virus can be detected in tissue culture by the use of the fluorescent antibody technic (40, 57).

HCV persists in cell cultures without a cytopathic effect. It is known to survive and multiply in leukocyte cultures for more than 2 months (22) and it persisted in subcultural leukocytes for more than 471 days (36).

**Immunity.** Animals that recover from an attack of HC have a long-lasting and durable immunity. It is generally accepted that a single immunological type of virus exists. In 1949 Dale *et al.* (14) described a variant strain that required larger doses of antisera produced against standard virus for protection against the variant strain than the normal homotypic virus strain. An encephalitic strain described by Dunne *et al.* (25) was only partially neutralized by commercial HC antiserum.

In preliminary tests with the PAV-1 cytopathic strain of HC virus, neutralizing antibody titers were correlated with resistance to hog cholera infection (45). This suggests that resistance is related to the presence of circulating antibody or to its rapid production. The neutralization test is accurate and specific. The presence of antibody appears to be indicative of resistance to HC. It can also be used to test the efficacy of vaccines. Immune serums to all strains of HC virus neutralize the PAV-1 cytopathic strain of virus. It has been used to study maternal and active immunity and also the relation of HC to virus diarrhea virus.

The newborn pig obtains most, if not all, of its antibody from the colostrum of its immune dam. Colostral antibody is lost from the young pig at a constant rate. Its half-life is 13 days, and pigs that have maternal antibody titers of 1:1,000 or above still have some antibody at 4 months. Pigs with maternal antibody titers in this range resist virulent HC virus at 4 months of age (10). Pigs that have sufficient antibody to resist virulent virus become solidly immune following challenge (10).

Colostral or serum antibody may interfere with the development of immunity following vaccination (21). In 1964 Coggins (11) showed that the interference is not an all-or-none phenomenon. Interference is dependent upon the amount of antibody in the host and the amount of virus in the vaccine. Tissue culture vaccine containing 10,000 immunizing doses of virus overcame maternal immunity at antibody levels of 1:1,000 or above. It was found that high levels of antibody did depress the antibody response to vaccine and such animals consistently developed lower titers. Thus, the amount of viable virus appears to be the most important single factor in overcoming maternal antibody interference.

**Transmission.** Hog cholera is transmitted principally by intimate contact with sick animals and directly or indirectly with fresh secretions and excretions. It is not known precisely how the virus is passed from farm to farm in every case. Birds have been suspected of carrying virus on their bodies, and undoubtedly virus may be carried on the shoes and clothing of persons and animals if they travel rather directly from infected to noninfected premises. The disease may be carried to new premises by the careless handling of blood virus, which is used for immunization, or of the bottles that have contained such virus.

Probably one of the most frequent ways by which hog cholera reaches isolated swine herds is through the practice of feeding kitchen scraps or garbage. Birch (5) in 1915 showed that many pigs were slaughtered for food while in the early stages of the disease when their tissues contain a great deal of virus, and that this virus persisted for considerable periods in fresh pork and even in pickled and smoked hams. Trimmings from such materials, finding their way into garbage, can readily start outbreaks. This work was amply confirmed by Doyle (20) in England. Claxton (9) points out that most English outbreaks are initiated in this way. During the period between 1944 and 1949, when World War II was raging, England imported very little pork from abroad and during this time the incidence of cholera (swine fever) fell far below the usual level.

Dunne *et al.* (24) showed that cholera virus, introduced in double gelatin capsules into the stomach, did not infect. Infection was readily accomplished through the tonsils and also through the respiratory tract when precautions were taken to avoid tonsillar infection.

Inasmuch as the virus does not persist on premises after swine have been removed, it has long been a mystery how the annual outbreaks of the disease were initiated. Cholera is largely a seasonal disease. It would be expected to be related to the farrowing seasons, because it is the new crops of pigs in which the disease occurs. Most of the sows are bred to farrow in the spring and fall of each year; hence most of the cholera outbreaks occur in those seasons. When new pigs have not been brought to the premises, or other obvious sources of virus have not been introduced, cholera outbreaks generally begin in a single, or at least a few animals, the main outbreak appearing some 10 days or more later.

Seeking an answer to the question of how and where virus persists in the relatively long periods which often intervene between frank outbreaks, Shope (56) reported some interesting observations which demonstrate that the virus may be harbored for substantial periods by animals other than swine. Shope showed that the swine lungworm could serve as a reservoir and intermediate host for the virus of hog cholera. Lungworms in affected pigs may acquire virus which is transmitted through their ova to succeeding generations of worms. The progeny of worms which had acquired virus may infect other swine, susceptible to cholera, without, in most instances, producing the disease. A provoking agent is needed to cause the "masked" virus to emerge as an actively pathogenic agent. One such agent was ascaris larvae. This provocation was effective only during the spring months of the year. Shope was also able to show that suspensions of adult lungworms which were derived from apparently normal, cholera-susceptible swine but which were the progeny of lungworms which had come from cholera-infected animals, could in some instances induce cholera when they were injected intramuscularly into susceptible animals.

The mechanism demonstrated by Shope may not operate frequently or effectively in the spread of the natural disease; however, it does mean that hog cholera may not be dependent wholly on a swine reservoir. It is entirely possible that other extraswine reservoirs of virus may be found. Certainly more information is necessary regarding the ecology of this disease.

The findings of Baker and Sheffy in 1960 (4) have far-reaching significance in the epidemiology of the disease. They reported that partially attenuated rabbit virus given to some young pigs caused stunting and reverted to virulence while persisting in the blood until the time of death 2 to 3 months later. Consequently, prenatal and neonatal infections that persist in immunologically tolerant piglets may be the principal and perhaps the main means by which HCV is maintained in nature. The success or failure of a HC eradication program probably hinges on this single factor.

**Diagnosis.** Prompt diagnosis of hog cholera is extremely important, because delays often mean the loss of entire herds when many animals might have been saved by prompt use of antiserum. If the diagnosis is in doubt, it is best to treat a disease as hog cholera rather than delay prophylactic treatment for a day or two until the nature of the disease becomes clearer. It is a case of risking the cost of unnecessary serum treatment against that of losing many of the herd.

The fluorescent antibody method is the preferred method with diagnostic laboratories for the detection of HCV. Direct examination of tissues from infected pigs makes a diagnosis possible within a few hours. It appears that field strains of HC virus grow in tissue culture without producing a cytopathogenic effect, but viral activity can be detected by the fluorescent antibody technic. This method provides a powerful tool for the diagnosis of this disease and its eradication. Solorzano et al. (58) tested specimens from 462 cases of suspected hog cholera utilizing the PK-15 cell line for viral propagation and the FA test for identification of viral replication. By this procedure 146 (32 percent) were positive, and 169 (37 percent) were positive when brain lesions were used as diagnostic criteria. The two methods agreed in 82 percent of the cases and disagreed in 18 percent. There were 32 cases (7 percent) positive by the FA that were negative for brain lesions and 53 cases (11 percent) with brain lesions were not confirmed by FA test. They concluded that the FA method is superior to conventional methods for HC diagnosis.

Teebken *et al.* (59) used the FA test to differentiate the effects of virulent, attenuated, and inactivated hog cholera viruses on tonsillar tissue in young swine. Bright cytoplasmic fluorescence was diffusely distributed throughout the epithelial and lymphoid tissues in tonsils of pigs given virulent HCV. After the injection of attenuated HC vaccines bright fluorescence was observed primarily in plaquelike areas in the tonsillar crypt epithelium. In pigs given either of two inactivated virus vaccines fluorescence was granular and limited to the tonsillar germinal centers.

The testing of acute and convalescent serum samples for antibody and the detection of a significant rise between the paired sera is another method that can be profitably used for the diagnosis of HC. The serum-neutralization test is usually used for this purpose (26).

The differential diagnosis between hog cholera and acute erysipelas infection often presents serious difficulties even to experienced veterinarians. In erysipelas infections it is not uncommon for several animals to die suddenly with few or no premonitory signs. This does not happen in cholera. In both infections the sick animals have high temperatures, but more animals are apt to develop signs about the same time in erysipelas than in cholera. The sick animals in both cases lie on their bedding, refuse food, and are reluctant to move, but whereas in cholera they are mentally depressed and sleepy, they are mentally alert in erysipelas. The joint swellings which appear in many cases of erysipelas are absent in cholera. Nausea and vomiting occur in both diseases. The characteristic "diamond skin" lesions of erysipelas appear most often in the chronic rather than the acute form of the disease, but they are sometimes seen in acute cases and may be helpful in diagnosis. In some cases of acute erysipelas infection, edema of the lungs develops and this causes the animals to pant and show evidence of shortness of breath. This is not seen in cholera.

The autopsy findings often are not very helpful in the more acute cases since these diseases may cause only minimal lesions. If facilities for blood counts are available, the leukopenia of cholera contrasts with the leukocytosis of erysipelas. The organism of erysipelas can usually be isolated from the spleen of affected animals, and this constitutes a method of confirmation of the field diagnosis.

**Immunization.** Several methods have been developed for the prophylactic immunization of swine against cholera. Passive immunity is accomplished with a hyperimmune antiserum made from swine. Active immunity may be conferred by the simultaneous injection of antiserum and active virus, with vaccines containing only inactivated virus, or with vaccines containing living, attenuated virus. The use of bovine viral diarrhea-mucosal disease virus of cattle as a means of protecting pigs against HC has been proposed by Atkinson *et al.* (1).

*Passive.* The value of the antiviral serum was demonstrated by a group of workers connected with the U.S. Department of Agriculture. The first report was by Dorset, McBryde, and Niles (19) in 1908. The serum is prepared from pigs. These either have acquired immunity naturally or they are first given virus with sufficient antiserum, simultaneously, to protect them. The immune animals are then given fresh, defibrinated blood taken at the height of the temperature reaction from young pigs that have been infected with cholera virus. This blood is injected into one of the ear veins at the rate of 5 ml per pound of body weight. This process is known as hyperimmunization. Large hogs are used for this purpose. After a period of 10 to 14 days these hogs are bled for their serum. After due processing the antiserum is preserved with 0.5 phenol, bottled in final containers, and held for potency testing under test procedures outlined by the U.S. Department of Agriculture.

Anti-hog-cholera serum is generally used for its prophylactic effect, but large doses sometimes are employed for treating animals very early in the course of the disease. As a prophylactic agent it is very effective, the immunity being established immediately. As a curative agent its usefulness is very limited, because most animals that show definite signs will die in spite of serum treatment. The principal use of serum alone is at the beginning of outbreaks to protect those animals that have not yet contracted the infection. It is very efficient for this purpose, but the immunity is short-lived.

Dosages of antiserum for hog cholera must be gauged to the body weight of the animal. Regulations of the U.S. Department of Agriculture have required manufacturers who sold in the United States to attach the following dosage table to the bottles.

Table XL.  THE DOSAGE LEVEL OF HOG CHOLERA ANTISERUM REQUIRED TO INDUCE PASSIVE IMMUNITY IN PIGS

| Pig weight | Minimum dose(ml) |
|---|---|
| Suckling pigs | 20 |
| 20 to 40 pounds | 30 |
| 40 to 90 pounds | 35 |
| 90 to 120 pounds | 45 |
| 120 to 150 pounds | 55 |
| 150 to 180 pounds | 65 |
| 180 pounds and over | 75 |

It is important that these dosage levels be not undergauged, particularly when serum is used simultaneously with virus. It is much better to give considerably more serum than needed, than too little.

*Active.* The simultaneous injection of antiserum and virus was the first method employed in the United States to protect pigs against hog cholera. This method sometimes caused a reaction in pigs and occasionally death, but the survivors were solidly immune. The use of virulent virus in the United States is prohibited since the inauguration of its eradication program.

When serum breaks occur they represent a failure of the antiserum to provide the expected protection against the virus administered. Serum breaks always occur within a few days. Virus breaks are cases in which pigs develop cholera several weeks or months following the simultaneous treatment. These failures occur when the virus lacks proper potency or when pigs fail to react properly to virus. Such animals are only passively immunized and become susceptible 2 to 3 weeks later.

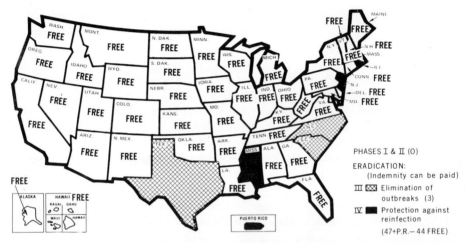

Fig. 251. Hog Cholera Eradication Program in the United States July 1, 1972. (Courtesy ARS, United States Department of Agriculture.)

Crystal violet vaccine is the most commonly used inactivated virus vaccine. It is prepared by mixing crystal violet and infectious defibrinated swine blood at 37 C (39). Live virus may survive vaccine production (48) so innocuity tests are essential because virulent virus is used in the product. Attenuated viruses prepared by this method are ineffective. In fact Mott (43) reported that a wide variation exists in the immunizing potential of blood from pigs infected with virulent virus and wide differences were encountered in the immune response of pigs in the field. Neutralizing-antibody titers following one injection of crystal violet vaccine are low or undetectable (10). A second injection improved its effectiveness (13). It takes longer to produce an adequate immunity with inactivated virus vaccine, more injections are required, and a dependable immunity does not persist any longer than 8 months. Undoubtedly it is safer than the attenuated virus vaccines because the virus will not spread and this makes inactivated vaccines useful in an eradication program. Another inactivated virus vaccine that has had wide usage is commonly known as *BTV* (Boynton tissue vaccine). Tissues that contain virus are treated with eucalyptol and otherwise processed until the virus is inactivated. A good article on the status of inactivated virus vaccines for HC is that of Sanders, Quin, and Mundell (47). Antiserum will interfere with the development of an active immunity from these vaccines and with certain attenuated virus vaccines (13). In the case of attenuated virus vaccines, this is probably related to the amount of virus in the vaccine.

The use of bovine viral diarrhea-mucosal disease virus of cattle for protection against hog cholera has been recommended (1). Vaccination with strain NY 1 of BVD-MD virus protects pigs against some HCV strains that were tested, but not all. This protection is based upon the secondary response since immunization with strain NY 1 produces BVD-MD antibody but no hog cholera antibody. Upon challenge with virulent hog cholera virus these pigs usually produce hog cholera antibody quickly, and this antibody may render clinical protection. Its potential use as an immunizing agent has certain advantages: its lack of pathogenicity for pigs; its safety factor, because hog cholera virus is not involved; and with no HC antibodies produced, HC antibody in a pig population can be related to field exposure of HC virus.

The most common vaccines formerly used in the United States were modified by rabbit passage (1). Certain modified vaccines are given simultaneously with HC antiserum. Serum use depends upon their degree of attenuation by rabbit passage or by tissue culture passage (27, 30). The tissue culture vaccines have largely replaced the rabbit-adapted virus vaccines. They cost less to produce and are reputed to contain more virus with higher antigenicity. The use of the cytopathic strain or the fluorescent antibody technic for the detection of noncytopathic vaccine strains makes production control and viral assay much simpler. There is evidence that the rabbit vaccines spread to susceptible pigs. Apparently tissue cultured vaccines also spread. The immunity derived from these vaccines lasts a long time and is quite durable. It may be necessary to revaccinate breeder stock. The use of rabbit vaccine virus is contraindicated in pregnant sows during pregnancy because the virus produces a variety of fetal abnormalities with fetal death and partial reabsorption sometimes occurring (49). Low passaged rabbit virus should not be used in young pigs because stunting and death may occur (4). It also would be well to avoid the use of tissue cultured virus vaccines in pregnant sows.

Vaccination shock. After pasteurization of anti-hog-cholera serum became a requirement, a type of shock occurring immediately after its injection came to notice. This occurs in only a few animals. The signs vary from animal to animal but usually consist of rapid respiration and prostration, and sometimes vomiting and convulsions. These signs are seen more often in young animals than in older ones. Deaths are rare; consequently the reactions are not considered to be serious enough to cause hesitancy in the use of serum. The shock-provoking principle can be precipitated from heated serum by ammonium sulfate in concentrations great enough to precipitate the euglobulin. Some evidence indicates that there is a relationship between serum shock and young pig anemia (42). For a discussion of the present status of this problem, see Mathews and Buthala (38).

**Control.** In the United States hog cholera has been the most important disease of swine. This is true despite the use of various types of biologics. At this writing (1971) a time-phased eradication program for hog cholera in the United States has been in effect for at least 6 years and notable progress has been made despite its complexity and wide distribution in the country (fig. 252). At present virulent virus, attenuated virus vaccines, and bovine viral diarrhea-mucosal disease vaccine virus are prohibited for use in swine as means for its eradication. The elimination of biologics and the cooking of garbage are not sufficient and certain rigid quarantine procedures and the slaughter program must be strictly adhered to for any reasonable chance for total success. It is already clear that the disease incidence has been markedly decreased. What other measures may be required depend upon what reservoirs exist outside of swine and how abundant they are. In Europe and Canada hog cholera outbreaks have been eradicated without great difficulty. It is not safe to conclude that methods used elsewhere will succeed in the United States because we may have virus reservoirs that do not exist elsewhere, but everyone is hopeful that this is not the case and that the eradication program is a complete success.

Hog cholera virus also is spread through fresh pork, the trimmings of which often find their way back to swine in garbage. When cholera appears in herds of swine of marketable size, farmers frequently rush their stock to market. In slaughtering establishments under federal meat inspection, efforts are made to prevent the slaughter of swine obviously ill from cholera, but very frequently such animals are not detected in the short time they are held in the yards. This means that many hogs that harbor active virus are slaughtered and enter the trade. Slaughtering establishments that are not under federal control probably distribute more virus through infected pork than those where some, but insufficient, control is exercised.

Laws requiring the cooking of all garbage fed to swine have long been in effect in many European countries and in Canada. These were enacted in most cases to reduce the hazards of foot-and-mouth disease transmission, but they also serve, of course, to reduce the hazards of other diseases including cholera. Such laws have been enacted in the United States only within the last decade to meet the emergency created by the rapid spread of another swine disease, vesicular exanthema, that has since been eradicated. Commercial garbage-feeding establishments in all states but one are now required to cook garbage before it is fed to swine. This has had a significant effect in controlling the spread of cholera in the United States.

**Relationship of Hog Cholera Virus to Bovine Viral Diarrhea-Mucosal Disease Virus.** Using the agar-gel-diffusion test Darbyshire (15) showed that the two viruses were related. The precipitation reaction was specific, and anti-body could be absorbed with heterologous antigen as well as with homologous antigen. In neutralization tests their respective antibodies did not cross-neutralize (54). Each virus is capable of stimulating a primary response for the other, and an accelerated antibody to the heterologous virus occurs in 5 to 7 days. In the case of HC in pigs this secondary response confers protection to virulent HC virus but apparently not against all strains (55). In calves, resistance was not clearly demonstrated because calves only have a mild clinical infection when given BVD-MD virus, making challenge evaluation difficult. Nevertheless, an anamnestic type of antibody response was found in these animals. HCV and BVD-MDV each multiply in the rabbit without the production of disease. In these animals hypertypic neutralizing antibody responses were seen irrespective of the virus injected (12).

Limited knowledge of the physical, chemical, and morphological features of both viruses show that similarities exist. They interfere with each other in tissue culture systems. There is cross-staining when immunofluorescence is employed. Furthermore, heterologous reactions indicate a common soluble antigen (40). This antigen has been used in a complement-fixation test to further characterize their relationship (29). Hyperimmune antiserums contain detectable levels of the heterotypic neutralizing antibody.

## REFERENCES

1. Atkinson, Baker, Campbell, Coggins, Nelson, Robson, Sheffy, Sippel, and Nelson.  Proc., U.S. Livestock Sanit. Assoc., 1962, 66, 326.
2. Bachmann, Sheffy and Siegl.  Arch. f. die Gesam. Virusforsch, 1967, 22, 467.
3. Baker.  Jour. Am. Vet. Med. Assoc., 1947, 111, 503.
4. Baker and Sheffy.  Proc. Soc. Exp. Biol. and Med., 1960, 105, 675.
5. Birch.  Rpt. New York State Vet. Coll., 1915–16, p. 60.
6. Bodon.  Acta. vet. Acad. Sci. Hung., 1965, 15, 471.
7. Boynton, Woods, Wood, and Castleberry.  Jour. Am. Vet. Med. Assoc., 1942, 101, 523.
8. Carbrey.  Ibid., 1965, 146, 233.
9. Claxton.  Agriculture (Gt. Brit.), 1954, 60, 473.
10. Coggins.  Cornell Univ. Thesis, 1962.
11. Coggins.  Am. Jour. Vet. Res., 1964, 25, 613.
12. Coggins and Seo.  Proc. Soc. Exp. Biol. and Med., 1963, 114, 778.
13. Cole, Henley, Dale, Mott, Torrey, and Zinober.  U.S.D.A. Inform. Bul. 241, 1963.
14. Dale, Schoening, Cole, Henley, and Zinober.  Jour. Am. Vet. Med. Assoc., 1951, 118, 279.
15. Darbyshire.  Vet. Res., 1960, 72, 331.
16. DeSchweinitz and Dorset.  U.S. Bur. Anim. Indus. Cir. 41, 1903.
17. Dinter.  Centrbl. f. Bakt., 1963, 188, 475.
18. Dinwiddie.  Ark. Agr. Exp. Sta. Bul. 120, 1914.
19. Dorset, McBryde, and Niles.  U.S. Bur. Anim. Indus. Bul. 102, 1908.
20. Doyle.  Jour. Comp. Path. and Therap., 1933, 46, 25.

21. Dunne.   Sympos. on Hog Cholera, Coll. of Vet. Med., Univ. of Minn., 1961, p. 161.
22. Dunne.   Diseases of swine, 3rd ed. Iowa State College Press, Ames, Iowa, 1970, p. 177.
23. Dunne and Clark.   Am. Jour. Vet. Res., 1968, *29*, 787.
24. Dunne, Hokanson, and Luedke.   *Ibid.*, 1959, *20*, 615.
25. Dunne, Smith, Runnells, Stafseth, and Thorp.   *Ibid.*, 1952, *13*, 277.
26. Gillespie, Sheffy, and Baker.   Proc. Soc. Exp. Biol. and Med., 1960, *105*, 679.
27. Gillespie, Sheffy, Coggins, Madin, and Baker.   Proc., U.S. Livestock Sanit. Assoc., 1961, *65*, 57.
28. Gustafson and Pomerat.   Am. Jour. Vet. Res., 1957, *18*, 473.
29. Gutekunst and Malmquist.   Canad. Jour. Comp. Med. and Vet. Sci., 1964, *28*, 19.
30. Hejl.   Sympos. on Hog Cholera, Coll. Vet. Med., Univ. Minn., 1961, p. 169.
31. Horzinek and Uberschär.   Arch. f. die Gesam. Virusforsch, 1966, *18*, 406.
32. Kernkamp.   *Ibid.*, p. 19.
33. Kumagai, Shimizu, Ikeda, and Matumato.   J. Immuno., 1961, 87, 245.
34. Lewis and Shope.   Jour. Am. Vet. Med. Assoc., 1929, *74*, 145.
35. Lin, Shimizu, Kumagi, and Sasahara.   Nat'l. Inst. Anim. Quart., 1969, 9, 10.
36. Loan and Gustafson.   Am. Jour. Vet. Res., 1961, *22*, 741.
37. Loan and Storm.   *Ibid.*, 1968, *29*, 807.
38. Mathews and Buthala.   *Ibid.*, 1958, *19*, 32.
39. McBryde and Cole.   Jour. Am. Vet. Med. Assoc., 1936, *89*, 652.
40. Mengling, Pirtle, and Torrey.   Canad. Jour. Comp. Med. and Vet. Sci., 1963, *27*, 249.
41. Millian and Englehard.   Am. Jour. Vet. Res., 1961, *22*, 396.
42. Mohler.   Rpt., Chief, Bur. Anim. Indus., U.S. Dept. Agr., 1931.
43. Mott.   Sympos. on Hog Cholera, College of Vet. Med., Univ. of Minn., 1961, p. 135.
44. Ritchie and Fernelius.   Vet. Rec., 1967, *69*, 417.
45. Robson, Coggins, Sheffy, and Baker.   Proc., U.S. Livestock Sanit. Assoc., 1960, *65*, 338.
46. Salmon and Smith.   Rpt., Chief, Bur. Anim. Indus., U.S. Dept. Agr., 1885.
47. Sanders, Quin, and Mundell.   Proc. U.S. Livestock Sanit. Assoc., 1950, *54*, 156.
48. Sato, Hanaki, Nishimura, and Kawashima.   Jap. Jour. Vet. Sci., 1962, *24*, 97.
49. Sautter, Young, Luedke, and Kitchell.   Proc. Am. Vet. Med. Assoc., 1953, p. 146.
50. Segre.   Am. Jour. Vet. Res., 1962, 95, 748.
51. Seifried.   Jour. Exp. Med., 1931, *53*, 277.
52. Seifried and Cain.   *Ibid.*, 1932, *56*, 345.
53. Sheffy, Bachmann, and Siegl.   Proc. U.S. Livestock Sanit. Assoc., 1967, *71*, 487.
54. Sheffy, Coggins, and Baker.   *Ibid.*, 1961, *65*, 437.
55. Sheffy, Coggins, and Baker.   Proc. Soc. Exp. Biol. and Med., 1962, *109*, 349.
56. Shope.   Jour. Exp. Med., 1958, *107*, 609, and *108*, 159.
57. Solorzano.   Penna. State Univ. Thesis, 1962.

58.  Solorzano, Thigpen, Bedell, and Schwartz.   Jour. Am. Vet. Med. Assoc., 1966,
     *149*, 31.
59.  Teehken, Aiken and Twiehaus.   *Ibid.*, 1967, *150*, 53.
60.  TenBroeck.   Jour. Exp. Med., 1941, *74*, 427.
61.  Urman, Underdahl, Aiken, Stair, and Young.   Jour. Am. Vet. Med. Assoc.,
     1962, *141*, 571.
62.  Young, Kitchell, Luedke, and Sautter.   *Ibid.*, 1955, *126*, 155.

## Bovine Viral Diarrhea-Mucosal Disease

SYNONYMS:   Mucosal disease, Virus diarrhea of cattle; abbreviation, VD,
BVD-MD

In 1946 Olafson, MacCallum, and Fox (30) described a disease of dairy cattle which had a striking resemblance to rinderpest except that it was much
milder. They had no difficulty in transmitting the disease with defibrinated
blood, spleen tissue, or other organ tissue by parenteral injection, and the disease proved highly contagious under natural conditions (31). In 1956 Pritchard, Taylor, Moses, and Doyle (34) described a similar disease in dairy and
beef cattle. It was thought that there were some immunological differences
and also some clinical variations between the New York and the Indiana diseases, and for a time they were identified as virus diarrhea—New York and
virus diarrhea—Indiana. The original Indiana strains have been lost, but Gillespie and Baker (8) made comparisons of other Indiana and New York
strains and found no differences between them. It is now assumed that there
is but one type of virus diarrhea in the United States.

All cytopathogenic strains of virus isolated from clinical cases of mucosal
disease first described by Ramsey and Chivers (35) are serologically and,
when tested, immunologically related to many available cytopathogenic
strains of VD virus. As these two entities are now considered clinical variations of the same virus disease, an Ad Hoc Committee on Terminology for the
American Veterinary Medical Association Symposium (2) named it bovine
viral diarrhea-mucosal disease. An awkward name, perhaps, but it clearly
states that the two disease conditions have a common etiology.

Virus diarrhea has been diagnosed in cattle in many countries of the world.
The only reported clinical cases of this disease involve cattle. The disease is
widespread and is found in the United States, Australia, Canada, Germany,
England, Scotland, Sweden, Japan, and Argentina. Strain NY 1 was isolated
by Baker, York, Gillespie, and Mitchell (1) from a New York herd and it was
the original type strain until the cytopathogenic strain Oregon (C24V) was
isolated by Gillespie, Baker, and McEntee in 1960 (9). The availability of
strain Oregon for comparative serological and virological studies has been
used by various investigators in the world to evaluate clinical entities that resemble VD (11, 24).

The clinical disease is most frequent in the late winter and spring. Serological surveys have been conducted in various parts of the United States and abroad. In a New York State survey 53 percent of cows selected at random within 500 herds (two cows per herd) distributed through 53 counties had antibodies (19). Serum samples from cattle in 22 counties of Florida showed that 65 percent of beef cattle and 61 percent of dairy cattle were positive for VD antibodies (22). In another survey of states where 100 or more cattle serums were tested, 59 percent in Illinois, 69 percent in Iowa, and 73 percent in Nebraska were positive (28). Incidence studies in Europe yielded similar results.

Neutralizing antibodies have been demonstrated in serums of white-tailed deer from New York State (19). A disease of white-tailed deer and mule deer in North Dakota with lesions similar to VD infection of cattle has been described by Richards *et al.* (36).

There is a suggestion that BVD-MD occurs as a natural infection without signs of illness in domestic swine in the United States (41).

**Character of the Disease.** The disease affects cattle of all ages, but young stock are more likely to show signs of illness. This may be related to the higher susceptibility rate of these animals.

The high incidence of cattle with antibodies suggests that most cattle experience a mild or inapparent infection. When the disease manifests itself in a herd, it may occur as a mild or severe acute infection or occasionally in a chronic form. As a herd disease it varies from one with a high morbidity and a low mortality to one with a low morbidity and a high mortality.

The severely affected cattle have a high temperature and a leukopenia. Other signs of illness include depression, anorexia, scouring, excessive salivation, recumbency, dehydration, reduced milk supply, cessation of rumination, conjunctivitis, congestion and ulcerations in the mucous membrane of the oral cavity, and possibly abortions in pregnant cows. These field observations of abortions were fortified by the isolation of BVD-MD virus from two aborted fetuses representing two New York State dairy herds (10). Lameness, probably caused by laminitis, occurs in some cases. Occasionally there is a mucoid nasal discharge which leads individuals to confuse it with infectious bovine rhinotracheitis, parainfluenza-3 infection, or some other respiratory illness.

The gross lesions associated with natural cases were first described in 1946 by Olafson, MacCallum, and Fox (30). The eyes were sunken and the carcasses gaunt and dehydrated. Erosions were found on the dental pad, palate, lateral tongue surface, around the incisors, and on the inside of the cheeks. Occasionally erosions were seen on the muzzle and at the entrance of the nostrils, and the nasal mucosa was reddened. Ulceration of the pharynx and larynx or diffuse necrosis of the mucous membranes in these regions occurred in some fatal cases. Secondary pneumonia was observed in some cows in one dealer's herd. Characteristic lesions were irregular, shallow, punched-out erosions of varying sizes and shapes in the mucous membranes of the esophagus, arranged in a linear fashion. Some of the ulcers coalesced, and sometimes the necrotic material remained intact. An occasional calf did not develop oral ulcers. The forestomachs may show small necrotic areas and a few ulcers. The small intestine may have a diffused reddened mucosa. The cecum often showed petechiae and small ulcers. Hemorrhages were sometimes seen in the subcutaneous tissue, in the epicardium, and in the vaginal mucosa. In subsequent descriptions of the disease other changes were mentioned (3, 33, 35). Hemorrhage, edema, necrosis, and ulceration of the pyloric portion of the abomasum were observed. Similar changes were occasionally noted in the small intestinal tract, with marked lesions in Peyer's patches (fig. 252). Other significant lesions were atrophic changes in lymphatic tissues and degenerative alterations in the kidney, skin, and adrenals. Erosions or ulcerations de-

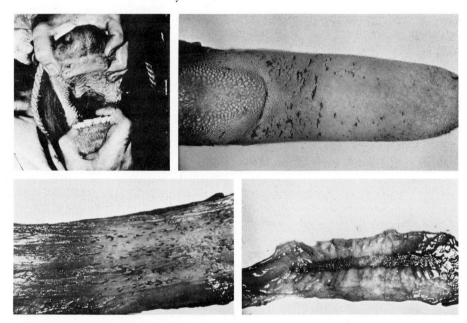

Fig. 252. Gross lesions in a severe case of MD-VD of cattle. (*Upper left*) Erosions and hemorrhages of gums. (*Upper right*) Erosions on dorsal surface on the tongue. (*Lower left*) Erosions and necrosis in esophagus. (*Lower right*) Hemorrhage and necrosis of Peyers patches of intestinal tract. (Courtesy K. McEntee.)

veloped in interdigital regions of some cattle, and extensive necrosis may have followed. The lymph nodes often appeared normal, but in some cases they were greatly enlarged and edematous.

Various investigators (3, 35, 42, 47) have reported on the microscopic changes allied with the natural and the experimental disease. The most striking changes occurred in the digestive system. Probably the first change in that portion lined by stratified squamous epithelium was the vacuolation of the cytoplasm in cells, particularly of the stratum germinativum and stratum spinosum. Destruction of the intercellular bridges occurred, and the nuclei became pyknotic. With cellular destruction lesions developed and coalesced with the formation of erosions. In the early lesions there was marked hyperemia with minimal infiltration of mononuclear cells. Some old lesions had deep ulcerations and a marked inflammatory cellular reaction because bacteria invaded the denuded epithelium.

Ulcers involving the fundus of the abomasum were formed by localized necrosis, erosion of the epithelium, and damage to the lamina propria. Accompanying changes were edema of the lamina propria and submucosa with moderate leukocytic infiltration and hemorrhage. Edema, hemorrhage, erosions, and ulcerations may occur in the pyloric mucosa. Sometimes the lesions were indicative of a necrotic abomasitis.

In severe cases marked changes occurred in the intestinal tract. The crypts of the intestinal glands were filled with mucus, necrotic cells, and varying numbers of leukocytes. Edema was evident in some cases. Destruction of the glandular epithelium occurred, especially in acute cases. In the submucosa lymphatic tissue, necrosis sometimes initiated changes which lead to erosion formation. Depletion of lymphocytes in Peyer's patches may be prominent. Ulcers were especially evident over Peyer's patches. Similar changes could be found in the colonic mucosa. Severe cecitis, colitis, and proctitis, varying from a catarrhal inflammation to a necrotic inflammation, were often found.

The thymus was smaller than normal and may contain grayish-white foci. There was a loss of differentiation between the medulla and cortex and a widespread depletion of thymocytes. Lymphocytes were replaced by large mononuclear cells in the tonsils.

There was a hyperplasia of the myeloid elements of the bone marrow with a decrease in the normal amount of fatty marrow.

Subepicardial and subendocardial hemorrhages were observed. Vessel changes only occurred in the media of the arterioles in the submucosa of the digestive tract where severe changes occurred, especially in the germinal centers. The subcapsular sinus may be extended and filled with leukocytes. Infiltration of neutrophiles in the cortex and the medulla occasionally happens. Similar histological changes occurred in the spleen and hemal nodes.

**The Disease in Experimental Animals.** Susceptible cattle are infected by mouth and parenteral injection. The incubation period is 2 to 3 days after parenteral injection. The first temperature response usually lasts for 1 to 2 days with the second response starting 2 to 3 days later and persisting 2 to 3 days with temperatures ranging from 104 to 107 F. A leukopenia occurs which may be followed by a leukocytosis. Diarrhea seldom is noted, and reddening and ulceration of the gums sometimes occurs (1).

Using a noncytopathic strain (Studdert) of BVD-MD virus isolated from an aborted fetus (10), Ward et al. (46) inoculated 11 pregnant dairy cows intravenously at varying stages of gestation (150 to 217 days). The fetus that was 150 days old at time of viral injection showed ataxia, blindness, and buccal lesions at birth. Two other neonatal calves had buccal lesions at birth and the eight other calves were normal. All 11 calves had BVD-MD antibodies at birth including four from whom blood samples were collected before suckling. The antibody levels persisted for 6 months without decline and six of these calves failed to develop signs of illness when given virulent virus at that time. This evidence gives substantial proof that the bovine fetus produces active antibody against BVD-MD virus as early as 5 months of embryo develop-ment. Subsequent experimental studies by Scott et al. (39, 40) extended these studies. These investigators gave the same Studdert strain intravenously to susceptible cows 3 to 5 months pregnant. Infection in the cows was followed by fetal death, fetal mummification, abortion, or birth at term of calves with cerebellar or ocular defects. Kahrs et al. (21) made similar observations in natural disease of a dairy herd: BVD-MD virus was isolated from one aborted fetus and rising serum-neutralizing antibody titers were demonstrated in some cows. These results suggest that BVD-MD virus causes abortions and congen-ital defects in the cattle populations. Sheep and goats are susceptible to ex-perimental inoculation with BVD-MD virus. An English strain produces a rise in temperature that occurs between the 5th and 8th day (17). Lack of ap-petite and diarrhea also were noted in the sheep. Ward inoculated pregnant sheep and reported the occurrence of congenital anomalies and antibody re-sponse in the fetus (45).

Strain NY 1 has been maintained in rabbits for more than 100 transfers and strain Indiana for more than 20 transfers without producing signs of illness in this species.

Experimental pigs given BVD-MD virus propagate the virus and specific antibodies are formed. No signs of illness occur.

The virus fails to elicit a response in white mice.

**Properties of the Virus.** BVD-MD virus is a RNA-helical-enveloped virus that presently does not fit in any recognized viral genus. Both 5 iodo-deoxyuridine and 5 bromo-deoxyuridine fail to inhibit the Oregon strain of BVD-MD (16). Inactivation occurs after treatment with chloroform and ether (13, 16). The sedimentation coefficient of the virus particle is 80 to 90 S. In a sucrose-den-sity gradient its buoyant density is 1.13 to 1.14 g per ml.

Electron photomicrographs of strain Oregon shadowed with chromium re-veal somewhat spherical particles that are 35 to 55 m$\mu$ in size (22). Ultrathin sections of viral pellets also reveal spherical particles approximately 40 m$\mu$ in diameter (16). In studies by Ritchie and Fernelius (37), three major size classes of particulate entities were observed by EM of negatively stained (phosphotungstic acid) crude and partially purified preparations of one non-cytopathic and two cytopathic (including strain Oregon) BVD-MD strains cultured in embryonic bovine kidney cells: (a) 15-to-20-m$\mu$ virus-specific pre-cursor particles considered to represent a ribosomelike soluble antigen—although quite similar in size to the 15 to 16 m$\mu$ unknown particlelike entities associated with the PAV-1 strain of hog cholera virus, these BVD-MD particles were different in appearance; (b) 30 to 35 mμ particles, a heterogenous population of three types of particulate entities; and (c) 80 to 100 mμ pleomorphic membrane-bounded particles. The two larger components had infectious particles and the surface of the largest unit generally was smooth with rare prominent projections. In other studies (26) with concentrated and purified strain Oregon involving the use of ultracentrifugation, density-gradient centrifugation in potassium tartrate, and rate-zonal centrifugation in sucrose, the virion of strain Oregon stained with uranyl acetate consisted of an envelope without projections and a nucleocapsid probably displaying a cubical symmetry. The particle was 57 ± 7 mμ with the core accounting for 24 mμ ± 4mμ. In general, the measurements from electron micrographs are in fair agreement among the various investigators, and the differences may be the result of different procedures of viral preparation for EM study.

Ultrafiltration experiments with Millipore filters indicate that some infectious particles are less than 50 mμ in size (16).

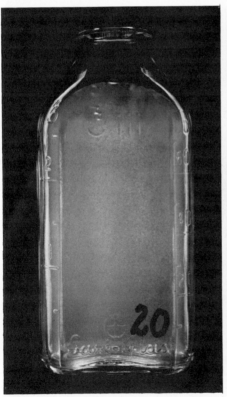 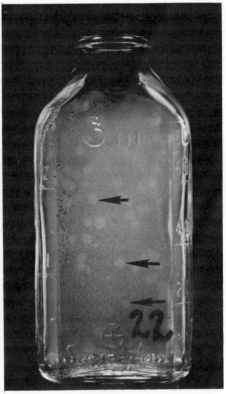

*Fig. 253.* Interference test for MD-VD virus. (*Left*) Culture first inoculated with noncytopathic virus followed by 50 PFU of cyopathic virus 3 days later. No plaques are visible as interference with viral replication occurred. (*Right*) Plaques (*arrows*) are clearly visible as this control culture was only inoculated with 50 PFU of cytopathic virus.

Gratzek (14) reported a tenfold loss of virus in 24 hours at 26 C or 37 C. Coggins (unpublished data, 1964) found no loss of strain Oregon virus in 24 hours at 25 C. The virus is readily maintained in lyophilized or frozen state ($-60$ to $-70$ C) for many years. Its density in a sucrose density gradient system is 1.13 to 1.14 (Coggins, unpublished data, 1964).

The virus produces neutralizing and complement-fixing antibodies. With the agar-gel-diffusion system either BVD-MD or hog cholera antisera produces a precipitation reaction with the VD antigen.

No hemagglutination has been associated with the BVD-MD virus particle.

**Cultivation.** Isolates of BVD-MD virus are either cytopathic or noncytopathic in various tissue culture systems. Strain NY 1 multiplies in bovine embryonic skin-muscle cells or embryonic bovine kidney cells without cytopathic changes (25). Similar results in embryonic bovine kidney cells were obtained with strain Indiana 46 and the Saunders strain (5). Noncytopathic virus is most conveniently demonstrated in tissue culture by the interference phenomenon (12, fig. 253), by the exaltation effect produced by the addition of Newcastle disease virus (18), or by the immunofluorescence test (15).

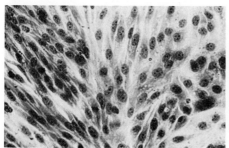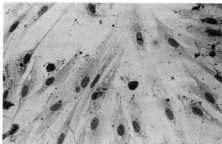

Fig. 254. (*Left*) Uninoculated 8-day-old tissue culture of embryonic bovine kidney cell. H and E. (*Right*) Eight-day-old virus diarrhea virus culture on embryonic bovine kidney cells. Note cytopathogenic effect. H and E. (Courtesy Gillespie, Baker, and McEntee, *Cornell Vet.*)

Noice and Schipper (29) and Underdahl, Grace, and Hoerlein (43) isolated cytopathogenic strains of virus from cases described as mucosal disease. Gillespie, Baker, and McEntee (9) isolated a cytopathogenic strain from the spleen of a calf supplied by investigators at Oregon State University which was designated strain Oregon of BVD-md virus. This strain produced experimental infection in calves and neutralized the homologous antiserum as well as antisera produced in calves that were inoculated with the NY 1 strain, Indiana strain, and others. These same investigators and additional ones soon isolated many cytopathogenic strains from field cases.

Some of the viruses produce a cytopathogenic effect quicker than others and completely destroy the cell sheet. Nuclei of bovine kidney cells become pyknotic and also marginated, and vaccuolization occurs. Various strains produce plaques, and this method can be used for more accurate viral titration (12, 23). Throughout the growth cycle the fluid phase of the culture has a greater concentration than the cells, and this suggests that the completely infective particle is formed in the cytoplasm (13).

Except for Darbyshire (6) other investigators have failed to propagate BVD-MD virus in hens' embryonated eggs. His strain produced pocks on the chorioallantoic membrane.

**Immunity.** THe high incidence of our bovine population with neutralizing antibodies and the viremic nature of the disease together suggest that animals develop a long and solid immunity after exposure to BVD-MD virus.

The MD England LS strain provided protection for two cattle that were challenged with virulent virus at 13 and 22 months following inoculation (17). Cattle immunized with strain Indiana 46, strain New York 1, or strain Oregon were resistant to virulent virus for at least 12 to 16 months (32). Calves that were infected with virus *in utero* had an active immunity at 6 months of age and were resistant to challenge (46).

After inoculation with BVD-MD virus no serum-neutralizing antibodies are detectable at 1 week postinoculation but the titers at 2 weeks ranged from 80 to 280 and at 4 weeks between 210 and 2,500 (38).

Maternal immunity studies were performed by Kahrs *et al.* (20) and Malmquist (27). Antibody titers persist for 6 to 9 months in calves whose dams are immune. For example, a new-born calf that has a titer of 1 : 1,024 after colostral feeding will have an antibody titer of approximately 1 : 16 when it is 28 weeks of age. Massive challenge with virulent virus can overcome maternal immunity as it approaches dimunition. This long duration of immunity must be taken into account in an incidence study or in a vaccination program.

Serum-neutralizing antibody is indicative of protection in cattle. The relationship between this test and immunity to challenge with virulent virus in a sequential experiment showed that the neutralization test is at least 95 percent accurate and thus is usable as a substitute for direct challenge (38). To assure reasonable accuracy the test was standardized by the use of 100 $TCID_{50}$ of cytopathic virus against serial three-fold dilutions of test serum (9). The serum titer varies according to the amount of virus in the test with an increase of 1 log of virus causing a decrease of 0.44 log of serum titer (4). The neutralization test is quite accurate, varying as little as 0.26 log within tests and 0.41 log between tests.

Calves given BVD-MD virus form complement-fixing antibodies before serum-neutralizing antibodies and the CF antibodies remained at high levels for at least 15 weeks (15).

Its immunological relationship to hog cholera virus was described earlier (p. 1280). Although rinderpest virus produces similar pathological changes, no immunological relationship between VD and rinderpest viruses could be established (7, 44).

**Transmission** Because this is a viremic disease it is assumed that the excretions contain infective virus during the acute stage of infection. Fecal material, blood, and splenic tissue contain virus during this state. Despite the presence of serum-neutralizing antibodies BVD-MD virus was isolated from buffy coat of cattle given virus 3 weeks before (15). Infection can be produced with infective virus by the oral route or by parenteral injection. There is excellent field evidence that the infection can be readily carried from one herd to another by mechanical means.

The natural occurrence of BVD-MD infection in sheep and goats is unknown, but they may play a role in transmission of the virus to cattle. There is strong evidence that it occurs as a natural infection in swine. Neutralizing antibodies have been found in a small percentage (3) of New York white-tailed deer (19). A disease resembling BVD-MD has been described in white-tailed and mule deer in North Dakota (36). One or more of these hosts may play a significant role in the ecology of this disease.

In order to understand the maintenance of this virus in nature, it is necessary to study the pathogenesis of the disease in cattle and to determine the role of the bovine species as a virus carrier. In addition, serious attempts to find an insect vector(s) should be made.

**Diagnosis.** The diagnosis generally is based upon clinical signs and more specifically upon lesions. This disease can be readily confused clinically with malignant catarrhal fever (p. 979) or rinderpest (p. 1053) in some instances and on occasions with bovine respiratory infections.

As far as we know, all noncytopathic and cytopathic field isolates replicate in tissue-culture systems including embryonic bovine cultures of kidney, spleen, testicle, and trachea. Virus has been isolated from the blood, urine, nasal, or ocular discharges of acute cases. At necropsy spleen, bone marrow, or mesenteric lymph nodes are good sources for virus. If cytopathic changes are not observed after three passages in cell culture, noncytopathic strains can be identified by the immunofluorescence test, by the END method, or by the cellular resistance test.

The demonstration of a rising titer with paired serums in the serum-neutralization or complement-fixation test constitutes good methods for diagnosis, but, in practice, the serum-neutralization test is preferred.

**Immunization.** No alteration in virulence in calves was noted with strain New York after 100 transfers in embryonic bovine kidney cells (Gillespie, 1965). In contrast, strain Oregon showed attenuation for calves by the 32nd passage in this same cell system and did not spread to a limited number of contact calves (5). Laboratory and field tests of this strain by other workers confirmed these observations and recommended its use in the field (48). This vaccine strain is now produced by commercial firms and probably produces a long-lasting immunity.

At an AVMA Symposium on Bovine Diseases in 1967 a Panel included BVD-MD vaccine in their recommendations in their herd health programs. In *beef cattle* a herd health program includes the following. In a preconditioning program for calves on the ranch BVD-MD modified living virus of tissue culture origin singly or in combination with *Leptospira pomona* bacterin, should be given to 5-month-old calves. Calves that arrive at feedlots without preconditioning should not be given BVD-MD vaccine unless a given feedlot has had previous problems with BVD-MD, and then only 48 hours or more after arrival, depending upon recovery from the stress of shipping. In the *self-contained dairy herd* inoculate calves with BVD-MD vaccine at 6 to 8 months of age only if the disease is prevalent in the area. Additions to the open herd should be kept in isolation for 30 days and immunized with BVD-MD vaccine if the disease is common in the herd.

The Panel (2) recognized that BVD-MD modified living vaccines are quite effective and relatively safe for most cattle under field conditions. Reports following field use indicate that in some cattle this vaccine may be a predisposing factor or possibly the primary cause of severe reactions. Such adverse reactions, which usually involve low morbidity and high mortality, are not clearly understood. In consideration of these reactions, BVD-MD vaccine is recommended only where previous or anticipated disease problems are of sufficient magnitude to warrant the risk involved. It should be recognized that BVD-MD antibody of maternal origin may persist in a small percentage of calves at detectable levels up to 9 months of age.

It is now known that BVD-MD virus causes abortions and congenital anomalies, so the use of vaccine in pregnant cows is ill advised.

**Control.** The economic importance of this disease in the United States has been reasonably well established, particularly in feedlot operations. Because it causes abortions and congenital anomalies there is little doubt of its economic significance in dairy cattle as well. Regular vaccination with the present vaccine is not advised despite the high incidence of infection in United States cattle populations unless it manifests itself as a serious disease malady in a given area or herd. An improved vaccine is highly desirable as there is a great need to vaccinate a greater proportion of the United States cattle population.

Great care should be exercised by individuals who go from one herd to another to avoid carrying the virus.

**The Disease in Man.** There is no evidence to suggest that man is infected with this virus.

## REFERENCES

1. Baker, York, Gillespie, and Mitchell.   Am. Jour. Vet. Res., 1954, *15*, 525.
2. Bovine Respiratory Disease Symposium.   Panel Report. Jour. Am. Vet. Med. Assoc., 1971, *152*, 940.
3. Carlson, Pritchard, and Doyle.   Am. Jour. Vet. Res., 1957, *18*, 560.
4. Coggins.   Cornell Univ. Thesis, 1962.
5. Coggins, Gillespie, Robson, Thompson, Wagner, and Baker.   Cornell Vet., 1961, *51*, 540.
6. Darbyshire.   Jour. Comp. Path. and Therap., 1963, *73*, 309.
7. DeLay and Knaizeff.   Am. Jour. Vet. Res., 1966, *127*, 512.
8. Gillespie and Baker.   Cornell Vet., 1959, *49*, 439.

9. Gillespie, Baker, and McEntee. *Ibid.*, 1960, *40*, 73.
10. Gillespie, Bartholomew, Thomson, and McEntee. *Ibid.*, 1967, *57*, 564.
11. Gillespie, Coggins, Thompson, and Baker. *Ibid.*, 1961, *51*, 155.
12. Gillespie, Madin, and Darby. Proc. Soc. Exp. Biol. and Med., 1962, *110*, 248.
13. Gillespie, Madin, and Darby. Cornell Vet., 1963, *53*, 276.
14. Gratzek. Univ. of Wis. Thesis, 1961.
15. Gutekunst and Malmquist. Canad. Jour. Comp. Med., 1963, *28*, 19.
16. Hermodsson and Dinter. Nature, 1962, *194*, 893.
17. Huck. Vet. Rec., 1957, *69*, 1207 and 1213.
18. Inaba, Omori, and Kumagai. Arch. f. die Gesam. Virusforsch., 1963, *13*, 245.
19. Kahrs, Atkinson, Baker, Carmichael, Coggins, Gillespie, Langer, Marshall, Robson, and Sheffy. Cornell Vet., 1964, *54*, 360.
20. Kahrs, Robson, and Baker. Proc. 70th Ann. Meet. U.S. Livestock Sanit. Assoc., 1967, 145.
21. Kahrs, Scott, and de Lahunta. Jour. Am. Vet. Med. Assoc., 1970, *156*, 1443.
22. Knaizeff. Quoted by Pritchard. Advances in veterinary science. Academic Press, New York, 1963, p. 8.
23. Knaizeff and Walker. *Ibid.*
24. Knaizeff, Huck, Jarret, Pritchard, Ramsey, Schipper, Stoeber, and Liess. Vet. Rec., 1961, *73*, 768.
25. Lee and Gillespie. Am. Jour. Vet. Res., 1957, *18*, 952.
26. Maess and Reczko. Arch. f. die Gesam. Virusforsch., 1970, *30*, 39.
27. Malmquist. Jour. Am. Vet. Med. Assoc., 1968, *152*, 763.
28. Newberne, Robinson, and Alter. Vet. Med., 1961, *56*, 395.
29. Noice and Schipper. Proc. Soc. Exp. Biol. and Med., 1959, *100*, 84.
30. Olafson, MacCallum, and Fox. Cornell Vet., 1946, *36*, 205.
31. Olafson and Rickard. *Ibid.*, 1947, *37*, 104.
32. Pritchard. Adv. Vet. Sci., 1963, *8*, 2.
33. Pritchard, Taylor, Moses, and Doyle. Ann. Rpt. Dept. Vet. Sci., Indiana Agr. Exp. Sta., 1954, p. 724.
34. Pritchard, Taylor, Moses, and Doyle. Jour. Am. Vet. Med. Assoc., 1956, *128*, 1.
35. Ramsey and Chivers. North Am. Vet., 1953, *34*, 629.
36. Richards, Schipper, Eveleth, and Shumard. Vet. Med., 1956, *51*, 538.
37. Richie and Fernelius. Arch. f. die Gesam. Virusforsch., 1969, *28*, 369.
38. Robson, Gillespie, and Baker. Cornell Vet., 1960, *50*, 503.
39. Scott, Kahrs, de Lahunta, Brown, McEntee, and Gillespie. Cornell Vet., 1973, *63*, (Oct).
40. Scott, Kahrs, and Parsonson. Jour. Am. Vet. Med. Assoc., 1970, *156*, 867.
41. Stewart, Carbrey, Jenny, Brown, and Kresse. Program, 108th Ann. Mtg., Am. Vet. Med. Assoc., 1971, 163.
42. Trapp. Iowa State Univ. Thesis, 1960.
43. Underdahl, Grace, and Hoerlein. Proc. Soc. Exp. Biol. and Med., 1957, *94*, 795.
44. Walker and Olafson. Cornell Vet., 1947, *37*, 107.
45. Ward. *Ibid.*, 1971, *61*, 179.
46. Ward, Roberts, McEntee, and Gillespie. *Ibid.*, 1969, *59*, 525.
47. Whiteman. Iowa State Univ. Thesis, 1960.
48. York, Rosner, and McLean. Proc. U.S. Livestock Sanit. Assoc., 1960, *64*, 339.

# LII | Tumor Viruses

In previous chapters it was clearly evident that some animal viruses in various genera are capable of producing malignant and benign tumors. Three other genera not previously mentioned include only viruses which are known principally for their oncogenic characters. The genus *Leukovirus* are RNA tumor viruses of leukogenic origin. The genera *Papillomavirus* and *Polyomavirus* are DNA tumor viruses and both are included in the family *Papoviridae*. Conspicuously lacking in previous chapters was mention of a virus of human origin that was definitely proved to induce a malignant tumor in man although it has been well established that benign warts and molluscum contagiosum of man are caused by viruses. It is reasonable to assume that man is not uniquely endowed in this regard and ultimately it will be shown that a virus(es) is capable of inducing malignancy in human beings.

## LEUKOVIRUSES

The animal RNA tumor viruses in the genus *Leukovirus* are similar in biochemical and biophysical properties, structure, and growth properties. These viruses produce tumors in their natural host.

Electron microscope photomicrographs show virus particles of these RNA tumor viruses only in the cell cytoplasm with budding forms at the cell membrane and mature particles in the intracellular spaces. The particles range in size from 70 to 100 mμ. The mature particles have an RNA electron-dense nucleoid, either central (type C particle) or acentric (type B particle). The nucleoid is separated from a single or double outer membrane (envelope) by an electron-lucid area (halo). The nucleoid of immature particles (type A) is electron-transparent since nucleic acid is lacking. Biological activity is associated only with type C virus particles in murine, avian, and feline leukemia viruses, and type B particles, in the case of murine mammary-tumor virus.

Most particles lack the internal helical structure typical for myxoviruses and only occasional particles have spikes on the outer member.

The nucleic acid is single-stranded RNA with a high molecular weight of above 1 by $10^7$ daltons. There is a suggestion that these RNA molecules may be composed of smaller subunits of 2 to 3 by $10^6$ daltons held together by heatlabile hydrogen bonds.

There are five principal groups based upon the type of tumor and host range, (a) avian leukosis complex, (b) murine leukosis complex, (c) feline leukosis complex, (d) murine mammary-tumor virus, and (e) bovine leukemia.

## Avian Leukosis Complex

SYNONYMS: Big liver disease, hepatolymphomatosis, diffuse osteoperiostitis, osteopetrosis gallinarum, marble bone, thick-leg disease.

In 1908 Ellermann and Bang (5) produced evidence to indicate that a leukemic condition of fowls could be transmitted to other fowls by the inoculation of cell-free filtrates. In 1910 Rous transmitted a spindle-cell sarcoma by inoculation and in the following year showed that cell-free filtrates carried the tumor-inducing agent. Up to 1933, when their paper was written, Claude and Murphy (4) reported that no less than 27 different types of tumors of chickens had been proved to be transmissible. Not all of these had been transmitted by filtrates, but the authors listed 19 instances in which they felt that evidence of filtrate transmission was satisfactory.

Many of the transmissible tumors of chickens may be regarded as laboratory curiosities rather than important economic problems. There are some, especially those of the so-called *leukosis complex,* that are of great economic importance because they behave like highly infectious diseases and thus involve large numbers of birds.

Earlier most pathologists refused to believe that the virus-induced tumors were true neoplasms. It is generally admitted now, however, that they may not be distinguished morphologically from the majority of tumors which have not been associated with viral agents. Recently there has been a growing conviction by many workers that it may eventually be shown that many, or perhaps all, malignant tumors are virus-induced. There is no proof for such a belief now. Virus-induced tumors occur in a number of mammals but none, except for some simple papillomas, have been identified in man.

The term *leukosis* is used to signify abnormal proliferation of primitive cells which are the precursors of leukocytes. The term is now favored over the older one, *leukemia,* which indicates that unusual numbers of such cells are found in the blood, for there are many forms in which such cells are found in the tissues but not in the blood stream. The terms *pseudoleukemia* or *aleukemic leukemia* are sometimes used to differentiate these forms. There is good evidence that two types of viruses are responsible for the production of tumors listed under the heading of the avian leukosis complex. There is

Marek's virus (see chapter on herpesviruses) and also the leukosis complex viruses included in this chapter.

**Character of the Disease.** The leukosis (ALV) viruses can be demonstrated in cell cultures of chick fibroblasts because they cause a cellular resistance, unrelated to interferon (8), to the Rous sarcoma virus which manifests itself as a cellular proliferation. This method has made possible many studies of the forms caused by the RIF viruses. Vertical transmission of the virus from the dam through the egg to the progeny occurs. The RIF viruses are antigenic and produce neutralizing antibodies that can be measured by the tissue culture neutralization test. Morphologically, these viruses are similar. The leukosis viruses are less pathogenic than the Marek virus types with slower horizontal transmission (bird to bird) and also slower development of lesions in the infected birds.

Erythroblastosis (AEV) and myeloblastosis (AMV) are produced by the RIF group of viruses. The terms erythroblastosis and myeloblastosis are applied to diseases in which leukemia develops, i.e., in which precursors of erythrocytes or of granulocytes occur in the blood stream. The disease is essentially one of the myeloid tissue of the bone marrow; the changes in the blood and other tissues are secondary. The air spaces and fatty tissue of the normal marrow are replaced with a grayish-red tissue consisting of proliferating myeloid cells. Sometimes the proliferating cells are precursors of erythrocytes, in which case the disease is called *erythroblastosis* or *erythroleukosis;* in other cases they are precursors of the granulocytes, in which case the disease is called *myeloblastosis* or *myeloleukosis.* The filterable agent that acts as the stimulant may cause proliferation of either type; hence if a number of susceptible birds are inoculated with the blood, or filtrates of plasma, of a single bird suffering from either type, some of them are likely to develop one type and some the other. Thus Stubbs and Furth (22) inoculated 25 birds with material from two chickens affected with leukosis, one of which was of the myeloid type and the other of the erythroid. Thirteen of these birds developed leukosis (52 percent). Both types were represented in this series, these being distributed through both groups of birds irrespective of the type used for inoculation. Ellermann and Bang (5) earlier had found that a single virus might produce both types of the disease. After passage in the laboratory they invariably produce one type.

The affected bird becomes weak and anemic. The comb and wattles are pale and the bird nearly always dies. The liver, spleen, and kidneys are found to be moderately enlarged and pale in color, the blood is thin and watery, and petechial hemorrhages are usually found in the loose areolar tissue and in the mucosa of the intestines. In practically every case, the immature myeloid cells, previously mentioned, are found in large numbers in the circulating blood, and the red cells are present in greatly reduced numbers.

*Visceral lymphomatosis.* This is a most frequently encountered type of tumor in chickens. Either the leukosis or Marek group of viruses can cause this form. It consists of infiltrations of lymphocytic or mononuclear cells in the organs. Usually the liver presents the most conspicuous lesions. These are of two kinds, the nodular and the diffuse. The liver generally is greatly enlarged and the body cavity may be filled with fluid (ascites). In the diffuse type the organ is grayish in color and granular in appearance. In the nodular form the areas of infiltration are in the form of discrete tumor masses of a grayish-white color. In the one case the infiltrations are small and scattered throughout, whereas in the other they are more localized. The tumor tissue has about the same consistency as that of the liver.

The kidneys, ovaries, heart, lungs, and, in fact, almost all structures of the body may be infiltrated with such tumors. There is a tendency for the Marek group to produce tumors in these organs, such as the gonads, heart, and others, which are richly supplied with nerves. The blood picture usually is normal but sometimes there may be a moderate increase in lymphocytic cells.

*Osteopetrotic lymphomatosis.* This condition has frequently been associated with other forms of lymphomatosis. Opinions differ as to whether it is etiologically associated but recent evidence suggests that ALV virus may be involved (23). It is a comparatively uncommon condition. It is manifested by bone deformities, especially of the long bones, but it sometimes involves the pelvis and shoulder girdle. It is essentially a condensing osteitis in which the bones become greatly swollen and very dense, and often the marrow cavity may be largely or completely obliterated. When the lesions occur in the long bones of the legs, the deformities can be seen or felt by palpation. There is no osteoporosis.

*Rous sarcoma virus.* Rous (15) in 1910 described the first of a series of transplantable, malignant sarcomas of the chicken. In 1911 (16) he showed that the tumor could be induced with dried cells, with cells that had been destroyed with glycerol, and with cell-free filtrates. The tumor is now known as the Rous sarcoma I. It is a spindle-cell sarcoma which metastasizes freely and usually destroys its host within 1 month. This tumor has been extensively studied. In 1912 Rous, Murphy, and Tytler (17) described another chicken tumor transmissible with filtrates, an osteochrondosarcoma, and a third, a spindle-cell angiosarcoma. A considerable number of additions have been made to the list in later years.

The active principle of these tumors, particularly of tumor I, has been extensively studied by Murphy and co-workers (13. 14) and by Sittenfield, Johnson, and Jobling (21). In recent years Rubin and co-workers have dealt with the problems of assay of virus and host-virus relations *in vivo* and *in vitro* (18).

**Properties of the Viruses.** The avian leukosis viruses have been classified into 5 antigenic subgroups (types) A, B, C, D, and E, each including different leukemia-inducing viruses and different sarcoma viruses. Subgroups A and B are the most important groups, and subgroup B shows serological evidence of heterogenicity within the subgroup and some cross-reaction with Group D.

This is probably explained by the fact that the classification is based upon the host range of genetically-defined chick embryo cells rather than upon serological composition.

RNA avian tumor viruses produce antibody. There is cross-reactivity by neutralization and precipitation tests among virus strains that cause lymphomatosis, myeloblastosis, and erythroblastosis.

Rous sarcoma virus (RSV) was originally thought to be an entirely defective virus (9). This is true in a quantitative sense only and a helper Rous associated virus (RAV) is required to make some RSV particles an infective virus. More than 90 percent of different NP (cells that fail to produce infectious virus or protein coat antigen) cell lines studied contained virus particles

Table XLI. AVIAN LEUKOSIS VIRUS GROUPS

| Subgroups (types) | Rous Sarcoma Virus Strains | | Leukosis viruses |
| | Nondefective | Pseudotypes | |
| --- | --- | --- | --- |
| A | SR-RSV-A | BH-RSV (RAV-1) | RAV-1 |
| B | SR-RSV-B | BH-RSV (RAV-2) | RAV-2 |
| C | PR-RSV-C | BH-RSV (RAV-49) | RAV-49 |
| D | SR-RSV-D | BH-RSV (RAV-50) | RAV-50 |
| E | RSV beta O | BH-RSV (RAV-60) | RAV-60 |

Abbreviations: RSV = Rous sarcoma virus; RAV = Rous associated virus. BH = Byran's high-titered virus; SR = Schmidt-Ruppin; PR = Prague C.

as detected by electron microscopy. These mature particles termed RSV-beta O were infectious for certain types of avian cells not used in past studies. More recently a second particle termed RSV-alpha O has been isolated from NP cells, and it is unable to replicate in any known avian cells by itself. Thus, it remains to be seen if the latter type of particle represents the RSV genome in the protein coat of another uncharacterized helper RAV virus or whether it represents a true nondefective RSV population in the Bryan's high-titered RSV strain.

Furth's leukosis virus was probably a resistance-inducing factor (RIF) type of virus (6). It was preserved by desiccation, and infective blood mixed with 50 percent glycerol remained active for at least 104 days. The virus survived for 14 days at 4 C but not at 37 C. He also found that 0.000,0001 ml of infective plasma was sufficient to produce the disease by intravenous injection.

A number of arboviruses injected into a lymphoid tumor lead to regression (20).

The Rous sarcoma virus is infectious for the rabbit and induces sarcomas in mice, rats, hamsters, primates, and chickens.

**Cultivation.** Most leukosis viruses multiply in cultures of chick embryo fibroblasts without causing a cytopathic effect or transformation. Virus replication can be detected by an immunofluorescence focal assay with type-specific chicken antisera or by failure of cells to transform when exposed to RSV, a phenomenon termed interference that is utilizable in a resistance-inducing factor test (RIF) as an assay procedure.

Morphologic transformation of mesenchymal target cells into myeloblast cells occurs only with AMV virus. The transformed cells multiply exponentially and produce new virus. This test is used to assay virus. The virus also incorporates the enzyme ATPase during replication, and there is relationship between this activity and viral infectivity.

The RSV readily and quickly transforms cells in culture with formation of foci of transformed cells. Virus activity is measured as the number of focus-forming units (FFU) per unit volume.

**Immunity.** Chickens that are immunologically competent develop neutralizing antibody after exposure to leukosis virus. These birds usually are not viremic but an occasional bird may harbor antibody and virus at the same time. Birds with antibody only do not develop tumors.

**Transmission.** Transmission experiments in the past were attended with great difficulties, not the least of which is that the disease appears spontaneously in many birds and the control birds frequently show appreciable numbers of cases, a fact which makes interpretation of the experiments subject to opinion. Careful culling of affected flocks generally has led to a reduction in the incidence of the disease. In areas where the incidence was previously high, usually it has decreased after a few years. Barber (1) found that when hatches of chicks were separated, some being reared where chickens had not previously been kept, the incidence of lymphomatosis varied according to the age at which such chicks were brought back to infected premises. Hutt and co-workers (11) found that divided lots of chicks brooded for the first 2 weeks at 40 and 200 feet away from infected pens showed a diminished incidence in those brooded at the greater distance.

Genetic factors undoubtedly influence susceptibility to lymphomatosis. The influence of these factors is summarized by Hutt (10) and Hutt and Cole (12), who point out that birds may be selected for resistance and that this process is occurring naturally in the field. Waters (24) and Waters and Prickett (25), working in experimental flocks which were kept under close quarantine, believe that they have shown that the disease is definitely infective and that the transmissible agent may be introduced into flocks in infected eggs used for hatching. Burmester (2) showed that adult hens could be immunized to the agent of lymphomatosis, that antibodies were produced, and that these were passed through the eggs to the newly hatched chicks.

The virus is transmitted horizontally through the feces and saliva. Vertical transmission occurs through the viremic hen but not the viremic rooster (18). Such hens and roosters usually fail to have antibody and are permanent shedders of the virus. The incidence of leukemia in vertical transmission is higher than in transmission by contact.

Ectoparasites could be involved in the transmission of leukosis viruses.

**Diagnosis.** At necropsy the various disease forms can be readily diagnosed. The isolation and classification of the leukosis viruses requires a competence that is limited to a few laboratories engaged in leukosis research.

**Control.** It is now possible to establish a breeder flock that is free of leukosis viruses. The procedure that will be described does not eliminate leukosis caused by the Marek virus.

Basically three steps are involved in this program as suggested by Hughes *et al.* (9). A limited number of hens are tested for neutralizing antibody by the use of a color test devised by Calnek (3) which is accurate and simple. The eggs laid by the selected hens which have neutralizing antibody are tested for virus by the RIF assay method. Chicks reared in isolation and from hens selected for freedom from transovarian passage of virus are tested for RIF antibody at 16 to 20 weeks of age. The birds without RIF antibody are then used as the breeders for an RIF free flock. With proper surveillance for RIF antibody and reasonable isolation it should be possible to maintain an RIF free flock.

**The Disease in Man.** It is not known to occur.

## REFERENCES

1. Barber.   Cornell Vet., 1943, *33*, 78.
2. Burmester.   Proc. Soc. Exp. Biol. and Med., 1955, *88*, 153.
3. Calnek.   Avian Dis., 1964, *8*, 163.
4. Claude and Murphy.   Physiol. Rev., 1933, *13*, 246.
5. Ellermann and Bang.   Centrbl. f. Bakt., I, Abt., Orig., 1908, *46*, 595.
6. Furth.   Jour. Exp. Med., 1932, *55*, 465 and 495.
7. Hanafusa, Hanafusa, and Rubin.   Proc. Natl. Acad. Sci. (U.S.), 1963, *49*, 572.
8. Hanafusa, Hanafusa, and Rubin.   Virology, 1964, *22*, 591.
9. Hughes, Watanabe, and Rubin.   Avian Dis., 1963, *7*, 154.
10. Hutt.   Brit. Vet. Jour., 1951, *107*, 28.
11. Hutt, Ball, Bruckner, and Ball.   Poultry Sci., 1944, *23*, 396.
12. Hutt and Cole.   Science, 1947, *106*, 379.
13. Murphy, Helmer, Claude, and Sturm.   *Ibid.*, 1931, *73*, 266.
14. Murphy, Sturm, Claude, and Helmer.   Jour. Exp. Med., 1932, *56*, 91.
15. Rous.   *Ibid.*, 1910, *12*, 696.
16. *Ibid.*, 1911, *13*, 397.
17. Rous, Murphy, and Tytler.   Jour. Am. Med. Assoc., 1912, *59*, 1793 and 1912.
18. Rubin.   Bact. Rev., 1962, *26*, 1.
19. Sevoian, Chamberlain, and Larose.   Avian Dis., 1963, *7*, 102.
20. Sharpless, Davies, and Cox.   Proc. Soc. Exp. Biol. and Med., 1950, *73*, 270.
21. Sittenfield, Johnson, and Jobling.   Am. Jour. Cancer, 1931, *15*, 2275.
22. Stubbs and Furth.   Jour. Exp. Med., 1931, *53*, 269.
23. Walter, Burmester, and Fontes.   Avian Dis., 1963, *7*, 79.
24. Waters.   Science, 1947, *106*, 246.
25. Waters and Prickett.   Poultry Sci., 1944, *23*, 321.

## Feline Leukosis Complex

In 1964 Jarrett and coinvestigators (17, 18) established that C-type viral particles were responsible for the production of feline lymphosarcoma in experimental cats. Later, Rickard *et al.* (23) observed C-type particles in a spontaneous case. Several investigators have now observed C-type particles in feline lymphosarcoma and have transmitted the disease with cell-free filtrates (12, 21, 24, 25).

Excellent papers of the feline leukemia complex are embodied in the proceedings issue of a feline infectious disease colloquium (1).

**Character of the Disease.** Leukemia disorders are among the most prevalent and devastating diseases of domestic cats and malignant lymphoma ranks first among all tumors of the cat (10). The true world-wide incidence of feline leukemia is difficult to assess as clinical diagnosis is difficult, but there is little doubt that the incidence and the mortality are high.

According to Schneider (30) malignant lymphoma is a tumor of young cats. His statement is based upon information established by a population-based animal neoplasm registry for the Bay Area of California that has been in existence since 1965. There also seems to be a predilection for males. Apparently, the disease also occurs in Siamese cats more frequently than in Persian cats, after adjustment for breed differences in the population. In contrast, a survey in the Boston area (10) indicates that age bears no relationship to the incidence of lymphoma in cats.

Excellent descriptions of the clinical signs and pathological lesions are presented by Gilmore and Holzworth (10) and Holzworth (13). The common signs of illness in all leukemic disorders are pallor of skin and mucosae, low-grade fever, and enlargement of the spleen and liver. There is often anorexia and occasionally enlargement of the lymph nodes. When malignant lymphoma is present in the form of solid tumors it causes a diversity of signs. Solid tumors have been found in almost every organ and tissue of the cat, either as single or multiple lesions. A common site is the kidney, usually bilateral, with the production of uremia in many cases. Lymphoma of the intestinal tract may lead to partial obstruction causing diarrhea and vomiting. Whenever lymphoma is elsewhere in the abdomen it often occurs in the liver, spleen and/or visceral lymph nodes to varying degrees.

It is a general impression among investigators that the disease in very young cats more often involves the anterior mediastinum or thymus than other organs. In these cases the lymphoma mass ultimately encases the heart, compresses the esophagus and trachea, and displaces the lungs. In addition there is a hydrothorax. Involvement of these organs leads to a myriad of signs referable to the respiratory, cardiac, and upper digestive disorders. Lymphoma occasionally involves the brain, spinal cord, and nasopharynx causing unusual signs in many instances. In the oral cavity it may mimic gingivitis, and on occasion involves the skin. Generalized lymphadenopathy occurs less often in cats than in dogs and cattle.

Sometimes malignant lymphoma manifests itself as a blood disease and it must be differentiated from other rarer leukemias by hematologic examinations (10). Furthermore, it must be recognized that blood and bone-marrow involvement does not always occur when solid tumors exist; perhaps less than 25 percent of cases have malignant cells in the blood. They are more likely to appear in the blood during the terminal stage of the disease. When neoplastic cells do occur in the blood, there may be more than 200,000 per mm³ or they may constitute only a tiny fraction of the cells in absolute lymphopenia. There is no typical hematologic picture with malignant lymphoma. While exceptions occur, basic indications of the disease are lymphoblasts in the blood, an absolute lymphocytosis of more than 14,000 per mm³, or more than 15 percent lymphocytes in the blood. Cats with lymphocytic leukemia usually lack specific clinical signs. Other than those associated with anemia and hepatosplenomegaly, cats may have hemorrhages, jaundice, or iridal discoloration and clouded anterior chambers. In these cats, an accurate diagnosis of leukemia and cell-type identification requires examination of blood and bone marrow, and perhaps of surgical biopsy material as well. For details about lymphocytic leukemia and less common hematopoietic malignancies of cat in order of their frequency—reticuloendotheliosis, mast-cell leukemia, and granulocytic leukemia—the reader is referred to the articles by Gilmore and Holzworth (10) and Schalm (29) and also the textbook by Schalm (28). Rare leukemias of the cat such as eosinophilic, plasma-cell, and stem-cell leukemias as well as erythemic myelosis and erythroleukemia also are described in these sources.

**The Disease in Experimental Animals.** Various strains of feline leukemia virus (FeLV) are known to produce malignant lymphomas in newborn kittens (fig. 255). Older cats presumably are infected but do not develop disease. At present very little is known about the replication of FeLV in experimental cats (16). It has been shown that the virus is present in tissues at 28 days after inoculation and persists throughout the disease process. Virus is detectable in the megakaryocytes of the spleen and bone marrow, which presumably leads to a viremia, since large numbers of viral particles are found in the blood platelets (21), and the viremia persists until death. Although Kawakami et al. (19) found virus in the blood of some cats in the terminal stages of spontaneous and experimental disease, others did not show a viremia.

The feline fibrosarcoma virus (FeSV) has been isolated from spontaneous cases of cats with fibrosarcoma. It has a rather broad experimental host-spectrum. This virus produces fibrosarcomas in experimental fetal and day-old kittens, fetal and day-old puppies (7, 8, 24), newborn rabbits, fetal sheep (31), and marmosets (4).

**Properties of the Virus.** The FeLV is similar in morphology to the viruses causing leukemia and sarcoma in the bird and mouse. The size of the virion is

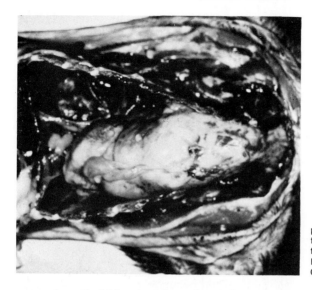

*Fig. 255.* Experimental lymphoma in a neonatal kitten. The
tumor mass principally involves
the thymus gland. (Courtesy C.
Rickard, J. Post, K. Lee, and J.
Gillespie.)

approximately 100 mμ, with an internal membrane about 60 mμ in diameter. It is
assembled by a process of budding from cell membranes. Type C particles
have been observed in spontaneous and experimental cases (fig. 256). It is an
RNA virus. Sodium dodecylsulfate releases viral RNA which can be resolved

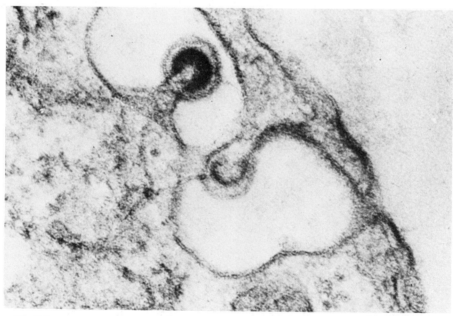

*Fig. 256.* Budding C-type feline leukemia virus particle characteristic of C-type oncogenic RNA
viruses. (Courtesy C. Rickard.)

by zone centrifugation into three components with sedimentation coefficients of 75 S, 35 S, and 4 S. In a sucrose gradient the bouyant density of FeLV is between 1.13 and 1.17 g per ml.

Viral interference patterns and neutralization tests were used by Sarma (27) to study the viral envelope antigens of several field strains of FeLV and 3 field strains of FeSV. Based upon these experiments the viruses were placed in three subgroups—A, B, and C. Viral interference studies suggest that subgroup A contains one antigenic type of virus whereas subgroups B and C contain two types with subgroup A as a component of each. Using this grouping procedure, several field strains of FeLV and the three strains of FeSV occur as virus mixtures. Purification of the field strains can probably be achieved by cloning and neutralization procedures.

Various serological methods are used to detect the various virion and non-virion antigens involved in FeLV infections (14). The type-specific antigen present in the envelope is ether-susceptible. It may contain two moieties and it can be detected by neutralization, complement-fixation, and immunofluorescence tests. There are two group-specific ether-resistant antigens (gs) in the virion: gs-1 is specific for the species and common within the species and the gs-3 antigen is shared by Type C virions of mice, hamsters, cats, and rats (fig. 257). The gs-3 antigen may be labile in the tissues. The gs antigens are detected and assayed by complement-fixation, immunodiffusion, and immunofluorescence tests. The nonvirion antigens associated with infected cells include the cell-surface antigens (CSA) and transplantation antigens (TSTA); although not well-characterized, they are believed to be specific. These cellular antigens are detected and assayed by cytotoxic colony-inhibition and transplantation-inhibition tests.

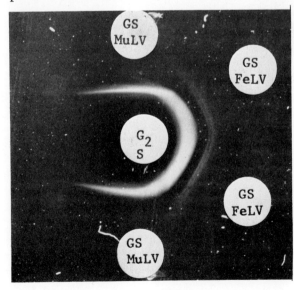

Fig. 257. Demonstration of gs-1 and gs-3 antigens by the immunodiffusion test. The broad band is the gs-3 (interspecies) antigen showing its presence in the murine leukemia virus (MuLV) and feline leukemia virus (FeLV). The lighter band demonstrates the species specific gs-1 antigens of FeLV. (Courtesy F. Noronha.)

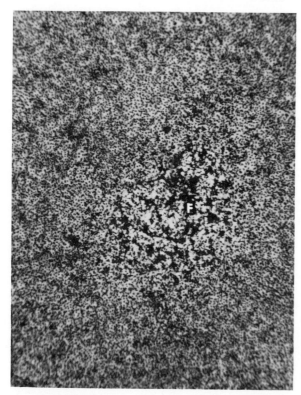

*Fig. 258.* A single focus (*F*) of transformed cells in the Crandell feline kidney cell line induced by the murine sarcoma—feline leukemia hybrid virus of Fischinger and O'Connor. May-Grünwald-Giemsa. X 23. (Courtesy K. Lee.)

Mammalian C-type particles, including the cat, contain three major structural polypeptides and 1 to 2 glycopeptides, presumably derived from the viral envelope (9). The third fastest migrating polypeptide in polyacrylamide gels contains the major group-specific (gs) antigenic determinants characteristic of the particular species of virus origin. This antigen has an apparent isolectric point near neutrality and clearly distinguishable from other viral components. The interspecies cross-reacting antigen still needs to be related to one of the structural components.

**Cultivation.** FeLV strains replicate in cell cultures of human, canine, and porcine origin but fail to replicate in selected cell-tissue cultures of bovine, murine, rat, or chicken origin. The virus grows as well in human cells as in feline cells, and virus recovered from both types of cultures was identical (16). Lee (22) found the murine sarcoma-feline leukemia hybrid virus of Fischinger and O'Connor (6) would replicate in many species of cells including dog, feline, cattle, and dolphin (fig. 258).

Feline embryonic cell cultures that were infected with a high multiplicity of FeLV virus ($10^3$ virus particles per tissue cell) yielded maximum titers of H-uridine-labeled particles at 24 hours (16). After this time there is a slight drop in virus titer to a level which is maintained indefinitely. Similar growth curves are reported for avian sarcoma viruses. Replication of virus can also be detected by production of foci of cell transformation.

**Immunity.** Prenatally inoculated kittens and kittens given FeLV and FeSV viruses within 1 week after birth usually develop tumors. Viral replication and tumor formation is probably caused by the inability of perinatal kittens to respond immunologically to the feline C-type viral and histocompatibility type cell-surface antigens or to the induction of immunologic tolerance in these individuals. On the other hand there is some evidence that immunologically mature cats do not develop tumors when given FeSV virus but are capable of producing antibodies against the viral envelope antigens (7). For example, in several adult cats with spontaneous lymphomas and others carrying FeSV sarcomas, positive reactions specific for the viral envelope antigens were detected in indirect fluorescent, ferritin antibody, and passive hemagglutination tests. Furthermore, serums from FeSV tumor-bearing kittens show neutralizing activity. The relationship between this neutralizing antibody and protection is yet to be established.

**Transmission.** Most investigators are in general agreement that feline leukemia and feline sarcoma viruses are transmitted vertically—from mother to progeny *in utero*, as a viral genome (virogene) that is repressed by the host throughout most of its life (15). The degree of virus expression or depression largely depends on host genetic factors, but carcinogens, concurrent viral infections, radiation, and the aging process can allow partial or complete activation of these virogenes with active disease ensuing.

Although most studies of avian and murine leukemia viruses have stressed the importance of vertical transmission, horizontal transmission of these viruses to virus-negative strains does occur. It is reasonable to assume that the same situation is true for feline leukemia.

The occurrence of FeLV gs antigen in feline fibrosarcomas is comparable to the murine leukemia-sarcoma complex (17). FeSV most likely arose from FeLV through some alteration. The occurrence of FeLV gs antigen in feline fibrosarcomas probably represents an excess of helper FeLV found in association with the FeSV. FeLV also is found in some cases of feline infectious peritonitis (16). At present it is difficult to determine the role of FeLV virus, if any, in the production of this rather common and invariably fatal disease of the cat (11).

Although FeLV replicates readily in human cell cultures, FeLV gs antigen has not been found in any naturally occurring human neoplasm (16). The search continues, however, as this is a most important area of concern—possible cross-species infection.

**Diagnosis.** Clinical diagnosis without the use of laboratory procedures is virtually impossible. The disease may involve so many different tissues, and produce a wide variety of clinical signs. Many diseases may be confused with feline leukemia, such as hemobartonellosis, toxoplasmosis, chronic bacterial infections, chronic viral infections, certain noninfectious disease processes, and other neoplasms. Lymphoma of the anterior mediastinum can be visualized by radiography after removal of fluid from the thoracic cavity. The presence of malignant lymphocytes in the fluid confirms the diagnosis. When lymphocytic leukemia is involved, study of blood smears may aid in the detection of feline leukemia and other rarer feline leukemias (28).

The agar-gel-diffusion test detects FeLV antigen in the solid tumor mass of approximately 70 percent of the lymphosarcoma cases. It also detects the FeLV gs antigen in most cases of feline fibrosarcoma. The indirect immunofluorescence test (26) can be used to find virus in infected cell cultures and also to detect antibodies in cat serums to FeSV antigen. The hemagglutination test is used to locate antibody in serums and appears to be more sensitive than the complement-fixation test (5). The serum-neutralization test can be used to detect specific antibody.

Electron microscopy also is commonly used in diagnosis and in research to show the C-type particles associated with the feline leukemia complex. In a study of 20 spontaneous cases of feline lymphosarcoma, type C particles were observed in 12 (20).

**Control.** As the infection in most instances is transmitted vertically, control measures are not useful in the prevention of the infection.

It was estimated that less than 10 percent of cats with feline leukemia are good candidates for treatment (3). Of the three forms of treatment currently available, surgery and irridation are of limited value. Chemotherapy for human leukemias is based upon vast clinical experience and utilizes a variety of drugs. Veterinary experience with antileukemic drugs is limited, and their expense great, so chemotherapy is rarely used; especially in the cat, as they are extremely sensitive to drugs. It is likely that feline leukemias will only be safely and effectively reduced through other approaches unavailable at present, such as immunotherapy or vaccination.

**The Disease in Man.** According to a Panel (2) there is no evidence at present to indicate the spread of feline tumor viruses to man. Whether cat tumor viruses contribute to the incidence of human lymphoma and sarcoma can only be determined by the carefully designed epidemiological studies now in progress. Preliminary reports of these studies indicate clearly that cats, with or without cancer, are not responsible for cancer in man.

## REFERENCES

1. American Veterinary Medical Association Colloquium. Jour. Am. Vet. Med. Assoc., 1971, *158*, 1013.
2. American Veterinary Medical Association Panel. *Ibid.*, 1971, *158*, 835.
3. Carpenter and Holzworth. *Ibid.*, 1971, *158*, 1131.
4. Deinhardt, Wolfe, Theilen, and Snyder. Science, 1970, *167*, 881.
5. Fink, Sibal, and Plata. Jour. Am. Vet. Med. Assoc., 1971, *158*, 1070.
6. Fischinger and O'Connor. Science, 1969, *165*, 714.
7. Gardner. Jour. Am. Vet. Med. Assoc., 1971, *158*, 1039.

8.  Gardner, Arnstein, Johnson, Rongey, Charman, and Huebner.  *Ibid.*, 1046.
9.  Gilden and Oroszlan.  *Ibid.*, 1099.
10. Gilmore and Holzworth.  *Ibid.*, 1013.
11. Hardy.  *Ibid.*, 1060.
12. Hardy, Geering, and Old.  Science, 1969, *166*, 1019.
13. Holzworth.  Jour. Am. Vet. Med. Assoc., 1960, *136*, 47.
14. Huebner, Sarma, Kelloff, Gilden, Meier, and Peters.  Ann. N.Y. Acad. Sci. 1971, *18*, 246.
15. Huebner and Todara.  Proc. Natl. Acad. Sciences, 1969, *64*, 1087.
16. Jarrett.  Jour. Am. Vet. Med. Assoc., 1971, *158*, 1032.
17. Jarrett, Crawford, Martin, and Davie.  Nature, 1964, *202*, 567.
18. Jarrett, Martin, Crighton, Dalton, and Stewart.  *Ibid.*, 566.
19. Kawakami, Theilen, Dungworth, Munn, and Beale.  Science, 1967, *158*, 1049.
20. Laird, Jarrett, Anderson, and Jarrett.  Jour. Am. Vet. Med. Assoc., 1971, *158*, 1109.
21. Laird, Jarrett, Crighton, and Jarrett.  Jour. Natl. Cancer Inst., 1968, *41*, 867.
22. Lee.  Jour. Am. Vet. Med. Assoc., 1971, *158*, 1037.
23. Rickard, Barr, Noronha, Dougherty, and Post.  Cornell Vet., 1967, 57, 302.
24. Rickard, Gillespie, Lee, Noronha, Post, and Savage.  Third Internatl. Sympos. Comp. Leukemia Res., Paris, France, S. Karger, Basel, 1967.
25. Rickard, Post, Noronha, and Barr.  Jour. Natl. Cancer Inst., 1969, *42*, 987.
26. Riggs.  Jour. Am. Vet. Med. Assoc., 1971, *158*, 1085.
27. Sarma.  Fifth Internatl. Sympos. Comp. Leukemia Res., Padova, Italy, S. Karger, Basel, Switzerland, 1972.
28. Schalm.  Veterinary hematology. 2d ed., Lea & Febiger, Philadelphia, Pa., 1965.
29. Schalm.  Jour. Am. Vet. Med. Assoc., 1971, *158*, 1025.
30. Schneider.  *Ibid.*, 1030.
31. Theilen, Snyder, Wolfe, and Landon.  Fourth Internatl. Sympos. Comp. Leukemia Res., Cherry Hill, New Jersey, S. Karger, Basel, 1970.

### Malignant Lymphoma of Cattle

SYNONYMS:  Bovine lymphomatosis, bovine lymphocytomatosis, bovine leukosis, cattle leukemia

This is a progressive, fatal disease of cattle manifested by enlargement of some or all of the lymph nodes. The glandular enlargements are preceded by blood changes. Many European workers believe that cattle may develop the blood changes without tumor formation.

The disease has been reported in the United States (9), Norway, Denmark, and Germany and probably exists elsewhere. In all the places mentioned it appears to be increasing rapidly in incidence. In the United States the records of the Meat Inspection Service of the Department of Agriculture suggest that the disease is becoming more prevalent. In all countries the disease appears to be distributed unevenly; that is, there are high and low incidence areas. In Denmark the incidence is reported to be as high as 40 cases per

100,000 cattle in some regions and as low as 1 in 100,000 in others. In the United States meat inspection statistics show a low of 5.3 and a high of 243.0 per 100,000 slaughtered cattle in different regions.

**Character of the Disease.** Affected cattle exhibit enlarged and firm superficial lymph nodes. Generally the disease progresses rapidly, emaciation develops, and death ensues. Sometimes an eyeball may protrude because of tumor formation in the orbit. Chronic bloating occurs in some because of enlargement of the thoracic nodes. Lameness and paralysis often occur because of pressures on parts of the spinal cord or peripheral nerves from the tumors. Lymphocytic infiltrations of some of the internal organs may result. Blood examinations may show as many as 50,000 large lymphocytes per mm$^3$.

**Etiology.** There is increasing evidence that a C-type virus may cause bovine leukosis (1, 6, 7, 10). Dutta and Sorensen (2) and Miller *et al.* (8) reported on the use of phytohemagglutinin (PHA) in cultured buffy-coat (BC) cells from cattle with persistent lymphocytosis or lymphosarcoma to enhance the appearance of C-type particles in these cell cultures. Ferrer *et al.* (3) enlarged upon these observations and found that PHA also uncovered type C particles in BC cultures from clinically normal cows without lymphocytosis, as well. The use of PHA certainly has given investigators a new technic that will assist them in efforts to establish the etiological significance of these type C particles in bovine leukemia.

Gillette, Olson, and Tekeli (4) reported on the use of the immunoflourescence test for detection of bovine lymphosarcoma antigen in diseased cattle. Specific staining was limited to the cytoplasm of tumor cells and usually was weak. Specific flourescence was observed in tumor tissues from 40 to 66 percent of other cattle, but it was not seen in lymph nodes of healthy cows.

**Immunity.** At present there is little information. One can only assume that its mechanism will be similar to avian and feline leukemia.

**Transmission.** Goetze *et al.* (5), in Germany, and others have carried out limited inoculation studies with inconclusive results; however, he and the Scandinavian workers are convinced that the disease is transmissible. Its localized occurrence, the occurrence of multiple cases in single herds, and its apparent rapid increase in recent years suggest, but do not prove the infectious theory.

Present epidemiological evidence indicates that either vertical or neonatal horizontal transmission may occur. This would be in keeping with the leukemias of other species about which we have more knowledge. This can only be proved when adequate assay methods are available for serological studies.

**Diagnosis.** It is accomplished by clinical, hematological, and necropsy procedures. Virological and serological methods for this disease are inadequate now to assist in making a diagnosis.

**Control.** Slaughter of affected animals is recommended.

**The Disease in Man.** There is no evidence that bovine leukemia produces disease in man, either by contact with leukemic cattle or consumption of milk from leukemic cattle.

### REFERENCES

1. Dutcher, Szekely, Larkin, Coriell, and Marshak. Ann. N.Y. Acad. Sci., 1963, *108*, 1149.
2. Dutta and Sorensen. Fourth Internatl. Sympos. on Comp. Leukemia Res., Cherry Hill, N.J. S. Karger, Basel, Switzerland, 1970.
3. Ferrer, Avila, Stock, Lin, and Guest. Fifth Internatl. Sympos. on Comp. Leukemia Res., Padova, Italy, S. Karger, Basel, 1972.
4. Gillette, Olson, and Tekeli. Am. Jour. Vet. Res., 1969, *30*, 975.
5. Goetze, Rosenberger, and Ziegenhagen. Monatsh. f. VetMed., 1954, *9*, 517.
6. Lee, Takahashi, and Gillespie. Cornell Vet., 1970, *60*, 139.
7. McKercher, Wada, Staub, and Theilen. Ann. N.Y. Acad. Sci., 1963, *108*, 1163.
8. Miller. Jour. Natl. Cancer Inst., 1970, *43*, 1297.
9. Monlux, Anderson, and Davis. Am. Jour. Vet. Res., 1956, *17*, 646.
10. Papparella, Cali, Rossi, and Lacobelli. Ann. N.Y. Acad. Sci., 1963, *108*, 1173.

### RNA Leukoviruses of Other Species

There is a great deal of information known about the murine leukosis complex (MLC). The reader is referred to other sources, such as the review article by Rich and Siegler (4), and the proceedings of the 4th (1970) and 5th (1972) International Symposia on Comparative Leukemia Research, published by S. Karger, Basel, Switzerland, for information about these important animal models for the study of cancer.

Spontaneous lymphomas occur in the dog. Generally speaking there is little information about them, but the incidence of spontaneous lymphomas in dogs does not appear to be as high as the incidence in cats and chickens. Limited trials to determine the transmissibility and etiology with cell-free extracts of these tumors has met with failure. Within the last 3 years various investigators were successful in transplanting a canine lymphosarcoma (3), canine osteosarcoma (3), mixed-cell tumor (2), radiation-induced canine myelomonocytic leukemia (5), and radiation-induced canine granulocytic anemia (1) in perinatal puppies. Quite obviously, the problem is more difficult than that encountered with the domestic cat, mouse, and chicken; but the degree of technical difficulty is similar to that encountered with studies of leukemia in humans and cattle.

### REFERENCES

1. Fritz and Norris. Fifth Internatl. Sympos. on Comp. Leukemia Res., Padova, Italy, S. Karger, Basel, Switzerland, 1972.
2. Jensen, Bowles, Kerber, Rangan, and Woods. *Ibid.*
3. Owen. *Ibid.*

4.  Rich and Siegler.   Ann. Rev. Microbiol., 1967, *21*, 529.
5.  Shifrine.   Fifth Internatl. Sympos. on Comp. Leukemia Res., Padova, Italy, S. Karger, Basel, Switzerland, 1972.

## THE GENUS *PAPILLOMAVIRUS*

The type-species for the genus *Papillomavirus* is *Papillomavirus* S-1 (Sylvilagus), commonly known as the Shope papillomavirus. Other members of the genus are the rabbit oral papillomavirus, human papillomavirus, canine papillomavirus, canine oral papillomavirus, and bovine papillomavirus. Probable members include the viruses causing papillomata of horses, sheep, goats, hamsters, monkeys, and other species.

The particles of viruses studied in this genus are 53 m$\mu$ in diameter. They contain double-stranded cyclic DNA with a GC ratio of 49 percent and a molecular weight of approximately 5 by $10^6$. The capsid is composed of 72 capsomeres in a skew arrangement. The buoyant density in cesium chloride is 1.34 g per ml. Particles are assembled in the nucleus. They are ether-resistant, acid-stable, and heat-stable. Several papillomata viruses hemagglutinate by reacting with neuriminidase-sensitive receptors. Each papovavirus is antigenically distinct and all those that have been studied differ in their base composition of their nucleic acid.

The principal viruses in the genus are oncogenic, especially in young or newborn animals. Nucleic acid extracted from these viruses is oncogenic. Subacute, latent, and chronic infections are commonly produced by these viruses. Papillomas, or common warts, occur in many species of animals. They seem to be most frequent in man, cattle, dogs, and rabbits. All of these tumors contain filterable agents with which the tumors may be induced in other individuals. They appear to have a high degree of host specificity, and some of them even have specificities for particular kinds of epithelium within a single host. Warts occur in epizootic form in herds of cattle and in kennels of dogs. All varieties are most prevalent in the young of the species.

### Bovine Papillomatosis

**Character of the Disease.** Warts frequently occur in calves and young stock less than 2 years old. They appear most often in the winter months when the animals are closely housed. The head, especially the region about the eyes, is most frequently involved, but they may appear on the sides of the neck and less commonly on other parts of the body. They usually do not occur on the legs. They appear first as small nodular growths, which develop slowly for a time and then often grow rapidly into dry, horny, whitish, cauliflowerlike masses, which finally fall off as a result of dry necrosis of their bases. Sometimes hundreds of these masses occur on a calf at the same time. The size varies from small ones no larger than a pea to confluent masses several inches in diameter. Such warts have been seen along the sides of the neck beginning at points where blood samples have been drawn from the jugular vein, an indication that an infected bleeding needle has been the transmitting agent. Warts have also been found in the nasal openings of many animals in the same herd, apparently transmitted by the fingers of persons who have held the animal or by a bull lead that has been used as a means of restraint.

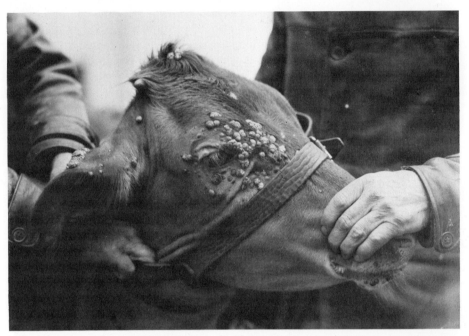

*Fig. 259.* Bovine papillomatosis (warts).

Occasionally infectious papillomas occur in dairy herds, the tumors appearing only on the teats. These cause difficulty in milking, and evidently are spread in the milking process. Whether they are caused by the same virus that causes general skin warts is not known. Another rather common papilloma of cattle is seen on the end of the penis of bulls and in the vagina of cows. Clinical evidence of transmissibility exists but experimental evidence is lacking (McEntee, 4).

The losses from warts are considerable. In young animals affected with many of these tumors, the general growth rate may be retarded. The greatest losses are in damages to the hides of slaughtered animals. Frequently the owner is most concerned by the reduction in the sales value of warty animals, especially in purebred stock.

**Properties of the Virus.** Very little is known about the causative agent of bovine warts except that it is filterable. Creech (3) inoculated 11 calves with ground unfiltered wart material and 11 additional with filtrates of the same materials from Berkefeld N filters. The filtrates were bacteriologically sterile. Eight "takes" were secured with the unfiltered material and seven with the filtered. The inoculations were made by scarification and intradermal injections.

**Cultivation.**   The virus of bovine papillomatosis can readily be cultivated on the chorioallantoic membrane of developing chick embryos. The presence of virus is indicated by marked epithelial thickenings which are rich in virus. It is the only member of the genus that grows in the embryonated hen's egg.

**Immunity.**   Although warts affecting animals always clear up spontaneously after a time, varying from one to several months, owners often demand curative treatment. Surgical removal of a few warts often leads to rapid regression and disappearance of the others. This has been interpreted as meaning that wart virus, escaping from the tumors during the operative procedures and absorbed in the wounds produced, has resulted in immunization. This explanation has not been confirmed by experimental proof, and it should always be kept in mind that warts retrogress spontaneously. All methods of treatment should be accepted with caution for this reason.

Artificial immunization of cattle with finely ground wart tissue suspended in a 0.4 percent formalin solution has been used for many years to combat wart outbreaks. In recent years, since it has been possible to propagate the virus on the membranes of embryonated eggs, most commercial companies have used the artificially-produced virus for vaccine manufacture. In many instances the results have appeared to be excellent; in others they were poor.

Experimentally, Bagdonas and Olson (2) and Olson and Skidmore (8) found that vaccines were of limited value. They agree that autogenous vaccines were more effective than stock vaccines. Olson, Segre, and Skidmore (6) found that inactivated bovine tissue vaccine did not produce complete immunity to all bovine virus strains and that vaccine produced by cultivation of the virus in eggs is worthless (7). On the other hand, Pearson et al. (9), working in the British Isles, found that autogenous vaccines made from bovine tissues gave protection to 87 percent of a large group of cattle, and nonautogenous, bovine tissue vaccines protected 76 percent. These were general body surface tumors. Teat wart vaccines were successful only in 4 out of 12 cases. Unvaccinated control cattle were kept on each of the farms where autogenous vaccines were used. These animals showed little change in their wart load while the vaccinated were showing wart regression.

Bagdonas and Olson found that animals that had been vaccinated with autogenous vaccines responded to inoculation with wart virus by connective tissue rather than epithelial growths. This was interpreted to mean that the vaccine had protected only against the epithelial elements of the warts.

**Transmission.**   The mode of natural transmission of warts is unknown. It has been pointed out above that there are indications that transmission may occur through the handling of animals by people and by needles used for breeding. Presumably they may be transmitted by friction between warty and normal animals. Often, in the same pens, animals may be found with extensive crops of warts and others of about the same age with few or none. Bag-donas and Olson (1) studied an extensive wart epizootic in a large herd of beef cattle in a feed lot. They discuss possible alternative routes of transmis-sion of the disease. The use of a tattoo instrument for placing an identification number in the ears of cattle causes a high incidence at this site in herds in-fected with this virus. This does not occur when metal ear tags are used.

Schultz (11) claims to have succeeded in transmitting bovine warts to man. Under natural exposure this seldom or never occurs. Olson and Cook (5) suc-ceeded in producing connective tissue tumors, resembling sarcoids, in horses by inoculation with bovine wart material. In studies by Ragland and Spencer (10), there was no evidence that the equine sarcoid and bovine papilloma agents were similar. Serums from horses with equine sarcoid failed to neutral-ize bovine papilloma virus. Furthermore, the response in horses with equine sarcoid to bovine papilloma virus was indistinguishable from that produced in normal horses.

## REFERENCES

1.   Bagdonas and Olson.   Jour. Am. Vet. Med. Assoc., 1953, *122*, 393.
2.   Bagdonas and Olson.   Am. Jour. Vet. Res., 1954, *15*, 240.
3.   Creech.   Jour. Agr. Res., 1929, *39*, 723.
4.   McEntee.   Cornell Vet., 1950, *40*, 304.
5.   Olson and Cook.   Proc. Soc. Exp. Biol. and Med., 1951, *77*, 281.
6.   Olson, Segre, and Skidmore.   Jour. Am. Vet. Med. Assoc., 1959, *135*, 499.
7.   Olson, Segre, and Skidmore.   Am. Jour. Vet. Res., 1960, *21*, 233.
8.   Olson and Skidmore.   Jour. Am. Vet. Med. Assoc., 1959, *135*, 339.
9.   Pearson, Kerr, McCartney, and Steele.   Vet. Rec., 1958, *70*, 971.
10.   Ragland and Spencer.   Am. Jour. Vet. Res., 1968, *29*, 1363.
11.   Schultz.   Deut. med. Wchnschr., 1908, *34*, 423.

### Equine Papillomatosis

Skin warts in horses have long been recognized, although they do not ap-pear to be as common as those affecting cattle. They develop most commonly on the nose and around the lips, appearing as small elevated horny masses which vary in number from a few to several hundred. Usually they remain quite small, but occasionally they may be large, especially when they are few in number. Generally they are not larger than 1 cm in diameter.

Cook and Olson (1) studied the transmissibility of equine warts, and also some of the characteritics of the virus. They had no difficulty in infecting horses, but they did not succeed in infecting calves, lambs, dogs, rabbits, and guinea pigs. Some degree of immunity was produced by experimental infec-tions. Natural infections produced solid immunity. The agent remained alive for 75 days when stored in 50 percent glycerol at 4 C but was inactive after 112 days. It remained viable in a frozen suspension at −35 C for 185 days but not for 224 days.

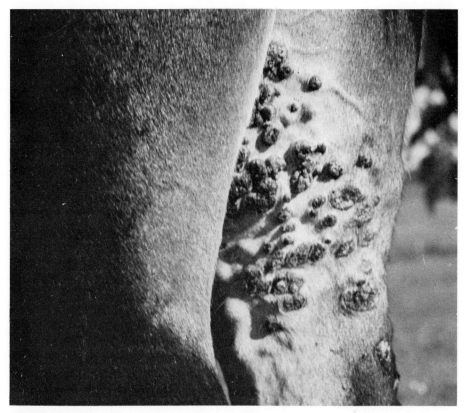

*Fig. 260.* Papillomas on leg of mule. (Courtesy W. Cameron and C. Milton.)

## REFERENCE

1. Cook and Olson. Am. Jour. Path., 1951, *27*, 1087.

### Caprine Papillomatosis

Warts in goats are not common; however, one outbreak in a herd was reported by Davis and Kemper (1). The tumors were located in various parts of the skin. They closely resembled those which occur in cattle. Although no transmission experiments were attempted, it is clear that they were infectious because the disease spread to many animals in the same herd. The herd was not in contact with cattle or other species of animals. It was believed that the disease had been introduced into the herd in purchased animals.

## REFERENCE

1. Davis and Kemper. Jour. Am. Vet. Med. Assoc., 1936, *88*, 175.

### Canine Papillomatosis

Benign epithelial growths, commonly called *warts,* are not uncommon in young dogs. The tumors usually are found around the lips and in the mouths of the animals, where they may cause serious inconvenience. The condition is highly contagious, often spreading through all the dogs in a kennel, according to Penberthy (3).

**Character of the Disease.** The warts begin around the lips, as a rule, as smooth whitish elevations, which later develop a roughened surface and appear as typical papillomas. Usually following the first one or two tumors, a secondary crop appears on the insides of the cheeks, the hard palate, the tongue, and even on the walls of the pharynx. The tumors have the appearance of cauliflowers. They may interfere considerably with mastication. After several months without any sort of treatment they disappeared spontaneously.

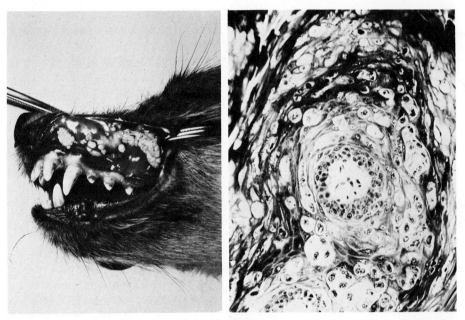

*Fig. 261.* Canine oral papillomatosis. (*Left*) Puppy's mouth showing the warts as they appeared 66 days after injection of a Berkefeld filtrate of tumor emulsion. In this case the incubation period was 33 days. (*Right*) A transverse section of a papilla of an actively growing wart. The inner core of Malpighian cells is approximately normal in size. They are surrounded by the enlarged, vacuolated wart cells. X 124. (Courtesy DeMonbreun and Goodpasture, *Am. Jour. Path.*)

**Properties of the Virus.** McFadyean and Hobday (2) showed that the warts were infectious by rubbing pieces of the tumors on the scarified mucous membranes of other dogs. DeMonbreun and Goodpasture (1) likewise found it easy to propagate the tumors in this way. McFadyean and Hobday state that the incubation period is from 4 to 6 weeks. DeMonbreun and Goodpasture found that it was about 30 to 32 days as a rule, but it was somewhat longer in malnourished dogs. The latter workers passed tumor suspensions through Berkefeld N and W filters and found that the virus was present in abundance in the filtrates. Wart material was dried while frozen and kept in this state for 64 days. At the end of this time it readily produced tumors, the incubation period being 32 days, an indication that there had not been appreciable attenuation of the virus. Wart tissue kept in glycerol for the same period likewise kept its virulence relatively unimpaired. Wart tissue that had been heated at 45 C for 1 hour retained its virulence but that heated at 58 C and 80 C proved inactive.

The attempts of DeMonbreun and Goodpasture to produce warts on the vaginal mucous membrane, on the mucous membrane of the conjunctiva, and on the skin of the abdomen proved unsuccessful, both with filtrates and with fresh unfiltered wart tissue. They also failed to infect the mouths of cats, rabbits, guinea pigs, and rats.

**Immunity.** Clinical experience indicates that dogs which recover from an attack of warts seldom or never are infected again. McFadyean and Hobday, also DeMonbreun and Goodpasture, found it impossible to reinfect, experimentally, dogs that had recovered.

Vaccines are sometimes used for treatment. These are made like those of cattle. Some veterinarians have reported good results from the use of these vaccines. Since the disease is self-curing, the results of the use of vaccines must be accepted with caution.

### REFERENCES

1. DeMonbreun and Goodpasture.  Am. Jour. Path., 1932, 8, 43.
2. McFadyean and Hobday.  Jour. Comp. Path. and Therap., 1898, 11, 341.
3. Penberthy.  Ibid., 363.

## PAPILLOMATOSIS OF RABBITS

Two kinds of virus-induced papillomas occur in rabbits. One, commonly known as the *Shope papilloma*, occurs on the skin and is never found on the mucous membranes of the mouth. The other occurs on the oral mucosa and is never found on the skin. The viruses of these tumors are not related to each other, serologically, and neither immunizes against the other.

### The Shope Papilloma of Rabbits

In 1933 Shope (9) showed that the common wart of the western wild cottontail rabbit was infectious and that the infectious agent was a virus. These warty growths are not uncommon among wild rabbits of the midwestern part of the United States. Usually there are from 1 to 10 of these tumors on the infected animal, but occasionally there may be hundreds of small tumors covering almost the entire body surface. Even when the tumors are numerous, they have little effect upon the general health of the rabbit. They are of little economic importance.

**Character of the Disease.** The naturally occurring tumors appear as tall, thin, horny structures, usually grayish or even black in color. Hunters sometimes refer to such animals as "horned" rabbits, especially when the warts occur upon the head. The sides of the neck, the shoulders, the abdomen, and the inside of the thighs are the sites of predilection.

Experimentally the disease may be transmitted easily by inoculating scarified skin areas with filtered or unfiltered tumor tissue. These tumors can be transmitted in series in the cottontail rabbit, but those produced in domestic rabbits by such inoculations are not transmissible although otherwise typical. Rous and Beard (8) showed that, if the tumor-bearing domesticated rabbits are kept for long periods (200 days or longer), a considerable number of the benign papillomas become transformed into malignant carcinomas. Kidd and Rous (5), studying the matter further, showed that the same thing was true of such tumors produced by inoculation in jack rabbits and snowshoe rabbits. In rabbit species in which the virus is foreign there apparently is virus variation which leads to malignancy. By gradual change in character, the malignant tumors arise from cells which are already neoplastic as a result of virus action.

**Properties of the Virus.** This is a double-stranded DNA virus (11) whose particles are icosahedral and 53 millimicrons in diameter. The virus starts its development in the nucleolus and shortly involves the rest of the nucleus.

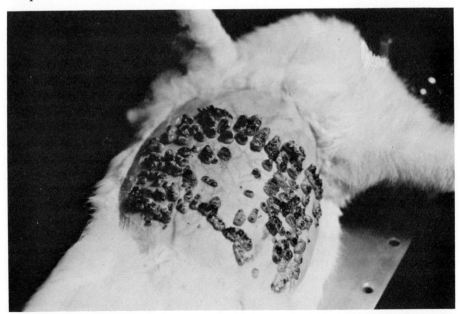

*Fig. 262.* Rabbit papillomatosis. Warts on the scarified skin of the abdomen of a rabbit were produced experimentally. The inoculation had been carried out about 1 month previously. (Courtesy R. E. Shope, *Jour. Exp. Med.*)

It is quite heat resistant requiring a temperature of 70 C for 30 minutes for inactivation. It survives for many years in glycerol and at low temperatures and is quite resistant to x-radiation and entirely resistant to ether. Purification can be accomplished with fluorocarbon or by precipitation with methanol (4).

The fluorescent antibody technic has shown that the viral antigen is located in the keratohyaline and keratinized layers of the skin (7). Rabbit red blood cells absorb the virus but the cells are agglutinated (2). Complement-fixing antigen is extractable from warts of cottontail rabbits, to a lesser degree from warts of domestic rabbits. No cross-neutralization or cross-immunity is demonstrable between the Shope papilloma and the papillomas of cattle and dogs or the rabbit oral papilloma (1).

**Cultivation.** Proliferation of epidermal cells was observed in skin organ cultures of newborn rabbits but propagation of virus was not proved (6).

**Immunity.** Shope (9, 10) has shown that rabbits carrying experimentally produced papillomas are partially or wholly immune to reinfection, and also that the sera of such animals are capable of partially or completely neutralizing the virus *in vitro*. Even though the tumors produced in domesticated rabbits contain no demonstrable virus, injections or suspensions of such tumors will actively immunize susceptible animals. Shope concluded that in the tumors of the domestic rabbit the virus is present but is masked in some unknown way. Bernheim and co-workers (3) claimed to have obtained the virus from cottontail rabbit tumors in the form of a homogeneous protein, but they were unable to find this protein in domesticated rabbit tumors. They did find in the latter, however, a noninfectious, antigenic protein that immunizes animals to the virus. They suggest that a factor exists, possibly enzymic in nature, in the domesticated rabbit which destroys the virus. They also speculate about the chance of the existence of such agents in other mammalian tumors and the possibility that this may explain why viruses have not been recognized in many of them.

**Transmission.** In view of the fact that animals can easily be infected through superficial scarifications of the skin, it is presumed that natural infections occur through direct contacts between infected and susceptible animals.

## REFERENCES

1. Andrewes.   Viruses of vertebrates. Williams and Wilkins, Baltimore, 1964.
2. Barabadze.   Virology, 1960, 5, 103.
3. Bernheim, Bernheim, Taylor, Beard, Sharp, and Beard.   Science, 1942, 95, 230.
4. Fischer.   Proc. Soc. Exp. Biol. and Med., 1949, 72, 323.
5. Kidd and Rous.   Jour. Exp. Med., 1940, 71, 469.
6. deMaeyer.   Science, 1962, 136, 985.
7. Noyes and Mellors.   Jour. Exp. Med., 1957, 106, 555.
8. Rous and Beard.   *Ibid.*, 1935, 62, 523.

9.   Shope.   *Ibid.*, 1933, 58, 607.
10.   *Ibid.*, 1937, 65, 219.
11.   Watson and Littlefield.   Jour. Mole. Biol., 1960, 2, 161.

## The Oral Papilloma of Rabbits

Parsons and Kidd (1) described oral papillomatosis of the rabbit in 1943. These are benign growths which were found in a rather high percentage of "normal" domestic rabbits in the New York City area. They are readily transmitted by filtrates to other domestic rabbits, to the cottontail rabbit and the jack rabbit of the midwestern states, and to the snowshoe rabbit of the north, although they apparently do not occur naturally in any but the domestic species. They are not transmissible to other species of animals.

**Character of the Disease.** The tumors consist of small, gray-white, sessile or pedunculated nodules found usually on the under surface of the tongue, occasionally on the gums, and rarely on the floor of the mouth. They often are multiple and sometimes quite numerous. The larger ones have cauliflowerlike surfaces and may be as large as 5 mm in diameter and 4 mm in height. The smaller ones usually are smooth and domelike.

Microscopically they are typical papillomas, the epithelial cells being swollen and vacuolated. In the cells near the surface, intranuclear inclusion bodies are found in about 10 percent of the lesions in the domestic rabbit. They are never found in lesions in other species.

The tumors are benign and cause little inconvenience to the host. Usually they are not noticed unless the oral mucosa is closely scrutinized.

Intranuclear inclusions were found by Parsons and Kidd in about 10 percent of the tumors in domestic rabbits, but none was found in the induced tumors in other species of rabbits. When present they were located in the outer 6 to 10 layers of epithelial cells. They varied greatly in size and shape. Some were hyaline and others showed a stippled structure. They were basophilic and located near the center of the nucleus, the chromatin being marginated. Such bodies were not found in normal oral epithelium of domestic rabbits.

**The Disease in Experimental Rabbits.** After inoculation on the tongue epithelium, tumors appear in from 6 to 38 days, depending upon the concentration of material used. The average, after applying virus with a tattooing needle, was 15 days. Following inoculation, the papillomas tend to increase in size for about 1 month, after which regression begins. In a few cases very little regression is noticeable for long periods. In most cases regression proceeds rather rapidly and no traces can be found after the second month. It is noticeable that when any tumors are present, the rate of regression tends to be faster than when there are few. The mortality from this disease is nil; in fact the affected animals are not noticeably inconvenienced by the presence of the tumors.

The disease is transmissible by scarification to rabbits that have not previously been infected. The lesions in experimental animals do not differ in appearance from those occurring naturally.

**Properties of the Virus.** The virus readily passes Berkefeld V and N candles. The average incubation period when unfiltered virus is used is 15 days; of Berkefeld V filtrates, 19 days; and of Berkefeld N filtrates, 23 days. The virus is a very stable one. Tissues stored in 50 percent glycerol at 4 C retain their pathogenicity relatively undiminished for 2 years and more. Those stored while frozen remain potent for long periods, and material dried, while frozen, remains potent many months. The resistance to heat is rather remarkable. Heating at 65 C for 30 minutes appears to do little injury. Some tumors were produced by materials heated at 70 C.

**Cultivation.** Reports of attempts to cultivate the virus of rabbit oral papillomatosis have not been found.

**Immunity.** After recovery from oral papillomatosis animals are solidly immune to reinfection for at least several months. There is no immunological relationship with the Shope papilloma. Animals affected with one type of tumor can readily be infected with the other, and animals solidly immune to one type as a result of regression are fully susceptible to the other.

**Transmission.** The disease does not appear to be particularly contagious because Parsons and Kidd observed no general spread among stock in the animal quarters of the Rockefeller Institute. It was noticed, however, that the tumor incidence of the litters from females which had papillomas was much higher (11.8 percent) than those from females free of tumors (1.3 percent). Virus was recovered in several instances from mouth washings of animals that had no papillomas. The authors believed that the virus is present in a dormant state in the mouths of many animals and that tumors are induced only when the mucous membrane is injured by rough feed or other agents. Several experiments in which coal tar was smeared on the skin of rabbits without tumors led to a higher incidence of tumors than in animals not so treated. Since the tar is licked off by the animals, it was thought that the tar was the precipitating factor. Abundant quantities of virus were recovered from the tar-induced tumors. The same tar did not induce tumors in wild rabbits, which do not carry this virus but are fully susceptible to it by inoculation. It was thought, too, that the virus might be transmitted from doe to offspring in the process of suckling.

### REFERENCE

1. Parsons and Kidd. Jour. Exp. Med., 1943, 77, 233.

### Genital Papilloma of Pigs

This condition was described by Parish in 1961 (1). He observed the natural occurrence of papillomas in the genital region of boars. The papilloma was transmissible by scarification or injection into the genital skin of adults. The warts appeared 8 weeks after injection. Cytoplasmic inclusion bodies were observed in the lesions.

This agent is inactivated readily by heat and survival at 4 C and −20 C is poor. It is resistant to ether. Neutralizing antibodies can be detected in the sera of hyperimmunized pigs and rabbits, but not in convalescent pig sera. Pigs that recover from the infection are resistant to challenge. Antigen can be demonstrated by the use of the gel-diffusion or conglutination complement-absorption tests (2).

## REFERENCES

1. Parish. Jour. Path. and Bact., 1961, *81*, 331.
2. Parish. *Ibid.*, 1962, 83, 429.

## TRANSMISSIBLE NEOPLASMS

### Transmissible Canine Mastocytoma

In 1959 and 1963 Lombard *et al.* (1, 2) reported the transmission of a canine mastocytoma with either cellular or cell-free inocula of tumor material in puppies from 1 to 30 days of age. The donor, an 11-year-old-female Doberman Pinscher, had a mast-cell leukemia and also neoplastic mast-cell infiltrations of spleen, liver, lymph nodes, kidney, and skin. Rickard and Post (3) also transmitted the disease with cellular and cell-free inocula from a spontaneous case in a 9-year-old Beagle which had leukemia and visceral mast-cell neoplasms but was conspicuously lacking in skin tumors. Both groups were able to maintain the infectious agent by serial passage in infant puppies, but not all experimental puppies developed the neoplastic growths.

As a rule, newborn puppies were injected either by the intravenous or intraperitoneal routes (1, 3). Mast-cell tumors developed at the subcutaneous inoculation sites and in the omentum following intraperitoneal injections. Marked mast-cell infiltrations occurred in most visceral organs and resulted in death. Practically all diseased puppies developed a mast-cell leukemia unless they died or were killed early in the course of the disease. Some developed gastric or duodenal ulcers, presumably from the pharmacological action of the histamine or serotonin in the mast-cell granules (3). The experimental dogs of Lombard *et al.* had dermal nodules like the dog from which the original material was derived. In contrast the isolate of Richard and Post failed to produce dermal lesions except at inoculation site, but then the spontaneous case from which the isolate was derived also was lacking in skin tumors.

Both groups prepared their cell-free inocula by ultracentrifugation. In addition, Lombard and Maloney (1) filtered some material through a Millipore HA or no. 12 Mandler filter. These treatments strongly support the idea that the infectious agent is a virus.

## REFERENCES

1. Lombard and Maloney. Fed. Proc., 1959, *18*, 490.
2. Lombard, Maloney, and Rickard. Ann. N.Y. Acad. Sci., 1963, *108*, 1086.
3. Rickard and Post. Third Internatl. Sympos. Compar. Leukemia Res., Paris, S. Karger, Basel, 1967.

## Canine Venereal Tumor

The canine venereal tumor was the first tumor transmitted by tissue transplantation (4).

**Character of the Disease.** The tumor affects both sexes and it has a worldwide distribution occurring as an endemic disease in some parts of the world.

In female dogs the tumor usually is found beneath the mucosa in any part of the vagina often extending to the adjoining vestibule and labia. In males, the tumors vary in appearance with small reddish nodules appearing on the affected part of the penis in the early stage of infection. They may become quite large with infiltration of tumor cells into the scrotum. The tumors usually persist for a long period of time and dogs rarely die as a result of these localized tumors. Histologically it has been characterized as a round-cell sarcoma while a few pathologists have termed it an endothelioma, contagious granuloma, or lymphosarcoma (1). A large number of tumor cells are found together with leukocytes and erythrocytes in the serous fluid exuding from the tumor surface. Tumor cells undergoing mitotic division probably are spontaneously transferred into the mucosa of the external genitalia of another dog during copulation. Metastates rarely occur.

Chromosome studies are often used in tumor investigations. Makino (3) studied 17 spontaneous cases of canine venereal tumors that were obtained from distantly separated localities and at different times. These tumors were uniformly characterized by tumor stem cells having a lower number of chromosomes (usually 59) than the normal dog tissue (78). In cells with well-delineated chromosomes there usually were 17 metacentric (J-shaped) chromosomes and 42 acrocentric (rod-shaped) chromosomes.

**Immunity.** Dogs that recover from the disease appear to be immune to some degree so the tumors seldom reoccur. Passive and active immunity studies to canine transmissible venereal sarcoma were reported by Powers (5). Passive immunity was substantiated by treatment of dogs with tumors and also by the inhibition of tumors in dogs that were given immune dog serum and inoculum at the same time. Dogs that recovered from neoplasma withstood challenge with infectious material demonstrating an active immunity. Tumor-specific antibody was demonstrated by the passive cutaneous anaphylaxis echnic in newborn littermate puppies.

**Transmission.** The disease has not been reproduced with cell-free extracts in the dog but transplantation attempts have succeeded. Sticker (7) produced tumors in foxes by the subcutaneous or intraperitoneal inoculation of tumor material. Shirasu (6) transplanted the tumor in the cheek pouch of the hamster. Forty successive transfers in dogs have been reported by Karlson and Mann (2).

**The Disease in Man.** There is no evidence that the disease is transmissible to man.

## REFERENCES

1.  Feldman.   Neoplasms of domesticated animals. W. B. Saunders & Co., Philadel-
    phia, Pa., 1932.
2.  Karlson and Mann.   Ann. N.Y. Acad. Sci., 1952, *54*, 1197.
3.  Makino.   *Ibid.*, 1963, *108*, 1106.
4.  Novinsky.   Zentbl. f. die Med. Wiss., 1876, *14*, 790.
5.  Powers.   Am. Jour. Vet. Res., 1968, *29*, 1637.
6.  Shirasu.   Jap. Jour. Vet. Sci., 1958, *11*, 245.
7.  Sticker.   Ztschr. f. Krebsforsch., 1904, *1*, 413.

## NEOPLASM OF UNKNOWN ETIOLOGY

### Ocular Squamous Carcinoma of Cattle

SYNONYM:   Cancer eye of cattle

Squamous cell carcinomas involving the conjunctival mucous membranes
and skin around the eyes of cattle are not uncommon, particularly in those
breeds or individuals in which the skin around the eyes is unpigmented. They
occur most frequently in the Hereford breed but are seen also in others. In
two studies made on large numbers of cattle presented for slaughter in the
midwestern part of the United States, about 0.5 percent in one case and 1.25
percent in the other were afflicted with this disease. In 40 percent of all these
cases there were metastatic lesions in other organs. The disease seems to be most
frequent in range cattle raised in hot, dry regions. The hot sun and the dust
have long been suspected of being contributing causes. The tumor is seen in
older animals, mostly in ones that are at least 4 years of age.

It has been suspected that an infectious agent may be involved in the causation of this tumor, but there is very little evidence to support such a hypothesis. Sykes, Dmochowski, and Russell (2) studied certain plaques occurring in the eyes of cattle which Russell, Wynne, and Loquavam (1)
considered to be precursors of the malignant growths. Growing cells from
these plaques in tissue cultures, they found inclusion bodies and other
changes which they believe indicate the presence of a virus.

## REFERENCES

1.  Russell, Wynne, and Loquavam.   Cancer, 1956, *9*, 1.
2.  Sykes, Dmochowski, and Russell.   Proc. Soc. Exp. Biol. and Med., 1959, *100*,
    527.

# LIII | Chronic and Degenerative Diseases Caused by Unclassified Viruses

There are a few diseases of the lower animals and man that are characterized by a long incubation period, insidious onset of clinical disease, protracted clinical course, high mortality, and pathologic changes different from acute viral disease (1). The conceptual approach of an infectious etiology, principally involving viruses, was developed by Sigurdsson (2) who coined the term "slow virus infections." In recent years there has been great interest in the United States, Canada, and England in the study of these animal viral diseases for two reasons: (1) the uniqueness of the lesions, suggesting immunopathic disease, and their similarity to certain human diseases, and (2) the unusual characteristics of some of these agents which appear to have properties unlike other viruses. At present the principal diseases in this category include visna and maedi viruses of sheep, equine infectious anemia of horses, Aleutian disease of mink, adenomatosis of sheep, lymphocytic choriomeningitis of mice, lactic dehydrogenase virus of mice, and a group of closely related agents causing scrapie in sheep, encephalopathy in mink, and Kuru, Jacob-Creutzfeld disease, and perhaps, multiple sclerosis of man. Adenomatosis of sheep is caused by a herpesvirus and thus placed in that chapter.

Lymphocytic choriomeningitis virus (LCM) is the type species for the newly designated genus *Arenavirus*. Because it is the only virus of this genus given treatment in this textbook the description of LCM is logically placed in this chapter as a chronic and degenerative disease but of a known classification.

## REFERENCES

1.   Abinanti.   Ann. Rev. of Microbiol., 1967, *21*, 467.
2.   Sigurdsson.   Brit. Vet. Jour., 1954, *110*, 7.

### Aleutian Disease in Mink

Parvo

SYNONYMS:   Plasmacytosis, Hypergammaglobulinemia; abb, AD

Aleutian disease (AD) in mink is characterized by genetic predisposition, presistent blood-borne infection, pronounced plasmacytosis, hypergammaglobulinemia, and other signs consistent with slow virus infections. The increased susceptibility of genetically defined types of mink appears to be associated with inheritance of a dysfunction of the protective mechanism, comparable to the Chediak-Higashi syndrome seen in man and in cattle.

The disease was first described by Hartsough and Gorham (8) and it has been reported in the United States, Canada, and Denmark.

**Character of the Disease.** It is a chronic progressive disease of high mortality and morbidity characterized by anorexia, loss of weight, lethargy, polydipsia, and hemorrages. It has a long incubation period and death usually occurs in a few to many months.

At necropsy the kidneys are enlarged, pale yellow, and mottled and the liver is slightly enlarged. Histological alternations are characterized by marked plasmacytosis of the lymph nodes, spleen, liver, and kidneys; marked rise in serum gamma globulin; hepatic degeneration with bile duct proliferation; and smudging of glomerular basement membranes (9). The severity of lesions are related to the degree of hypergammaglobulinemia. In one quarter of natural cases there are vascular lesions consisting of segmental periarteritis and fibrinoid degeneration of small and medium-sized arteries. There are many points of histochemical similarity to human connective tissue diseases, but also differences (14). The serum protein alterations and pathologic changes are similar to those seen in certain human connective tissue disorders such as disseminated lupus erythematosus, rheumatoid arthritis, and plasma cell hepatitis. The intercapillary nodular lesions are similar to those found in diabetes mellitus. The presence of a monoclonal type of gamma globulin late in the disease is comparable to changes seen in multiple myeloma or monoclonal gamma globulin production in man.

**The Disease in Experimental Animals.** The disease is readily produced in genetically susceptible mink. Although the Aleutian type of mink develop lesions more quickly and die sooner after injection, other genotypes are also susceptible (16, 19). The virus can be serially transferred in mink (7).

Overt signs of Aleutian disease are not seen in naturally or experimentally infected ferrets (13). The infection produced a systemic proliferation of lymphoid elements in association with a hypergammaglobulinemia and vasculitis. Most ferret sera examined electrophoretically had gamma globulin levels about 20 percent, considered to be the upper normal limit for most domestic animals (1). A monoclonal type of hypergammaglobulinemia was frequently found in ferrets; usually observed only in mink that survive early AD. Natural subclinical infection also occurs in ferrets maintained on ranches where AD is found in mink.

**Properties of the Virus.** In 1962 Russell (17), Karstad and Pridham (11), and Trautwein and Helmboldt (19) independently reported that Aleutian disease is caused by a virus. The disease is reproducible with filtrates of infected tissues or with pellets after ultracentrifugation. Fluorocarbon extraction fails to reduce appreciably its infectivity (4). The virus is present in blood, serum, bone marrow, spleen, feces, urine, and saliva of infected mink (7).

Millipore filtration experiments suggest that the size range of the infective agent is 10 to 50 millimicrons (2). AD virus passed a 50 m$\mu$ Millipore filter and a <100 m$\mu$ Gradocol membrane, but did not pass Gradocol membranes of smaller average pore size (5). It was unaffected by treatment with ether. Its resistance to formalin was not remarkable, but its resistance to heat was greater than that of most known animal viruses. There is a suggestion that it is a DNA virus, and extracted DNA from spleens of mink with viral plasmacytosis is infective for mink (3). This may account for the unusual heat-resistance of the infective agent. Indeed, there are others who suggest that the infective agent is devoid of nucleic acid and is similar to other infectious agents termed "slow viruses."

**Cultivation.** Specific morphological alterations are produced by the agent in cultures of mink testis and mink kidney cells (2).

**Immunity.** Although plasmacytosis and hypergammaglobulinemia are characteristic of the disease, there is no evidence of natural or acquired immunity. Gamma globulin from infected mink fails to neutralize virus. This indicates that virus and gamma globulin can exist together in a cell-free environment (6) and also in the serum of affected mink. Circulating infectious antigen-antibody complexes have been detected and it is probable that these complexes deposited in blood-vessel walls cause the hyaline degeneration associated with disease (10). These same lesions are seen during late stages of lymphocytic choriomeningitis of mice. It appears that antiglobulin antibodies (positive Coombs test) are produced as a result of AD infection (18).

Karstad et al. (12) produced an inactivated vaccine by treating tissues of infected mink with 0.3 percent of formalin at 37 C. Vaccinated mink maintained in contact with infected mink failed to develop the disease, but they succumbed to injection with infective tissue suspension—even after vaccination with three doses.

**Transmission.** Because the virus is present in various body excreta two routes of transmission are possible; (1) fecal-oral and (2) saliva-aerosol-respiratory circuits. Indeed, mink were infected experimentally by both routes (7). These experimental studies do not entirely fit the pattern of natural infection (7). Often only certain individuals in litters show signs of illness. The isolation of virus in the saliva of mink 4 months after exposure suggests an extended infectious period (7).

Vertical transmission of infection from the dam to its progeny does occur.

Although the agent was isolated with equal facility from both susceptible and resistant breeds of pregnant females, the fetal mortality was greater in the genetically susceptible mink (15).

**Diagnosis.** This can be established by three means: (1) a series of positive iodine agglutination tests of increasing activity, (2) clinical signs, and (3) typical lesions at necropsy. The iodine test reveals an increase in gamma globulin, a decrease in albumin, an increase in total serum proteins, and a change in the A : G ratio (7). The cytoplasmic inclusion bodies of Aleutian disease stain strongly by the periodic acid-Schiff (PAS) method differentiating them from distemper inclusions.

**Control.** No adequate control measures have been devised. More information must be accumulated about the pathogenesis of the disease before this will be possible.

**The Disease in Man.** This agent is not known to cause infection in man. It has been compared with periarteritis nodosa in humans.

## REFERENCES

1. Abinanti. Ann. Rev. Microbiol., 1967, *21*, 467.
2. Bosrur, Gray, and Karstad. Canad. Jour. Comp. Med. Vet. Sci., 1963, *27*, 301.
3. Bosrur and Karstad. *Ibid.*, 1966, *30*, 295.
4. Burger, Gorham, and Leader. Quoted by Leader. Arch. Path., 1964, *78*, 390.
5. Elklund, Hadlow, Kennedy, Boyle, and Jackson. Jour. Inf. Dis., 1968, *118*, 510.
6. Gorham, Leader, and Henson. Fed. Proc., 1963, *22*, abstract 627.
7. Gorham, Leader, and Henson. Jour. Inf. Dis., 1964, *114*, 341.
8. Hartsough and Gorham. Natl. Fur News, 1956, *28*, 10.
9. Helmboldt and Jungherr. Am. Jour. Vet. Res., 1958, *19*, 212.
10. Karstad. Canad. Vet. Jour., 1970, *11*, 36.
11. Karstad and Pridham. Canad. Jour. Comp. Med. and Vet. Sci., 1962, *26*, 97.
12. Karstad, Pridham, and Gray. *Ibid.*, 1963, *27*, 124.
13. Kenyon, Williams, and Howard. Proc. Soc. Exp. Biol. and Med., 1966, *123*, 510.
14. Leader. Arch. Path., 1964, *78*, 390.
15. Padgett, Gorham, and Henson. Jour. Inf. Dis., 1967, *117*, 35.
16. Padgett, Leader, and Gorham. Quoted by Leader. Arch. Path., 1964, *78*, 390.
17. Russell. Natl. Fur News, 1962, *34*, 8.
18. Saison, Karstad, and Pridham. Canad. Jour. Comp. Med. and Vet. Sci., 1966, *30*, 151.
19. Trautwein and Helmboldt. Am. Jour. Vet. Res., 1962, *23*, 1280.

## Scrapie

SYNONYMS: *Tremblant du Moulton,* Rida

Scrapie is a disease of sheep, occasionally of goats, characterized by a very long period of incubation, pruritus, nervous signs, and, nearly always, death. The disease is obviously infectious and is generally considered to be of viral origin. If the causative agent is, indeed, a virus, it is a most unusual one. It has long been thought that the disease had hereditary features, and there is evidence to indicate that certain kinds of sheep are more susceptible than others.

Scrapie has existed in Europe for 200 years or longer, particularly in England and Scotland, but it is also known on the continent. The first case in the United States was diagnosed in 1947 in Michigan in an animal which had been imported from Great Britain by way of Canada. In 1952 cases were recognized in California (12). Shortly afterward positive diagnoses of scrapie were made in Ohio, Illinois, New York, and Connecticut (22). Most of these cases occurred in the Suffolk breed, and most of them were traced to Canada, thence to importations from the British Isles. In 1952 isolated cases were reported in Australia and New Zealand in sheep imported from England.

It was originally believed that visna was the same disease as scrapie. Subsequent studies have shown visna to be a distinct and separate virus (the same as maedi—see p. 1336) which also produces a nervous syndrome in sheep.

**Character of the Disease.** The earliest sign frequently noticed is pruritus, although it is probable that more careful observation would detect certain nervous signs before the onset of pruritus. The itching is manifested by the animal's rubbing against objects and biting the itching areas, particularly the flanks. When rubbing, the animal draws back its lips, showing its teeth, and runs its tongue in and out. These signs can usually be elicited by rubbing or lightly pinching the skin over the lumbar region or in the flanks. Tremors of the muscles may be elicited in the same way. This sign has caused the French to call the malady *trembling disease*. Rubbing of the skin usually pulls out the wool, and the first impression is that the animal suffers from scabies. The skin is not encrusted, however, as it is in scabies, furthermore no mites can be found in scrapings. As the case advances, motor disturbances become more pronounced; the gait is affected, the animal weaves as it walks, the head is carried higher than normal, and the eyes assume a staring appearance. If the animal is frightened by being chased, it may fall down repeatedly because of its inco-ordination of locomotion, and sometimes the animal goes into convulsions. Paralysis, particularly of the hind quarters, then occurs in many cases, and finally the animal becomes recumbent and is unable to rise. Affected animals usually lose weight rapidly. Fever is not observed in any stage of the disease. It may possibly occur in an otherwise presymptomatic stage of the disease and escape attention.

Scrapie has an extraordinarily long incubation period. In the natural disease it is believed to be from 1 to 4 years. By inoculation it can be produced in 6 months or less, if the inoculum is given intracerebrally to day-old lambs. Older animals will generally have a longer period, that is, up to 1 year or longer, but some will develop signs in less than 6 months. In goats the period of incubation is about the same as in sheep.

Most animals die in from 4 to 6 weeks after developing signs, but some survive considerably longer. The death rate in scrapie is essentially 100 percent.

There are no gross lesions in this disease and even the microscopic lesions are controversial. Some French authors and Parry (15) in Great Britain claim to have demonstrated muscular lesions which they believe to be partly responsible for the signs. Other workers have not been able to find such lesions.

Because the signs of illness are definitely related to the nervous system, lesions have been sought there. No evidence of encephalitis has ever been found. The pathologic changes are more degenerative than inflammatory, and are found only in the central nervous system. The earliest lesion is an astrocytosis, later neuronal degeneration. Neurons in the gray matter of all parts of the brain except the cerebral cortex are involved.

It is believed by most who have worked with this disease that brain vacuoles are more numerous and more constant in scrapie than in normal animals. Zlotnik and Rennie (24), reviewing the matter, studied normal sheep from breeds that were known to be highly susceptible to scrapie and found vacuoles in all breeds and nearly all animals, but the numbers were always small, averaging about one to a microscopic field. In scrapie sheep they were identical in appearance but much more numerous. For more information about pathological changes see Abinanti (1).

**The Disease in Experimental Animals.** Scrapie has been transmitted by inoculation to mice, goats, mink, rats, hamsters, gerbils, and sheep. Wilson, Anderson, and Smith (23) passed the disease through nine generations of sheep by intracerebral inoculation. In some passages no more than 25 percent of the inoculated animals developed the disease. In some cases animals exhibited signs of pruritus, which was considered as evidence of infection, and later became well. This raises the question of whether or not natural cases of scrapie may sometimes be nonfatal.

Cuile and Chelle (3), working in France, believed they were successful in transmitting scrapie to sheep and goats by inoculation. Greig (8) alternated scrapie-infected and normal sheep on the same pasture, taking care that there were no direct contacts between the two groups. Ten of the 26 normal sheep eventually developed the disease, the first cases after about 3 years, the last after about 5 years. Greig concluded that the incubation period of the natural disease was very long and that the infective agent could persist for a time on grasslands.

There is now good evidence that scrapie can be transmitted by intracerebral, subcutaneous, and intradermal inoculation of filtered brain material, although not all sheep will become infected (21). Pattison, Gordon, and Millson (17) succeeded in infecting all of 10 goats with brain material of a Welsh mountain sheep affected with scrapie, whereas no disease was produced in another lot of 10 goats injected in the same way with brain material from a normal animal of the same breed. The incubation period is reduced by serial goat passage of the agent. Virus has been segregated into itching and sleepy strains which breed true (18).

Chandler (2) transmitted an agent from a sleepy strain to Swiss mice by intracerebral injection, and after serial transfers, the incubation period was reduced to 3 to 4 months. The mice showed signs referable to the central nervous system. The agent withstood boiling and was similar to scrapie in this respect. Elkund *et al.* (4) extended these studies and showed that first passage mouse brain produced scrapie in goats injected intracerebrally.

Rennie and Zlotnick (20) reported the experimental transmission of mouse-passaged scrapie to goats, sheep, rats, and hamsters producing comparable brain lesions in all species. It is known that scrapie spreads from inoculated to uninoculated mice.

Recently Hanson *et al.* (10) reported on the experimental transmission of the scrapie agent to mink producing a disease with clinical signs and pathological lesions indistinguishable from the naturally occurring transmissible encephalopathy of mink (TEM), a disease of undetermined origin. The most striking lesion observed in electron micrographs was a spongiform polioencephalopathy of the cerebral cortex and round-shaped lesion of electron lucent appearance surrounded by processes of nerve cells and glial cells. Mink that were given scrapie-infective brain from Suffolk sheep developed mink encephalopathy within 12 to 14 months. Mink given the Cheviot sheep infective brain remained normal for 20 months. Both inocula produced scrapie in mice after incubation periods between 15 and 16 months. The scrapie and TEM agents have a different host spectrum based upon production of disease (10) but perhaps no differences in infection susceptibility. The TEM agent causes disease in three species of subhuman primates (16), in raccoons, and striped skunks.

Eklund *et al.* (5) reported on a pathogenesis study in mice given the scrapie agent subcutaneously. The agent first appeared in the lymphatic tissues and over a period of many weeks spread slowly to the other tissues. It finally reached the spinal cord by the 12th week, and the brain by the 16th week. The highest concentrations of infective agent occurred in the CNS. Histological lesions were not detected until 8 weeks after the brain reached its maximum titer of the agent and clinical signs appeared 9 weeks later.

**Properties of the Virus.** The infectious particle is apparently smaller than 50 $m\mu$. The agent withstands boiling for 30 minutes without losing infectivity (21). Previous reports that it withstands boiling were not confirmed by a test that employed a Seitz filtrate of a 0.1 suspension of infected mouse brain (4). The suspension did withstand 80 C for 30 minutes, so it is unusually resistant to heating. It survived 0.35 percent formalin for 3 months (8) and also 10 to 12 percent formalin for periods ranging from 6 to 28 months at room temperature (16). Discrepancies exist regarding its ether-resistance. The present attitude is to accept the idea that the infectious agent is viral, recognizing that it has features different from other conventional viruses, especially the experiments that suggest it is dialyzable (19). These experiments have not been confirmed but the results are intriguing.

Attempts to demonstrate the infective agent in the animal tissues by the fluorescent antibody technic have failed (11). No serological procedure is now available.

**Cultivation.** The 23rd cell subculture of midbrain from an infected sheep produced scrapie in mice. The 23 subcultures of the midbrain tissue required 14 months (9). No cytopathic effects were noted, but in comparison with normal cultures, the astrocytes had a wider range of cell and nuclear size and a greater order and intensity of multinucleation. The cells developed a tendency to proliferate and overlap as in cell cultures infected with certain oncogenic viruses.

**Immunity.** Little is known about immunity in scrapie. Attempts to demonstrate circulating antibody and/or specific antigen in scrapie disease in sheep have not met with success (5, 7).

Various reasons are given for the probable lack of protection against the scrapie agent (1). One theory suggests that the agent's initial affinity for lymphocytic tissue destroys its capacity to produce antibody and permits the virus to persist and eventually invade the CNS. The second concept embraces the idea that the slow production of the agent in the defense cells causes gradual disturbance of their function and hence the body does not recognize the agent as a foreign antigen and does not produce antibody. The third idea, and perhaps the one most readily accepted today, suggests that the agent initiates subtle changes in the host tissues, particularly the CNS, making them unusually antigenic; and the ultimate damage is typical of an immunopathic disease where the antigen-antibody complexes disrupt the normal physiological function of these cells. There is experimental evidence to support the latter concept (1).

**Transmission.** Artificial transmission has been discussed under the heading, "The Disease in Experimental Animals." The means of natural transmission is unknown. Reference has already been made to the possibility that genetic factors influence susceptibility. Stamp (21) states that the disease is found more often in some breeds of sheep than in others, and that purebred sheep appear to be more susceptible than crossbred.

**Diagnosis.** The diagnosis of scrapie at present rests largely on identification by the rather characteristic signs of illness. The vacuolization of the medullary neurons may be used as confirming evidence.

**Control.** In Europe, where the disease has long existed, no serious efforts to control it have been made. Some have suggested the slaughter of all animals in infected flocks and starting new flocks from uninfected sources. Greig denies that this will succeed, because he thinks that premises may remain infective for long periods.

Because the infection has only recently been introduced into the United States and is not widespread, attempts to control and eradicate it here are being made. It remains to be seen whether these will succeed. The long incubation period of scrapie makes the task unusually difficult, since it is obvious that before clinical signs are apparent many animals will have been exposed and many of these will have been distributed to other flocks, carrying the disease with them. Infected flocks have been slaughtered and the owners indemnified from public funds, and attempts are made to trace all stock sold to other flocks, with particular emphasis on blood lines, and to keep these under surveillance by means of periodic inspections. It is hoped by this means to detect newly infected flocks early and to eliminate them before they spread the disease. Because it appears that all cases have been imported, directly or indirectly, from the British Isles, quarantine restrictions have been established which, it is hoped, will prevent importation of additional cases.

**The Disease in Man.** There is increasing concern that the scrapie agent may cause disease in man. A few years ago 4 of 7 workers engaged in research on a neurological disease of sheep (swayback) developed a disease diagnosed as multiple sclerosis. Icelandic sheep inoculated with brain material from a patient that died with multiple sclerosis developed a disease clinically and histopathologically indistinguishable from scrapie (13). Subsequent studies with similar human brain material yielded comparable results (14).

In 1957 Gajdusek and Zagas (6) described a degenerative disease of the CNS in human beings called kuru. The lesions of CNS are quite similar to those described for scrapie in sheep. There is increasing evidence that kuru, mink encephalopathy, scrapie, and Jacob-Creutzfeld (spastic pseudosclerosis) agents have many similarities and may be closely related and also that their host spectrum may be broader than it was originally thought. Kuru is known to produce a lethal infection in chimpanzees, spider monkeys, and mice, and the Jacob-Creutzfeld agent causes death in chimpanzees.

The public health significance of the two agents that naturally infect nonhuman animals is obscure at present and the problems of their importance to man are compounded by their long incubation period, genetic predisposition, and probable remission of clinical disease.

## REFERENCES

1. Abinanti.   Ann. Rev. Microbiol., 1967, *121*, 467.
2. Chandler.   Lancet, 1961, *1*, 1378.
3. Cuile and Chelle.   Comp. rend. Acad. Sci., 1938, *206*, 78. Vet. Med., 1939, *34*, 417.
4. Eklund, Hadlow, and Kennedy.   Proc. Soc. Exp. Biol. and Med., 1963, *112*, 974.
5. Eklund, Kennedy, and Hadlow.   Jour. Inf. Dis., 1967, *117*, 15.
6. Gajdusek and Zagas.   New Engl. Jour. Med., 1957, *257*, 974.
7. Gardiner.   Res. Vet. Sci., 1966, 7, 190.
8. Greig.   Jour. Comp. Path. and Therap., 1950, *60*, 263.
9. Gustafson and Kanitz.   Slow, latent, and temperate virus infections. NINDB Monograph 2, U.S. Publ. Health Service Publ. 1378, 1965, p. 221.
10. Hanson, Eckroade, Marsh, Rhein, Kanitz, and Gustafson.   Science, 1970, *172*, 859.

11.   Moulton and Palmer.   Cornell Vet., 1959, *49*, 349.
12.   News Item.   Jour. Am. Vet. Med. Assoc., 1952, *121*, 263.
13.   Palsson, Pattison, and Field.   Slow, latent, and temperate virus infections. NINDB Monograph 2, U.S. Publ. Health Service Publ. 1378, 1965, p. 49.
14.   Palsson.   Quoted by Abinanti. Ann. Rev. Microbiol., 1967, *121*, 467.
15.   Parry.   Vet. Rec., 1957, *69*, 43.
16.   Pattison.   Jour. Comp. Path., 1965, *75*, 159.
17.   Pattison, Gordon, and Millson.   Jour. Comp. Path. and Therap., 1959, *69*, 300.
18.   Pattison and Millson.   *Ibid.*, 1961, *70*, 182.
19.   Pattison and Sansom.   Res. Vet. Sci., 1964, *5*, 340.
20.   Rennie and Zlotnik.   Vet. Rec., 1965, *77*, 984.
21.   Stamp.   Vet. Rec., 1958, *70*, 50.
22.   Wagner, Goldstein, Doran, and Hay.   Jour. Am. Vet. Med. Assoc., 1954, *124*, 136.
23.   Wilson, Anderson, and Smith.   Jour. Comp. Path. and Therap., 1950, *60*, 267.
24.   Zlotnik and Rennie.   *Ibid.*, 1958, *68*, 411.

## Lymphocytic Choriomeningitis (LCM)

This disease of mice has great historical importance, as it was the first virus disease in which immunological tolerance was observed. Traub (4) showed that newborn mice or mice infected *in utero* with LCM developed such a state. Such tolerant mice continued to harbor the virus in high titers in the blood and organs, but no antibody was produced. In mouse colonies with this infection, birth and growth rates are lower and mortality is higher (3). Mice infected as newborns show no signs of illness, but develop a runting condition later in life (2). This chronic infection apparently leads to the production of an autoimmune disease (3). Depending upon the disease form that the infection assumes in mice, the pathologic picture is one of a meningoplexal and perivascular infiltration by lymphoid cells, plasmacytes, macrophages, and other cells, with occasional areas of focal gliosis. There is often serous pleurisy and peritonitis, hepatitis, and also necrosis, hemorrhage, and serofibrinous exudate in lymphatic organs. Lymphoid cell infiltrations are present in the kidney, salivary gland, and pancreas. The renal lesions in this disease are comparable to those seen in Aleutian disease in mink, lupus glomerulitis in man, and a spontaneous glomerulonephritis found in sheep in the United States and England (1). There is a proliferation of the mesangial and endothelial cells with occasional thickening of the basement membrane.

## REFERENCES

1.   Abinanti.   Ann. Rev. Microbiol., 1967, *21*, 467.
2.   Hotchin.   Cold Springs Harbor Sympos. Quant. Biol., 1962, *27*, 479.
3.   Seamer.   Arch. f. die Gesam. Virusforschung, 1965, *15*, 169.
4.   Traub.   Science, 1935, *81*, 298.

## Lactic Dehydrogenase Virus of Mice (LDV)

LDV infection has received a great deal of attention as an animal model because it is the first virus that produces an increase in enzyme activity in the peripheral circulation of an animal by decreasing the rate of enzyme clearance (7). A number of other viruses are known to cause cell damage with an ensuing release of intracellular enzymes (2-4). Evidence suggests that LDV impairs the clearance of enzymes by its action on the reticuloendothelial system (7).

LD infection in mice is characterized by a persistent viremia and enzyme elevation, a high virus titer, persisting neutralizing antibody, and the lack of clinical disease. This virus is known to be widely disseminated in mouse populations and many stocks of mouse tumor viruses and others were contaminated with this virus.

The size and structure of the agent are uncertain as round particles, 40 to 57 m$\mu$ in diameter, and elliptical particles, 30 x 60 m$\mu$, have been described in association with infectious material; rod-shaped forms also have been seen in electron-microscope photomicrographs (8). The particles appear to be surrounded by a dense double membrane (8). It appears to be an RNA virus with susceptibility to ether. The virus propagates in cell cultures of mouse peritoneal macrophages and mouse-embryo cells without an apparent cytopathic effect (1, 7). Rats are not susceptible to infection with the virus (7) and this fact offers a possible means by which LDV can be eliminated from murine tumor viruses contaminated with this agent. The agents fail to elicit antibody production in rabbits or guinea pigs (7).

It would seem that LDV has an affinity for the cells of the reticuloendothelial system (RES). Electron photomicrographs of peritoneal macrophages reveal virus particles within these cells. Consequently, the virus appears to be growing in or damaging the RES cells, which play an important role in host defense. This may also account for the reduced rate at which LDV and LDH are cleared from the circulation. It has been shown that the titer of Semliki forest virus was increased in the plasma of mice after blockade of RES with thorotrast (6) and Mahy (5) has made a similar observation with LDV. Initial plasma titers of LDV are about $10^{10.5}$ ID$_{50}$ per ml of blood but as the functional capacity of RES returns to normal the blood viral titer persists at levels approximating $10^4$ to $10^6$ ID$_{50}$ per ml. The immune mechanism in this disease presumably is similar to some other degenerative viruses discussed in this chapter where persisting virus and antibody occur in the host (9).

## REFERENCES

1.   DeBuy and Johnson.   Jour. Exp. Med., 1966, *123*, 985.
2.   Gilbert.   Virology, 1963, *21*, 609.
3.   Kelly and Greiff.   Jour. Expt. Med., 1961, *113*, 125.

4.   Latner, Gardner, Turner, and Brown.   Lancet, 1964, *1*, 197.
5.   Mahy.   Quoted by Notkins. Bact. Rev., 1965, *29*, 143.
6.   Mims.   *Ibid.*, 1964, *28*, 30.
7.   Notkins.   *Ibid.*, 1965, *29*, 143.
8.   Prosser and Evans.   Jour. Gen. Virol., 1967, *1*, 419.
9.   Rowson, Mahy, and Bendinelli.   Virol., 1966, *28*, 775.

## Visna-Maedi

The viruses known as *visna* and *maedi* are so similar that it is agreed to regard them as a single virus capable of producing nervous or respiratory manifestations. It is generally believed that the virus resembles oncogenic RNA viruses.

Visna and maedi were present in Iceland and may also occur in Texel and in India. Maedi, progressive pneumonia of sheep in the United States, and lung disease (*zwolgerziekte*), in Holland, are the same disease or very closely related.

**Character of the Disease.** *Maedi (respiratory form).* Sheep that are 2 years or older in age are affected with emaciation and dyspnea. The disease is highly fatal. The incubation period is 2 years or longer, but sheep inoculated by various routes have lung lesions 1 month later. Infection also occurs after feeding or by contact.

At necropsy the lungs are much enlarged, weighing as much as double the normal. There is diffuse perivascular and peribronchiolar infiltration with mononuclear cells but little fibrosis.

*Visna (nervous form).* Early signs of illness in the disease are abnormal head posture and lip trembling. Other nervous manifestations lead to paraplegia and total paralysis. The incubation period is measured in months and this slow demyelinating disease persists for weeks or months, terminating in death. Pleocytosis in the cerebral spinal fluid may appear 1 month after injection with clinical signs appearing as long as 18 months later.

The lesions are typical of a diffuse encephalomyelitis with demyelination (4). In early reports visna was confused with *Rida*, a disease probably identical to scrapie in sheep (3).

The nervous disease is transmissible to sheep by intracerebral inoculation whereas the respiratory form (maedi) occurs after intranasal exposure. Present evidence suggests that visna is an encephalitic form of the lung disease (6).

**Properties of the Virus.** Visna and maedi viruses are antigenically related (7). Slight antigenic differences have been noted. In cross-neutralization tests in cell culture, maedi virus has a somewhat broader antigenic structure than visna virus (7).

The viruses are inhibited by the DNA inhibitors, 5-bromodeoxyuridine and actinomycin D. This doesn't necessarily imply that they are DNA viruses, only that cellular DNA is required for their synthesis (7). In fact it has been established that visna virus contains RNA (1). The analogy between visna virus and oncogenic RNA viruses has been extended by the demonstration of reverse transcriptase in purified visna virus (2). The morphology and maturation of the visna virus particle is somewhat comparable to the type C-oncogenic virus particle observed in feline, murine, and avian leukemia. The visna virus particles vary in diameter from 60 to 90 m$\mu$, with a central core of 30 to 40 m$\mu$. Surface projections 10 m$\mu$ in length have been observed (7). There is a suggestion of a concentric arrangement with the core and a few helical rods 9 m$\mu$ are seen. Particles appear to be released at the cell surface from two walled buds (5).

The virus particles are ether- and chloroform-sensitive, and inactivated readily by heat. Most are stable between pH 7.2 and 9.2 and survive storage for months at $-70$ C. Phenol (4 percent), formaldehyde (0.04 percent), and ethanol (50 percent) readily inactivate the virus. In the presence of toluidine blue, visna is sensitive to light.

Neutralizing antibodies are formed to visna and maedi virus strains with cross-neutralization generally resulting. Inhibitory substances have been found in the sera of cattle and other species. Most human sera of all ages inhibit these viruses; it is a heat-stable serum component believed to be a nonspecific inhibitor.

**Cultivation.** The virus strains are isolated from sheep tissues such as blood, spinal fluid, and saliva and propagated in cell cultures derived from ependyma or choroid plexus of sheep brain. Multinuclear giant cells are formed with subsequent cell destruction; cytopathic changes occur in 2 to 3 weeks. By serial transfer the time is shortened to 3 to 15 days depending upon the viral dose. Virus can persist in cultures for at least 4 months.

**Immunity.** Sheep that show clinical signs die with the disease. There is no evidence that inapparent infections occur in sheep, but there is a suggestion of it in other species, such as cattle, that have a viral-neutralizing substance in their sera.

**Diagnosis.** Visna can be distinguished from Rida (scrapie) by clinical signs and pathological changes. Maedi can be differentiated from ovine adenomatosis by pathological changes (see respective sections on Character of the Disease for distinguishing features).

**Control.** A slaughter policy in 1951 in Iceland was apparently successful in eliminating both disease forms; however, the respiratory form reappeared in 1965.

**The Disease in Man.** The significance of a viral-neutralizing inhibitor in human sera is unknown.

## REFERENCES

1. Harter, Rosenkranz, and Rose. Proc. Soc. Exp. Biol. and Med., 1969, *131*, 297.
2. Lin and Thomar. Bact. Proc., 1970, *6*, 702.
3. Sigurdsson. Brit. Vet. Jour., 1954, *110*, 255.

4. Sigurdsson, Palsson, and van Bogaert. Acta Neuropath., 1962, *1*, 343.
5. Thomar. Virology, 1961, *14*, 463.
6. Thomar. Zeitschr f. Neurol., 1971, *199*, 155.
7. Thomar and Helgadottir. Res. Vet. Sci., 1965, *6*, 456.

## Equine Infectious Anemia

SYNONYMS: Swamp fever, equine malarial fever

This is a disease of horses characterized by a diversity of signs and an exceedingly variable course. An excellent detailed account of the disease will be found in the monograph of Dreguss and Lombard (5) and the papers presented at the American Veterinary Medical Association Symposium on Equine Infectious Diseases (1).

Members of the horse family are the only known natural hosts. European workers have reported limited success in obtaining multiplication of the virus, sometimes accompanied by mild signs in sheep, goats, pigs, rabbits, and some other species, including man. Workers in the United States generally have not been able to confirm these findings. It seems safe to say that the susceptibility of species other than the equine is slight.

Infectious anemia of horses has been recognized in practically all parts of the world where horses are raised. It occurs mostly in rather small areas from which it shows little tendency to spread. The name *swamp fever* is derived from the fact that the disease is most frequent in animals pastured in low-lying areas. This is not always the case, however. Scott (17) saw the disease on lands in Wyoming which were 9,000 feet above sea level. Even at high altitudes, flat, swampy lands are found, and such lands apparently favor the disease. The disease has been seen in the United States for more than 60 years. It has been reported at one time or another from 42 of the 50 states. Formerly it was common in the Mississippi Delta region in mules that worked in the cotton fields, but tractors have now largely replaced work animals. Udall and Fitch (26) recognized a focus of the disease in northern New York in 1914. In 1947 an outbreak occurred in Thoroughbred horses at the Rockingham Race Track in Salem, New Hampshire. At least 47 cases were definitely diagnosed and about 15 deaths occurred (Stein and Mott, 22).

In 1970 Coggins and Norcross (3) reported on an immunodiffusion test which is remarkably accurate in its detection of virus carriers. It has become apparent that certain breeding establishments had the infection on the premises without being aware of its presence. Through the use of the test as a diagnostic procedure, it is evident that the disease is more prevalent in the United States than clinical reports would indicate.

The greater number of acute and subacute cases are seen during the late summer and early fall months, a circumstance which fits in well with the idea that most initial infections occur from the bites of bloodsucking flies and mosquitoes.

**Character of the Disease.** Infectious anemia may appear in an acute, subacute, or chronic form. The acutely ill animal develops signs suddenly. A temperature of 105 to 108 F commonly appears; the horse is very dejected, refuses feed, becomes anemic, and shows congested and even icteric mucous membranes. It often sweats profusely in warm weather and frequently develops a serous discharge from the nose. These attacks often last for 3 to 5 days, after which the animal appears to recover. It may be free of signs for many days, weeks, or months, but usually, sooner or later, other acute attacks occur. In any of these attacks, death may come.

The chronic form of the disease consists, essentially, of a series of short acute attacks, between which the normal intervals may be very long. Such animals may show no signs whatsoever, but most of them develop anemia and hypergammaglobulinemia, the sedimentation rate of their corpuscles is greatly increased, the heart action becomes irregular, edematous swellings appear and disappear, and muscular weakness varies from slight to so much that the animal cannot stand or walk, or if it can walk, the gait may be very uncertain and wobbly. Such animals gradually become emaciated in spite of the fact that their appetite is often very great. Chronically infected animals have been kept under constant observation for periods in excess of 18 years (23), during which time their blood was constantly infective for other horses. With the availability of test procedures such as immunodiffusion and immunofluorescence tests, it should be possible to determine whether some virus carriers are completely asymptomatic.

When horses are inoculated subcutaneously with infected blood, the incubation period generally is from 12 to 15 days. Occasionally it is shorter and frequently it is considerably longer—as long as 90 days in a few cases.

As has already been said, one of the striking features of this disease is the great variability in its duration. Acute episodes usually last from 3 to 5 days. Periods between episodes may be months or years.

In all likelihood most infected animals eventually die of the disease unless their life span is terminated otherwise before the disease has run its full course. Experimentally it has been found that some animals, after carrying active virus for long periods, eventually become free of it. These recoveries apparently are the exceptions.

Animals dying of the acute form of the disease exhibit lesions of general septicemia. Hemorrhages occur in most of the parenchymatous organs; the spleen generally is enlarged and softened and its capsule is hemorrhagic. The lymph nodes of the abdominal cavity are swollen, and their peripheries generally are infiltrated with blood originating in hemorrhages in the organs from which their lymph sinuses drain. Splotchy hemorrhages occur on the serous membranes and in the mucous membrane of the intestines. The kidneys and liver show evidence of parenchymatous degeneration. Subcutaneous edema, emaciation, and evidences of anemia usually are apparent.

Animals which die after suffering from the chronic form of this disease show lesions similar to those described, but in addition there usually are characteristic changes in the liver and bone marrow. If the long bones are split lengthwise, the yellow marrow frequently is found to have disappeared more or less completely and to have been replaced with red marrow, an indication of tremendous stimulation of hematopoiesis in an effort on the part of the blood-forming tissues to compensate for the loss of red blood cells destroyed by the virus. The liver in such cases usually is reddish brown in color and enlarged because of great proliferation of the endothelial cells of the sinusoids, many of which are loaded with the brownish iron-containing pigment (hemosiderin) derived from destroyed blood cells. Other microscopic alterations include generalized lymphoproliferative changes with perivascular and hepatic lymphoid infiltrations, lymphoid hyperplasia in the lymph nodes and spleen; hepatic cell necrosis and glomerulitis (7). The mononuclear infiltration and necrosis in the liver are usually quite prominent in the disease. A proliferative glomerulitis with increased cellularity and thickening of glomerular tufts is prominent. The kidney lesion appears to be the result of immune complex deposition because the capillaries contain granular deposits of C'3 and IgG (7). A vasculitis has been described but it is not a common finding. Inclusion bodies have not been demonstrated.

Information about the pathogenesis of the disease is rapidly developing, because assay procedures for viral assay and antibody detection now are available. At the end of 1 week after subcutaneous inoculation of the horse, the agent is detectable in the serum and leukocytes (7). During the first febrile period, the virus titer in the serum increases, probably reaching its peak. After the fever subsides, the titer decreases only to rise again during subsequent fever episodes. More recently McGuire et al. (15) used the direct immunofluorescence test in a study of EIA viral antigen in tissues of 24 experimentally infected horses. Virus-infected cells were found in horses examined 6 to 40 days after inoculation. Horses examined for fluorescence before the 6th day after inoculation were negative and those examined at 98, 218, and 915 days had no demonstrable fluorescence. Fluorescence was noted in the spleens of all 18 positive horses while fluorescence was seen in the splenic nodes of 14, livers of 12 and kidneys of 9. Fluorescence was observed occasionally in a number of other lymph nodes, various visceral organs, and the brain. Kupffer cells were infected with virus in the liver and macrophages in all other organs. EIA antigen also was observed in mononuclear cells in blood vessels of many organs. In all instances the antigen was located in the cytoplasm. The type of cell that was infected, and its distribution, are similar to those observed in certain other persistent virus infections (15).

**The Disease in Experimental Animals.** The only dependable animals for experimentation with this disease are members of the equine family.

Various European workers claim to have produced thermal reactions and even fatal terminations in swine with this virus. Virus multiplication has also been obtained in rabbits, chickens, and pigeons, and there are some records of the finding of virus in naturally infected birds on farms where the disease occurred in horses. Köbe (9) reports that small splenectomized pigs are especially suitable subjects for inoculation. Stein (19) reports that his attempts to infect calves, sheep, swine, dogs, cats, rabbits, guinea pigs, rats, mice, and pigeons were unsuccessful.

**Properties of the Virus.** The virus nature of the causative agent was determined by Carré and Vallée (2) in 1904 and has been amply confirmed by many others. The blood is infectious in all stages of the disease, and filtrates of Berkefeld or porcelain filters are about equally infectious. Virus is also found in washed blood cells, all parenchymatous organs, milk, urine, saliva, and feces. The particulate size of the virus has been reported as 18 to 50 millimicrons in diameter. It is inactivated by ether treatment. It is made inactive by heating at 58 to 60 C for 1 hour, by phenol, formalin, and other chemicals (5, 24). It survives lyophilization and freezing for long periods of time. The virus contained in blood is quite resistant to heat, chemicals, and putrefaction. Dried blood retains virulence for some months if protected from sunlight. In thin layers the virus is quickly destroyed by sunlight, and thus it is believed that infected secretions, such as urine, will not long remain virulent on pastures. The infective agent can be separated from serum proteins and concentrated by DEAE cellulose chromotography (25). Chromatography and other methods were used in combination to purify and concentrate the virus.

Electron photomicrographs of tissue-cultured preparations containing the EIA agent display a viruslike particle, which buds from the cell surface, has a relatively translucent core with a laminated outer membrane, and is approximately 70 m$\mu$ in diameter (7). Additional studies are required to establish that the viruslike particle is the EIA agent.

The EIA agent can be detected in horse-leukocyte cell cultures by the indirect immunofluorescence test and in infected horse tissues by the direct immunofluorescence test (15).

Coggins and Norcross (3) described an immunodiffusion test for EIA which detects specific antibody in chronically infected horses for long periods of time. In an experiment to determine correlation between presence of antibody and infection with EIA virus blood from 84 serologically test-positive horses representing acute, chronic, and inapparent EIA infection, was induced in 84 experimental ponies as determined by clinical signs of illness and production of EIA antibody (4). Blood from 77 serologically test-negative horses did not infect ponies and EIA antibody was not produced. Consequently the immunodiffusion test is accepted as being at least 95 percent accurate for the diagnosis of EIA infection.

The complement-fixation test described by Kono and Kobayashi (11) has been used to study various isolates of EIA virus. These isolates, made in Japan, the United States, and Germany, share common CF antigens. There is no evidence to suggest that EIA virus shares a common CF antigen with other equine viruses.

The EIA virus is presumably capable of producing neutralizing antibodies in horses as assayed by the cell culture technic (12). The method has not been adequately investigated as yet, especially as it relates to protection.

Interferon is not produced in the serum of infected horses or in cell cultures infected with three different strains of EIA virus (13).

**Cultivation.** Primary peripheral horse leukocyte cultures are used for the propagation of the virus (10). A cytopathic effect may occur, but the changes are similar to spontaneous changes occurring in culture. To detect virus the CF test is applied utilizing a standard antiserum (11) or the indirect immunofluorescence test is utilized (27). Exacting procedures and proper source of biological materials are essential to the success of a horse-leukocyte culture system.

Although reports in the literature might suggest otherwise, it is presently accepted that laboratory animals are insusceptible to EIA virus. Attempts to propagate the virus in the hen's embryonated egg have failed.

**Immunity.** Until recently all evidence suggested that only one immunological type of EIA virus existed. Kono *et al.* (12) reported that two strains used in their studies were immunologically heterologous by protection tests in horses and by reciprocal serum-neutralization tests performed in cell cultures. In the course of these experiments it also was shown that repeated inoculations of an attenuated horse leukocyte cell culture strain failed to produce disease or a viremia and withstood protection against its virulent parent strain. Furthermore, virus failed to replicate in these horses after challenge, but these same horses were not protected against a heterologous virulent horse virus. These experiments must be viewed with caution until confirmed, because of the impact this newer knowledge may have on the control and prevention of EIA.

Obviously, there is still a great deal to be learned about the mechanism of immunity, or the lack thereof in the form of protection. It is clear that in natural infections the virus persists in most horses for long periods of time despite the presence of antibody in the form of precipitating, complement-fixing and even neutralizing antibody. Chronically infected horses will not react to the injection of fresh virus. In a few animals that freed themselves from virus after a long course of infection, inoculation of virulent virus caused disease in some animals but not in others.

Many experiments have been directed toward prophylactic immunization (2) but these have usually been unsuccessful. The report of Kono *et al.* (12) is encouraging and undoubtedly calls for more study in this area.

There are no biological products now available in the United States for immunization against EIA.

**Transmission.** Infectious anemia is believed to be spread principally through the agency of insects, particularly of bloodsucking flies. *Stomoxys calcitrans,* the common stable fly, is capable of transmitting the disease and perhaps is the principal agent. Scott (18), who studied the disease in Wyoming, believed that this fly was the principal agent concerned, and in this the Japanese Commission (8) concurred. Lührs (14) in Germany believes that mosquitoes, particularly *Anopheles maculipennis,* are the chief offenders. Other bloodsucking flies, particularly tabanids, probably are involved at times. Scott showed that infections in horses could be produced by a single prick with a hypodermic needle which had been infected by pricking an infected horse. This finding suggests that any type of insect which feeds first upon one animal and then another at short intervals could carry the disease. In the outbreaks at the New England race tracks in 1947 it was noted that there had been an influx of horseflies from nearby marshes shortly after sick horses had arrived.

There seems to be sufficient evidence to indicate that the disease may spread from one animal to another by simple contact without the intervention of insects. Fulton (6) believed that he had produced cases by injecting horses with water from swampy areas in pastures where infected horses were kept, and there are accounts of infections in horses kept within screened buildings with infected animals, all animals being watered out of common containers and all being fed from the floor, so there was ample opportunity for contamination of food and water with infectious secretions. Inasmuch as infections can be produced, although somewhat irregularly, by feeding infectious material, it is reasonable to believe that natural infections can occur more or less directly.

Several authors have suggested that some of the roundworms parasitic in horses might play a part in the transmission of the disease. Stein, Lucker, Osteen, and Gouchenour (20) tested this hypothesis by injecting emulsions of washed parasites from animals suffering from infectious anemia. Out of a number of such experiments they succeeded only once in obtaining an infection. In this case the infecting material consisted of an extract prepared from strongyles.

Stein and Mott (21) state that it is difficult to transmit the disease by administering infective material *per os* or by direct contact. They were unable to obtain definite evidence that foals contracted the disease by suckling their infected dams or by associating with them. It was shown that the milk of infected mares sometimes contains virus, that the foals may be inapparent carriers, and that suckling foals may be infected artificially.

Rather conclusive evidence has been obtained that equine infectious anemia has been transmitted to susceptible horses by careless use of hypodermic syringes, tattooing needles, and other piercing instruments. Such instruments should be sterilized by boiling after they have been used on one animal and before they are used on another. Biological supply houses in the United States licensed to do interstate business by the U.S. Department of Agriculture are required to heat all antisera prepared from horses at 58 to 59 C for 1 hour to destroy any virus which may be present. This should eliminate the possibility of transmitting this disease by antitoxins or other antisera made in horses. As an added safeguard it is recommended that each horse be tested for antibody by the immunodiffusion test that detects viral carriers.

The persistence of the virus in the blood of chronically affected, apparently normal, animals is astonishing. Schalk and Roderick (16) have published an account of one case which, after a number of acute attacks during a period of 3 months following inoculation with infected blood, lived in apparent health for 14 years, then suddenly developed acute signs and died. During this apparently normal period 18 other horses were inoculated with its blood at intervals of about 1 year and all but one of these developed acute signs of infectious anemia. During the first 3 years after inoculation there were occasional febrile periods, but during the remainder of the time until the final illness there were only rare febrile periods, which may or may not have been due to the infection. The persistence of virus in the horse offers a mechanism which virtually assures its maintenance on premises unless carrier horses are eliminated by the immunodiffusion test procedure.

**Diagnosis.** Clinical pathological procedures and pathological alterations can be utilized as a means to assist in the diagnosis of EIA. Clinical pathological alterations are related to the activity of the disease in a horse. Asymptomatic carriers have few detectable changes. The packed-cell volume and RBC counts decline during active disease. The hemolytic anemia probably is immunologically related. Sideroleukocytes are found in variable numbers in active disease. Hypergammaglobulinemia occurs. The WBC cell count varies, but associated with a decrease is a relative lymphocytosis as a result of a decrease in granulocytic type cells. There is a deranged coagulation hemeostatis, so liver biopsies are ill-advised during active disease. Tests for liver changes are indicated. The principal distinctive alterations then are hepatic changes associated with periodic pyrexia, sideroleukocytosis, and anemia.

The only dependable animals for diagnostic inoculations are members of the equine family. Young animals are preferred to old, and individuals should be sought that lack precipitating antibody. Blood or tissue extracts may be injected parenterally. The test animals should be kept indoors and given good care; their temperatures should be taken twice daily. If the animals have not been previously exposed, they usually respond with a temperature reaction and other signs of the acute form of the disease. This reaction may be expected in most instances during the 2nd or 3rd week, but in a few cases the interval is much longer—sometimes as much as 3 months.

Various laboratory tests have been advocated from time to time by different workers, but none has proved to be reliable. The immunodiffusion test described by Coggins and Norcross (3) is rapidly gaining acceptance in the United States as a valid test for the diagnosis of EIA (fig. 263). It seems only a matter of time before the direct (15) and indirect immunofluorescence tests gain comparable support for the diagnosis of the disease.

The complement-fixation test has only limited value as CF antibodies do not persist beyond 2 months after an initial exposure to the virulent virus regardless of the existence of persisting virus or the reoccurrence of clinical disease (7). An occasional horse will have a response to second CF antibody to an attenuated strain of EIA (12), but the titer only persists for a few days.

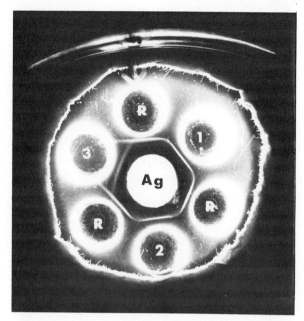

*Fig. 263.* A typical immunodiffusion test for diagnosis of equine infectious anemia (EIA). The antigen (*Ag*) is in the center well. The outer wells contain serums from horses labeled R (positive reference serum), 1 and 2 (positive suspect horses), and 3 (negative EIA horse). There is a single line of identity except for well 3 indicating that all sera are positive except from horse 3. The single line of nonidentity by well 3 is a nonEIA reaction. (Courtesy L. Coggins.)

Too little is known about the serum-neutralization test to evaluate its use in diagnosis.

**Control.** Because the immunodiffusion test (3) detects viral carriers, officials have an accurate method for the control of the disease. Positive animals should be eliminated. In certain instances confirmation of the test may require the inoculation of a horse. This horse test necessitates a waiting period of 45 days combined with bidaily temperature readings on the animal. If there are no signs of illness or a rise in temperature the test is considered to be negative.

Many breeding farms in New York State are using the test for detecting carrier animals and eliminating the positive reactors. Certain racetracks in the United States are requiring horses stabled at the track to have a negative immunodiffusion test result for EIA. Recent surveys have indicated that the incidence of infection at racetracks in New York and other northeastern states is about 1 percent.

The Equine Practice Committee of the New York State Veterinary Medical Society prepared a set of guidelines for use by veterinarians and horse-industry officials until such time as the immunodiffusion test is officially recognized by the federal and state control officials and regulations for the control of EIA are introduced. Annual testing of horses for carriers is the principal feature of the guidelines and a 90 to 120 day retest recommendation on premises, especially breeding farms, where infection exists until a complete negative testing is achieved.

In areas where the disease occurs, the use of common equipment—bridles, currycombs, and brushes—should be avoided. Surgical instruments, needles, and syringes should be thoroughly sterilized before use on each animal. Flies and insects should be controlled and the horses should be kept from infected pastures.

## REFERENCES

1. American Veterinary Medical Association Symposium. Jour. Am. Vet. Med. Assoc., 1969, *155*, 327.
2. Carré and Vallée. Comp. rend. Acad. Sci., 1904, *139*, 26.
3. Coggins and Norcross. Cornell Vet., 1970, *60*, 330.
4. Coggins, Norcross, and Nusbaum. Am. Jour. Vet. Res., 1972, *33*, 11.
5. Dreguss and Lombard. Experimental studies in equine infectious anemia. Univ. of Penn. Press, Philadelphia, 1954.
6. Fulton. Jour. Am. Vet. Med. Assoc., 1930, 77, 157.
7. Henson, McGuire, Kobayashi, Banks, Davis, and Gorham. Proc., 2nd Internatl. Conf. Equine Infec. Dis., S. Karger, Geneva, 1970, 178.
8. Japanese Commission. Review of report, Vet. Jour., 1914, *70*, 604.
9. Köbe. Arch. f. Tierheilk., 1938, *73*, 399.
10. Kobayashi. Virus, 1961, *11*, 249.
11. Kono and Kobayashi. Natl. Inst. Anim. Health Quart., 1966, *6*, 194.
12. Kono, Kobayashi, and Fukunaga. *Ibid.*, 1970, *10*, 113.
13. Ley, Burger, McGuire, and Henson. Jour. Inf. Dis., 1970, *12*, 10.
14. Lührs. Zeitschr. f. Tierheilk., 1919, *31*, 369.
15. McGuire, Crawford, and Henson. Am. Jour. Path., 1971, *62*, 283.
16. Schalk and Roderick. N. Dak. Agr. Exp. Sta. Bul. 168, 1923.
17. Scott. Univ. Wyo. Bul. 121, 1919.
18. Scott. Jour. Am. Vet. Med. Assoc., 1920, *56*, 448.
19. Stein. Infectious anemia. U.S. Dept. Agr., Farmers Bul. 2088, 1955.
20. Stein, Lucker, Osteen, and Gouchenour. Jour. Am. Vet. Med. Assoc., 1939, *95*, 536.
21. Stein and Mott. Vet. Med., 1946, *41*, 274.
22. Stein and Mott. Proc. U.S. Livestock Sanit. Assoc., 1947, *51*, 37.
23. Stein, Mott, and Gates. Jour. Am. Vet. Med. Assoc., 1955, *126*, 277.
24. Stein, Osteen, Mott, and Shahan. Am. Jour. Vet. Res., 1944, 5, 291.
25. Tanaka and Kirasawa. Natl. Inst. Anim. Health Quart., 1962, *2*, 108.
26. Udall and Fitch. Cornell Vet., 1915, 5, 69.
27. Ushimi, Nakajimi, and Tanaka. Natl. Inst. Anim. Health Quart., 1970, *10*, 90.

# LIV | Infectious Diseases of Domestic Animals Caused by Unclassified Viruses

**Borna Disease**

SYNONYM: Enzootic encephalomyelitis; Near East equine encephalomyelitis

This disease is an encephalomyelitis of horses, and occasionally of sheep, which has occurred annually for a century or more in certain localities in Saxony. There are no characteristic gross lesions but microscopically the usual lesions of virus encephalitis and myelitis are exhibited. These consist of perivascular infiltrations of lymphocytes (blood vessel "cuffing"), degeneration of ganglion cells, neuronophagia, and multiplication of neuroglia cells. The lesions are most marked in the brain stem. Lesions in the spinal cord are much less severe than those in the brain. A characteristic feature of Borna disease is the intranuclear bodies, commonly called *Joest* bodies, which were first described by Joest and Degen (1) in 1909. These inclusion bodies are seen in the ganglionic cells in the hippocampus and in the olfactory lobes, more rarely in other parts of the brain and cord. With the Giemsa stain they appear as reddish, round or oval bodies, varying in size, embedded in the nuclei, which are stained a light-blue color. Each of the bodies is surrounded by an unstained halo. They can be found in nearly all cases of Borna disease. In 1927 Zwick, Seifried, and Witte (2) isolated a virus from the brains of naturally infected horses and demonstrated its causal relationship to the disease.

**Character of the Disease.** The period of incubation of this disease is at least 4 weeks, in this respect differing from the other forms of virus encephalomyelitis in which it is very much shorter. The initial signs consist of a low fever, difficulty in swallowing, salivation, hyperesthesia, reflex irritability, spasms of

1347

the neck muscles, and other signs of cerebral irritation. These terminate in drowsiness and paralysis, either localized or general. The signs vary greatly. The course of the disease is also varied. Many cases die within 1 week after the appearance of the first signs; others may not die for 3 weeks. The mortality averages 90 percent.

Borna disease can be transmitted from horses to rabbits by intracerebral, intraocular, corneal, nasal, intravenous, intraperitoneal, or subcutaneous inoculation of brain material. Guinea pigs, rats, hens, and sheep can be infected by inoculation, but these species are not so susceptible as rabbits. The virus can be propagated indefinitely in rabbits by brain-to-brain inoculation. The incubation period in rabbits is from 3 to 4 weeks, and the period of signs is from 1 to 2 weeks. Death occurs in nearly all cases. A variety of nervous signs are exhibited by the animals, and general paralysis occurs before death ensues. Zwick and co-workers produced two cases of the disease in monkeys. Human infections have not been recognized.

**Properties of the Virus.** Elford and Galloway estimate its size as between 85 and 125 millimicrons. It is much more resistant than the other encephalitis viruses. In 50 percent glycerol, brain virus can be kept for at least 6 months. Zwick and Witte found that dried virus kept its virulence for more than 3 years.

Neutralizing antibodies are not readily detected in serum of immune animals. The brain of infected rabbits contains a complement-fixing antigen.

**Cultivation.** Successful propagation of the virus on the chorioallantoic membrane of the embryonated hen's egg maintained at 35 C is described. No reports on propagation in tissue culture have been seen.

**Immunity.** Zwick, Seifried, and Witte (3) report the successful immunization of horses with lapinized virus. The method has been used successfully in the field.

**Transmission.** The mode of transmission of this disease is not known with certainty. Unlike the other forms of virus encephalitis of horses which occur almost wholly during the warm periods of the year, Borna disease occurs throughout the year. Most of the cases are seen from February to July. About the time of year when the other forms of encephalitis appear, Borna disease cases become less frequent. The seasonal occurrence suggests that insects play no part in its transmission. According to Joest and Degen, the virus is present in the salivary glands, in the saliva, and in the secretions of the nasopharynx. The fact that lesions may be demonstrated regularly in the olfactory tract is suggestive of an entry path here by way of the nasopharynx. Successful feeding experiments have been reported; hence the digestive tract may be a portal of entry.

### REFERENCES

1. Joest and Degen.   Zeitschr. f. Infektionskr. Haustiere, 1909, 6, 348.
2. Zwick, Seifried, and Witte.   *Ibid.*, 1927, 30, 42.
3. Zwick, Seifried, and Witte.   Arch. f. Tierheilk., 1929, 59, 511.

## Ulcerative Stomatitis

In 1947 Gibbons *et al.* (3) described an ulcerative stomatitis in calves. This could be reproduced in normal calves by blood transfer or scarification in some instances (1). The experimental animals showed a temperature, leuko-penia, and diarrhea. Diarrhea was not a common sign in natural outbreaks, however. The investigators indicated that the disease was not like virus diar-rhea-mucosal disease but cross-immunity tests were not done.

In natural cases ulcerative stomatitis in calves is usually mild, but calves that are debilitated by parasitism, malnutrition, or hyperkeratosis may be se-verely affected with death ensuing. Ulceration and redness of the oral cavity characterize the disease.

In 1958 Pritchard *et al.* (8) reported on an infectious ulcerative stomatitis of cattle which they called bovine infectious ulcerative stomatitis. The disease does not cause mortality, but the morbidity may be 100 percent in some herds. It is characterized by erosions and ulcerations of the oral mucosa. The lesions are quite similar to those observed in ulcerative stomatitis of calves. The virus particle is spherical with a diameter between 125 to 150 millimi-crons. This agent has not been compared in cross-immunity tests with bovine viral diarrhea-mucosal disease virus or Gibbons' ulcerative stomatitis virus of calves, so its immunological relationship to these diseases is unknown.

## Bovine Papular Stomatitis

It was first described in the United States by Griesemer and Cole in 1960 (4). It had been described earlier in various countries in Europe and also in East Africa and Australia which suggests that it is worldwide in distribution. The disease is caused by a virus that usually produces a mild infection in calves characterized by proliferative papular lesions in and around the mouth. The course is prolonged but afebrile, and recovery ensues without treatment. In experimental calves the lesions persisted as long as 98 days.

Virus grows in bovine kidney cells without the production of a cytopatho-genic effect (5).

In natural and experimental cases lesions were limited to the oral cavity, esophagus, and the forestomachs. The principal microscopic changes were focal hydropic degeneration, hyperplasia of the mucosa or epidermis, and the formation of intracytoplasmic inclusion bodies (6).

The gross lesions may be confused with the early changes of foot-and-mouth disease, vesicular stomatitis, bovine viral diarrhea-mucosal disease, the oral form of infectious bovine rhinotracheitis in young calves, and other types of stomatitis occurring in cattle.

## Proliferative Stomatitis

According to Olson and Palionis (7) this condition is caused by a filterable agent. It is rarely seen as a primary disease but usually accompanies condi-tions such as hyperkeratosis (chlorinated naphthalene poisoning) and avitaminosis A. It has been said as a primary condition in one large herd of Hereford calves that had a severe ulcerative and proliferative stomatitis. A few of the cows had proliferative lesions on the teats (2). Very young calves that are healthy are susceptible to injection with infective material. Immunity follows an active infection. The virus appears to be different from that of vesicular stomatitis, cutaneous papilloma of cattle, and oral papilloma of the dog.

The virus produced localized papular lesions on the hands of two attendants who were working with the experimental calves (7).

## REFERENCES

1. Gibbons. Quoted by Gibbons. Diseases of cattle. 2d ed., Am. Vet. Publications, Inc., Santa Barbara, Cal., 1963.
2. *Ibid.*
3. Gibbons, Lee, Johnson, and Robinson. *Ibid.*
4. Griesemer and Cole. Jour. Am. Vet. Med. Assoc., 1960, *137*, 404.
5. Griesemer and Cole. Am. Jour. Vet. Res., 1961, 22, 473.
6. *Ibid.*, 482.
7. Olson and Palionis. Jour. Am. Vet. Med. Assoc., 1953, *123*, 419.
8. Pritchard, Claflin, Gustafson, and Ristic. *Ibid.*, 1958, *132*, 273.

## Contagious Pneumonia of Young Calves

SYNONYM: Calf pneumonia

Calf pneumonia in many large breeding herds is one of the most serious of the disease problems. The disease occurs in animals as old as 6 months and perhaps even older but generally is seen in calves from 10 days to 4 months old. It is not usually a serious problem in small herds where the annual calf crop is small and where many young calves are not kept in close association. Larger establishments frequently maintain special calf barns, or nursery units, where the young calves are kept together for the first several months of their lives. Often these are models of construction but it is in such units that the infection usually takes its greatest toll. The disease is highly contagious, and the fresh calves that are brought in from time to time serve as fuel to keep the fire going.

It is generally believed that there is a direct connection between a common diarrheal disease of young calves, known as *white scours* or *calf scours*, and this highly contagious pneumonia. The diarrheal disease usually precedes the pneumonia, since it ordinarily occurs when the calf is from 1 day to perhaps 10 days old. Scours, however, occurs in calves which do not later have pneumonia, and pneumonia occurs in animals that have not previously scoured.

An etiological connection between scours and pneumonia has not been certainly established. For many years strains of *Escherichia coli* have been isolated from the intestinal discharges and tissues of calves dying of scours, and this organism was regarded as the causative agent by the earlier workers even though it was not usually possible to reproduce the disease by feeding large quantities of such cultures. From the lungs of calves dying from pneumonia a miscellaneous collection of bacteria have been isolated, streptococci, *Coryne-bacterium pyogenes*, and *Pasteurella multocida* being the most frequent. Since it has never been possible to reproduce the characteristic pneumonia in calves with such cultures, it has been assumed that they were secondary invaders. The fact that the pneumonia spread so readily among groups of animals has suggested to many that a viral agent might be the initial pathogen which paved the way for the bacteria which are so prominent in the fatal lesions. In 1942 Baker (1, 2) described a virus which he regarded as the primary agent in this disease. Moll (3) in 1952 was able to reproduce and extend Baker's work. It is presumed that the virus with which he worked was the same as the one which Baker described, although no comparisons of them were made.

**Character of the Disease.** The disease is seen at all times of the year but is most prevalent during the winter months when animals are kept closely crowded in weather-proof buildings in which the ventilation often is very faulty. The disease is manifested by loss of appetite, high fever, unthriftiness, prostration, a scanty nasal discharge, and rapid breathing. The older and stronger the animal is originally, the better it will withstand the disease, and the more likely it is to recover. The younger, weaker calves may die after a course of only a few days; the larger, stronger animals may run a course of several weeks. If recovery from the acute phase of the disease occurs, permanent unthriftiness often remains because of the damage to the lung tissue from the bacterial agents which invariably accompany the virus.

The lesions are found most commonly in the anterior and ventral lobes. Usually the lesions occur bilaterally. The pneumonic tissue is dark red, or dark red mottled with gray. The affected tissue is firmer than normal and is not dry like hepatized tissue but is rather moist. Fibrinous exudate is sometimes found on the pleura but this is exceptional. Usually the pleura over the pneumonic areas is smooth, moist, and glistening. The nonpneumonic areas frequently show emphysema. If the disease has been protracted, small abscesses commonly are found in the pneumonic areas, and the bronchi are filled with thick mucopurulent exudate. The pneumonic tissue in these cases is practically always mottled with grayish areas made up of large collections of neutrophilic leukocytes. When diarrhea accompanies the disease, the small intestine, especially the mucosa of the ileum, is covered with a sticky mucus.

**The Disease in Experimental Animals.** Baker found that a transmissible pneumonia of white mice could be produced by introducing calf lung filtrates into their air passages. Filtrates of mouse lung virus readily produced disease in calves when it was introduced into their air passages, and the disease was transmitted by pen contact from artificially inoculated calves to normal ones.

The disease was typical in every way of natural infection. Artificially inoculated calves developed fever in from 2 to 4 days, and this lasted for 3 to 5 days, the peak usually being from 104 to 106 F. Diarrhea usually appeared the day after fever began and signs of penumonia about the 5th day after inoculation. The pneumonic signs usually were mild and the calves ordinarily recovered. Destroyed animals exhibited evidence of catarrhal enteritis, and pneumonic foci occurred in the ventral lobes of the lung. Calves that had recovered from the disease were resistant to reinfection, and their serum contained neutralizing antibodies. Neutralizing antibodies for the mouse virus also developed in calves that suffered from the naturally occurring disease.

**Properties of the Virus.** Early in the course of the disease the virus is found only in the lungs and intestines, but 3 to 4 days from the onset of fever the virus is generally distributed throughout the body. It readily passes a Berkefeld N filter and can be recovered from infected tissues by introducing filtrates into the air passages of etherized white mice in the manner used to recover influenza viruses of man and swine.

Frozen and dried virus specimens were active after storage for 4 months. Specimens frozen at −4 C remained active for longer than 1, but less than 4 weeks, and storage in 50 percent glycerol for a week resulted in complete loss of virulence (2).

**Cultivation.** No attempts to cultivate this virus on artificial media have been reported.

**Immunity.** Clinical experience and Baker's work both indicate that one attack of this disease confers immunity to reinfection.

**Transmission.** It is quite clear that natural transmission of this disease commonly occurs through inhalation of infective droplets projected into the air of the calf quarters through the coughing of affected animals.

### REFERENCES

1.  Baker.   Cornell Vet., 1942, 32, 202.
2.  Baker.   Jour. Exp. Med., 1943, 78, 435.
3.  Moll.   Univ. Wis. Thesis, 1952.

# LV  Infectious Diseases of Domestic Animals of Uncertain Viral Etiology

Since Pasteur and Koch laid the groundwork for determining the causative agents of infectious diseases, research workers have identified these agents in most of our better-known diseases of man and animals. In the beginning workers generally tried to incriminate bacteria, but gradually it was learned that other kinds of agents were responsible for many diseases; hence we now recognize pathogenic protozoa, fungi, rickettsiae, and viruses. We also know that many clinical entities are caused by the action of two or more of these types operating in conjunction. The causative factor or factors of a few of the well-known infectious diseases still remain to be elucidated, and new entities appear from time to time, the causes of which are not always determined immediately. Thus we always have a certain number that cannot be accurately assigned to any etiological group. This chapter is devoted to brief descriptions of a few important diseases of domestic animals that at present are in this category.

In addition to those described, references will be found throughout the text to others, described under specific agents, for which the etiological evidence is not very convincing. Thus Hjarre's disease (p. 142) is mentioned under coliform organisms, winter dysentery of cattle (p. 130) and a virulent dysentery of swine (p. 130) under *Vibrio*, shipping fever of cattle (p. 178) under *Pasteurella*, atrophic rhinitis (p. 195) of swine under *Bordetella bronchiseptica*, and edema disease of swine under *Escherichia coli* (p. 142).

### Infectious or Epizootic Infertility of Cattle

SYNONYMS: Epivaginitis (epivag), specific bovine venereal epididymitis and vaginitis, catarrhal vaginitis of cattle

Epivaginitis is a chronic disease of cattle transmitted by coitus. It occurs in East, South, and Central Africa (1, 2, 3). A clinically similar disease has been described by Kendrick et al. (4) in California.

It is generally believed that epivaginitis is viral in etiology, although this has not been established. McIntosh et al. (5) have cultivated in mice and embryonated hens' eggs a virus associated with vaginitis of cattle. Cows and heifers infected with material from both the mouse- and egg-propagated lines of this strain showed definite, though mild, signs of vaginitis. Daubney et al. (2) have suggested that there may be two types of infectious vaginitis and that the virus of McIntosh et al. may be the cause of the milder form. The agent isolated by Kendrick and co-workers in California was more pathogenic for chick embryos than the McIntosh strain; it also differed from the latter in being more difficult to adapt to mice. Serum-neutralization tests were not done to establish the identity of the two agents.

The incubation period in cattle is about 2 to 8 days. The vagina is affected and there is a vaginal exudate. Examination reveals diffusely reddened areas in the anterior part of the vaginal mucosa and cervix but no ulcers, vesicles, or granular lesions. The acute infective stage may last for 2 weeks to 9 months. Most cows and heifers recover eventually, but 15 to 25 percent may become permanently sterile. In bulls the characteristic lesion is an enlargement and hardening of the epididymis. Occasionally an orchitis may develop and result in degeneration and atrophy of the testes.

Transmission is by coitus and the disease can be controlled by artificial insemination.

### REFERENCES

1. Anderson, Plowright, and Purchase. Jour. Comp. Path. and Therap., 1951, 61, 219.
2. Daubney, Hudson, and Anderson. East African Agr. Jour., 1938, 4, 31.
3. Henning. Animal diseases in South Africa. 2d ed. Central News Agency, South Africa, 1949, p. 863.
4. Kendrick, McKercher, and Saito. Jour. Am. Vet. Med. Assoc., 1956, 128, 357.
5. McIntosh. Onderstepoort Jour. Vet. Res., 1954, 26, 479.

### Sweating Sickness of Cattle

This is an acute disease of unknown etiology which is known to occur only in certain parts of the southern part of the continent of Africa. It is manifested by characteristic signs among which is a moist eczema that sometimes involves the entire body. The name is a misnomer; the victims do not sweat.

The disease is tick-transmitted. A good general account of this disease may be found in Henning's textbook (2).

The disease is important only in cattle, particularly calves. It also occurs in sheep and swine.

**Character of the Disease.** The disease is occasionally seen in older animals but most cases are in animals less than 1 year old, and the most severe cases are usually in young calves. Following an incubation period of 4 to 7 days, anorexia and fever suddenly appear. The temperature may reach 108 F, but later in the disease the fever disappears. The affected animal is depressed and listless. A moist eczema soon appears, sometimes in restricted areas but often involving the skin of the entire body. The skin feels cold and the hair becomes matted with the moist secretions. The hair in the eczematous areas may easily be pulled out leaving raw places, and often the victim loses a great deal of its hair. The skin is very sensitive to touch and to hot sunlight. The body develops an unpleasant sourish odor. The ear tips and the end of the tail may become necrotic and slough off. Screwworms often invade the exposed tissues and greatly complicate the condition. The mucous membranes of the mouth develop necrotic areas from which the epithelium easily peels off. The mouth becomes so sore that the animal may refuse to eat, and there may be a copious flow of saliva, which causes frothing of the mouth. There may be severe conjunctivitis and keratitis with the development of corneal opacities. The nasal and vaginal mucosae develop lesions like those of the mouth. Nervous signs sometimes are evident.

Sweating sickness generally leads to death in 2 to 4 days when the animal is severely affected. Less severe cases may recover after a course of 1 to 2 weeks.

The mortality varies greatly in different areas and in different age groups. It is greater in the younger victims. The mortality rate according to different observers varies from 10 to 50 percent and higher. The pathological changes are confined to the skin and mucous membranes, as already described.

**Etiology.** The cause of this disease is unknown. Some have doubted its infectiousness but most workers long ago agreed that its epizootiology strongly indicated an infectious disease (Du Toit, 1). Inoculations of blood and tissues have failed to produce the disease in the hands of all who have tried them. In 1954 Neitz (3) supplied evidence that the disease was transmissible and that at least one vector is the tick, *Hyalomma transiens*. The disease agent apparently undergoes biological changes in this arthropod, and it is transmitted transovarially through at least five generations without loss of virulence for cattle.

No effective method of treating affected animals has been developed, other than supportive measures and force-feeding of victims that will not eat voluntarily. Because the tick is the only known transmitter, preventive measures lie in eradicating the vector or adopting other measures of protecting cattle from its bites.

## REFERENCES

1. Du Toit.   9th and 10th Rpt., Director Vet. Educ. and Res., Union of So. Africa, 1924, p. 233.
2. Henning.   Animal diseases in South Africa. 3d ed. Central News Agency, So. Africa, 1956.
3. Neitz.   Jour. So. African Vet. Med. Assoc., 1954, 25, 1.

### Atrophic Rhinitis of Swine

Atrophic rhinitis (AR) of swine is a condition that affects the young chiefly and is characterized by sneezing, nosebleed, stunted growth, and dissolution of the turbinate bones. It is prevalent in Canada and in the midwest and it is quite certain that the diseases known in Sweden and Germany under the names *Schnüffelkrankheit* and *Niesenkrankheit* are similar to atrophic rhinitis. It has been suggested that inclusion body rhinitis is caused by the same agent or agents.

**Character of the Disease.** Atrophic rhinitis usually affects young pigs. Violent sneezing accompanied by a nasal discharge of blood, rubbing the nose against hard objects, holding the head to one side, and coughing is a common sign of the disease, although in some individuals the most conspicuous sign may be a distortion of the snout. This is brought about by involvement and dissolution of the turbinate bones.

Doyle *et al.* (1) distinguish between so-called *bull nose* and atrophic rhinitis of swine. The former is characterized by granulomatous swelling with necrosis in the central portion and with rarely any distortion of the snout other than that which results from the swelling. On the other hand, unilateral or bilateral dissolution of the turbinate bones at the point of transection halfway between the end of the nose and the eyes indicates atrophic rhinitis.

**Etiology.** Numerous causes for this condition have been proposed. At one time it was believed that a combination of *Pseudomonas aeruginosa* and *Spherophorus necrophorus* produced the infection. This view is no longer held. Schofield and Jones (10), who studied the pathology and bacteriology of the disease in 1950, were not able to find the infectious agent either by bacteriologic examination or by search for a virus but were able to transmit the disease to control pigs by means of unfiltered emulsions from typical lesions. In 1953 Spindler *et al.* (11) stated that there was an etiological relationship between trichomonads and rhinitis of swine, but Fitzgerald *et al.* (2) were unable to show that bacteria-free cultures of these protozoa caused rhinitis of swine. In the same year Gwatkin *et al.* (3) presented evidence that nasal instillation of pure cultures of *Pasteurella multocida* produced rhinitis in baby pigs. The importance of this organism in atrophic rhinitis has not been established at this time. Attempts to establish pleuropneumonialike organisms or a virus as the cause have also failed.

Investigators at Iowa State University have studied the etiology and pathology of AR for a number of years, and it is their belief that the natural disease is infectious. Various bacteria, principally *Bordetella bronchiseptica,* have been suggested as the etiology of AR (4, 8). The production of disease in pigs is influenced by the strain virulence of *B. bronchiseptica* (9), by complication with other microorganisms and with environmental stresses (9), and by possible immune status and age of pigs (5).

In 1965 Krook, Pond, and Brown (7) did two experiments with virus pneumonia-free Yorkshire pigs and showed that atrophic rhinitis can be reproduced by feeding diets low in calcium or by imbalance in calcium and phosphorus. Furthermore, their data suggested that the dietary calcium for the fast-growing pig should be increased above the currently recommended level of 0.8 percent calcium and 0.6 percent phosphorus to 1.2 percent calcium and 1.0 percent phosphorus in order to promote higher bone ash and better integrity of the nasal turbinates.

In 1970 Kemeny *et al.* (6) in a study on the experimental transmission of AR concluded that gross atrophy of the turbinates could be produced experimentally only by nasal instillation of infectious material, and that the dietary factors studied were of little or no importance. They did not associate a specific microorganism with the disease, but found many microorganisms in the nasal tissue material used for exposure of the pigs. In a subsequent study with a culture of *B. bronchiseptica,* Kemeny (5) was able to produce AR in most experimental pigs.

Until the etiology of this disease can be clearly established, it is logical to consider AR as an infectious disease, but also to establish clearly that swine herds are receiving adequate levels of calcium in the proper ratio with phosphorus.

**Control.** The only known means of controlling this disease is by disposing of the entire herd, cleaning and disinfecting the premises, and restocking from clean herds after a few months. Inasmuch as the disease has become so common in the United States it is difficult to procure stock that is known to be free of the disease. Many are now starting clean herds from pigs that are removed from the dam by Caesarean section and raising them by hand from the very beginning on clean ground away from all older stock. This procedure also provides a means of obtaining herds free from virus pneumonia. If the primary cause proves to be a lack of calcium, this will change management practices now in effect for the control of this malady.

## REFERENCES

1. Doyle, Donham, and Hutchings.   Jour. Am. Vet. Med. Assoc., 1944, *105,* 132.
2. Fitzgerald, Hammond, and Shupe.   Cornell Vet., 1954, *44,* 302.
3. Gwatkin, Dzenis, and Byrne.   Canad. Jour. Comp. Med. and Vet. Sci., 1953, *17,* 215.
4. Harris and Switzer.   Am. Jour. Vet. Res., 1968, *29,* 777.
5. Kemeny.   Cornell Vet., 1972, *62,* 477.
6. Kemeny, Littledike, and Cheville.   Cornell Vet., 1970, *60,* 502.

7.  Krook, Pond, and Brown.   Proc. Cornell Nutr. Conf. for Feed Manufacturers, 1965, p. 18.
8.  Ross, Duncan, and Switzer.   Vet. Med., 1963, *58*, 566.
9.  Ross, Switzer, and Duncan.   Canad. Jour. Compar. Med. Vet. Sci., 1967, *31*, 53.
10.  Schofield and Jones.   Jour. Am. Vet. Med. Assoc., 1950, *116*, 120.
11.  Spindler, Shorb, and Hill.   *Ibid.*, 1953, *122*, 151.

## Feline Infectious Peritonitis (FIP)

This disease was first described in 1963 by Holzworth (2). Sixteen naturally occurring cases, coupled with transmission studies, were described 3 years later (6). In the last few years the disease has been diagnosed with increased frequency. The affected cats range in age from 3 months to 17 years. The proportion of males to females is significantly higher. The occurrence of the disease does not vary significantly with the season of the year. There is insufficient evidence to suggest if certain breeds of cats are more susceptible to the disease. The disease is widespread in domestic cats located in the United States, and also occurs in large wild cats in the United States and Europe.

**Character of the Disease.** FIP is a chronic debilitating disease characterized by fibrinous peritonitis and often pleuritis (3). Other clinical signs of illness include peritoneal and pleural effusion, depression, persistent or recurrent fever, inappetence, wasting, and anemia. Less common signs are thirst, constipation, iritis, or hypopyon, harsh lung sounds, ventral edema, and bleeding gums. Masses occasionally are palpable in the abdomen, and these presumably are enlarged nodes or viscera with adhesions. Pain is noted in some cases. Most affected cats die within 5 weeks after diagnosis and treatment is almost never effective. Often there is a relative or absolute hypergammaglobulinemia.

The macroscopic lesions in cats with spontaneous disease are characterized by excessive abdominal fluid and diffuse fibrinous peritonitis (7)(fig. 264). Histopathologically, characteristic lesions include a layer of fibrinous exudate that is distributed on the peritoneal serous surfaces, subserosal and subcapsular inflammation and necrosis, and periorchitis. Focal necrosis, pleuritis, and meningitis are present in 20 to 40 percent of the cats with natural disease.

**The Disease in Experimental Domestic Cats.** The lesions in experimental cat, the only species known to be susceptible at present, vary in severity depending in all likelihood on the amount of infectious agent in the batch of infective material used for production of infection. When the dosage of the infective agent is high, the disease is more acute and the chronic type of disease observed in the field is not seen (5). Dilutions of the same inoculum produce the typical syndrome observed in practice. As the etiology is obscure, the pathogenesis of the disease is poorly understood.

**Properties of the Agent.** The infectious agent responsible for this disease remains an enigma. Most investigators are convinced that it is caused by a

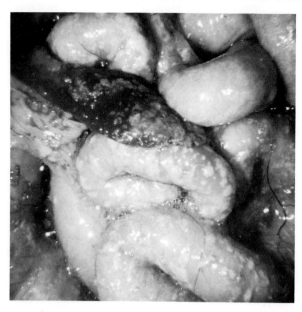

*Fig. 264.* Elevated fibrinous plaques on the visceral and parietal peritoneum observed in a typical case of feline infectious peritonitis. (Courtesy J. Gaskin.)

virus because bacteria-free, *Mycoplasma*-free material and also filtrates of organ extracts from cats with naturally occurring disease produce FIP in experimental cats. Viral particles have been observed in lesions of experimental cats but not of spontaneous cases. The viral particles of the experimental disease have not been isolated, purified, or shown to produce the disease, so the case for a viral etiology is still circumstantial.

The viruslike particle associated with experimental FIP has an average diameter of 75 to 90 mμ and is probably an RNA virus, since it replicates by budding from the endoplasmic reticulum (8). It is morphologically similar to feline leukemia virus, which also is found in some experimental and spontaneous cases of FIP (1).

**Cultivation.** Attempts to grow this infectious agent *in vitro* have not succeeded (1).

**Immunity.** This is a completely unknown area. There is no evidence that cats recover from this malady, but then it is possible that subclinical cases do occur. It is rare indeed that the mortality of any disease is 100 percent. Obviously, additional work must be done to clarify any immunity associated with this disease.

**Transmission.** The natural route of transmission of FIP is unknown. The lesions involve most of the body systems so the agent conceivably is present in exudate from the respiratory, gastrointestinal, and urinary tracts. Cats can be infected by many routes of inoculation, such as the intraperitoneal, intravenous, intracerebral, subcutaneous, oral, intranasal, and the intrathoracic (4).

**Diagnosis.** The best aid to diagnosis in the live cat is laboratory examination of the syrupy, hazy, golden-colored fluid exudate from the abdominal or thoracic cavity (3). The exudate has a high specific gravity and protein content, often contains fibrin strands, and may coagulate rather swiftly. Bacteria are rarely seen or isolated and white blood cells are not numerous.

**Control.** Cats are not responsive to antibiotic therapy—additional evidence that the infectious agent may be virus-induced.

In a cattery it may be well to isolate ill cats from the others if possible.

**The Disease in Man.** It is not known to occur.

## REFERENCES

1. Hardy. Jour. Am. Vet. Med. Assoc., 1971, *158*, 994.
2. Holzworth. Cornell Vet., 1963, *53*, 157.
3. Holzworth. Jour. Am. Vet. Med. Assoc., 1971, *158*, 981.
4. Ward. Univ. Calif. Thesis, 1970.
5. Ward and Pederson. Jour. Am. Vet. Med. Assoc., 1969, *154*, 26.
6. Wolfe and Griesemer. Path. Vet., 1966, *3*, 255.
7. Wolfe and Griesemer. Jour. Am. Vet. Med. Assoc., 1971, *158*, 987.
8. Zook, King, Robison, and McCombs. Path. Vet., 1968, *5*, 91.

# Index

**HAGAN'S INFECTIOUS DISEASES
OF DOMESTIC ANIMALS**

Designed by R. E. Rosenbaum.
Composed by Vail-Ballou Press, Inc.,
in 10 point linofilm Caledonia, 2 points leaded,
with display lines in Helvetica.
Printed offset by Vail-Ballou Press
on Allied Laurel Text, 50 pound basis.
Bound by Vail-Ballou Press
in Columbia book cloth
and stamped in All Purpose foil.

Library of Congress Cataloging in Publication Data
(For library cataloging purposes only)

Hagan, William Arthur, 1893–1963.
  Hagan's infectious diseases of domestic animals.

  Previous editions published under title: The infectious diseases of domestic animals.
  Includes bibliographies.
  1. Communicable diseases in animals.
2. Veterinary microbiology. I. Bruner, Dorsey William, date. II. Gillespie, James Howard.
III. Title.
SF781.H3   1973      636.089'69     72-12909
ISBN 0-8014-0752-4